Core Concepts in

ADVANCED PRACTICE NURSING

Core Concepts in

ADVANCED PRACTICE NURSING

Denise Robinson, PhD, RN, FNP

Professor and Director, MSN Program
Northern Kentucky University
Highland Heights, Kentucky
Family Nurse Practitioner
Northern Kentucky Family Health Centers
Covington, Kentucky

Cheryl Pope Kish, EdD, RNC, WHNP

Professor and Coordinator
Graduate Programs in Health Sciences
Director, FNP Program
Women's Health Nurse Practitioner
Student Health Services
Georgia College and State University
Milledgeville, Georgia

with 100 *illustrations*

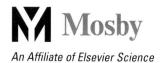

An Affiliate of Elsevier Science

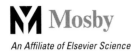

Vice President and Publishing Director, Nursing: Sally Schrefer
Executive Editor: Barbara Nelson Cullen
Associate Developmental Editor: Stacy Welsh
Project Manager: Catherine Jackson
Production Editor: Clay S. Broeker
Designer: Julia Ramirez

NOTICE

Pharmacology is an ever-changing field. Standard safety precautions must be followed, but as new research and clinical experience broaden our knowledge, changes in treatment and drug therapy may become necessary or appropriate. Readers are advised to check the most current product information provided by the manufacturer of each drug to be administered to verify the recommended dose, the method and duration of administration, and contraindications. It is the responsibility of the licensed prescriber, relying on experience and knowledge of the patient, to determine dosages and the best treatment for each individual patient. Neither the publisher nor the editor assumes any liability for any injury and/or damage to persons or property arising from this publication.

Permissions may be sought directly from Elsevier's Health Sciences Rights Department in Philadelphia, USA: phone: (+1)215-238-7869, fax: (+1)215-238-2239, email: healthpermissions@elsevier.com. You may also complete your request on-line via the Elsevier Science homepage (http://www.elsevier.com), by selecting 'Customer Support' and then 'Obtaining Permissions'.

Mosby, Inc.
An Affiliate of Elsevier Science
11830 Westline Industrial Drive
St. Louis, Missouri 63146

Printed in the United States of America

Library of Congress Cataloging in Publication Data

Core concepts in advanced practice nursing / [edited by] Denise Robinson, Cheryl Pope Kish.
     p. ; cm.
  Includes bibliographical references and index.
  ISBN 0-323-00897-6
    1. Nurse practitioners. 2. Nursing ethics. 3. Nursing. I. Robinson, Denise L. II. Kish, Cheryl Pope.
  [DNLM: 1. Nursing Theory—United States. 2. Delivery of Health Care—United States.
3. Ethics, Nursing—United States. 4. Health Policy—United States. 5. Health Promotion—United States. WY 86 C7968 2001]
RT82.8 .C67 2001
610.73—dc21
                                                                00-067868

03 04 05 GW/MV 9 8 7 6 5 4 3 2

Section Editors

Margaret M. Anderson, EdD, RN, C, CNAA
Associate Professor and Chair
Department of Nursing
Northern Kentucky University
Highland Heights, Kentucky

Anne M. Dollins, MPH, MSN, CNM, PhD
Assistant Professor and Assistant Dean
College of Professional Studies
Northern Kentucky University
Highland Heights, Kentucky

Cheryl Pope Kish, EdD, RNC, WHNP
Professor and Coordinator
Graduate Programs in Health Sciences
Director, FNP Program
Women's Health Nurse Practitioner
Student Health Services
Georgia College and State University
Milledgeville, Georgia

Ann Schmidt Luggen, PhD, RN, ARNP, CS, CNAA
Professor of Nursing
College of Professional Studies
Northern Kentucky University
Highland Heights, Kentucky

Cheryl McKenzie, RN, C, MN, FNP
Associate Professor of Nursing
Northern Kentucky University
Highland Heights, Kentucky

Sue E. Meiner, EdD, RN, CS, GNP
Assistant Professor
University of Nevada, Las Vegas
Las Vegas, Nevada

Louise M. Niemer, PhD, ARNP, CPNP
Associate Professor, Nursing
Northern Kentucky University
Highland Heights, Kentucky

Alice G. Rini, JD, MS, RN
Associate Professor of Nursing
Northern Kentucky University
Highland Heights, Kentucky

Contributors

Karen D. Agricola, MSN, RN, CRNP
University of Cincinnati
Department of Family Medicine
Cincinnati, Ohio

Margaret M. Anderson, EdD, RN, C, CNAA
Associate Professor and Chair
Department of Nursing
Northern Kentucky University
Highland Heights, Kentucky

Janet L. Andrews, PhD, WHNP, RNC
Associate Professor
School of Health Sciences, Nursing
Georgia College and State University
Milledgeville, Georgia

Linda Baas, PhD, RN, CS-ACNP, CCNS
Associate Professor
College of Nursing
University of Cincinnati
Cincinnati, Ohio

Theresa Beery, PhD, RN
Assistant Professor, Adult Health
College of Nursing
University of Cincinnati
Cincinnati, Ohio

Sue A. Blevins, RN, MS, MPH
President
Institute for Health Freedom
Washington, DC

Lisa Bradshaw, RN, MSN, FNP
Nurse Practitioner
Community Medical Professionals
North Andover, Massachusetts

Leslie Cooper, MSN, RN, CS, FNP
Director of School Health Services
Boone County Board of Education
Florence, Kentucky
Family Nurse Practitioner
Warsaw Family Medicine
Warsaw, Kentucky

Sandra L. Cromwell, PhD, RN
Assistant Professor
College of Nursing
University of Arizona
Tucson, Arizona

Jean E. DeMartinis, PhD, APRN, FNP-C
Assistant Professor and Director
Cardiac Health and Rehabilitation/NP
MS in Nursing Program
Creighton University School of Nursing
Omaha, Nebraska

Anne M. Dollins, MPH, MSN, PhD, CNM
Assistant Professor
Assistant Dean
Northern Kentucky University
Highland Heights, Kentucky

Jacqueline Fawcett, PhD, FAAN
Professor
College of Nursing
University of Massachusetts, Boston
Boston, Massachusetts

Diane Eigsti Gerber, MS, RN
Foodnet Surveillance Officer
Emerging Infections Program
Communicable and Environmental Disease Services
Tennessee Department of Health
Nashville, Tennessee

Mary Gers, MSN, CNS, RNC
Assistant Professor
Northern Kentucky University
Highland Heights, Kentucky

Patricia M. Gray, BSN, MEd, PhD
President, PMG Consulting
Cleveland, Ohio
Clinical Instructor
Francis Payne Bolten School of Nursing
Case Western Reserve University
Cleveland, Ohio

Ann W. Keller, RN, BSN, MEd, MSN, EdD
Assistant Professor
Northern Kentucky University
Highland Heights, Kentucky

Cheryl Pope Kish, EdD, RNC, WHNP
Professor and Coordinator
Graduate Programs in Health Sciences
Director, FNP Program
Women's Health Nurse Practitioner
Student Health Services
Georgia College and State University
Milledgeville, Georgia

Kathy Kolcaba, PhD, RN
Associate Professor, College of Nursing
The University of Akron
Akron, Ohio

Linda LaCharity, MN, PhD, RN
Assistant Professor
College of Nursing
University of Cincinnati
Cincinnati, Ohio

Pamela C. Levi, EdD, MSN, RN
Dean and Professor
School of Health Sciences
Georgia College and State University
Milledgeville, Georgia

Alice B. Loper, MN, RN, FNP
Assistant Professor of Nursing
Director, Student Health Services
Georgia College and State University
Milledgeville, Georgia

Elizabeth A. Lorenzi, MSN, RN, CHTP
Associate Professor
Northern Kentucky University
Highland Heights, Kentucky

Ann Schmidt Luggen, PhD, RN, ARNP, CS, CNAA
Professor of Nursing
College of Professional Studies
Northern Kentucky University
Highland Heights, Kentucky

Cheryl McKenzie, MN, RN, C, FNP
Associate Professor of Nursing
Northern Kentucky University
Highland Heights, Kentucky

Sue E. Meiner, EdD, RN, CS, GNP
Assistant Professor
University of Nevada, Las Vegas
Las Vegas, Nevada

Irene S. Morgan, PhD, RN, FNP
Professor of Nursing
California State University, Chico
Chico, California

Margaret R. Murphy, MSN, RN, FNP, CS
Instructor/Clinical
UTHSCSA School of Nursing
San Antonio, Texas

Louise M. Niemer, PhD, ARNP, CPNP
Associate Professor, Nursing
Northern Kentucky University
Highland Heights, Kentucky

Carol Ormond, MSN, RN, CS, FNP
Assistant Professor
Georgia College and State University
Milledgeville, Georgia

Mollie R. Poynton, MSN, RN, ARNP
Doctoral Student
Indiana University
Indianapolis, Indiana

Alice G. Rini, JD, MS, RN
Associate Professor of Nursing
Northern Kentucky University
Highland Heights, Kentucky

Denise Robinson, PhD, RN, FNP
Professor and Director, MSN Program
Northern Kentucky University
Highland Heights, Kentucky
Family Nurse Practitioner
Northern Kentucky Family Health Centers
Covington, Kentucky

Lisa Spangler Torok, MSN, PhDc, RN
Assistant Professor
Thomas More College
Crestview Hills, Kentucky

Gracie S. Wishnia, PhD, MSN, RN-C (Gerontology)
Spalding University
Louisville, Kentucky

Reviewers

Sue Adams, MS, RN
President
Healing Interventions of Scottsdale, PC
Scottsdale, Arizona

Patricia H. Arford, PhD, RN
Associate Professor
College of Nursing
Medical University of South Carolina
Charleston, South Carolina

Kathleen D. Becker, MS, CRNP
Assistant Professor
Coordinator, Adult Nurse Practitioner Program
The Johns Hopkins University
School of Nursing
Baltimore, Maryland

Pat Bradley, MSN, DNS, RN
Associate Professor
Texas Christian University
Fort Worth, Texas

Joan K. Carter, PhD, RN
Associate Dean
Saint Louis University
School of Nursing
St. Louis, Missouri

Esther H. Condon, PhD, RN
Associate Professor of Nursing
Hampton University
Hampton, Virginia

Linda Curry, PhD, RN
Associate Dean, Harris College of Nursing
Texas Christian University
Fort Worth, Texas

Nancy J. Fishwick, PhD, RN, CS
Associate Professor
University of Maine
School of Nursing
Orono, Maine

Joyce Newman Giger, EdD, RN, CS, FAAN
Professor, Graduate Studies
School of Nursing
University of Alabama at Birmingham
Birmingham, Alabama

Thomasine D. Guberski, PhD, CRNP
Associate Professor
University of Maryland
School of Nursing
Baltimore, Maryland

Mary Reuther Herring, MSN
Hypnotherapist
Healing Interventions of Scottsdale, PC
Scottsdale, Arizona

Kathleen Huttlinger, PhD
Professor and Director, FNP Program
Director, Grants and Sponsored Programs
Samuel Merritt College
Oakland, California

Rhonda Johnston, MS, PhD, FNP-C, ANP-C, CNS
Associate Professor
Director of the School-Based Wellness Centers
University of Southern Colorado
Parkview Medical Center
Pueblo, Colorado

Patricia S. Jones, PhD, RN
Professor
Loma Linda University
Loma Linda, California

Karen Anderson Keith, PhD, RN, CS, FNP
Associate Professor and Chairperson
Department of Graduate Studies
Lienhard School of Nursing
Pace University
Pleasantville, New York

Judy A. Lidy, FNP, RNC
Dr. Roger Bishop and Associate Staff
Effingham, Illinois
Southern Illinois University, Edwardsville
Edwardsville, Illinois

Ann B. Mech, MS, RN, JD
Assistant Professor and Coordinator, Legal Services
School of Nursing
University of Maryland
Baltimore, Maryland

Jayne F. Moore, PhD, RN
Assistant Professor
Orvis School of Nursing
University of Nevada
Reno, Nevada

Louise C. Selanders, EdD, RN
Associate Professor
Michigan Sate University College of Nursing
East Lansing, Michigan

Jeanne M. Sorrell, PhD, RN
Coordinator, PhD in Nursing Program
Professor
College of Nursing and Health Science
George Mason University
Fairfax, Virginia

Thanks to my son and daughter-in-law, Brian and Angela, and my grandsons, Morgan and Andrew, for their love and encouragement throughout this project. "Boys, now Tiggy can come out and play!" To Denise, thanks for asking me to be a part of this incredible journey! Working with you has been very special indeed.

CPK

Thanks to my family, John, Kristin, and Callie, who knew when to get me out of my office and when I needed to be left alone. I am so glad that you are with me on my journey. Thanks also to Cheryl—what a team we made! I could not have done it as well without you.

DR

Preface

Master of Science in Nursing (MSN) programs have increased by 7.6% over the last 5 years, in large measure because of renewed interest in advanced practice nurse (APN) roles (American Association of Colleges of Nursing [AACN], 1996). The majority of MSN programs require specific core content before a student may take specialization courses in his or her respective focus area, and this book was developed because of our desire to have all of the core content for MSN education for advanced practice represented in one source. This idea was based on the AACN's definition of core curriculum content, or those curriculum topics that are considered foundational for all MSN programs irrespective of specialty. In its book *Essentials of Masters Education in Nursing* (1996), the AACN has laid out recommendations for any APN who provides direct patient care. Once this core content is mastered, students can them complete specialization courses for their specific clinical focus.

The core curriculum content areas are very broad, so it is difficult to find a text that addresses all areas. Certainly, there are excellent individual books on theory, health promotion, role development, diversity, health care delivery, ethics, and health policy, but it is unlikely that one book would include all these topic areas. More often, faculty select a book that addresses only part of the content, relying on extensive outside readings as supplements, because no book is an ideal match for all course content. However, graduate students need the opportunity to explore their attitudes and make decisions regarding the incorporation of diverse concepts into their personal and professional value systems. Texts exploring all sides of the issues create more tolerant APNs. Because no currently available book seemed to capture all the information needed, we wrote *Core Concepts in Advanced Practice Nursing*. This book, while not totally inclusive of all content related to the core curriculum, will serve well as a basis for most core courses. Since this content is included on many certification examinations, it should also serve as a resource for preparing for certification.

To help the reader better understand the foundation of *Core Concepts in Advanced Practice Nursing*, the AACN's core curriculum areas are presented, with the goals for inclusion in the curricula, in the following list:

- *Research*—The goal of research is to prepare a clinician who is proficient at the use of research, including skills in evaluation, problem identification, awareness of practice outcomes, and clinical application. This includes practice outcomes and the use of the findings for clinical and organizational decision-making.
- *Health care policy*—The purpose of health care policy is for an APN to develop a comprehensive knowledge of how health policy is formulated, how to affect the process, and how it affects clinical practice and health care delivery.
- *Organization of the health care delivery system*—The organization of health care provides an understanding of community and the organization of community-based and acute care delivery systems. This understanding contributes to efficient functioning and the ability of an APN to serve in the role of leader.
- *Health care financing*—Knowledge of health care financing helps an APN develop an understanding of and familiarity with health financing as a foundation for the delivery of health care services.
- *Ethics*—Ethical decision-making provides an understanding of principles, personal values, and beliefs that provide a framework for nursing practice.
- *Professional role development*—Content related to the area of speciality practice provides a clear understanding of the nursing profession, APN roles, requirements for and regulation of these roles, and the necessary professional behaviors.
- *Theoretical foundations of nursing practice*—Knowledge about theory helps an APN be prepared to critique, evaluate, and utilize appropriate theory within his or her practice; the theoretical foundations of nursing are based on a wide range of theories.
- *Human diversity and social issues*—Diversity provides an understanding and appreciation of human diversity in health and illness and the foundation needed to provide culturally sensitive care.
- *Health promotion and disease prevention*—Information related to health promotion, illness prevention, and maintenance of function across the health-illness continuum serves and influences the goal of achieving health for patients.

What is different about *Core Concepts in Advanced Practice Nursing*? This book addresses all of the core content areas identified in the previous list in one reference source. While the core content area of research is not treated as a separate topic (there are many excellent research texts available), research is emphasized in every topical area. In addition, because the aim of this text is to provide an overview of MSN core curriculum topics, readers are referred to additional readings for more in-depth information on each topic.

Specific features of the text in each content area include definitions related to the topic; application of the content to APNs; and implications for research, MSN education, and clinical practice. Suggestions are provided for class discussion and critical thinking and analysis. Internet topics and resources are provided for each area, as are suggestions for further learning and a thorough bibliography. Specific practice-related examples are included throughout the text, including examples from the professional arenas of the clinical nurse specialist (CNS), nurse practitioner (NP), certified registered nurse anesthetist (CRNA), and certified nurse midwife (CNM). Each section of the text stands alone so the book does not have to be read from cover to cover in any particular order. Faculty and students can select sections useful for their own courses or that they find most compelling.

The contributors to this book were recruited from across the United States and bring their own expertise and diversity to the content. Many of them are in the forefront of nursing practice and research. In addition, nursing faculty reviewers from across the nation also shared their recommendations to make this book the best it can be.

We hope that these core concepts serve as your milestones for advanced practice and that *Core Concepts in Advanced Practice Nursing* serves you well, making a positive contribution to both your journey and your final APN destination.

American Association of Colleges of Nursing (1996). *Essentials of Masters Education in Nursing*. Washington, DC: American Association of Colleges of Nursing.

ACKNOWLEDGMENTS

Thanks to our nursing faculty colleagues who shared their expertise through both writing and reviewing parts of this manuscript—they helped to make this a thorough and complete reference. We also want to thank Stacy Welsh, Developmental Editor, for her superb organizational skills and multiple contributions to this book.

Contents

Core Concepts in

ADVANCED
PRACTICE
NURSING

Section I

Health Care Policy

Alice G. Rini

Health care policy is continuously changing. In the past decade, it has been characterized by rapid, dramatic transformation in several directions. One change comes from the forces of the economic market, which affect policy and the law arising from such policy. Competition among care providers has permitted the emergence of a variety of health care professionals and others who offer different aspects of care to individuals seeking such care. Regulations at federal and state levels attempt to control the entry of health care practitioners into the health care system and then control their practice. Much of this regulation is promoted and demanded by existing health care providers, and such competition has changed the health care environment, yielding both accommodation and control.

Federal and state governments are changing too. In some cases, existing government programs are responding to market forces by restructuring health care programs. In other cases, the government has resisted the market and the consumer demands and tried to institute a single-payer system.

This change raises serious policy issues related to the control of decision-making regarding the quality and cost of health care, what individuals and organizations make decisions, what providers are available to offer care, and how access to care is addressed. Much of this decision-making is driven by people's beliefs about health and its care. How much of health is determined by behavior and lifestyle, and how much can traditional allopathic medical care affect it? How can advanced practice nurses (APNs) use knowledge of the political system to achieve the best approach to the health care that Americans want?

Chapter 1 presents a scholarly and critical introduction to the organization of health care, its regulation, the concern for quality, and the issues of individual freedom in the health care market. Health care policy concerns some of the most important political, legal, and philosophical issues in the lives of American (and international)

citizens. Health care is not only an important issue, it is one of the most expensive. Costing more than a trillion dollars, or at least 15% of the gross national product, it deserves attention from APNs who, as administrators of health care entities and as direct care providers, are major players in the health care industry. Chapter 1 also addresses who and what should determine how access to health care is managed, how health care is financed, what policies and practices are most beneficial to American citizens and communities, and how this affects the interests of providers, consumers, and institutions of care. APNs need to be competent in understanding the origin and structure of health care policy, its players, and how they may interact with these players. Nurses need to be able to critically analyze existing and new policies in terms of their effect on consumers and providers, while also understanding that the United States has a constitution which should (and generally does) guide the policies that are developed.

There is little mention of nursing in much of the health policy literature. However, nurses are contributing to policy in major ways. Chapter 2 includes extensive references to health policy–analysis organizations and government and independent Internet sites, where there is a vast amount of information about laws and regulations related to health policy. This information will facilitate the ability of APNs to familiarize themselves with health policy literature and assist them to analyze and contribute to that policy.

Chapter 3 discusses how to influence healthy policy through lobbying and educating policy-makers. Specific information is provided on how to communicate confidently and competently with legislators and policy analysts. APNs must be able to articulate their roles and contributions to consumers and the health care system in terms of the quality and extent of care they provide. Chapter 3 stresses the important components of how to present data in a way that is logical and understandable to all involved parties.

Chapter 1

Evolution of Health Care Policy in the United States

Alice G. Rini

A nation's health policy is a function of its beliefs about health, the role of government in the lives of citizens, and the demands of people as reflected in their behaviors and use of health care services. Health plays an important part in the social and economic life of society. One's physical and psychological health is a determinant of many social and economic opportunities (i.e., participation in work, recreation, and human relationships). Social and economic factors also have an effect on individual health. Reasonably, then, the health of each individual and the population as a whole is important to the functioning of society. Longest (1998) defines *health policies* as authoritative decisions by governmental bodies which direct or influence actions and decisions of organizations and individuals in the health care system. Policies are actually made in both the public and private sectors. Significant and influential private organizations that make authoritative decisions in the United States include the Joint Commission on the Accreditation of Healthcare Organizations (JCAHO), the American Hospital Association (AHA), and the National Committee for Quality Assurance (NCQA). On a smaller scale, managed care organizations (MCOs) and professional associations also develop policies that influence the behavior of their members (Longest, 1998).

Policy-making is influenced by the society it affects. American people value freedom, autonomy, self-determination, and privacy. These values are evident in the movement to gain control over health care decisions at the end of life, the activities of the United Seniors Association in combating laws that prevented Medicare beneficiaries from privately contracting for their health care (*United Seniors Association, Inc. v. Shalala*), and the resistance to the universal health identifier proposed by the Health Care Financing Administration (HCFA). Because proposed and existing health care policies often interfere with these values, there is an ongoing conflict between the efforts of public (or governmental) policy-makers and the independence of the American people.

There is no universal agreement on the definition of health. The World Health Organization (WHO, 1958) defines *health* as "a state of complete physical, mental, and social well-being, and not merely the absence of disease or injury." Taken at face value, such a definition has appeal; however, this definition does not consider how well-functioning people with mild to moderate impairments or controlled chronic conditions could be healthy. Brook and McGlynn (1991) propose a broader conceptualization that considers the diversity of the population, the inevitability of aging and change, and the reality that health and adaptation to one's environment and to life itself are unique and individual. Their definition views health as a condition of the maximum functioning of biological capacity and the everyday life role as measured by certain well-accepted indicators. In addition to managing one's own life tasks, such as work, recreation, interaction with family and friends, and spiritual activities, certain biological markers have been identified with good health. Ten biological characteristics are described that are indicative of health status. They are muscle mass, strength, basal metabolic rate, body fat percentage, aerobic capacity, blood sugar tolerance, cholesterol level, cholesterol/high-density lipoprotein (HDL) ratio, blood pressure, and temperature regulation (Evans & Rosenberg, 1992).

The way a society or culture conceptualizes health reflects the values of that society with regard to the abilities and functioning of its individuals. It may also determine what support society may provide to its citizens in their pursuit and maintenance of health. Health care or (more accurately) medical care tends to provide acute care, drug therapy, and surgery. Although these therapies are quite useful in many circumstances, there seems to be little offered that is directed toward improving the ten aforementioned biological characteristics. Research shows that such improvement would have a significant effect on an individual's ability to engage in life tasks important to them (Evans & Rosenberg, 1992).

Advanced practice nurses (APNs) might do well to consider a holistic approach to patients (an approach that has long been an important nursing function) rather than rely exclusively on a medical model of care. Lobbying for

3

policy changes that would alter the way health promotion and maintenance are defined could also be a valuable activity.

Since society is affected by both public and private policy-making, it is important to understand the difference between them. Both play an important role in the functioning of health care systems. This means not only lobbying for appropriate public policy, but also lobbying with the private organizations that are intimately affecting health care.

DEFINITIONS

A *constitution* is the fundamental law of a nation or state, generally written, which establishes the character of its government; determines the principles to which the nation or state conforms; organizes the government; regulates, distributes, and limits the functions of its various parts; and prescribes the extent and manner of exercise of its sovereign power (Black, 1991).

Legislation pertains to state and federal legislatures making, altering, amending, and repealing laws and programs, which, by constitutional mandate, they have the authority to do (Black, 1991). A *bill* is a draft of a proposed law from the time of its introduction in one of the houses of Congress or state legislature, through committee hearings, and through to its final consideration. If not passed, a bill dies at the end of a Congressional or state legislative session and must be reintroduced at the next session if it is to be reconsidered (Black, 1991). An *appropriations bill* addresses the raising and expenditure of public funds; at the federal level, such bills originate in the House of Representatives. Once a bill has been acted upon and passed into law by a legislature it is know as an *act* (Black, 1991).

Some composites of laws are called programs. *Programs* are legislative enactments that stand independently and are aimed at specific legislative objectives (Longest, 1998). Legislation related to health care, the industry that provides it, and the practitioners who make up the health care work force is generated at both federal and state levels. Legislation starts with a bill, introduced in one of the houses of the federal or state legislature—Senate and House of Representatives in Washington, DC, and Senate and House or Assembly at the state level. (Names vary by state for the lower chamber.)

Policy refers to the general principles by which a government is guided in its management of public affairs; it also means the general purpose or tendency of a law, ordinance, or rule (Black, 1991).

Police power is the authority conferred to the states by the Tenth Amendment of the U.S. Constitution, through which they are able to establish laws and regulations that preserve the public order and generally secure the comfort, safety, morals, health, and prosperity of the citizens; states may place restraints on the personal freedom and property rights of persons in order to promote public safety. Police power is subject to the limitations of federal and state constitutions and the requirements of due process (Black, 1991).

Due process is provided for by the federal Constitution in the Fifth Amendment, which protects citizens from actions by the federal government, and in the Fourteenth Amendment, which protects individuals from state action. Procedural due process guarantees fair procedures, while substantive due process protects a person's property from unfair governmental interference or seizure. The Fifth Amendment demands that laws be reasonable (not arbitrary or capricious) and have a substantial relation to the end being sought by the enactment of the law. Essential elements of due process are notice and the opportunity to be heard, the chance to defend oneself in an orderly proceeding adapted to the nature of the case or problem, and the characteristics of fairness and justice (Black, 1991).

Health insurance is a contract or agreement whereby one party, for the agreed-upon payment of a premium, is obligated to pay or provide a benefit to another party should there be bodily injury, illness, disability, or some other affliction that falls under the contract's enumerated risks. Group insurance for persons with something in common, such as place of employment, fraternal organization, or student body, provides coverage for the enumerated casualties to the specified group; group insurance remains in effect only as long as a person remains affiliated with the group.

CRITICAL ISSUES: HEALTH POLICY ISSUES FACING ADVANCED PRACTICE NURSES

The composition and power of a legislative body is mandated by a federal or state constitution. Each body (House or Senate) has a presiding officer. At the federal level, the Vice President presides in the Senate (there is also a majority leader) and the Speaker of the House presides in the House of Representatives. The majority party in either house holds majority officer status, this officer being elected by the other members of the party. Both houses also have party minority leaders. State legislative bodies are organized in a similar manner.

When there is a perceived need for a law or a change in a current law, a bill is introduced. The impetus for the bill may come from many sources—the President or Governor, a member of the legislature, an interest group, or an individual. For example, the Kentucky Coalition of Nurse Practitioners and Nurse Midwives (KCNPNM) decided that further clarification and mandate was needed for nurse practitioners (NPs) to dispense samples. The rules and regulations related to prescribing talked about samples but were unclear. The Board of Pharmacy felt that the ability to dispense samples was not implicit in the advanced practice act. The KCNPNM approached a sympathetic representative and broached the idea of the needed legislation.

When it is determined that an idea needs action, one of the representatives (called *assemblymen* or some other appropriate name) or senators drafts and introduces a bill. Other representatives and senators are asked to participate as sponsors; sponsors are critical to the success of a bill. Each bill is numbered, with the designation S. for Senate or H.B. for House Bill; this designation identifies the bill throughout its transit in both houses and the committees, and on to passage or defeat.

Bills are assigned to committees in the house of origin based on the subject matter of the proposed law. In committee, the bill is discussed, altered, approved, or discarded, then reported to the respective legislative body for consideration. If there are to be hearings on the bill, they are done through the committee. Once back in the originating legislative body, the bill is voted upon. If passed, it goes to the other legislative body, where a similar pattern is followed. If a bill passes both houses, it goes to the executive (President or Governor) for a signature or veto. If signed, the bill becomes law; if not signed or if vetoed, it does not become law unless the legislative bodies override the veto. Such an override requires a two-thirds vote of each house. Bills do not always become laws, and if they do, they may not become effective immediately; the draft of a law may indicate a future time that the provisions become effective.

In the case of the sample dispensing, a legislator (who also happened to be a nurse) drafted the bill and gained support from other legislators. The bill was assigned a number for both houses. The lobbyist of the KCNPNM and many of the APNs in Kentucky worked hard to get the bill passed. This meant contacting legislators to describe how important sample dispensing is for their practice, having patients write letters to support the bill, and attending sessions in the capital. The bill was passed, and APNs in Kentucky were able to dispense samples beginning in July 2000.

Once a bill becomes law, it gets a new number. The number has a public law designation and is named for the number of the Congress that passed it and the chronological number of the passed bill. The new law must be carried out in a manner consistent with the purposes Congress has stated. This is the responsibility of the administrative agency, which has jurisdiction over the subject matter of the law or act. The agency enacts rules and regulations that implement the provisions of the law. Bills, rules, and regulations may be challenged in court by agencies or individuals affected by them.

Examples of federal legislation are Medicare (Public Law 89-97, Title XVIII; health insurance for the aged) and the Nurses Training Act (Public Law 88-581, Title VIII; construction grants for schools of nursing, academic projects, and student loans). Examples of state legislation include licensing of health care providers, certification of need programs to control institutional expansion, and certification of long-term care (LTC) facilities.

Laws that Affect Advanced Practice Nurses

APNs are affected by laws, regulations, policies, and court decisions that address APN practice related to scope of practice, reimbursement, qualifications for licensure, delegation of authority from physicians, quality of care, and requirements for collaboration (Buppert, 1999). Many APNs believe that many such laws, regulations, and policies are barriers to APN practice. Anderson, Gillis, and Yoder (1996) identified numerous barriers for APN practice in the state of California, two of which were legal barriers: lack of prescriptive authority and reimbursement problems. Many APNs get involved in the health policy arena when they find that a statue, regulation, or policy keeps them from doing something to improve the quality or viability of their practice. For example, many states are using Medicaid managed care plans to help control expenses for Medicaid patients. APNs were not admitted to the provider panels, which meant they could not serve as primary care providers (PCPs) for their patients. In some states, NPs are requesting clarification of the state law so that they are specifically identified as PCPs (Buppert, 1999).

Financing of New Legislation

One of the major problems in enacting new laws is financing their implementation. Every time a law is passed, the cost must be considered. Many federal laws have been criticized because they are officially passed, but when certain actions are required by states or other entities, no sources of funds are identified or made available. Another possibility is a possibly significant cost to citizens and taxpayers. The array of proposals for Medicare prescription drug coverage currently in Congress illustrates the issue of financing programs. Congress has, in the past, considered adding a prescription drug coverage provision to Medicare; however the projected cost has been a major deterrent (O'Sullivan, 1999). (Chapter 11 provides information on the cost of implementing laws and the programs they establish.)

At present, Medicare is in financial peril, particularly considering the aging of the "baby boomer" generation, the first of whose retirees will be eligible for Medicare coverage in 2008, just as the program becomes insolvent. A new program, which could be extremely expensive, will significantly increase the cost of Medicare and the taxpayers' cost to maintain the program. There are only two means to manage the increase—raising taxes, which currently pay for 75% of the ongoing program, or raising the premiums or cost-sharing for Medicare beneficiaries.

A Senate bill (S. 841) suggested the use of tobacco tax funds to finance the projected $20 billion a prescription drug program will cost taxpayers. However, with the number of smokers declining, it is not likely the expected tax revenue will be generated. Furthermore, the government has consistently underestimated the costs of running its programs, so the $20 billion estimate may be far less than the proposed drug program will actually cost (Frogue, 1999).

In 1988 to 1989, the Medicare Catastrophic Coverage Act appeared to have widespread support until beneficiaries found out the cost of such a program. Outpatient prescription drugs were to be covered. However, when it was determined that the federal law implementing the Act would require states to pay Medicare premiums, deductibles, and coinsurance for millions of low-income older adults and disabled persons, and that those not classified as low income would be subject to higher premiums, new taxes, and higher deductibles and co-payments, there was a massive response from seniors. Congress repealed the Act (Moffit, 1994). At the time the Act was passed in 1988, the Congressional Budget Office (CBO) estimated the costs (in terms of prescription drugs) for the program for fiscal years (FY) 1990 to 1993 to be $5.7 billion. By 1989, the CBO had revised its estimate to $11.8 billion (O'Sullivan, 1999).

In President Bill Clinton's health care reform proposal of 1994, a similar situation existed. The Health Security Act proposed by the Clinton administration was estimated to cost $69.1 billion for FY 1996 to 2000. The CBO estimated that for 2000 alone, the cost of the Clinton program would be $19 billion, $2 billion higher than the administration's estimate (O'Sullivan, 1999).

In terms of the current prescription drug proposal, there are similar concerns about cost. Medicare Part B spending for prescription drugs in 1997 was about $2.75 billion. The Balanced Budget Act of 1997 called for payments for drugs at 83% of the average wholesale price. It was believed that Medicare was paying more for the limited number of drugs it covered than were physicians and prescription drug suppliers. Even with a decrease in the wholesale price of drugs, the estimate for a new prescription drug benefit with a $250 deductible, 20% coinsurance, and a $1000 cap on out-of-pocket expenses would be $22.5 billion in 2000. This amount is after beneficiaries have paid their premiums, which cover only 25% of costs (Crippen, 1999).

The National Academy on Social Insurance estimates that a drug benefit would add 7% to 13% to the cost of Medicare over the next 10 years. This figure assumes that deductibles, coinsurance, benefits, and maximum out-of-pocket amounts rise at the same level as the consumer price index (Gluck, 1999). In the past, drug costs have increased at a rate almost three times that of health care in general. From 1992 to 1998, spending on pharmaceuticals doubled. The HCFA suggests that this increase is due to the number of new, high-priced drugs becoming available, as well as increased consumer demand for them.

The Pharmaceutical Research and Manufacturers of America reported in an industry profile that the 15.7% increase in spending in 1998 was due to a 12.5% increase in the volume of purchases and a 3.2% increase in prices (Pharmaceutical Industry Profile, 1999). This long-term change is likely due to the effectiveness and quality of available and near-available medicines and to the public's trust in the medicines, a trust earned over time. A government program disturbing this progress would not be well received by either the public or the health care providers that participate in the drug market.

Rules and Regulations that Affect Advanced Practice Nurses

Rules and regulations provide for policy implementation. This begins with rule-making by the agencies, which are part of the executive branch of government and responsible for implementation of laws passed by the legislature. In the rule and regulation formulation phase, agencies are expected to make their proposals public. They do this by publishing an initial draft of the proposed rules called an *advance notice of proposed rulemaking* (ANPR) in the *Federal Register* (which is published daily). Generally, organizations, associations, and even individuals affected by the regulations comment, suggest modifications, and provide information on the effect of the regulation on the operation of the affected industry.

For example, if state regulations addressing nursing homes do not address APN practice, the state NP organization would want to make changes. First, the organization could ask the director of the appropriate state agency for a change in regulations to include APNs as providers in nursing homes. Secondly, the group could ask legislators for a regulation change and, if necessary, for a statute requiring the agency director to change the regulations regarding APNs (Buppert, 1999).

Health care, including LTC, is heavily regulated. There are many complex regulations that affect the industry and those who work within it or provide services for patients seeking care. Health care agencies are subject to regulations promulgated by federal agencies and state agencies.

Rules and regulations promulgated by administrative agencies have the same legal effect as any other laws and are actually governmental policy. These laws are found in the *Code of Federal Regulations* (CFR). Although the administrative agency is responsible for implementation of policy, the legislative branch (Senate and House) maintains oversight responsibility to ensure that legislative intent is fulfilled and the final rules and regulations reflect the public interest (Longest, 1998). The oversight function is important because the representative body at the federal or state level is elected and represents the people or electorate. Agency personnel are appointed or merely hired as employees, usually by or through the executive (President or Governor), and have little accountability to the citizens. To maintain a truly representative government, such oversight is imperative.

Rules and regulations are implementation details for enacted laws or modifications of earlier laws and acts. A recent example is a proposal by the HCFA to require home care agencies to collect and report sensitive personal information from care recipients to develop a database for use by government agencies to assist in the management of the Medicare program. This proposal has generated significant controversy and is currently challenged by the Heritage Foundation (a health policy research organization), the American Civil Liberties Union (ACLU), and other organizations. Another example from the HCFA is the Medicare prospective payment system, which sets an amount of reimbursement to hospitals for patient care based on the final diagnosis at the time of discharge. Provider payment schemes (through the HCFA and private MCOs) are also classified as policies; these influence the caregiving behavior of physicians and other providers using a series of rewards and punishments.

Legislative oversight is a complex process that includes committee action, receipt of reports, and other involvement with administrative agencies. (An overview of legislative oversight is provided in Box 1-1.) Citizens and organizations affected by the implementation of policies may appeal to administrative courts, where their complaints are heard by administrative law judges (ALJs). While this is not direct legislative oversight, the provision of such hearings is mandated by the legislature to provide a judicial remedy for problematic policy implementation.

Regulation of health care personnel
The health care industry is one of the nation's largest employers. In 1993 the U.S. Department of Labor reported that more than 10% of the U.S. workforce, or 11 million people, were employed in health care positions. This is due to a variety of factors, including the expansion of health care technology; the population increase, especially among older adults; a tax policy favoring partially employer-funded health insurance; treatment advances from research; federal support for education of health care personnel; and public financing of the building of hospitals and nursing homes (Sultz & Young, 1997).

Recently, the growth trend has changed. An effort to contain growth and costs has altered the mix of personnel sought and supported. There is a shift of employment from hospitals to outside service settings and an emphasis on lower-level personnel to provide care in all areas. At the same time, the expansion of technology requires personnel to possess specialized knowledge and skills. It is likely that much experimentation with the mix of skills and education of personnel will be needed before the ideal balance is found.

As the health care industry is highly regulated, so too

Box 1-1

Overview of Legislative Oversight

Congress achieves its responsibility to oversee the function of administrative agencies through:

1. Sustaining, reducing, or eliminating funding appropriations (money to implement programs) by Congressional committees that provide for the continuing implementation of the laws to which the regulations apply; annual funding decisions are made based on:
   a. The performance of the agency implementing the policy
   b. The continued need for the policy
   c. Inadequacies in the implementation
   d. Any negative effect of the regulations on the regulated industry, inconsistent with the goals of the law.
2. Direct contact with personnel involved in policy implementation; this includes:
   a. Agency personnel providing testimony before Congress
   b. Use of oversight agencies specifically organized to provide services, such as the CBO and the GAO (Longest, 1998)
3. Reviewing and evaluating the application, administration, and effectiveness of a policy and its implementation; this is:
   a. Accomplished by each Congressional committee for which the subject matter of the law is within that committee's jurisdiction (Longest, 1998)
   b. Required by the rules of the Senate and House of Representatives (Rule X, Clauses 2b [1] and 2d [1] in the Rules of the House; there is a similar rule in the Senate)

---

are the health professions. Education and licensure are regulated at the state level. Because of this, there is variation among states in titles, scopes of practice, licensure requirements, and other factors. State governments claim to regulate the health professions in order to protect the public from unprepared, incompetent, and malpracticing practitioners, but there is controversy about this regulation. Critics assert that regulation excludes practitioners who do not meet the established criteria, criteria that were promulgated by members of the professions themselves. The criticism is basically about currently established practitioners protecting their own turf, when in fact, research has shown that for some lay practitioners, the overall safety of their patients is similar to that of licensed practitioners. Blevins (1995) describes how state practice laws and federal reimbursement policies limit patient access to the full range of available health care providers, including nurse (or other) midwives and NPs. Regulatory restrictions also limit the manner in which health care institutions can use personnel. Such restrictions may interfere with innovation and new strategies to deliver care (Sultz & Young, 1997). However, many of the strategies proposed and implemented by hospitals and LTC facilities have been criticized as unsafe and significantly understaffed with professional personnel, and such strategies are risky; there are several court cases involving patient injury that were decided on the basis of inadequate staffing.

Through licensure of health occupations, state law regulates the education and testing requirements for practice. Some states regulate only prelicensure programs; others regulate all programs, including those that advance the education of health care personnel beyond the first professional degree. State law also restricts the use of the professional title to those who have met the state standard; it is illegal for anyone not so credentialed to use a professional title. State boards of licensure, composed of members of the profession (and sometimes others, including consumers of health care), set standards for entry into the profession, mandate (or choose not to mandate) continuing education requirements, and censure practitioners who practice while impaired or in a manner inconsistent with set standards. There is criticism of professional licensing boards over their monitoring of continued professional competence. Although boards are vigilant when reports of malpractice or failure to meet standards are made, there is no regular assessment of continued competence and often no content requirement in the continuing education mandates. This permits or even encourages members of the profession to take continuing education courses that are not job specific, are nontechnical, or are merely convenient in time or place. Other professions, such as accounting, require specific content areas to ensure continued technical and substantive competence (Personal communication, Arthur Anderson Consulting, March 19, 2000).

Certification and licensing of health care personnel

Certification is a process by which a state or professional organization recognizes educational achievements and professional competence in a particular health field or specialty. Certification means that the person holding the title has obtained advanced and specialized education. Professional certifying bodies do not censure or probate practitioners for malpractice or practicing while impaired (Sultz & Young, 1997). Certification status may be lost if certain educational and practice requirements are not met. Certifying bodies include the American Nurses Credentialing Center (ANCC) and certain specialty nursing associations.

Nurses and most other professionals are licensed in a particular state. Most of the time, one can obtain licensure in more than one state, but for some professions, one can only maintain active licensure in the state where the majority of one's practice is performed. The National Council of State Boards of Nursing (NCSBN) has proposed a mechanism to permit interstate practice for

nurses. Such multistate practice agreements would permit nurses to practice in several states while maintaining licensure in their home states only. It is expected that such a plan would facilitate obtaining work and limit the need for relicensure each time a nurse accepts a position in a new state. This is particularly an issue for those living near the borders of states and for persons who move their residence frequently. There is already precedent for such agreements; nurses who work for the Veterans Administration or are in the military carry their home state licensure to their assigned location without seeking licensure in a new state.

The American Nurses Association (ANA) has some concerns about multistate licensure. The ANA suggests that boards of nursing need adequate mechanisms to ensure knowledge of who is practicing within a state. At the same time, nurses need mechanisms designed to provide them with practice-related information particular to that state. One suggestion is for a registry, so that any nurse practicing within a state is registered with the appropriate agency in that state. That state could then provide the nurse with current practice laws and other necessary information (ANA, 2000). Such interstate mechanisms need to provide for action taken on complaints about practitioners as well, because such action is within the purview of the board. The state interest in the safety of its citizens, which is the function of licensure, must be preserved in any interstate practice pattern (ANA, 2000).

Role of Consumers in Health Care Policy

What is the role of the consumer in health care? Much of the history of health care in this country and others is of paternalism by health care providers toward health care consumers. From the mid-1800s through the mid-1900s, there was fairly strong control of health care by the medical profession. This control was supported by government legislation and judicial decisions. The purpose was to guarantee the authority and autonomy of physicians, and this purpose was evident in patient consent to treatment, liability for malpractice, professional licensure and control of the health care situation, and publicly funded programs, all of which promoted the individual physician in private practice (Rosenblatt & Rosenbaum, 1997). In the mid-1900s, a shift began toward a more egalitarian perspective—the notion that patients and other health care providers have a legitimate interest in the health care system and should have equal protection. There is little question that there are still very unequal relationships between physicians and patients, insurers and health care consumers, and hospitals and both consumers and health care employees (Rosenblatt & Rosenbaum, 1997). More recently there has been a movement to equalize power among these parties by strong support for such things as consumer education, legal protection of a patient's right to consent to or refuse treatment, standards of care, and consumer-centered choice regarding health care insurance, its provider, and health care itself.

Evolution of consumer power

As far back as the twelfth century, the majority of health care providers, or *healers* as they were known then, were women. Although there were some well-known names in early medicine (such as Maimonides, Semmelweis, and Locke), most healers had little or no formal training, nor were they organized as a "professional" group. Until the 1800s, most care was provided in a patient's home, which, at the time, was a far safer place than the hospital for care of the sick. The hospitals that were available were unsanitary and generally provided care only to those who were unable to be cared for in their homes. Some cities provided care for the very poor in publicly supported hospitals that were little more than prisons meant to control and reform patients. For others such as seamen, urban workers, poor people who were neither criminals nor mentally ill, and travelers who were not economically destitute, voluntary or charitable hospitals were established. These hospitals were later used for medical education and advanced medical practice (Starr, 1982). Consumers had little choice regarding care because they knew little about physiology, pathology, and the cure of disease. Even wealthy, educated health care consumers had little or no power in the health care system; they may have had some influence on their choice of physician, but only if they lived in an urban area.

There was a definite improvement in health outcomes in the nineteenth and twentieth centuries. Although medical advances in sterilization, anesthesia, and surgical techniques had an effect on a patient's well-being, public health measures had a more far-reaching effect on overall societal health. Public sanitation, nutrition, immunizations, health education, and isolation of those with contagious diseases promoted the health of all members of society (Rosenblatt & Rosenbaum, 1997). However, governmental regulation and legal decisions continued to support the authority and income of physicians in the patterns of reimbursement provided by governmental and private entities and the access that patients had to information and choice about their health care problems, the remedies available, and the quality of the physicians they might select to address the problem. This situation continues today.

However, several events have contributed to an improvement in consumer power, including increased belief in quality of care and informed consent. The concept of quality of care is based not only on the technical competence and judgment of physicians, but also on promoting the well-being of patients. What this means is that one kind of medicine does not fit all patients; a patient's own goals and values are important in determining what treatment is appropriate. A therapy that causes pain, discomfort, disfigurement, or disability may be the most common treatment, but it may not be of "quality" to

a patient who prefers a less aggressive treatment that interferes less with the quality of life. However, there are situations in which medical personnel might determine that an older adult (for example) would not choose aggressive treatment and do not offer it; such generalization is not appropriate.

Quality seems to be a changing entity. Until recently, physicians generally believed that patients should be minimally informed about their illnesses and proposed treatments. Hippocrates probably originated this approach; he advised that a physician's most important characteristic was confidence and therefore he or she should have the goal of inspiring a patient's confidence in the physician's knowledge and skill. Without such confidence, a patient might not stay with the treatment (Konner, 1993). In theory, consent has been an important legal principle since 1914, at which time New York State Supreme Court Justice Benjamin Cardozo indicated that a patient was an autonomous person who had "the right to determine what would be done with his own body; and a surgeon who performs an operation without his patient's consent, commits an assault, for which he is liable in damages" (*Schloendorff v. Society of New York Hospital*, 105 N.E. 92, 93 [N.Y. 1914] J. Cardozo).

However, consent was not clearly defined for many years after 1914. If a patient did not actively object to treatment, this was considered consent, but certainly treating without consent is assault and/or battery. However, more recent interpretations of consent refer to its adequacy—does the patient have the information he or she needs to make an informed and intelligent decision about the care proposed? If consent is not adequate or is misleading, the situation becomes a negligence issue. Consent issues are addressed by state law, and the way any failure to obtain informed consent is handled varies by state. The responsibility for providing informed consent resides with the provider who will provide the care, treatment, or procedure, although this task can be delegated. It is not uncommon for physicians to delegate the function of providing appropriate information to registered nurses (RNs). Legislation and judicial opinions in this area maintain the accountability of the health care provider to provide appropriate information with regard to a proposed treatment. Even if this task is delegated to another provider, the one who undertakes to provide information or complete a program of teaching before a patient's acceptance of treatment assumes the responsibility for adequacy.

Another issue of informed consent is whether the standard of consent should be a professional one (i.e., what similarly situated, reasonably prudent physicians or other health care providers would do) or a patient-centered one (i.e., what a reasonable patient would find material to his or her decision to undergo or forego a treatment). A slight majority of states have adopted the professional standard, either by legislation or court decision. So, although the principle of informed consent contributes to consumer power and autonomy, it is still somewhat constrained by medical standards that may deny patients all the information they might desire regarding treatment. Consent-to-care laws generally provide protection for informed consent before instituting treatment unless there are certain extenuating circumstances. Such circumstances include an emergency so critical that there is no time to obtain consent; unconsciousness or incompetence of a patient in the absence of anyone else who could consent; and court orders.

Consumers of health care have also achieved some consideration in determining standards of care. At one time, acceptance of local standards was the norm. It no longer is, and a national standard has emerged in medical, nursing, and other health care provider practices because the professions themselves have accepted such a standard. There is national accreditation of schools of medicine, nursing, and other professions. Nationwide dissemination of knowledge is available to practitioners via journals and other media, including the Internet. There are also easy lines of communication with professionals in academic medical centers who can provide consultation using a variety of methods, including those that transmit voice, real-time photographs and video, and diagnostic information. However, critics of this national standard assert that the problem is not lack of information about technology or inability to find consultation; it is the unfamiliarity that practitioners in small towns and rural areas have with newer technology because of a lack of regular exposure to such technology. Those who herald the demise of the locality rule point out that it was unfriendly to consumers. It permitted possibly incompetent practitioners to establish the local standard. Experts on local standards to testify against even gross negligence were also difficult to find (Walz, 1969). However, some local standards may still operate since the policy of most courts is to allow for evidence of whether a practitioner was a generalist or specialist; the idea of the "same or similar circumstances"; and local factors such as the availability of certain resources.

One of the developments within the health care system that supports consumer autonomy and self-determination is the changing education of nurses. In their philosophies and curricula, most schools of nursing address their relationship with consumers of health and nursing care. Many of the theories of nursing practice focus on the importance of the patient as the locus of decision-making regarding care, either independently or in consultation with the nurse (see Section VI, Theoretical Foundations of Nursing Practice). Furthermore, since the development of the NP role, the APN is now established in providing primary care, managing the care of patients with chronic illnesses, and working in other care settings within industry, schools and colleges, clinics, primary and specialist physicians' offices, LTC, and psychiatric practice. This type of practitioner provides another choice for the health care consumer, and many consumers have chosen to have their care provided by a NP. Also very successful is the certified nurse midwife (CNM), who provides care during the prenatal, birth, and postpartum periods of a woman's pregnancy. Bullough and Bullough (1994) describe research that shows a woman with a healthy pregnancy, labor, and delivery is as safe in the care of a CNM as in the care of a physician. Nurse midwives are particularly effective in managing prenatal care so that women experience better outcomes in terms of minimizing the incidence of premature or underweight babies. Nurse midwives have been providing such care for most of the twentieth century in the United States and for a longer time in Europe.

Consumers are protected in terms of quality of care by the requirement of advanced testing and national certification and recertification of competency at specified intervals. Such recertification requires regular practice for a specified number of hours to remain certified. NPs tend to focus on promotion of wellness, patient education and counseling, health assessment, and health maintenance. Their care is holistic in that the patient as a whole is considered. This is different from traditional medical care, which is episodic and focuses on a particular health problem, possibly to the exclusion of a patient's need to incorporate normal life with the health problem and treatment.

Insurance and consumer behavior

Consumers in the health care system behave in a similar manner to any other consumer in any other market. The assumption in consumer behavior is that each consumer calculates the value of consuming a product or service and determines whether or not the value received is equal to the cost. If the price is borne directly by the consumer, then generally the lower the cost, the more the consumer will use the service. With the current kinds of health insurance available, consumers are shielded from the real cost of their consumption of medical care because most insurers cover costs from the first dollar of expenditure. This is typical of health maintenance organizations (HMOs), MCOs, and any other insurance that relies on copayments as risk-sharing by consumers and insurers. A copayment is a cost- or risk-sharing agreement between the insurer and the consumer (the insured) (Phelps, 1997). When the consumer obtains health care, he or she pays the amount of the copayment to the provider at the time of service. This keeps the consumer aware that there is a cost to the care received. The more the consumer is aware of the actual cost of care, the more he or she will consider value versus cost before consumption. Critics of insurance that provides first dollar coverage claim that since the consumer has no idea of the cost of care (merely paying a small payment at the time of the visit), there is a tendency to overconsume care. Phelps (1997) demonstrates that consumer behavior is affected by the amount of the

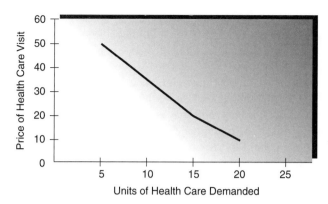

Figure 1-1 Demand for health care. The curve reveals that the number of visits to health care providers decreases as the price of the visits increases.

copayment; if copayments increase, consumption (or *demand*, as economists describe it) decreases. (Figure 1-1 shows the relationship between price and consumer behavior in terms of visits to physicians or other health care providers; the lower the price, the more visits are made.)

Consumers who have insurance plans with a deductible behave in two ways. Before spending the amount of the deductible, the consumer behaves as if he or she had no insurance (i.e., he or she carefully considers the cost of a visit to a health care provider) (Phelps, 1997). For example, a consumer with a health plan that carries an annual deductible of $500 must spend $500 of her own funds before the insurance pays anything. Suppose the consumer breaks a wrist while bicycle riding in March and visits the physician's office, where she receives a brace, some pain medication, and instructions on how to treat the wrist. She pays $100 for this treatment. Although the insurance company is notified of the visit and the payment, it takes no action except to record that the insured has satisfied $100 of the $500 deductible. For this problem the consumer chose to visit the physician because she knew she was injured, had considerable pain, and was concerned about the future use of the wrist. The consumer behaves as if she had no insurance because she was responsible for the full amount of the visit and treatment. She has considered the value received in relation to the cost expended. There is another economic value to the visit besides the care and treatment—the deductible has also been decreased to $400. If the consumer has no other health problems during the year except a bad cold on December 28th of the deductible year, it is likely that she will avoid seeing the physician until January 1st, the start of another deductible year. These are economic decisions that consumers make.

If, however, a consumer has several visits to physicians, he or she may satisfy the entire deductible, after which the insurance pays for care (this is possibly subject to a copayment). Phelps (1997) indicates that early in the deductible year, consumers behave as if they had no insurance. As the full deductible amount is approached,

the consumer begins to view things as if insurance was paying, except at the end of the deductible year. Once the deductible is completely satisfied, consumer behavior changes to that of other consumers with insurance (i.e., displaying less consideration for price and value).

People purchase insurance because they tend to be uncomfortable with risk. Since the threat of ill health is so unpredictable, insuring against the financial loss associated with illness or injury is a logical act on the part of the risk-averse consumer of care. How much and what kind of insurance is purchased is often a function of how much disposable income a person has and how much he or she is willing to risk. Such a model of consumer behavior is the basis of economic interpretation of such decisions. Economists predict that the higher the value or utility of insurance to the consumer, the more likely that consumer is to purchase insurance against financial risks (Hershey, Kunreuther, Schwartz, & Williams, 1984).

The demand for medical or health care is a function of the desire for health. As long as care produces better health, rational economic decision-making by health care consumers yields the common demand curve (as shown in Figure 1-1). As can be seen, the demand curve slopes upward, revealing that less care is demanded as the price increases, all other factors being equal. If there is serious illness, the demand curve is more vertical—more medical care is demanded by the seriously ill person, with less consideration of price.

Much of this consumer behavior is the result of the way health insurance is provided. Most people are covered for health insurance through their employers, although this is changing to some degree. For many years, however, the tax policy of the United States encouraged consumers to pay as much as possible of their health care costs through employer-based health care insurance, because this was paid with untaxed dollars. This situation started during World War II at a time when the government enacted wage and price controls as part of the war effort. Employers, in an attempt to attract and keep employees, added benefits in place of salary increases. The employers were able to take a tax deduction as a business expense on their income tax returns equal to the cost of the health insurance premiums paid on behalf of their employees. Employees did not have to count the value of the premiums paid as income, nor did they pay tax on it. However, this advantage was only for people employed by companies that purchased group insurance for their employees, not for self-employed persons or employees of small businesses that did not provide health insurance. Therefore consumers who purchased their own health insurance for any reason did not have the same tax advantage as those employed by companies that purchased it for employees; this is still partially the case.

People have long sought employment on the basis of the benefits offered; this means making employment decisions based on tax advantage and perhaps not on the basis of the best job. Furthermore, when choosing health insurance coverage, there is a tendency to choose coverage that is more comprehensive than is likely to be needed. By insuring against relatively predictable and manageable health care expenses, there is little incentive to control lifestyle and behavioral factors and hazards that might temper the use of health services (Havighurst, Blumstein, & Brennan, 1998). The tax subsidy has had adverse consequences. Long experience with employer-based health insurance and the tax advantages it enjoys has changed insurance from a protection against unmanageable risk to something consumers view as an entitlement. This is no different in a population that has government-paid insurance, such as Medicare or Medicaid.

These programs are also helped by certain laws passed by the U.S. Congress, such as the Emergency Medical Treatment and Active Labor Act (EMTALA) (42 U.S.C.A. sect. 1395dd, 1995). This law requires the provision of emergency medical treatment to any individual who has an emergency medical condition or is in active labor. The health care institution may not deny care based on the patient's kind of insurance or lack of it. While this law had good intentions at the time of its passage, there have been unintended consequences that actually interfere with the intent of the act—to provide immediate care for all persons who have life-threatening illnesses or women who are in labor without consideration of the ability to pay. Emergency departments report women requesting pregnancy testing and parents appearing with children with colds or ear infections of several days duration who refuse care at a primary care site, even if it is immediately available. The emergency department is improperly used, wasting resources that might be needed for true emergencies and costing a great deal for little or no value. Hospitals fear denying any kind of care because of the severe penalties provided for in EMTALA, which can run to $50,000 for each violation.

Sociologist Talcott Parsons (1951) describes what he calls a *sick role*, a set of behaviors that are relatively predictable and seem to be based on the history of health care provider–consumer relations in the past. Parsons identifies four elements of patient behavior/belief in cases of illness: (1) the patient is not responsible for the illness, and it is not within his or her power to get well, (2) the patient is not expected to assume his normal personal and social obligations, based on the severity of the illness, (3) the patient should take action to obtain treatment for the illness from appropriate health care providers, and (4) the patient should comply with the treatment prescribed. This description of the sick role may help to explain the behavior of some patients who abdicate personal responsibility for their conditions and submit to authority for treatment. More recently, provider-patient relationships are based on the recognition and acceptance of more proactive and responsible roles for patients and a

role for providers that diminishes authoritarianism and embraces partnership (Sultz & Young, 1999).

APNs will see the kind of "sick" behavior described above and must take steps to discourage it. Education regarding the use of the emergency department is critical (e.g., letting the patient know when it is appropriate to go and when it is not). This may even mean denying approval for a visit to the emergency department, if the APN could see the patient in the primary care setting but the patient chooses not to because there might be a wait or it is inconvenient. Another important piece of the process is to track the emergency visits of patients within the practice, particularly Medicaid patients. It is difficult for an APN on call to make a decision regarding a patient needing emergency care. It is prudent to err on the conservative side. However, it is important to follow up (at the next primary care visit) on why an emergency department visit is inappropriate and on how the patient can take self-care measures at home instead of choosing the emergency department.

Health Care Fraud and Abuse

With nearly $1 trillion being spent on health care, there has been heightened scrutiny of waste, fraud, and abuse of the system that would increase the already escalating costs. According to the United States General Accounting Office (GAO) (1996), 10% of every health care dollar is lost to waste, fraud, and abuse. *Waste* is the incurring of unnecessary cost as a result of inefficient practices and poor systems or controls by management. *Fraud* is the deliberate misrepresentation of material facts for financial gain. *Abuse* is any practice inconsistent with accepted regulations or ethical principles that yields unfair gains to persons in positions of responsibility. It is difficult to determine how much is lost to each of these problems. One estimate found between 10% and 25% of Medicaid program costs to be attributable to fraudulent billing (Jesilow, 1991). There has always been fraud and abuse of the system, but as the system changes, so do the strategies used to defraud payers. It is often difficult to ascertain whether claims are for services that have actually been rendered.

There are several federal laws that prohibit false claims against the government for Medicare and Medicaid payments. They include criminal prosecution and civil penalties for certain acts that violate provisions of the Social Security Act (42 U.S.C.A. sections 701 et seq., 2001 et seq., 1128 [various parts], and 1320 [various parts]). Criminal false claims include knowingly and willingly making (or causing to be made) false statements or representations of material facts in order to obtain payment or benefit under federal or state health care programs. Conviction of health care providers for a felony carries fines of not more than $25,000 and imprisonment for not more than 5 years. If another person (a nonprovider) makes the false statements, it is a misdemeanor carrying fines of up to $10,000 and imprisonment for not more than 1 year. In addition, there are several other laws pertaining to defrauding the government and the acts surrounding such fraud; these have additional penalties.

Civil false claims cover any person or organization presenting (or causing to be presented) any claim for a medical item or service that is known or should be known to be false, not provided as claimed, or not for a person or service included in the program. Civil penalties of up to $2000 per incident may be assessed, as well as up to twice the amount claimed for the item or service in lieu of damages sustained by the government in prosecuting the fraud (42 U.S.C.A. section 1128a, 1320a-7a). The government is quite serious about prosecuting false claims. It is an abuse of taxpayer money and a cause of concern for patients either not receiving care or receiving unnecessary care. There have been some very high fines assessed for fraudulent claims, including $250,000 for "inartfully" describing services provided or not providing services as claimed (*Anesthesiologists Affiliated v. Sullivan*, 941 F.2d 678 [8th Cir. 1991]), $79 million against one health care provider (*United States v. Diamond*, No. Civ. 2121 [S.D.N.Y. 1987]), and $19 million against a dentist who fraudulently billed for oral cancer screenings provided to nursing home residents whose physicians had not ordered the screenings (*United States v. Lorenzo*, 768 F. Supp. 1127 [E.D. Pa. 1991]). The statutes provide that the same fraudulent act can give rise to both criminal and civil actions. In *United States v. Halper* (490 U.S. 435 [1989]), the Supreme Court determined that a manager of a laboratory that provided services to New York City Medicare patients overcharged the government fiscal intermediary 65 times for a total overpayment of $535. Halper was criminally convicted on all 65 counts as well as 16 counts of mail fraud because he used the U.S. Postal Service to forward his fraudulent claims. He was sentenced to 2 years in jail and fined $5000. The government then brought a civil action, which provided for a $2000 penalty for each of the 65 offenses, an amount totalling $130,000. Although the federal District Court ruled that such a high penalty would violate the double jeopardy clause of the U.S. Constitution (in the Fifth Amendment), the Supreme Court determined that a civil action following a criminal action in this case did not constitute double jeopardy. The purpose of a civil penalty in any legal proceeding is to make the plaintiff *whole* (i.e., put him or her in the position he or she would have been in if the fraudulent act had not taken place). Of course, in addition to overpaying $535, the government expended taxpayer funds to investigate, find, and prosecute the case. Some critics believe that such high penalties are indeed additional

punishments, perhaps serving as a deterrent to others who might seek to defraud government health insurance programs.

A related opportunity to find and convict parties who attempt to defraud the government is called a *qui tam action*. The Federal False Claims Act (31 U.S.C.A. sections 3729-3733) permits private individuals who have knowledge or evidence of fraud or abuse of the government to report such action and participate in the prosecution of the case. The *relater*, or reporting person, who provides substantial assistance in prosecuting a false claim case may receive 15% to 25% of the final judgment or settlement. There has been a significant increase in qui tam actions against health care providers in recent years. Most of the relaters are former employees of agencies or competitors. Because many of the claims yield thousands of dollars, there is great incentive for relaters to report suspected false claims. Unfortunately, many health care providers have settled for large dollar amounts rather than defend the action in court, which might be significantly more expensive and could secondarily exclude them from further participation in government health programs. Even when the government's case has been weak, it has often been able to receive settlement funds (Manning, 1996).

Health care providers who refer a patient to another provider for care and services paid by Medicare, Medicaid, or any other government-funded health care program in exchange for some benefit or remuneration may be guilty of criminal action. Although there are some exceptions to the law, it is a very complex one and exposes health care providers to significant legal risk. The statute (42 U.S.C.A. sections 1128B, 1320a-7b) provides that any health care provider who knowingly and willfully receives any remuneration for referrals of patients for which payment is made through a government program, or who offers any remuneration (including kickbacks, bribes, or rebates) to induce such a referral, is guilty of a felony and can be fined up to $25,000 and imprisoned for up to 5 years. The purpose of the statute is to ensure referrals are made on the basis of the best interests of a patient rather than the monetary reward for the referring provider. It is further based on the belief that permitting referral fees would result in overutilization of care. However, this position is not universally held; there are some who believe that referral fees and fee-sharing might override the incentives of fee-for-service providers treating patients themselves rather than making a referral that would be more appropriate for a patient (Rosenblatt & Rosenbaum, 1997). The statute also prohibits referrals to any health care provider or entity in which the referring provider has a financial interest.

Fraud issues related to APNs usually revolve around the issues of documentation of health care visits and inappropriate coding based on that documentation, seeing Medicare patients "incident to" when the physician has not

Table 1-1

Agencies Responsible for Enforcing Medicare Rules

AGENCY	FUNCTION
Health Care Financing Administration	Drafts the rules governing Medicare.
	Conducts the process of review and finalization of rules and regulations.
	Must follow the laws written by Congress.
	May write rules and regulations that build on statutory law.
	Oversees Medicare carriers.
Office of the Inspector General	Audits and investigates.
Department of Justice	Prosecutes fraud cases for the government. The investigative arm of the Department of Justice is the Federal Bureau of Investigation (FBI).
Medicare carriers	Pay, on behalf of HCFA, the claims submitted by health care providers.
	Are private contractors.
	May identify cases of suspected fraud and initiate investigations through referrals to the Office of the Inspector General.

Data from Buppert, C. (2000). *The primary care provider's guide to compensation and quality.* Gaithersburg, MD: Aspen Publishers.

seen the patient, and not following the complicated rules and regulations related to Medicare reimbursement. Buppert (2000) recommends knowing which agencies are charged with enforcing the law on Medicare. There are three government agencies and a regional network of private contractors charged with enforcing Medicare rules. (Table 1-1 identifies these agencies.)

Areas that have been traditionally identified as problematic include home health care (e.g., prevalent abuse) or medical groups (e.g., improper documentation of office visits, hospital visits, and other services). Abuse can also include billing errors such as *upcoding,* or billing for a higher level of service (and higher reimbursement) than what the documentation of the visit dictates. (See Chapter 13 for specific details on documentation and coding.) APNs can expect private insurers to follow the policies of government auditors when they conduct their own audits.

It is important for APNs to learn and apply the rules to prevent the potential for fraud. Not knowing the laws, rules, and regulations is not an excuse in the eyes of the law.

Health Care Access and Opportunity

While a right to health care has never been established for a variety of ethical, political, and ideological reasons, it is evident in U.S. laws that there is agreement that some level of care in particular times of need should be provided. The core question has been: if there is a right to medical or health care, who has the duty to provide it? In the latter half of the twentieth century, the government encouraged the provision of necessary care by requiring that organizations and other providers who receive benefits from the government agree to provide services to people who need them but may not be able to pay for them. Most people obtain health care by purchasing health care insurance via some mechanism. Others are covered voluntarily or involuntarily by government insurance, and some people are uninsured, at least temporarily. As has been indicated elsewhere, the most important determinant of possessing health insurance is being employed, and the decline of the number of people who are continuously insured is primarily due to the decrease in the availability of employment-based coverage. An increase in the number of small firms, an increase in the number of self-employed persons, and other factors enhance this (Crippen, 1994).

One of the problems relating to care for the uninsured population is the refusal of some private or not-for-profit institutions to care for them beyond minimal efforts. Transfers of patients who visited emergency departments or had urgent medical needs from such institutions to public ones increased markedly in the 1980s. The transferring hospitals cited lack of insurance or other ability to pay for care as the reason for such transfers. Hospitals claimed that rendering more care would be economically impossible (Hospitals in cost squeeze dump more patients who can't pay bills, 1985; Schiff, 1986). While some critics claimed that transfers were harmful to patients, others indicated that most patients benefit from transfer to an institution that has better surgical coverage and a full-time special care staff (Jonasson & Barrett, 1987).

Several cases brought this issue to the attention of the public and legislature. The cases addressed the need to provide emergency treatment that is "immediately and reasonably necessary for the preservation of life, limb, or health" (*New Biloxi Hospital v. Frazier,* 146 So.2d 882 [Miss. 1962]). Professional organizations defined what constituted a medical emergency (Wing, 1985). To recover damages under common tort law, a patient/plaintiff had to demonstrate that there was a duty to provide care and that the refusal of care by a certain health care provider caused an injury. Over time, the law has evolved from a "no duty" perspective to one that recognizes that inequalities in power and the ability to bargain or contract in the midst of a critical illness may require societal support for some level of care that does not abandon the sick person. In the 1980s, many states enacted emergency care requirements; statutes generally include that no transfer may be made by one hospital to another unless the patient has been stabilized, the receiving hospital must be willing and able to take the patient, medical care must be available during the transfer, and medical records must be sent with the patient. A good example may be found in Texas Administrative Code, title 25, section 133.21 (1986). The number of deaths reported following the transfer of patients from one hospital to another decreased dramatically after the adoption of this law, and it served as the model for federal legislation in 1986. The federal EMTALA of 1986 (42 U.S.C.A. section 1395dd) set standards for the emergency treatment of emergency department patients and transfers and provided remedies for denial of care or improper transfer.

Two other important federal laws affect health care insurance. The Employee Retirement Income Security Act of 1974 (ERISA) and the Consolidated Omnibus Budget Reconciliation Act of 1986 (COBRA) provide federal oversight of employee health insurance plans. ERISA (ERISA section 514; 29 U.S.C.A. section1144a) was primarily concerned with protecting employee pensions, but it was then expanded to require any employer who provides health care coverage to meet the provisions of the statute. It also exempts such organizations from state insurance law. Critics have said that the standards and remedies under the federal law are more limited than state law. The COBRA (ERISA section 601 et seq.; 29 U.S.C.A 1161) law provides for the continuation of health insurance coverage when a person loses an attachment to employer-provided or other private coverage.

The federal and state governments, as well as private industry, are significantly involved in health care in the United States. Despite the belief that it is a primarily private system, the influence of public law and policy cannot be denied.

IMPLICATIONS FOR MSN EDUCATION AND ADVANCED PRACTICE

Most Master of Science in Nursing (MSN) programs have trends and issues courses, legal ethical courses, or advanced practice role courses that discuss how a bill becomes a law. Milstead (1997) proposes that the study of health policy includes more than knowing how a bill becomes a law. She feels it is important for APN students to know that the public policy process is made up of several components and is much broader in scope than a legislative approach. APN students must become knowl-

edgeable about the entire policy process in order to function appropriately in the advanced role. Milstead identifies the components of policy that an APN should be familiar with: agenda-setting; government response in the form of laws, regulations, and programs; and the design and implementation of policies and programs.

APNs are required to work within the policy environment at the time and location of their practice. The evolution of policy toward a more consumer-centered orientation has significant implications for nursing. Although the education of nurses generally supports patient-centered care, the workplace may not be so supportive. Differences with physician providers with whom APNs may work can make the practice setting difficult. Nurses are advised to be familiar with the legal decisions that reflect the state of the law as it affects patient-provider relationships.

Knowledge of the structure and processes of government is important to nurses. Passive acceptance of the current status of health policy is not the goal to which APNs should aspire. Nurses can participate effectively in the political process, and APNs can not wait for others to alert the government to serious health problems. Elected and appointed officials are not "experts" in health; they rely on professionals to let them know what issues are important. As health care providers, APNs know "not only about the biological and physiological significance of problems, but also the psychosocial, community and environmental impacts" (Milstead, 1997).

Cohen, Mason, Kovner, Leavitt, Pulcini and Sochalski (1996) list four levels of nursing's political development: (1) buy-in, (2) self-interest, (3) political sophistication, and (4) leading the way. Leading the way is based on the premise that participation of nurses in policy-making is vital not only to serving self-interests but also to enhancing the health of individuals and the nation. The authors identify activities that might take place during stage 4, such as leadership in agenda-setting or the attainment of high-level positions in various agencies that are accountable to constituencies besides nursing. Recommended strategies to enhance activities include coalition-building, leadership development, involvement in political campaigns, and development of public media expertise.

APNs must also recognize that sometimes the battle is lost but the war is won. APNs must not feel it is a personal failure when a vote is lost. In some cases, APNs must support policy that in the short term may seem deleterious for the profession but in the long run could create a winning situation. It is also vital for APNs to realize that although the detailed work of forming policy and taking policy positions is important, the ability to form relationships, alliances, and partnerships necessary to achieve or advance policy positions may be even more critical. Issues are too complex, with too many implications, for any unilateral solution to predominate. Nurses must concentrate on building partnerships and coalitions. As APNs participate in the energetic, conflict-laden dialogue process, utilizing a variety of perspectives, they will be a part of developing a meaningful agenda for health care. Beyers, Gunn, Egging, and Thomas (1997) express the opinion that "policy involvement demonstrates caring, a willingness to stand up to values, and a belief that the nursing profession's mission and work are necessary to health care."

PRIORITIES FOR RESEARCH

Historical study of the important health policies, acts, and laws yields interesting information. Often those affected by policy and law are only aware of the outcome (i.e., the final iteration of an act or program). However, all of the information about the formative processes are available to the ambitious researcher. All of the preliminary bills, reports from committees, and actual hearings and discussions in the houses of Congress are published. Much is available on the government's Internet sites or in the documents section of university and college libraries.

Another avenue for research is the effect of certain policies, acts, or laws on the activities of APNs. What support or barriers are created by new laws? A nurse can review one or more cases of fraud and abuse. What are the elements that reveal fraud or abuse of the health care reimbursement system? Are those elements fair? Issues of access to health care can be identified. Are there any strategies available to APNs that could affect access without resorting to more central control of payment for care?

Study of the evolution of certain standards of care provides an interesting look at trends in practice. One can also analyze the manner in which patient education and consent to treatment is managed and what kinds of information patients want, need, and use.

The more APNs can identify and reveal their essential character in the health care system, the more their value will be evident. Research might look at how involved APNs have been in health care policy formulation. Program evaluation should also be a part of research. Information related to incidence, prevalence, at-risk populations, and sensitivity and specificity are important variables to include in program evaluation. Issues related to chronic illness, access to primary care, and the effect of primary care on patients (especially the underserved and uninsured) serve as ways to promote agenda items where nursing can make a difference, particularly when outcomes are documented through research. Milstead (1997) recommends that APNs contribute to the knowledge base of policy analysis through well-designed research directed toward program implementation. She expresses her opinion that APNs have a social mandate to move health issues onto the national agenda and create, design, implement, and research policies and programs that can address these issues. Nursing has effective leadership that can help move policy, and therefore people, toward a healthier society.

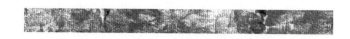

DISCUSSION QUESTIONS

These questions can be used to promote critical thinking and encourage discussion.

1. There are conflicts among the American values of freedom, autonomy, self-determination, and privacy. From your understanding of national health policy initiatives, how are the values affected by the initiatives? Can the conflict be resolved?
2. Rules and regulations provide for policy implementation. Review a federal public law and the regulations that support it. Discuss how the regulations affect the health care organization against which they are directed or the population on which the law has its effect. Some good examples include the Managed Care Act of 1973, Medicare, the Family and Medical Leave Act, and the Orphan Drug Act.
3. Evaluate the state's regulation of health care providers in terms of choices for patients, quality of care, safety of the public, and cost of care. Discuss the issues concerning the delivery of nursing care in a variety of settings. Are there enough nurses at varying levels of practice to provide safe, effective, and meaningful care? What are the legal ramifications of an inadequate number of nurses? Read some of the case law on inadequacy of staffing and its effect on institutional and agency liability for patient injury. Discuss how nursing leaders can address this issue in an environment of cost containment.
4. Evaluate the current certification process for APNs in a variety of specialties. What is the value of certification to patients, the health care system, the health care agencies for which nurses work, and the nurses themselves.
5. Discuss the relationship between consumers and providers of health care. What strategies can you identify to make the relationship more equal so consumers can be legitimate participants in the health care system? Why should there be a more equal relationship? Should health care providers take a leadership role in reducing costs and conserving resources for the good of society, or is this kind of leadership not a societal good? What is the role of the APN in this leadership?
6. Trace the evolution of informed consent (or refusal) to health care. What is the role of the APN in ensuring that informed consent law is observed? In terms of informed consent, what is the difference between the professional-centered and the patient-centered standard? With which standard are you more comfortable or more satisfied?

7. How does a national standard of care affect the practice of nurses in small institutions, rural areas, or inner-city health care settings? Do you believe that a local standard of care is fair to providers? To patients?

8. Discuss the effect of the following situations on demand curves (representing consumer behavior):

   • Discuss the effects of visits to a physician by a consumer who has insurance that pays a flat $25 for each office visit and requires the consumer to pay nothing until the insurer has spent $200 on his or her behalf.

   • Assuming the quality of medical care has improved for a particular illness, how, if at all, will consumer behavior change if the consumer has knowledge of the change before needing the service or learns of it after first needing the service?

   • Describe the change, if any, in consumer behavior when the health care consumer has a significant increase in income but little change in health status.

   • Discuss the possible consumer behavior of a population that previously had no health insurance but now has an insurance plan with a deductible of $100 per family member, after which the insurance company pays 80% of all covered medical and dental expenses.

9. What should a hospital's duty be to a patient coming to an emergency department who has a health problem that is not an emergency? What should that duty be if there is an emergency illness but the legally required treatment has been completed? Discuss why a hospital may choose to provide continued care for an uninsured person even though it is not legally mandated.

10. Discuss the principle of economically based consumer decision-making with regard to health care. What are the important factors in making such decisions? What are your thoughts about the cost-sharing features of most health insurance policies?

11. Suppose you are a midwife or women's health NP working at a community clinic. You suggest an arrangement with a local hospital that would permit

Suggestions for Further Learning

• Go to the website of the JCAHO or the NCQA. What is the philosophy and purpose of the organization? Discuss the policies that determine the actions and activities of those organizations.

• Using a state or federal government website or your university library government documents department, review the legislative history and text of a law relating to health care policy or health care delivery. Keep a log of your search. Discuss the findings with your class.

• Using the Internet or the government documents section of your university library, find and study the various provisions and amendments to the EMTALA law. Discuss how it affects the use of emergency care. Does this law define a "right" to some level of health care? What is the effect of that "right," if any, on the behavior of health care providers?

• Find and review the antikickback and COBRA laws. What effect do antikickback and referral limitations have on practice? Is there a better way to minimize fraudulent claims? What would you do if you had knowledge of such actions? Determine the process of reporting fraud and abuse of government or private insurers.

• Get the article: Palmer, S., Sabo, D., & Wertz, B. (1997). Community health care: servicing Colorado's uninsured: a health policy legislative proposal. *Advanced Practice Nursing Quarterly, 3,* 69-76. What lessons do you learn from this hypothetical proposal? How effective do you think this proposal would be in the development of public and private initiatives for the provision of health care for the uninsured and indigent in the state of Colorado, or in any state?

• Get the articles: Frogue, J. (1999, June 16). How to provide prescription drug coverage under Medicare. *Backgrounder.* Washington, DC: The Heritage Foundation; and O'Sullivan, J. (1999, April 19). *Medicare: prescription drug coverage for beneficiaries* (CRS report for Congress). Congressional Research Service, The Library of Congress. These two publications provide interesting analysis of policy-making and the activities of health policy analysis organizations. They also provide a meaningful review of a major policy issue.

• Visit the website for the Cato Institute at www.cato.org. Cato is a free-market policy analysis organization. Their Policy Analysis, Regulation, and Commentary sections are useful for very current and informative material on health policy. All articles and research are well documented and contain extensive bibliographies. They provide a somewhat different point of view than most texts and commentary from popular media sources. Their website is easy to navigate and has a search feature.

• Visit the Heritage Foundation at www.heritage.org. This policy-analysis organization publishes *Backgrounder* and texts of its testimony before Congress on a variety of subjects, including health care policy. The articles are well researched and provide extensive bibliographies. Some of their publications make recommendations and provide analysis to Congress on certain policy matters. Their website is easy to navigate.

• Visit the National Center for Policy Analysis at www.ncpa.org. This policy-analysis organization publishes policy reports, brief analyses, and policy backgrounders. One of the organization's major interests is health policy. The website is easy to navigate.

referral of all the clinic's Medicare and Medicaid patients who need the hospital's services in exchange for the hospital's agreement to set aside two of its obstetrical beds for the clinic's uninsured maternity patients. Would such an arrangement violate antikickback legislation? Why or why not? Although the arrangement probably does not give the hospital any fraudulent income since reimbursement for Medicare and Medicaid patients is set by the HCFA, and since patients who might not get adequate care would be able to get it, why might this arrangement be prosecuted? Review the legislation to answer these questions.

12. Review the antikickback statute. Discuss how it might affect MCOs that require participating patients to use only providers who are part of an MCO or HMO. Are there provisions that permit these entities to avoid the referral problems of fee-for-service providers? Does it give them an unfair advantage?

REFERENCES/BIBLIOGRAPHY

1999 Pharmaceutical industry profile. (1999, March). Washington, DC: Pharmaceutical Research and Manufacturers of America.

Acs, G., Long, S.H., Marquis, M.S., & Short, P.F. (1996, Summer) *Self-insured employer health plans: prevalence, profile, provisions, and premiums,* Health Affairs.

American Medical Association (1994). *The future of medical practice* (Order No. OP211594). American Medical Association.

American Nurses Association. Accessed online on 6/14/2000 at www.nursingworld.org.

Anderson, A., Gillis, C., & Yoder, Y. (1996). Practice environment for nurse practitioners in California: identifying barriers. *Western Journal of Medicine, 165*(4), 209-214.

Anderson, O.W. (1990). *Health services as a growth enterprise in the United States since 1875.* Ann Arbor, MI: Health Administration Press.

Beyers, M., Gunn, I., Egging, D. & Thomas, K. (1997). Policy: advanced practice nursing issues and challenges: specialty association viewpoint. *Advanced Practice Nursing Quarterly, 3*(3), 31-35.

Black (1991). *Black's law dictionary.* St. Paul, MN: West Publishing.

Blevins, S. (1995). *The medical monopoly: protecting consumers or limiting competition?* (Cato Policy Analysis No. 246). Washington, DC: The Cato Institute.

Brook, R.H., & McGlynn, E.A. (1991). Maintaining quality of care. In E. Ginzberg (Ed.), *Health services research: key to health policy* (pp. 784-817). Cambridge, MA: Harvard University Press.

Bullough, B., & Bullough, V. (1994). *Nursing issues for the nineties and beyond,* New York: Springer Publishing.

Buppert, C. (1999). *Nurse practitioner's business practice and legal guide.* Gaithersburg, MD: Aspen Publishers.

Buppert, C. (2000). *The primary care provider's guide to compensation and quality.* Gaithersburg, MD: Aspen Publishers.

Bureau of National Affairs (1997, August 11). School-based centers gaining attention for providing access for uninsured kids. *Health Care Policy Report 5*(32).

Cantril, H. (1991). *Public opinion 1935-1946.* Princeton, NJ: Princeton University Press.

Chapman, C.B., & Talmadge, J.M. (1970). Historical and political background of federal health care legislation. *Law and Contemporary Social Problems 35*(2): 334-47.

Cihak, R., Williams, B., & Ferrara, P.J. (1997, June 11). The rise and repeal of the Washington State Health Plan: lessons for America's state legislatures. *Backgrounder, 1121/S.* Washington, DC: The Heritage Foundation.

Cohen, S., Mason, D., Kovner, C., Leavitt, J., Pulcini, J., & Sochalski, J. (1996). Stages of nursing's political development: where we've been and where we ought to be. *Nursing Outlook, 44,* 259-266.

Cohen, W.J., & Ball, R.M. (1965). Social Security Amendments of 1965: summary and legislative history. *Social Security Bulletin, 28*(9), 3-21.

Commonwealth of Pennsylvania House of Representatives (1996, November). *Findings of fact and report* (Committee on Education, Select Subcommittee on Education, Select Subcommittee on House Resolution No. 37).

Corning, P.A. (1969). *The evolution of Medicare: from idea to law* (Research report no. 29). US Department of Health, Education, and Welfare, Social Security Administration, Office of Research and Statistics. Washington, DC: US Government Printing Office.

Crippen, D. (1994). *Sources of health insurance and characteristics of the uninsured: analysis of the March 1993 current population survey.* Washington, DC: House Committee on Ways and Means, Employee Benefit Research Institute.

Crippen, D. (1999, March 8). *Health care and Medicare spending.* Washington, DC: U.S. Congressional Budget Office for the Subcommittee on Health.

Evans, & Rosenberg (1992). *Fraud and abuse in Medicare and Medicaid: stronger enforcement and better management could save billions.* House of Representatives 104-161, 104th Congress, 2nd session.

Friedman, E. (1995). The compromise and the afterthought: Medicare and Medicaid after 30 years. *Journal of the American Medical Association, 274*(3), 278-282.

Frogue, J. (1999, June 16). How to provide prescription drug coverage under Medicare. *Backgrounder.* Washington, DC: The Heritage Foundation.

Gluck, M.E. (1999, April). *A Medicare prescription drug benefit* (Medicare brief no. 1). National Academy of Social Insurance.

Havinghurst, C.C., Blumstein, J.F., & Brennan, T.A. (1998). *Health care law and policy* (2nd ed.). New York: The Foundation Press.

Health Care Financing Administration (1997, January 28). *Managed care in Medicare and Medicaid* (Fact sheet).

Hershey, J., Kunreuther, H., Schwartz, J.S., & Williams, S.V. (1984). Health insurance under competition: would people choose what is expected? *Inquiry, 21*(4).

Hospitals in cost squeeze "dump" more patients who can't pay bills. (1985, March 8). *Wall Street Journal.*

Iglehart, J.K. (1992). Health policy report: the American health care system. *New England Journal of Medicine, 327,* 742-747.

Jesilow, P. (1991). Fraud by physicians against Medicaid. *Journal of the American Medical Association, 266,* 3318.

Jonasson, O., & Barrett, J. (1987). Editorial: transfer of unstable patients: dumping or duty, *Journal of the American Medical Association, 257,* 1519.

Kingdon, J. (1995). *Agendas, alternatives and public policies* (2nd ed). New York: Harper Collins.

Konner, M. (1993). *Medicine at the crossroads.* New York: Pantheon.

Lipson, D.J. (1997). State roles in health care policy: past as prologue. In T.J. Litman & L.S. Robins (Eds.), *Health politics and policy.* Albany, NY: Delmar Publishers.

Liu, J.C., & Moffit, R.E. (1995). *A taxpayer's guide to the Medicare crisis.* Washington, DC: The Heritage Foundation.

Longest, B.B. (1998). *Health policymaking in the United States.* Chicago: Health Administration Press.

Lopez, N. (1998). *Are American children being lured into socialized medicine?* Washington, DC: Institute for Health Freedom.

Making the Grade (1997). *National survey of state school-based initiatives: school year 1995-96.* Washington, DC: George Washington University Press.

Manning, M, (1996, August). Recent developments in federal false claims cases, *Health Law Digest, 24,* 8. National Health Lawyers Association.

McCubbin, R. (1997, June 6). The Kentucky health care experiment: How managed competition clamps down on choice and competition. *Backgrounder, 1119/S.* Washington, DC: The Heritage Foundation.

Milstead, J. (1997). A social mandate: APN leadership for the whole policy process. *Advanced Practice Nursing Quarterly, 3*(3), 1-8.

Moffit, R. (1994, August 4). The last time Congress reformed health care: a lawmaker's guide to the Medicare catastrophic debacle. *Backgrounder, 996.* Washington, DC: The Heritage Foundation.

National Center for Policy Analysis (1997). *State health care reform briefing book.* Washington, DC: Idea House, National Center for Policy Analysis.

National Governors' Association for Best Practices (1998, May 7). *How states can increase enrollment in the state children's health insurance program* (NGA Center for Best Practices Issue brief).

O'Malley, J. (1997). The art and science of shaping public policy. *Advanced Practice Nursing Quarterly, 3*(3), v-vi.

O'Sullivan, J. (1999, April 19). *Medicare: prescription drug coverage for beneficiaries* (CRS report for Congress). Congressional Research Service, The Library of Congress.

Palmer, S., Sabo, D., & Wertz, B. (1997). Community health care: servicing Colorado's uninsured: a health policy legislative proposal. *Advanced Practice Nursing Quarterly, 3*(3), 69-76.

Parsons, T. (1951). *The social system.* New York: The Free Press.

Phelps, C.E. (1997). *Health economics.* Reading, MA: Addison Wesley.

Poen, M.M. (1979). *Harry Truman versus the medical lobby: the genesis of medicare.* Columbia, MO: University of Missouri Press.

Porter-O'Grady, T. (1997). Influencing policy: foreign territory for nurses. *Advanced Practice Nursing Quarterly, 3*(3), 79-80.

Rosenblatt, S.A., and Rosenbaum, S. (1997). *Law and the American health care system.* Westbury, NY: The Foundation Press.

Schiff, R. (1986). Transfers to a public hospital: a prospective study of 467 patients. *New England Journal of Medicine, 314,* 552.

Schriver, M.L., & Arnett, G.M. (1998, August 14). Uninsured rates rise dramatically in states with strictest health insurance regulations. *Backgrounder.* Washington, DC: The Heritage Foundation.

Selden, T.M., Banthin, J.S., & Cohen, J.W. (1998, May/June). Medicaid's problem children: eligible but not enrolled. *Health Affairs, 17,* 3.

Shi, L., & Singh, D.A. (1998). *Delivering health care in America.* Gaithersburg, MD: Aspen Publishers.

Starr, P. (1982). *The social transformation of American medicine.* Cambridge, MA: Basic Books.

Sultz, H.A., & Young, K.M. (1999). *Health care USA.* Gaithersburg, MD: Aspen Publishers.

Twight, C. (1997). Medicare's origin: the economics and politics of dependency. *The Cato Journal, 16,* 3.

United States General Accounting Office (1995, June 12). *Health insurance regulation: variation in recent state small employer health insurance reforms* (GAO/HEHS-95-161FS).

United States General Accounting Office (1996, June 27). *Fraud and abuse.*

United States General Accounting Office (1997, July). *Private health insurance: continued erosion of coverage linked to cost pressures* (GAO/HEHS-97-122).

United States General Accounting Office (1998, March 9). *Testimony before the Special Committee on Aging, U.S. Senate.*

Walz, X. (1969). The rise and gradual fall of the locality rule in medical malpractice litigation. *DePaul Law Review, 18,* 408.

Wing, K.R. (1985). The emergency room admission: how far does the open door go? *University of Detroit Law Review, 63,* 119-24.

World Health Organization (1958). *The first ten years of the WHO.* New York: World Health Organization.

Chapter 2

The Study of Health Policy

Alice G. Rini & Denise Robinson

Health policy refers to public policies that influence the pursuit of health (Shi & Singh, 1998). Health policy may be studied using a variety of sources. However, since policy is dynamic, the best way to understand it is to use as many primary sources as possible. Students of health policy will want to become familiar with the unique, possibly unknown resources available to them. These resources are readily available in university and other libraries, on the Internet, at government agencies, and through certain private agencies. The thing that characterizes primary sources is that no one has previously digested the material for the reader and then written about it from his or her own point of view. In such secondary sources, the bias of the writers becomes evident. The meaning of a written work should be analyzed using the original material, instead of basing the analysis only on another person's interpretation. This is not to say that analysis by policy experts is not valuable; however it remains important to review what policy-makers say in hearings, as well as the exact text of bills and public laws.

Secondary sources are useful after one reviews the primary material. Sometimes using primary sources requires persistence. Available resources for locating primary sources are helpful in this effort; such tools provide outlines and guides to access material often not organized in a familiar manner. This chapter documents the tools and resources available for studying and researching health policy (Chart 2-1). While this chapter concentrates primarily on public policy, one must also be aware of private policy because of the many powerful private organizations whose health policies affect health care and its practitioners. The chapter also addresses some of the issues and concerns through which policy may be analyzed.

DEFINITIONS

Rights are something to which one has a just claim, or a power or privilege to which one is entitled. They are also considered a capacity, residing in one individual, of controlling, with the assent of the state, the actions of others (Black, 1991). *Natural rights* are those rights that are part of human nature, as distinguished from those created by law and dependent on civil society; natural rights are generally identified as life, liberty, privacy, and good reputation (Black, 1991). *Civil rights* are those rights that belong to every member of a civilized society by virtue of citizenship and are not connected with the organization or administration of government; these include the rights of property, marriage, contract, equal protection of law, and trial by jury—essentially those rights capable of being enforced by civil law (Black, 1991).

Negative rights are essentially a condition of being free from interference with one's activities and ideas. The Constitution of the United States is said, in its Bill of Rights, to expound such rights in terms of being free from governmental interference with certain specified actions. Negative rights also refers to the right to be left alone. *Positive rights* are affirmative rights to act or make agreements that are enforceable by law.

The *Congressional Record* is the proceedings of the activities of Congress, published daily when Congress is in session. The first series, officially reported, printed, and published by the federal government, began March 4, 1873 (Black, 1991). Members of Congress are permitted to edit their speeches before publication and may add material that was never actually spoken in a Congressional session as long as the latter is agreed to by the respective house from which it becomes public (Black, 1991).

A *bill* has many meanings in law. In this chapter, it means the draft of a proposed law from the time of its introduction through its enactment as a law. Once introduced, a federal bill may be considered in any session of Congress, but it dies at the end of a Congressional session and must be reintroduced as a new bill if a succeeding Congress is to consider it (Black, 1991).

The *United States Code* is the systematic collection or compendium of laws in force, including revisions, and rules and regulations that support the laws. The *Federal Register* is the vehicle that publishes, on a daily basis, federal agency regulations and other legal documents of the executive branch of government. The *Federal Register* includes proposed changes to rules, regulations, and standards of governmental agencies and also includes an invitation to submit written commentary, criticism, and arguments for or against such proposed regulation (Black,

Chart 2-1

Tools for Studying Health Policy

1. Congressional Information Service (CIS) (web.lexis-nexis. com). The CIS, using Lexis-Nexis, provides online access to information on the Congressional Universe. Lexis-Nexis and the CIS are licensed services and must be accessed at a library, university campus, or other site that subscribes to the service. It generally requires a password for access. The CIS provides the following kinds of documents:
   - Full text of Congressional reports, including the entire report as generated by one of the houses of Congress or a committee
   - Other Congressional documents
   - Prints
   - Full texts of bills before Congress
   - The *Congressional Record*
   - Congressional testimony before committees and in other meetings
   - Bill-tracking reports that follow bills through Congress
   - Texts of public laws
   - The United States Code
   - The *Federal Register*
   - The *Code of Federal Regulations* (CFR), which are rules promulgated by administrative agencies
   - Biographical and financial information for members of Congress
   - Voting records of members of Congress
   - Congressional Committee rosters, charters, and schedules of committee meetings
   - Full text articles from *National Journal* and *Congress Daily*
   - Full text news articles on important and emerging policy topics
   - Links to related websites

   The CIS, using Lexis-Nexis, also provides online access to the following on the Academic Universe:
   - Full-text articles from major national newspapers and international news sources
   - Broadcast news transcripts (radio and television)
   - Articles from popular magazines, news magazines, and major trade journals
   - Current events and business news
   - Annual financial reports from many national and international corporations
   - Current company information from the Disclosure database
   - Hoover's Company Reports
   - EDGAR filings
   - Stock reports
   - Access to Medline, health news, accounting and tax sources, and legal resources
   - Full text of federal and state court cases, which includes case law
   - Full-text law review articles and other legal news sources
   - Full text of the United States Constitution
   - European and other foreign law and policy

   The Congressional Universe and Academic Universe sites are very valuable sources of information. They are also very user-friendly. The How Do I section provides guidance to new and returning users. The Help area is clear and provides direction for navigating the site.

2. Specific government sites
   - THOMAS (thomas.loc.gov). This very user-friendly site provides access to legislation, the *Congressional Record*, and information about committee activities. It is searchable by bill number or certain key words. Also included is a directory of Congress and the schedules and home pages for committees and individual senators and representatives.
   - GOVBOT (ciir2.cs.umass.edu/govbot). This site provides web pages from United States government and military sites. It claims to have more than 1.5 million pages of data and provides a form to search by word and terms from document titles or web addresses.
   - Library of Congress (www.loc.gov). This online catalog of twelve million records and documents includes books, serials, computer files, manuscripts, maps, sound recordings, and a gallery of exhibits. It also includes links to other sites. Many of the cataloged items are available online, or the library may direct a researcher to a site where an item is available.

3. Professional, policy, and research organizations
   - Joint Commission on Accreditation of Healthcare Organizations (JCAHO) (jcaho.org). The mission of the JCAHO is to continuously improve the safety and quality of care provided to the public through the provision of health care accreditation and related services that support performance improvement in health care organizations. Its site can be searched for a variety of documents associated with the organization.
   - National Committee on Quality Assurance (NCQA) (www.ncqa.org). This is a private not-for-profit organization that has as its primary mission assessing and reporting on the quality of managed care plans. It partners with the state and federal governments, employer and consumer groups, and business groups. It also provides information to consumers and purchasers of managed health care and encourages plans to compete on quality and value. The website provides information about the activities of the organization.
   - American Hospital Association (AHA) (www.aha.org)
   - American Medical Association (AMA) (www.ama-assn. org). The AMA site provides information on the organization's activities, news and features from scientific journals (including *JAMA*, its own journal) and links to other medical sites.
   - American Nurses Association (ANA) (www. nursingworld.org)

Continued

Chart
2-1

Tools for Studying Health Policy—cont'd

- The Cato Institute (www.cato.org). This policy analysis organization does research and analysis of public policy, primarily of federal-level policy. Publications that are generally available in full online include *Policy Analysis, Regulation,* and *Commentary.* The site also has a search feature that can be utilized by topic or key words.
- National Center for Policy Analysis (www.ncpa.org). See Chapter I for information.
- Pacific Research Institute for Public Policy (www. pacificresearch.org). This organization focuses on public policy issues such as education, the environment, law and economics, and social welfare. A California-based organization, it also concentrates on issues concerning Californians. The website is easy to use.
4. Other Internet sites
   - HealthSTAR with MeSH (available via search.epnet.com or other commercial databases to which libraries may subscribe). This requires access to a library or other organization that subscribes to EPSCO or another similar service; it will likely require a password as well. The site permits research of clinical and nonclinical aspects of health care delivery, including administration, health planning, health services, clinical practice guidelines, and health care technology assessment. The site is provided by the National Library of Medicine and includes medical subject headings.
   - Health Business FullTEXT (available via search.epnet.com or other commercial databases to which libraries may subscribe). This requires access to a library or other organization that subscribes to EPSCO or another similar service. It includes information on the business of health care administration and other nonclinical aspects of health care and its institutions. It supports Library of Congress subject headings and contains full text for administrative journals, magazine, and monographs; it also includes abstracts and indexing of other titles.
   - Alt-Health Watch (available via search.epnet.com or other commercial databases to which libraries may

subscribe). This requires access to a library or other organization that subscribes to EPSCO or another similar service. It is a full-text database focusing on complementary, holistic, and integrated approaches to health care and wellness. One-hundred sixty international journals, magazines, reports, proceedings of meetings, newsletters, original research, and other publications are available. It is an easy-to-use site that also has graphics and links to other sources of information.
   - Cumulative Index to Nursing and Allied Health Literature (CINAHL) (available via search.epnet.com or other commercial databases to which libraries may subscribe). This requires access to a library or other organization that subscribes to EPSCO or another similar service. It is a source for health literature for nursing and allied health students and professionals. The database includes nursing, biomedical issues, allied health disciplines, and consumer health, with indexing for more than 900 nursing publications, 250,000 records, journals and abstracts, dissertations, conference proceedings, standards of practice, and audiovisual material.
   - MEDLINE (available via search.epnet.com or other commercial databases to which libraries may subscribe). This requires access to a library or other organization that subscribes to EPSCO or another similar service. It is a database of medical information from more than 3800 U.S. and international biomedical journals, 9 million records, and tables of contents for an additional 2400 titles.
   - Comprehensive MEDLINE with FullTEXT (available via search.epnet.com or other commercial databases to which libraries may subscribe). This requires access to a library or other organization that subscribes to EPSCO or another similar service. This site joins the National Library of Medicine with complete text of articles. The database includes information in medicine, nursing, dentistry, the health care system, and preclinical sciences. It can also be accessed via Pubmed from National Library of Medicine (www.nlm.gov), which is a free service.

1991). The **Code of Federal Regulations** (CFR) is the annual accumulation of executive agency regulations published in the daily *Federal Register* and previously issued regulations that are still in effect. The CFR is divided into fifty titles, each representing a broad subject area (Black, 1991). The **United States Constitution** serves as the organic and fundamental law of the country that describes the basic principles by which the country is structured, organizes the government, limits its functions, and prescribes the extent of its sovereign powers. The

government derives all its authority from the consent of the governed—that is, the people (Black, 1991).

Police power is the authority that is conferred (by the Tenth Amendment of the U.S. Constitution) upon individual states and can be delegated to the local governments. Police power permits the establishment of police departments and the adoption of rules, regulations, and ordinances that secure the safety, health, morals, and prosperity of citizens by preserving public order and preventing conflicts of rights among the citizens (Black, 1991). Police power gives the public health department the ability to enforce immunizations or quarantine those with highly contagious diseases.

CRITICAL ISSUES: HEALTH POLICY AND POLITICS— IS THERE A RIGHT TO HEALTH CARE?

When studying health policy, one must understand that political ideology and the intense interest in health care and policy inherent in the social agenda of the United States have an enormous effect on the way policy evolves. The working assumption about health care is that it is a "right" and should be made available to all (Epstein, 1997). Such an assumption leads to the discussion about what policy direction is needed to implement such a right. Typically, the answers tend to lie in the direction of a larger and enduring government role in policy-making. Little discussion in Congressional or executive branch proposals address individual rights, personal responsibilities, or alternative ways to address the problems in the health care system.

It is helpful to understand the conception of *rights* as evidenced in the common law and the Constitution to make sense of the debate about rights and health care. This conception drives the discussion of health care policy and will assist advanced practice nurses (APNs) in comprehending the differing opinions of how the health care policy situation should be solved. The Constitution and common law describe what are often called *negative rights*. Examples of negative rights can be found in the Bill of Rights. At the time of the adoption of the Constitution in 1787, the representatives to the first Constitutional Convention expressed concern that the Constitutional articles alone might be inadequate "to prevent misconstruction or abuse of [governmental] powers, that further declaratory and restrictive clauses should be added." The Amendments restrict the activities of government and seek to prevent its intrusion into the lives of the citizens. In fact, the First Amendment of the Bill of Rights begins with the words, "Congress shall make no law." Other Amendments deal with prohibitions against the government requiring citizens to quarter soldiers, interfering with the possession of firearms, and entering private dwellings or examining private papers or effects, as well as citizens' rights within the criminal justice system.

The concept of *positive rights* deals with "rights to" have or do something. These rights, by virtue of their construction, elicit correlative duties to provide the things to which others already have rights. Unlike private contracts and other agreements, which confer certain positive rights between and among individuals, the positive

rights asserted in a society target the government or state for their fulfillment. This can only be accomplished by taxation of some to provide certain rights to others.

One's perspective on rights affects policy-making and implementation. Although there has never been a national policy in this country that claims health care is a "right," there have been actions by the federal and state governments that appear to provide a "right" to some forms of health care. In 1946, Congress passed the Hospital Survey and Construction Act (42 U.S.C., various sections), also known as the Hill-Burton Act. The purpose of the Act was to assist states in constructing and modernizing public and not-for-profit hospitals and other medical facilities to encourage provision of care to all the citizens of that state. States that wanted federal funds submitted a plan for the use of the funds that included assurance that the institutions benefiting from the construction and modernization would provide care to all persons residing in the area, including a reasonable volume of services to persons unable to pay for them (Havighurst, Blumstein, & Brennan, 1998). Although the history of care provision by funded institutions is spotty, eventually the Department of Health, Education, and Welfare (DHEW) set standards for compliance with the care requirements. Litigation by some public interest groups yielded (at least in one court) a potential standing by plaintiffs to enforce a free-care requirement (*Euresti v. Stenner*, 458 f.2D 1115 [10th Cir. 1972]). The question of whether there was a right to free care from hospitals that had received Hill-Burton funds was also addressed in *Newsom v. Vanderbilt* (653 F.2d 1100 [6th Cir. 1981]), a case holding that neither the statute nor the regulations provided any certain right to a particular individual. The court suggested that to meet the objective of free health care, the government needed to arrange enforcement through appropriate regulations. The Hill-Burton program had a 20-year limit, so that hospitals and other agencies that benefited from the funds no longer have an obligation to provide free care based on their subsidy (42 C.F.R. sect. 124.501[b][I] [1996]). The idea of a right to health care through Hill-Burton was never clear. Although the law required that subsidized hospitals and health care agencies provide care at no cost to those residents of the area who could not afford to pay, there was no mechanism for enforcement, so compliance was inconsistent.

There was also a community service obligation in the Hill-Burton Act (42 U.S.C. sect. 300s—1[b][1][k] [1994]) that required hospitals to make their services, including emergency services, available to all persons in the facility's area. The hospitals were prohibited from requiring preadmission deposits and could not discriminate against Medicare beneficiaries and Medicaid recipients. There were, however, no sanctions for noncompliance, and the Department of Health and Human Services (DHHS) did not enforce the law (Havighurst et al, 1998). The

Hill-Burton requirements were of the "rights to" genre in that the obligation to provide the free care fell to the hospitals and other health care agencies without any concomitant obligation on the part of the recipient of care or any other entity. Hospitals asserted that after so many years of providing free care as required in the original Hill-Burton Act, they had more than paid their debt related to the construction funds they received.

At the state level, there are also mandates that require local governments to provide health care to indigent persons. The requirement to provide care may be expressed in specific terms (California Welfare and Institutional Code, sect. 17000 [1991]) or merely authorize a locality to provide such care (Arizona Revised Statutes, Ann. Sect. 11—251[5] [1990]). Some courts have interpreted the statutes to indicate that indigent health care is mandatory, while other courts have held that states could choose not to provide certain types of care, such as abortions. It is possible to construe that such laws do confer a "right to" health care.

The Joint Commission on the Accreditation of Healthcare Organizations (JCAHO) addresses patients' rights. Its guidelines require that hospitals avoid denying access based on the financial resources of a patient (Havighurst et al, 1998).

In 1986 Congress passed the Emergency Medical Treatment and Active Labor Act (EMTALA) (42 U.S.C., sect. 1395dd). This act requires that any hospital with an emergency department provide appropriate medical screening within that institution's capacity and determine whether an emergency exists. If an emergency exists, the institution must provide sufficient medical treatment to stabilize the condition if facilities are adequate to do so, or transfer the patient to another appropriate medical facility if the attending physician determines that the medical benefits of transfer outweigh the risks. Consent for the transfer must be obtained from the patient if at all possible. Violation carries severe penalties—$25,000 per violation for hospitals with fewer than 100 beds and $50,000 for larger institutions. Patients injured by violations of this act may sue the institution in civil court for damages incurred as a result of an inappropriate transfer or substandard care. With such sanctions, there is stronger evidence of some right to a certain level of health care. In fact, EMTALA was clearly intended to provide all citizens with initial care for emergency health problems regardless of ability to pay (131 Congressional Record S13904 [Oct. 23, 1985]).

EMTALA was passed as part of a budget reconciliation act (the Consolidated Omnibus Budget Reconciliation Act [COBRA]). Interestingly enough, unlike other major legislation, there were no public hearings before its passage (Havighurst et al, 1998). Two years later, however, there was a hearing, during which allegations and anecdotes about inappropriate transfers (so-called "patient dumping") of indigent patients were largely disproved. Furthermore, empirical studies revealed that patients did

not suffer damage because of transfers, which were often to a more appropriate facility (Havighurst et al, 1998). Yet there has been no change in EMTALA, even though it was based on apparently false information. EMTALA requires that emergency services be provided to all patients who present themselves with a medical emergency but makes no provision for payment for such services. Since hospitals that participate in Medicare are obligated under EMTALA, some critics have suggested that Medicare funds be provided for at least some of the expenses of complying with EMTALA, but this has not happened. Morreim (1995) asserts that there seems to be a pervasive policy of "coerced private altruism that requires private citizens to make up for others' misfortunes that they in no way caused." There is also anecdotal evidence that inappropriate care is provided to persons who present themselves with obviously nonemergent conditions and demand care from emergency personnel fearful of sanctions under EMTALA.

The Medicaid program also provides evidence that there is some right to health care. Of course, Medicaid does not provide that everyone has access to health care, only those who meet certain criteria. However, the program does serve those who normally would not be able to pay for care, providers may not discriminate against those persons who use Medicaid, and states must follow federal guidelines (although the better a state does economically [as measured by per-capita income], the less it gets in federal matching funds). This situation seems to militate for a "right to" health care no matter what the goals or economic viability of a state. Nevertheless, APNs need to be aware that there is no explicit "right" to health care.

The Constitution and Declaration of Independence

The Constitution was enacted to prevent unbridled use of power by the central government. The founders of the United States were all too conscious of what an overweening government could do from their experience with the oppression of Great Britain before the Revolutionary War. Many people believe that in the more than 200 years since the Revolution, things have changed and no one need fear abuse of government power. However, one need only observe the news of the day to see things differently— international news of abuse of regular citizens by governments around the world, national news of attempts to pass laws that restrict the exercise of freedoms that Americans have enjoyed for decades, and national and local news of the abuse of police power regarding rights to privacy and autonomy.

It is occasionally worth reading these documents again to understand the foundation from which policy about other issues, including health care, arises. To start from a familiar area, one should consider that nursing curricula always require internal consistency—the mission gives rise to a philosophy, and the philosophy gives rise to goals and objectives, which in turn prescribe the concepts and content of a program. Health policy, therefore, must be consistent with the Constitution, and one should attempt to analyze policies, laws, and regulations or practices resulting from laws in light of Constitutional principles.

In the United States, the political order originated with the 1776 Declaration of Independence, in which the idea of an autonomous population and the notion of power resting with the people was stated:

> We hold these truths to be self-evident, that all Men are created equal, that they are endowed by their Creator with certain inalienable rights, that among these are Life, Liberty, and the Pursuit of Happiness—that to secure these Rights, Governments are instituted among Men, deriving their just Powers from the Consent of the Governed, and that whenever any form of Government becomes destructive to those ends, it is the Right of the People to alter or abolish it.

When exploring the concept of personal autonomy, it is also instructive to examine Article I, Section 8 of the Constitution, which provides the government power to collect taxes to support the military and provide for the general welfare. This means that government spending may be done only for the enumerated purposes found in the Constitution and for the general welfare, not the welfare of specific groups or persons. Another area of interest is the power given to Congress, also in Article I, Section 8 (the Commerce Clause), to regulate commerce. This section promotes the free flow of goods and services among the states and with foreign governments and is limited by the Necessary and Proper Clause, which directs Congress to avoid making laws that are unnecessary or improper in exercising the enumerated powers.

The Amendments to the Constitution are also important. Many are cited in explaining and examining the rights and responsibilities of patients and health care providers. The Bill of Rights, included in the Constitution in 1791, was added because the founders wanted to prevent any misconstruction or abuse of governmental powers. Furthermore, because it was impossible to enumerate everything that might become an issue in the years to come, the Ninth Amendment provides that such enumeration "shall not be construed to deny or disparage [other issues] retained by the people" (Ninth Amendment, Bill of Rights, Constitution of the United States).

A way a patient might use the rights and responsibilities given by the Bill of Rights is as follows: Geri is a woman who did not give up. Her struggles and triumphs were once described in a woman's magazine, and she epitomizes the ability of all people to influence the development of health policy. Her first personal encounter with the health care system came when her son was diagnosed with Hodgkin's disease at the age of 13. When he was admitted to an unclean hospital without a special pediatric waiting room, she worked with other parents on the unit and confronted the hospital administrator. She also contacted the local paper. By the end of the week, all of Geri's concerns were addressed. She became aware that many people might label her an "activist," although she was just fighting for her son's health. Eventually, Geri also had to fight for her own needs, because shortly after her son died, she began her own battle with breast cancer. As her own health improved she began to work for other women with breast cancer. She helped establish a breast cancer action coalition in New York. This group persisted in getting their voices heard regarding the high rate of breast cancer on Long Island; they received federal funding for breast cancer research and cancer studies. Now Geri Barish is regarded as one of the country's foremost advocates for breast cancer awareness and research (Saslow, 2000). When she started campaigning, Geri said she was "terrified and did not know how to lobby or negotiate." However, she learned how to listen, identify the most important issues, and be patient and persevere for what she believed. Her story shows the power of demanding to be heard for what you believe. To improve community health care, APNs will need such dedication and commitment.

Congressional Role in the Construction of Health Policy

Policy and law generally arise in the legislature—either the houses of Congress or the state legislature. Presidents, governors, and other public officials may also recommend or suggest policy. The executive branch of the federal or state government is able to manipulate and influence legislators to do its bidding through threats of veto or promises of compromise.

At the federal level, much of the work of Congress occurs in committee. Shi and Singh (1998) identify at least 14 committees and subcommittees in the House of Representatives and 24 committees and subcommittees in the Senate that have an influence on legislation; however, a mere 5 of these control most of the legislation. If a bill involves taxation, Constitutional law requires that it begin in the House of Representatives. The Ways and Means Committee, according to House rules, has the most influence on bills that call for taxation of the populace. For example, the Ways and Means Committee was responsible for the origination of much of the health financing legislation of the 1960s and 1970s (Shi & Singh, 1998). Currently, this committee has responsibility for Medicare Part A, Social Security, unemployment compensation, public welfare, and health care reform measures. It shares responsibility with the House Commerce Committee for Medicare Part B. The Commerce Committee itself is responsible for Medicaid, public health, mental health, health personnel, health maintenance organizations (HMOs), foods and drugs, air pollution, consumer products safety, health planning, and biomedical research. It is important to know the jurisdictional areas of the committees so that research into pending bills and their passage through Congress can be easily followed. Furthermore, if it is of interest to attend hearings of House committees, one would at least need to know what committee was dealing with an issue of interest and when hearings open to the public would be held. It is also possible to communicate with committees to provide input and opinion for their deliberations. A very important committee in the House is the Committee on Appropriations, which is responsible for providing for (or not providing) funding of other legislation. This includes appropriations or funding for health-related legislation (except that regarding Medicare and Social Security, which are funded through the Social Security Trust Fund).

In the Senate, committees important to health care issues include the Committee on Labor and Human Relations, which is responsible for the Public Health Service Act, the Federal Drug and Cosmetic Act, HMOs, health care personnel, and mental health legislation (Shi & Singh, 1998). Bills dealing with taxation and revenue generation are the responsibility of the Committee on Finance. This committee has a subcommittee on health; it has jurisdiction over Medicare, Medicaid, professional standards review organizations, and laws affecting hospitals and nursing homes.

Current bills, both those that have been considered and not passed and those that have become law, may be researched using the tools available in libraries, on the Internet, through governmental and private sources, through publications by private and public organizations, and by contact with legislators' offices. Other sources of information are compiled and available to organizations that subscribe to certain services; these may be available to students who have affiliations with larger health care institutions and other organizations, but they are generally not easily available to private individuals because they are a paid subscription service or a privilege of membership. (For more information about the Congressional process of creating and instituting health policy, see Chapter 3.)

Professional, Policy, and Research Organizations and the Formation of Health Policy

There are countless organizations that conduct research, analyze policy and policy proposals, and represent professional groups. These organizations provide a great deal of information about policy, including commentary on bills in Congress and the effect of laws on certain societal functions or professional practices. Although this information comes from the point of view of the organization, it provides valuable insights. Research and analysis organizations employ professional staff who study all aspects of bills, laws, and policies. They often have easier access to information, of which there is more than is possible to study in a reasonable amount of time; their condensation of such data into manageable forms is helpful to the APN researcher. Furthermore, if there is interest in looking at the original data, much of the organizations' work is heavy with references to which the APN can go whenever it is necessary or desirable.

Professional organizations produce publications, maintain Internet websites, and sometimes conduct research, often found in abstract form, full-text articles, or references on their Internet sites. Other organizations that provide much the same service include policy analysis organizations, corporations involved in health care and related endeavors, and others. Many individuals and groups conduct research or analyze policy and publish it in the journals of universities, colleges, and professional organizations (including small, specialty organizations) and publications of commercial publishing houses.

A useful source for a fairly comprehensive listing of professionally related organizations on the Internet, with evaluations and descriptions of the sites, is the publication *Healthcare Guide to the Internet* (Wayne-Doppke, 1998), which is now available online (for a fee). (See Chart 2-1 for a list of other Internet sources that are useful for the study of health policy.)

Executive Branch, Administrative Agencies, and the Implementation of Health Policy

In the implementation phase of establishing laws and policies (after the legislature or Congress has enacted them), responsibility shifts to the various administrative agencies that are part of the executive branch of government. There are major departments, such as the DHHS, and independent agencies, such as the Environmental Protection Agency (EPA) and the Food and Drug Administration (FDA) (Longest, 1998). An important subdivision of DHHS is the Health Care Financing Administration (HCFA), which is responsible for Medicare, Medicaid, and other federal health programs. These administrative agencies can be accessed directly on their own Internet sites (at their [acronym].gov locations). While these are primary sites not filtered by a third party, a researcher should understand that governmental agencies present information that depicts themselves in the most positive light; their material should be read objectively.

IMPLICATIONS FOR MSN EDUCATION AND ADVANCED PRACTICE

The importance of primary sources in the study of and research into health policy cannot be overestimated. The one difficulty is the volume of data available regarding policy-making. It can be overwhelming and somewhat daunting to find hundreds or thousands of pages of testimony, commentary, Congressional pronouncements, drafts of bills, and other material about just one act or law. Before and after enactment one also finds critical or analytical articles (the secondary sources) by researchers, policy analysts, academic faculty, attorneys, and students.

Once APNs become involved in the study of policy, reading and studying the available resources have the effect of making the law a living entity rather than a dry, remote subject. Nurses familiar with the processes and outcomes of policy development are able to negotiate and navigate health care systems to the benefit of their own practice and of the institutions and agencies in which they are employed.

The state of Kentucky provides a clear example of how APNs can become involved in policy-making. The Kentucky Coalition of Nurse Practitioners and Nurse Midwives (KCNPNM) had tried numerous times in the past to get prescriptive authority. According to Partin (1996), Kentucky nurse practitioners (NPs) began seeking prescriptive privileges in 1980. While their efforts were not successful, each time members learned a little more about what it would take to attain prescriptive authority. The early endeavors were not successful in part because of "political naïveté," but by 1992 things looked promising. By 1994, a bill was actually introduced and passed in the House, only to die in a Senate committee. The KCNPNM vowed that the next time it would be different. Several factors led to the passage of the prescriptive authority bill in 1996. One was the collaboration of KCNPNM with the Kentucky Nurse Association (KNA) and the Kentucky Nurse Anesthetist Association. These organizations worked together to educate the people who were able to influence the making of health policy in Kentucky. Legislators were invited to come and visit NPs in the clinical area to see firsthand what services NPs could provide. In addition, both the KCNPNM and the KNA hired an attorney/lobbyist. All three organizations had their members write letters to their legislators.

Information regarding successful and unsuccessful attempts to gain prescriptive privileges was obtained, and numerous negotiations took place with the Kentucky Medical Association (KMA) to write mutually agreeable language for all four organizations (Partin, 1996). Having KMA support was an important part of the bill's success. Many physicians in practice with NPs wrote letters supporting the endeavor. The sponsor of the bill was a nurse legislator who also worked very hard for its passage.

Important points in the drafting of the bill's language included the following:

- General language was to be used for the prescriptive authority so no unnecessary constraints were put on practice.
- The word *supervision* was not acceptable in the bill, and no concessions would be made that restricted advanced registered nurse practitioner (ARNP) practice more

than it already was. The KCNPNM agreed to kill the bill (if necessary) if this language was inserted.
- Prescriptive authority was to be granted for nonscheduled legend drugs.
- Continuing education requirements every 2 years would be put in place.
- A collaborative practice agreement with a physician for prescriptive privileges would exist; this agreement pertained only to prescriptive authority and not practice as a whole.
- The collaborative practice agreement did not need to be filled with the KMA.

The legislative journey began in January 1996, first in the House and then the Senate. It passed unanimously in the House Health and Welfare Committee, and 90 to 1 on the House floor (Partin, 1996). The committee in the Senate was the Licensing and Occupations Committee. This committee had more questions, and it was obvious that some senators were intent on either slowing the bill or stopping it. After debate, it passed with only the addition of the word *nonscheduled* to make it clear the Bill did not include controlled substances. In the Senate, one senator actually proposed 38 amendments to the bill! The amendments included things such as decreasing reimbursement or restricting the ability to diagnose patients; these amendments would have made NP practice in the state of Kentucky very difficult, if not impossible. After debate, the bill was passed by a vote of 31 to 6. After the addition of the word in the Senate version, the bill had to return to the House for approval on the language change. At this time, the KCNPNM thought there would be no difficulty with passage. However, the senator who had proposed all the amendments requested that the House majority leader not bring the bill forward for a vote on the word change. Nurses, physicians, NPs, certified registered nurse anesthetists (CNRAs), the KNA, and even patients began bombarding the House majority leader with letters, faxes, and phone calls to bring the bill forward for a vote. This involvement on the part of nurses and others continued throughout the month of March (Partin, 1996). ARNPs in Kentucky met with the governor to enlist his support. Finally, on the last day of the session, the bill was brought forward and passed. Unfortunately, the next venture with the legislature in 2000 to clarify the sample dispensing language met with similar obstacles and difficulties. While a bill that outlined dispensing abilities was finally passed, it was not the one the KCNPNM wanted. Once again, various amendments were attached by the Senate, affecting the intent of the bill. The original bill was abandoned after negative amendments were attached.

APNs can influence the passage of local, state, and national health policy. It takes the belief in what is being done, as well as perseverance in the system. It also requires the art of persuasion. Conger (1999) discusses the need for people to learn the fine art of persuasion. Most people see persuasion as a skill to help sell things or coerce someone to do something they do not want to do. However, it is more than this. If persuasion is used constructively and for full effect, it becomes "a negotiating and learning process through which a persuader leads colleagues to a problem's shared solutions." Conger agrees that persuasion does mean leading other people to a position they currently do not hold through proper framing of arguments, supporting evidence, and a "correct emotional match" with the audience. If APNs can appeal to colleagues, legislators, and physicians and demonstrate how to get from here to there, establish credibility, support a position with data, and enlist support, the world is their oyster! Learning about the audience, attaining supporting evidence, researching other states' endeavors, and considering the ultimatum and alternative options—these were all stages undertaken before the KCNPNM began their journey toward prescriptive authority.

Conger (1999) identified the essential steps in effective persuasion (Table 2-1). Conger says "the most valuable lesson I've learned about persuasion over the years is that there's just as much strategy in how you present your position as in the position itself. In fact, I'd say the strategy of presentations is the more critical."

The study of rights is often neglected in the curricula for any level of nursing practice. Too frequently the concept of rights is misunderstood and misused. APNs should be familiar with the ideas of natural rights and constitutionally or legally enforceable rights, as well as the notion that some rights engender obligations in others.

PRIORITIES FOR RESEARCH

Longest (1998) feels that the research community can influence health policy through documentation, analysis, and prescription. The first step in researching policy is documentation; this means gathering information, cataloging it, and describing the state of the world and its health. Ideally, research is able to influence health policy by identifying what does and does not work. Pilot or demonstration projects help provide substantiated data for determining how well a program or policy intervention will work. This analysis can provide insight for policy-makers.

Table 2-1	

Steps to Effective Persuasion

STEPS TO EFFECTIVE PERSUASION	CHARACTERISTICS/GOALS
Establish credibility	• Credibility comes with expertise in an area. • One must honestly assess where one stands in terms of credibility by asking questions such as: How is my track record? How will others perceive the change I am proposing? Do people see me as trustworthy and supportive? How do I stand in comparison with them (emotionally, intellectually, and politically)?
Frame goals in a way that identifies common ground with those they intend to persuade	• Illuminate the advantages of your position. • Identify shared benefits • Give details (e.g., details that show increased sales or increased quality). • Identify objectives and tangible benefits. • Know all the facts about your audience. • Brainstorm with others for arguments and perspectives.
Reinforce positions using vivid language and compelling evidence	• Use language in such a way as to supplement numbers with examples, stories, and analogies to make your point. • Paint a "word picture" of your position.
Connect emotionally with the audience	• Be aware of the underlying emotions of your audience and adjust your presentation accordingly. • Match your style of presentation to the audience's ability to receive the message. • Use informal conversations to give insight into reactions. • Too much emotion is as bad as too little; judge what is needed based on your knowledge of the audience.

Data from Conger, J. (1999, January 1). The necessary art of persuasion. *Health Forum Journal*. Available online at www.healthforum.com/thfnet.thfimenu.htm.

One health care policy that has influenced a number of pilot projects is the DHHS campaign to introduce healthier communities in the United States. For example, five hospitals joined forces to create Lancaster Healthy Communities, a public service organization. This organization has as its goal the improvement of the quality of life for residents. The Lancaster organization held forums regarding health and quality of life; this information was then shared with county commissioners. Six key areas were identified related to health, and a comprehensive plan was developed to address them, including partnerships among schools, civic organizations, and businesses and citizens getting involved in the planning process for changing health policies. A similar initiative was started in California and called the California Healthy Cities and Communities program. This program helps fight the health hazard of secondhand smoke. The program supported the passage of smoke-free ordinances in local cities. Future research will analyze the health effects of this legislation; early results indicate that cancer incidence and deaths are declining in California faster than in the rest of the nation. Because smoking-related diseases occur years after the initial exposure to smoke, the true effect of the antismoking legislation will be felt in the long run.

APNs who contribute to this type of research are indirectly having an influence on the development and revision of health policy. For example, any research that provides data related to Healthy People and its goals serves to affect subsequent revisions of the policy. APNs are intimately involved with many of the Healthy People Objectives; collecting data to substantiate nursing interventions and outcomes would provide needed data.

Lamm (1994) makes the case that the current health system is not healthy for our country. He stresses that people need to look at the ways decisions about health care spending are made. Health policy research can start by defining an adequate level of care for people. The United States cannot afford to deliver all beneficial care; instead, one must start asking what the benefits are, given the costs of a particular service. An example of health policy outcomes research occurred in the state of Oregon. The state decided not to fund transplants under its Medicaid program and instead chose to fund basic health care for the people currently outside the health system (Lamm, 1994). They effectively shifted payment from the expensive transplant system to coverage of every person with an income less than the poverty level. Oregon argues that it is better to address the identified priorities in services and procedures, based on the benefit to the population. At some point, the United States will probably decide that basic health care is the first priority that needs to be addressed. Most other countries have emphasized public health and preventive care, which may also be described as basic health care.

Few nurses are involved in health care policy research. Sue Blevins is the President of the Institute for Health Freedom, one of the few nurse-run health care policy agencies. Other well-known nurses in the field include

Suggestions for Further Learning

- Go to THOMAS (thomas.loc.gov; see the site description in Chart 2-1). Use THOMAS to research a particular law related to health care. Find the committee hearings and discussion, as well as the comments and testimony that might have occurred on the floor of the Senate or House. An interesting commentary to read as a beginning is that of Representative Ron Paul, who is also a physician, speaking about the Patient's Bill of Rights and the Medicare prescription drug proposals.
- Go to the CIS (Lexis-Nexis). This is such a comprehensive service that it is worth navigating just to see what kinds of information are available. Aimless or non–goal-centered perusal is sometimes enlightening, but it may consume many hours. It is generally more useful to have an idea in mind when you search; you will still find material that is unrelated and interesting, material that will perhaps be useful at another time or with another topical study.
- Get the book: Litman, T. (1997). *Health politics and policy* (3rd ed.). Albany, NY: Delmar. Read the discussion titled "Contributing factors to the failure of Clinton's health care reform initiative: a policy perspective." Do you think these factors did contribute to the demise of the health care reform? What role did APNs or nurses play in its demise?
- Get the article: Christenson, M. (1999, July 1). No shots, no school. *Health Forum Journal.* Accessed online at www.healthforum.com/thfnet.thfimenus.htm. What message does this article present that is related to the ability to influence health policy at the local community level?
- Another article describes the role of the community in changing policy: Adams, C. (2000, January 1). Changing public policy. *Health Forum Journal.* Accessed online at www.healthforum.com/thfnet.thfimenu.htm. Is the presence of nurses/nursing visible in these articles? If not, why not? What should the nurse's role be in influencing health policy?
- Go to www.healthcommunities.org. This site includes policies and actions that will help communities improve their health and quality of life. Identify policies on strategies that APNs can implement. Where could you start in getting your community interested in initiating such a program?

Charlotte Twight and Grace Arnett. As more nurses recognize the power of their voices, both individually and collectively, the number of nurses involved in health policy research will increase.

DISCUSSION QUESTIONS

These questions can be used to promote critical thinking and encourage discussion.

1. Using one of the government ([acronym].gov) websites, enter key words or other information about a policy issue of particular interest to you. Keep the topic narrow. What kind of responses did you receive? Is the site helpful in finding information about your topic? Keep a record of your activities.

2. Using the same topic, search one or more of the professional, policy, or research organization's sites. Which of them is most useful for your topic? Can you find articles or commentary with different points of view about your policy issue? Keep a record of your activities or make copies of useful articles by downloading them to your computer or floppy disk or by making a paper copy.

3. Read the U.S. Constitution and the Amendments. Where can you find a copy of this document? Discuss your policy topic (from the previous exercise) in light of the provisions of the Constitution or Bill of Rights. This might be a useful classroom exercise to promote critical analysis of ideas.

4. Read or review Epstein's book *Mortal Peril* (1997). Discuss the concepts of rights and health care from Epstein's view. What are his main arguments for or against a right to health care. Defend or refute his assertions using legal and/or ethical arguments.

REFERENCES/BIBLIOGRAPHY

Adams, C. (2000, January 1). Changing public policy. *Health Forum Journal*. Available online at www.healthforum.com/thfnet.thfmenu.htm.

Anderson, A., Gillis, C., & Yoder, Y. (1996). Practice environment for nurse practitioners in California: identifying barriers. *Western Journal of Medicine, 165*(4), 209-214.

Beyers, M. (1997). Moving nursing forward. *Advanced Practice Nursing Quarterly, 3*(3), vii.

Beyers, M., Gunn, I., Egging, D., & Thomas, K. (1997). Policy: advanced practice nursing issues and challenges: specialty association viewpoint. *Advanced Practice Nursing Quarterly, 3*(3), 31-35.

Black, H.C. (1991). *Black's law dictionary*, St. Paul, MN: West Publishing.

Buppert, C. (1999). *Nurse practitioner's business practice and legal guide*. Gaithersburg, MD: Aspen Publishers.

Buppert, C. (2000). *The primary care provider's guide to compensation and quality*. Gaithersburg, MD: Aspen Publishers.

Cohen, S., Mason, D., Kovner, C., Leavitt, J., Pulcini, J., & Sochalski, J. (1996). Stages of nursing's political development: where we've been and where we ought to be. *Nursing Outlook, 44*, 259-266.

Conger, J. (1999, January 1). The necessary art of persuasion. *Health Forum Journal*. Available online at www.healthforum.com/thfnet.thfmenu.htm.

Epstein, R. (1997). *Mortal peril*. Reading, MA: Addison-Wesley Publishing.

Havinghurst, C.C., Blumstein, J.F., & Brennan, T.A. (1998). *Health care law and policy* (2nd ed.). New York: The Foundation Press.

Kingdon, J. (1995). *Agendas, alternatives and public policies* (2nd ed). New York: Harper Collins.

Lamm, R. (1994). The brave new world of health care. In P. Lee & C. Estes (Eds.), *The nation's health* (4th ed.). Boston: Jones and Bartlett.

Longest, B.B. (1998). *Health policymaking in the United States*. Chicago: Health Administration Press.

Milstead, J. (1997). A social mandate: APN leadership for the whole policy process. *Advanced Practice Nursing Quarterly, 3*(3), 1-8.

Morreim, H. (1995). Futilitarianism, exoticare, and coerced altruism: the ADA meets its limits. *Seton Hall Law Review 25*, 883.

O'Malley, J. (1997). The art and science of shaping public policy. *Advanced Practice Nursing Quarterly, 3*(3), v-vi.

Palmer, S., Sabo, D., & Wertz, B. (1997). Community health care: servicing Colorado's uninsured: a health policy legislative proposal. *Advanced Practice Nursing Quarterly, 3*(3), 69-76.

Partin, E. (1996). Prescriptive authority for Kentucky advanced registered nurse practitioners. *Nurse Practitioner, 21*(8), 15-16.

Porter-O'Grady, T. (1997). Influencing policy: foreign territory for nurses. *Advanced Practice Nursing Quarterly, 3*(3): 79-80.

Saslow, L. (2000). Never give up. *Family Circle, 113*(9), 13-14.

Shi L., & Singh, D. (1998). *Delivering health care in America*. Gaithersburg, MD: Aspen Publishers.

Twight, C. (1997). Medicare's origin: the economics and politics of dependency. *The Cato Journal, 16*(3).

Wayne-Doppke, J. (1998). *Healthcare guide to the Internet*. Santa Barbara, CA: COR Healthcare Resources.

Chapter 3

Influencing Health Policy

Sue A. Blevins

Today's health care providers are subjected to thousands of federal and state regulations that directly affect the nursing profession and patient care. For example, there are more than 111,000 pages of rules and regulations pertaining to Medicare alone (Moffit, 1999). As the nation's largest group of health care providers, nurses are well positioned to monitor the effects of government regulations and make recommendations for improving them. Therefore it is important for nurses to understand how to influence health policy—that is, how to turn recommendations into law. This chapter explains how to influence health policy through lobbying and educating policy-makers in order to improve the delivery of nursing care and, ultimately, enhance the quality of patient care in the United States.

DEFINITIONS

Lobbying is one of the most widely used techniques for influencing health policy. Simply put, lobbying is advocating a point of view. It is a way for people to voice their opinions and convince lawmakers to accept their positions on a particular issue. Lobbyists serve the primary function of bringing about the passage of laws favorable to an organization's mission or defeating laws contrary to its interests (Chronicle Guidance Publications, 1998). The activity of petitioning lawmakers is as old as government itself. The word *lobby* was first recorded in 1808 when it appeared in the annals of the Tenth Congress (Congressional Quarterly, 1990). By 1929, the term *lobby-agent* was applied to petitioners who hung out in the lobby of the New York State Capitol waiting to address legislators.

CRITICAL ISSUES: LOBBYING TO CHANGE HEALTH POLICY

Most people think lobbying is something only large organizations do. However, small volunteer groups and individuals can and do lobby Congress, the White House, and state legislators. In fact, all Americans have a Constitutional right to influence lawmakers. The First Amendment states

that "Congress shall make no law . . . abridging the freedom of speech, or of the press; or of the right of the people peaceably to assemble, and to petition the Government for a redress of grievances."

Today there are more than 106,000 persons employed as lobbyists, representing some 20,000 organizations and firms (Chronicle Guidance Publications, 1998). In 1998, total expenditures on federal lobbying amounted to $1.42 billion. In all, there were more than 38 registered lobbyists and $2.7 million in lobbying expenditures for every member of Congress in 1998 (Shuldiner, 1999).

While there are no licensing or certification requirements for lobbyists, nearly 17,000 (of the 106,000) lobbyists are registered under the Federal Lobby Disclosure Act (P.L. 104-65). According to the Act, *lobbyists* are legally defined as persons who spend at least 20% of their time for a particular client on lobbying activities; have multiple contacts with legislative staff, members of Congress, or high-level executive branch officials (including the Vice President and President); and work for a client paying more than $5000 over 6 months for that service. Additionally, organizations employing in-house lobbyists whose expenses exceed $20,500 for a semiannual period must register (Shuldiner, 1999). Persons or organizations meeting these criteria must register with the Secretary of the Senate's Office of Public Records and the Clerk of the House's Legislative Resource Center. Additionally, they must file reports twice a year, providing both midterm and end-of-year reports of lobbying activities and expenditures. The reports are open to the public. Individuals wanting to view the information must visit the Senate's Office of Public Records and the House's Legislative Resource Center. However, the Senate plans to make the information available on the Internet, and the House is considering doing so too. Currently there are several organizations that track federal lobbying expenditures and post the information on the Internet.

Most registered lobbyists are college graduates, and many have advanced degrees; nearly one third of all lobbyists have a law degree (Chronicle Guidance Publications, 1998). To be effective, lobbyists must possess the following qualifications: (1) training or experience in a particular field, (2) a good understanding of the legislative and political process, (3) above-average oral and written communication skills, and (4) the ability to conduct research and organize findings. Some of the most influential lobbyists are former members of Congress who, upon leaving office, join a private law firm or association. They are viewed as highly effective because they know the legislative process and have many personal contacts on Capitol Hill. They know which members to contact on a specific issue and how to approach various important committee members.

However, it is important to recognize that one does not need to be a registered lobbyist to lobby Congress. Individual citizens, Hollywood actors, prominent businessmen, and even active members of Congress all commonly work to influence legislation. The First Amendment right to petition Congress applies to all citizens. However, only those who meet the previously mentioned criteria must register as official lobbyists.

One of the best ways to learn about influencing health policy is to serve an internship with Congress or state legislature. Graduate nursing students can obtain assistance in seeking such internships through their school's department of health policy or by contacting their U.S. representatives and senators, as well as their state lawmakers. Many lawmakers welcome the input and assistance of experienced health care providers.

What Does Lobbying Entail?

Businesses, professional organizations, nonprofit associations, and community organizations all hire lobbyists to advance their agendas. Lobbyists serve the interests of the organizations or associations they represent. They communicate their client's needs to Congress, the executive branch, state legislatures, and regulatory agencies at both the federal and state levels. Lobbyists often provide lawmakers with data and assistance in interpreting and explaining technical and complex issues.

Lobbyists are paid to closely monitor legislation and regulations for the clients they represent. They conduct research and write reports on how new or proposed laws and regulations could affect their clients. They also help prepare for Congressional hearings by nominating witnesses, preparing written testimony, and crafting pro and con position papers on the issue at hand. They help organize coalitions to work together on the same policy or law. Finally, and most importantly, lobbyists play an important role in helping to draft the bills that become the nation's laws. Of course, although lobbyists play an integral role, the final responsibility for drafting bills rests with legislators. Once a law is passed, lobbyists communicate and work closely with regulatory agencies to influence how final regulations are written.

There are pros and cons to lobbying. The public benefits from the research and analysis provided by the thousands of registered lobbyists. On the other hand, some argue that politicians bow to special interest groups to the detriment of the general public's interest. While there is no doubt that wealthy organizations are a powerful force on Capitol Hill, one must consider that they represent the voices of many individuals. Organizations such as the American Association of Retired Persons, National Rifle Association, and National Organization of Women are examples of associations that wield significant influence on Capitol Hill because of their large membership base. The lobbyists they employ speak for many individuals. Most people are too busy to monitor legislation and prefer to join an organization that represents their particular interests. The groups, in turn, hire lobbyists to carry their message to Washington and state capitols. The alternative is that individuals would not get to voice their opinions through private associations.

Over the past 100 years, the nursing profession has become aware of the importance of influencing health policy and has begun to build an effective lobbying base for nurses. Nurses realize that if they want to turn their recommendations into policies, they too must employ the efficient methods used by other organizations to communicate their needs to Congress and state lawmakers. Furthermore, as more Americans rely on Medicare and Medicaid for financing their health care, advanced practice nurses (APNs) need to gain a thorough understanding of how these programs work in order to effect positive change.

Ways to Lobby

The most common forms of lobbying involve supporting lawmakers with campaign contributions, applying pressure through grassroots activities, and directly lobbying via face-to-face communications. Any American citizen (except federal contractors) can contribute money to political parties or candidates running for elected federal office. Foreign citizens who are not permanent residents in the United States are prohibited from contributing to any U.S. candidate, including those running for federal, state, or local offices.

Campaign contributions serve two primary functions: to make sure a group's legislative interests are represented and to help ensure that a member of Congress friendly to an organization's issues remains in office. Influencing members of Congress directly with money dates back to the 1830s and has been well documented during the nineteenth and twentieth centuries. However, grassroots lobbying and political action committees (PACs) became more prevalent during the 1940s. Although corporations have been barred from making direct contributions to campaigns for federal office since 1907, labor unions were not barred until 1943 (Congressional Quarterly, 1990). However, organized labor responded to the new restriction by creating a political financing mechanism known as the PAC. The PAC system allowed labor unions to bypass the 1943 federal law that banned direct contributions to campaigns. Instead of contributing money from dues

Table 3-1

Federal Campaign Spending Limits

	TO A CANDIDATE OR CANDIDATE'S COMMITTEE (PER ELECTION)	TO ANY NATIONAL PARTY OR PARTY'S COMMITTEE (PER CALENDAR YEAR)	TO ANY PAC OR OTHER POLITICAL COMMITTEE (PER CALENDAR YEAR)
Individuals can give:	$1000	$20,000	$5000
PACs can give:	$1000	$20,000	$5000

Data from Center for Responsive Politics (1996). *Open secrets*. Washington, DC: Center for Responsive Politics.

Box 3-1

Writing an Effective Lobbying Letter

- Send a typed or neatly handwritten letter, including your complete return address and telephone number.
- Do not send a form or duplicated letter.
- Address your correspondence to a specific legislator (see the addresses below).
- Reference the name and number of the bill you are concerned about at the beginning of your letter.
- Keep your letter short (one to two pages) and get to the point immediately. For example, state up front if you want your legislator to support or oppose a specific bill and why.
- Include reliable, current data to support your position.
- Include any newspaper clippings that support your position.
- Explain how the proposed legislation will affect costs and access to health care in the legislator's district.
- State that you are a RN, give your current position, and note any professional affiliations (such as being a member of the ANA). Be sure to make it clear for whom you are speaking.

- Stress that you are a registered voter residing in the legislator's district.
- If the letter concerns a critical issue, consider sending it as a certified letter and requesting a returned receipt.
- Ask your legislator to vote in a specific way. For example, ask, "Can I count on you to support H.R. 100?"
- Request a written response to the question(s) you pose.
- If the legislator does what you ask, be sure to send a thank-you letter.

Include the same information in an e-mail message. Be sure to request verification that the e-mail letter was received.

Address correspondence to:

The Honorable (full name)
United States Senate
Washington, DC 20510

Dear Senator
(last name):

The Honorable (full name)
U.S. House of Representatives
Washington, DC 20515

Dear Representative
(last name):

directly to political campaigns, the new system used voluntary contributions to the union PAC, which in turn gave the money to political campaigns and candidates.

Over the next 30 years, the number of PACs grew, and by 1974 there were some 608 PACs in the United States. Today there are more than 4000 PACs that greatly influence the political process (Center for Responsive Politics, 1996). There are no limits on the amount of money that candidates running for office can spend on an election. However, the 1974 Federal Election Campaign Act limits the amount a candidate or national party may receive from individuals and organizations. (Those limits are summarized in Table 3-1.)

Another important method of lobbying is grassroots activism. This involves coordinating the efforts of many individuals to get them to phone, write, or e-mail their elected officials. Other methods for influencing health policy include contacting the media, sponsoring public forums and rallies, and starting petitions. Organizations

such the AIDS Coalition to Unleash Power (ACTUP) and the National Taxpayers Union often use grassroots lobbying to influence lawmakers.

Letters are one of the best methods for influencing lawmakers. Writing an effective lobbying letter is quite easy, but it must include some key information (Box 3-1). The letter should be addressed to a specific legislator, typed, and include the writer's return address and telephone number. The writer should be sure to reference the name and number of the pending bill they are concerned about; this information should appear at the very beginning of the letter. Additionally, the writer should get to the point immediately. For example, the letter should state a desire up front for the legislator to support or oppose a specific bill and why. It is also important to include reliable, current data, including recent newspaper clippings, to support a position. An effective lobbying letter should explain how a proposed bill would affect costs and access to health care in the legislator's district. An APN

Table 3-2

Lobbying Techniques Used by 174 Sampled Interest Groups

TECHNIQUE	PERCENTAGE OF GROUPS USING THE TECHNIQUE
Testify at hearings	99
Contact government officials directly to present a point of view	98
Engage in informal contacts with officials (e.g., at conventions, over lunch)	95
Present research results or technical information	92
Send letters to members of an organization to inform them about activities	92
Enter into coalitions with other organizations	90
Attempt to shape the implementation of policies	89
Talk with people from the press and media	86
Consult with government officials to plan legislative strategy	85
Help to draft legislation	85
Inspire letter-writing or telegram campaigns	84
Shape the government's agenda by raising new issues and calling attention to previously ignored problems	84
Mount grassroots lobbying efforts	80
Have influential constituents contact their congressman's office	80
Help to draft regulations, rules, or guidelines	78
Serve on advisory commissions and boards	76
Alert congressmen to the effects of a bill on their districts	75
File suit or otherwise engage in litigation	72
Make financial contributions to electoral campaigns	58
Do favors for officials who need assistance	56
Attempt to influence appointments to public office	53
Publicize candidates' voting records	44
Engage in direct-mail fundraising for an organization	44
Run advertisements in the media about a specific position on issues	31
Contribute work or personnel to electoral campaigns	24
Make public endorsements of candidates for office	22
Engage in protests or demonstrations	20

Data from Davidson, R.H., & Oleszek, W.J., (1990). *Congress and its members.* Washington, DC: Congressional Quarterly Press. Originally published in Schlozman, K.L., & Tierney, J.T., (1986). *Organized interests and American democracy.* New York: Harper & Row.

should state that he or she is a registered nurse (RN), give his or her current position, and note any professional affiliations (such as being a member of the American Nurses Association [ANA]). However, the APN should make it clear for whom he or she is speaking. Finally, if a legislator does what the concerned citizen requests, that citizen should be sure to send a thank-you letter. Several advanced practice organizations are utilizing a grassroots campaign of letter writing to oppose HR 1304, the Quality Health-Care Coalition Act of 1999. While this bill sounds like the kind of legislation that nurses typically would support, this act may in fact lead to antitrust issues. Several nursing organizations have combined their voices, via letters, expressing concerns about the legislation.

The next best approaches for contacting legislators include sending e-mail messages or faxes and placing telephone calls. Although legislators are increasingly relying on e-mail, some Congressional staffers have stressed that letters are taken more seriously than e-mails because writing a letter takes a greater effort, including more time and resources, than sending an e-mail message.

Much lobbying is still carried out by direct communication with elected officials. This involves scheduling appointments and meeting face-to-face with lawmakers or their staff members. The main purpose of these meetings is to inform policy-makers by providing research and analyses on particular issues. Lobbyists also serve as expert witnesses and can help find cases to present at Congressional hearings. This is a very effective way to inform lawmakers, the media, and the public about an issue at hand.

All three of these lobbying techniques are used by thousands of organizations to influence national polices. In order to maintain access to elected officials, lobbyists must be certain the information they give a staff member is accurate and complete. Also, it is very important to explain both sides of an issue, as members do not appreciate being uninformed about how their opposition views a particular issue. (Table 3-2 shows lobbying techniques used by 174 sampled interest groups.)

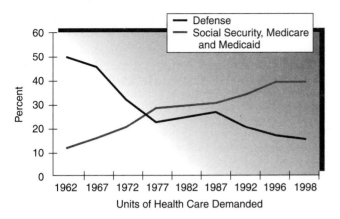

Figure 3-1 Share of federal spending (1962-1998).

Why Do Organizations Lobby?

The majority of organizations that lobby are groups that rely heavily on federal funds. Congressional historian George B. Galloway wrote that "perhaps nine-tenths of the work Congress is concerned . . . with is the spending of public money" (Congressional Quarterly, 1990). In 1997, the most heavily lobbied issues were the federal budget, taxes, health, transportation, and defense. Some 42% of lobbyists listed the federal budget as one of their interests that year (Salant, 1998).

Nurses petition Congress, the White House, and state legislators primarily to influence bills related to the practice of nursing. For example, state practice acts directly affect nurses; thus nurses work to make sure state laws allow nurses to practice fully according to their educational training. Nurses also lobby legislators to help patients gain access to care through government health insurance programs.

Government spending on social insurance programs has increased significantly since the New Deal era. In 1935, the government spent $31 million, or less than 1% of total federal revenues, on social insurance programs. By 1990, spending on such programs amounted to $380 billion, or 36.9% of federal revenues (Congressional Quarterly, 1990). The percentage of federal spending on health care has increased dramatically over the last 30 years. In 1962, the government spent the greatest share of federal dollars on defense. However, by 1998, Medicare and Medicaid represented the largest share of federal spending. (Figure 3-1 shows trends in federal spending between 1962 and 1998.)

As a greater number of patients enroll in government health care programs, APNs need a better understanding of the federal rules and regulations that affect the patients they serve. Moreover, Congress is likely to tighten Medicare regulations in the coming years in order to maintain the program's solvency. Many nurses, like other health care professionals, will likely take an active part in ensuring the program is managed fairly and efficiently in the coming years.

Lobbying Expenditures

U.S. organizations and associations spent $1.42 billion on federal lobbying in 1998. The top five contributors by industry include insurance ($77.2 million), pharmaceutical and health products ($73.8 million), telephone utilities ($67.9 million), tobacco ($67.4 million), and electric utilities ($63.7 million). The health professions industry ranked as the seventh largest contributor ($45.8 million).

The five largest individual organizations include British American Tobacco ($25 million), Phillip Morris ($23 million), Bell Atlantic ($21 million), the U.S. Chamber of Commerce ($17 million), and the American Medical Association (AMA) ($16.8 million). There is no question that physicians represent the largest share of lobbying expenditures by health professionals. However, nurse anesthetists rank second, spending some $1.7 million on lobbying during 1998. (The top ten health professions' lobbying expenditures are presented in Table 3-3.)

The ANA spent $540,180 on lobbying during 1998. Other nursing organizations with significant lobbying expenditures during 1998 included the American Organization of Nurse Executives ($200,000), the American College of Nurse Midwives ($134,773), and the National Association of Pediatric Nurse Associates ($120,000). All told, nursing organizations spent $3,078,953 on lobbying during 1998 (Table 3-4). This represents approximately 6.7% of total lobbyist spending ($45,839,289) by all health professionals during that year.

Nonprofit organizations such as hospitals and universities also spend money on lobbying. For example, the National Committee to Preserve Social Security and Medicare spent some $6.78 million on lobbying expenditures during 1998, contributing 70% of that amount to Democrats (Shuldiner, 1999). Economics America, an organization that tracks expenditures according to political affiliation, reports that liberal nonprofit groups (including charities) outspend their conservative counterparts on lobbying by a ratio of two to one. Liberals also maintain more total revenues; in 1996, politically active groups on the left had revenues of nearly $4 billion, compared with less than $900 million for their counterparts on the right (Lenkowsky, 1999).

Role of Think Tanks

Besides lobbyists, legislators have traditionally relied on trade associations, government agencies, and academia for information to guide political decision-making. However, over the past few decades, lawmakers have begun to turn to "think tanks" for data and analyses on a myriad of issues. Think tanks are nonprofit organizations that were established to conduct research and policy analyses on timely national issues. Typically, they do not lobby, although by law they can spend a small amount of their total expenditures on direct and grassroots lobbying. Think tanks tend to employ academicians and former govern-

Table 3-3

Top Ten Health Professions by Lobbying Expenditures

RANK/ORGANIZATION	LOBBYING EXPENDITURES (1998)	CAMPAIGN CONTRIBUTIONS (1998)*
American Medical Association	$16,820,000	$2,701,607
American Association of Nurse Anesthetists	$1,735,000	$645,369
American Society of Anesthesiologists	$1,537,015	$961,726
American College of Physicians	$1,200,000	$1,000
College of American Pathologists	$1,120,000	$242,788
American College of Emergency Physicians	$1,020,584	$387,675
American Occupational Therapy Association	$960,000	$255,445
American Academy of Family Physicians	$936,993	$500
American Society of Internal Medicine	$908,142	$82,970
American Psychological Association	$880,000	$1,950

*Campaign contributions include individuals, PACs, and soft money to federal campaigns and party committees; this information is obtained from the Federal Election Commission.

Data from Shuldiner, A. (1999). *Influence Inc.: the bottom line on Washington lobbying.* Washington, DC: Center for Responsive Politics.

Table 3-4

Lobbyist Spending by Nursing Organizations

NURSING ORGANIZATION	LOBBYIST SPENDING (1998)
American Academy of Nurse Practitioners	$29,000
American Association of Critical-Care Nurses	$80,000
American Association of Nurse Anesthetists	$1,735,000
American Association of Occupational Health Nurses	$60,000
American College of Nurse Practitioners	$40,000
American College of Nurse Midwives	$134,773
American Nurses Association	$540,180
American Organization of Nurse Executives	$200,000
Association of Operating Room Nurses	$40,000
Emergency Nurses Association	$40,000
National Association of Pediatric Nurse Associates	$120,000
National Association of School Nurses	$40,000
Wound Ostomy Continence Nurses	$20,000
Total	$3,078,953

Data from Shuldiner, A. (1999). *Influence Inc.: the bottom line on Washington lobbying.* Washington, DC: Center for Responsive Politics.

ment officials from many fields, including economics and law. They differ from academia, however, in that they focus more on practical solutions than theories. However, most think tanks do incorporate academic theories into their analyses and policy proposals.

Think tank experts are often invited to testify before Congress and speak on national television and radio programs across the country. While many think tanks claim to be nonpartisan and therefore not beholden to any particular political party, most of them do support a specific ideology. For example, the Brookings Institution is one of the nation's largest think tanks. It tends to advocate liberal approaches for solving the nation's social and economic problems. On the other side, the Heritage Foundation has become the nation's largest conservative think tank. The libertarian Cato Institute's policies tend to be liberal when pertaining to social issues, but conservative when pertaining to economic ones. Liberal think tanks typically support government intervention for social and economic problems (such as universal health care); conservative groups advocate reducing government spending (such as tax cuts) and controlling some behaviors (such as illegal drug use); and libertarian think tanks advance a position that favors allowing individuals to pursue personal choice, while advocating that individuals must take responsibility for their lives, including financial responsibility. Libertarians are opposed to government-mandated universal health care, but they support a universal tax credit for health insurance so that all Americans can receive the same tax break that employers enjoy today (Box 3-2).

How a Bill Becomes a Law

Health policy in the United States is determined by our laws and regulations. APNs can take an active role in

Box 3-2

National Think Tanks that Influence Health Policy

Alpha Center	www.ac.org
American Enterprise Institute	www.aei.org
Brookings Institution	www.brookings.org
Cato Institute	www.cato.org
Center for Policy Alternatives	www.cfpa.org
Children's Defense Fund	www.childrensdefense.org
Commonwealth Fund	www.commonwealthfund.org
Competitive Enterprise Institute	www.cei.org
Families USA	www.familiesusa.org
Heritage Foundation	www.heritage.org
Institute for Health Freedom	www.forhealthfreedom.org
National Center for Policy Analysis	www.ncpa.org
Pacific Research Institute	www.pacificresearch.org
Public Citizen	www.publiccitizen.org
RAND	www.rand.org
Urban Institute	www.urbaninstitute.org

shaping laws by first understanding the process through which they are developed.

The first step of federal lawmaking is drafting a bill. This involves turning an idea into a legislative format. Anyone can present an idea for a bill: an individual, a member of Congress, a special interest group, or the President. However, only a member of Congress can introduce the bill. The particular senator or representative that introduces a bill is referred to as its *sponsor*. After a bill is introduced into the Senate or House it is given a number and officially starts the legislative process. The steps are similar in both the Senate and House. Lack of action at any step can cause a bill to die.

- *Introduction:* The first step involves the formal introduction of a bill in either the House or Senate. A bill originating in the House is designated by the letters H.R., signifying House of Representatives. A Senate bill is designated by the letter S. followed by its number. The Library of Congress currently maintains a database of all bills introduced in Congress (thomas.loc.gov).
- *Referral to Committee:* Next, the bill is referred to a committee, then (in most situations) a subcommittee. The bill is examined carefully at this point. If the committee or subcommittee does not act on a bill, that bill goes no further in the process and dies. Most bills get this far and no further.

- *Subcommittee Hearings:* The subcommittee next holds hearings about the bill. At this time, witnesses for the administration, lobbyists, experts, supporters and opponents of the bill, and other interested parties can have their opinions heard by the subcommittee.
- *Mark Up:* After the hearings are completed, the subcommittee marks up—that is, makes changes and adds amendments to—the bill. The subcommittee next refers the bill to the full committee. The full committee can hold further hearings at this point. The committee votes on whether the bill should be presented to the full Senate or House.
- *Report:* If the committee votes to proceed, a written report is prepared that summarizes the legislation, its effect on existing laws, and the views of opponents. This report is distributed to members of the Senate or House.
- *Floor Action:* When a bill reaches the floor of the Senate or House, it is open for debate by all members. The Senate and House have specific rules as to how this debate takes place.
- *Voting:* The bill is voted on by all members of either the Senate or House. If the bill is passed by the Senate or House, it must go through all the previous steps in the other chamber of Congress.
- *Conference Committee:* If the bill is altered significantly by the other chamber of Congress, a conference committee is formed. This committee attempts to reach a compromise on both versions of the bill.
- *Final Vote:* The revised bill is sent back to the floor of both the Senate and House for final vote. No changes are allowed at this point.
- *Referral to the President:* If the bill (in the same form) passes both chambers, it is sent to the President for signature or veto.
- *Overriding a Veto:* If the bill is vetoed, it goes back to Congress where a two-thirds majority can override the veto. The bill would then become law.

When the President receives the bill, it is either signed into law or vetoed. The President can also choose to do neither, and if Congress is in session, such a bill will automatically become law after 10 days. A "pocket veto" occurs when the President takes no action on a bill when Congress is adjourned, and the bill dies. (Figure 3-2 graphically depicts the legislative process at the federal level.)

Role of Committees

It is important to note that one of the most important steps in the political process involves influencing committee members. A former member of Congress stated that "the committee system is still the crux of the legislative process and is still the basis for congressional action. Laws are not really made here on the floor of the House or on the floor of the other body [the Senate]. They are only revised here.

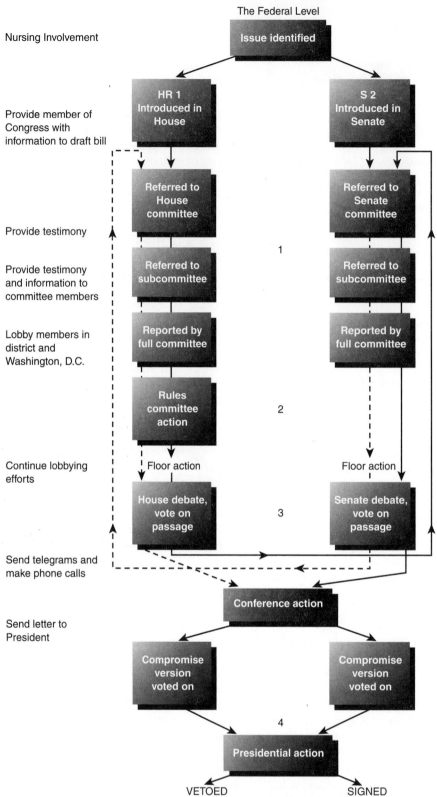

The Federal Level

Nursing Involvement — Issue identified

HR 1 Introduced in House S 2 Introduced in Senate

Provide member of Congress with information to draft bill

Referred to House committee Referred to Senate committee

Provide testimony

Provide testimony and information to committee members

Referred to subcommittee Referred to subcommittee

1

Lobby members in district and Washington, D.C.

Reported by full committee Reported by full committee

Rules committee action

2

Continue lobbying efforts

Floor action Floor action

House debate, vote on passage Senate debate, vote on passage

3

Send telegrams and make phone calls

Conference action

Send letter to President

Compromise version voted on Compromise version voted on

4

Presidential action

VETOED SIGNED

[1] A bill goes to full committee first, then to special subcommittees for hearings, debate, revisions, and approval. The same process occurs when it goes to full committee. It either dies in committee or proceeds to the next step.

[2] Only the House has a Rules Committee to set the "rule" for floor action and conditions for debate and amendments. In the Senate, the leadership schedules action.

[3] The bill is debated, amended, and passed or defeated. If passed, it goes to the other chamber and follows the same path. If each chamber passes a similar bill, both versions go to conference.

[4] The President may sign the bill into law, allow it to become law without his signature, or veto it and return it to Congress. To override the veto, both houses must approve the bill by a $2/3$ majority vote.

Figure 3-2 The legislative process. (From Mason, D.J., Talbott, S.W., & Keavitt, J.K. [1993]. *Policy and politics for nurses: actions and changes in the workplace, government, organization, and community* [2nd ed.]. Philadelphia: WB Saunders.)

Ninety percent of all legislation that has been passed was passed in the form reported by the committee to the floor" (Congressional Quarterly, 1990). In other words, committees are most responsible for influencing the final form of most laws in the United States.

There are several important committees that affect nursing care. The Senate Health, Education, Labor and Pensions Committee (HELP) has jurisdiction over health and labor issues, including biomedical research and public health. The Senate Finance Committee oversees the Medicare and Medicaid program. In the House, the Ways and Means Subcommittee on Health has jurisdiction over Medicare (the nation's largest insurer), while the Commerce Committee oversees health programs and health facilities not supported by payroll taxes. Finally, the Senate and House Appropriations Committees oversee federal revenues and the passage of appropriations bills.

Congress must pass 13 general appropriations bills to fund the federal government annually. Each February, the President is required by law to submit a budget proposal to Congress for the following fiscal year. Congress has the Constitutional authority to increase or decrease funding levels, eliminate funding for programs, or add funding for new programs not requested by the President. Ultimately, Congress has the power to accept or deny the President's spending requests. About one half of federal spending each year is funded through the appropriations process, including funding for nursing research (Congressional Quarterly, 1990).

Federal Rule-Making

Getting a law passed is really only the beginning of influencing health policy. Oftentimes laws are drafted in purposefully vague language to give federal agencies plenty of room to modify rules according to changes in society. The real nuts and bolts of policy-making occur during this rule-making stage. Thus nurses should become informed about the rule-making process and learn about opportunities to comment on proposed rules. APNs would benefit from practicing "preventive politics" by making sure regulations friendly to nursing are drafted when permitted by law. It is easier to prevent being left out of a program, then to try to amend a government regulation, such as a Medicare regulation, to include nurse practitioners (NPs) or other APNs in a new rule.

In addition to drafting regulations for new laws, government agencies also have the authority to change existing rules as long as they stay within the wide statutory framework they are often provided. This authority derives from the Administrative Procedure Act (APA). Under this act, federal agencies can change rules by placing a notice of proposed rule making (NPRM) in the *Federal Register* at least 30 days before the rule is to take effect. The notice includes a description of the rule, its terms, and information on to whom to submit comments. It also includes a time limit in which interested parties must respond. This is referred to as the *open public comment period*. Organizations and individuals are encouraged to share their comments on how the proposed rule will negatively or positively affect them—personally, professionally, and within society as a whole. The governing federal agency then modifies the proposed rule, with consideration given to the many comments it receives from the public at large. Regulations issued through the APA process (with notice and comment) have the force and effect of law.

Code of Federal Regulations

Once a new law's regulations are finalized, they are published in the *Code of Federal Regulations* (CFR). The purpose of the CFR is to present a complete guide to permanent government regulations. The full set of the CFR consists of approximately 200 volumes that provide the text of final regulations. The 200-volume CFR is revised at least once a year. A reference copy of the CFR is available at any federal depository library. CFR regulations can also be accessed on the Internet.

IMPLICATIONS FOR MSN EDUCATION AND ADVANCED PRACTICE

Since nursing practice and patient care are greatly affected by many national and state regulations governing health care, it is imperative that APNs learn how to influence health policy in order to ensure quality patient care and access to all health care providers. Examples of recent health policy issues affecting APNs include Medicare reimbursement for NPs, the national nursing shortage, and the epidemic of prescription drug errors. NPs have fought hard for Medicare reimbursement by utilizing many of the lobbying techniques listed in Table 3-2. The American College of Nurse Practitioners continues to monitor legislation affecting NPs.

All types of APNs are qualified to provide information about how the national nursing shortage affects the quality of patient care across the country. This issue could also be an important one for building a coalition among various APN specialty organizations. Moreover, those APNs with prescribing privileges are well positioned to serve on advisory commissions that are examining ways to reduce prescription drug errors. Such an activity is an important way to educate policy-makers and the public.

One of the techniques less commonly used by APNs is the filing of lawsuits to exercise legal rights. APNs may be hesitant to engage in contentious litigation due to high legal costs or because of the general sensitivity to frivolous lawsuits. Nevertheless, they should not overlook this effective technique for upholding certain legal rights, including workplace safety codes and adequate nurse-to-patient ratio workloads.

All told, using the lobbying and educational techniques described in this chapter, APNs can take an active role in utilizing hands-on experience to inform policy-makers and the public about the important role of APNs in delivering high-quality, cost-effective care and monitoring drug errors. Turning recommendations into policy is a key to improving health care in the United States.

PRIORITIES FOR RESEARCH

Information is one of the important keys to persuading policy-makers and public opinion. APNs could benefit greatly by researching and communicating the ways in which various laws and regulations affect nursing practice and (ultimately) patient care. Examples of current health policies that could be researched include: How does the delivery of primary care delivered by NPs compare to care delivered by general practitioners (GPs) in terms of quality and costs? What are the trends in hospital nurse-to-patient ratios, and how do those trends compare to hospital reports of medication errors? What role do nurses play in preventing medication errors, and how has the recent nursing shortage affected their role? How many APNs get involved in legislative issues? How many have contacted their legislators about health policies important to them? How many APN programs teach about the legislative process and encourage Master of Science in Nursing

(MSN) students to contact their legislator as part of the course requirements? How effective are nursing grassroots efforts?

Another important issue for future research is to examine how the globalization of health care is going to affect state laws. Historically, nurses have been licensed at the state level. However, with recent developments in telemedicine, the United States is likely to see a trend toward international regulation of general health care. Nurses, especially APNs, must examine how the globalization of health care will affect their ability to practice independently in the United States.

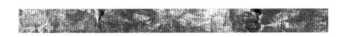

DISCUSSION QUESTIONS

These questions can be used to promote critical thinking and encourage discussion.

1. What is your understanding of how federal laws are made and subsequently drafted into regulations?
2. Using the CFR website, identify a federal regulation that affects your ability to practice nursing (e.g., identify a particular Medicare regulation stipulating the amount of reimbursement for NPs). Read the regulation in its

---

Suggestions for Further Learning

- There are several key sources of information for understanding how health policy is influenced in the United States. The Library of Congress maintains a computerized database of bills introduced in Congress (thomas.loc.gov). At this website, citizens can access a more detailed explanation of how a bill becomes a law.
- Another important source of information is a report titled *Influence Inc.: The Bottom Line on Washington Lobbying*. It was published by the CRP, a nonprofit research organization that tracks expenditures for lobbying Congress. The report can be accessed at CRP's website (www.crp.org).
- All professionals who must abide by thousands of pages of federal rules and regulations should familiarize themselves with the *Federal Register* and the CFR (both can be accessed at www.access.gpo.gov/su_docs/aces/aces140.html). These important federal websites provide a detailed listing of the many rules and regulations affecting APNs and (ultimately) the quality of patient care in the United States.

- Visit one of the following websites to learn more about influencing health policy:
  - Center for Responsive Politics at www.crp.org
  - Congressional database at thomas.loc.gov
  - *Federal Register* at www.access.gpo.gov/su_docs/aces/aces140.html
  - How a Bill Becomes a Law at thomas.loc.gov/home/lawsmade.toc.html
- Go to the websites of various nursing organizations and find out if they have legislative information. Such information might include how to contact your legislator, how to write effective letters, and how to determine who your representatives are. Which website includes the most information about legislative efforts? Which site includes the least? Some possible sites include:
  - American Nurses Association at www.nursingworld.org
  - American Academy of Nurse Practitioners at www.aanp.org
  - American College of Nurse Practitioners at www.acnp.org

entirety. Using the electronic version of the *Federal Register* (www.access.gpo.gov/su_docs/aces/aces140.html), examine the history of the regulation, including the initial NPRM and the final rule published in the *Federal Register*. According to public comments about the regulation, can you identify which groups supported the regulation and which opposed it?

3. Visit the Center for Responsive Politics' (CRP's) website (www.crp.org) to examine the lobbying influence of various health care professionals. How much money did various groups (those who supported and those who opposed the regulation) spend on lobbying Congress during the past year?

4. Do you think APNs should pursue a greater role in influencing federal and state health policy through lobbying Congress and state legislatures? Why or why not?

5. If you had the opportunity to change only one health policy in the United States, what policy would you change and why?

REFERENCES/BIBLIOGRAPHY

Center for Responsive Politics (1996). *Open secrets*. Washington, DC: Center for Responsive Politics.

Chronicle Guidance Publications (1998). *Lobbyists*. Moravia, NY: Chronicle Guidance Publications.

Congressional Quarterly (1990). *CQ guide to current American government*. Washington, DC: Congressional Quarterly Press.

Davidson, R.H., & Oleszek, W.J. (1990). *Congress and its members*. Washington, DC: Congressional Quarterly Press.

Kelly, L. (1996). *The nursing experience* (3rd ed.). New York: McGraw Hill.

Lenkowsky, L. (1999, April 8). Seeing through the left's false lament. *The Chronicle of Philanthropy, 11*(12), 39-40.

Mason, D.J., Talbott, S.W., & Keavitt, J.K. (1993). *Policy and politics for nurses: actions and changes in the workplace, government, organization, and community* (2nd ed.). Philadelphia: WB Saunders.

Moffit, R. (1999). *Setback for Medicare reform*. AAPS News.

Salant, J.D. (1998). *$1.17 spent to lobby Congress*. Associated Press.

Schlozman, K.L., & Tierney, J.T. (1986). *Organized interests and American democracy*. New York: Harper & Row.

Shuldiner, S. (1999). *Influence, Inc.: the bottom line on Washington lobbying*. Washington, DC: Center for Responsive Politics.

Section II

Organization of the Health Care Delivery System

Margaret M. Anderson

Health care organizations are experiencing rapid change. The only stable element is the notion that things will continue to change. Change is constant, pervasive, inevitable, and unpredictable. Chaos theory has been proposed as a way to approach this constant change. Since changes in one part of the health care system influence the other parts, most organizations are influenced by external environmental changes. Organizations that are able to react to these changes are flexible, with mature systems that allow them to react responsibly; such organizations have learned from past changes. This continuous change in the health care delivery system affects nursing. In the past, nursing has evolved in response to need, but today, nurses have an extraordinary opportunity to serve as leaders in the efforts for change.

To serve as leaders, advanced practice nurses (APNs) must have a clear understanding of the health care delivery organization; therefore concepts of reengineering, change, leadership, quality, and managed care are essential components of the nursing curriculum. This section provides a view of the health care delivery system, and important components of the system are presented.

Chapter 4 discusses health care delivery in the United States. This view of the organization of the health care delivery system includes the history of the system, as well as current and future perspectives. Information is presented for gaining an understanding of the totality of health care systems, especially within the integrated care systems of today.

As a more specific view of the organizations that provide care, Chapter 5 delves into the individual components that make up the health care system. Both public and private organizations are described. Community-based systems of care, such as rural health clinics, community health centers and public health organizations, are examined in detail.

As a concept, managed care is congruent with the nursing philosophy, involving preventive care, cost-effectiveness, efficiency, and evaluation of care on patient outcomes. Chapter 6 is concerned with not only describing managed care so as to provide an understanding of how it works, but also with giving a historical perspective and a view of where managed care may be developing. The role of APNs in managed care is stressed, with particular emphasis on areas where nursing must make the most of its position.

The notion of quality care is discussed in Chapter 7. As the health care system changes, one issue remains at the forefront of discussion: quality care. Consumers are becoming more empowered, and health care plans are utilizing quality outcome data to promote care providers. Everyone is asking how to deliver quality care in a cost-efficient manner. This chapter elaborates on how APNs can gather data to show quantitatively and qualitatively the extent to which nursing can provide quality, holistic care.

Given the rapid changes in health care in the last 15 years, it is critical to examine what could have been done differently. Chapter 8 elaborates on how to reengineer health care, which involves reexamining how things have always been done (i.e., "looking outside the box"). This chapter describes the general nature and innovation of change, the process of and responses to change, and strategies to create and lead change in health care organizations.

As the health care delivery system reacts and changes, APNs are in a position to serve as leaders. No matter the position, APNs must be effective leaders and followers to function optimally in today's clinical settings. Chapter 9 presents a theoretical background to guide APNs in this process, with emphasis on the essential tasks and characteristics of leadership. Transformational leadership theory is emphasized as the process that produces the best results. This chapter also stresses that leadership and vision are important components of successful APN practice.

Chapter 4

Health Care Delivery in the United States

Margaret M. Anderson & Denise Robinson

Understanding the evolution of the health care delivery system in the United States and its effect on the development of the involved professions helps explain where health care is today, as well as exposing the dilemmas that face it. Even though health care is not guaranteed by the Constitution of the United States, it has often been considered an inherent right for all Americans. Now, when debates rage as to whether health care is a right or a free market commodity, the history of care delivery helps one understand why health care is considered a right. The question is: to what extent is there a right to health care and who should pay for that right?

CRITICAL ISSUES: ASSESSING THE "RIGHT" TO HEALTH CARE

The history of the system provides some insight into why Americans believe that health care is a "right." American health care followed the European model for delivery and evolution. Images of the local country doctor and his nurse-wife providing services and care to people in their community and receiving food, services, goods or farm animals in return for those services are alive and well in the romantic lore of the nation. This was the common model; the establishment of an American hospital did not occur until 1751, in Philadelphia. Before that, lay or untrained nurses delivered health care in the home. Families were expected to care for their own ill (Doheny, Cook, & Stopper, 1997). The wealthy paid for someone to help with that care; the poor made do with what resources they had. Americans went to hospitals for the salvation of their soul, since most hospitals were controlled by religious orders who were as concerned with salvation as they were restoration of health (Catalano, 1996). Hospitals were places to die, not organizations for the healing and treatment of the ill.

As science and civilization developed with the advent of the Civil War, health care improved dramatically. Before that, most doctors were poorly trained, and most nurses were apprentice-trained. The need for health care in the Civil War brought about changes in medical and nursing education. Hospital environments were improved, sanitation was augmented, and health care delivery to large numbers of ailing, injured, and dying in the hospital setting became the most efficient use of medical and nursing care. Intensive courses of training for doctors and nurses, as well as the knowledge that germs caused infection, brought about sweeping reforms in health care (Doheny et al, 1997).

Government gradually became more involved in both the structure and development of cities. As cities grew rapidly, with heavy immigration from Europe, so did the numbers of problems related to environmental sanitation (Roemer, 1986). By the end of the nineteenth century, boards of health had been established within the governments of most large cities; there were also similar boards at the state level. The scope of health departments did not broaden until the turn of the century, and for the most part, voluntary groups of citizens were the driving force for these changes. Milk stations were set up in New York City for poor mothers who could not nurse their babies. The New York City Health Department organized a Bureau of Child Hygiene, staffed by nurses. These nurses provided care to newborn babies and their mothers in tenements, and they conducted child health clinics. Development of tuberculosis clinics followed a parallel path in terms of extension of health department activities. Public health agencies became more widely established between 1910 and 1935; however, their main focus was on environmental sanitation and preventive control of communicable diseases. These agencies were "weak" when compared to boards of education or police departments (Roemer, 1986). Public health nursing first appeared in the largest cities, in which concentrations of people led to the spread of communicable diseases.

The increased use of health care organizations (hospitals and offices) was inspired by the medical profession's need and desire to treat and care for larger numbers of people than could be handled through the old house call method. Hospitals facilitated the education of physicians by serving as places to learn about treatment and observe patient progress. Sick individuals came to the physician rather than the physician making a series of house calls. The burden of getting the patient to the physician then became the responsibility of the patient or family. Other systems focused on the essential need of the patient to get medical care—ambulances, clinics, offices and hospitals—grew up in populated areas such as towns, cities, and villages. It was often necessary for small villages to join together to create a hospital to meet the needs of their citizens. The education and role of nursing then became organized around hospitals rather than the home. (Kalisch & Kalisch, 1995)

Development of Health Insurance

In the early 1900s, health care was free to the poor; the wealthy paid for service and made donations to hospitals to provide care for those less fortunate. During the Great Depression, the wealthy were unable or unwilling to make large donations to public hospitals for the care of the poor. In place of health insurance, the Social Security Act of 1935 was implemented; it included two titles designed to strengthen public health services by federal grants-in-aid to the states. Title V provided support for maternal and child health services, as well as the diagnosis and treatment of crippled children. Title VI provided for general public health under the administration of the U.S. Public Health Service. These federal grants greatly strengthened public health agencies. A National Health Survey conducted in 1935 and 1936 revealed a large number of untreated diseases in the population, particularly in the low-income groups. Senator Robert Wagner (sponsor of the Social Security Act) introduced an amendment to the Social Security Act that would have supported federal grants to the states for the organization of health insurance plans covering workers and their dependents. However, the onset of World War II interfered with the serious consideration of this amendment (Roemer, 1986). In 1943, legislation was introduced into Congress for launching a federally administered national health insurance program. The American Public Health Association did not support this legislation because it focused only on prevention; the new leaders in the public health field felt that public health service should include all aspects of health care delivery, including medical care.

Hospitals began providing health care in return for premiums, which was the beginning of insurance as it is known today. In other words, a system of paying in advance to health care organizations to cover the costs of hospitalization before it was needed was developed. The Blue Cross/Blue Shield Company became the first company to offer insurance and became a major player in the financing of health care. Budgets of health care organiza-

tions needed approval by "The Blues" before charges for services could be raised.

The movement for health care insurance as a benefit for the employed became prevalent after World War II. As wage freezes limited monetary increases, labor unions pressed for benefits in lieu of increased wages. Where increased wages might mean higher taxes for employees, increased benefits did not necessarily result in higher taxes. In addition, health benefits were tax deductible for employers. Thus the employer (usually a large, powerful company) became the gatekeeper of health care access through the provision of health insurance benefits for employees and their families. Employees usually did not have to pay for health care benefits until the inflation-plagued 1970s and 1980s. Before that time, it was not difficult to meet health care costs from either side of the equation. When health care costs rose, health care organizations raised their rates. When health care organizations raised their rates, employers raised the consumer cost of their goods and services. A circle was invented; an increase in one area led to an increase in the other. In the middle to late 1970s, employers began requiring employee contributions for the health care insurance benefit (Catalano, 1996).

Employers also began to screen employees for preexisting health conditions that may lead to increased health care costs or use of the health care system. During this time, very little emphasis was placed on disease prevention or health promotion. Annual exams, well-baby checks, and other health promotion activities were rarely covered services. Treatment of disease was covered, but health promotion services were not.

Establishment of Medicare and Medicaid

In the 1960s, against the backdrop of the Vietnam conflict, President Lyndon Johnson's administration turned its attention to providing health care for older adults and the poor. This drew public attention (at least for a while) to a domestic issue. In 1965, the federal and state governments initiated the Medicare and Medicaid insurance programs through Social Security amendments as an attempt to alleviate the health care access issues for the poor and older adults. Little strategic planning was used in the development of these programs, and this has caused problems in the long term. It is important to keep in mind that without a plan there is no way to evaluate the success of the program or how well it meets its goals (Harrington & Estes, 1997). However, these programs had a dramatic effect on expansion of health care in the United States.

Medicare is a federally funded program financed through employee payroll taxes. Older adults and the disabled are eligible to benefit from Medicare. Medicare Part A is for hospital, nursing home and home care

System	Characteristics	System goals		
		Costs	Access	Quality
Pre-1970	Low direct consumer prices; cost base and fee for service reimbursement	↑	↑	↑
1970s	Same as above but with regulatory controls	↑	↑	↑
1980s	Increasing direct prices, prospective reimbursement, per capita (HMOs) increasing	↓	↓	?

Figure 4-1 Overview of economic characteristics of the health care system in three periods and their influence on goals of the system. (From Delougherty, G.D. [1995]. *Issues and trends in nursing*. St. Louis: Mosby.)

services; Part B is for physician, laboratory, outpatient, and other services. Part A is free; Part B is available for a monthly premium. Medicaid is an individual state-run entitlement program for the poor and uninsured. Both of these programs were designed to pay for the required medical care of older adults and the poor. Under the retrospective payment system, the government paid whatever the health care organization charged. Basically, this system encouraged greater costs, greater access, and greater quality.

Shortly after Medicare and Medicaid were instituted, it became evident that the programs were going to be costly, and a method of cost control was needed. Capital expenditure review was instituted. This included reviews of major equipment purchases (computed tomography [CT] and magnetic resonance imaging [MRI] scanners) and additions or renovations to the facility (e.g., adding facilities for open heart surgery). A Certificate of Need would be issued certifying that the hospital's plans were in accordance with the regulatory agency's guidelines. Certificate of Need regulations first appeared in New York in 1964, but it was not until the middle 1970s that a full-scale federal effort at capital expenditure planning (via the National Health Planning and Resources Development Act in 1974) was implemented. Although regulation seemed like a means to decrease spending, it did nothing to change the costs, access, or quality prior to 1970. The good old days of retrospective payment and its resultant rising costs ran unchecked until 1983, when the prospective payment system was phased in over several years to contain costs. With the retrospective payment system, fraud was rampant on both the provider and patient sides. Under the prospective payment system, the government

used a number of criteria and historical data to determine a fair payment based on diagnostic-related groups (DRGs). If a health care organization could perform the needed services for the payment, they broke even. If they could perform the services and discharge the patient in less time, the organization made money and could keep the profit. If they overran the cost, the organization lost money. There has been a growing concern that having incentives to curtail resources may in fact affect quality. In addition, hospitals have been forced to carry the burden of nonpayment for those patients who have no health insurance coverage and can not afford to pay for the high cost of hospitalization. In the 1980s and afterward, decreasing costs, decreased access, and questionable quality became evident. (Figure 4-1 shows an overview of economic characteristics of the health care system in three periods, based on reimbursement.) This highlighted the need for, and was the beginning of, health care reform in the United States (Catalano, 1996).

Evolution of Health Care Delivery Systems

The onset of health care reform caused the evolution of different kinds of health care delivery systems. Ludwig von Bertalanffy originally described *systems theory* in 1968 as a complex feedback system of inputs, throughputs, and outputs. Systems theory can be used to examine health care delivery systems. According to systems theory, a health care delivery system, seen as a large medical care organization, would be one with various entry and exit points. It would contain multiple subsystems such as hospitals, clinics, and physicians' offices. The managed care organization (MCO) would exist within a suprasystem of the health care system at large. Environmental influences change systems and theoretically make them more responsible to the larger society. Some of the environmental influences on health care systems include financial issues, technological advances, and social policy. The accessing of a system, especially in health care, is a point of issue today. Systems are defined as open or closed depending on the essential nature and business of the system. Health care is considered an open system, implying its reliance on others (e.g., individuals, systems, suppliers) outside the system to maintain its status within society as well as its continued existence (Catalano, 1996). Figure 4-2 identifies the components of a health services system. The graphic shows the interaction between the persons and care providers, as well as the various factors that affect that relationship. However, more recently, the question being asked is: to whom is the health care system open and at what cost?

Economic Flow Analysis

The amount spent on health care would not be a problem in and of itself if more people felt they were getting "benefits" for the large expenditures. There is a current feeling that medical care is subject to diminishing returns. This means that as more and more is spent on medical care, the effectiveness or outcomes of additional expenditures diminishes (Jacobs, 1995). If this hypothesis holds true in most circumstances, it is vital that a careful examination of increasing medical expenditures be conducted. Economic flow analysis is helpful to look at how the money and services flow between all those involved in the financing of health care. Figure 4-3 shows a simplified version of how the money flows from the ultimate payers (consumers and employers) through two key groups of provider-physician practices and hospitals (Jacobs, 1995). The role of advanced practice nursing (APN) in the economic flow diagram is not clearly defined at this point.

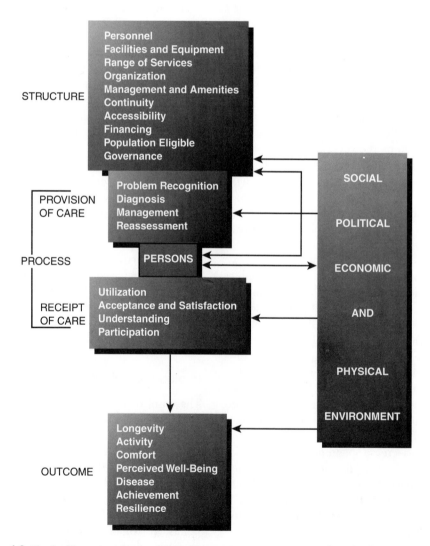

Figure 4-2 The health services system. (From Clawson, D., & Osterweis, M. [1993]. *The roles of physician assistants and nurse practitioners in primary care.* Washington, DC: Association of Academic Health Centers.)

For many years, APNs did not bill independently for their services, and so the true picture of nursing in health care costs is not evident. This is one of the many reasons why APNs need to actively participate in getting reimbursement for their services. APNs have traditionally been "shadow providers" because they have been holistically caring for patients within the shadow of physicians who have prescribing and reimbursement capabilities (Wilcox, 1995). The lack of reimbursement abilities by APNs may be the major constraint to advanced practice in the United States. Clearly, APNs must be paid for services rendered for health care regardless of whether they are working independently, in a group practice, in a rural setting, or within a managed care system.

Rising Health Care Costs

After the introduction of the prospective payment system for Medicare, the states followed the federal government's lead with Medicaid, and the private insurance companies saw an opportunity to save money. Private insurers began to require hospitals and (later) physicians to decrease costs and improve quality through a number of changes. These changes included decreased numbers of laboratory and diagnostic tests, increased numbers of patients seen in an hour, formal referrals for specialists, and monetary incentives for decreasing costs. Opponents of these drastic changes in health care delivery and financing expressed concern that the prospective payment systems would force hospitals (primarily) to focus on money rather than quality of care (Kovner, 1995). Older adults would be forced to go home before they were ready and then return to the hospital or simply die at home. The care in hospitals would be sloppy, uncaring, and bordering on neglect and malpractice. Another concern was that the poor would be denied health care except in the most emergent of circumstances (United States General Accounting Office, 1991). The answer to these fears was the implementation, by the federal government, of the Medicare Utilization and Quality Peer Review Organization (PRO). This group is charged with ensuring quality care and preventing misuse of the prospective payment system. The changes requested by the private insurers included preauthorization or certification for admission to acute care organizations; decreased lengths of stay through changes in hospital systems and practices; improved documentation of patient needs and progress; and early ambulation and emphasis on self-care or family care. At the same time that insurers and major employers were demanding decreased use and proliferation of medical care, physicians and hospitals were beginning to see an increase in litigation for mistakes and perceived malpractice on the part of consumers.

It provides an interesting dilemma for health care organizations, physicians, health care workers, and patients. On one hand, there is a need to decrease costs and increase efficiency; on the other, there is the need to not miss a diagnosis (regardless of its obscurity) or make a mistake in the care of a patient. On the primary care side, consumers have failed to demand data on quality. In some states, however, employers and states have combined to provide consumers with quality data. The National Committee for Quality Assurance (NCQA) was formed by the health maintenance organizations (HMOs) to combat the public perception that the quality of care in HMOs was poor (Buppert, 2000). This organization has emerged as the leader in health care quality.

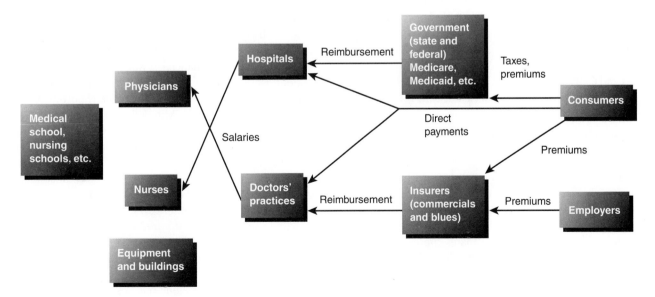

Figure 4-3 Simplified presentation of financial flows in the health care system. (From Deloughery, G.D. [1995]. *Issues and trends in nursing.* St. Louis: Mosby.)

Current Status of the Health Care System

It was clear that a "bandaid" approach to fixing the health care system was not going to work. The Clinton administration proposed a "crosscutting" federal role in the organization and financing of health care, which was rejected by the legislators. Consequently the nation embraced the notion of competition in the marketplace as a way to manage growing problems with quality and cost. However, even if competition does deal effectively with these things, Fletcher (1999) identifies some aspects of health care that he predicts will not be addressed. Areas such as care of disadvantaged and vulnerable people, as well as care of communities themselves, are essential to a sound, compassionate health care system. Teaching and research will likely not be addressed by a competitive market system. Current research reveals that as the managed care penetration increases, it is less likely that physicians will provide charity care or find time for teaching; hospital resources are also becoming less available to sponsor research (Cunningham, Grossman, St Peter, & Lesser, 1999; Fletcher & Fletcher, 1996; Weissman, Saglam, Campbell, Causino, & Blumenthal, 1999). Fletcher (1999) believes that "not only are these areas social responsibilities, they are investments in the health of each of us over the long term."

The most recent changes in the health care delivery system have had an effect on APNs. The decrease in the number of family practice and primary care providers (PCPs) and the changes in the market have provided opportunities. Currently only one third of the physician workforce is in primary care, providing ample opportunities for APNs to practice in the primary care arena (Clawson & Osterweis, 1993). Restrictive scope-of-practice laws for nonphysician PCPs also has played a role in the numbers and location of APN practices. Projections of dramatic increases by 2015 in nonphysician clinicians may have major ramifications for health care delivery. Some groups, such as the National Organization of Nurse Practitioner Faculties (NONPF) (Harper & Johnson, 1996), as well as Jones and Cawley (1994), have presented strategies relative to the role of these clinicians in health care reform.

Primary Care in the Health Care Delivery System

Primary care is that level of service that provides the vast majority (approximately 99%) of care for health problems. Primary care has four unique functions: (1) it is first-contact care, (2) it is longitudinal over time, (3) it is comprehensive, and (4) it coordinates the care a patient receives (Starfield, 1992). It is vital that APNs are active participants in primary care. To enhance primary care, APNs must contribute to one or more of the four elements. There is evidence that APNs perform somewhat better than physicians in recognizing certain kinds of problems experienced by patients, such as those that require

counseling (Office of Technology Assessment, 1986). Some advocates of APNs assert that primary care should be a nursing specialty rather than a physician specialty in light of the declining interest in primary care practice among physicians. Stafford, Seglam, Causino, Starfield, Culpepper, Marder, and Blumenthal (1999) analyzed a sample of adult office visits from 1978 to 1981 and 1989 through 1994. They found that visits to primary care physicians decreased from 52% in 1978 to 41% in 1994, while the average age of the patient increased from 49 to 52 years. More substantial changes were noted in the proportion of visits of patients ages 65 and older and 85 and older. Trends included dramatic growth in the ethnic diversity of patients, doubling of HMOs, increased provision of prevention services, and an 18% increase in the duration of visits. So while the number of visits has decreased, the length of visits has increased, perhaps reflecting the increased complexity of aging patients and the need to balance both acute and preventive care. This is in direct odds with the emphasis on increased productivity that is so common in managed health organizations. The changes noted for physician visits will probably also hold true for APNs. As the complexity of the patients' needs increases, it will be more difficult for APNs to incorporate preventive services, education, and counseling—all typically thought of as benefits of seeing an APN—within a brief office visit.

Health Care Reform and the Health Care Delivery System

Another factor prompting reform is the fragmentation of the health care system at all levels. The system faces opposing incentives of financial reward and provision of quality care. One physician office has to make choices for individual patient treatment from several insurance providers, which offer differing monetary rewards. Capitation, fee-for-service, and per diem payment systems offer the physician different financial rewards and incentives. The patient is often caught in the middle between quality care and insurance payment incentives (Shortell, Gillies, Anderson, Erickson, & Mitchell, 1996). Shortell et al further offer that the health care system will remain fragmented and out of balance until Americans can balance "the traditional values of autonomy, individuality, self-determination and diversity with an increase in solidarity, greater attention to the common good, promotion of other-directedness and the development of community."

The onset of reform required hospitals to rethink their basic mission and become more diverse in their services. They expanded their core enterprise to include outpatient, home care, exercise, nursing home, residential care, and durable medical equipment businesses. The health care organizations had for-profit arms in addition to their traditional not-for-profit arms. Health care became big business. Local organizations merged, national organiza-

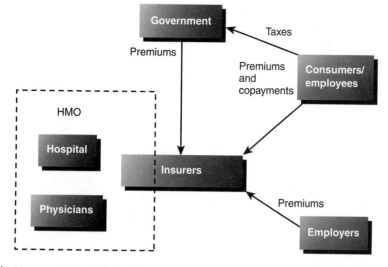

Figure 4-4 Flow presentation of the health maintenance organization. (From Deloughery, G.D. [1995]. *Issues and trends in nursing.* St. Louis: Mosby.)

tions moved into new markets, and new methods for saving money and increasing profit for survival were invented. HMOs were formed to manage the health of patients. (Figure 4-4 shows the economic flow of HMOs.) In the early- to mid-1990s, the downsizing or rightsizing of health care organizations began in earnest. Layers of management and nonessential employees were eliminated. Efforts to consolidate jobs and make care less expensive resulted in many types of health care workers, including unlicensed technicians and multifunctional workers. Over the years, Americans have become less and less content with the present health care system and its continually increasing costs. This discontent has resulted in discussion of a national health care system (Lee & Estes, 1994).

Access to Primary Care for Uninsured and Underinsured Persons

Lee, Soffel, and Luft (1994) believe that in addition to Medicare and Medicaid fraud, the most fundamental factors driving health care reform are rising costs and the uninsured and underinsured. They note that the United States does not "compare well with other industrial democracies in universal coverage, cost containment, and health status." The cost of health care will soon be 16% of the gross national product (GNP), and it continues to rise. It is the fastest-rising cost sector in the United States (Lee et al, 1994). The cost for senior citizens is increased premiums in Medigap insurance, which covers the gap between out of pocket copayments and what Medicare pays for service. Since Medicare does not cover prescription drug costs, prescriptions account for much of the increase in cost for older Americans. Some of the factors cited by Lee et al as contributing to rising costs include "technology, administrative costs, defensive medicine and productivity." Each of these factors is compounded by

several other factors, making the issue of rising costs very complex and seemingly without end. No one group or service is responsible for the rise, but the rapid escalation of cost is proving detrimental to both the industry and consumers.

The issue of cost raises the problem of preexisting conditions. Often, when the employee changes jobs or the employer changes insurance plans, there is a preexisting condition clause. This clause prohibits a number of costly chronic conditions from being covered by the insurance plan until time has elapsed, with varying restrictions. While the employee may not be directly affected, members of the dependent family might be. Conditions often subject to preexisting clauses include diabetes, asthma, hypertension, cancer, multiple sclerosis, cystic fibrosis, cerebral palsy, heart disease, peripheral vascular disease, and mental illness.

As of 1998, 48 million Americans were uninsured, and this number is expected to rise (Gundersen, 1998). An uninsured American may be working, but if the employer is small (less than six employees), the company may not provide health insurance coverage as a benefit, or the premiums may be so cost prohibitive that the employee forgoes coverage. Without insurance, dealing with the health care system is difficult. An important entry point is the PCP. Without insurance, a PCP may not be selected, so use of emergency or urgent services becomes the only option for treatment. Even low-cost clinics require some type of payment, which the uninsured may not have. These clinics are often federally funded and rely on grants and individual donations to remain open.

Although precise numbers are not available, it is thought that several million Americans are underinsured (Gundersen, 1998). The underinsured American is one that is only covered for serious illness or hospitalization. Routine visits to the physician for health maintenance, such as lab screening, radiology, or annual mammograms, are not covered; therefore the patient does not go until a true emergency arises. Children may not receive necessary immunizations and health care screenings because well-child or preventive services are not covered. These trips to the physician often are very costly, so the underinsured do not go. Sometimes the employee portion of the insurance premium is so high, the employee must choose the cheapest "no-frills" plan. This is typically the plan in which preventive, health promotion services are not provided.

Although all of the reasons for increases in sheer numbers of uninsured and underinsured are not clear, a contributing factor is the amount of the premium cost the employer is shifting to the employee to pay. The employee's premium cost may be prohibitive. Recent statistics indicate that cost-shifting of the premium burden to an employee means that if the employee was at the federal poverty level, the premium cost for health insurance would use one quarter of his or her gross income and one third of the income of a family of four (Gundersen, 1998). This would prove quite a burden for even the most frugal of families.

In 1997, President Bill Clinton signed into law a program of federal matching grants for the states to develop the State Children's Health Insurance Program (SCHIP). This is designed to provide health insurance coverage for uninsured children. The eligibility level is 200% of the federal poverty level. The SCHIP program went into effect in March 2000. Even though 2 million children have been covered by this program, the highly positive reception that was originally expected has not been realized (Health Care Financing Administration [HCFA] Press Office, 2000).

In the United States, there seems to be a disproportionate number of poor persons, African-Americans, and Hispanics in the ranks of the uninsured or underinsured (Lee et al, 1994). Gundersen (1998) reports that "1.4 million Hispanic families have difficulty obtaining health care and 70% of those families attributed the problem to cost." Without health insurance, the family or individual probably does not have a relationship or regular contact with a health care provider. The plight of the uninsured and underinsured brings up the issue of access. If a person has little or no insurance, how does he or she access the health care system? That again throws the burden of care back on the family or acute care emergency department. Lack of access is often associated with decreased health status and, of course, with raising the cost of health care (Lee et al, 1994).

The problem of the uninsured and underinsured continues, even though the economy is strong and unemployment is low. The cost of premiums is often not affordable, and many employers simply do not provide benefits. Part-time employment is also a problem because employers do not generally provide health insurance for part-time employees. Therefore many Americans work two or more jobs, with none of them providing health insurance benefits.

Many states have instituted stricter guidelines for eligibility, making some individuals and families no longer eligible for Medicaid. The income eligibility for children to receive Medicaid is higher in some states than for families. Once a family goes off welfare, children are frequently still eligible for Medicaid despite the increased income. Yet parents may be uninformed of their children's eligibility, and so the children become uninsured. Often, uninsured Americans simply wait until illness is intolerable and then arrive for treatment in an urgent care or emergent setting. They are unable to pay for the services but are treated anyway. Efforts are often made to find lower-cost alternative clinics (as opposed to urgent settings), but the uninsured continue to use the emergency department in acute care facilities (Lee et al, 1994).

Health Care Delivery Systems and the Continuum of Care

Nursing models often define *health* as a point on a continuum between perfect health and illness (Catalano, 1996). People can be at any point along the continuum at any time. In the health care delivery system, people usually enter the system as either healthy patients seeking checkups or ill persons seeking treatment for discomfort. Patients are assigned to or select a PCP as the one to perform checkups or to treat discomfort and disease. Referral to specialists may indicate movement along the continuum into a less healthy state and then, with treatment, back to a more healthy state. Patients seek a balance in health.

Current lifestyles and changes in lifestyle cause a patient to move up and down the continuum. The continuum is not linear but rather multidimensional. Patients define a healthful state in relative terms of feeling better or worse depending upon the tension between their physical, mental, spiritual, and emotional states. PCPs and other health care workers help patients achieve the best state of health possible. However, a patient is the one who defines health for himself or herself, despite what a PCP may think.

The continuum of care results in more or less care, as described previously. The health care delivery system forces a patient to assume responsibility at some points along the continuum and forces his or her family to assume responsibility for the patient at other points. As the delivery system has evolved, the cost of caring for patients as a whole is balanced with caring for individuals. The issue becomes: who can afford to pay for health care, and what can they afford (beyond the basics) compared to what can be guaranteed for most Americans? The direction of the health care system currently forces an employer to assume more costs for health care but does not require them to pay for high-end health care. Whatever contract the employer negotiates with the insurance carrier is what the employees get. Under federal law (the Consolidated Omnibus Budget Reconciliation Act [COBRA]), if an employee leaves the work place, he or she can pay for insurance coverage for up to 6 months; however the cost is often prohibitive. Leaving for a new position or being laid off requires the worker to pay to continue the old insurance plan before the new plan is implemented. Failure to pay the premiums results in lack of insurance coverage for a time. While this is agreeable to some, it is simply not an option for others. An employee's decision is often dependent on where the employee and family members are on the health care continuum.

Current Problems in the Health Care Delivery System

A historical perspective provides some insight into the current problems of health care delivery. There are numerous critical issues affecting the evolution of the delivery system. Perhaps the most critical of these is whether Americans have a right to health care, and if they do, at what level? Assuming all rights carry some responsibility, what personal responsibility do people have for their own health? Who should pay for smoking-related illnesses and complications of diabetes due to self-neglect or illegal drug use?

In addition, one needs to consider what can and should be done about the continued rise in health care costs. As premiums rise and employers pick up less of the total cost of benefits, what can be done to alleviate the burden on employees? With the rise in costs, more and more people fall into the categories of the uninsured and underinsured. What can be done to provide access to primary care for these groups? These questions need to be answered, particularly if a type of national health insurance is proposed as an answer to the issue of inadequate insurance coverage.

Current health care reform proposals do place greater emphasis on the delivery of primary services; however the issue of nonphysician providers and fragmented care is not adequately addressed. The Pew Commission recommends interdisciplinary collaboration to help with the problem of fragmented care (Pew Health Professions Commission, 1995). With all the questions that remain unanswered, discussion of the national health care reform is sure to continue.

PRIORITIES FOR RESEARCH

The future of health care delivery and the role of nursing within the system offer opportunities for growth. The nursing profession stands to benefit from continued reform as nursing is sorted out from other fields. The opportuni-

ties for advanced, as well as different, practice will be overwhelming. Research priorities in health care delivery should focus on outcomes. Research areas would include the effect of Medicare and Medicaid on the health of older adults and the poor. Medication costs for older adults are a hot topic. Research relating to the use of formulary drugs, drug foundations, and the amount of support provided for indigent drug programs by pharmaceutical companies, as well as potential solutions to the problems, would assist legislators and care providers in knowing the extent of the issue.

Appropriate use and responsibility in primary care by Medicaid patients is another issue that warrants research. While Medicaid patients are eligible for health benefits based on their income level, it appears that for many patients, there is no incentive for cost-saving. Research evaluating the best way to offer health care to Medicaid patients would be beneficial. Areas such as a small copay, effectiveness of managed care plans for decreasing fragmented care, and the amount and quality of care provided by nonphysician clinicians seem particularly relevant.

Research as to the quality of care provided in all realms of the health care system is vital. Annual increases in health care costs have flattened with the use of a gatekeeper system. Administrative and regulatory burdens became increasingly larger. Most consumers recognize that they will be asked to bear some of the cost increases in managed care, and they seem willing to do so to get what they want (Vinn, 2000). APNs need to be at the forefront in collecting quality data regarding their practice. They need to proactively identify potential problem areas and work to improve quality. Most PCPs believe they give good care to their patients. Buppert (2000) reported that when the California Board of Health asked physicians to estimate the percentage of patients in their practices who were appropriately immunized against communicable diseases, they estimated the number to 90%. Yet, when the actual rate of immunizations were assessed, only 52% of children had been immunized. APNs can not fall into this same level of complacency. To be admitted to care provider panels, APNs must share their successes related to quality outcomes.

IMPLICATIONS FOR MSN EDUCATION AND ADVANCED PRACTICE

Since nursing is primarily a middle-aged, white female profession, the key is for nursing to embrace reform and change; diversify the profession by race, gender and practice specialty; and continuously improve the opportunities for success of its members. Nursing administration education will be important to the health care delivery organizations for providing leadership when change is a constant. Continued curriculum development should occur at this level.

Nurse practitioners (NPs) will continue to be an important provider in the health care system. Their education should focus on health care reform, with a major emphasis on the need for their voices in shaping health policy. Content related to reimbursement and disease management will be vital components of the curriculum. Educating the public will become an even more important part of the APN role.

Practice management will assume an even greater significance in the future. PCPs must satisfy the needs of patients for information, access, and convenience because consumers will become a driving force in the market. An emerging new model of delivery is the employer-provider coalition. Features include contracting between providers and employers, open access, and no fee restrictions. These coalitions measure patient perceptions about outcomes, cost, and customer service, in addition to collecting data on the percentage of patients who received the screening for which they are eligible. The public likes this type of data; providers who have high scores in the listed areas attract more enrollees than groups that scored low (Larkin, 1999). APNs need to emphasize quality monitoring and develop ways of measuring performance. It will be important to maintain a focus on patients despite the distractions of the health care payment system.

All PCPs must focus on controlling costs while increasing quality. The emergence of the consumer as an active partner in his or her care will become commonplace. Electronic medical records will become the standard, and patients will even be able to access their providers via the Internet to schedule appointments and view lab results.

It will also be important for APNs to be courageous, maintaining an open-minded attitude and a willingness to try new ideas. Coping with constant change requires a willingness to let go of a relatively stable environment and embrace a new ambiguous environment. According to Trofino (1997), keys to organizational success will include accepting change, encouraging good performance, and fostering a sense of team learning and commitment. As one can see, these changes in health care delivery all provide new options for APNs.

DISCUSSION QUESTIONS

These questions can be used to promote critical thinking and encourage discussion.

1. Discuss how health care reform has affected various professions: medicine, dentistry, rehabilitation, nursing

---

Suggestions for Further Learning

- For additional information related to personal satisfaction and service to the under-served read the material at archfami.ama-assn.org/issues/v9n3/full/foc8074.html. What are the implications for APNs?
- Read the article: Doescher, M.P., Franks, P., Banthin, J.S., & Clancy, C.M. Supplemental insurance and mortality in elderly Americans: findings from a national cohort. *Archives in Family Medicine.* Available online at archfami.ama-assn.org/issues/v9n3/full/foc9054.html. What are the implications for APNs who care for older adults?
- Read any of the following articles regarding nonphysician clinicians: Cooper, R.A., Laud, P., & Dietrich, C. (1998). Current and projected workforce of non-physician clinicians. *Journal of the American Medical Association, 280,* 788-794; Cooper, R., Henderson, T., & Dietrich, C. (1998). Roles of non-physician clinicians as autonomous providers of patient care. *Journal of the American Medical Association, 280,* 795-802; Flanagan, L. (1998). Nurse practitioners: growing competition for family physicians? *Family Practice Management, 5*(9). Available online at www.aafp.org/fpm/980100fm/nurse.html; Grumbach, K., & Coffman, J. (1998). Physicians and non-physician

clinicians: complements or competitors? *Journal of the American Medical Association, 280,* 825-826; and Family physicians and nurse practitioners: a perfect team. *Family Practice Management, 5*(6). Available online at www.aafp.org/fpm/980600fm/spectrum.html. What are the implications for the health care delivery system if the projected workforce of nonphysician clinicians proves to be accurate? How would you address the issue of curtailing the production of health care professionals (both nonphysician clinicians and physicians) given that past calls for a reduction in the output of graduates have gone unheeded?
- How do the articles in the previous point compare to this report by the NONPF: Haper, D., & Johnson, J. (1996). *NONPF workforce policy project technical report: nurse practitioner educational programs 1988-1995.* Washington, DC: National Organization of Nurse Practitioner Faculty.
- Evaluate the website at www.consumerchoice.com. Look at survey data pertinent to a health care plan. What implications do the data hold for the health care delivery systems and APNs?

homes, and so on. Brainstorm on the impact of reform within the next 20 years.

2. Discuss the effect of new medical technology on health care reform, treatment, and cost of health care.

3. Discuss the issue of personal responsibility related to health care. Who should pay for the health care needs of individuals who choose unhealthy lifestyle behaviors or individuals who ignore complication prevention strategies for chronic conditions such as diabetes, heart disease, and obesity?

4. Respond to the following phrase: Value is defined as outcome divided by cost. What implication does this have for both the patient and the APN?

5. Describe how APNs contribute to the four components of primary care.

REFERENCES/BIBLIOGRAPHY

Barer, M., Evans, R., Holt, M., & Morrison, J. (1994). It ain't necessarily so: the cost implications of health reform. *Health Affairs, Fall,* 88-99.

Berwick, D. (1994). Eleven worthy aims for clinical leadership of health system reform. *Journal of the American Medical Association, 272,* 797-802.

Blumenthal, D. (1996). Effects of market reforms on doctors and their patients. *Health Affairs (Millwood), 15,* 170-184.

Blumenthal, D., & Rizzo, J. (1991). Who cares for uninsured persons? *Medical Care, 29,* 502-520.

Bodenheimer, T. (1999). The American health care system: the movement for improved quality in health care. *New England Journal of Medicine, 340,* 488-492.

Brook, R., Kambers, C., & McGlynn, E. (1996). Health system reform and quality. *Journal of the American Medical Association, 276,* 476-480.

Buppert, C. (2000). *The primary care provider's guide to compensation and quality.* Gaithersburg, MD: Aspen Publishers.

Catalano, J.T. (1996). *Contemporary professional nursing.* Philadelphia: FA Davis.

Clawson, D., & Osterweis, M. (1993). *The roles of physician assistants and nurse practitioners in primary care.* Washington, DC: Association of Academic Health Centers.

Cunningham, P., Grossman, J., St. Peter, R., & Lesser, C. (1999). Managed care and physician's provision of charity care. *Journal of the American Medical Association, 281,* 1087-1092.

Doheny, M.O., Cook, C.B., & Stopper, M.C. (1997). *The discipline of nursing* (4th ed.). Stamford, CT: Appleton & Lange.

Fletcher, R. (1999). Editorial: who is responsible for the common good in a competitive market? *Journal of the American Medical Association, 281.*

Fletcher, R., & Fletcher, S. (1996). Managed care and medical education. *Lancet, 348,* 1003-1004.

Franks, P., Nutting, P., & Clancy, C. (1993). Health care reform, primary care and the need for research. *Journal of the American Medical Association, 270,* 1449-1453.

Gundersen, L. (1998, September 15). Number of uninsured continues to rise. *Annals of Internal Medicine.* Available online at www.acponline.org/journals/annals/15sep98/currunin.htm.

Harper, D., & Johnson, J. (1996). *NONPF Workforce policy project technical report: nurse practitioner educational programs 1988-1995.* Washington, D.C: National Organization of Nurse Practitioner Faculty.

Harrington, C., & Estes, C. (1997). *Health policy and nursing* (2nd ed.). Boston: Jones and Bartlett Publishers.

Hastings, K. (1994). Health care reform: we need it but do we have the national will to shape our future? *Nurse Practitioner, 20*(1), 52.

Health Care Financing Administration Press Office (2000). *State children's health insurance program now reaching two million.* Available online at www.hcfa.gov/init/20000111.html.

Herzlinger, R. (1997). *Market driven healthcare.* New York: Perseus Books.

Jacobs, P. (1995). Economics of health care. In G. Deloughery (Ed.), *Issues and trends in nursing* (2nd ed.). St. Louis: Mosby.

Jones, P., & Cauley, J. (1994). Physician's assistants and health system reform. *Journal of the American Medical Association, 271,* 1266-1272.

Kalisch, P., & Kalisch, B. (1995). *The advance of American nursing* (3rd ed). Philadelphia: JB Lippincott.

Kassirer, J. (1999). Hospitals, heal yourselves. *New England Journal of Medicine, 340,* 309-310.

Kovner, A. (1995). *Health care delivery in the United States* (5th ed). New York: Springer.

Kuttner, R. (1999). The American health care system—employer-sponsored health coverage. *New England Journal of Medicine, 340*(3). Available online at www.nejm.org/content/1999/0340/0003/0248.asp.

Larkin, H. (1999). Doctors starting to feel report cards' impact. *American Medical News, 42*(28), 1.

Lasker, R., & Lee, P. (1994). Improving health through health system reform. *Journal of the American Medical Association, 272,* 1297-1298.

Lee, P., & Estes, C.L. (1994). *The nation's health* (4th ed.). Boston: Jones and Bartlett.

Lee, P., Soffel, D., & Luft, H. (1994). Initiative for reform. In P. Lee & C. Estes, *The nation's health* (4th ed.). Boston: Jones and Bartlett.

Lee, P.R. (1995). Health system reform and the generalist physician. *Academic Medicine, 70*(suppl), S10-13.

Newacheck, P., Stoddard, J., Hughes, D., & Pearl, M. (1998). Health insurance and access to primary care. *New England Journal of Medicine, 338,* 513-519.

Office of Technology Assessment (1986). *Nurse practitioners, physician assistants and certified nurse midwives: a policy analysis* (Case study no. 37). Washington, DC: US Government Printing Office.

Pew Health Professions Commission (1995). *Critical challenges: revitalizing the health profession for the twenty-first century.* San Francisco: Pew Health Professions Commission.

Roemer, M.I. (1986). *An introduction to the US health care system* (2nd ed.). New York: Springer.

Shortell, S.M., Gillies, R.R., Anderson, D.A., Erickson, K.M., & Mitchell, J.B. (1996). *Remaking health care in America: building organized delivery systems.* San Francisco: Jossey-Bass, Inc.

Snyder-Halpern, R. (1995). Health care system innovation: a model for practice. *Advanced Practice Nursing Quarterly, 1*(4), 12-19.

Stafford, R., Saglam, D., Causino, N., Starfield, B., Culpepper, L., Marder, W., & Bllumenthal, D. (1999). Trends in adult visits to primary care physicians in the United States. *Archives in Family Medicine, 8,* 26-32.

Starfield, B. (1992). *Primary care: concept evaluation and policy.* New York: Oxford University Press.

Taylor, D. (1998). Crystal ball gazing: back to the future. *Advanced Practice Nursing Quarterly, 3*(4), 44-51.

Trofino, J. (1997). The courage to change: reshaping health care delivery. *Nursing Management, 28*(11), 50-54.

United States Department of Health and Human Services (1996). *Health United States 1995* (DHHS publication [PHS] 96-1232). Hyattsville, MD: National Center for Health Statistics, Centers for Disease Control and Prevention, US Department of Health and Human Services.

United States General Accounting Office (1991). *Health insurance coverage: a profile of the uninsured in selected states.* Washington, DC: US General Accounting Office.

Vinn, N. (2000). The emergence of consumer-driven health care. *Family Practice Management, 7*(1), 96.

Weissman, J., Saglam, D., Campbell, E., Causino, N., & Blumenthal, D. (1999). Market forces and unsponsored research in academic health centers. *Journal of the American Medical Association, 281,* 1093-1098.

Werning, S., & Lederman, P. (1995). Advanced practice nursing: new challenges in a changing healthcare system. *Advanced Practice Nursing Quarterly, 6*(5), 10-16.

Wilcox, P. (1995). *Advanced practice model response to needs of women at risk for female malignancies* (Abstract presentation). Anaheim, CA: Oncology Nurses Society National Conference.

Chapter 5

Institutions Providing Health Care Delivery

Margaret M. Anderson & Denise Robinson

Health care is delivered to the consumer by a variety of organizations. This chapter presents an overview of the health services systems in the United States as a framework to help understand the intricacies of the health care delivery method. *Health care delivery* refers to the system, its components, and the process that enables people to receive health care.

CRITICAL ISSUES: UNDERSTANDING THE HEALTH CARE DELIVERY SYSTEM

Health care delivery is more than just the act of providing health services to patients. Most developed countries have some form of national health insurance program that is financed by taxes and administered by the government (Shi & Singh, 1998). However, the United States does not have insurance coverage for all Americans. In fact, Wolinsky (1988) argues that the United States does not have a true health care delivery system at all; a single unified system that regulates health services does not exist. Such a system would be expected to function in an integrated and organized manner. Unfortunately, the United States health care system is made up of a variety of delivery, insurance, payment, and financing mechanisms, so that the system is composed of several fragmented service components. There are some government programs that offer services for select population groups meeting specific criteria. However, the bulk of the services available in the United States are provided by private organizations. In the current health care marketplace, multiple organizations are encouraged to participate. Cost containment, quality assurance, and resource planning are all mandatory elements. As the complexity of the health care system increases (with the integration of public and private involvement), duplication, overlap, and waste become prevalent, driving the cost of health care even higher. With the lack of central planning and an office to oversee

health care, it is probably impossible for any one organization to impose order and control. (Box 5-1 identifies the strengths and the weaknesses of the current health care system in the United States.)

Health Care Delivery Systems in Other Countries

The United States' health care delivery system is unlike those in other developed countries. In the U.S. system, no national health insurance plan exists, no overseeing agency governs the system, no single organization provides payment for services rendered, practice behavior is influenced by the fear of litigation, and access to health care is selectively based on insurance coverage (Shi & Singh, 1998). (Table 5-1 provides a visual comparison between the United States and the health care delivery systems in other developed countries.)

The health care system in the United States can be frustratingly complex. Many organizations and individuals are involved in the delivery of health care, with numerous types of care provided. The health care components range from educational institutions to suppliers, insurers, and providers. Many organizations have merged or forged alliances to contend with soaring costs. As these organizations merge, they are able to offer a multitude of services within an integrated network. Integrated delivery organizations such as regional health alliances are beginning to dominate the market in some areas of the country.

The United States' health care system is huge. It is the largest and most powerful employer in the country, employing about 700,000 doctors of medicine (MDs), about 33,500 doctors of osteopathy (DOs), and about 1.9 million nurses, 140,000 of which are advanced practice nurses (APNs) (Shi & Singh, 1998). (Table 5-2 provides a closer look at APNs.)

Approximately 3% of the total labor force works in the health care service industry. The majority of health professionals are employed in hospitals (40.9%) (US Bureau of the Census, Bureau of Labor Statistics, 1996).

Box 5-1

Characteristics of the U.S. Health Care System

STRENGTHS

Uses the latest technology.
Excellent medical and nursing educational programs.
Focused on research.
Sophisticated institutions, products, and processes.
Focused on treatment of illness.
No central agency to govern.
Free market; one single player does not dominate the system.
Legal risks influence practice behavior.
Certification standards set minimum quality.

WEAKNESSES

Fragmented, with no central agency to govern.
Complex.
Mammoth.
Access based on insurance coverage.
Expensive.
Not cost-effective.
Lack of focus on health promotion and maintenance.
Private financing, primarily through employers.
Legal risks influence practice behavior.
Health plans are "real" buyers in the market.
High administrative costs for billing, collections, and debts.

Table 5-1

Health Care Systems of Selected Industrialized Countries

	UNITED STATES	CANADA	GREAT BRITAIN	GERMANY
Type	Pluralistic	National Health Insurance	National Health service	Socialized insurance
Owner	Private	Private	Public	Private
Finance	Voluntary, multipayer system (premium or general taxes)	Single payer (general taxes)	Single payer (general taxes)	Single payer (payroll and general taxes)
Reimbursement (Hospital)	Varies (DRG, negotiated fee for service, per diem, capitation)	Global budgets	Global budgets	Per diem payment
Reimbursement (MDs)	Resource-based relative value scale (RBRVS), fee for service	Negotiated fee for service	Salaries and capitation payments	Negotiated fee for service
Consumer Payment	Positive, small to significant	Negligible	Negligible	Negligible

From Shi, L., & Singh, D. (1998). *Delivering health care in America: a systems approach.* Gaithersburg: MD: Aspen Publishers.

Currently there is an imbalance between primary and specialty care. In addition, geographically, there are areas of the country that do not offer the same level of health care delivery due to a shortage of health care providers. Institutions include more than 6500 hospitals, 16,000 nursing homes, 5000 facilities for mental health, and 19,000 home health agencies and hospices. This does not even include the many primary care programs, such as migrant health centers, community health centers, human immunodeficiency virus (HIV) programs, and substance abuse programs, all of which create employment opportunities for APNs.

It is essential for APNs to understand the health care delivery system. Changes within the system require adap-

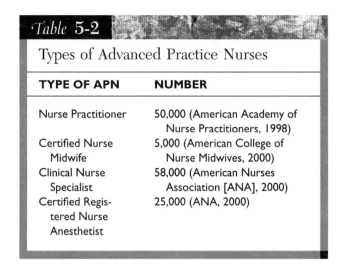

Table 5-2

Types of Advanced Practice Nurses

TYPE OF APN	NUMBER
Nurse Practitioner	50,000 (American Academy of Nurse Practitioners, 1998)
Certified Nurse Midwife	5,000 (American College of Nurse Midwives, 2000)
Clinical Nurse Specialist	58,000 (American Nurses Association [ANA], 2000)
Certified Registered Nurse Anesthetist	25,000 (ANA, 2000)

tation. Although the system is complex, an understanding will help APNs anticipate change and plan for its potential effects. This understanding is especially important if critical decisions related to strategic planning and the mission of the organization must be made. For those APNs who provide care to patients, the information is just as important. Knowing the ins and outs of insurance payment criteria, billing, and the income and expenses of the practice can make a difference in terms of employment.

Inpatient Institutions and Hospitals

Inpatient institutions are divided into public and private institutions. They can be further subdivided into categories by length of stay (i.e., short vs. long term) and type of service provided (e.g., psychiatric, rehabilitation, children's hospital). Sometimes hospitals can be classified by their degree of access or location (e.g., urban or rural). In general, hospitals are defined by the American Hospital Association (AHA) as institutions of at least six beds whose primary functions are to "deliver patient services, diagnostic and therapeutic, for particular or general medical conditions" (1994). They must be licensed, have an organized physician staff, and offer 24-hour nursing services under the supervision of registered nurses. General hospitals are those that offer a variety of services, including services necessary to meet the needs of the community, such as surgery or obstetrics. Most of the hospitals in the United States are general hospitals.

The primary purpose of hospitals changed dramatically from 1840 to 1900, during which they were transformed from places that provided custodial care to places that provided skilled medical and nursing care. Most hospitals in the United States were developed by voluntary organizations (led by influential physicians and philanthropists) rather than by religious orders, as was the case in Europe. Most hospitals in Europe that were church associated became tax-supported government institutions. In the United States, most voluntary hospitals were owned by

private organizations when the wealthy were not able to continue financial support. By the middle of the nineteenth century, hospitals had become centers for new medical knowledge. Training of new physicians became a major factor in the establishment of voluntary hospitals (Shi & Singh, 1998). The Hill Burton Act of 1946 provided grants for the construction of new hospital beds after World War II. This program assisted in the building of nearly 40% of the beds in acute care hospitals during the 1950s and 1960s (Haglund & Dowling, 1993). Even small communities were able to have their own hospitals. The creation of Medicare and Medicaid also had an indirect effect on increasing the number of hospital beds. The number of community hospitals increased from 741,000 beds to 988,000 beds from 1965 to 1980 (AHA ,1996). However, things changed during the mid-1980s, and the number of beds declined. Three forces have influenced the decline: reimbursement, the growth of managed care, and economic constraints faced by small hospitals, especially those in rural areas. In addition, many services were switched from an inpatient to an outpatient basis, further decreasing the need for hospital beds. The average daily census declined from 73.8% of capacity in 1983 to 62.8% in 1995 (AHA, 1996). (Figure 5-1 shows the growth and decline in the number of beds of acute care hospitals, while Figure 5-2 shows the proportion of United States hospitals by size.) There are a variety of types of hospitals in the United States, both public and private. The majority (85%) are voluntary, nonprofit, short-term, general hospitals. Hospitals owned by state and local governments are the next most common, followed by for-profit agencies and then federal hospitals. (This distribution is shown in Figure 5-3.)

Voluntary hospitals

Most health care in the United States is delivered through the private sector. These organizations are divided into not-for-profit (voluntary) and proprietary or for-profit organizations. The not-for-profit hospitals must have a single mission (generally to serve the community where they are located) and are expected to demonstrate fiscal responsibility. Funding for these agencies comes from revenue from third-party payers, commercial insurers, Medicare and Medicaid, endowments, donations, and private payers. If a for-profit arm exists, revenue can come from that area also. Profits are turned back into the organization for improvements. Voluntary hospitals are exempt from taxes and must demonstrate their ability to meet their mission. Church-affiliated hospitals were established during the latter half of the nineteenth and twentieth centuries. A number of different Catholic sisterhoods established the first church-sponsored hospitals in the United States. These organizations are different from the rest of the types of voluntary hospitals only by the influence of the church groups that sponsor them. (Box 5-2 shows some characteristics of the voluntary, nonprofit institutions.)

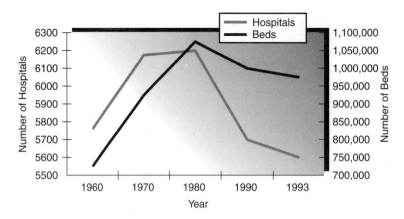

Figure 5-1 The growth and decline of short-stay hospitals. (Data from the National Center for Health Statistics [1995]. *Health, United States*. American Hospital Association.)

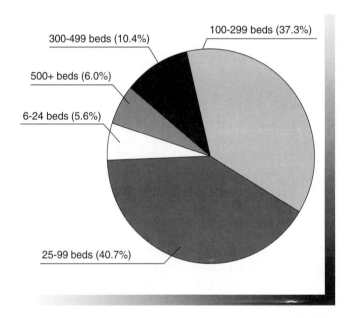

Figure 5-2 Proportion of U.S. hospitals by size: 1995. (Data from American Hospital Association [1996]. *Hospital statistics* [1996-1997 ed.]. Chicago: American Hospital Association.)

Public hospitals

Public hospitals are owned by agencies of federal, state, or local governments. These hospitals developed from almshouses and pesthouses. Federal hospitals are limited to special groups of federal beneficiaries, such as Native Americans, military personnel, or veterans. Of these federal agencies, the Veterans Affairs hospitals make up the largest percentage. State governments usually are the owners of mental or tuberculosis hospitals, since the role of such hospitals was to protect the general public by isolating these patients. As fewer mental and tuberculosis patients were institutionalized, the numbers of these state hospitals shrank dramatically. Local governments tend to operate large general hospitals that generally serve urban, indigent, and minority patients, with most of these hospitals in large urban areas (Kassirer, 1995). These hospitals are supported

by tax levies and in many situations are associated with medical schools and residency training. (A *teaching hospital* is defined by the presence of a training program for physicians only).

Proprietary health care systems

Proprietary hospitals are owned by individuals, partnerships, or corporations (Shi & Singh, 1998). This means that the companies are accountable to their stockholders. For-profit or proprietary organizations are health care agencies who do not have to put profits back into operating revenues but rather can use stock options and financial incentives to encourage cost-cutting. For-profit agencies have revenue from commercial insurers, Medicare and Medicaid, third-party payers, and all other departments that produce revenue (e.g., pharmacy, physical therapy,

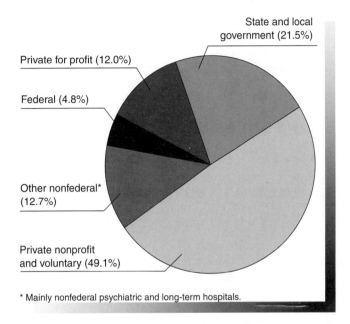

Figure 5-3 Proportion of U.S. hospitals by type of hospital: 1995. (Data from American Hospital Association [1996]. *Hospital statistics* [1996-1997 ed.]. Chicago: American Hospital Association.)

Box 5-2

Characteristics of Voluntary, Nonprofit Hospitals

- Must have open access to and unrestricted use of the emergency department.
- Must provide emergent care regardless of payer status.
- In recent years, may have developed for-profit arms for the purpose of offering financial incentives to management for increased productivity and cost containment, including durable medical equipment stores, adult day cares, child day cares, home care, and pharmacy services for other organizations.
- Make up the largest portion of hospitals in the United States (Catalano, 1996).

Box 5-3

Characteristics of Proprietary Hospitals

- Must pay taxes at the local, state, and national levels.
- Operate as a business and have many tax cuts, benefits, and write-offs.
- Have no requirements for humanitarian purposes but often feel pressured by communities to give something back, which they generally do.
- Include hospitals, nursing homes, and clinics as well as home care agencies and outpatient services.
- Must render emergency services and stabilize patients before transfer to another health care agency, regardless of a patient's ability to pay.

---

occupational therapy, laboratories). They may also have stocks, endowments, or donations. These companies are often publicly traded. (Box 5-3 shows some characteristics of proprietary agencies.)

It is sometimes difficult to tell not-for-profit agencies from proprietary agencies. The integration of services and mergers of organizations have made the governance structure of agencies difficult to navigate. All organizations must make a profit in order to survive; this is true for nonprofit organizations too. However, the major difference between voluntary hospitals and proprietary hospitals is tax status. Nonprofit hospitals are formed for the good of the public and cannot distribute any of the profits to any shareholder or individual whereas the goal for the profit

hospitals is to make a profit or return for its shareholders. Both types of organizations have as their goal to deliver the highest quality of care at the most reasonable cost (Shi & Singh, 1998).

Changes in Health Care Institutions

Since the change in Medicare payment from retrospective to prospective, health care delivery organizations have begun offering a variety of services in different settings. Often these settings are defined by function. Acute care hospitals have established subacute units to provide care to patients too sick for home or long-term care (LTC) but not sick enough for the acute care setting. Hospice units and freestanding sites have been established for end-of-life palliative care. Rehabilitation units and hospitals have opened for the care of patients requiring extensive rehabilitation following postorthopedic surgery, stroke, or other traumatic injuries. The purpose of these units or agencies is to return a patient to as functional a status as possible in the shortest time possible. When these "new concept" arenas were first established, it was a financial boon to the acute care hospital. They often were not subject to diagnostic-related groups (DRGs), and they offered an alternative to nursing homes and home care by families already overwhelmed by financial woes, emotional shock, and worry. Eventually these health care settings would also be subject to cost containment, decreased length of stay, and other managed care requirements. The success of some subacute units, hospice units, and rehabilitation facilities rests in part with the shift in attitude about health for consumers. Consumers are beginning to see that wellness is preferable to illness and are willing to support agencies providing wellness care or care that promotes a patient's resources to the best of that patient's ability. A lot of the day-to-day care of ill persons has been transferred to the home care setting (Shi & Singh, 1998).

Another recent change that has occurred is the multihospital affiliation. Many institutions have merged to help with saving costs. This way, duplication of services and personnel can be avoided, while these systems also gain the ability to provide a wide spectrum of care and increased access to capital markets (Snook, 1995). Religious orders are frequent owners of these multiunit affiliations. For example, the Daughters of Charity National Health System in St. Louis owns 41 hospitals. Overall, the largest multiunit organization is the proprietary organization Columbia/Health Care of America (HCA) chain, which owns 304 hospitals. This merging process has affected many of the personnel who work in these organizations. Layoffs and elimination of jobs has occurred in many of these organizations when mergers are finalized. APNs have been affected as specialty programs have been combined and jobs have been eliminated. These affiliations have made APNs realize that even positions in primary care are vulnerable during the merging process.

Rural Health Agencies

Rural health care agencies face unique difficulties. Catalano (1996) believes that rural health care presents a challenge because of health care provider shortages, lack of access to the latest technology, and expenses that outpace revenues. Shortell, Gillies, Anderson, Erickson, and Mitchell (1996) point out that no one solution is effective for all rural areas. Some are more remote than others, some are contiguous to large metropolitan centers, and some are so remote and sparsely populated that health care services simply can not be provided to meet individual health care needs. Both Shortell et al (1996) and Catalano

(1996) believe that the only solutions for rural areas are to continue their current pattern and seek government aid, join with a suburban-urban center for the services needed, or form some type of rural cooperative to provide necessary services. The access issues for rural areas are steadily increasing as the rest of America enjoys advanced health technology and treatments. In addition, there are disproportionate numbers of older adults and poor persons in rural areas, so rural community hospitals frequently find themselves in financial difficulties. Approximately 43% of rural hospital revenue is accounted for by Medicare, an increase of more than 5% in 5 years (Cys, 1999). If a rural hospital in financial trouble is part of a large multihospital system, it is likely to be converted to a primary care clinic or other facility. If the rural hospital is owned by investors, it is more likely to be closed (Alexander, 1996).

Recruitment and retention of care providers in rural areas has been difficult. In rural counties with fewer than 50,000 inhabitants, the ratio of generalist physician to population has been decreasing since 1990 (Shi & Singh, 1998). Most rural hospitals use both nurse practitioners (NPs) and physician assistants (PAs) to provide outpatient care. The Rural Health Clinic Program, which requires employment of a midlevel provider to be a certified rural health clinic, is a major factor in the employment of NPs and PAs by rural hospitals (Krein, 1997). While NPs can prescribe medications and other therapeutic tests, considerably fewer NPs have admitting or discharge privileges. PAs seem to provide a more expanded scope of services in rural hospitals. Both types of primary care providers (PCPs) are hired because physicians are unavailable or too difficult to recruit and because nonphysician providers are considered cost effective or more economical for rural areas.

Outpatient Services

Outpatient care does not require an overnight stay in an institution, and it has typically been considered ambulatory care. *Ambulatory care* is care given to a person who can ambulate into the office. The terms *outpatient care* or *outpatient service* are theoretically more correct, since they refer to "any health care services that are not provided on the basis of an overnight stay in which room and board costs are incurred" (Shi & Singh, 1998). Historically, outpatient care has been separate from inpatient care. In recent years, hospitals have gradually become the dominant players in both the outpatient arena and the inpatient arena. Hospitals were able to capitalize on their technology for lab services and other diagnostic testing. State and local governments have sponsored outpatient services but on a limited scope and separate from the private system.

Primary care has served as the cornerstone for ambulatory care (see Chapter 4 for a discussion of the components of primary care). (Figure 5-4 shows a comparison of the number of ambulatory visits in 1992 and 1995.) Most basic outpatient care (80%) still takes place in a provider's office (Shi & Singh, 1998). However, that office

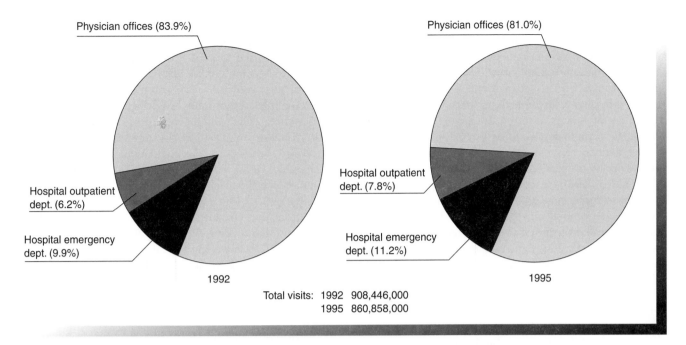

Figure 5-4 Ambulatory care visits. (Data from National Center for Health Statistics [1996]. *Health, United States 1995*. US Department of Health and Human Services; and National Center for Health Statistics [1997]. *Health, United States 1996-1997*. US Department of Health and Human Services.)

is more than likely going to be part of a larger group practice or a subsidiary of a hospital alliance. Outpatient services are a key component in the profits for hospitals, and many see this as the future of health care in the United States. Approximately 37% of a hospital's total gross revenue is constituted by outpatient revenues (HCIA, Deloitte, & Touche, 1997). Services such as home health care, urgent care clinics, dental care, optometry, women's health centers, and alternative care are included in the clinical services of outpatient care.

The goal of primary care is to optimize health. Unfortunately, many people in the United States do not have access to primary health care due to being uninsured or underinsured. (Chapter 4 discusses this issue in depth.) Secondary and tertiary services can also be provided in an outpatient setting (or inpatient setting), but they typically include more specialized services than those provided in primary care. General physicians provide primary care in Europe. In the United States, primary care providers include general and family medicine, along with internal medicine, pediatrics, obstetrics, and gynecology. In addition, APNs and PAs provide primary care for patients.

Public Health Care Delivery

The public health care system is established by law and consists of agencies supported by the government through taxes collected from the citizenry. These agencies are broad in scope and function to "administer and coordinate programs, conduct research, analyze statistics and set

> ### Box 5-4
>
> ## Characteristics of Public Health Service
>
> - Made up of local, county, and state health departments and the U.S. Public Health Service (USPHS), which houses the Centers for Disease Control and Prevention (CDC)
> - At each level, shares responsibility for part of the data collection for the agency at the next higher level.
> - Active in disease prevention and reporting, tracking trends, and developing national policy for dealing with health care issues at the local, state, and national levels.
> - Includes county-, city-, and/or state-supported acute, chronic or LTC facilities that focus on health promotion and disease prevention.
> - Supported by taxes and may use some form of third-party payment, fee-for-service, donations, or endowments as financial support (Catalano, 1996).

standards and qualifications" (Doheny, Cook, & Stopper, 1997). However, public health services have no consistent pattern for services offered, so the scope of service may vary drastically from one part of the country to another. In most cases, public health programs are limited to the following services: well-baby care, sexually transmitted disease clinics, family planning, tuberculosis screening, and ambulatory mental care services. (Box 5-4 shows the characteristics of the public health service.)

Public and Voluntary Clinics

Some other settings for health care delivery include nurse-run clinics, community centers, school-based clinics, adult day care centers, and outpatient centers. These areas have a clearly defined set of services to offer. When a patient presents with something outside their service block, he or she is referred to another setting. The advantage of these service areas is that the service block is well defined and can be provided as efficiently and inexpensively as possible. These public and voluntary clinics also offer services at the site where it is most needed (i.e., where the patient base is located). Immunizations and flu shots are offered at school clinics. Help with food stamps or welfare forms is offered at the school with the neediest patients. Flu shots, occupational therapy, and exercise may be offered at adult day care centers where adults at risk are located. (Catalano, 1996).

The Neighborhood Health Center (NHC) Program originated in the 1960s under the Economic Opportunity Act. They were set up to provide comprehensive ambulatory care to the indigent living in underserved areas, primarily inner-city and rural locations. These clinics were among the first to participate in the training and employment of NPs and PAs (Mezey & Lawrence, 1995). The NHC program was renamed the Community Health Center (CHC) Program and is operated under the auspices of the Bureau of Primary Health Care, U.S. Public Health Service. CHCs serve as the "safety net" for the poor and underserved in inner-city and rural areas. Migrant health centers are also included in the CHC designation. The majority of patients seen by CHCs are Medicaid recipients. As of 1996, there were 685 CHCs nationwide, serving approximately 8 million people (30% of the indigent population) (St. Martin, 1996). Funds come from the federal government via Title III of the Public Health Service Act and constitute approximately 25% to 28% of CHC budgets. The remaining funds come from Medicaid, Medicare, private insurance, and charges paid by patients. All CHCs must offer sliding-scale fees based on a patient's income.

Long-Term Care

LTC includes care provided in nursing homes, but it also includes noninstitutional services such as care provided by family members, foster care, and board and care facilities. (Figure 5-5 shows the ideal characteristics of a well-designed LTC system.) While the thought of LTC brings older adults to mind, it is not confined to them. LTC is care provided to a chronically impaired person over an extended period of time (Shi & Singh, 1998). The same categories of institutional and community-based services apply to LTC and hospitals. A wide variety of services is needed because no two individuals are exactly alike. Frequently the care overlaps with other services, such as primary care or acute care. As a person becomes

functionally impaired and can not maintain activities of daily living, the need for LTC increases; this may range from monitoring to a long-term stay in a nursing home. APNs are becoming more involved in LTC, especially the care of older adults. As reimbursement for APNs becomes more defined, the number of APNs working in this arena will increase. The need for more providers for older adults will continue to grow as the number of older adults increases to 20% of the population by the year 2030 (Satariano, 1997). The "old-old" portion of the older adult population is the most rapidly growing segment of the U.S. population.

Throughout the history of health care, services have gradually shifted from the inpatient setting to the outpatient setting. As economic, social, and technological forces continue to affect care, more change is forthcoming. APNs must be aware of the large variety of services available to positively affect patient health.

Continued Challenges Facing the Health Care Delivery System

The health care delivery system continues to evolve and change. Hospitals need to continue to respond to the need for cost containment. The structure of the health care delivery system may change even more drastically as care continues to move from an inpatient to an outpatient focus. Hospitals may strive to offer one-stop shopping for all types of services, blurring the status of not-for-profit and proprietary health care institutions. The nonprofit designation will probably continue to be challenged as nonprofit agencies engage in the same aggressive marketplace behaviors once reserved for the proprietary chains. Wolfson and Hopes (1994) found that for-profit hospitals offer the same level of charity as nonprofit institutions. Not all nonprofit agencies offer charity care. Large hospitals are more likely to provide uncompensated care than smaller agencies. Some states are already demanding that nonprofit hospitals contribute to the community to retain their state and local tax exemptions (Morrisey, 1996)

It is expected that the merging of health care delivery systems into large conglomerates will continue. Communities and care providers need to be closely involved in determining the effect on health care for the community in these situations. This is particularly true for underserved populations; they may be easily ignored when changes are proposed but may also be the most adversely affected groups.

The special needs of rural health agencies and areas experiencing health care provider shortage must be addressed in a more systematic manner. One of the reasons why the APN program was developed was to improve access for medically underserved populations and expand the availability of primary care. Data regarding the employment of NPs reveals that the majority (91%) work in metropolitan counties. NPs prepared in certificate

Health Care Delivery System

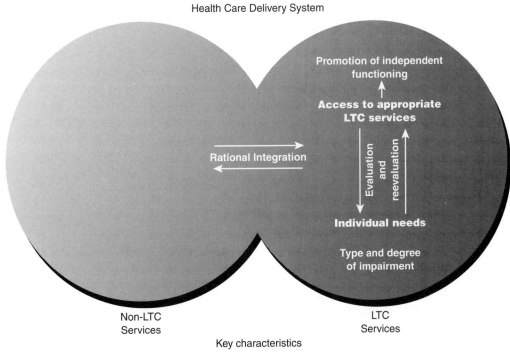

1. The LTC system is rationally integrated with the rest of the health care delivery system. This rational integration facilitates easy access to services between the two components of the health care delivery system.
2. Appropriate placement of the patient within the LTC system is based on an assessment of individual needs. For example, individual needs determine whether and when institutionalization may be necessary.
3. The LTC system accommodates changes in individual needs by providing access to appropriate LTC services as determined by a reevaluation of needs.
4. LTC services are designed to compensate for existing impairment and have the objective of promoting independence to the extent possible.

Figure 5-5 Key characteristics of a well-designed long-term care system. (From Shi, L., & Singh, D.A. [1998]. *Delivering health care in America: a systems approach*. Gaithersburg, MD: Aspen Publishers.)

programs appear to be more likely to work in rural and small towns than Master's level practitioners (Clawson & Osterweis, 1993). Clawson and Osterweis (1993) note that NPs have provided services to the underserved in settings where physicians are less likely to practice, such as community, school, or migrant health centers. One recent study found that CHCs average 2.2 full-time equivalent nonphysician PCPs per site, with plans to increase this number substantially in the future (Samuels & Shi, 1991). Dobin, Gelber, and Freeman (1992) identify the following factors as important in retaining NPs in CHCs: links to community, spouse employment, availability of continuing education, positive work environment, and the ability to serve as student preceptors. The majority of homeless clinics funded by the McKinney Act employ NPs as PCPs.

Other critical areas include the widening gap between urban and rural access to health care services and technology. Even within hospitals, an "e-commerce" gap is emerging (Solovy, 2000). A group of the "most wired"

hospitals are submitting about 16% of their health plan claims online, and these same institutions are using the Internet to verify eligibility for insurance plans. However, few of the remaining hospitals submit their claims online (3%) or verify eligibility online (3%). Using electronic claims creates a significant reduction in manual labor and increases the ease of confirming eligibility. Another area where the "most wired" hospitals lead is in terms of clinical practice. About 27% of these institutions have physicians and nurses perform order entry. More and more institutions are using technologies such as electronic medical records, Palm Pilot, and disease management databases. Some experts even predict that patients will eventually be able to access their records from home, with the ability to schedule appointments and procedures (Solovy, 2000); consultation with a PCP for advice and lab results will occur sooner rather than later. APNs need to participate in the development of these systems to ensure effective development and serve as patient advocates in the process.

IMPLICATIONS FOR MSN EDUCATION AND ADVANCED PRACTICE

Given the multitude of organizations within the health care system, multiple opportunities abound for APNs. Educational programs need to discuss role options for APNs and emphasize that there are no limits in the available positions. APNs are limited only by their own creativity and energy.

To increase the number of APNs who work in rural areas or serve the underserved populations, a number of strategies need to be implemented. First, a number of studies have found that health professionals from the same cultural background as their patients are better able to communicate with patients and have a positive influence on health outcomes (Agency for Health Care Policy and Research, 1990). Minority students still make up a small number (< 15%) of APN students. Ways to increase their representation in the profession should be encouraged. Most colleges of nursing wish to increase the diversity within their programs, but without specific goals this will be difficult.

Schools that increased the number of graduates who worked in underserved areas were examined by Fowkes, Gamel, Wilson, and Garcia (1993). The most successful programs were those who had "comprehensive strategies related to the goal of deploying graduates to work with under-served populations that were interwoven throughout their selection and educational processes, programs that had adapted their structure and function to fit their chosen missions" (Clawson & Osterweis, 1993). Programs that were either located in or near an underserved area had the ability to recruit students from the area and could utilize local clinical sites, thus increasing their chance of deploying graduates in the region. Some programs that matched a preceptor and student together before admission to the program had higher levels of success in placing graduates in underserved areas. Strategies to recruit students from underserved areas include financial assistance, flexible admission requirements, part-time programs, extra academic support, offering outreach programs, having faculty from ethnic minorities, and recruiting in underserved areas. Financial aid is a particularly important factor since many students have family and financial obligations that must be lessened if they hope to attend school. PA programs had more evidence of successful outcomes than NP programs. One limiting factor in this study was the lack of data regarding the employment of graduates for both PA and NP programs.

Fowkes et al (1993) caution that the higher the degree attained, the further away from the patient the practitioner becomes. It will be important for APN faculty to model the importance of providing care for the underserved. Colleges of nursing that value only scholarship and research may be limiting for clinicians willing to teach; APNs must continue their practice to stay current, and they may choose to practice rather than to teach. APNs who are Master's-prepared clinicians tend to have "lower status" than those who are doctorally prepared. APNs with doctoral degrees and clinical experience are very scarce, although this is changing as many programs have added NP programs; doctorally prepared faculty returned for additional schooling and experience to meet the need for these positions (Margolius & Sneed, 1999).

Another factor limiting the availability of clinical experiences in an underserved area is the lack of clinical sites. Many medical schools and PA programs now require their students to rotate into primary care sites, specifically underserved settings. Area health education centers (AHECs) have personnel who arrange clinical rotations for these medical and PA students. This makes it competitive for APNs to secure clinical experiences in these "desirable" locations. These programs will need more government and institutional funding as well as more clinical opportunities as students arrange for access to these sites.

Limitation on scope of practice is a large issue that affects the ability of APNs to practice autonomously in underserved areas. Those states with restrictive nurse practice acts will have greater difficulty in recruiting APNs to practice within the state. APNs will find themselves increasingly more in direct competition with physicians for the same primary care positions. This will require a market-driven pricing of services if APNs are going to compete successfully (Harris, 1998). The Pew Commission is predicting that many of the nation's hospitals will close, with a resulting surplus of 200,000 to 300,000 nurses. The Commission is also predicting that there will be an oversupply of physicians. This prediction is supported in research done by Cooper, Laud, and Dietrich (1998). In such cases, nurses may be in the best position to know what works in the health care system and what does not (Hoyt, 1991).

As more and more health care delivery institutions emerge, it is important for nurses to remember the needs of older adults, the poor, and the underserved. These institutions may have more of a profit motive than an outreach motive. Nurses must advocate for all patients—those that can pay and those that can not. There is also some concern that the health care system is so complex, it is too difficult for the average American to navigate. The proliferation of freestanding services and mergers, as well as insurance changes, make the system very complex during a stressful time in a patient's life. It is the nurse's role to advocate for those who are unable to advocate for themselves.

PRIORITIES FOR RESEARCH

The effect of consistency and quality of care on the health of the public will continue to be an important research topic. APNs need to welcome the opportunity to show, via hard data, how critical the issue of quality is. Patients and politicians want more "bang for the buck." It goes without

Suggestions for Further Learning

- Go to the School-Based Health Center Model at www.gwu.edu/mtg/mtg/sbhcmodel.html, which is supported by the Robert Wood Johnson Foundation. Discuss what insight and guidelines it provides on the issue of school health.
- Obtain the following article: Nichols, L. (1992). Estimating costs of under-using advanced practice nurses. *Nursing Ecnomics, 10,* 343-351. What implications does it have for the use of APNs in various roles in the health care delivery system?

- Read the article: *Americans as health care consumers: the role of quality information.* Available online at www.ahrq.gov/qual/kffhigh.htm. What implications does it have for APNs?
- Read the article: *Advanced nursing practice in the 21st century: do we want to be right or do we want to win?* Available online at www.nursingworld.org/ojin/tpc6/tpc6_2.htm. Do you agree with the author's stance of being right versus winning?

saying that containment of costs while maintaining quality is a critical issue for APNs in the future. This is a time for APNs to demonstrate how evidence-based care is an integral part of advanced practice. Ample evidence exists from more than one million clinical trials of the last 30 years. APNs who practice using the existing data will find themselves at the head of the pack, especially if positive outcomes are documented. While most Americans view quality as the most important factor when choosing a health plan, many make their decision based on personal recommendations from their doctors, family members, and friends. Seven out of ten people regard their family and friends as "good sources" of information about health plans (Agency for Health Care Research and Quality [AHRQ], 1996). This survey has implications for APNs. It becomes even more crucial for APNs to be active in the community, provide quality care to their patients, and make sure that those patients are willing to share their views with family members and friends. According to the survey by the AHRQ (1996), Americans are most concerned with how well a provider communicates with patients and shows a caring attitude. This is one of the strengths of APNs—sharing information with patients and families.

DISCUSSION QUESTIONS

These questions can be used to promote critical thinking and encourage discussion.

1. Examine the mergers, closures, and expansions of health care organizations in your local area. Which services are similar? Which are different? Why do some organizations survive and some flourish? How has this changed the character of the American health care delivery system? Is it different?

2. What are the effects of mergers, closures, and openings on APNs and their patients?
3. How can the plight of rural health care be best addressed?
4. What is the explanation for the disparities in health morbidity and mortality between urban and rural areas?
5. What are strategies that would increase APN representation in rural, urban, and low-income areas?
6. Identify strategies that would help promote the image of APNs as caring and communicative providers.

REFERENCES/BIBLIOGRAPHY

Agency for Health Care Policy and Research. (1990). *Annotated bibliography of AHCPR research on nonphysician primary care providers 1969-1989.* Rockville MD: US Department of Health and Human Services.

Agency for Health Care Research and Quality (1996). *Americans as health care consumers: the role of quality information.* Available online at http://www.AHRQ.gov.

Ahmed, K., & Muus, K. (1991). Comparison of metro and non-metro nurse practitioner characteristics. *Journal of Rural Health, 8,* 6-7.

Alexander, J. (1996). Determinants of profound organizational change: choice of conversion or closure among rural hospitals. *Journal of Health and Social Behavior, 37*(3): 238-251.

American Academy of Nurse Practitioners (2000). Accessed online at www.aanp.org.

American College of Nurse Midwifery (2000). Accessed online at www.acnm.org.

American Hospital Association (1994). *AHA guide to the health care field* (1994 ed.). Chicago: American Hospital Association.

American Hospital Association (1996). *Hospital statistics* (1996-1997 ed.). Chicago: American Hospital Association.

American Nurses Association (2000). Accessed online at www.nursingworld.org.

Bergeson, J., Cash, R., Boulger, J., & Bergeron, D. (1997). The attitudes of rural minnesota family physicians toward nurse practitioners and physician assistants. *Journal of Rural Health, 13*(3), 196-205.

Brown, S., & Grimes, D. (1993). *Nurse practitioners and certified nurse midwives: a meta analysis of studies on nurses in primary care roles.* Washington DC: American Nurses Association.

Catalano, J. T. (1996). *Contemporary professional nursing*. Philadelphia: FA Davis.

Clawson, K., & Osterweis, M. (1993). *The roles of physician assistants and nurse practitioners in primary care*. Washington, DC: Association of Academic Health Centers.

Community health centers need more resources to provide proper care to high risk asthma patients. *Research Activities, 231*, 6-7.

Cooper, R., Laud, P., & Dietrich, C. (1998). Current and projected workforce of non-physician clinicians. *Journal of the American Medical Association, 280*(9), 788-794.

Cys, J. (1999). AHA survey shows patient margins plummeted at rural hospitals in 1998. *AHA News*. Available online at healhforumprod.genpublishing.com/news/doc16230.htm.

Dobin, B., Gelber, L., & Freeman, H. (1992). Patient care and professional staffing patterns in McKinney Act clinics providing primary care to the homeless. *Journal of the American Medical Association, 267*, 698-701.

Doheny, M.O., Cook, C.B., & Stopper, M.C. (1997). *The discipline of nursing* (4th ed.). Stamford, CT: Appleton & Lange.

Drevdahl, D. (1999). Meanings of community in a community health center. *Public Health Nursing, 16*(6), 417-425.

Dunn, E., & Higgins, B. (1993). Comparisons of two types of non-physician providers using episode based data. *Journal of Rural Health, 3*(2), 11-22.

Edelman, M., & Menz, B. (1996). Selected comparisons and implications of a national rural and urban survey on health care access, demographics and policy issues. *Journal of Rural Health, 12*(3), 197-205.

Foster, P. (1995). School based clinics: overcoming the obstacles. *Kansas Nurse, 70*(6), 1-2.

Fowkes, V., Gamel, N., Wilson, S., Garcia, R. (1993). *Assessment of physician assistant, nurse practitioners and nurse midwife training on meeting health care needs of the under-served*. (Final report of HRSA contract no. 240-91-0050). Stanford, CA: Health Resources and Service Administration.

Hacker, K. (1994). A nationwide survey of school health services delivery in urban schools. *Journal of School Health, 64*(7), 279-283.

Hacker, K., & Wessel, G. (1998). School based health centers and school nurses: cementing the collaboration. *Journal of School Health, 68*(10), 409-414.

Haglund, C, & Dowling, W. (1993). The hospital. In S. Williams & P. Torrens (Eds.), *Introduction to health services* (4th ed.). Albany, NY: Delmar.

Harris, M. (1999). The development of a hospital sponsored community based, nurse managed health center. *Family and Community Health, 21*(4), 63-73.

Harris, R. (1998). Advanced nursing practice in the 21st century: do we want to be right or do we want to win? *Online Journal of Issues in Nursing*. Available online at www.nursingworld.org/ojin/tpc6/tpc6_2.htm.

HCIA, Deloitte, & Touche (1997). *The comparative performance of US hospitals: the sourcebook*. Baltimore, MD: HCIA.

Hoyt, M. (1991). A health quiz. *Columbia Journalism Review, 30*(2), 14.

Kassab, C., Luloff, A., Kelsey, T., & Smith, S. (1996). The influence of insurance status and income on health care use among the non-metropolitan elderly. *Journal of Rural Health, 12*(2), 89-99.

Kassirer, J. (1995). Our ailing public hospitals: cure them or close them? *New England Journal of Medicine, 333*, 1348-1349.

Kiefe, C., & Hyman, D. (1995). Do public clinic systems provide health care access for the urban poor? A cross sectional survey. *Journal of Community Health, 21*(1), 61-70.

Krein, S. (1997). The employment and use of nurse practitioners and physician assistants by rural hospitals. *Journal of Rural Health, 13*(1), 45-58.

Lee, P., & Estes, C.L. (1994). *The nation's health* (4th ed.). Boston: Jones and Bartlett Publishers.

Lynch, J., Kaplan, G., Pamuk, E., Cohen, R., Heck, K., & Balfour, J. (1998). Income inequality and mortality in metropolitan areas of the US. *American Journal of Public Health, 88*(7), 1074-1080.

Margolius, F., & Sneed, N. (1999). From expert to novice: doctorally prepared nursing faculty retooling for the future. *Nurse Educator, 24*(1), 9-11.

McKnight, J. (1994). Two tools for well being: health systems and communities. *American Journal of Preventive Medicine, 10*(3), 23-25.

Mezey, A., & Lawrence, R. (1995). Ambulatory care. In A. Kovner (Ed.), *Health care delivery in the United States*. New York: Springer.

Mitchell, J., & McCormack, L. (1997). Access to family planning services: relationship with unintended pregnancies and prenatal outcomes. *Journal of Health Care for the Poor and Underserved, 8*(2), 141-152.

Morrisey, M. (1996). Do non-profit hospitals pay their way? *Health Affairs, 15*(4), 13-144.

Muus, K., Geller, J., Williams, J., Ludtke, R., Knowlton, D., & Hart, L. (1998). Job satisfaction among rural physician assistants. *Journal of Rural Health, 14*(2), 100-108.

National Center for Health Statistics (1998). *Health United States: 1998 with socioeconomic status and health chartbook*. Hyattsville, MD: National Center for Health Statistics.

Pathman, D., Williams, E., & Konrad, T. (1996). Rural physician satisfaction: its sources and relationship to retention. *Journal of Rural Health, 12*(5), 366-377.

Ricketts, T. (1990). Education of physician assistants, nurse midwives, and nurse practitioners for rural practice. *Journal of Rural Health, 6*(4), 537-543.

Rust, G., Murray, V., & Octaviani, H. (1999). Asthma care in community health centers: a study by the southeast regional clinicians' network. *Journal of the National Medical Association,, 91*(7), 398-403.

St. Martin, E. (1996). Community health centers and quality of care: a goal to provide effective health care to the community. *Journal of Community Health Nursing, 13*(2), 83-92.

Samuels, M., & Shi, L. (1991). *Report on the survey of community and migrant health centers regarding utilization of nurse practitioners, physician assistants and certified nurse midwives*. Columbia, SC: Department of Health Administration, School of Public Health, University of South Carolina.

Satariano, W. (1997). Editorial: the disabilities of aging: looking to the physical environment. *American Journal of Public Health, 83*(3), 331-332.

Shi, L, Samuels, M., Konrad, R, Ricketts, T., Stoskopf, C, & Richter, D. (1993). The determinants of utilization of non-physician providers in rural community and migrant health centers. *Journal of Rural Health, 9*(1), 27-39.

Shi, L., & Singh, D.A. (1998). *Delivering health care in America: a systems approach.* Gaithersburg, MD: Aspen Publishers.

Shortell, S.M., Gillies, R.R., Anderson, D.A., Erickson, K.M., & Mitchell, J.B. (1996). *Remaking health care in America: building organized delivery systems.* San Francisco: Jossey-Bass Company.

Snook, I. (1995). Hospital organization and management. In C. Wolper (Ed.), *Health care administration: principles, practices, structure, and delivery* (2nd ed.). Gaithersburg, MD: Aspen Publishers.

Solovy, A. (2000). Is an e-commerce gap emerging among the nation's hospitals? *Hospitals & Health Networks.* Available online at www.healthforumprod.genpublishing.com/hhn/doc 16428.htm.

Strickland, W., Strickland, D., & Garretson, C. (1998). Rural and urban non-physician providers in Georgia. *Journal of Rural Health, 14*(2), 109-120.

United States Bureau of the Census, Bureau of Labor Statistics (1996). *Statistical abstracts of the United States.* Washington, DC: US Government Printing Office.

White, S. (1997). Schooled in primary care. *Hospitals and health networks, 7*(17), 80.

Whiteis, D., & Salmon, J. (1992). Public health care delivery in 5 US municipalities: lessons and implications. *Henry Ford Hospital Medical Journal, 40,* 16-25.

Wolfson, J., & Hopes, S. (1994, July). What makes tax exempt-hospitals special? *Healthcare Financial Management,* 56-60.

Wolinsky, F. (1988). *The sociology of health: principles, practitioners and issues* (2nd ed.). Belmont, CA: Wadsworth Publishing.

Wolper, L., & Pena, J. (1995). History of hospitals. In L. Wolper (Ed.), *Health care administration: principles, practices, structure and delivery* (2nd ed.). Gaithersburg: MD: Aspen Publishers.

Zapka, J., Pbert, L., Stoddard, A., Ockene, J., Goins, K., & Bonollo, D. (2000). Smoking cessation counseling with pregnant and postpartum women: a survey of community health center providers. *American Journal of Public Health, 90*(1), 78-84.

Chapter 6

The Role of Managed Care in Health Care Delivery

Margaret M. Anderson & Denise Robinson

Managed care is here to stay. Current estimates suggest that 100 million Americans are insured under some version of managed care. Pressure from employer groups and government will continue to move patients out of traditional indemnity plans into those that are more closely managed (American College of Physicians [ACP]–American Society of Internal Medicine [ASIM], 2000). Managed care is the most significant recent development in America's health care delivery services, though many of the factors influencing managed care were in place even as far back as the 1970s (Shi & Singh, 1998). However, it was not until the 1980s that the controls over health care utilization and care of patients within preexisting prepayment arrangements came together. At the time, many leaders in nursing looked at managed care's emphasis and the focus of nurse practitioners (NPs) and concluded that this may be a prime opportunity for advanced practice nurses (APNs) to find their niche in the delivery system. However, anecdotal reports from APNs have suggested that this is not happening; in fact new barriers to APN practice may be developing (Cohen, Mason, Arsenie, Sargese, & Needham, 1998). This chapter discusses the *ins* and *outs* of the managed care system and presents critical issues related to APN practice.

DEFINITIONS

Managed care "is the process of the application of standard business practices to the delivery of health care in the tradition of the American Free enterprise system" (Hughes, 1994). Rather than the typical definition of managed care, which lists its components, this definition indicates that managed care is a process. The components of managed care, such as health maintenance organizations (HMOs), are the result of the process. Hughes feels that the health care industry is going through the same economic disciplining that other industries have gone through. This means eliminating economic waste, excess, and surplus and turning it into something more productive.

He reflects that this is in the tradition of the American free enterprise system—a capitalistic process and not necessarily "warm and fuzzy." There *are* winners and losers. Hughes believes two groups have driven the process to where it is now. The first is the "chance to do better" group, usually made up of the professionals. The second group believes that they can make money from the process. These two forces are linked, but they frequently disagree on issues related to managed care. Each group needs the other. In an organization, it is important to determine which force is dominant. APNs may choose to work within a system that focuses on a chance to do better rather than one whose only focus is on the bottom line.

The ultimate goal for managed care is to achieve the best quality product for the least cost, while continuously striving to improve the outcomes of the product (Hughes, 1994). Shi and Singh (1998) define managed care in two different contexts. The first is the process of providing health care via two main features: (1) integration of the functions of insurance, delivery, and payment within one organization, and (2) exercising formal control over use. The second context refers to managed care organizations (MCOs), which have a variety of different forms and types. All managed care plans try to integrate the delivery and financing of care while applying constraints on encounters between providers and patients. A MCO is an organization that delivers health services without having to use the services of an insurance company. The MCO functions like an insurance company in that the employer pays a monthly premium to the MCO, and the MCO delivers a comprehensive set of services while assuming all the risk. Feldstein (1994) indicates that approximately 15% of the fee is spent on insurance and administration, 40% on facilities, 40% on physicians, and 5% on pharmacy services.

Terms commonly used in MCOs include ***gatekeeping***, which refers to the coordination of health care services needed by a patient. This gatekeeping is generally done by the primary care provider (PCP). The gatekeeper controls access to other health care services such as specialists or testing. In effect the gatekeeper controls the patient's

---

Table 6-1

Information Requested for Credentialing of Advanced Practice Nurse and Physicians

ADVANCED PRACTICE NURSE	PHYSICIAN
• Transcripts showing graduation from nursing school and a NP program • Certification as an APN • Previous experience as an APN • References • License history • Teaching appointments • Professional organizations • Professional liability history, including insurance carrier and malpractice suits • Disciplinary procedures • Disclosure of criminal convictions	• Transcripts showing graduation from college and medical school • Licensure and certification history • Previous experience • Teaching appointments • Disclosure of criminal convictions • Disciplinary procedures and complaints of any nature, including loss of employment privileges, license, or certificate • History of physical, mental, or chemical dependency • Performance data, including intensity of service, charge per encounter, frequency of visits by diagnosis, use of x-rays, mortality rates, and Hedis data • Financial factors • Visits per hour, appointment waiting times, and after hours coverage

Data from Rustia, J., & Bartek, J. (1997). Managed care credentialing of advanced practice nurses. *Nurse Practitioner, 22*(9), 90, 92, 99-103.

access to the whole health care delivery system. **Case management** is a type of gatekeeping. A case manager serves as a monitor and facilitator for services needed and helps the patient access those services in a cost-effective manner. **Credentialing** is an administrative process that collects and profiles information on a provider's training and experience to determine that the person is qualified to perform specific clinical activities (Rustia & Bartek, 1997). This process was developed to identify physician competence, avoid liability issues, and determine the effect a physician's practice would have on the MCO (Table 6-1). However, if APNs were expected to provide the amount of data required by physicians, many would not be able to do so. Most APNs have not kept that kind of data regarding their practice. **Privileging** is "the process through which the employing organization grants a professional specific authority to perform the designated clinical activities" (Rustia & Bartek, 1997). The decision to give a provider privileges is a professional peer judgment. As these peer committees are presently configured, decisions are generally made by physicians. It can be expected that APNs will be subjected to the same degree of scrutiny that physicians have experienced in the past. This scrutiny may increase as competition develops and more nonphysician providers enter the market.

In a MCO environment, both credentialing and privileging may be repeated every 2 years. Buppert (1999) suggests the following steps if provider status is denied. First the APN should ask if the MCO admits APNs to provider panels; if not, he or she should ask "why not?" Then the APN should find out who the company decision-maker is that could change the policy. If a state

law is identified as the reason for not being accepted, Buppert recommends asking "which law precludes APNs being PCPs?" From there the APN should strategize with the state advanced practice organization and hire an attorney to analyze the alleged legal barrier. If the MCO itself has a policy against APNs, then the APN should write letters to the MCO president specifically stating how APNs can satisfy the business needs of the organization. Data supporting APNs as PCPs should be presented in the letters and in any face to face meetings. Patients can write to both their employer and MCO requesting the services of NPs as PCPs. Physician colleagues can write letters of support too. Finally, the APN should persevere and request another application packet in 6 months.

Utilization review is another common term used in conjunction with managed care. It refers to the process of "evaluating the appropriateness of the services provided" (Shi and Singh, 1998). Some people see this utilization review as a way to deny requests, but the main objective is to review each case and determine the appropriate level of services and cost-effective health care delivery.

Practice profiling is another term that developed based on managed care. It refers to the development of using practice patterns or data to allow comparison of providers. This profiling can serve as a way for providers to get a sense of how they are doing in terms of care (e.g., in numbers of patients seen per year, percentage of referrals, most common diagnoses). However, this profiling can also be used to discipline or eliminate providers who do not fit the norm or who are not producing at an acceptable level. For APNs this profiling may serve a wonderful purpose in that it will help provide data to increase APN visibility.

APNs should know how many patients they see, what their rate of no-shows are, the most common diagnoses, and their cycle times to be able to promote and explain their practice. This data also gives APNs the ability to compare their care to national statistics. For example, Cheryl, an APN who works in a community health center, conducted a profile of how many of her 2-year-old patients had been immunized. Using the computer-assisted self-assessment (CASA) program developed by the Centers for Disease Control and Prevention (CDC), her practice pattern was 73%. This is higher than the national average for complete childhood immunizations at 2 years old (64.8%). Cheryl is pleased that the CASA program gives feedback about missed opportunities for immunization; in that area she had a 100% for not missing opportunities. Pulling the charts, she identified that getting the patients back in the center to complete the immunization series was the real problem area. Cheryl was not happy with the percentage immunized, so she and the care team instituted various interventions to improve these patterns. If Cheryl were looking for a position and shared how well her practice patterns were for childhood immunizations, glycosylated hemoglobin (HgbA1C) with diabetics, or hospitalizations for asthma patients, it would be clear to potential employers that Cheryl was providing quality patient care.

CRITICAL ISSUES: UNDERSTANDING THE ADVANCED PRACTICE NURSE'S ROLE IN MANAGED CARE

The beginnings of managed care can be traced to back to the Great Depression. In Oklahoma, citizens developed a prepay system for hospital surgical services and a copay system for house calls and dental services (ACP-ASIM, 2000). Baylor Hospital offered a predetermined fixed-fee-per-month prepaid plan back in 1929, and other hospitals started offering inpatient services (Shi & Singh, 1998). Interestingly enough, this first insurance by Baylor was a capitation plan, with all risk being borne by the providers.

Before MCOs became prominent, the major type of insurance existing in the United States was fee-for-service. Patients believed this care to be of high quality, and competition was driven. In these situations, MCOs were at a disadvantage because the fee-for-service plans allowed the patients to choose their own physician or hospital. Why would a patient choose a plan that restricted their choices? Providers also were not interested in plans that restricted potential income or controlled the type of care they provided. Kaiser Permanente may have served as the prototype of HMOs. It was an independent prepaid group practice started in 1942. It provided comprehensive care; its managed care concept began when the organization began to exercise control over hospitals by contracting for

---

Box 6-1

How Managed Care Plans Control Costs

- Networks of providers
- Integration of financing and delivery of medical care (i.e., financing, payment, and insurance)
- Obtainment of discounts from providers
- Sharing of risks with providers
- Utilization control and management
- Coordination of a broad range of services
- Monitoring to determine if care is appropriate
- Increased use of outpatient services rather than inpatient services
- Restricted access to providers
- Gatekeeping (i.e., case management)
- Capitation fees and salaries for providers

---

their services. It also penalized physicians for excessive use of hospital services.

The Health Maintenance Act of 1973 stimulated some growth of HMOs by providing federal funds for the establishment and expansion of new HMOs. Employers with more than 25 employees were required to offer an HMO as an alternative if one was available in the area. This was the first attempt by the government to sponsor an alternative to fee-for-service plans. HMOs were seen as a way to stimulate competition among health plans and encourage efficiency, and as a way to slow the increase in health care costs (Davis, 1990). However, the Act of 1973 was not very successful in stimulating the development of HMOs. By 1976, only 174 HMOs had formed, and even by the end of the 1970s, fewer that 10 million people were enrolled in HMOs. It was not until the 1980s that employers began seeking alternatives to the expensive, cost-escalating fee-for-service model as a way to provide employee health benefits. As the health care costs continued to escalate, many employers took control of their health benefit plans. Between 1981 and 1987, HMO enrollment tripled from 10 million to approximately 30 million (Kraus, 1991). By 1990, more than one third of employees were enrolled in managed care plans. (Box 6-1 identifies reasons why managed care plans were able to control costs.)

Competition among MCOs led to the many types of MCOs that exist today. It is important for the APN to get an idea of "where it started" to get a sense of appreciation for how the organizations operate. There is no doubt that management of utilization makes up the "managed" part of MCOs. The latest change on the horizon is the notion of managed competition. Iglehart (1994) states that the central idea of managed competition "is to divide physicians and hospitals into competing economic units, called 'accountable health partnerships,' that would contract with insurance-purchasing cooperatives (health insurance purchasing cooperatives [HIPCs]) to provide standardized packages of medical benefits for fixed per capita

Table 6-2

Benefits and Burdens for Managed Care Organization Parties

PARTY	BENEFITS	BURDENS
Patients	Discourages overtreatment, encourages preventive care, and attempts to promote cost containment and quality health care delivery; copayments are usually low; study by Udvarhelyi et al (1991) showed that quality and quantity for HMO patients is similar or better than fee-for-service patients.	Restrictions on care; questions about the ability of a provider to answer to both a patient and the MCO; patient autonomy; limited access to particular providers and services not covered by the plan.
Providers	Limits practice startup costs and offers dependable incomes, regular practice hours, and structured practices; minimum standard for credentialing of providers; financial incentive to deliver care in a efficient, cost-effective manner; accessible patient population.	Moral and professional challenges; changes provider-patient relationships; provider caught between expectations of higher-technology care and MCO cost-containment expectations; less autonomy in diagnosis and treatment.
Payers	Equal access for all members; provides financial incentives for administrators and others; payers can use business principles and test principles in new markets (e.g., quality improvement [QI] being applied to health care).	Financially risky enterprise; little outcome data available; may be liable in some situations, creating increased litigation potential.

rates." The HIPCs would serve as purchasing agents on behalf of the consumer. Managed competition assumes that money, or profit, is the most important determinant of how patients, payers, and providers behave when they seek, finance, or render medical care (Iglehart, 1994). It is hoped that health care reform can be achieved by changing the roles of the patients, payers, and providers and reworking their relationships with one another. The focus of the relationship would be the price of the package of health care services, not the cost of each individual service. The concept of managed competition was advanced during President Bill Clinton's first campaign in 1991 and 1992. After the failure of his health care reform plan in 1993, the term is not used as frequently. Nevertheless, the concept is still a viable option. By managing the competition and encouraging economic incentives for reform, the responsibility for stemming costs in health care continues to rest with the payers, patients, and providers. These three groups still have the major responsibility for making health care reform work.

Managed care is a slightly different concept that assumes cost savings can be realized by abandoning the traditional fee-for-service approach to health care. Managed care restrains autonomy in clinical decision-making. The patient's choices in treatment and plan of care may also be restricted so that the cheapest method of care is often the preferred option. Patients are limited to physicians within the plan or network of the managed care company (Iglehart, 1994).

Characteristics of Managed Care Systems

As managed care becomes more complex, some researchers have developed a typology to help explain the differences between managed care systems (Welch, Hillmna, & Pauly, 1990). There appear to be five distinguishing characteristics:

1. The basic method by which providers are paid for primary care services (ie, salary, capitation or fee-for-service)
2. Whether the providers can see other patients with traditional indemnity insurance besides HMO patients
3. The nature of the HMO's financial contract with any middle tiers
4. The nature of the risk or reward to providers (physicians) in addition to the basic payment method
5. The size and nature of the risk pool used to share the risk or reward.

These characteristics can help determine the differences between various MCOs.

In addition, there are three basic ethical assumptions on which managed care was founded: (1) equality of access for all MCO members; (2) a trusting and covenant-based provider-patient relationship, even when it is contractually based; and (3) the use of quality assurance activities and utilization management issues to promote quality care rather than to punish patients or providers. Given these founding principles, there are benefits and constraints for all involved in MCOs. (Table 6-2 identifies both benefits and burdens for providers and patients.)

It is important for APNs to recognize the differences between the various organizations and understand the ethical principles on which they are based. Many times, an APN needs to be familiar with referral policies of various MCOs, and he or she may have to serve as a patient advocate when services are not approved. For example, Steve was seeing a 17-year-old patient complaining of acne. She had no cystic lesions, but she did have active comedones on her face. She had been treated for 2 weeks with conventional therapy, but she wanted to be referred to a dermatologist. By HMO rule, referral to a dermatologist could be done only when the patient has cysts or the acne is unresponsive to conventional treatment. What should Steve have done? Should he have referred her to the dermatologist and broken the rules of the MCO or made a special effort to get her covered? Steve discussed with his patient that any treatment takes approximately 6 weeks to see improvement and convinced her to wait a few more weeks. When the patient returned, there had

been some improvement, but the acne had not resolved. In this case, Steve then made the appropriate referrals to the dermatologist (LaPuma & Schiedermayer, 1994).

Types of Managed Care Organizations

There are a number of types of MCOs. Many of the differences between types of MCOs have become blurred in the past 5 years because they may offer different types of managed care products. The most common and oldest are the HMOs. According to Shi & Singh (1998), there are five types of HMOs. (The types are presented in Table 6-3.) In addition, there are four main characteristics of HMOs:

Table **6-3**

Types of Health Maintenance Organizations

MODEL	CHARACTERISTICS
Staff model	Physicians employed by the HMO; salary may be increased by bonuses for performance; all common specialists employed; physicians may only provide services to enrolled patients; utilization management easier based on the amount of control the HMO has over physician practice patterns; large number of enrollees are required to support the high salaries of physicians; HMO contracts separately with one or more hospitals, and employee physicians must use and be privileged in those hospitals.
Group model	HMO contracts with a large, multispecialty group practice of physicians; group practice and not the HMO is the employer of the physicians; an inclusive capitation fee per enrollee is paid to the group practice for services for the enrollees; since the group practice is independent and contracts with the HMO, the practice may also contract with other HMOs or see nonenrolled patients; exclusive contract with the HMO gives the HMO more control, but most large group practices are not exclusive contractors; the number of enrollees still gives the HMO a degree of control over practice habits and patterns; practice is responsible for quality control; HMO also uses one or more area hospitals.
Network model	More common in large metropolitan areas; HMO contracts with several group medical practices and may have several contracts with primary care practices, paying a capitated fee to the practice selected by the enrollee; PCP is responsible for the enrollee's medical care and pays the specialist directly, or the HMO may contract with groups of specialists to whom the PCP must refer; this model offers a wider choice of PCPs, but this increased choice also means less utilization control.
Independent Practice Association (IPA) model	IPA is an independent organization that contracts with individual and group practices for services; HMO then contracts with the IPA instead of individual and group practices; IPA pays the physician a capitated fee per enrollee per HMO and is responsible for quality control; HMO is still responsible for providing health care for enrollees, but the IPA secures the physician services for the HMO; essentially, the IPA serves as an intermediary or agent for the physicians to the HMOs; majority of growth has occurred in the IPA/HMO model in the last few years.
Direct contract model	HMO bypasses the IPA and contracts directly with large numbers of individual and group practices for services for enrollees; gatekeeping method of care coordination and utilization control is used, so PCPs use HMO-contracted specialists; HMO has little control over utilization management; HMO reimburses physicians at an agreed amount per patient or service.
Mixed model	Have various combinations of small and large group medical practices as well as independent practitioners; usually have contracts with a number of MCOs.

Data from Shi, K., & Singh, D.A. (1998). *Delivering health care in America: a systems approach*. Gaithersburg, MD: Aspen Publishers; Iglehart, J.K (1994). In P.R. Lee & C.L. Estes (Eds.), *The nation's health* (4th ed.). Boston: Jones and Bartlett Publishers; and Reres, M. (1996). *Managed care: managing the process*. Glencoe, MO: National Professional Education Institute.

1. Services are emphasized.
2. Access to services is based on a fixed monthly fee per enrollee with control for utilization maintained by the HMO.
3. Care can only be provided by participating organizations, physicians, and other service providers.
4. The HMO is responsible for ensuring quality control for services provided.

The major disadvantage of the early HMOs was the limited choice of physician providers. Using that as a standard, other types of MCOs were designed to overcome the obstacle and provide the delivery of services promised. The barrier the early MCOs faced was the organization of health care delivery into networks that adequately provided access for the enrollee and still left adequate control to the MCO for utilization of the services. The issue was not that the enrollee should not have the service, but rather did the enrollee need the service? The risk-sharing and payment for services made the development of MCOs move in different directions, so that different managed care plans and models of HMOs have emerged in today's market (Shi & Singh, 1998).

Preferred provider organizations (PPOs) are the second most common type of MCO (Figure 6-1). They began appearing on the market in the late 1970s but were not common until the mid- to late-1980s (Shi & Singh, 1998). These plans offer discounted fee-for-service to organizations, rather than capitation. The advantage of these organizations is that the patient has larger choice of physician and hospital selections. The assumption is that the discount is made up in volume by the organization. Set

fees are contracted for diagnostic-related groups (DRGs), bundled services, specific services, or any other arrangement one can conceive. A patient can see physicians and obtain services outside the PPO list, but the provider is reimbursed at the discounted rate and the patient is responsible for the rest of the fee. Other costs to the consumer such as copays and deductibles are also higher if service is obtained outside the PPO list. There are two types of PPOs available, and these plans are discussed in Table 6-4. (Table 6-5 shows the intensity of managed care and influence on health care for six of the most common types of MCOs.)

Medicaid, Medicare, and Managed Care Organizations

Medicaid and Medicare both have MCO options. Medicaid has made the most strides in enrolling patients, with almost one third of all beneficiaries enrolled by 1995 (Priester, 1997). The Balanced Budget Act of 1997 gave states the authority to implement managed care programs without federal waivers (Moscovice, 1998). Some states, such as New Jersey, have used the services of an enrollment broker to encourage Medicaid recipients to join managed care plans. New Jersey achieved almost 90% enrollment. The enrollment brokers earn incentive fees based on the number of people who enroll.

Medicaid managed care is a type of care that many providers now want to access after years of avoiding it. As more states turn to Medicaid managed care as a strategy to cut costs, many providers see increased income from monthly capitation fees. It will be important for all

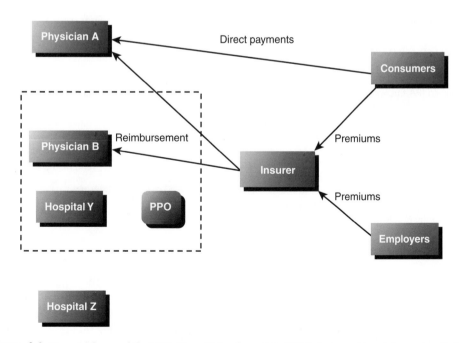

Figure 6-1 Financial flows and the PPO (From Deloughery, G.D. [1995]. *Issues and trends in nursing.* St. Louis: Mosby.)

Table 6-4

Types of Preferred Provider Organizations

TYPE	CHARACTERISTICS
Exclusive provider organization (EPO)	EPOs resemble PPOs, except that enrollees are not allowed to use providers not on the EPO's list; gatekeeping may be used in that the patient must see the PCP before obtaining other services; PCP coordinates services and controls utilization.
Point of service (POS)	POS plans attempt to combine the best features of HMOs with the patient choice of PPOs; capitation and gatekeeping are employed; even though enrollee selects a PCP, enrollee can use any provider for service; enrollee does pay higher copays and deductibles, but a wide choice of providers is available; PCP must authorize in-network treatment and (often) out-of-network treatment, but patient has the perception of choice (patients may never exercise choice, but they want the option of choice) (Shi & Singh, 1998)

Table 6-5

Control of Managed Care for Managed Care Organizations (from Least to Most Control)

TYPE OF ORGANIZATION	MANAGEMENT CONTROL	EFFECT ON MEDICAL CARE
Fee-for-service: Complete freedom of choice to patients; reimbursement on a fee-for-service basis	None	None
Managed indemnity plan: Free choice and fee-for-service; insurer imposes some utilization control	Utilization review (UR)	External
PPO: Patients choose from "preferred providers"; insurer has financial risk for performance	UR and discounted fees	External
IPA: Insurer directs patients to provider in small or independent practice who has agreed to some financial risk; payment is capitation or fee-for-service, with incentive based on performance	UR and financial risk	Financial risk based on performance
Network IPA: Similar to IPA but with larger group practices; payment is capitation	Group, business, and social structures in addition to UR and financial risk	Indirect, through management personnel and cultural and financial risk
Staff/group HMO: Prepaid, large group multi-speciality practice; patients can only get care at HMO; providers are salaried	Group, business, and social structures in addition to UR and financial risk	Direct, through coordination, systems, and structural design and financial risk

Data from American College of Physicians–American Society of Internal Medicine (2000). *Primary care in managed care*. Available online at www.acponline.org/mgdcare/primary.htm.

---

providers, including APNs, to realize that most Medicaid patients differ from those in commercial plans. Most Medicaid patients have complex issues, including homelessness, teen pregnancy, human immunodeficiency virus (HIV), abuse, and single-parent households. These are issues that frequently can not be solved in short 10-minute visits, and many times they may require the assistance of social service. Three groups typically make up the Medicaid population: (1) poor children and families, including single parent families who qualify for Aid to Dependent Children; (2) chronically ill and disabled individuals who are under 65 year of age and qualify for

Medicaid due to their disabilities; and (3) people who qualify for both Medicaid and Medicare (i.e., over 65 and below the federal poverty level). This last group tends to have even more complex problems, with more chronic illnesses. Flanagan (1997) recommends several strategies for providers to use when converting to a Medicaid managed care plan. Most importantly, the APN should be familiar with the state provisions for Medicaid managed care. Information that will affect care includes regulatory requirements and eligibility. Also important for the APN to determine is the population to be served. Collection of data is crucial to keep track of fees, costs, and patient outcomes. Reengineering the APN practice for Medicaid managed care patients might include some changes to make the site more friendly, such as evening hours, open schedule access, and providing services directly in the neighborhood. Patient education is even more vital for Medicaid patients because many of them need to learn basic self-care skills.

Medicare has not had the same numbers of beneficiaries enroll in managed care plans as Medicaid; the majority are still enrolled in fee-for-service plans. Only about 13% were enrolled in MCOs by the end of 1996 (Georges & McGinley, 1997). As in commercial MCOs, there are wide differences between urban (over 20% enrolled) and rural (only 1% enrolled) beneficiaries. This issue was also addressed in the Balanced Budget Act of 1997, so that more enrollment opportunities will be available for those who live in rural areas. Shi and Singh (1998) note that one of the big advantages of a MCO plan for seniors is more plan for less money. Most MCOs cover medications, preventive services, and eye and hearing examinations, and they offer lower copayments. When surveyed, the majority of Medicare MCO enrollees were satisfied with their plan and would recommend it to others.

Issues for the Future of Managed Care Organizations

Trends in managed care are mostly financial in nature. Patients want choice and employers want low cost. Employers spend $18 billion annually on health benefits. Often an employer will charge an employee more for plans with a higher cost than the base plan the employer offers at a modest cost to employees. There is considerable blurring between PPOs and MCOs. The PPO is a managed care plan but not necessarily a MCO. MCOs often offer plans similar to PPOs that are not HMOs. More and more reliance on gatekeeping is evident in the health care insurance plans available to the consumer. The consumer wants more choice in their health care, but he or she does not want to pay for higher premiums. However, the consumer may pay higher premiums if offered more choices. The MCO market is currently dominated by for-profit companies rather than not-for-profit ones. This puts a different slant on the makeup of the managed care

market and the choices employers and employees have for health care. Employers are continuing to pass the increased cost of health care off to their employees. Consumers will be paying more out of pocket in the form of deductibles, copayments, and three-tiered formularies. Generic medications cost $5 to $10 dollars in the first tier of the formulary. Brand-name, sole-source drugs require a $15 to $20 copayment, while the third tier "lifestyle" drugs such as Viagra are available for a $35 to $50 copayment. Patients are becoming increasingly savvy about health care. Morrison (2000) noted that 70 million people can access information via the Internet, with 91% of them finding information pertinent to what they were looking for.

It is also becoming increasingly common that PPOs are sponsored by hospitals and groups of physicians. Integrated delivery systems (IDSs) are becoming more prevalent in recent years. An IDS is a network of organizations that provides services to a defined population. The IDS is financially and clinically responsible for outcomes and costs related to the care of this population. A provider-sponsored organization (also known as a provider-service organization [PSO]) is a type of IDS. A physician-hospital organization (PHO) is very similar to a PSO except that it includes hospitals as well as physicians and gives them the legal ability to negotiate with MCOs. PHOs offer the benefits of integration while preserving the autonomy of physicians. For this reason, many cost-cutting measures and utilization monitoring are not very successful in these organizations. While the integration of services may seem like a good cost-cutting strategy, many of the hospital and organization mergers have not reduced excess capacity or produced efficiency (Alpha Center, 1998). Many of these organizations have had to close facilities and lay off personnel.

In some cases, the result of managed care is a great disruption in continuity of care. If employers or patients change insurers frequently, then a new PCP may need to be selected annually. If a plan of care is in force or treatment for serious illness has been initiated and is not accepted by the new insurer, then valuable treatment time and money are lost. This may also be a point in the ethics of preexisting condition clauses. What options does the patient have?

Because of ethical issues that have been raised regarding the withholding of treatment, denial of claims, and misuse and abuse of power, the HMOs get mixed reviews. Some have saved money and reduced costs; others have not. Employers are still the ones demanding lower costs for health care because they are paying the health care bill, but they also are exposed to a lot of dissatisfaction and distrust about HMOs from their employees. The conflict between a satisfied employee group and reduced health care costs rages on. Large employers typically pay a major part of the costs associated with both low-end and high-end health care plans, so they end up substantially supporting the health care system more than they would like (Iglehart, 1994). (The evaluation and assessment of quality, including the Henry Ford Balance Sheet, the Donabedian method, and the HEDIS Report Card, are discussed in Chapter 7.) A recently released report compares health care quality among nations. The United States ranks as 37 out of 191, despite being first in health care spending (World Health Organization, 2000). The report addresses the issue of value for money. The United States excels at expensive, heroic care, but it is less effective at providing the low-cost preventive care that keeps people in other countries healthy.

Other critical issues still need to be resolved relative to MCOs. One important issue is access. While most people who are enrolled in a plan can be seen on a timely basis, there has been a tremendous increase in the number of people who are uninsured. While there is no relationship between increased numbers of people in MCOs and uninsured persons, one factor influencing the high numbers of uninsured may be the cost. More employers are offering health insurance benefits, but in most cases the benefits require a fairly substantial contribution on the part of the employee. For example, Teri, an APN at a community health center, heard one of her patients say at the last visit that she could not afford $68 a month for health insurance coverage. While to many that does not seem like a large amount, for those with incomes barely above poverty, it is not affordable.

Community health centers and other public hospitals and clinics that serve the uninsured or underinsured also have been affected by the increased competition. These agencies are having a more difficult time serving all the patients who need their services. In Kentucky a welfare plan has increased numbers of single mothers working, but as the mothers work, they lose their own medical coverage. Now only the children are covered. Mothers put off their own care until they have no other options. Community health centers are frequently dependent on pharmaceutical samples for the uninsured; this may be the only way to know that a patient is getting the required treatment. APNs are then forced to choose between what samples they have on hand and other more efficacious treatments. Either way, the options are not attractive.

Gag rules are clauses in MCO contracts that prohibit providers from speaking to patients about options, coverage, and treatment determinations about the plan (Shi & Singh, 1998). Legislation has been passed in numerous states to prevent "drive-by births", giving mothers an option for 48-hour hospitalization after delivery. There are several cases pending that challenge the inability of an individual to sue a MCO for poor quality or lack of appropriate or timely referrals. All are issues that will have a great effect on the future of MCOs.

Legislation also has been passed in a number of states related to *any willing provider*. This means that physicians can not be excluded from a MCO when the physician meets the qualifications for participation. These laws have proven to be beneficial for APNs since they are also considered in the "any willing provider" category.

Additional issues in managed care include the viability of managed competition and managed care's business and decision-making practices. MCOs in California are struggling with inadequate income; many of the practices are going bankrupt (Parrish, 2000), and a number of HMOs and MCOs are having difficulty remaining financially solvent. This raises several issues. Should a provider serve as gatekeeper when the provider also serves to gain when services are limited? What is the industry average in terms of treating preexisting conditions? Do patients have difficulty when they switch MCOs? Frequent switching of MCOs seems to be the norm today, and patients could be penalized if they have a preexisting disease. Other issues to address include the degree to which nonphysician providers are included as PCPs in MCO provider panels and their ability to obtain direct reimbursement.

PRIORITIES FOR RESEARCH

Cook, Ingersoll, and Spitzer (1999) have identified research priorities related to managed care. They identify five trends that are defining the shift in health care delivery; these areas can be used to develop a research agenda. The first trend is population-based care. Some providers are looking at the effectiveness of population-based services as a way to manage risk and increase access. Important information affecting population-based care includes demographical trends, epidemiological data, and population trends. Questions that need to be addressed include: What are the best methods for identifying and defining populations? What are the services that MCOs must offer to maintain the health of certain populations? What are nursing interventions that are effective for delivering cost effective, high quality care for all ages?

A second trend in managed care is the change from illness to wellness care. Care needs to emphasize the prevention or postponement of illness, with education leading to patient self-management. Appropriate research questions for this trend include: How can health promotion be accomplished with various populations? What early intervention activities are the most effective? What services do APNs provide that match this change from illness to wellness perspective? Data supporting the focus of APNs is needed.

The third trend influencing managed care is the increased involvement of consumers. This ranges from consumers demanding a voice in decision-making to providers being aware of consumer expectations. Knowing the best way to keep consumers informed would be helpful for APNs providing care. Knowing what level of involvement patients want in terms of decision-making for the plan of care would help APNs improve relationships with patients.

The fourth trend is the changing relationships between care providers. There is more interdependence of professionals. Research that focuses on how best to promote this interdependence would help increase collaboration between all involved parties.

The fifth and final trend is care management and delivery systems reengineering. Questions pertinent in this area include: What are the boundaries observed by MCOs? Who are the stakeholders involved in health policy issues? How can ambulatory practice reengineer to most economically and efficiently meet population needs? APNs need to be involved with the reengineering processes that promote cost and treatment efficiency.

A number of studies have been done indicating that HMOs provide care that is as effective or more effective than that of fee-for-service providers (Brook, Kamber, Lohr, Goldberg, Keeler, & Newhouse, 1990; Hornrook & Berki, 1985; Murray, Greenfield, Kaplan, & Yano, 1992; Udvarhelyi, Jennison, Phillips, & Epstein, 1991; Yelin, Shearn, & Epstein, 1986). Gold, Hurley, and Lake (1995) conducted a study looking at the arrangements that MCOs had with physicians. Cunningham, Grossman, St. Peter, and Lesser (1999) looked at the relationship of managed care and physician provision of charity care. Their findings indicate that physicians who practice in a highly managed practice provide fewer hours of charity care than those physicians who had little involvement with managed care. All these studies looked at the role of physicians in managed care, with no mention of APNs.

A few studies have been conducted looking at APNs and managed care plans. Dial, Palsbo, and Bergsten (1995) found that only half of staff and group HMOs include NPs as PCPs on provider panels. This was similar to the data collected by Weiner, Steinwachs, and Williams in 1986; they found that HMOs made limited use of NPs. Sekscenski, Sansom, and Basell (1994) showed that supportive state practice environments increase the number and use of nonphysician providers. Research needs to look at the practices of MCOs in collaboration with APNs: what is the level of employment of APNs in MCOs?

An important study looking at the role of APNs in managed care was conducted by Cohen et al (1998). Their research reveals a number of important trends for APNs in managed care. The purpose of their study was to explore NP experiences and perspectives on arrangements they had with MCOs. The authors used focus groups of 27 NPs to identify facilitators and barriers for credentialing as PCPs in managed care plans. Results of the research indicate that the majority of the NP subjects were female, with Master's-level preparation and an average of 10 years in practice. Of the 27 NPs, 8 were listed on a primary care panel of an MCO, and most practiced in sites affiliated with MCOs. The majority of the NPs lacked a Medicaid billing number and did not receive reimbursement in their own names. The major perception of the focus group participants was a sense of *invisibility*. Most felt like invisible providers because they were not recognized by the MCOs, even though they brought in considerable revenue. Invisibility was also a term used by Fagin (1987) when describing nursing's status, but it is particularly applicable when describing APNs and managed care. This invisibility is promoted when patients are tracked using a physician's name or number, as well as when prescriptions are written only using the physician's information.

Another important consequence of this invisibility is the inability for patients to locate APNs if they are not listed in managed care directories. A grounded theory study by Martin and Hutchinson (1997) looked at the world of NPs. The subjects in this study identified the "marginalized position" role that NPs frequently assume. Being in a marginalized position meant that many of the NPs were discounted in their roles as PCPs. It also meant that in many situations, they were working from a disadvantaged position when dealing with many different groups. This marginality and discounting contribute to making NPs invisible.

Table 6-6 describes identified barriers to being listed as PCPs by MCOs. In some cases this barrier was imposed by the MCOs; in others, it was imposed by NPs. The NPs also identified facilitators to being listed on MCO panels. Physicians, hospital administrators, and employers all assisted NPs in getting added to MCO panels. Medicaid waivers that include NPs as PCPs also help in getting MCOs to credential NPs. Patients may be the most important supporters for APNs in getting listed by MCOs as PCPs. Having patients write or call and request APNs as PCPs may be one of the most important steps to getting added to the list. A majority of the NPs agreed that persevering in the credentialing process is critical, even if the initial response is less then optimistic.

An issue that affected NPs in the Cohen et al (1998) study was the issue of reimbursement. There appear to be two sides to the issue of reimbursement. On the one hand, to get the highest percentage of reimbursement, bills need to be submitted in the physician's name. This practice increases an NP's cost-effectiveness as a provider. However, once again the NP is invisible because there is no record that the patient was seen by an APN. On the other hand, if the NP uses her or his own name for reimbursement, the practice revenue could potentially decrease. However, the APN would no longer be invisible and could track outcome data. This dilemma brings up the question of the rate of APN reimbursement when compared to the rate for physicians. Some NPs express the view that APNs can not afford to remain invisible and bill under the physician's name. This invisibility leads to loss of power and perhaps to the loss of PCP status on MCO provider panels. Research by APNs related to the above issues is critical. Studies similar to that by Cohen et al (1998) need to be conducted in other states to assess the extent of MCO involvement across the United States.

Research needs to evaluate the role of NPs in managed care and their contribution to health outcomes and quality. How do providers, patients, practitioners, and payers define quality care? The Agency for Health Care Quality and Research has defined *quality* in two ways: consumer ratings and clinical performance measures. Consumer

Table 6-6

Perceived Barriers to Being Listed a Primary Care Provider by a Managed Care Organization

	BARRIER	SPECIFIC INFORMATION
Nurse practioner	Lack of knowledge about MCO issues	Capitation and financial arrangements (how MCOs pay clinic or agency, how much the capitated payment is); little understanding of how bonus or withholds calculated or the implications of these arrangements on APNs
	Lack of interest in applying to be on MCO panels	More concerned about job security; "not my problem"; no desire to disturb status quo; apathy; satisfied with current arrangement
	Inability to articulate contributions to quality and cost-effectiveness	Lack of research related to outcomes of quality and cost-effectiveness; no documentation of the benefits to patients or MCO
	Lack of practice-based data	Most NPs unsure of how much revenue they generated for practice; identified need for NPs to have their own provider codes so all encounters are counted and therefore show how much money is generated
MCO	Resistance of MCOs to the use of NPs	Prevalence of the medical model; not recruiting or approving nonphysician providers
	Lack of understanding on the part of MCOs about credentialing	No idea that certification is similar to credentialing of physicians
Other	State practice acts	Some nurse practice acts act as barriers to MCO use and credentialing (may include physician collaboration or direction); issue of physician cosignature a turn-off to MCOs
	Hospital privileges	Lack of hospital privileges may be a barrier in getting credentialed; having them certainly a facilitator

Data from Cohen, S., Mason, D., Arsenie, L., Sargese, S., & Needham, D. (1998). Focus groups reveal perils and promise of managed care for nurse practitioners. *Nurse Practitioner, 23*(6), 48-77.

ratings look at health care from the consumer's point of view. Two ratings that measure consumer satisfaction are the Consumer Assessment of Health Plans (CAHPS) and the Health Plan Employer Data and Information Set (HEDIS) member satisfaction survey (which includes CAHPS questions). HEDIS is based on information such as medical records. These outcome measures may be helpful for APNs to use when performing self-evaluation of the care they provide. The measures may also be useful when researching the effectiveness of various nursing interventions. (These measures of quality are discussed further in Chapters 7 and 46.) Important questions to research related to patients and managed care include: Has the cost of health care been reduced or maintained? Do the patient outcomes equal the cost to provide them? What is a consumer's concept of health care and quality?

A number of research projects are being conducted by the Agency for Health Care Policy and Research. The Expansion of Quality of Care Measures (Q-SPAN) is a project designed to strengthen the scientific base of quality measurement. It also will expand the scope and availability of validated, ready-to-use measures. One of the projects is concentrating on a Global Quality Assessment Tool for Managed Care (QSPAN, 1998). APNs need to be aware

of the quality research outcomes and initiate research projects that validate and confirm the high quality of care that APNs deliver.

IMPLICATIONS FOR MSN EDUCATION AND ADVANCED PRACTICE

Students in graduate programs need to understand managed care and its potential long-term effects on health care delivery. Graduate education for APNs needs to focus specifically on the effects of managed care on advanced practice. This includes the number of patients seen, tests ordered, and prescriptions ordered, as well as how nursing at this level is practiced. Some NPs are not independent practitioners and must have a collaborative physician. The decisions that the physician collaborators make will affect the autonomy, income, and practice of the NPs. NP students need to carefully evaluate the process of interdependent practice; observations of how their preceptors interact with other care providers are important pieces in forming their own practice model (Doheny, Cook, &

Suggestions for Further Learning

- Go to the Agency for Health Care Policy and Research website at www.ahcpr.gov. Look at the information available to help patients choose a quality health care plan. How helpful would it be for a person who wanted to know what to look for when choosing both a health plan and a provider? Is this information supportive of APNs as PCPs?

- Read the article: Light, D. (1999). Good managed care needs universal health insurance. *American College of Physicians–American Society of Internal Medicine, 130,* 686-689. The author makes the point that to have good clinically managed care, one needs four elements: continuity of care, stable teams to develop and deliver integrated care programs, a patient population that remains in place long enough to develop a working relationship with providers, and health insurance coverage that does not change or evaporate for the entire population. He feels that the health insurance coverage supports the other three. Do you agree with his view? Why or why not?

- Go to the Effective Medical Practice and Managed Care Site at www.acponline.org/mgdcare/emptest.htm. Each month this site poses two questions that pertain to primary care in a managed care environment. A critique follows each question so that your responses can be compared to the experts.

- Find the article: Ground rules for dealing with health care plans. (1999, February). *Family Practice Management.* Available online at www.aafp.org/fpm. What guides does it give related to dealing with MCOs? These guidelines are meant to serve as the basics for interacting with health care plans. Do they have relevance for APNs?

- Look for the following resources for more information:
  - The American Association of Health Plans (AAHP) has a standard application that it encourages health plans to use for credentialing. Examine this form so you will know what is expected when you apply to become part of a MCO's provider panel. This is available at www.aahp.org.
  - Medicare Compare, available at medicare.gov/comparision, is an interactive database with detailed options on Medicare's health plan options.
  - "How to Choose a Health Plan and Straight Talk about Health Plans" is available free from the American Association of Health Plans at www.aahp.org.
  - The Health Insurance Association of America offers a "Guide to Health Insurance" at www.hiaa.org.
  - The National Committee for Quality Assurance Publications Center offers information on finding quality in health plans at www.ncqa.org.
  - The American Accreditation Health Care Commission (also known as URAC) develops accreditation standards and programs for managed care addressing five general areas: network management, utilization management, quality management, credentialing, and member participation and protection. It may be accessed at urac.org.
  - The American Association of Retired Persons (AARP) has information on how to get the most from your managed care plan. It is available at aarp.org.
  - Health Pages offers information on choosing managed care and may be accessed at www.thehealthpages.com/armanag.html.
  - Families USA offers information related to managed care at www.familiesusa.org/managedcare.

Stopper, 1997). APN students should learn about the credentialing and privileging process and begin collecting data about their effectiveness. Even data collected as a student will provide some indication of levels of care and quality.

Morrison (2000) gives some predictions of how physician roles will change to address the changes in the health delivery system. He predicts that physicians will need to be clinical data collectors, healers, heath advisors and coaches, knowledge navigators, proceduralists, diagnosticians, managers, and quality assurance specialists in order to survive in the future. Morrison recommends that physicians develop a future that moves beyond the "good old days." These roles sound similar to those currently held or recommended to APNs. The majority of APNs have received their education in the last 10 years; so most of them do not have the "good old days" mentality. In fact, these new roles sound suspiciously like the roles nursing has occupied for years. APNs should look at future roles for

nursing and set the pace for innovation. This innovation will help organize and lead future changes in health care delivery.

The Cohen et al (1998) study gives several messages for APN practice. The good news is the sense by NPs in the focus groups that they can carry on in the manner they had in the past when faced with opposition and challenge. They describe ways to get around the system and get the best they could for their patients. However, while using past techniques may be helpful in day-to-day work, the issue of becoming involved with needed policy changes cannot be ignored. It will be critical for APNs to be involved in collective or organized action. Organized groups need to raise consciousness about issues of APN credentialing. The past involvement of APNs in legislative and policy issues is not sufficient in this era of managed care. Cohen et al (1998) recommend that APNs continue their efforts to reshape policies related to APNs and MCOs.

Questions related to ethical and legal implications of

MCOs need to be answered. For example, if an NP sees a patient but the physician is required to sign the chart, who is legally accountable? What about when an APN seeing a patient means that the MCO can not be billed? What if the APN writes a prescription that will not be reimbursed because it is not cosigned by a physician? Issues similar to these come up on a daily basis, and APNs need to decide how to legally and ethically address them.

Based on the research by Martin and Hutchinson (1997) APNs need to work toward gaining "symbolic space." The successful negotiation of symbolic space means "NP acceptance as PCPs, including the ability to practice independently in a collaborative role with physicians, unencumbered by discounting and the constant struggle for acceptance and recognition." Ways that APNs can begin to negotiate symbolic space include establishing role responsibilities and role boundaries. This may mean negotiating the role in every setting, depending on with whom they interact. The gaining of symbolic space occurs over time. Factors such as respecting self and others, acknowledgment of professional limitations, recognizing gender influences on the APN role, collegial support, and displaying consistent knowledge and skills assist in gaining symbolic space. Strategies that APNs use to gain symbolic space include cultivation of connections between NPs and others, bargaining for financial equity, confrontation in conflict situations, and disengaging from highly frustrating situations (Martin & Hutchinson, 1997).

Simpson (1997) feels that managed care is a prime opportunity for nursing and APNs to demonstrate the value of the nursing approach: longitudinal care, patient education, prevention of problems, and a holistic family approach. APNs need to take a strong position on how MCOs should be organized and managed. Simpson feels that information systems will be an important part of this vision. APNs need to utilize advanced information systems to track patient care, incorporate patient education, and quantify outcomes. Rather than fighting managed care, APNs need to embrace the opportunities and make them work for the advancement of the profession.

DISCUSSION QUESTIONS

These questions can be used to promote critical thinking and encourage discussion.

1. What is the possible effect of managed care on society?
2. Discuss how influential managed care will be on health care for the underinsured and noninsured. What effect do you think managed care will have on the development of social policies for older adults and the poor?

3. Can a balance exist between cost-containment and managed care so that Americans receive appropriate health care at a reasonable cost? Why or why not?
4. What is your sense of the quality of managed care in the United States today? Evaluate the care you have seen provided in acute care settings for you or your family members. How would you rate it?
5. What strategies did you use to cultivate your "symbolic space"? What strategies were successful or unsuccessful for you, and under what conditions? Self reflection can actually help promote or contribute to the acquisition of symbolic space.

REFERENCES/BIBLIOGRAPHY

Alpha Center (1998, April). *A tale of two cities: hospital mergers in St. Louis and Philadelphia not reducing excess capacity* (Health Care Financing and Organization findings brief).

American College of Physicians–American Society of Internal Medicine (2000). *Primary care in managed care.* Available online at www.acponline.org/mgdcare/primary.htm.

Archibald, P., & Bainbridge, D. (1994). Capacity and competence: nurse credentialing and privileging. *Nursing Management, 25*(4), 49-56.

Aymond, R. (1999, September). 22 tips for improving your practice. *Family Practice Management.* Available online at www.aafp.org/fpm/990900fm/20.html.

Baker, S. (1998). Improving service and increasing patient satisfaction. *Family Practice Management, 5*(7). Available online at www.aafp.org/fpm.

Bindman, A., Grumbach, K., Vranizan, K., Jaffe, D., & Osmond, D. (1998). Selection and exclusion of primary care physicians by managed care organizations. *Journal of the American, 279,* 675-679.

Blum, J. (1994). The evolution of physician credentialing into managed care selective contracting. *American Journal of Law and Medicine, 12*(2&3), 173-203.

Blumenthal, D. (1996). Effects of market reforms on doctors and their patients. *Health Affairs, 15,* 170-184.

Brook, R., Kamber, C., Lohr, K., Goldberg, G., Keeler, E., & Newhouse, J. (1990). Quality of ambulatory care for fee for service and prepaid patients. *Annuals of Internal Medicine, 115.*

Brown, R., & Biancolillo, K. (1996). The integral role of nursing in managed care. *Nursing Management, 27*(4), 22-24.

Buerhaus, P. (1994). Economics of managed competition and consequences to nurses: part 1. *Nursing Economics, 12*(1), 10-17.

Buppert, C. (1995). Justifying nurse practitioner existence: hard facts to hard figures. *Nurse Practitioner, 20,* 43-48.

Buppert, C. (1999). *Nurse practitioner's business practice and legal guide.* Gaithersburg, MD: Aspen Publishers.

Catalano, J.T. (1996). *Contemporary professional nursing.* Philadelphia: FA Davis.

Cohen, S., & Juszcak, L. (1997). Promoting the nurse practitioner role in managed care. *Journal of Pediatric Healthcare, 9*(3), 3-11.

Cohen, S., Mason, D., Arsenie, L., Sargese, S., & Needham, D. (1998). Focus groups reveal perils and promise of managed care for nurse practitioners. *Nurse Practitioner, 23*(6), 48-77.

Conway-Welch, C., & Harshman-Green, A. (1995). At the table: nursing in managed care. *Nursing Policy Forum, 1*(5), 11-16.

Cook, J., Ingersoll, G., & Spitzer, R. (1999). Managed care research, part 1. *Journal of Nursing Administration.* 29(11), 23-30.

Cunningham, P., Grossman, J., St. Peter, R., & Lesser, C. (1999). Managed care and physician's provision of charity care. *Journal of the American Medical Association, 281*(12),1087-1092.

Curtin, L. (1997). Managed care pure and simple. *Nursing Management, 28*(3), 7-8.

Davis, K. (1990). *Health care cost containment.* Baltimore, MD: Johns Hopkins University Press.

Dial, T., Palsbo, S., & Bergsten, C. (1995). Clinical staffing in staff and group model HMOs. *Health Affairs, 14*(2), 168-180.

Doheny, M.O., Cook, C.B., & Stopper, M.C. (1997). *The discipline of nursing* (4th ed.). Stamford, CT: Appleton & Lange.

Emanuel, E., & Dubler, N. (1995). Preserving the physician-patient relationship in the era of managed care. *Journal of the American Medical Association, 25*(1), 35-38.

Expansion of Quality of Care Measures (QSPAN) (1998). *Agency for health care policy and research.* Rockville, MD. Accessed on January 12, 1998 at www.ahrq.gov/qual/qspanovr.htm.

Fagin, C. (1987). The visible problem of an "invisible" profession. *Inquiry, 24,* 19-26.

Feldstein, P. (1994). *Health policy issues: an economic perspective on health reform.* Ann Arbor, MI: Alpha/Health Administration Press.

Felt-Lisk, S. (1996). How HMOs structure primary care delivery. *Managed Care Quarterly, 4*(4), 96-105.

Fiesta, J. (1997). Managed care liability update. *Nursing Management, 28*(3), 20-22.

Finger, A. (1999, December 20). Caring for the uninsured: how America's doctors are making a difference, *Medical Economics.* Available online at www.pdr.net/memag/public.htm?path=docs/122099/article1.html.

Finger, A. (1999, December 20). Caring for the uninsured: will the problem ever be solved? *Medical Economics.* Available online at www.pdr.net/memag/public.htm?path=docs/122099/article2.html.

Flanagan, L. (1997). Keys to success in Medicaid managed care. *Family Practice Management, 4*(2). Available online at www.aafp.org/fpm.

Flarey, D. (1997). Managed care: changing the way we practice. *Journal of Nursing Administration, 27*(7/8), 16-20.

Fletcher, R. (1999). Who is responsible for the common good in a competitive market? *Journal of the American Medical Association, 281*(12).

Frary, T. (1998). Managed health care and rural America. *Journal of the American Association of Physician Assistants, 11*(9), 43-49.

Georges, C., & McGinley, L. (1997, June 30). Primer on how the Medicare overhaul is shaping up. *Wall Street Journal,* A16.

Ginzberg, E., & Ostow, M. (1997). Managed care—a look back and a look ahead. *New England Journal of Medicine, 336,* 1018-1020.

Gleason, S., Sokolov, J., & Henshaw, C. (1998). Provider sponsored organizations: a golden opportunity in Medicare managed care. *Family Practice Management, 5*(3). Available online at www.aafp.org/fmp.

Gold, M., Hurley, R., & Lake, T. (1995). A national survey of the arrangements managed care plans make with physicians. *New England Journal of Medicine, 333,* 1678-1683.

Goldberg, J. (2000, May 22). Group practice economics: is primary care paying its way? *Medical Economics.* Available online at www.pdr.net/memag/public.htm?path=docs/article1.html.

Ground rules for dealing with health care plans. (1999). *Family Practice Management, 6*(2). Available online at www.aafp.org/fpm.

Guanowsky, G. (1995). Liability in managed care for the health care provider. *Nursing Management, 26*(10), 24.

Hall, J., Palmer, H., & Orav, E. (1990). Performance quality, gender, and professonal role: a study of physicians and non-physicians in 16 ambulatory care practices. *Medical Care, 28,* 489-501.

Haven, D., & Evans, E. (1995). A future for nurse practitioners in managed care. *Journal of Pediatric Healthcare, 9*(3), 88-91.

Havens, D., Ronan, J., & Hannan, C. (1996). Maintaining the nurse practitioner identity in a world of managed care. *Journal of Pediatric Healthcare, 10,* 86-88.

Hicks, L., Stallmeyer, J., & Coleman, J. (1992). Nursing challenges in managed care. *Nursing Economics, 10,* 265-276.

Hoffman, C. (1994). Medicaid payment for nonphysician practitioners: an access issue. *Health Affairs, 13*(4), 140-152.

Hornrook, M., & Berki, S. (1985). Practice mode and payment method: effects on use, costs, quality and access. *Medical Care, 23,* 484-511.

Hughes, E. (1994). Foreword. In D. Nash (Ed.), *The physician's guide to managed care.* Gaithersburg, MD: Aspen Publishers.

Iglehart, J.K. (1994). In P. Lee & C.L. Estes (Eds.), *The nation's health* (4th ed.). Boston: Jones and Bartlett Publishers.

Jones, W. (2000). Economics and delivery: health in 2025. *Health Forum Journal, 43*(1). Available online at www.healthforum.com.

Kerekes, J., Jenkins, M., & Torrisi, D. (1996). Nursing managed primary care. *Nursing Management, 27*(2), 44-48.

Kletke, P., Emmons, D., & Gillis, K. (1996). Current trends in physicians' practice arrangements: from owners to employees. *Journal of the American Medical Association, 276,* 555-560.

Kongstvedt, P. (1995). *Essentials of managed care.* Gaithesburg, MD: Aspen Publishers.

Kraus, N. (1991). *The interstudy edge: managed care: a decade in review 1980-1990.* Excelsior, MN: Interstudy.

LaPuma, J., & Schiedermayer, D. (1994) Ethical issues in managed care and managed competition: problems and promises. In D. Nash (Ed.), *The physician's guide to managed care.* Gaithersburg, MD: Aspen Publishers.

Larkin, G. (1999). Ethical issues of managed care. *Emergency Medicine Clinics of North America, 17*(2), 397-415.

Loewy, E., & Loewy, R. (1998). Ethics and managed care: reconstructing a system and refashioning a society. *Archives of Internal Medicine, 158*(22). Available online at archinte.ama-assn.org/issues/v158n22/full/ilt80612.html.

Loewy, E., & Loewy, R. (1999). Ethics and managed care can coexist with a free market. *Archives of Internal Medicine, 159*(12). Available online at archinte.ama-assn.org/issues/v159n12/full/ilt0628-6.html.

Long, S., & Marquis, S. (1999). Geographic variation in physician visits for uninsured children. *Journal of the American Medical Association, 281*(21), 2035-2040.

Long, S., Marquis, M., & Rodgers, J. (1998). Do people shift their use of health services over time to take advantage of insurance? *Journal of Health Economics, 17,* 105-115.

Martin, P., & Hutchinson, S. (1997). Negotiating symbolic space: strategies to increase NP status and value. *Nurse Practitioner, 22*(1), 89-102.

Moore, K., & Coddington, D. (1999). The next wave of infusion. *Health Forum Journal.* Available online at www.healthforum journal.com/asp/ArticleDisplay.asp?PubID=7&ArticleID=559.

Morrison, I. (2000). The future of physicians' time. *Annals of Internal Medicine, 132*(1): 800-884.

Moscovice, L. (1998). Expanding rural managed care: enrollment patterns and prospectives. *Health Affairs, 17* (1), 172-179.

Mundinger, M. (2000, first quarter). Now and future primary care. *Reflections on Nursing Leadership,* 12-14.

Murray, J., Greenfield, S., Kaplan, S., & Yano, E. (1992). Ambulatory testing for capitation and fee for service patients in the same practice setting: relationship to outcome. *Medical Care, 30,* 252-261.

Nash, D. (1994). *The physician's guide to managed care.* Gaithersburg, MD: Aspen Publishers.

Newacheck, P., Stoddard, J., Hughes, D., & Pearl, M. (1998). Health insurance and access to primary care. *New England Journal of Medicine, 338,* 513-519..

Nichols, L. (1992). Estimating costs of underusing advanced practice nurses. *Nursing Economics, 10,* 343-45, 348-351.

Parrish, M. (2000, January 24). The California nightmare: is this where managed care is taking us? *Medical Economics.* Available online at www.pdr.net/memag/public.htm?path=docs/012400/artiacle5.html.

Pennachio, D. (1995). The midlevel provider: colleague or competitor? *Patient Care, 29*(1), 20-37.

Priester, R. (1997). Does managed care offer value to society? *Managed Care Quarterly, 5*(1), 57-63.

Reres, M. (1996). *Managed care: managing the process.* Glencoe, MO: National Professional Education Institute.

Robinson, J. (1998). Consolidation of medical groups into physician practice. *Journal of the American Medical Association, 279,* 555-560.

Rustia, J., & Bartek, J. (1997). Managed care credentialing of advanced practice nurses. *Nurse Practitioner 22*(9), 90, 92, 99-103.

Sekscenski, E., Sansom, S., & Bazell, C. (1994). State practice environments and the supply of physician assistants, nurse practitioners, and certified nurse midwives, *New England Journal of Medicine, 331,* 1266-1271.

Serb, C. (1999, December 1). Branding: the key to luring new customers. *Hospitals and Health Networks.* Available online at healthforumprod.gcnpublishing.com/hhn/doc16188.htm.

Shi, K., & Singh, D.A. (1998). *Delivering health care in America: a systems approach.* Gaithersburg, MD: Aspen Publishers.

Simpson, R. (1997). Take advantage of managed care opportunities. *Nursing Management, 28*(3), 24-25.

Spicer, J. (1998). Coping with managed care's administrative hassles. *Family Practice Management, 5*(3). Available online at www.aafp.org/fpm.

Stahl, D. (1995). Managed care credentialing. *Nursing Management, 26*(6), 18, 20.

Swansburg R., & Swansburg, R. (1999). *Introductory management and leadership for nurses.* Sudbury, MA: Jones and Bartlett.

Terry, K. (2000, May 22). Discounted Medicare: it's already here. *Medical Ecnomics.* Available online at www.pdr.net/memag/public.htm?path=docs/article2.html.

Terry, K. (2000, April 10). Managed care 2000: where's managed care headed? *Medical Economics.* Available online at www.pdr.net/memag/public.htm?path=docs/041000/article1.html.

Tottenham, T., Wilson, R., & Jewell, C. (1998). Leveling the playing field? The nation's first managed care liability law. *Journal of Health Hospital Law, 31,* 14-22.

Udvarhelyi, I., Jennison, K., Phillips, R., & Epstein, A. (1991). Comparison of the quality of ambulatory care for fee for service and prepaid patients. *Annals of Internal Medicine, 115,* 394-400.

Vinn, N. (2000). The emergence of consumer driven health care. *Family Practice Management, 7*(1). Available online at www.aafp.org/fpm.

Warren, M., Weitz, R., & Kulis, S. (1999). The impact of managed care on physicians. *Health Care Management Review, 24*(2), 44-56.

Weber, D. (1997, September/October). The empowered consumer. *Health Forum Journal.*

Weiner, J., Steinwachs, D., & Williams, J. (1986). Nurse practitioner and physician assistant practices in three HMOs: implications for future US health manpower needs. *American Journal of Public Health, 76*(5), 507-511.

Welch, W., Hillmna, A., & Pauly, M. (1990). Toward new typologies for HMOs. *Millbank Quarterly, 68,* 221-243.

World Health Organization (2000). *France rated no. 1 in health care.* Available online at news.excite.com/news/ap/000621/01/news-best-health-systems.

Yelin, E., Shearn, M.A., & Epstein, W. (1986). Health outcomes for a chronic disease in prepaid group practice and fee for service settings: the case of rheumatoid arthritis. *Medical Care, 24,* 236-247.

Chapter 7

Quality Management: Implications for Nursing

Patricia M. Gray, Margaret M. Anderson, & Denise Robinson

Cost, access, and quality are considered the three cornerstones on which health care delivery is built. Cost and access have held center stage for many years, primarily because it has been difficult to define and measure quality. However, members of the health care community are increasingly interested in the concept of quality because of concerns that the focus on cost may have had a negative effect on quality. Each stakeholder in the process has a differing idea of quality, and patients, payers, and providers all define quality differently, introducing differing expectations and thus differing ways to evaluate the concept (McGlynn, 1997). The Institute of Medicine (IOM) has defined *quality* as the "degree to which health services for individuals and populations increase the likelihood of desired health outcomes and are consistent with current professional knowledge" (McGlynn, 1997). This definition implies that quality performance is measured on a continuum; that quality performance focuses on health care services; that quality may be measured from a variety of viewpoints, focusing on health outcomes and with the goal to improve them; and that professional consensus can be used to determine the definition and measurement of quality since scientific evidence is lacking. The IOM definition does not address either cost or access, both critical issues, particularly when the United States does not have universal access to basic health care.

High quality can be achieved when care is provided in an efficient, cost-effective, and accessible manner (Al-Assaf, 1993a, 1993b). All health professionals want to provide clients with the highest quality health care. However, they are faced with questions concerning how to achieve desired levels of quality care and continuously improve services without it becoming cost prohibitive. Shi and Singh (1998) propose looking at the issue of quality from both a micro and macro view. The micro view focuses on services at the point of delivery and their subsequent effects. It is associated with the performance of individual providers and health care organizations. The macro view looks at quality in terms of affecting the population. It reflects the performance of the entire health care delivery system.

The micro view of quality includes the clinical aspects of care delivery, the interpersonal aspects of care delivery, and the quality of life (Shi & Singh, 1998). Clinical aspects of care deal with technical quality, including where the care is delivered, qualifications of the caregivers, cost, efficiency of care, and the end results on patients' health. From the patient's perspective, quality must also include the various interpersonal relationships. Things such as caring, personal attention, time spent with a patient, and the demeanor of the provider all influence the patient's perception of the interaction. All people within an organization have an effect: the person who answers the phone, the nursing personnel, the housekeeper, and the provider. The quality of life aspect is particularly important when more people are living longer, but with more chronic illnesses and declining health.

The macro view encompasses systemwide effects on quality, including the concepts of quality assurance (QA) and quality assessment. Because it applies to the entire health care delivery system, it is the focus of most of research and development.

DEFINITIONS

Quality is a combination of product features with a freedom from deficiencies, as defined by the customer (Juran, 1989). This definition, while not in opposition to the definition proposed by the IOM, is certainly more "businesslike." ***Quality assessment*** is the measurement of quality against an established standard (Shi and Singh, 1998).

Quality assurance is the process of establishing a target degree of excellence for nursing interventions and taking action to ensure that each patient receives the agreed-upon level of care (Gillies, 1994). QA is a step beyond quality assessment because the process does not stop just with comparison against the established standard; steps are taken to make changes to improve the quality of the process.

There are those that believe QA and quality improvement (QI) are one and the same. QI is similar to QA but with the addition of institutionalizing quality through ongoing assessment and using the results of the assessment to improve a variety of processes. **Outcomes** are the final effects or results of the health delivery process. Many people believe outcomes are the bottom-line measure of the effectiveness of the health care delivery system (McGlynn & Brook, 1996).

Continuous quality improvement (CQI) is an ongoing process of innovation, prevention of error, and staff development that is used by corporations and institutions who adopt the quality management philosophy (Wendt & Vale, 1995). **Quality improvement** is a way of continuously examining processes and making them more effective (Coleman & Endsley, 1999). QI is used today by most health care organizations to decrease costs, increase productivity, improve processes, decrease waste, and increase efficiency. It involves changing the corporate culture, including "customers" in problem-solving, training and involving all employees in its methodology, and requiring committed organizational leadership. Because it is a new way of doing business, it takes much work and time— approximately 5 to 10 years (Schaffner, 1997)—to change a health care organization and its members into dedicated QI proponents. For many nurses, the words *quality improvement* means extra work and a way to identify the people who are not during their job. However, QI can be more rewarding and positive than most nurses realize. QI can help to empower advanced practice nurses (APNs) and others to strive for quality; it will hopefully energize the process and help decrease inefficiencies, while boosting the satisfaction of everyone, including patients (Coleman & Endsley, 1999).

Total quality management (TQM) is an integrative management philosophy that involves cultural change and a commitment to quality from all employees, with the goal of continuously improving the quality of delivered goods and services through the participation of all levels and functions of the organization. (Table 7-1 provides a summary of all of these terms of quality.)

It is important to differentiate between QA, CQI, and TQM. QA monitors care through indicators to identify improvement opportunities. CQI "builds on quality assurance methods by emphasizing the organization and focuses on processes . . . data driven analysis and decisions" (Lancaster, 1999). TQM is a total management system that achieves total quality by focusing on employee empowerment and customer satisfaction. Improved revenues and reduced costs result from becoming a TQM organization (Lancaster, 1999). (Table 7-2 summarizes the differences between QA and CQI.)

Donabedian (1980) developed a model to define and

Table 7-1

Terms and Definitions

TERM	DEFINITION
Quality	Services that are free from deficiencies and meet customer needs
Quality assurance (QA)	Monitoring of care provided through measurement of indicators (level and incidence) to identify necessary improvements
Continuous quality improvement (CQI)	Building upon QA methods by emphasizing the organization; focus on processes (not individuals); customer-focused; requires that analysis and decisions be data driven
Total quality management (TQM)	Management system to achieve total quality as evidence by satisfied customers, empowered employees, reduced costs, and higher revenues

From Lancaster, J. (1999). *Nursing issues in leading and managing change.* St. Louis: Mosby.

assess quality care in health care organizations using a structure, process, and outcomes framework. Later the model was applied to most of the programs or services a patient might encounter. It was a guide to measuring quality care to the extent it could be evaluated. **Donabedian's model** (Shi & Singh, 1998) focused on evaluating the domains of structure, process, and outcomes as a way to evaluate the quality of the care provided. **Structure** evaluations focused on the physical aspects of the program or service, such as the setting of the program, the adequacy of equipment, organizational components, and appropriate qualifications of staff presenting the program. The goal was to compare the structure of the program with the program objectives for consistency and adequacy. Appropriate structure should support the program or service to meet the objectives of the project.

Process is the actual delivery of the services in terms of quality of the service, number or quantity of services available to meet program goals, and types of service offered. In medical care, process indicators of waiting time, appropriateness of diagnostic tests, and application of diagnostic reasoning are evaluated.

As previously mentioned, outcomes are the results of a program or service. Did the patient benefit from the care, service, or program provided? Did the program or service

Table 7-2

Differences between Quality Assurance and Continuous Quality Improvement

QUALITY ASSURANCE	CONTINUOUS QUALITY IMPROVEMENT
Uses external determinants	Uses internal determinants
Detects errors and deficiencies	Determines requirements and expectations
Fixes blame and responsibility	Identifies process improvement opportunities
Uses postevent investigation	Focuses on prevention
QA department responsible	All members in organization responsible
Inspires fear	Inspires hope and energy

From Lancaster, J. (1999). *Nursing issues in leading and managing change.* St. Louis: Mosby.

produce the desired results? Were the outcomes the ones anticipated during program development and design? The structure, process, and outcome evaluation process is similar to the research process and the nursing process. (Lancaster, 1999; Shi & Singh, 1998)

Managed care has initiated a **quality report card** from health provider organizations. The report card serves to indicate how well an organization does at meeting the quality indicators assigned. The best known of these report cards is the HEDIS. This report card is the result of a collaborative effort among insurers, employers, and the National Committee for Quality Assurance. The report card contains 71 indicators of performance for a plan covering eight areas of concern for quality care. The same criteria, data collection methods, and definitions are used to collect information for commercial, Medicare, and Medicaid members (Shi and Singh, 1998). (This topic is discussed further in Chapter 45.)

The Health Care Financing Administration (HCFA) requires a QA review on an annual basis for Medicare-certified facilities. This review is an assessment of how well the facility meets the standards established for certification. HCFA assumes that the agency meeting the standards provides quality care. Shi and Singh (1998) believe this is a form of quality monitoring rather than QA. These authors equate QA with QI, and quality assessment is defined as "the measurement of quality against an established standard." An agency not meeting the standards established by HCFA faces stiff penalties and possible loss of certification. In many agencies, meeting these standards is a paper trail rather than real movement toward the improvement of patient care.

The **Henry Ford Balance Sheet** is another effort made to assess and balance quality outcomes with financial risks and responsibilities (Henry Ford Health System, 1995). The Henry Ford Balance Sheet has a series of qualitative and quantitative criteria that are rated for achievement. Obviously, the standard is to look for balance between qualitative and quantitative goals. This is a good method for countering the notion of finances as the whole measure of quality performance.

Benchmarking is a newer concept for quality evaluation that is based on the comparison of an organization deemed "great" at what it does and an organization making an effort to improve. Benchmarks are targets in the industry that all others may want to achieve. Lancaster (1999) defines benchmark as the "overall performance of an individual or organization that is judged to represent the best achievable standard for a product or service." A **world class benchmark** is "a comparison from outside the industry . . . usually in administrative and business processes," and **competitive benchmarks** are "comparisons derived from inside the health care industry" (Lancaster, 1999). The organization wanting to benchmark itself selects other organizations with which to compare, based on selected criteria. The criteria may include similarities in type of health care system, number of beds, payer mix, service or product lines, culture, and inner city versus rural location. The organizations chosen as the benchmark institutions may not know they are considered benchmarks. Data is collected by the organization hoping to improve, then compared with their current situation. Plans are then made to make changes to reach the benchmarks. This is usually a long process, but goals are established and planning is always focused toward the goals (Lancaster, 1999). For example, federally funded community health agencies are compared against one another. The data is published by region and nationally, giving community health centers (CHCs) data for the same type of agencies around the United States. Each agency can then compare how well they do in comparison to other similar agencies. Because CHCs are so different from private organizations, comparison with them is invalid.

CRITICAL ISSUES: IMPLEMENTING QUALITY MANAGEMENT IN THE HEALTH CARE DELIVERY SYSTEM

The quality movement began after World War II when Dr. W. Edwards Deming and Dr. J.M. Juran, two engineers, were invited to Japan to assist in their postwar development, using statistical process control methods (Juran, 1989; Walton, 1986). During World War II, Japan's manufacturing plants had been destroyed, severely hampering the nation's ability to compete in world markets. American manufacturers rebuffed Juran and Deming, so

Table 7-3

Comparisons among Quality Management Approaches

CROSBY (14-STEP QUALITY IMPROVEMENT PROCESS)	DEMING (14 POINTS OF MANAGEMENT)	JURAN (UNTITLED)
1. Management commitment	1. Maintain constancy of purpose (i.e., have a vision)	1. Quality triology: • Quality planning (meeting consumer needs) • Quality control (measurement) • Quality improvement (change)
2. Improvement teams	2. Adopt a new philosophy	2. Broad operational perspective
3. Quality measurement	3. Cease dependence on inspection	3. Focus on external and internal customers expectations and targets
4. Cost of quality evaluation	4. Award business contracts on various factors, not just price	4. Institutionwide planning and strategy development
5. Quality awareness	5. Improve continuously	5. Employee involvement
6. Corrective action	6. On-the-job training	6. Group problem-solving
7. Zero-defects planning committee	7. Leadership for system improvement	
8. Supervisory training	8. Drive out fear	
9. Zero defects day	9. Break down departmental and program barriers	
10. Goal setting	10. Eliminate arbitrary quotas and slogans without resources	
11. Error/cause removal	11. Cease numerical quotas	
12. Recognition	12. Remove barriers to "pride of workmanship"	
13. Quality council	13. Educate everyone	
14. Do it all over again	14. Transform all jobs and the organization	

From Lancaster, J. (1999). *Nursing issues in leading and managing change.* St. Louis: Mosby.

they were pleased to go to Japan to assist in the rebuilding. During the late 1940s and 1950s, goods manufactured in Japan were considered poor in quality. They were poorly constructed and did not last when used (Walton, 1986). After Deming and Juran went to Japan, the quality of Japanese products soared. Japanese products were in great demand around the world by the late 1960s. The goods, including high-tech devices, cars, toys, and many other common consumer products, were well made, durable, reasonably priced, and attractive. The postwar economy boomed in Japan.

The quality movement in the United States was delayed until 1980, when competition from Japan's manufacturing industries threatened the American economy. Soon, both Deming and Juran were solicited to work with industries in the United States to improve the quality of their products.

Innovators in Total Quality Management

Philip Crosby was a student of TQM and refined and modified the principles espoused by Deming and Juran. (Table 7-3 compares these experts' TQM processes.)

TQM is a management philosophy as well as a method of QI. It must start with the chief executive officers and vice presidents and trickle down to the employees. In other words, quality must permeate everything the organization is and does. While employee training is necessary to implement TQM, it must first be demonstrated at the highest administrative levels. TQM is a philosophy in which employees know how to make improvements in the production of goods and services and want to do a good job and be proud of their work. In TQM, the employees are the most important resource in the organization; listening to them and their ideas results in a better product. The philosophy is as important as the processes of improvement utilized. Cost control (and therefore increased profit) is a byproduct of the TQM process and philosophy, but it is not the primary reason for instituting TQM; QI as a product of process improvement is the main goal (Juran, 1989; Walton, 1986). A TQM organization is committed to ongoing improvement, and the process does not stop after the problem area is fixed. The goal is not static, and higher goals can be set if the previous ones are obtained. A TQM organization is customer driven, directing all efforts toward customer satisfaction. *Customer* refers to both internal and external customers of an organization. For example, a pharmacy has both external customers (the community) and internal customers (hospital units or nurses). Both internal and external customers need to be satisfied, and both are critical to the success of an organization.

Juran (1989) identifies a trilogy of processes necessary for a quality management organization: quality planning, quality control, and QI. He recommends changing the corporate culture of an organization to one that advocates

Table **7-4**

Deming's 14-Point Philosophy of Management

DEMING'S POINT	EXPLANATION
Create constancy of purpose for service improvement.	Leadership is responsible for setting the vision and improvement goals for an organization.
Adopt the new philosophy.	All employees must be intolerant of poor workmanship. Everyone must strive to do his or her job right the first time.
Cease dependence on inspection to achieve quality.	Do not rely on a measurement of performance that falls below a predetermined level. Build in measures that will allow changes in the process.
End the practice of awarding business based on price alone.	Low prices frequently mean poor quality. Partnerships should be formed with suppliers for long-term relationships that will ensure quality products.
Constantly improve every process for planning, production, and service.	Improvement is continuous. Everyone in an organization must be familiar with the improvement process and allowed to use it.
Institute training on the job.	For employees to do their jobs correctly and effectively, trained preceptors must teach them.
Adopt and institute leadership.	Managers must adopt leadership skills that will assist people to do their jobs. Management is responsible for improving the systems and processes within which employees work.
Drive out fear.	Workers must not be afraid to make suggestions for improvement. When an organization's culture does not support suggestions from employees, the organization loses valuable insight into process improvement.
Break down barriers among staff.	Typically, organizational sections and departments have goal conflicts that prevent them from working together. These barriers must be lowered and common goals established for crossfunctional processes to be improved.
Eliminate slogans, exhortations, and targets for the workforce.	Arbitrary goals and slogans assume that employees are not doing a good job and make no difference in improving performance.
Eliminate numerical quotas for the workforce and numerical goals for management.	When emphasis is placed on numerical goals and quotas, quality is sacrificed. People will focus on achieving the numerical goal with little regard to quality of service or product.
Remove barriers that rob people of pride of workmanship.	Sometimes it is impossible for people to do their jobs effectively because of faulty or missing equipment, defective materials, and unwieldy processes.
Institute a vigorous program of education and self-improvement for everyone.	All employees must be educated in the new methods of statistical techniques and the improvement process. The organization should support employee learning and development outside the institution.
Put everyone in the company to work in accomplishing the transformation.	It will take a team effort to accomplish organizational transformation. Leaders must determine the vision of quality and set the course to accomplish it, while employees must understand and use the quality process. Neither group can succeed by itself.

and values QI, a culture led by quality leaders. Deming's 14 points (1986) identify a quality philosophy that requires changes in management style and helps to empower employees (Table 7-4). (Table 7-5 shows a comparison of these conceptual differences.)

Quality Evaluation and the Health Care Delivery System

QA departments once shouldered the burden of ensuring quality for health institutions. The evolution from a focus on quality control and QA to one of QI in health care occurred as a result of increasing health care costs, third-party payer involvement, increased competition, consumer demands, improved technology, and requirements by regulatory agencies. It was not until the late 1980s that health care found itself in a similar situation to the American manufacturing industries earlier in the decade; health care providers increased price to cover cost without controlling quality. Health care was in crisis and chaos (Walton, 1990). The cost of health care was escalating at an alarming rate, and third-party payers were pressuring health care providers to do more for less money. Emphasis was placed on shortening the patient's length of stay, and

Table 7-5

Conceptual Differences of Quality Management Experts

CONCEPT	DEMING	CROSBY	JURAN
Definition and measurement of quality	Definition of quality deals with predicting uniformity of the product (conformance to standards), largely established by use of statistical process methods; incorporates customers through the concept of extended process; calls for deriving the dollar value of concerns such as customer dissatisfaction.	Definition of quality based on conformance to customer need–based requirements; specifies a zero–defects standard in meeting these set requirements; measures quality by way of costing the lack of quality.	Defines quality by the fitness of services for their intended use in meeting customer expectations; Juran's is the most explicitly customer-focused approach to quality; also calls for incorporating the quantification of "reducing production costs" in delivering services and increasing revenue.
Management commitment	Deming's first and second points define the tasks of management; indeed, all of the articulated points are aimed at management, implying the necessity for its undivided attention toward creating a total quality system.	Crosby's first point deals explicitly with management commitment; stresses the importance of communication, understanding, and commitment; most focused on creation of a quality culture.	Quality planning, control and improvement process seeks management support at all levels; a project approach to improvement activities, which assigns management involvement and responsibility, is used.
Continuous system	Establishes the continuity of the quality system by repeating the 14 steps; advocates use of the PDSA cycle to sustain the process.	Recommends repetition of the cycle of quality planning, control, and improvement.	Use of the trilogy concept requires continuous assessment and subsequent and neverending organizational response.
Human resource capacity	Discusses the training of all employees in his sixth point and the need for retraining to keep pace with changing customer needs in his thirteenth point.	Eighth point specifically deals with quality education; however, emphasis on developing a quality culture also implies a commitment to developing capacity.	Does not explicitly address education or training, which is implicitly contained in the execution of the trilogy (knowledge is required by all employees on a project by project basis to diagnose defects and determine remedies).
Elimination of problem-causers	Uses statistical techniques to identify special causes or chance causes; identifies variation outside of control limits as a special cause variation (workers are responsible to eliminate these); variation that falls within control limits (common causes) is the responsibility of management to eliminate.	Eleventh point addresses a course of action for removal of causes of error; also uses zero-defects standard.	Differentiates common from special causes and categorizes error sources; operator error is categorized as inadvertent, willful, or resulting from improper or inadequate training or improper technique; Juran provides specifics for achieving the zero-defects performance standard.

From Lancaster, J. (1999). *Nursing issues in leading and managing change.* St. Louis: Mosby.

hospitals were forced to provide more services on an outpatient basis, with expectations of similar or improved outcomes. At the same time, consumers were becoming more conscious of their rights and more knowledgeable about health care. They demanded more and better health care services. Members of the health care industry began exploring the use of QI methods to gain a competitive edge.

In 1994 the Joint Commission on Accreditation of Healthcare Organizations (JCAHO) published its *Framework for Improving Performance: From Principles to Practice*, which outlines the JCAHO's methods for continuous improvement for health care. By including standards for improving organizational performance in their accreditation manual, the JCAHO emphasized the necessity for health care organizations to pay attention to QI in all aspects of their business (especially in matters of patient care). Their framework consists of enhancing outcomes, patient satisfaction, quality of care, and value through improvement of an organization's functions and processes (JCAHO, 1994). Today, most heath care organizations have QI among their strategic initiatives.

Nurses have always been concerned with improving quality of care and have used various methods to independently evaluate its three elements: structure, process, and outcome. Currently, to be effective, improvement efforts must be focused on all three of these interdependent frameworks (Gillies, 1994). Since TQM embraces employee empowerment and employee contributions to the organization, it is a philosophy that nursing can also embrace. Whether the nurse is a manager or a NP seeking to continuously improve processes for patient care and employees, being an integral part of QI is worthwhile. CQI enables APNs to seek and use patient and employee input into improving care. The work environment is more pleasant and productive, and the care the patient receives is of higher quality. Nursing is very good at balancing those qualitative measures of patient care with the fiscal issues. CQI and TQM provide the management and philosophical framework for this to happen.

Tools used in quality improvement

Following a standard method of QI necessitates the use of proven tools for teamwork and data collection and analysis. (Some of the tools consistently used in QI are shown in Chart 7-1.) Team process tools may be used with a large group of people from whom input is desired. For example, if someone was seeking input from a group of patients, he or she might have them divide into age groups and then brainstorm to identify areas they believe warrant improvement. The use of small groups helps ensure that people who do not feel comfortable speaking in a large group share their thoughts. Then each small group could report their findings to the whole group, and a list could be generated. This allows all people to participate; in a large group, it is likely that not all would be able to share their opinions. A vote could then be taken to have the participants identify areas with the highest priority. Once the focus of the process is identified, the data need to be

---

Chart 7-1

Team Process Tools

Brainstorming

This is a technique for generating list of ideas. No idea is rejected, regardless of how off the wall or out of the mainstream it may be. Team members present their ideas in random fashion, often shouting out spontaneous ideas. Ideas are listed on the blackboard or flip chart until everyone has exhausted their ideas or the preset time limit has expired (usually not more than 20 to 30 minutes, depending on the topic). This technique is used to generate ideas in all stages of the improvement process (e.g., generation of problems to study, generation of solutions).

Nominal Group Technique

This technique is used with brainstorming to provide every participant the opportunity to participate. The group leader or facilitator asks each person their ideas or suggestions in an orderly fashion. If a participant does not have an idea for their turn, the participant responds with "pass" and the leader moves to the next person. This lacks some of the spontaneity of brainstorming but gives each member an opportunity for participation. After two rounds of each participant saying "pass," the session ends.

Multivoting

This technique is used with brainstorming and nominal group technique to actually select a topic for data collection, a problem, a solution, or an item to monitor. Each team member is assigned points to use in voting. The member can assign as many points as he or she wants to a selection. The item with the highest number of points is the item selected for the project.

For example, there are eight members on a QI team. Each team member is given eight points to use for three solutions proposed for a specific problem, a total of 64 points to be spread over the solutions. The first person assigns three points to solution C, one to solution B, and four to solution A, the second person assigns two points to solution A, three to solution C, and three to solution A, and so on. At the end of the voting, the solution with the highest number of points is selected. In event of a tie, the process is repeated.

collected and then analyzed. (Chart 7-2 contains data that can provide graphic assistance during the process.)

Methods for improving quality

There are a number of QI methods available for process improvement in health care: Juran's QI process, the Hospital Corporation of America's FOCUS-PDSA model, Joiner's Seven-Step Method, and the JCAHO's Cycle for Improving Performance. Whichever method is used by the APN or health care organization, several key concepts (outlined in Box 7-1) are universally associated with QI.

Whichever improvement method is chosen by an organization, the steps are similar. If an APN chooses to implement QI within a patient care organization, the following principles apply:

- Remember who the customer is—the patient.
- Focus on continuous improvement of all processes.
- Involve the whole office (or organization, depending on size) in the process.
- Use the strengths of all teams members to improve decision-making.

There are many processes involved with ambulatory practice, such as triage, medical records, scheduling, and test results. Not everyone in the practice knows all about every process. The skills and strengths of each individual should contribute to the process, and the purpose or change to be accomplished should be clearly established. The FOCUS-PDSA model works well when implementing the QI process (Walton, 1990) (Box 7-2).

The first step in the FOCUS model is to *find* a process that needs improvement in relation to the goals of the organization. Patients, staff, and colleagues can be asked for ideas about how the practice could be improved. What makes the day more difficult than it should be? Why do some days flow smoothly and others not? What are things that you have noted when we have increased no-shows? Another way to find processes to improve is to identify any activity that has no value. The office can be examined from a patient's or staff member's point of view. Internal reviews, chart audits, and external reviews such as HEDIS might also provide data related to areas that could be improved. A literature review might identify people who are doing well in a particular area. The idea is to list all possibilities, with some ways to make potential changes. The list of potential change projects should be prioritized.

Once a list of potential projects has been generated, one should *organize* a team and its resources. People who are involved in the process and represent all vital steps should be chosen. The team should identify which projects they feel are the most pressing and establish what the team is to accomplish and why. It is helpful to have clear parameters and goals for the QI project. Six people is generally the maximum number of people on a team, and it helps if people are willing to volunteer to serve on the committee

rather than being drafted. Each member's role should be clarified. Having team "ground rules" related to the decision-making model (a consensus); team etiquette; and good listening skills are helpful. An APN must run effective meetings, so planning and preparation are vital.

Next, one must *clarify* current knowledge about the process. The current process should be charted to collect baseline data. Good data collection is essential; it provides feedback to the team and reinforces the intervention. Collection of data may require the use of manual systems to gather it; a computer system that collects this information makes the process go more quickly. The data collection plan needs to be very specific. What population is being studied (e.g., all patients, active patients, random sample)? What defines the population being studied (e.g., age, sex)? What is the time frame of the study?

After the data collection, one must *understand* sources of process variation. What are the customer needs and how well does the process meet them? Data should be collected to identify the process. A key premise of QI is that one can not begin to improve the process until the process is fully understood. A flow chart can assist in identifying the major steps to the process and the normal sequence of the process. Flow charting also helps stimulate discussion and identify problem areas.

Last, one must *select* an improvement or intervention. From the list of possible solutions, the best one should be chosen. Flow charting should help identify which part of the process is the best place to start in terms of intervention.

Before a team is assembled, one must ensure that the infrastructure of the organization will support the QI efforts. Teams must be actively supported. In a large group, it may be more efficacious to have a quality council that can oversee the QI momentum. Glasser (1994) feels the workers must trust management for the process to work best. All people on the team should be asked to do only useful or purposeful work. They should feel that they are making a worthwhile contribution to the process. The APN should serve as a lead manager in the process, as well as a role model in that he or she will settle for nothing less than quality work. Glasser's last point is that quality work always feels good.

Once the problem and a potential intervention have been identified, one begins the process of *plan-do-study act* (Box 7-3). The planning step concentrates on how to implement the intervention that was identified.

The City Heights Family Health Center used the FOCUS-PDSA process to address one of their problem areas. (The components of the model are identified in parentheses.) Rachel was a family nurse practitioner (FNP) interested in QI and patient outcomes. She worked in a small, federally funded CHC in a housing project with another part-time nurse practitioner (NP), a registered nurse (RN), and a patient service representative (PSR).

Chart
7-2

Data Collection and Analysis Tools

Flow Chart

This is a schematic drawing that demonstrates the steps of a work process in the sequence in which they occur. This tool leads to an understanding of the work process so improvement is possible. The individuals who are actually involved in the process should diagram it. This group decides where the process begins and ends; they brainstorm the main activities and decision points in the process and then arrange these activities and decision points in their proper order using arrows to show the direction of flow. As it becomes necessary, the main activities are broken down to show the complexity of the process. The group may discover steps in the process that have nothing to do with the process or cause the process to bog down. A good "practice process" is the admission of a patient to an ambulatory care office, hospital, or long-term care (LTC) facility. Typically, certain symbols are used to identify elements in the chart, and there are computer software programs available to help with the diagramming process. (Symbols used to graph the data are identified in Table 7-6. An example is provided in Figure 7-1.)

Pareto Chart

This is a bar chart used to visually represent the distribution of occurrences or situations being studied by a team (Figure 7-2). The most frequent occurrence is represented at the far left, with the other occurrences in descending order to the right. This tool is used to identify the one or two situations or categories in which most problems occur. The appropriate categories are found by asking questions regarding what, where, who, why and how. The typical Pareto pattern indicates that the highest categories are responsible for most of the effects. More than one Pareto is often required, with each one exploring a different question.

Cause-and-Effect Diagram (Fishbone Diagram)

This is a diagram that demonstrates a large number of possible causes for a problem (Figure 7-3). Detailed causes are attached to a small number of main causes so that the completed diagram looks something like the skeleton of a fish. This tool is used to establish the bigger picture of a problem, help team members use their knowledge of the causes of the problem, and provide ideas for data collection and solutions. Usually the problem is written on the right side of a flip chart or board with a large arrow pointing toward it. Arrows are drawn toward the main arrow to indicate main causes or contributing factors.

Specific causes are brainstormed and attached to the main causes or factors. Subcauses may also be identified. The most common categories for this tool include people, machines, methods, and materials. This diagram only shows possible causes; data is needed to determine the actual causes.

Control Chart

This is "a run chart with statistically determined upper and lower limits drawn on either side of the process average (Figure 7-4). The upper and lower control limits are determined by allowing a process to run untouched and then analyzing the results using a mathematical formula. Every process has variation. The more finely tuned a process, the less deviation there is from the average" (Walton, 1986).

Frequency Distribution

Also called a *histogram*, this tool graphically demonstrates the relative frequency with which a variable occurs and the relationship between the value of the variable and frequency of occurrence (Figure 7-5) (Lancaster, 1999).

Checksheet

This is a form for recording data that indicates how many times something has happened. This tool provides a record of data gathered and ensures that all team members receive comparable data. To use a checksheet, the team must know the data needed. An individual sheet should be designed for each data collector. A tally checksheet is then used to collate the results of the individual checksheets.

Run Chart

This is a chart that displays the results of a process in the order they are produced. Each result is plotted in sequence and then connected to form a line graph. The graph is helpful in identifying trends (Figure 7-6).

Gantt Chart

This is a chart that identifies all the activities required for a project and the time frame assigned to each activity. These are often called *activity charts* and *project management charts* (Lancaster, 1999).

Decision Matrix

This is a technique that helps evaluate all potential solutions for a quality project in an organized and objective manner, facilitating selection of the best possible solution for implementation. The criteria for solution are placed across the top of the matrix, with the solutions down the left side. The criteria are coded to from 1 to 10 or 1 to 3, or by whatever rating the committee determines. The solution that achieves the highest number on the criteria is selected as the solution for implementation.

Box 7-1

Universal Concepts Associated with Quality Improvement

- To be successful, quality improvement must flow from the top of an organization to the bottom.
- Improvement is continuous and never ending.
- Processes are improved through teams.
- Interdepartmental processes are best improved through crossfunctional teams.
- Decisions are based on data.
- Outcomes are key measures of improvement and organizational performance.
- The emphasis is on customers and their definition of quality.
- Improvement teams are composed of those involved in and closest to the process under assessment.
- Partnerships are formed with suppliers.
- Variation is reduced.
- The focus is on improving processes, not improving individuals.
- The focus is on improving processes, not inspecting the product.

Box 7-3

The PDSA Model

Plan

Analyze the process, determine what changes would most improve it, and establish a plan for making the improvement. Target such areas as irritations, slow processes, or costly issues.

Do

Put the changes into motion on a small scale or trial basis. (A pilot basis may be the way to start.) Change the process until there is 80% compliance. Share the data with those doing the work.

Study

Check to see if the change is working and check the results and lessons learned from the team effort. Check the results of the implementation against the original expectations. Identify variations, both positive and negative (i.e., performing better or worse than the system performs).

Act

If the change is working, implement it on a larger scale. If the change is not working, refine it or reject and begin the cycle again.

Box 7-2

The FOCUS Model

- **F**ind a process to improve.
- **O**rganize a team and its resources.
- **C**larify the current knowledge about the process.
- **U**nderstand the sources of process variation.
- **S**elect an improvement or intervention.

Table 7-6

Elements of a Flow Chart

	Activities that occur
	Decision points
	Direction of flow from one activity to the next
	Input points
	Beginning or end of the process

The center's staff held quarterly meetings to discuss issues pertaining to the practice. The HEDIS data revealed that their child immunization rates were not as high as they could or should be *(find a process to improve)*. The team discussed this issue *(organize)* and decided this was a priority that they wanted to work on. Baseline data revealed that the immunization rates were 70%; their goal immunization rate was 95% *(clarify current knowledge)*. Barriers to completing the required immunizations included the following:

- Poor documentation of previous immunizations
- Inability to get records of prior immunizations from some agencies
- Missed opportunities during acute visits
- One-time-only visits from one of the other offices of the organization
- Inadequate well-child visits
- Changing immunization requirements every year

After reviewing the above barriers, the team decided to concentrate on immunizations for 2-year-olds and younger

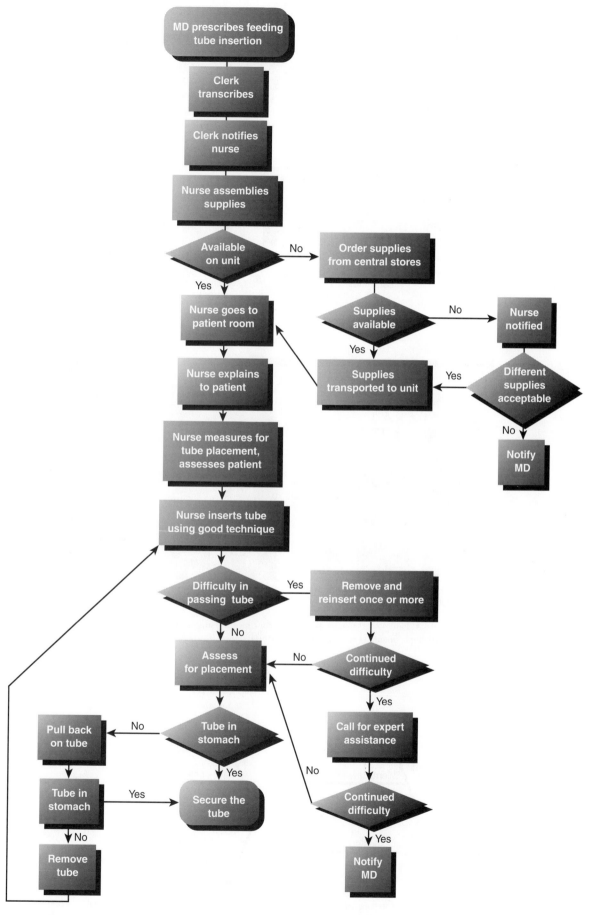

Figure 7-1 Example of a detailed flow chart. (From Schroeder, P. [1994]. *Improving quality and performance*. St. Louis: Mosby.)

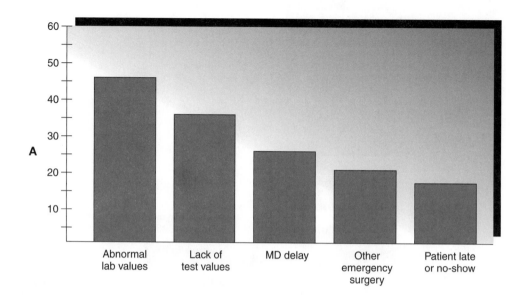

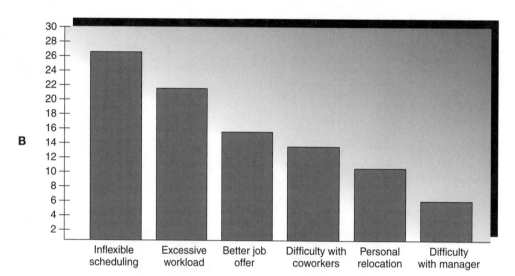

Figure 7-2 Pareto charts. **A,** Pareto chart ranking the reasons for canceling surgery. **B,** Pareto chart ranking nurses reasons for leaving hospital employment. (From Schroeder, P. [1994]. *Improving quality and performance.* St. Louis: Mosby.)

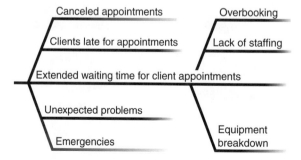

Figure 7-3 Fishbone diagram showing possible causes of extended waiting time for clinic patients. (From Yoder-Wise, P. [1999]. *Leading and managing in nursing.* St. Louis: Mosby.)

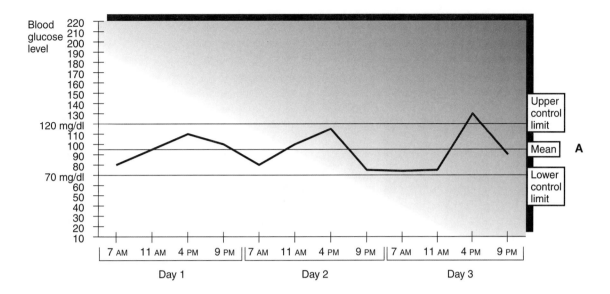

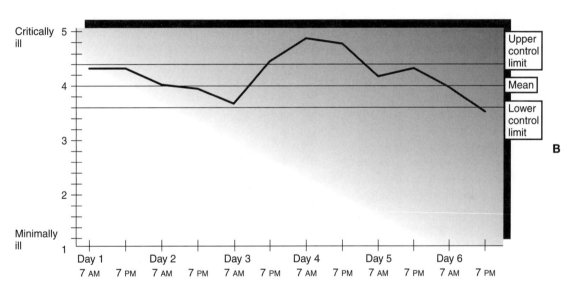

Figure 7-4 Control charts. **A,** Blood glucose control chart for a person with diabetes. **B,** Control chart for acuity level of patients cared for on the unit. (From Schroeder, P. [1994]. *Improving quality and performance.* St. Louis: Mosby.)

children *(data collection plan).* While immunization of preschool children and adolescents is important, lack of immunizations is solved when the children can not attend school without them, providing an impetus for parents to complete the needed immunizations. Children 2 years old and under have to meet no such requirements, so it is more likely the immunizations may be delayed.

The process, as it related to immunizations, was flow charted (Figure 7-7) revealing a number of missed opportunities for immunizations *(understand variance).* The process was clearly defined and the data and literature were assembled; now the team felt they were able to choose an intervention. The team felt they could improve immunization rates by addressing all missed opportunities; all team members would be involved *(select an improve-*

ment). No new forms were needed—only a way to remind the team to look at the immunization record *(plan).* In this case, because it was a small office and the process was well defined, it was implemented for the whole team *(do).* The plan included the following:

- The PSR would check for the presence of an immunization record.
- If it was not present, she would call the other office to get a copy of the immunization record or call the previous provider's office to obtain the records.
- The RN would assess the immunization record for missing immunizations and identify which ones needed to be given, noting the needed immunizations on a sticky note in the chart.

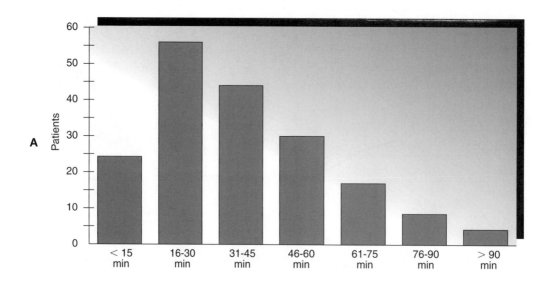

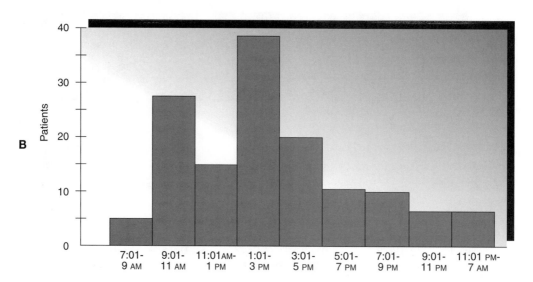

Figure 7-5 Histograms. **A,** Histogram of waiting time in clinic. **B,** Histogram of time of day of patient admissions to unit during two weeks of the month. (From Schroeder, P. [1994]. *Improving quality and performance.* St. Louis: Mosby.)

• The NP would also check the immunization record and order the missing immunizations if there were no contraindications.

After implementing the QI process for 1 month, a quick chart audit revealed that 93% of the children seen in the last month had up-to-date immunizations. This was a great start, and the team planned on continuing the process. They also planned for times when they could not comply with the new process. The one area that still seemed to be a problem was getting immunization records from other provider practices. In some cases, the organizations refused to send a copy of records. The team planned to address this issue in 6 months by talking with the other centers within the organization for ideas. The team also

planned to continue the process; while it was working, they were concerned that patients they did not see often still might be missed. An audit of all children between the ages of 18 months and 36 months was planned to determine if all immunizations were up to date. If they were not, they planned on sending a card or calling to remind the parents that immunizations were needed.

The Advanced Practice Nurse's Role in Quality Improvement

Although in health care, quality becomes the responsibility of all employees, nurses are particularly important in improving the quality of care. Nursing leadership must be involved in the organization's QI planning and implemen-

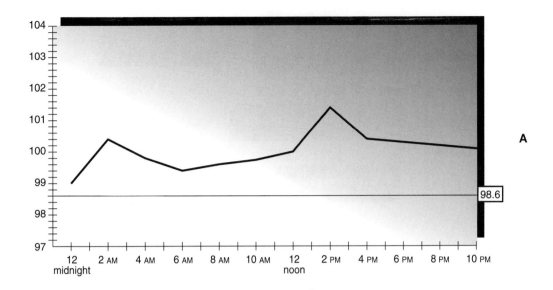

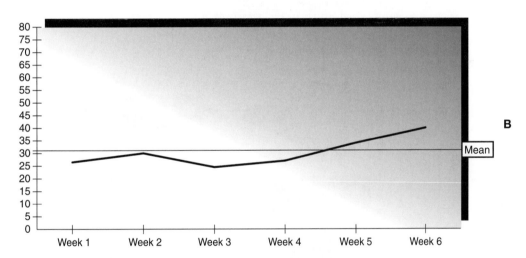

Figure 7-6 Run charts. **A,** Run chart of temperature. **B,** Run chart of number of infiltrated peripheral intravenous lines requiring restarts. (From Schroeder, P. [1994]. *Improving quality and performance*. St. Louis: Mosby.)

tation. In addition, nursing leaders are responsible for ensuring that members of the nursing department are knowledgeable in and able to utilize QI methods.

Individual nurses may be asked to participate on interdepartmental, crossfunctional teams. They can also improve processes in their own area of work. By following the prescribed steps in the QI method, they can select and analyze processes in which they are involved. Teams can be formed to solve problems, but individual APNs can also use the method for problem-solving and process improvement in his or her own nursing practice.

As an interdisciplinary team member, a nurse not only contributes the viewpoint of a health professional, but also that of an advocate for patients. Using QI, each team member is chosen because he or she is intricately involved in the process being assessed, and each brings a different

perspective to problem-solving; every team member's opinion are equally important. For example, a perioperative nurse may be asked to join a crossfunctional team charged with improving the flow of surgical patients through the operating room or of ambulatory patients through a clinic. The nurse is asked to participate (as are the other team members—surgeon, anesthesiologist, housekeeper, and scheduler for the operating room; scheduler, provider, medical assistant, receptionist for the clinic) because of his or her unique role in the process. While patient input is desirable, the nurse, who spends the most time with the surgical patient before, during, and after the surgical procedure, would have a good understanding of the patient's perspective on the issues discussed. Using the old system of problem-solving, the nurse, and possibly all of these team members, would not

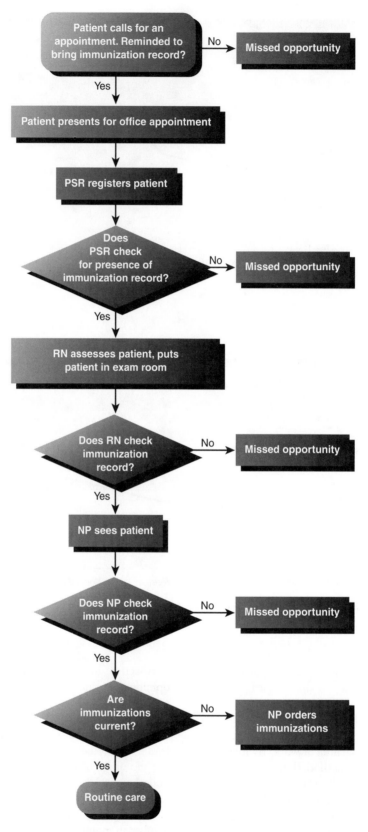

Figure 7-7 Flow chart for the immunization problem.

have been involved in process improvement. Management would have made all the decisions.

During the last couple of decades, the role of the professional nurse has evolved and now includes the use of QI in the delivery of care. Professional nurses at all levels of the organization must be knowledgeable of and participate in continuous QI activities. A nurse has the opportunity to identify quality issues or points of friction because of his or her role as patient advocate. The nurse usually has an overview of all processes pertaining to patient care in any setting. For example, a NP may notice that too many new physicals are scheduled in one day or at the beginning or end of a day, causing increased waiting times and often throwing off the schedule for the whole day. The NP could get the involved people together (e.g., receptionist, scheduler) to talk about improving the process. The first meeting could be spent identifying when, what, why, and how often the problem occurs. They could then collect data on the problem using some of the CQI tools to see if it is really a process problem or a management problem. Management problems can not be solved with CQI—only process problems can. Is the problem a scheduling problem? Scheduling problems are management problems that can be solved with only one or two people. If the problem is the process by which patients are brought in and readied for the physical, it is a problem that needs to be solved using QI. A solution can be selected for implementation and then evaluated for results. It is important that once a new process is implemented, time for inclusion in the daily activity must be allowed. The learning curve for a new process is about 6 months. Change in QI is slow and can not be hurried. If the planned solution is modified too early, the results are never truly known.

PRIORITIES FOR RESEARCH

The emphasis on QI in health care has gained popularity over a very short time. Although some research has been conducted to evaluate the benefits of QI methods, further research is needed to assess such areas as the effect of the QI process on patient outcomes. Since most managed care companies and other payers want to see necessary improvements made without sacrificing quality, research on how patients fare in new processes is most important. If the quality of the care does not improve, the process needs to be investigated again. One should remember that the cost-saving is a byproduct of process change. One process that addresses patient outcomes is the disease management process. It identifies the criteria and data that needs to be collected but does not identify what processes need to be improved or changed to help improve patient outcomes. (The disease management process is discussed in depth in Chapter 46.) The disease management process can serve as a way to identify what problems need to be addressed; it fits nicely into the QI process.

Time is another area of research related to QI. Can the QI process be shortened and have similar positive results? There has not been much research on this in health care, but the results of shortening the whole QI process or not incorporating the philosophy of TQM has rated disappointing results in business (Collins and Porras, 1997; Hagan, 1994; Hunt, 1993; Lawler, 1995; Phillips, 1997). Processes take time, and QI does not lend itself to shortcuts.

An applicable framework for QI research is the model proposed by Watson, Bulechek, and McCloskey (1987). The quality assurance model using research (QAMUR) is based on the assumption that QA studies must be conducted in the form of scientific inquiry and can serve as the bridge between nursing practice and nursing education. Evaluation of the quality of patient care is essential in the nursing process. All too often, the effectiveness of interventions has not been taken into account in a systematic model. QA can help determine the effectiveness of care. The QAMUR model incorporates both problem-solving through research utilization and problem-solving through research conduction (Figure 7-8). For both sides of the model, the beginning is ongoing QA that leads to the identification of a clinical practice problem. QA and QI process can both identify and address problem areas. Research related to this process will contribute to the advancement of scientific knowledge for nursing.

Solberg, Kottke, Milo, Brekke, Magnan, Davidson, Calomeni, Conn, Amundson, and Nelson (2000) evaluated how a CQI program could improve the delivery of eight clinical preventive services (blood pressure monitoring, Pap smear, cholesterol monitoring, tobacco use/cessation, breast examination, mammography, influenza vaccine, and pneumococcal vaccine). Forty-four primary care clinics in Minneapolis were randomly assigned to CQI for preventive services or usual care. The main outcome measure was the proportion of patients who were up to date for the eight preventive services. Compared to the control group, only one preventive service (pneumococcal vaccine) was increased significantly in the intervention group. In addition, patients in the intervention group reported being offered only one preventive service (cholesterol screening) when compared with the control group. This study did not show the results expected when using the CQI approach. The researchers identified barriers of CQI to be its long lead-time and the large effort needed to implement projects. Possible explanations for the failure of this controlled trial include atypical clinics, inadequate measurement and analysis of preventive services, inadequate delivery of the interventions, and CQI being an inappropriate mechanism for making preventive improvements. The study results are similar to those found by Goldberg (1998) when CQI failed to show improvements with cases of depression and hypertension. APNs would be well advised to use newer, more rapid cycles and tests over the traditional

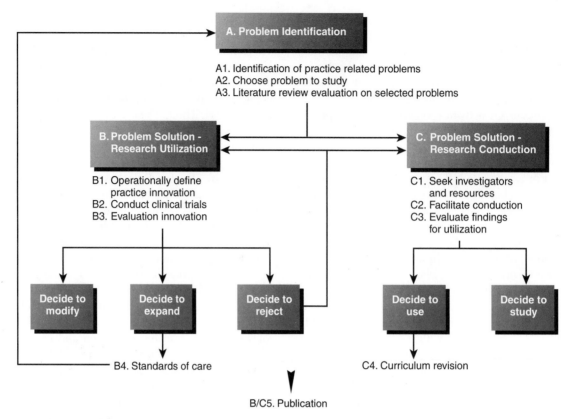

Figure 7-8 Quality assurance model using research. (Reprinted with permission from Watson, C., Bulechek, G., & McCloskey, J. [1987]. QAMUR: A quality assurance model using research. *Journal of Nursing Quality Assurance, 2*[1], 21-27. Aspen Publishers.)

approach for CQI (Alemi, Moore, Headrick, Neuhauser, Hekelman, & Kizys, 1998; Berwick, 1998). However, additional testing of the newer, faster version of CQI is badly needed.

IMPLICATIONS FOR MSN EDUCATION AND ADVANCED PRACTICE

Graduate education in nursing has not spent time or placed emphasis on the importance of QI and its effects on all areas of nursing practice. Nurses often seem removed from the improvement process when it should be a cornerstone of nursing practice in every specialty. An increased emphasis could be placed on QI by applying the Deming method to the development of interdisciplinary TQM projects within the curriculum. Another area where QI or TQM could be implemented is via a change project or project during a clinical practicum. APN students could use flow charting to help analyze how they perform in a clinical situation (e.g., how they access reference materials when in the middle of seeing patients). Students could also collect data on the types of patients seen during the clinical practica, examining factors such as ages and diagnoses. A

histogram could then be used to identify where the bulk of the student's experience has been, perhaps identifying areas that needed more exposure.

APNs need to realize that the QI process is here to stay and should plan on using this method to offer patients optimal care and service. The QI process provides an opportunity to APNs willing to explore patient care issues and possible solutions. The data is already being collected by HEDIS and other managed care companies. The prudent APN will take advantage of the identification of problems and use the QI process to make changes. There will be no choice in the issue; consumers and other agencies are currently able to see data regarding provider patterns—there is a new Internet-based system that allows patients to complete a clinical evaluation on their providers and compare it to what other providers did for their patients. In the long run, this Internet program is expected to supply overall ratings of doctors' clinical performances (Terry, 2000). While the online rating at this point does not mention APNs or other providers, they will be included as the process picks up steam.

The system is being propelled by a group called the Foundation for Accountability (FACCT), which is a nonprofit coalition of large corporations, government agencies, and consumer groups representing about 80 million people. FACCT sees these evaluations as being more impor-

Suggestions for Further Learning

- Access the Institute for Healthcare Improvement at www.ihi.org. Its mission is to identify and disseminate information about innovations that have improved health quality. Describe two of their current initiatives: the Breakthrough Series Collaboratives and the Idealized Design of Clinical Office Practices.

- Get the following articles: Coleman, M., & Endsley, S. (1999). Quality improvement: first steps. *Family Practice Management, 6*(5), 29-34; Schwarz, M., Landis, S., & Rowe, J. (1999). A team approach to quality management. *Family Practice Management. 6*(4), 25-32; and Giovino, J. (1999). Holding the gains in quality improvement. *Family Practice Management, 6*(5), 29-34. These provide more specific details on how to implement quality improvement within an ambulatory setting. Identify a process within your clinical practice setting that would benefit from a quality improvement evaluation and process.

- Get the article: Thurston, N., Watson, L., & Reimer, M. (1993). Research or quality improvement. *Journal of Nursing Administration, 23*(7), 46-49. What are your views on the issue of quality improvement as a form of research? Support your view.

- Go to the FACCT website at www.facct.org. How would you feel if a patient presented this information? What is your reaction to this web page?

- To learn more about quality management and quality improvement, the following books are recommended: Mears, P. (1994). *Healthcare teams: building continuous quality improvement.* Delray Beach, FL: St. Lucie Press; Scherkenbach, W.W. (1991). *The Deming route to quality and productivity: road maps and roadblocks,* Washington, DC: CEEPress Books; and Senge, P.M. (1990). *The fifth discipline: the art & practice of the learning organization.* New York: Doubleday.

tant to consumers than the report cards published by health maintenance organizations (HMOs), which focus more on information collected from claims and not patients. Patients believe that the only way they can ensure quality is through their relationship with individual providers, which is good news for APNs. While not supported by large amounts of scientific data, the data do reveal that close APN/patient relationships may be the reason many patients prefer APNs as providers (Campbell, Mauksch, Neikirk, & Hosokawa, 1990).

The online evaluation asks questions related to the following:

- Are practice guidelines followed?
- Is the patient involved in making decisions about care?
- Are the communication skills and trustworthiness of the provider satisfactory?
- How does the patient rate their symptoms and quality of life?

For example, for patients with diabetes, the questions revolve around having their feet, blood sugar, and eyes checked. If these examinations were not performed, the patients would be cued to ask their providers why these have not been done. The evaluation empowers patients to know what to expect and what to ask about during their visits. The initial online evaluations concentrate on several chronic conditions, as well as early childhood care and end-of-life care. Terry (2000) predicts that while initially the evaluations just coach patients on what to expect, in the future the FACCT data might profile physicians for provider groups, health plans, or employers. Feedback from physicians regarding this new evaluation system is mixed. Many have reservations about a rating system based

on patient reports, especially when issues such as patient compliance and episodic care (instead of well visits) are the domain of patients and out of the control of providers. Others feel that having patients assume more self-care and reminding physicians about things that need to be done are not all bad. It might even weed out incompetent physicians. APNs should watch the development of this evaluation system in the next few years. Chances are all primary care providers (PCPs) will be rated using this system. It is always better to be in front of the curve and anticipating future changes. QI helps contribute to this anticipation by identifying processes that are not contributing to optimal patient care and service.

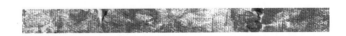

DISCUSSION QUESTIONS

These questions can be used to promote critical thinking and encourage discussion.

1. Choose a process for improvement in your work setting.

- Discuss the reason for your selection of this process for improvement.
- Select members for the multidisciplinary team.
- Create a flow chart for the current process.
- Discuss data you would collect to evaluate the current status.
- Identify the next steps the team should take in the improvement process.

2. Discuss the important issues involved in TQM or CQI as they relate to health care. These issues may include:

- Cost-containment versus decreasing costs
- Deming's principles of driving out fear, instituting a program of education, and self improvement

REFERENCES/BIBLIOGRAPHY

Abel, E. (1994). Productivity vs. quality of care: ethical implications for clinical practice during health care reform. *Nurse Practitioner Forum, 5*(4), 238-242.

Agency for Health Care Policy and Research–Kaiser Family Foundation (1996). *Americans as health care consumers: the role of quality information.* Washington, DC: Agency for Health Care Policy and Research.

Al-Assaf, A. (1993a). Introduction and historical background. In A. Al-Assaf and J. Schmele (Eds.). *Textbook of total quality management* (pp. 3-12). Delray Beach, FL: St. Lucie Press.

Al-Assaf, A. (1993b). Outcome management and TQ. In A. Al-Assaf and J. Schmele (Eds.). *Textbook of total quality management* (pp. 221-237). Delray Beach, FL: St. Lucie Press.

Alemi, F., Moore, S., Headrick, L., Neuhauser, D., Hekelman, F., & Kizys, N. (1998). Rapid improvement teams. *Joint Commission Journal of Quality Improvement, 24*, 119-129.

Anctil, B., & Winters, M. (1996). Linking customer judgment with process measures to improve access to ambulatory care. *Joint Commission Journal of Quality Improvement, 22*(5), 345-357.

Anderson, C. (1994). Advanced practice: quality control. *Nursing Outlook, 42*(2), 54-55.

Berwick, D. (1998). Developing and testing changes in delivery of care. *Annals of Internal Medicine, 128*, 651-656.

Buppert, C. (1999). *Nurse practitioner's business practice and legal guide.* Gaithersburg, MD: Aspen Publishers.

Buppert, C. (2000). *The primary care provider's guide to compensation and quality.* Gaithersburg, MD: Aspen Publishers.

Campbell, J., Mauksch, H., Neikirk, H., & Hosokawa, M. (1990). Collaborative practice and provider styles of delivering health care. *Social Science Medicine, 30*, 1359-1365.

Careu. R. (1995). *Measuring quality improvement in healthcare: a guide to statistical process control applications.* New York: Quality Resources.

Cesta, T. (1993). The link between continuous quality improvement and case management. *Journal of Nursing Administration, 23*(6), 55-61.

The challenge and potential for assuring quality health care for the 21st century (Publication No. OM 98-0009 for the Domestic Policy Council). (1998, June 17). Washington, DC: Department of Health and Human Services. Available online at www.ahcpr.gov/qual/21stcena.htm.

Chassin, M. (1997). Assessing strategies for quality improvement. *Health Affairs, 16*(3), 151-161.

Coleman, M., & Endsley, S. (1999). Quality improvement: first steps. *Family Practice Management, 6*(5), 29-34. Available online at www.aafp.org/fpm/990500fm.

Collins, J., and Porras, J. (1997). *Built to last: successful habits of visionary companies.* New York: Harper Business.

Cumberland, A. (1993). Making the transition to a TQM system. *Nursing Management, 24*(8), 62-63.

Del Bueno, D. (1993). Outcome evaluation: frustration or fertile field? *Journal of Nursing Administration, 23*(7), 12-13, 19.

Deming, W.E. (1986). *Out of the crisis,* Cambridge, MA: Massachusetts Institute of Technology, Center for Advanced Engineering Study.

Donabedian, M. (1980). *Explorations in quality assessment and monitoring: the definition of quality and approaches to its assessment* (vol. 1). Ann Arbor, MI: Health Administration Press.

Enns, S. (2000). Measuring practice performance: are you providing quality care? *Clinician Reviews, 10*(5), 132-138.

Fiesta, J. (1992). Cost standards, quality and technology. *Nursing Mangement, 23*(2), 16-17.

Gaucher, E., & Coffey, R. (1993). *Total quality in health care: from theory to practice.* San Francisco: Jossey-Bass Inc.

Gillies, D. A. (1994). Quality improvement. In D.A. Gillies (Ed.), *Nursing management: a systems approach.* Philadelphia: WB Saunders.

Giovino, J. (1999). Holding the gains in quality improvement. *Family Practice Management, 6*(5), 29-34.

Glasser, W. (1994). *The control theory manager.* New York: Harper Business.

Goldberg, H., Wagner, E., & Fihn, S. (1998). A randomized controlled trial of CQI teams and academic detailing: can they alter compliance with guidelines? *Joint Commission Journal of Quality Improvement, 24*, 130-142.

Hagan, J. (1994). *Management of quality: strategies to improve quality and the bottom line.* New York: Business One Irwin.

Henry Ford Health System (1995). *Henry Ford balanced scorecard measures.* Detroit, MI: Henry Ford Health System.

Hunt, V. (1993). *Managing for quality: integrating quality and business strategy.* Homewood, IL: Business Irwin.

Joint Commission on Accreditation of Healthcare Organizations (1994). *Framework for improving performance: from principles to practice.* Oakbrook Terrace, IL: Joint Commission on Accreditation of Healthcare Organizations.

Juran, J.M. (1989). *Juran on leadership for quality: an executive handbook.* New York: The Free Press.

Kennedy, M. (1992). Combining the best of QA and TQM. *Quality Management Update, 2*(1), 1, 10-14.

Kirk, R. (1992). The big picture—total quality management and continuous quality improvement. *Journal of Nursing Administration, 22*(4), 24-31.

Lancaster, J. (1999). *Nursing issues in leading and managing change.* St. Louis: Mosby.

Langley, G., Nolan, K., & Nolan, T. (1996). *The improvement guide: a practical approach to enhancing organizational performance.* San Francisco: Jossey-Bass Inc.

Lawler, E., Mohrman, S., & Ledford, G. (1995). *Creating high performance organizations: practices and results of employee involvement and TQM in fortune 1000 companies.* San Francisco: Jossey-Bass Inc.

Leshan, L., Fitzsimmons, M., Marbella, A., & Gottlieb, M. (1997). Increasing clinical prevention efforts in a family practice residency program through CQI methods. *Joint Commission Journal of Quality Improvement, 23*(7), 391-400.

MacIsaac, A. (1991). Quality assurance welcomed as nurse practitioners begin to write prescriptions. *Journal of Nursing Quality Assurance, 5*(3), 52-58.

McGlynn, E. (1997). Six challenges in measuring the quality of health care. *Health Affairs, 16*(3). 7-21.

McGlynn, E., & Brook, R. (1996). Ensuring quality of care. In R. Anderson, T. Rice, & G. Kominski (Eds.), *Changing the US health care system: key issues in health services, policy and management*. San Francisco: Jossey-Bass Inc.

Nelson, E., Batalden, P., & Ryer, J. (1998). *Clinical improvement action quide*. Oakbrook Terrace, IL: Joint Commission on Accreditation of Healthcare Organizations.

Ornstein, S., Jenkins, R., & Lee, F. (1997). The computer based medical record as a CQI tool in a family medicine center. *Joint Commission Journal of Quality Improvement, 23*(7), 347-361.

Phillips, J. (1997). *Return on investment training and performance improvement programs*. Houston, TX: Gulf.

Schaffner, L.D. (1997). Total quality management: impact on the executive nurse. In S.R. Byers (Ed.), *The executive nurse: leadership for new health care transitions* (pp. 113-133). Albany, NY: Delmar.

Schroeder, P. (1994). *Improving quality and performance*. St. Louis: Mosby.

Schwarz, M., Landis, S., & Rowe, J. (1999). A team approach to quality management. *Family Practice Management. 6*(4), 25-32.

Sherman, J., & Malkmus, M. (1994). Integrating quality assurance and total quality management/quality improvement. *Journal of Nursing Administration, 24*(3), 37-41.

Shi, L., and Singh, D. (1998). *Delivering healthcare in America*. Gaithersburg, MD: Aspen Publishers.

Solberg, L., Kottke, T., Milo, L., Brekke, M., Magnan, S., Davidson, G., Calomeni, C., Conn, S., Amundson, G., & Nelson, A. (2000, May/June). *Failure of a continuous quality improvement intervention to increase the delivery of preventive services*. American College of Physicians–American Society of Internal Medicine. Available online at www.acponline.org/journals/ecp/mayjune00/solberg.htm.

Terry, K. (2000). Now patients will rate you online. *Medical Economics Magazine*. Available online at www.pdr.net/memag/public.htm?path=docs/042400/article6.html.

Walton, M. (1986). *The Deming management method*. New York: Putnam.

Walton, M. (1990). *Deming management at work*. New York: Perigee.

Watson, C., Bulechek, G., & McCloskey, J. (1987). QAMUR: a quality assurance model using research. *Journal of Nursing Quality Assurance, 2*(1), 21-27.

Wendt, D., & Vale, D. (1995). Managing quality and risk. In P.S. Yoder-Wise (Ed.), *Leading and managing in nursing* (pp. 185-205). St. Louis: Mosby.

Western, P. (1994). QA/QI and nursing competence: a combined model. *Nursing Management, 25*(3), 44-46.

Wheeler, D. (1998). *Building continual improvement*. Knoxville, TN: SPC Press.

Williams, S., & Torrens, P. (1993). Influencing, regulating and monitoring the health care system. In S. Williams and P. Torrens (eds.), *Introduction to health services*. Albany, NY: Delmar.

Zazove, P., & Klinkman, M. (1998). Developing a CQI program in a family medicine department. *Joint Commission Journal of Quality Improvement, 24*(8), 391-406.

Chapter 8

Redesign and Reengineering of the Health Care Organization

Margaret M. Anderson & Denise Robinson

Capitated payments and managed care are here to stay. "Do more with less" is a need and goal for most health organizations. To reduce the cost of delivering health care, health care organizations are reorganizing, restructuring, redesigning, or reengineering to decrease waste and inefficiency. The health care delivery system and insurance industry answer to higher health care costs is to reengineer or redesign health care. While redesign and reengineering are appropriate processes for industry, it is sometimes difficult for health care workers to think of providing health care differently than the way it is currently and always has been done. Flarey (1995) indicates that redesign is a radical departure from the norm. It may involve multiple and complex changes in a system, that prepare the organization to respond effectively to what he calls the "real revolution."

DEFINITIONS

Hammer and Champy (1993) define **reengineering** as "the fundamental rethinking and radical redesign of business processes to achieve dramatic improvements in critical measures of performance." It is the opposite of tinkering, bandaiding, and fixing. Hammer and Champy believe it is returning to the basic core business of the enterprise and rethinking how it is done in light of culture, technology, and change. Redesign and reengineering is the "re-invention" of an organization.

Hammer and Champy state that the key terms in reengineering are *fundamental, radical redesign, dramatic,* and *processes*. **Fundamental** refers to asking the basic questions about the business (e.g., why do we do what we do?). These fundamental questions make people look at the rules (written or implicit) and assumptions that direct the way business is conducted. Reengineering begins with no assumptions or premises—it takes nothing for granted.

Radical redesign means getting to the bottom of things—not making choices that just fix up things, but actually disregarding present ways of doing things and inventing new ways of accomplishing the work (Hammer & Champy, 1993). The third key word is **dramatic**. This refers to making a large change in performance, not marginal improvements. Reengineering is only needed when a "heavy blast" is the only thing that will change things. Traditional methods can address a 10% hole. Reengineering should be saved for those times when the hole is deep. Finally, the most important key word is **processes**. This refers to a collection of activities that takes one or more kinds of input and creates an output that is of value to customers (Hammer & Champy, 1993). Many business people are focused on tasks, people, jobs, or structures, but not processes. In most businesses, people focus on the individual tasks in the process (all of which are important) and in so doing, lose sight of the larger objective—to get the product into the hands of the customer. Businesses have been influenced by task-based thinking for the last 200 years; however, the shift to process-based thinking is here, and a number of blue chip companies have made radical changes based on this shift.

Nursing redesign is defined by Flarey (1995) as "an evolving methodology focused on producing fundamental and radical changes within a system. Its sole purpose is to ensure survival in a threatened environment." Flarey believes that nursing redesign is a radical departure from how things have always been done, creating new and innovative ways and means of delivering nursing care. The whole paradigm of health care and nursing care delivery must be changed to ensure survival of the profession and the health care system in general. Nurses can and should be the health care leaders of the future. The unique ability of nurses to serve as patient advocates, care for the public's health, and interact and connect with other health care professionals gives nurses the opportunity to be leaders. To assume this leadership role, nurses must be willing to redesign the delivery of health care and nursing care and change the entire culture of nursing. Nursing must "transform systems in order to respond effectively to a real revolution" (Flarey, 1995). (While there are fine differences in the terms, *reengineering* and *redesign* are used interchangeably for purposes of this discussion.)

CRITICAL ISSUES: APPLYING REENGINEERING TO HEALTH CARE

Most companies can trace their work styles and organizational structure back to the prototypical pin factory described in 1776 by Adam Smith in *The Wealth of Nations*. Smith explained the principle he called the *division of labor*. This principle was based on the premise that many workers, each performing a single step in the production of the pin, could make more pins than a person who made the whole pin. The division of labor increased the productivity of the workers many times over. Many factories today utilize the principle of division of labor. This principle encourages specialization and fragmentation of labor, particularly for large corporations. This division applies not only to manufacturing jobs, but also to secretarial and other jobs. The railroads set up organizational frameworks by formalizing operating procedures and structures. Contingencies were identified for any problems that might occur, and workers were to act only in accordance with the rules. The command and control system in place in most companies reflects the systems developed by the railroads 150 years ago.

Henry Ford took the concept of fragmentation even further, dividing work into tiny, repeatable tasks. He initially had workers go to the parts, but then he developed the assembly line to bring parts to the workers. Because management of these many workstations was complex, Alfred Sloan created smaller, decentralized divisions, overseen by managers. This meant the principle of division of labor was now applied not only to manufacturing, but management as well (Hammer & Champy, 1993). This concept can be applied to nursing; in functional nursing, each nurse is responsible for a portion of patient care, depending on his or her job skills and educational level. This is particularly true with the use of unlicensed personnel.

The last evolutionary step in the development of today's corporations came during a period of tremendous economic expansion. Senior managers planned how much business they wanted to have and what returns they should expect, making changes as needed to keep the business going. This was a great model for the boom time after World War II because of growing demand and accelerating growth. Customers were willing to buy whatever was offered after suffering during the Depression and the war (Hammer & Champy, 1993). Quality and service were not big issues; keeping up with the demand was the big issue during the 1950s and 1960s, and the organizational structure was ideally suited to the high-growth environment.

As the number of tasks grew, so did the complexity of managing these processes. An increased layer of middle managers were needed to keep up with all the numbers of workers who did the simple, repetitive jobs. As this happened, the hierarchical structure of the companies continued to enlarge, separating the senior management from the customers and service.

American companies are now beginning to realize that organizational structure, fragmentation of jobs, and division of labor does not work in today's different world. Today, nothing is constant. Doing business through the division of labor is using yesterday's paradigm (Hammer & Champy, 1993). The three forces that are driving today's business world are customers, competition, and change. Customers are not the passive, accepting people they were in the 60s. Customers now demand products and services specific to their own unique needs. They expect to be treated individually, and their expectations have soared mainly because they know that they can get more. Once customers experience superior service, they are not willing to accept less.

The second force is competition. It used to be that the best price determined the sale. Now it is not as simple. Technology has changed the nature of the competition, as U.S. firms are competing head to head with companies from other parts of the world.

The last force influencing the changes in business is the notion of change. Change has become constant and normal, and the pace of change has accelerated. This means that the time available to develop new products has diminished as products become obsolete in shorter periods of time. Consider the life cycle of a computer, which becomes obsolete almost as soon as it is purchased. Companies that do not plan for these changes and "move quickly" will soon be not moving at all. The changes demand that companies constantly look in many directions at once. It is difficult to anticipate changes if one does not know what to look for. If a person is looking for what is expected, he or she will not see anything but what is expected. Keeping up with the multitude of changes means American businesses must take another look at how they get their work done. It is no longer necessary to organize jobs and work around the outdated principle of division of labor. Division of labor stifles creativity and innovation. Instead companies must organize around processes (Hammer & Champy, 1993). If processes cannot be fixed, they must be reinvented.

In the early 1980s, American car manufacturers were in difficult straits. The foreign car market had greatly expanded because total quality management (TQM) had made a radical difference in Japan. American companies could not match their quality or service. American car manufacturers decided to radically change the process of building and buying cars. Reengineering was required to renew the organization. The processes involved in making cars did not have to be dramatically changed from car to car because the same manufacturer may produce a number of models that are essentially the same. However, the processes involved in making and selling cars did affect the way customer service is perceived. A customer does not care how the car is made; a customer only cares that the car is well made and will not be a problem (or if it is a problem, that it can be fixed). In other words, customers are demanding high quality with outstanding service, both when they buy their cars and when the cars need to be fixed.

The automotive industry was not the only industry suffering from a poor image and poor quality. Many industries and companies such as Disney, the airline industry, Harley-Davidson, and others radically redesigned their organizations to make higher quality, cheaper products using the methods advocated by Hammer and Champy. These industry giants researched their core enterprise and redesigned their business practices and processes so customers felt confident in the products. Using the radical methods of including employees in planning, using investment capital, and including customers in the focus of the enterprise, they reengineered their corporations to be better, faster, and smarter, with added value.

Application of Reengineering to Health Care

In health care, the processes are more convoluted and complex. There is more than one way to enter the health care delivery system, more than one way to deliver patient care, and more than one category of worker to deliver that care. Patients have multiple needs and periods of remission and exacerbation. Because of the complexity of the human system, the patient has multiple methods of entering and exiting from one health care environment into another, and the lines for admission and discharge processes are ambiguous and transient. Health care professionals make an effort to keep patients from falling through the cracks, but the multiple entries and exits, care providers, organizations, and networks make it impossible to attend to every possible situation. Unfortunately, the stakes are higher in health care if care is not provided; the patient can become sicker or even die if not provided the right care. When one redesigns health care delivery, all the methods of entering and exiting the system, treatment sites, care providers, and cultures of the area must be taken into account.

As was true of TQM, reengineering is seen as a way to transform health care, improving profits and decreasing costs. While TQM is a management philosophy, reengineering is the method to achieve the goals. Key areas in reengineering include getting employees involved in the process of reinventing the corporation or system and changing the focus back to the core enterprise of the organization. TQM as a management philosophy is first implemented; then reengineering or reinventing of the large corporation begins.

The onset of the prospective payment system necessitated hospital and health care reengineering in the early 1980s. During the retrospective payment era, there was no need to do things differently just to save costs. With the advent of prospective payment, the margin of profit grew slimmer. It was time to do things differently. During the early 1980s, there was also a nursing shortage—not as pervasive as what exists in the late 1990s and 2000s but certainly critical for the time. Nursing care delivery had to be redesigned to ensure appropriate use of the nursing resources available.

Implementation of Reengineering in Health Care

Reengineering has been implemented in several health care organizations with varying results. It has often been done in conjunction with a TQM approach, with no disruption of the quality of care provided to patients as a goal. Flarey (1995) states that redesign in nursing has as its sole purpose to "ensure survival in a threatened environment." Nursing is threatened by health care reform. Yet the basic work of nursing, the provision of nursing care to the ill, the prevention of illness, and the meeting of unmet needs has not changed. Since the charge from society is to advocate for patients, the basic work of providing care in conjunction with patient wants and needs remains the same. The variety of settings and the wide diversity in scopes of practice for varying levels of nursing practice do not change the basic work or charge of nursing. However, the technology and methods used to deliver nursing care have seen some radical improvements in the way care is delivered.

The American Nurses Association (ANA) has entered into the reengineering discussion with a professional advocacy initiative. This includes examining nurse health and safety issues, work environment issues, and legal issues that affect every nurse in every state. If the work of nursing is to be reengineered, then reengineering should be done by nurses with expertise in the targeted areas. Health care organizations cannot change the work of nurses to achieve goals that may be to contrary to the goals and practice of nursing.

The Process of Reengineering

The foundation of effective reengineering is to involve everyone in the organization in the changing and learning process. This requires a radical change in how both leaders and employees view their jobs, how they interact with each other, and their mission or vision of the organization. These radical changes can not happen if the whole community is not involved in the process. This process is a big challenge for any organization, but particularly for hospitals (Jaffe & Scott, 1997). Many places that go through reengineering are not totally prepared for the process, so managers are afraid to give up their "power" and employees are hesitant to take on new responsibilities. People like having structure, defined roles, and limited risks; they like things to be safe (even though this might be boring). Those people who have been traditionally considered experts are not the key. This process requires the discovery of new ways of thinking and working by people in the organization. It requires open systems and the full sharing of information across boundaries, not limitations on information by level of position or a "need to know" (Jaffe & Scott, 1997). According to Jaffe and Scott, true reengineering is built on the cooperation of people representing different roles, responsibilities, and tasks in making the needed changes. (Box 8-1 shows some important leadership concepts that lead to successful reengineering.)

The most important part of the redesign process is the appointment of a group of core people who will design and implement the change. This core group should be dedicated and diverse, representing different areas and levels of the organization. This is not a group of "experts" who have gone through reengineering before. These are people with leadership qualities who are committed to the process. This change team should not be a committee of established leaders—the very nature of the appointment of this committee signifies to the rest of the organization that status quo will not be the goal. Jaffe and Scott (1997) recommend that this change group be treated as the learning group. The group should go through a learning process on how to do its work. This means setting the scope and direction of their activity and identifying the root causes of the challenges and difficulties the organization may be facing. The change group also needs to combine

learning with doing and to build engagement with the whole system; there is a real danger for the change team to become isolated and lose touch.

As reengineering is accomplished, it becomes evident that there is a new work outlook in place. It is a shift away from the expectations of security and dependency and is based on the principle of mutual maturity. This means that every employee, no matter his or her job, must take on a larger, more responsible role. Even though the role has expanded, certain benefits come along with expansion, including:

- Greater decision latitude and the ability to exercise individual judgment with fewer established guidelines or policies in place
- A broader job description with more strategic responsibility
- Individual responsibility to solve customer problems directly
- Responsibility for continuous improvement of skills
- A need to demonstrate team and interpersonal skills
- Less certainty and more ambiguity, because change is the norm (Jaffe & Scott, 1997)

Rules for Successful Reengineering

Certain assumptions exist related to what is needed for successful reengineering. Some of these ideas include the use of the computer as the major vehicle for managing information; the use of the information as a way to link people together, no matter where they are physically located; the need for fewer, but new leadership roles; and a higher expectation of all workers within the system. Porter-O'Grady (1996) identifies seven basic rules that contribute to successful redesign. The first rule is that there are no exceptions. He goes on to explain that "the change the world is experiencing leaves no one untouched." This change affects the way people do things and the way in which they interact with the world. No one is exempt from the nature of change. Since no one knows what will happen in the future, the ability to predict the future is not important. It is, however, important to be able to read the "signposts," to be able to get a sense of where the change is leading (Box 8-2).

Another rule to successful reengineering is the construction of a vision. This helps give meaning to what people do. A vision is full of meaning and purpose. It tells what an organization is about. The vision is never permanent; it should be periodically reevaluated for relevance and updated as needed. Empowerment is another rule of a successful redesign venture. It is the "recognition of the power already present in a role and allowing it to be appropriately expressed" (Porter-O'Grady, 1996). People need to make their own decisions and be accountable for their actions. This is true "point of care" decision-making. Empowerment transfers ownership of work from the

---

Box 8-1

Leadership Concepts that Contribute to Successful Reengineering

- The process starts at the top.
- The leader of the process needs to first show that changes have been made in his or her own behavior. If a leader can not change, how can anyone else be expected to?
- The leader must not show any signs of political discord, inadequate commitment, or ambivalence about the change.
- The leader needs to be open, direct, visible, and honest. Everyone is a stakeholder—no more secrets!
- The leader must walk the walk and talk the talk. He or she must show no incongruity between what is said and what is done.
- The leader and others must learn to let go.
- The leader must remember that everyone needs options.
- The leader must not allow people to "escape." Everyone needs to respond to the changes that confront them.

How to Determine Where Change Is Leading

- Look beyond health care. Read about and visualize trends in a global context that affects how things are done. Read futurist health care authors so that the future geography may begin to take shape.
- Identify the driving forces of the changes (e.g., social, financial, economic, cultural).
- Make changes specific and personal to the organization. Ask the question: how well do organizational practices reflect the changes?
- Develop a leadership group to discuss the future and its effects on the organization.
- Translate these views of the future into action plans and work processes. It is important to be guided by future indicators and build on those indicators.

organization to the employee. It demands performance, so roles and expectations must be clear for all people within the organization.

In order to empower, a new management structure or architecture needs to be in place (the fourth rule). The structure of the organization must be designed such that the employees are empowered. The role of a manager is to support the staff, not be a parent to the staff. Another rule is that the staff needs to become self-directed. The structure should be lean and trim; more than two layers of structure diminishes the effectiveness of the organization.

The next rule for a successful reengineering event is to always have a plan of action. Goals should be developed to indicate when the activities and processes are contributing to the success of the system. Everyone is a stakeholder; if the system does not succeed, all fail. There should be few goals; those goals that are developed should be clear and understandable. These goals serve as the foundation for all plans and action. Strategies should reflect the goals toward which they are headed.

The last rule is to evaluate, adjust, and evaluate again. All too often, the whole process of change becomes a living entity in and of itself. Staying focused on the reason for the change and the desired outcomes can be difficult. It is important for all people to focus on the desired outcome. Data should be collected that evaluates progress toward that outcome. It is important to plan for time in advance so the evaluation can take place; it provides a map to where the whole process stands. Staff members should define and conduct the evaluation because ownership is essential to accountability. The seven rules should be a way of approaching the work and not work in and of themselves. The rules help to provide a context for reengineering.

Technology and Changes in Health Care Delivery

A major iunfluence on redesign and reengineering in health care has been the technology explosion—not just in biomedical engineering but in the ability of organizations to communicate with one another and employees. Patients who used to travel several miles for treatment can be treated by telemedicine from the armchair of their home. Supervisors can talk with staff through the use of cell phones and e-mail. While the conventional telephone is still a good means of communication, decision-making is facilitated by the rapid improvement of technology via computers and teleconferencing, telemedicine, cell phones, and e-mail. Data is readily retrievable and can be used to improve treatment and decision-making. Technology will continue to improve and become more affordable, so that an organization's redesign plan will be almost obsolete before it is implemented.

For patients with reduced access to care, access will be improved as communication technology becomes less expensive and more refined. As urban areas spread into rural areas, the benefits of technology will penetrate to previously underserved areas. This penetration of rural areas by urbanites will improve the opportunity for health care access because available technology will move with the urban population. There will always be isolated areas in the United States, but the opportunities for access provided by technology will be of great benefit.

The other issue technology raises is the role of the rural health care center in the care of patients. Patients in urban areas have access to large research-oriented medical centers. These centers are often on the cutting edge of health care. In times of health care reform, even these centers are forced to restructure, decrease costs and length of stay, and improve efficiency. As more health care resources are diverted to rural areas, what will the effect be on medical centers? Can rural health care centers provide the type of care necessary for their populations? If more resources are diverted to medical centers and research, will there be resources to support rural access to care? The two issues are related due to the smaller number of health care dollars, but the needs are not mutually exclusive. The rural population certainly benefits from the research of medical centers.

Reengineering may ultimately decide these issues. If medical centers radically change the way patient care is delivered, that care may be brought to rural areas. If rural health care centers return to their core enterprise, the need for more research dollars for the medical centers may be apparent. The resources may be used in areas that will serve the greater good.

A good example of reengineering health care in larger organizations is the organization of different tasks among multifunctional workers. Rather than a patient going to an electrocardiogram (ECG) technician for an ECG and a

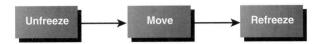

Figure 8-1 Process of change. (From Marriner-Tomey, A. [2000]. *Guide to nursing management and leadership* [6th ed.]. St. Louis, Mosby.)

laboratory technician for phlebotomy, the ECG technician can be trained in phlebotomy so this multifunctional worker could go to the bedside for procedures. In some organizations, the respiratory technician is trained to perform ECGs, blood draws, and respiratory therapy, as well as administer medications; this is the *technical* multifunctional worker. The *nontechnical* multifunctional worker might set patients up for meals, feed patients, perform housekeeping duties, and change beds. The idea is that every worker have transferable knowledge from one situation to another and that each worker can perform more than one task. It is reengineering because it is a radical departure from how health care has been delivered. This is also a good TQM project because it involves systemwide processes for delivering services.

Change and Reengineering

Going through a reengineering process, no matter how large or small, means change. The process of maintaining the integrity of boundaries (homeostasis) means that people and organizations resist attempts to change (Jaffe & Scott, 1997). The old way is the comfortable way; the new way is unknown and scary. This is particularly true if employees are asked to question the very foundation of what they do and how they do it. Lewin's theory of change (Lancaster, 1999) can be used to implement redesign. Lewin identified three steps in the change process, and most of the other change theories are based on Lewin's theory, simply amplifying or expanding the steps so the process is clearer. (For purposes of this discussion, Lewin's theory is applied.)

Lewin's steps are unfreeze, move, and refreeze (Figure 8-1). Essentially, unfreezing means that employees must be aware of the need for change, identify the process or object of change, and plan what the new process will be. This often includes decision-making processes and ethical concerns. Political and social forces are examined to determine if the proposed change can be successful. Lewin calls these *driving and restraining forces*. The driving forces must be stronger than the restraining forces in order for change to be successful (Figure 8-2). Once a plan is determined, the next stage is move. This is the stage where the proposed change is implemented. Depending on the complexity of the change, the learning curve for the change to be accepted may take longer than anticipated. A change agent in charge of the process spends a lot of energy smoothing out rough spots, communicating with the

people affected by the change, and generally making the change a success. The last step is refreezing. In this step, the change is evaluated and modified if necessary. It is incorporated into practice, or the process is incorporated into the larger system. The change agent then steps out of the process, leaving the employees to own the change and the new process or practice.

It is important to realize that change is not always welcomed by employees; therefore it needs to be clear that a change is needed or relevant. Employees are the ones most affected by a change, so their input and support is most important. The employees who resist change need time to get used to the idea and understand the need for this new innovation. Change should be approached in a positive and enthusiastic manner. The change agent needs to be a good communicator and a good listener.

The change must be well planned, and employees need to be prepared for the start date. Education and training is important to ensure success. Many of the "what if" questions (what if this happens, or what if this occurs?) need to be addressed in the plan. One of the biggest reasons change is not successful or not fully implemented is because the plan is not well thought out and employees are not invited to participate. The driving and restraining forces need to be identified and examined early in the process. If more planning and preparation is done on the front end, more success will be experienced on the back end. Ongoing evaluation of a project is necessary until the change has been fully incorporated into the normal way of doing things.

Too many quick changes to the same kind of processes doom future projects. Humans can only tolerate so much chaos and disruption in their lives before they become hardened by new projects and continue to do things their way. This is especially true in health care where the work itself is so stressful that the way the work is delivered becomes paramount to maintaining some semblance of order. Too much change too fast is often given as the reason nurses leave acute care to further their education and move into different positions, find jobs in less-stressful organizations, or leave nursing altogether.

An example of a smaller scale reengineering took place within a community health center (CHC) organization. Cycle times for seeing patients were too long; it was taking too long from the time patients signed in until they were examined by providers. The question was, "How can the appointment and check-in process be changed to reduce wait time, increase efficiency for staff, and maintain quality care?" The staff most affected by this redesign process served as the change team; they included a nurse practitioner (NP), the nursing staff, a patient service representative (PSR), and a physician. Using Lewin's model, the change team began talking about the need and relevance for changing the current process and solicited input from the whole center. The goal was to get patients into and out

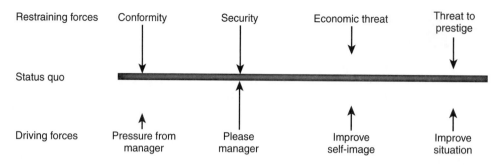

Figure 8-2 Strength of driving and restraining forces. (From Marriner-Tomey, A. [2000]. *Guide to nursing management and leadership* [6th ed.]. St. Louis, Mosby.)

of the system within 45 minutes. Once the goal was determined, the change team began to look at the current process and determine how it should be changed, modified, or developed from ground zero (remember reengineering means "radical" change) to achieve the goal. The driving and restraining forces were identified, and their ability to support or thwart the process was evaluated. The driving forces were the patients, physicians, NPs, and office nurses. Another driving force was the opportunity to work with a team that was self-chosen, giving the team some autonomy and accountability. The restraining forces were the office manager (who designed the process originally and felt it suited the billing process), the medical assistants (who were concerned for how their role might change), and the receptionists (who were resistant to change). In this case, the driving forces (power forces) outweighed the restraining forces, so the change went forward. The change team came up with the idea of care teams. Each team was composed of one provider, one nurse, and one PSR. A team would work the same schedule (i.e., if one was on vacation the others were off, or if the provider went to another site, the whole team went). After discussion with the whole center, the next step was to determine teams. Everyone had to identify the people they wanted to work with. Interviews were held, and the teams were decided based on input from potential team members. Each team would greet their own patients, register them, and triage them back to the provider's room. In this way each individual member had more accountability for getting the team's patients in and seen. Education of all staff was carried out. Construction of individual team cubicles helped facilitate the move to teams. An implementation date was determined and then the project was implemented.

Some adjustment was necessary and some negotiating occurred. For example, working in teams emphasized the need for clear communication between team members. If there was an issue, it needed to be dealt with immediately. In some cases, the team did not function well. One licensed practical nurse (LPN) did not take responsibility for her role in the patient cycle times. She did not seem comfortable making decisions about the patient flow. She preferred the "old" stable process of the past. Continued

work on improving her ability to feel empowered did not help, and she ended up being removed from the team. Once the change was going smoothly, the refreezing began. The project was evaluated, modified and then incorporated into the processes and practices of the CHC. In this case, the reengineering was also started at other sites. One of the reengineered sites was not successful in the process, and analysis is currently underway to determine what went wrong; then the process will begin again.

While this was a simple example, it is a very realistic explanation of how change occurs and redesign can be implemented. The role of the change agent is to keep the project in the forefront and moving smoothly. The change agent could be a staff member, a physician, or an advanced practice nurse (APN). Legitimate authority must be given to the change agent to make sure the change is an authorized and legitimate project. One can assume that if patient waiting times are decreased and overtime reduced, the change was a radical departure from the norm. Checking the outcomes of the project against the goals ensures that the change project did accomplish what was intended.

Barriers for Implementing Reengineering

There are numerous barriers to a redesign of the health care system. One of the concerns in reengineering health care is the sheer size of the industry, which makes the redesign process more difficult. There is still a lot of competition for services and survival among health care systems in urban areas and a lack of any services in some rural areas. Nurses can not decide if health care is a business or a semibusiness (i.e., a service with business aspects). The insurance industry has a lot of power over the health care system, but it can not be allowed to dictate medical and health care for vast numbers of people. Very few people can go through life without any contact with the health care system. So how can health care be reengineered to meet the needs of all at the least expense? The answer to that question will be the solution for health care. Unfortunately, it was probably not as difficult for Ford to redesign car manufacturing processes as it will be for health care to redesign health care delivery.

Opportunities Provided by the Health Care Reform Movement

The reform movement in health care is an opportunity to accomplish some of the long-standing long-term goals of the nursing profession. These include differentiated practice, recognition of the professional nurse as a knowledge worker, the leadership role of the professional nurse in various settings, and the opportunity for APNs to assume an important role in primary health care delivery. Other new roles for nurses include occupational health, entrepreneurial health care businesses, integrated therapies, medical and bioengineering, law, and wellness promotion.

For several decades the issue of differentiated practice has been discussed. There is some consensus that there are differing levels of nursing knowledge. However, there still appears to be reluctance to differentiate the practice of the Associate Degree in Nursing (ADN) graduate and the Bachelor of Science in Nursing (BSN) graduate. The BSN graduate and the ADN graduate do possess similar skills and a similar knowledge base. The BSN graduate possesses more knowledge about the larger issues of patient care, and the 4-year graduate has more to offer an employer. They have benefited from different experiences and educational opportunities. They have a better understanding of the profession and the larger issues surrounding the health care delivery system. Health care reform offers the opportunity to implement differentiated practice and then evaluate the outcomes. One may imagine the radical and dramatic change in care delivery if BSNs and ADNs determined their scopes of practice and implemented them in a health care setting.

Redesign offers the opportunity for nurses to collectively make their role felt. If nurses take a leadership role in redesigning in the health care system, then the amount and usefulness of the nurses' knowledge would be highlighted. Nurses could spearhead redesign efforts and contribute (from a nursing perspective) to the changes made in patient care and the health care system.

The importance of APNs to health care has already been demonstrated. There is plenty of research to support their roles as primary health care providers. Reengineering also offers APNs the opportunity to expand their roles in primary care. Because of their unique knowledge bases in nursing as well as medicine, they could function in expanded roles in acute care, long-term care (LTC), home care, mental health facilities, community agencies, and emergency departments. Even though APNs have expanded their practices into these areas, they could identify other ways to contribute to the redesign of the organization and expand their roles even further.

These opportunities also contain threats from the health care system at large. The growth of unlicensed personnel in the acute care setting; the locus of control regarding decision-making about roles and supervision of these workers; and the dependence of acute care and LTC on paraprofessional workers are a result of health care redesign and reengineering that could threaten the survival of the nursing profession. It is important for nurses to take a strong stand in the redesign of the role of nursing in various health care delivery organizations. If health care organizations can use uneducated, unlicensed, more compliant personnel in structured settings for less money, it is only logical that these uses be explored. Unless nursing is willing to voice its collective disagreement with these measures, then fewer nurses may be needed in these settings. Also, the issue of supervising employees without having authority for discipline and training has been voiced as a concern in most settings. Nursing needs to advocate for one another to lessen the effect of these issues on the individual practice of nursing.

PRIORITIES FOR RESEARCH

Little in-depth objective information is available about the process or outcomes of restructuring or reengineering. Effken and Stetler (1997) identify some reasons why data are lacking. First, it is difficult to conduct research in a traditional manner within the context of a dynamic and changing organization. It can be difficult to collect baseline data or establish adequate research controls when the pace of change is so rapid. Another factor is the nature of the topic. A broad redesign effort is very complicated; therefore the study of the effort is very difficult. Taking a good hard look at the process and outcomes can be risky for administrators; they must be willing to learn that the outcomes may not be what they wanted. The American Organization of Nurse Executives has identified the effect of redesign on patient care outcomes as a research priority. Research related to changes in work roles, work flow, clinical support, and management needs to be evaluated for its effect on both organizational and patient outcomes (Urden & Roode, 1997).

Effken and Stetler (1997) used an alternative approach to assess organizational change in an acute care medical center. Some key aspects of their plan included formative evaluations with an exploratory summative evaluation and use of a large, interrelated set of data from a variety of sources (e.g., managers, staff, patients, physicians) to answer the following question, "To what extent did the new delivery system continuously improve quality and use resources effectively?" Highly specific questions across each level (e.g., organization, clinical service, patient care unit) were used by the authors. Because of the high degree of interrelatedness and a nonlinear process, no causal questions were posed. Their conclusion, based on a preponderance of evidence, "was that the patient-centered redesign had made significant progress in creating an innovative, patient-centered, hospital wide delivery system within the organization that was continuously improving quality and using resources effectively." The use of an organizational culture survey showed a more patient-centered, decentralized culture than existed before the redesign. Several factors have bearing on this study. First, an information system that is adequate for measuring what is needed is critical. Second, this elaborate research was funded by grants from several charitable trusts and foundations; having program staff funded by grant money gives an organization the opportunity to have people specifically designated for research activities. The lack of a designated person to design and lead a research project would make it very difficult for most organizations to consider and gather the needed data. A similar study by Kinneman, Hitchings, Bryan, Fox, and Young (1997) reported evaluation outcomes research related to a systematic program of "reengineering, reconfiguring and reeducating its personnel" using a quasi-experimental/longitudinal repeated measures design. The major research focus was on patient satisfaction, along with other major components: staff satisfaction, physician satisfaction, efficiency of care, cost of care, and quality of care. The researchers felt that the evaluation needed to include both the process and the outcomes to give a true reflection of the redesign. The researchers found significant changes in patient satisfaction on two of the evaluated units. In addition, the perceptions of registered nurses (RNs) indicated that the practice environment also was improved. These initial results were positive, so additional units have gone through the redesign process as research continues related to the effect of the nursing staff mix on safety and quality of care.

Even though TQM is often the philosophy and method used to achieve reengineering projects, there have not been research studies to support the combination of these concepts. Research on the compatibility of TQM and redesign is necessary for confirmation of the importance of these concepts and their ability to achieve desirable outcomes for patients and nurses.

It is known that the work environment for nurses is frequently stressful and chaotic. While this can be confirmed through anecdotal evidence, research is necessary to support this observation. The work environment should improve if one of the goals of redesign is to make the work environment more compatible with quality patient care. If one dramatically and radically changes how care is delivered, regardless of setting, one would not expect the work environment to be worse; rather, the goal of the design project would include a better work environment for nurses. The use of chaos theory might be an appropriate framework to test during the process of reengineering. Chaos theory proposes that the universe is not an orderly place and can not be predicted (Bergquist, 1993; Kellert, 1994; McDaniel, 1996; Priesmeyer, 1992; Thietart, & Forgues, 1995). Instead it is filled with chaos, unpredictability, and uncertainty. As organizations strive to create more permanent organizational structures, they are doomed to fail because the assumptions on which the organizations were built become irrelevant. As an organization grows it loses its ability to adapt and respond to the environment. While chaos theory is still in its infancy, it might serve to explain what happens in organizations that go through reengineering.

Another theory that may be applicable for use with reengineering is the concept of innovation and its diffusion. Rodgers' (1995) model focuses on individual change. He has identified six patterns of how people adapt to new innovations (Box 8-3). Knowing how people adapt to change may be helpful in both research toward and planning of changes. (This is discussed more in Chapter 31.)

The ultimate goal of redesign is the conservation of money and resources. Radical redesign does carry a cost, but is the cost worth the benefit achieved? Outcome research on the cost and benefit of redesign is necessary to justify such continuing efforts.

The work environment that nurses foster for each other has a definite effect on recruitment and retention in the profession. While efforts toward both recruitment and retention in the employment setting have been initiated, there is little documentation of what might happen if the profession of nursing fails to replenish itself. The current

---

Box 8-3

How People Adapt to New Innovations

- *Innovators* are the first ones to adopt new innovations. They like adventure and are usually very technologically inclined.
- *Early adopters* are open and receptive to new ideas, but they are less obsessed with seeking out changes than innovators.
- *Early majority* people like being in the middle of a new innovation; they are neither the first nor the last to adopt something new. These folks like the status quo, but they adopt new ideas shortly before the average person.
- *Late majority* people tend to be followers, skeptical of innovation, and likely to express negative views on changes. These people adopt change only after the majority of people have adopted it.
- *Laggards* are the last people to adopt a new innovation. They are dedicated to tradition and highly suspicious of new innovations.
- *Rejectors* openly oppose innovation and change, encouraging others to oppose them as well. Rejectors may completely immobilize the change process, the system, or the change agent, and they may even sabotage the whole process.

Data from Bushey, A., & Kamphuis, J. (1993). Response to innovation: behavioral patterns. *Nursing Management, 24*(3), 62-64; and Rodgers, E. (1995). *Diffusion of innovation* (3rd ed.). New York: The Free Press.

nursing shortage and the impending faculty shortage could require radical redesign in how education for nurses is conducted and how nurses could be replaced in employment settings. This is an important area for research in the very near future.

IMPLICATIONS FOR MSN EDUCATION AND ADVANCED PRACTICE

Nursing education has not changed substantially in the last several years. The growth of associate-degree programs barely maintained the number of students needed for employment up until 1995. Now the nation is experiencing a major nursing shortage. This shortage also exists at the faculty level. The average age of faculty in the United States is 52 (American Association of Colleges of Nursing [AACN], 1999). As faculty ages and nursing shortages occur at all levels of the profession, redesign in education will be necessary (AACN, 1999). There have already been major redesign efforts in nursing staff development. As technology and distance learning become more common, nursing education will be forced to rethink how education is done.

At some point, nursing education as a whole may need to be transformed and redesigned to better meet the needs of society and continue to be a key player in the health care arena. One way of doing this is to make better use of preceptors and compress the educational timeline. At this time, nursing programs are becoming longer instead of shorter, and it takes a long time to move from one degree to another. Preceptors in both educational and employment settings can help new students and new nurses orient in shorter periods of time. There should be tracks that help students move from the BSN degree to the PhD degree in less than 6 years. Better use of technology means that more students can be taught using fewer faculty members.

As nursing at the Master's level continues to become more specialized, the role of the ANA in the representation of all nurses will be challenged. At present, the ANA is an inclusive organization that purports to represent all nurses. However, the number of common issues for different specialties is decreasing as nursing roles expand. The ANA needs to study its own mission to determine if redesign would make it more or less representative of nurses.

Although the redesign movement offers several opportunities for and threats to nursing, the effect of redesign on nursing and health care is more profound. Nursing redesign should occur in conjunction with other redesign plans for a health care organization. In most health care organizations, nursing plays a key role in achieving the core business of the institution. Health care reform is important to nursing, but nursing should not forget that it is important to health care reform. Health care and nursing are integral to one another and therefore should work together to achieve the goals of redesign and reengineering.

Using a quality management design for nursing redesign may help with the integration of quality into nursing care and aid in goal-achievement for the profession. Flarey (1995) offers some important suggestions for this:

- Examine how nurses' skills are being used in light of quality improvement.
- Maintain quality of care as the focus for redesign.
- Achieve job satisfaction, retention, and productivity through redesign, not in spite of redesign.
- Ensure that the financial goals of the organization are achieved, keeping in mind that compromise here is less expensive than compromise in the other points.
- Tailor redesign for each organization, rather than for many organizations. Redesign programs may be similar in process but not in result.
- Redesign and reengineering efforts must be agency wide. All departments or divisions of an agency must be included in the redesign.
- Apply the principles of TQM and quality improvement to the redesign efforts.
- Review the organization's philosophy, mission, and objectives to make sure the redesign effort is in agreement with the essential work of the organization.
- Engage nursing leadership and administration to be key players in redesign plans and demand their support of nurses in the organization.
- Educate the workforce on the plans and goals for redesign so that their participation is voluntary and enlightened.

Nurses should embrace the opportunities redesign offers at every level and in every health care setting. Using the principles just outlined, nurses can have more effect than other professions at aiding an organization to examine its core values and radically change how care is delivered. Nursing must raise the consciousness of the organization in order to redesign it with the quality health care needs of patients in mind.

In their practices, APNs may want to consider the future in terms of scheduling patients. Open access scheduling is a form of practice reengineering that calls into question everything about a practice, from staff roles to how rooms are stocked. The basic premise is to start the day with mostly open appointment slots. Open access appears to boost provider efficiency and builds trust with patients because appointments are available when they need them (Grandinetti, 2000b). The flow of making appointments improves because there are only two types of appointments: same day and next day. Open access also improves the no-show rate. Patients are more likely to keep appointments that they make on the same day. Because access has been shown to be a vital component in how consumers choose providers, having an open access schedule can help increase the number of patients enrolled in a practice's panel. To start open access scheduling, the backlog of patient appointments needs to be worked down, which means putting in more hours. It also means addressing multiple problems in each visit so a patient does not have to return often. Also, it is necessary to track patient phone calls to determine how many patients a day wanted an appointment and how many could come for an appointment if it was available. The Institute of Healthcare Improvement is helping practices that are interested in trying open access scheduling. Implementing open access scheduling is challenging because of the resistance from colleagues when the system is first proposed. The CHC discussed previously was investigating open access scheduling. When providers first heard about the concept they were resistant to the idea. All they could envision was more patients added to their already full schedules. It also can take up to a year to work out the problems of open access scheduling. (Disease trends change with the seasons, influencing the number of people who need to be seen in a day.) Incentive pay to help work through the schedule backlog might be one answer to the resistance. Another is to involve all providers and staff in the planning process so the benefits of the system are clear to all.

Other innovative changes anticipated in future practice sites include e-mail communication between APNs and patients, the use of headsets to improve communication among team members, no waiting rooms (because patients will be triaged and registered in the examination room), and a patient registry for those with chronic diseases (Kilo & Endsley, 2000). Anything is possible if APNs dismiss any preconceptions about what a "medical office" looks like or how it works. What would an office system that allows APNs to give patients the best possible health care, while being a joyful place to work and producing efficient and high-quality outcomes, look like? The sky is the limit on innovation and creativity as long as APNs are not locked into old preconceived notions.

A final idea on redesign for nursing might be for each individual nurse to reexamine his or her response to peers and new graduates. Meissner (1986) reported that experienced nurses were not supportive of new nurses and often behaved in an impatient, irritated, and hostile manner toward new graduates or nurses new to the employment setting. She also found that nursing faculty were hostile and demeaning to nursing students. In 1999 Meissner repeated her study and found that faculty and experienced nurses are behaving better toward new nurses and students, both in educational and employment settings. However, she believes nurses have more to do to be truly supportive and collegial with one another. In dealing with the effects of reengineering, each nurse should revisit the impact he or she might have on new employees and students. Nurses are aging, and faculty are aging. Now is the time to preserve the profession for the future by restructuring individual attitudes and behaviors toward those with less experience. Nurses should respect one another for what they know and the achievements they have accomplished. Nurses with a higher educational level should remember where they came from, and nurses who have not achieved a higher level should offer respect and support for those who have. Helping and supporting one another demonstrates to other health care professions that nursing is a caring, supportive profession that advocates for patients and respects all of its members for the roles they serve in the care of patients. This is a professional redesign effort all nurses could undertake and achieve on their own.

DISCUSSION QUESTIONS

These questions can be used to promote critical thinking and encourage discussion.

1. Discuss redesign and reengineering success stories and horror stories in class. Why were some situations successful and some not? Identify barriers and supporters in the process. If the reengineering was unsuccessful, what would you do differently?

2. Using the principles already discussed, develop a new way for students to get clinical experiences, knowing that hospital patients are getting sicker and sicker. What would be an alternate way to get health assessment skills?

3. Discuss the advantages and disadvantages of redesign and reengineering on the nursing profession. How might nursing make this an opportunity to shine?

4. What is the effect of telemedicine on patient care across state lines? Discuss if telemedicine should be regulated across state lines. If telemedicine capability is added to a physician practice, what effect would it have on how that practice works? Would the practice need to be redesigned? Is this a project for which redesign is needed, and why or why not?

5. Determine how a nursing unit or any work group would change how care is delivered. For example, if a unit is moving from primary nursing to team nursing, who and how are the tasks and knowledge work of nursing affected? How is the role of the professional nurse changed?

6. React to the following statement: Hammer and Champy (1993) believe that most businesses are not process oriented but rather people, customer, task or structure oriented. It is the process that is most often tinkered with and not radically and dramatically redesigned. Do you agree or disagree with this statement? Discuss the rationale for your view.

Suggestions for Further Learning

- Get one of the following articles: Effken, J., & Stetler, C. (1997). Impact of organizational redesign. *Journal of Nursing Administration, 27*(7/8), 23-32; and Kinneman, M., Hitchings, K., Bryan, Y., Fox, M., & Young, M. (1997). A pragmatic approach to measuring and evaluating hospital restructuring efforts. *Journal of Nursing Administration, 27*(7/8), 33-41. What can you learn related to research of redesign or reengineering efforts? Think about how you would gather the enormous amount of data needed to support the redesign efforts. Identify some of the research instruments that you think might be appropriate.

- Another article to find: Houston, S. (1994). Getting started in outcomes research. *American Association of Colleges of Nursing Clinical Issues, 7*(1), 146-152. This can provide some specific details on how to get started with outcomes research.

- A new concept was discussed previously related to patient scheduling—open access. How would you envision reengineering a practice to make this access possible? Consider the following articles: Grandinetti, D. (2000). Re-engineering your practice: you mean I can see the doctor today? *Medical Economics.* Available online at www.pdr.net/memag/public.htm?path=docs/032000/article5.html; and Kilo, S., & Endsley, S. (2000). As good as it could get: remaking the medical office. *Family Practice Management, 7*(5).

- For more information on care teams, see: Grandinetti, D. (2000). Re-engineering your practice: making the most of your staff, *Medical Economics.* Available online at www.pdr.net/memag/public.htm?path=docs/042400/article5.html. While this article is written from a physician viewpoint, what implications does it have for APNs?

- Get the books: Ackoff, R. (1981). *Creating the corporate family.* New York: John Wiley; and Flarey, D. (1995). *Redesigning nursing care delivery,* Philadelphia: JB Lippincott. Use Ackoff's phases of interactive planning to help in redesign efforts. Do you think this model is appropriate and helpful in the process, or does it just create more work?

- For more information on redesign and reengineering, obtain the following resources: Flarey, D.L. (1995). *Redesigning nursing care delivery.* Philadelphia: JB Lippincott; Hammer, M., & Champy, J. (1993). *Re-engineering the corporation.* New York: HarperBusiness; Ciancio, J. (1998, September). Organizational restructuring and the psychologic contract, *Nursing Management, 29,* 81-82; Coccia, C. (1998, May). Avoiding a "toxic" organization. *Nursing Management, 29,* 32-33; and Pritchett, P. (1994). *New work habits for a radically changing world.* Dallas, TX: Pritchett & Associates.

REFERENCES/BIBLIOGRAPHY

American Association of Colleges of Nursing (1999, April). *Faculty shortages intensify nation's nursing deficit.* Washington, DC: American Association of Colleges of Nursing.

Barton, A.J. & Russin, M.M. (1997, May). Re-engineering intensive care: The role of informatics. *American Association of Colleges of Nursing Clinical Issues: Advanced Practice in Acute and Critical Care, 8*(2), 253-261.

Bergquist, W. (1993). *The post modern organization: mastering the art of irreversible change.* San Francisco: Jossey-Bass.

Brett, J. (1989). Organizational integrative mechanisms, and adoption of innovations by nurses. *Nursing Research, 38*(2), 105-110.

Bushey, A., Kamphuis, J. (1993). Response to innovation: behavioral patterns. *Nursing Management, 24*(3), 62-64.

Chesanow, N. (2000a, February 21). Re-engineering your practice: pick the team and write the game plan. *Medical Economics.* Available online at www.pdr.net/memag/public.htm?path=docs/022100/article3.html.

Chesanow, N. (2000b). Re-engineering your practice: easy ways to track your progress. *Medical Economics.* Available online at www.pdr.net/memag/public.htm?path=docs/article3.html.

Ciancio, J. (1998, September). Organizational restructuring and the psychologic contract, *Nursing Management, 29,* 81-82.

Coccia, C. (1998, May). Avoiding a "toxic" organization. *Nursing Management, 29,* 32-33.

DeLellis, A.J. (1997). Creating a climate of mutual respect among employees: a workshop design. *Health Care Supervisor, 15*(4), 48-56.

Dianis, N., Allen, M., Baker, K., Carledge, T., Gwyer, D., Harris, S., McNemar, A., & Swayze, R. (1997). Merger Motorway: giving staff the tools to reengineer. *Nursing Management, 28*(3), 42-47.

Effken, J., & Stetler, C. (1997). Impact of organizational redesign. *Journal of Nursing Administration, 27*(7/8), 23-32.

Flarey, D.L. (1995). *Redesigning nursing care delivery.* Philadelphia: JB Lippincott.

Flower, J. (1996). We are what we can learn. *Healthcare Forum, 39*(4), 35-41.

Gelinas, L.S., & Manthey, M. (1997, October). The impact of organizational redesign on nurse executive leadership. *Journal of Nursing Administration, 27,* 35-42.

Gerteis, M., Edgeman-Levitan, S., & Daley, J. (1993). *Through the patient's eyes: understanding and promoting patient centered care.* San Francisco: Jossey-Bass.

Gotler, R., Kikano, G., & Valancy, J. (1999). Re-engineering a family practice center. *Family Practice Management, 6*(9).

Grandinetti, D. (2000a, April 24). Re-engineering your practice: make the most of your staff. *Medical Economics.* Available online at www.pdr.net/memag/public.htm?path=docs/042400/article5.html.

Grandinetti, D. (2000b, March 20). Re-engineering your practice: you mean I can see the doctor today? *Medical Economics*. Available online at www.pdr.net/memag/public.htm?path=docs/032000/article5.html.

Hammer, M., & Champy, J. (1993). *Re-engineering the corporation*. New York: HarperBusiness.

Hammer, M., & Stanton, S. (1995). *Re-engineering revolution*. New York: HarperBusiness.

Herriott, S. (1999). Reducing delays and waiting times with open office scheduling. *Family practice management, 6*(4), 38-43.

Hodgetts, R., Luthans, F., & Lee, S. (1994). New paradigm organizations: from total quality to learning to world class. *Organizational Dynamics, 22*(3), 5-18.

Jaffe, D., & Scott, C. (1997, September-October). The human side of re-engineering. *Health Forum Journal*, 1-9.

Kellert, S. (1994). *In the wake of chaos*. Chicago: University of Chicago Press.

Kenney, J.W. (1996). *Philosophical and theoretical perspectives of advanced nursing practice*. Sudbury, MA: Jones and Bartlett Publishers.

Kilo, S., & Endsley, S. (2000). As good as it could be: remaking the medical practice. *Family Practice Management, 7*(5).

Kinneman, M., Hitchings, K., Bryan, Y., Fox, M., & Young, M. (1997). A pragmatic approach to measuring and evaluating hospital restructuring efforts. *Journal of Nursing Administration, 27*(7/8), 33-41.

Lancaster, J.C. (1999). *Nursing issues in leading and managing change*. St. Louis: Mosby.

Lutjens, L., & Tiffany, C. (1994). Evaluating planned change theories. *Nursing Management, 25*(3), 54-57.

Mateo, M., Newton, C., & Wells, R. (1997). Making planned and unplanned role transitions. *Journal of Nursing Administration, 27*(9), 17-23.

McCloskey, J., & Grace, H.K. (1997). *Current issues in nursing* (5th ed.). St. Louis: Mosby.

McCloskey, J., Mass, M., & Huber, D. (1994). Nursing management innovations: a need for systematic evaluation. *Nursing Economics, 12*(1), 35-44.

McDaniel, R. (1996). Strategic leadership: a view from quantum and chaos theories. In W. Duncan, P. Ginter, & L. Swayne (Eds.), *Handbook of healthcare management*. Oxford, England: Basil Blackwell Publishing.

Meissner, J.E. (1986, March). Nurses: are we eating our young? *Nursing 86*, 51-53.

Meissner, J.E. (1999, February). Nurses: are we still eating our young? *Nursing 99*, 42-43, 51-53.

Minnick, A., Pischke-Winn, K. (1996). Work redesign: making it a reality. *Nursing Management, 27*(10), 61-66.

Porter-O'Grady, R. (1996). The seven basic rules for successful redesign. *Journal of Nursing Administration, 26*(1), 46-53.

Priesmeyer, H. (1992). *Organizations and chaos: defining the methods of nonlinear management*. Westport, CT: Quorum Books.

Rodgers, E. (1995). *Diffusion of innovation* (3rd ed.). New York: The Free Press.

Stetler, C., Creer, E., & Effken, J. (1996). Evaluating a redesign program: challenges and opportunities. In K. Kelly & M. Maas (Eds.), *Outcomes of effective management practice (SONA 8: series on nursing administration)* (pp. 231-244). London: Sage.

Taylor, D. (1998). Crystal ball gazing: back to the future. *Advanced Practice Nursing Quarterly, 3*(4), 44-51.

Thietart, R. & Forgues, B. (1995). Chaos theory and organization. *Organization Science, 6*(1), 19-31.

Torres, G. (1992). A reassessment of instruments for use in a multivariate evaluation of a collaborative practice project. In O. Strickland & C. Waltz, (Eds.), Measurement of nursing outcomes (vol. 2: *Measuring nursing performance*) (pp. 381-391). New York: Springer.

Trofino, J. (1997). The courage to change: reshaping health care delivery. *Nursing Managment, 28*(11), 50-54.

Urden, L., & Roode, J. (1997). Work sampling: a decision making tool for determining resources and work redesign. *Journal of Nursing Administration, 27*(9), 34-41.

Werning, S., & Lederman, P. (1995). Advanced practice nursing: new challenges in a changing healthcare system. *Healthcare Trends and Transitions. 6*(5), 10-16.

Chapter 9

Leadership in the Health Care Delivery System

Margaret M. Anderson & Denise Robinson

Many nurses believe that if they are not managers, they do not need to be concerned about leadership behaviors or responsibilities. However, during this era of health care change, it is vital for all nurses to engage in leadership roles whether they are involved in direct patient care, work in a consultant position, or serve in positions of formal authority. It takes effective leadership to function optimally in today's clinical settings (Yoder-Wise, 1999). There are increased opportunities and expectations for nurses, especially advanced practice nurses (APNs), to influence the delivery of patient care. These opportunities are available when providing patient care, serving on quality assurance (QA) teams, maintaining medical records, serving on research committees, and acting as leaders of APN organizations. Actually, it takes both management and leadership to accomplish organizational goals. There are many management styles available and many leadership theories in current practice. In today's health care environment, a manager must be a leader and a leader needs to know something about management. This chapter addresses leadership theory and the issues of leadership involved in the current health care environment.

DEFINITIONS

Leadership and *management* are not synonymous terms. While one person may be both a leader and a manager, leadership is often described as "pushing from behind" and management as "pulling forward." **Management** can be defined as the act, art, or manner of managing, handling, controlling, or directing careful, tactful treatment. A **manager** is one who manages a business or institution, affairs or expenditures, and is generally employed by an institution. The manager is held responsible and accountable for accomplishing the goals of an organization (Sullivan & Decker, 1997). The manager focuses on planning, supervising, evaluating, and coordinating resources. Swansburg and Swansburg (1999) refer to management as the body of

knowledge that is the foundation for the art of managing. In effect, management is a process to get the essential work of an organization done. A **leader**, by comparison, is anyone who "uses interpersonal skills to influence others to accomplish a specific goal. The leader exerts influence by using a flexible repertoire of personal behaviors and strategies" (Sullivan & Decker, 1997). The leader may not have a formal position of leadership. **Formal leadership** is when a leader has legitimate authority (such as that of a manager or supervisor) delegated by his or her organization. **Informal leadership** occurs when there is not a specified management role. The informal leader uses his or her knowledge, skills, and interpersonal influence to accomplish a particular goal that may or may not coincide with the organization's goals. (Table 9-1 clarifies the differences between managers and leaders. Table 9-2 compares various definitions of management and leadership.)

When discussing leadership and management, **administrators** are often mentioned. In health care and business, *administrator* is often the term applied to the person who manages the direct supervisors of groups of employees. It refers to the highest echelon of an organization. In the current management environment, the manager is responsible for several areas, so the term *administrator* includes middle management. **Administrate** means to oversee or manage areas of responsibility. The terms *manage* and *administrate* and *manager* and *administrator* are used interchangeably in the current literature. This chapter uses *leader* and *manager* interchangeably because APNs need to possess the characteristics of both leaders and managers.

Another key word associated with both leadership and management is *power*. **Power** is "the capacity to produce or prevent change" (Sullivan & Decker, 1997). A leader may use power to influence the attitudes and behaviors of individuals. There are various types of power that can be used to influence others (Table 9-3). **Positional powers** are based on the position a person holds. These powers include reward, coercive, and legitimate power and relate directly to the power and job held within an organization. **Personal powers** are based primarily on a

Table 9-1

Differences Between Leaders and Managers

KEY AREA	LEADER	MANAGER
Definition	One who "uses interpersonal skills to influence others to accomplish a specific goal. He or she exerts influence by using a flexible repertoire of personal behaviors and strategies" (Sullivan & Decker, 1997).	One who manages a business or institution, affairs, or expenditures and is generally employed by an institution. He or she is held responsible and accountable for accomplishing the goals of the organization.
Power	Relies primarily on personal power sources to develop interest, inspire commitment, instill confidence, and motivate followers.	Has legitimate power arising from the position. He or she tends to use positional power to promote compliance with standards and policies and facilitate orderly operation in areas of responsibility. Managers may also use personal power to sustain commitment and interest in jobs and boost the morale of employees.
Position	Does not have to occupy formal managerial position, and may be appointed by a group of followers.	Occupies a formal position within an organization and is usually appointed by someone higher in the hierarchy.
Traits	Inspires, develops, and relies on people, which requires trust.	Administrates, maintains, and relies on the system, which requires control.
Focus	People.	Systems and structure.
Freedom	Not limited by organizational position of authority.	Tied to a designated position within an organization.
Actions	Does the right thing (Bennis & Nanus, 1985).	Does things right (Bennis & Nanus, 1985).

Data from Sullivan, E., & Decker, P. (1997). *Effective leadership and management in nursing* (4th Ed.). Menlo Park, CA: Addison Wesley; Grossman, S., & Valiga, T. (2000). *The new leadership challenge*. Philadephia: F.A. Davis; and Marriner-Tomey, A. (2000). *Guide to nursing management and leadership* (6th ed.). St. Louis: Mosby.

person's reputation, expertise, and ability to build trust. Expert, referent, information, and connection power are all types of personal power. The individual with positional power can use those types of power to enhance or effect his or her power.

A manager or leader must use power judiciously; improper use of power can destroy a manager's effectiveness. Power should be seen as a valuable resource to be acquired, conserved, and invested with care. Shortell and Kaluzny (1994) recommend that power be used to support organizational priorities, facilitate important decisions and activities, and help with the relationships of various organization members. A competent leader or manager with good interpersonal skills is more likely to get the assistance of coworkers or employees than someone only using rewards and punishments. (Table 9-4 shows the effect of managerial power.)

For example, an APN serving as chair of the medical records committee of a community health center (CHC), could find that commitment and interest on the part of the other committee members is best obtained by asking for input on a list of goals or objectives for the committee to work on during the year. Each committee member would feel that his or her input was important and contributing to the work of the committee. If work assignments were made based on the priority list, it would make sense for the chair of the committee to have the member who had personal or vested interest in an item work on the development of the item. An APN who works in the women's health center and does many pelvic examinations would logically be the best person to develop a new pelvic examination charting form. Similarly, a physician who sees most of the back injury patients would be the best choice to develop a back pain/musculoskeletal charting form. In this way, the leader uses the strengths of each committee member in delegating tasks, tasks that each committee member wants to accomplish given their area of practice and expertise.

Managers have traditionally served four functions: planning, organizing, directing (command and coordination), and controlling. (Table 9-5 describes the characteristics of these four functions.) Many health care organizations use this systematic and organized approach to management. Others feel that a behavioral approach to management is much more appropriate for health care organizations. Mintzberg (1973) stated that much of a manager's role involves dealing with human relations or interactions. This premise was supported through research done by Dienemann and Shaffer (1992) that found that

Table 9-2

Definitions and Concepts of Leadership and Management

AUTHOR	DEFINITION
H. Fayol	Management can be taught, and the need for managerial ability increases in importance as an individual advances in the chain of command. Principles include division of work, authority, discipline, unity of command, unity of direction, subordination of individual interests to the general interest, remuneration, centralization, scalar chain, order, equity, stability or tenure of personnel, initiative, and *esprit de corps* (Farley, 1990; Marriner-Tomey, 2000).
L. Urwick	Administration is a practical art that improves with practice and requires hard study and thought. Three principles of administration are the investigation of facts, as well as research that results in planning; appropriateness, which underlines forecasting, organization, and coordination; and resource appropriation and allocation (with effective control of each) (Swansburg, 1990).
R. Stogdill	Leadership is a "process of influencing the activities of an organized group in its efforts toward goal setting and achieving" (Farley, 1999). There are differences in responsibilities among group members, but followership is voluntary. Both the leader and the members influence the group's activities (Farley, 1999).
J. Gardner	Leadership is "the process of persuasion and example by which an individual (or leadership team) induces a group to take action that is in accord with the leader's purposes or the shared purposes of all" (Farley, 1999).
R.K. Merton	Leadership is a social transaction in which one person influences other. People in authority are not necessarily good leaders; effective people in authoritative positions combine authority and leadership to assist an organization to achieve goals. Leaders receive and understand communication, and the resources necessary to meet the communication request are available or obtainable. Communication is consistent with the receiver's personal interests and values, as well as the organization's purposes and values (Farley, 1990).
D. McGregor (1960)	Leadership is a highly complex relationship that changes with time and outside forces (a theory developed from the managerial implications of Maslow's theory). Four variables involved in leadership are the characteristics of the leader; the attitudes, needs, and personal characteristics of the followers; the characteristics of the organization, such as purpose, structure, nature of tasks, and cultural values; and the social, economic, and political milieu.
C.M. Talbott	Leadership is "the vital ingredient that transforms a crowd into a functioning useful organization" (Farley, 1990).

more than 50% of a manager's time is devoted to human resource management and nursing services.

In addition to the historical functions of leadership, managers must also manage time effectively, make decisions, communicate with others inside and outside of the organization, plan staff development activities, motivate employees, and formulate and achieve goals. A manger or leader serves as a coach for employees and guides them in meeting organizational goals. The number of managers within organizations has generally been reduced, so managers now have responsibility for several areas. The amount of time each manager spends with each employee is therefore greatly reduced, and a manager may be learning about new areas of responsibility as well as managing. It is helpful for APNs to learn about the numerous leadership theories and apply the appropriate ones to his or her practice. A model proposed by Mintzberg (1994) brings together the need for both leadership and management roles in the Model of Managerial Work (Figure 9-1). In this model, managerial work in five roles—communicating, controlling, leading, linking, and doing—occurs in three concentric circles: information (communication), people, and action. Mintzberg found that when used for an analysis of nursing management, this model served as a way to blend various roles into a "caring management" style.

CRITICAL ISSUES: LEADERSHIP AND THE ORGANIZATIONAL REALIGNMENT OF HEALTH CARE

As the current health care crisis looms, changes in organizational structure to reduce the cost of health care have become prevalent. Rather than the pyramidal shape of past organizational charts, today's chart is linear (Figure 9-2). First-line and middle managers have a responsibility for a wider range of units of productivity. Direct supervision

Table 9-3

Types of Power and Guidelines for Use

TYPE OF POWER	CHARACTERISTICS	GUIDELINES FOR EFFECTIVE USE
Positional Power		
Reward	Goods or benefits that can be offered in exchange for help towards the goal *Example:* Giving approval to a sought-after vacation request if the goal is supported	• Encourage mutual loyalty and teamwork without rewards. Using incentives all the time promotes the expectation of incentives for everything. • Do not use incentives as a bribe for future performance; these effects generally do not last for long. • There are a variety of rewards; money may be the least effective. • Avoid appearing manipulative.
Coercive	Penalties that can be imposed if individuals do not help in moving the goal toward its completion *Example:* Sticking an individual who does not support the goal with more off shifts during the next work schedule	• Use coercion and punishment only when absolutely necessary. • Punish only to deter extremely negative behavior. • Discipline promptly and consistently. Make the punishment appropriate to the infraction. • Give employees responsibility in solving problems. • Use a system of warnings before punishment; if punishment is necessary, always follow through with the consequences.
Legitimate	Associated with the specific job or rank in an organization	• Make requests in a polite manner with clear direction. • Explain the reasons for the request. • Follow-up to see if a request is carried out.
Personal Power		
Expert	Based on the nurse's expertise, skill, and knowledge in a particular area	• Maintain credibility at all costs; avoid careless statements. • Keep up with changes within the field. • Act calmly and decisively in a crisis. • Do not appear superior. • Garner coworkers views and support for ideas. • Serve as a good role model.
Referent	Based on admiration and respect for an individual	• Treat all coworkers as you would want to be treated. • Serve as a good role model by "walking the talk."
Information	Based on the access of information. *Example:* If a person withholds information, power is gained; if a person knows information before the rest of the people, power is gained	• Share information to allow sharing of power. • Do not hold information to the detriment of coworkers.
Connection	Based on connections or links to other people who are powerful or influential	• Avoid "name-dropping." • Do not over exploit connections; recognize the limits of connections. • Use connections only when needed and not for coercive purposes.

Table 9-4

Effects of Managerial Power

TYPE OF POWER	OVERUSE OR MISUSE LEADS TO	UNDERUSE LEADS TO	PROPER USE LEADS TO
Positional Power Reward Coercive Legitimate	Jealousy Distrust	Lack of decision making Failure to achieve goals and objectives Loss of credibility Perception of incompetence	Commitment is possible if a request is polite, reasonable, and nonthreatening. Compliance is likely if a request is legitimate and impersonal. Compliance is possible if coercion is used in a motivational way.
Personal Power Expert Referent Connection Information	Perception of manipulation, overstepping of bounds, and interference Appearance of indecisiveness Accusation of unfairness Lack of objectivity Supervisor hostility Loss of confidence	Perception of unapproachability Lack of concern Being out of touch	Commitment is likely if a request is persuasive or important to the leader and is shared. Compliance is likely if leader is credible. Compliance is possible if a request is persuasive and perceived to be important to the leader.

From Sullivan, E., & Decker, P. (1997). *Effective leadership and management in nursing* (4th ed.). Menlo Park, CA: Addison-Wesley. Reprinted by permission of Prentice-Hall Inc., Upper Saddle River, NJ.

of every employee by a first-line manager is no longer feasible. As health care agencies merge or close and organizations realign to accomplish new goals while staying fiscally viable, employees must adjust to a variety of management styles and behaviors. Sometimes, nonnurse managers are supervising traditional nursing units. The reasoning behind this trend is that the units will be administered or managed as a business unit rather than a patient unit. The hope is that physical, human, and material resources will be used more judiciously than in the traditional nursing model (where a nurse is the manager).

As one can imagine, some approaches are more successful then others. For example, perhaps a vice president for nursing in an acute care organization used to be responsible for nursing units only. With the onset of cost-cutting and realignment, he or she now has responsibility for patient services and carries the title of vice president of patient services. This includes such areas as clinical laboratory, pharmacy, physical therapy, radiology, outpatient services, and operating rooms. The person put in this position may or may not be a nurse, and to learn about these diverse areas and then manage them is quite a task. The vice president may have area directors reporting to him or her, instead of nurse managers or pharmacy managers. In

such a case, the breadth and depth of responsibility for each layer of administration is increased, and the number of layers of administration is decreased.

There are instances where this organizational model is not successful. Very large or very traditional organizations may not function well outside of traditional models of health care. This may be due to a lack of knowledge about how to make changes or a lack of trust for a new administration. In one case, a very small hospital hired someone who was not a nurse as vice president for clinical services. This particular individual did not have any clinical background and did not seem inclined to learn the clinical aspects of patient care. This person made some very poor organizational decisions due to ignorance about the clinical course of illness and the clinical nature of the care provided. Over time, the clinical staff lost faith in this individual's ability to make appropriate decisions; they rebelled, and the vice president was removed from the position. The organization returned to a traditional model of organization, with a nurse as vice president of nursing.

For most APNs, their organizations are not large. In some instances, ambulatory care offices may not even have an organizational chart, depending on the number of people employed within the office. There is usually one

Table 9-5

Characteristics of Management Functions

FUNCTION	CHARACTERISTICS	EXAMPLE
Planning	Four stage process: 1. Establish objectives. 2. Evaluate the present situation and predict future trends. 3. Develop a planning statement (i.e., how the plan will be carried out). 4. Develop an action statement. Addressing how, what, why, when, and who. Making strategic plans (for long-term objectives) and contingency plans (for problems that arise or interfere with getting the work done).	Sherri and Diane, the APNs at Redbud Community Health Center, noticed that many of their patients were obese. They worked on planning a way to address this issue. First they used *Healthy People 2010* to develop their goal. Then they conducted a survey of the adults and found that 75% of them were considered overweight and obese. The APNs then talked with patients about what would assist them in losing weight. After gathering data for 3 to 4 months, the APNs developed two ways to address the issue. First, they offered healthy diet information in a class session one time a month. Second, they offered a beginning exercise class one time a week to help patients get started. The goal of the staff was to have five people attend the healthy diet class and five people attend the exercise class.
Organizing	Coordinating to get the work done. Identifying the work of the organization and who does what within the organization. Developing the chain of command and assigning authority for each position. Developing policies and job descriptions.	Each APN concentrated on one topic. Sherri offered the healthy diet class and Diane coordinated the exercise class. The RN at Redbud developed a poster to advertise the classes and distributed it to patients' homes.
Directing	Getting the organization's work done. (Note that things such as power, leadership style, delegation skills, interpersonal skills, and authority all influence a leader's ability to get work done.)	Since this was a topic near and dear to Sherri, she assumed the leadership portion. With only four people involved, the issue of leadership was not as critical. All four members of the staff worked well together and divided the work according to expertise.
Controlling	Determining outcomes and standards of performance. Evaluating performances and giving feedback. Implementing quality improvement and peer review.	The classes were offered at Redbud. Six people came to the healthy diet class, and fifteen people came to the exercise class the first week. Only eleven came the second week. Sherri and Diane discussed ways to keep attendance steady. They decided to use a contract system to help keep the patients motivated and offered free magazines that stressed health. They considered writing a grant request to obtain funds to support their efforts.

person considered to be in charge or serving as the medical director. In some cases, a nonclinician will serve in the role of the office manager. Depending on the complexity in the office and who the employer is, the organizational charts can look very different. In situations where a nurse practitioner (NP) is an employee of a physician and there is a medical director, the organizational chart would look like that in Figure 9-3. In a situation where all providers are considered equal, it would look like Figure 9-4. When a NP is independent and has a physician collaborator, the organizational chart would look like Figure 9-5. No organizational chart is strictly right or wrong; the chief

function of such charts is to clearly indicate lines of command.

There are some traditional positions that are still in vogue, such as director of nursing and nurse manager. However, most titles, including the traditional ones, now reflect a broader range of responsibility. There is still a chief executive officer (CEO) as the head of a corporation and all of its component parts. A chief financial officer (CFO) is responsible for the financial health of the organization. The chief nursing officer (CNO) is responsible for nursing and most allied health or patient care activities, generally at the corporate level. The chief

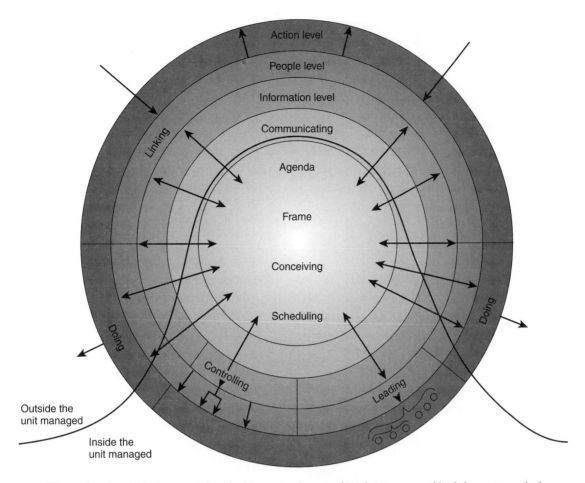

Figure 9-1 A model of managerial work. (From Mintzberg, H. [1994]. Managing as blended care. *Journal of Nursing Administration, 24,* 30.)

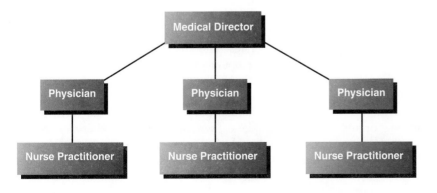

Figure 9-2 Flat organizational structure. (From Yoder-Wise, P. [1999]. *Leading and managing change in nursing.* St. Louis: Mosby.)

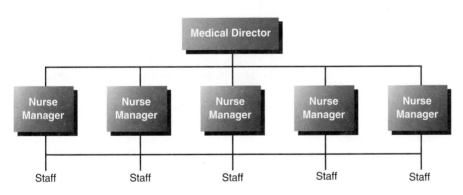

Figure 9-3 Organizational chart depicting the nurse practitioner as the employee of a physician group.

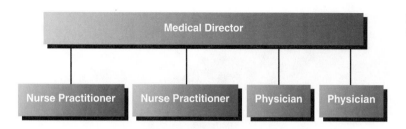

Figure 9-4 Organizational chart showing all providers on equal status.

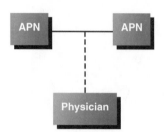

Figure 9-5 Organizational chart for independent practice of advanced nurse practitioners with a physician collaborator.

information officer (CIO) is responsible for the management of the information of the corporation. Other titles include director, assistant administrator, assistant director, executive vice president, vice president, and assistant vice president. A title is dependent on the breadth and depth of responsibility in an individual organization or system. Titles can be misleading, so it is important to clarify what a title means, the breadth and depth of responsibility, and the placement on the overall organizational chart. In realigning the organizational charts with current organizational thought, a new type of structure has evolved. This is known as *matrix management*. Matrix management is organized around the goals of an organization so that the manager of a unit may report to more than one person (Figure 9-6). A nurse manager may have responsibility for three units, all of which have a service or product line. The nurse manager may then report to the vice presidents for each service line, as well as the vice president of patient services. For example, Sally is responsible for the cardiac step-down unit, a general medical-surgical unit that houses all the orthopedic patients and the older adult mental health unit. Under matrix management, Sally reports to the vice president for patient services regarding the overall productivity of each unit and to the service line vice presidents for cardiac care, orthopedic services, and the mental health program for older adults.

Depending on the organizing framework of a corporation, there may be a chief operating officer (COO) at the agency level, or there may be a mid-level COO who has responsibility for more than one agency. In this latter case, there may be a director or administrator at the agency level who has responsibility for the activities of a building or a range of functions related to some organizing property. The work of the organization is still accomplished through

workers at the line level. The line level is where customers needing care interact with employees of the organization. Part of the current chaos in health care is a result of many organizational changes brought on by changes in management or ownership.

Many people are needed to maintain the health of an organization. In a physician's office, the financial officer pays the bills and personnel and manages the revenue to maintain the fiscal health of the organization. The office manager gets patients into the rooms, handles scheduling errors, and generally maintains order. This is helpful to an APN when he or she is providing client care. Although the other people may not be involved in direct care of patients, they are important to the overall health of the organization. (Figure 9-7 shows the organizational chart of a community health center with several different offices.) Private ambulatory care offices that are all owned by an organization or alliance may have an APN that serves as the "chief" APN and oversees hiring and other policy issues related to APNs.

Analysis of Health Care Organizations

Health care organizations can be analyzed using a systems theory loosely analogous to the biological theory of evolution. That is, an organization attempts to secure its viability by responding to changes in the environment. An organization's response to the environment produces further changes in the environment; thus an evolution occurs, with the environment forcing organizational response and the organization forcing environmental response. This occurs in organizations in much the same way that organisms change their biology to meet new challenges, thus ensuring their place in nature. Of course, biology does not usually change as quickly as the health care environment has changed in recent years. The health care organization is considered an open system; it has permeable boundaries that are affected by the society in which it operates. The changes in society force internal changes in the operation of an organization. The rapidity with which these changes have occurred recently is responsible for the chaos about which most health care workers and administrators complain (Yoder-Wise, 1999).

An example of systems theory in operation is the rapidity with which the health care environment responded to changes in the payment system. Once health

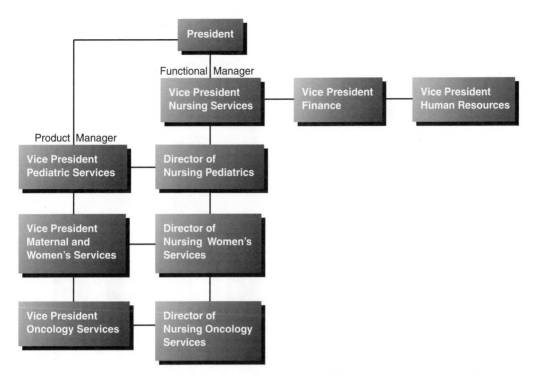

Figure 9-6 Matrix organizational structure. (From Yoder-Wise, P. [1999]. *Leading and managing change in nursing*. St. Louis: Mosby.)

care organizations became convinced that payers would no longer tolerate such rapidly rising costs, the agencies began a series of measures designed to maintain or reduce costs. These measures included reductions in force, flattening of the organizational chart, and investigation of the use of unlicensed personnel. In other words, the health care system responded to a threat to its viability through cost reduction measures. These changes also can affect APNs. For example, a large physician group owned by a hospital organization is overextended due to expansion. A few of the offices are closed, and personnel are moved to different offices. Several APNs lose their positions due to these changes. Therefore APNs need to be aware that as the system is affected by a change in one area of the system, the change will frequently be felt in other parts of the organization.

Role of Knowledge Workers in the Health Care Arena

The business of health care agencies is the provision of health care services. This business is accomplished through the use of health care workers, such as nurses and other professional workers, who provide the services or care necessary to meet the needs of patients (the clients). Thus an agency hires knowledge workers to meet their goals. One of the conflicts that often arise is that managers often do not understand the difference between knowledge workers and skilled workers. Knowledge workers use a professional framework to gather data, make a diagnosis, or determine a problem or conclusion and then plan and implement interventions to solve the problem, alleviate the diagnosis, or meet a need. Knowledge workers have a special set of skills to support clinical decision-making. The organizing professional framework calls for evaluation of the plan and intervention and then modification based on actual results versus desired results. In nursing this organizing framework is the nursing process. The APN uses this framework in assessment, planning, and intervention for patients.

Skilled workers have learned skills but limited knowledge with which to use those skills in the care or servicing of customers. For example, the licensed practical nurse (LPN) may hold a license, but his or her knowledge base is limited when compared with the registered nurse (RN). The LPN has many skills for giving treatment and even providing data for assessment. However, the ability of the LPN to critically evaluate patient data is limited due to the knowledge base he or she possesses. That is not to imply that a skilled worker does not add to his or her knowledge base through training and experience, but the breadth and depth of his or her beginning knowledge base limits ability. Skilled workers are important to the health care system for delivery of patient care, but what they can do is limited.

If health care management does not understand the differences between knowledge and skilled workers, there is a danger that neither will be used to the fullest extent or that they will be considered equal and the cheapest used to meet important high-level organizational goals. This is

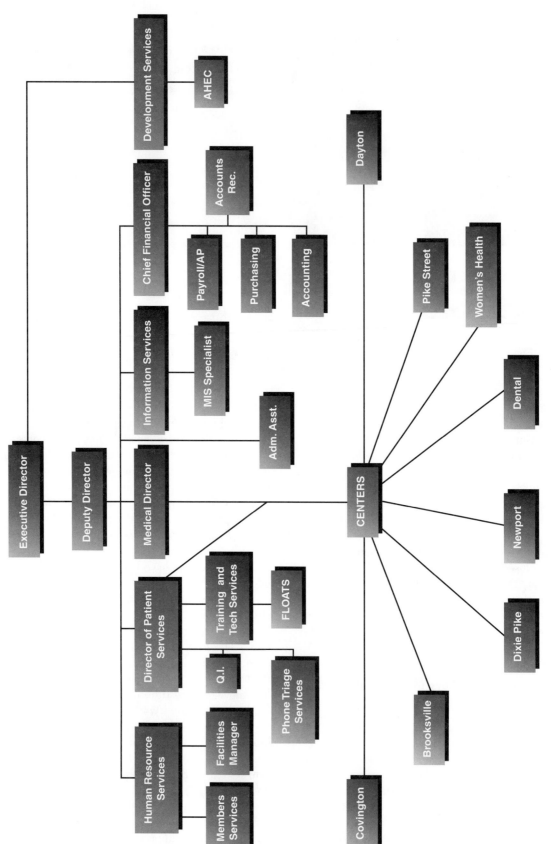

Figure 9-7 Organizational chart for a community health center with several offices.

especially a danger in rapid change organizations. Professional nurses are still the best resource for providing competent patient care. Failure to use professional nurses (knowledge workers) to the best advantage in delivering patient care in any setting decreases the quality of care provided and the benchmark standard of care. In physician offices, a medical assistant can not assess the patient at the same level as a RN. However, a RN can not assess and treat the patient at the same level as a NP. Each worker has a role in patient care, but those roles increase in responsibility, accountability and knowledge as the transition from skilled worker to knowledge worker progresses.

The concept of knowledge worker can go beyond individuals. Organizations are striving for a knowledge-based stance with the focus on applied knowledge and service. This means that the natural asset of the organization will be its workers and people. Organizations want a design that makes them flexible and resilient to support innovation and address market demands. The preferred organization is made up of teams, preferably of knowledge workers. The new definition of manager is "one who is responsible for the application and performance of knowledge" (Weaver & Sorrells-Jones, 1999). Organizations that have adopted this format have few layers of management between the patient level and senior leadership, with the preferred method of work done through teams. Each team member is a vital part of the team, offering unique knowledge and skills. Teams are flat and not hierarchical, possessing the power to accomplish their goals. The operating premise for knowledge organizations is that knowledge can be managed. This model is drastically different from other models; the emphasis is on "achieving results rather than performing activities" (Weaver & Sorrells-Jones, 1999). The primary role of the leader is to present and support the broad vision of the organization, working strategically to support teams' efforts to work creatively and innovate. Another role of the leader is to manage the environment, giving teams leeway to focus on the essential jobs. Health care organizations, especially hospitals, are "among the most rigidly bureaucratic and hierarchical, discipline fragmented institutions in America" (Sorrells-Jones, 1999). This does not come as any surprise to most APNs. In these types of organizations, it is critical to create an organizational design that supports and encourages knowledge work. No matter the ultimate organizational design, the leader must support both knowledge work and knowledge workers. A leader serves in the role of integrator and facilitator for the knowledge teams. This focus on results and not processes may require a shift in thinking for some, but APNs are in the habit of looking at patient outcomes, so the resulting shift may not be drastic. It will require risk-taking on the parts of all involved; however the risk may be to not take the risk and therefore miss the opportunity for knowledge workers to gain intrinsic rewards from the completion of the work. A knowledge-based environment has the poten-

tial for high performing results, and APNs will want to be involved in the process of transformation.

Leadership Theory and Transformational Leaders

There are many theories of leadership and management that have been popularized over the years. (The most common theories and their basic tenets are included in Table 9-6.) These theories often conflict with individual philosophy or values. Nevertheless, individual managers have wrestled with the conflict of personal values versus professional values or expectations over the years. (This conflict is more fully explored in Chapter 14.) When an individual is asked or expected to compromise personal values for the sake of an organization, it is a dilemma that causes great personal stress and anger. The anger is a result of having to make a choice between personal beliefs and organizational necessity. An example is the expectation or request that a manager lie to an employee. If the manager values truth, honesty, and sincerity, a request to lie is unacceptable. However, to not lie may place the manager's job in jeopardy. The manager may feel some disillusionment if he or she believed the organization valued honesty in dealing with employees.

The newest and perhaps the most viable theory being proposed is the concept of transformational leadership. This theory has as its core concept the idea of trust and honesty on the part of both employer and employee. This theory works well with systems theory because it assumes common or shared goals on the part of employee and employer. It assumes that both employer and employee will do what ever is ethically and legally necessary to meet the goals of the organization and employees and ensure the survival of the organization. Transformational leadership is the result of movement from an industrial orientation to a service orientation. This leadership model is based on a new view of leadership, management, and the world of work. Its absolute application to health care is difficult because the work unit for health care is a human one as opposed to an object, but the principles are applicable.

The theorists commonly associated with the evolution of transformational leadership are James McGregor, James Burns, Peter Drucker, Tom Peters, Peter Senge, Warren Bennis, and (more recently) Stephen Covey. In nursing, Ann Marriner-Tomey and Ann Barker have laid the groundwork for application of transformational leadership in nursing. It is within the discussions of these leadership experts that it becomes apparent that leadership is an art distinguished by ethical principles and open, honest communications, and that management functions may occur within the leadership activity but are not necessarily a distinguishing characteristic (Farley, 1999). Although it is true that *managers* are appointed and *leaders* may or may not have formal appointments within an organization, most managers are appointed for their leadership potential as

Table 9-6

Common Leadership Theories

Trait Theories

Great Man Theory (McGregor, 1960)	Wanted to identify intellectual, emotional, physical, and other personal traits of effective leaders. His assumption was that leaders are born and not made, with few people being born with all the needed characteristics. No particular traits were ever identified, although some traits appeared to be common.
Unnamed (Stogdill)	Developed a profile of successful leaders and traits: drive for task completion, responsibility, vigor, persistence, creativity in problem-solving, social initiative, self-confidence, accountability of actions, stress resistance, tolerance of frustration, and ability to influence the behaviors of others.
Unnamed (Bass)	Identified three categories of traits for a leader: intelligence (judgment, decisiveness, knowledge and fluency), personality (adaptability, alertness, integrity, and nonconformity) and abilities (cooperativeness, popularity, and tact).
Unnamed (C.R. Hollomon)	Believed that leaders are born as such and meet the personal needs of groups. True leadership results when the appointed head causes group members to accept directives without any apparent exertion of authority or force. A leader is sufficiently popular and prestigious enough to deepen collective unity in the group (Farley, 1990).

Leader-Constituent Interaction Theories

Leadership Task Theory (J.W. Gardner)	Identified tasks performed by leaders: envisioning goals, affirming values, motivating, managing, achieving work unity, explaining, serving as a symbol, representing the group, and renewing (Farley, 1990).
Leader-constituent interaction (J.W. Gardner)	Noted that charismatic leaders emerge in troubled times and that crowds follow them because of a belief that the leaders are endowed with qualities that set them apart from others. Leaders can be evil. Gardner also assumed that leaders and constituents have equal influence on each other, and that the constituents select the leader. Leaders want to be leaders. Transforming leaders respond to the desire among constituents for a positive goal (Farley, 1999).

Behavioral Theories

Theory X and Theory Y (McGregor, 1960)	Related to Maslow's motivation theories and based on the premise that security is a need of constituents and that a leader must provide security in the form of fair pay and fringes. An atmosphere of approval must be provided for subordinates, and they need to know what is expected of them. Discipline must be consistent, and employees need to feel independent so they will accept responsibility to perform tasks to meet the organization's goals. Theory X, a conventional view of the 1950s, said that management is responsible for organizing work and that employees do the work. Managers direct the work and control the actions of workers. Workers are passive and therefore in need of active intervention by management. Workers lack ambition and prefer to be told what to do. Theory Y, the suggested replacement for Theory X, says that management organizes work and workers do the work. Management and employees are motivated to get the work done because of positive regard for the goals of the organization and employees. Management must develop employees for higher and more responsible positions and work. Employees are motivated to do good work and desire approval from their supervisor (Farley, 1999).
Systems of leadership (R. Likert)	Identified four systems of leadership. Leadership effectiveness improves as it approaches System IV. • *System I*—Exploitative-authoritative: Decision-making and communication are top down; motivation is coercive; review and control functions are centered on the top management. • *System II*—Benevolent-authoritative: Decision-making and communication mostly top down; ego and economics are motivating factors; review and control functions mostly centered at the top. • *System III*—Consultative-democratic: Some delegated decisions made at lower levels; communication is up and down; motivation is based on ego, economics, and other concepts, such as a desire for new experiences; review and control functions primarily centered at the top, but input is sought from lower levels. • *System IV*—Participative-democratic: Dispersed decision-making; communication up, down, and lateral; motivation by economic rewards established by the group; review and control functions shared by all employees (Farley, 1999).

Data from Swansburg, R., & Swansburg, R. (1999). *Introductory management and leadership for nurses* (2nd ed.). Sudbury, MA: Jones and Bartlett; Sullivan, E., & Decker, P. (1997). *Effective leadership and management in nursing* (4th ed.). Menlo Park, CA: Addison-Wesley; and Marriner-Tomey, A. (2000). *Guide to nursing management and leadership* (6th ed.). St. Louis: Mosby.

Table 9-6

Common Leadership Theories—cont'd

Behavioral Theories—cont'd

Managerial Grid (R. Blake & A. McCanse)	Described a two-dimensional leadership model with dimensions of tasks or production and employee orientations of managers. The concern for the people dimension is on the vertical axis; the concern for production is on the horizontal axis. Five leadership styles are plotted in four quadrants of a two-dimensional grid. This grid uses a nine-point scale with 1 being low concern, 5 being average, and 9 being high concern. The assumption is that a concern for both people and production is integrated in a manager's thinking so that both are present to some degree. The belief is that the manager can use the grid to sort out various possibilities, attitudes, values, and beliefs. Shared 9,9 status is assumed to achieve the highest quality results over time because no conflict exists between employee needs and organizational needs for production.
Studies of leadership styles (Lewin and Lippett, 1938)	Identified three common leadership styles related to forces within the leader, group members, and situation. • *Autocratic*— Leaders make all decisions; more concern with task achievement than people; promotes hostility, aggression, apathy, and decreased initiative. • *Democratic*—Employees involved in decision-making; people oriented, with a focus on human relations and teamwork; results in increased productivity and job satisfaction. • *Laissez-faire*—Leaders are loose and permissive and tend to abdicate leadership responsibilities; fosters freedom for creativity and a "feel good" atmosphere; results in decreased production and frustration.
Ohio State Studies (I. Myguire, D. Mosley, and P. Pietri)	Use a quadrant approach that relates leadership effectiveness to structure initiation, with an emphasis on the task or production process and consideration for employees. The studies identified four primary leadership styles (Farley, 1999).

Leadership Style Theories

Contingency Model of Leadership Effectiveness (Fiedler, 1967)	Identified three classifications that measure how much power and the type of power and influence a group gives to a leader. Classifications include the relationship between the leader and the group members; the task to be performed (the more highly structured the assignment, the less power the leader has); and the positional power of the leader. Various combinations of these factors result in situations that are favorable, moderately favorable, or unfavorable for manager effectiveness. A leadership style is most effective when matched to the situation.
Situational Leadership Theory (Hershey & Blanchard, 1988)	Developed and based around the Contingency Model. Four distinct leadership styles are based on the readiness and ability of the followers: participating, delegating, telling, and selling. This is based on the developmental level of the group members, individually and collectively. The more immature the followers, the more task oriented a leader must be for employees to remain passive. As followers mature, a leader can focus on relationships and growth and development of the followers.
Expectancy Model (Vroom & Yetton, 1973)	Developed as a model that helps managers know how much employee involvement is needed in decision-making. The creators identified five leadership styles: tell, sell, consult, join, and delegate.
House-Mitchell Path-Goal Theory (House & Mitchell, 1974)	Applied the theory of human motivation and task performance to leadership effectiveness. It uses the method of removing obstacles in the way of goal attainment. There are four kinds of leadership behavior: supportive leadership, participative leadership, achievement-oriented leadership, and directive leadership.
Three-Dimensional Theory of Management (W.J. Reddin)	Created as a combination of Blake's and Mouton's theory, Fiedler's theory, and Effectiveness Theory. The result is four basic leadership styles. These are: • *Separated*—Task and relationship orientations are low. • *Dedicated*—Task orientation is high and relationship orientation is low; leaders are dedicated to the job. • *Related*—Relationship orientation is high and task orientation is low, leaders relate to subordinates. • *Integrated*—Task and relationship orientations are high, leaders focus on managerial behavior combining task orientation and relationship orientation. One dimension of effectiveness is a leader's degree of achievement of position objectives. Also, an effective leader applies a particular style based on the situation (Farley, 1999).
Theory Z Organizations (W. Ouchi)	Focused on consensual decision-making. The style is democratic, decentralized, and participatory. It encourages employee involvement. Leaders and managers concentrate on interpersonal skills. Quality-of-life issues are important to the organization (Farley, 1999).

Continued

Table 9-6

Common Leadership Theories—cont'd

Contemporary Theories

Transactional leadership (Homans, 1958)	Based on the premise that people interact based on expected rewards or benefits. Interaction continues until it no longer is valuable. Therefore leaders need to know what rewards employees want and use incentives to keep employees motivated and loyal.
Transformational leadership (Bass, 1985)	Based on going beyond the status quo. It aims to change interactions based on major changes going on within organizations. An example would be to include both the leader's and employees' needs and goals in one common goal. The focus is on higher values and causes, with the leader inspiring the followers.
Transformational leadership (Bennis & Nanus, 1985)	Based on the idea that "leaders do the right things; managers do things right" (Marriner-Tomey, 2000). Four strategies for taking charge are: attention through vision, meaning through communication, trust through positioning, and deployment of self.
Connective leadership (Klakovich, 1994)	Based on collaboration and teamwork. As health care organizations become more complex, more and more collaboration and cooperation will be needed to accomplish the goals of an organization.
Shared leadership	Based on empowerment principles of participative and transformational leadership (Sullivan & Decker, 1997). This theory describes the belief that each group is composed of many leaders so that all involved may get a chance to serve in a leadership capacity. It encompasses self-directed work teams and shared governance.
Servant leadership (Greenleaf, 1991)	Based on the notion that leadership comes from a desire to serve; one outcome of serving may be leading. It is also based on the concepts of caring, service, and the welfare of others.

Data from Swansburg, R., & Swansburg, R. (1999). *Introductory management and leadership for nurses* (2nd ed.). Sudbury, MA: Jones and Bartlett; Sullivan, E., & Decker, P. (1997). *Effective leadership and management in nursing* (4th ed.). Menlo Park, CA: Addison-Wesley; and Marriner-Tomey, A. (2000). *Guide to nursing management and leadership* (6th ed.). St. Louis: Mosby.

well as their management skills. Bennis (1989) asserts that to transform means to fundamentally change in design, character, shape, purpose, or use. Transformational leadership exists in organizations and is a philosophical approach to leadership, a moral edict for fundamental change. Bennis acknowledges how hard it is but says that with effort and study it can be done.

Marriner-Tomey (1993) defines transformational leadership in nursing as "a relationship grounded on the leader's values." She further asserts that transformational leadership is not a series of techniques but rather visionary leadership. Change at a higher level is transformation. While it is not a religious experience, transformation is a higher order of change, and transformational leadership is a higher order of leadership. It is leadership grounded in principle and guided by vision. For nursing, this means a transformation of the profession into leadership roles in the health care system. Four cognitive skills are required to be a visionary (transformational) leader (Marriner-Tomey, 1993). These skills involve the ability to express the vision, explain the vision, extend the vision, and expand the vision. This would imply that a transformational leader has a vision of where the organization is headed and how it can get there, shares the vision with others through verbal and written communication, broadens the vision beyond the

executive suite, and ensures that the vision pervades the organizational culture. It is often said that the transformational leader "walks the talk," accomplishing what he or she says will be accomplished.

Leadership in the Health Care System

Leaders must possess personal qualities that make them want to be leaders. One of the distinguishing characteristics of transformational leaders is the ability to envision the direction or collective purpose of the agency, or to have a vision of where the organization (or smaller division) is headed. The transformational leader can communicate that vision and garner the resources necessary to achieve the goal. This type of leader addresses goals with whatever form and structure are necessary to achieve the collective purpose of the organization. This means that not all organizations or agencies within a large system may be organized exactly the same. Room for growth or development is encouraged. One outstanding characteristic is trust. Trust begets trust, and distrust begets distrust. Honesty and trust are expected, practiced, and rewarded; lying and distrust are discouraged, dispelled, and eventually "punished." Transformational leaders have a lot of positive regard for self and others. This is not the same as self-confidence or self-esteem; it is regard and respect for oneself and one's employees. Bennis (1989) identifies five characteristics for the transformational leader. These characteristics are vision, passion, integrity, trust and curiosity, and daring. Bennis says curiosity and daring involve lifelong learning and risk-taking. These are characteristics to be nurtured and cultivated in the leaders of tomorrow's health care organizations.

It is difficult to find these qualities in today's health care managers and leaders. Part of the reason for this might be that these characteristics have not always been desirable in the "good" manager or administrator. In the past, more emphasis was placed on the need to get the job done with the smallest number of people at the lowest cost; this does not require as much leadership skill as the ability to see the short term, the upcoming shift or week. Currently, power is withheld or used in less than appropriate ways to achieve organizational goals. The vision of the organization's goals is often lost in the mire of sculpting a healthy bottom line. Every new administration means a new method of management. Being a truly transformational manager/leader in health care today requires a lot of risk-taking and the legitimate use of power to achieve higher goals. There is not a lot of trust in health care, so the first job is to rebuild trust and integrity as desirable and rewarded characteristics for managers. Bennis suggests that transformational leaders keep an eye on the horizon as well as the bottom line and seek a good balance between the two. There are currently some transformational leaders in health care, in places such as magnet hospitals. Other locations for transformational leaders include CHCs and even office locations.

Farley (1999) points out that in health care, there are more men in positions of leadership then women. Men tend to be direct and autocratic leaders and believe what is objective and fair. On the other hand, women tend to be more democratic and participative by sharing power and information, encouraging consultation and enhancing group members' self-worth (Marriner-Tomey, 2000). Women are more likely to have leadership styles similar to transformational leadership because women tend to be concerned with relationships and preserving self-esteem. Women are historically outnumbered in health care management at the higher echelons. In the last 10 years, women have been promoted to high level positions in health care, but they do not appear to have the same level of power as their male counterparts (Farley, 1999). Also, nursing remains primarily a female occupation, as well as being the largest employment unit in most health care agencies. Nursing has not asserted its potential power for health care change in most organizations. Nurses tend to view their work as a job rather than a meaningful and important professional endeavor. However, nurses are important knowledge workers in all facets of health care and can be the leaders of the future.

Nursing's Role in Changing the Health Care System

Now is the time for nursing to exercise its potential to make important changes in health care and to assert its leadership for the health of the society. How this is accomplished is up to the professional organizations within the profession. Rather than fighting the same old battles, nursing organizations should work together to create dynamic change in the whole health care system. Keeping in mind that the health care system reacts to changes in the environment, now is the time to make that system react to changes the nursing profession is willing to sponsor and achieve to provide better, more accessible health care for the nation. For example, nurses from all practice settings and all levels of practice could unite on the need for nurses at the bedside and the need for that work to be rewarded and respected.

It is also important to note that all nurses are both leaders and followers. There are distinct times for all nurses, from the staff nurse to the doctorally prepared nurse, to exercise their leadership skills, and there are distinct times for them to follow the nursing leadership available. Marriner-Tomey (2000) indicates that the industry needs great followers as well as great leaders, because followers contribute about 80% to the success of organizations. They do utilize independent and critical-thinking skills. The American Nurses Association (ANA) is an inclusive organization that is the voice of the profession. The ANA is well acquainted with nursing issues, and they have lobbyists available to help support change at the national, state, and local levels. The ANA is involved in securing prescription privileges for APNs, as well as discussing staffing and work environment issues in acute and long-term care (LTC) settings. There are other APN organizations that also function as voices of the profession, such as the American College of Nurse Practitioners.

There are some highly critical issues related to leadership in health care organizations. These issues are complex and interrelated, and they include the continual change in philosophy and personal values required as organizations merge, close, and change their relationships with one another. When organizations merge or purchase other organizations, there is a tendency for the dominant organization to disregard and disrespect the other. However, each organization brings its own unique set of cultural behaviors and values to the new organization. A transformational leader merges the cultures into one with integrity, respect, and open communication with the new corporate culture, whereas a traditional leader might require cultural changes without respect to the merged organization's history or traditional values.

Another issues involves an organization's stated management philosophy, compared with the actual practiced behavior and the cognitive dissonance in employees and consumers resulting from what is said and what is done.

Cognitive dissonance is a concept that implies that what is expected is not what actually exists. An example might be the image of nurses, portrayed on television, as dressed in white uniforms and high heels, which is not what a patient sees in the hospital; a patient's nurse might be dressed in scrubs and certainly not in high heels. Cognitive dissonance also results when an employee observes that management does not practice what it preaches (i.e., employees not being treated the way they expect). In advanced practice, a practitioner may not have the autonomy he or she expected.

The effect of education and training on the behavior of managers is a critical issue. More education on leadership theory and practice and more training in management techniques creates a better manager/leader. Advanced education also helps a manager become a critical thinker who questions higher management. Advanced education could create a horde of transformational leaders in health care that can solve some of the problems inherent in the system.

Another critical area is the notion of paradoxes in the leadership of health care organizations and the stated goals of these organizations. It seems that health care organizations are confused about their primary business. While health care certainly has business aspects to it, the fact that it deals with human lives actually makes it a semibusiness. Health care organizations should come to some consensus about what is business and what is health care. How do organizations meld the need for financial survival with the charge to protect the nation's health?

PRIORITIES FOR RESEARCH

Research priorities include leadership preparation for health care leadership positions. Research on the necessary educational preparation for nurse administrators and clinical specialists as well as other advanced practitioners is needed. Further research is still needed on the expectations of employers for employees and the leadership skills needed to be a leader. Research that continues to evaluate the applicability of Mintzberg's Managerial Model is also needed.

The Northwestern University Graduate School developed the Manager as Developer Model to provide a framework for leadership development. It was developed in reference to the acute care setting, but Aroian, Meservey, and Crockett (1996) see its applicability in community-based primary care. The concept of manager as developer is based on the notions that professionals must "guide their own work, maintaining autonomy and responsibility for their own practice" (Aroian, Meservey, & Crockett, 1996), while also maintaining links with other organizations. The Manager as Developer Model (Bradford & Cohen, 1984) implies a search for excellence as leaders move from strategy to action. It is a process-

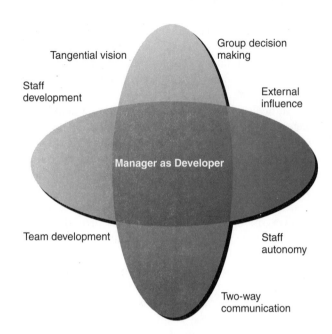

Figure 9-8 Manager as Developer Model. (From Aroian, J., Meservey, P., & Crockett, J. [1996]. Developing nurse leaders for today and tomorrow: part one. *Journal of Nursing Administration, 26*[9], 18-26.)

oriented model with seven major concepts (Figure 9-8). Research by Aroian (1990) and Gilbert (1986) provided research data and support for the model. The *Guidelines for Essentials for Nursing Education for Nursing Administration* identify critical content area for nursing administrators and are integrated into Figure 9-9. This model is also appropriate for APNs in the community. In order to survive in today's health care environment, the APN role needs to encompass much or all of the model as presented. The APN is not and should not be limited to only patient care; to strive for excellence and change, areas such as marketing, finance, and communication must be considered. Future research looking at the components of the APN role in the community is needed to help define and explain the leadership traits that APNs exhibit.

Leadership is not a fine science, but further research on the application of transformational leadership to nursing and the health care system may greatly enhance the role nursing can play in the advancement of the health care system. Boston and Forman (1994) conducted a study of nurse executives across the United States to identify specific motivational and demotivational factors that influenced them to apply for middle-management positions. The primary motivational factors were individual empowerment, recognition, respect, autonomy, and participation in decision-making. They said that job satisfaction came from having the power to effect change and enjoying a sense of personal accomplishment, as well as

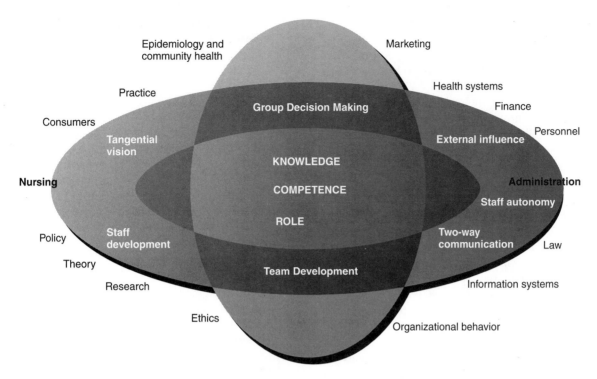

Figure 9-9 Nursing administration in community health. (From Aroian, J., Messervey, P., & Crockett, J. [1996]. Developing nurse leaders for today and tomorrow: part one. *Journal of Nursing Administration, 26*[9], 18-26.)

their ability to influence and develop staff. Demotivational factors included fiscal constraints, uncompensated time, and accountability without authority. This study notes that factors that support nursing leaders are important for job satisfaction. It also builds on the work on motivational factors by Maslow (1970) and Herzberg (1977). Further research that examines both types of factors to help plan strategies that recruit and retain good leaders/managers is important.

Other research needs to center around the role that APNs play as leaders. Busen and Jones (1995) evaluated the relationship of personal variables (e.g., personality type, self-esteem, learning style) on the leadership potential of pediatric NP graduates over a 3-year period. Significant results were found to relate those students who learned abstractly and the ability to function effectively as a change agent after graduation. Other research looking at APNs' leadership potential or skills is woefully lacking. Using the Leadership Performance Competence Profile (Desimone, 1996) may be one way to identify leadership behaviors and competence in APNs. It would be interesting to use this instrument in the context of novice-to-expert role attainment to see if the leadership scores would increase over time or in different APN positions. Jones, Guberski, and Soeken (1990) looked at APN perceptions of the leadership climate in their organizations, as well as the APNs' self-reported formal and informal leadership behaviors. A 37-item questionnaire to measure self-reported leadership behaviors and a 50-item questionnaire

to measure organizational climate were given to a random sample of NPs. The findings indicate that the dimensions of the organizational climate predicted the NPs' perceptions of their leadership behaviors. Those areas with a negative relationship indicate areas where nurse practitioners need more self-direction. The factors that most influenced self-reported leadership behaviors were risk, structure, reward, and responsibility. A positive organizational climate and manager can support both formal and informal leadership behaviors in NPs. This research is a start; however, no further research related to the leadership of APNs was found. While most research is focused on patient outcomes, nursing interventions, and quality of care, there is still a place for research related to leadership traits and behaviors of APNs.

IMPLICATIONS FOR MSN EDUCATION AND ADVANCED PRACTICE

Nursing education is at the cutting edge for health care leadership change. The complexity and rapidity of the changes make the crystal-ball approach to education more complex than ever before. Nurse educators must study the trends and patterns in business and health care and the political winds to determine the skills that new APNs, staff nurses, and nurse leaders need to influence and lead in the future. Nursing can continue to be an important force in health care if nurses assume the leadership roles necessary to affect health care delivery. Some very important decisions must soon be made for the profession to move into the future.

One area that needs to be addressed regarding the preparation of health care professionals is the provision of information about knowledge-intense organizations, knowledge workers, and integrative teams. Many professionals work hard during their careers, and most of these have been successful. This success means that it is likely these individuals never learn from failure; when things go wrong, they are likely to blame others. The Pew Health Professions Commission issued its report *Recreating Health Professional Practice for a New Century* in 1998. In the report they identify 21 competencies that health care professionals need to be successful in the twenty-first century (Box 9-1). One competency relating to interdisciplinary interaction was so important that it is one of four focused recommendations (Sorrells-Jones & Weaver, 1999b). Interdisciplinary practice needs to be emphasized in APN programs so that all health care professionals have the opportunity to study and work together. This also implies the need for APNs to learn about other health care professionals and the skills and competencies they bring to patient care.

For APNs to be equal partners within the interdisciplinary team, it is vital for them to have the same educational credentials. As it stands, nurses are the least educated professionals on the team. Pharmacists are moving toward the doctorate (Pharm D), and in social work, a Master of Social Work degree is the norm. APNs need the added boost that the Master's degree brings, along with a strong professional self-concept. APNs need to believe that they contribute to the work of the group and that their input is unique and valuable. Pike (1997) describes how the poor self-concept of many nurses inhibits their ability to function as full colleagues or collaborators with other health care professionals. APNs must be willing to share their voice on the knowledge team or risk losing their "seats at the table." Pike (1997) goes on to say that "when a nurse makes the choice to define herself as a colleague, participating in patient care as an integral and equal member of the health care team, she seizes opportunities for professional fulfillment while affording patients the benefits of integrated care." APNs are likely in a better position than RNs in regard to speaking out as members of a knowledge team, but this is an anecdotal conclusion only. This information is very pertinent to Master of Science in Nursing (MSN) programs. It behooves programs to present information about knowledge workers and the necessity for APNs to function as knowledge workers. APNs need to know that they fill a unique role on the knowledge team. Since technology will be at the center of any interdisciplinary team, APNs need to be comfortable

Box 9-1

Twenty-One Competencies for the Twenty-First Century

- Embrace a personal ethic of social responsibility and service.
- Exhibit ethical behavior in all professional activities.
- Provide evidence-based, clinically competent care.
- Incorporate the multiple determinants of health in clinical care.
- Apply knowledge in the new sciences.
- Demonstrate critical thinking, reflection, and problem-solving skills.
- Understand the role of primary care.
- Practice preventive care religiously.
- Integrate population-based care and services into practice.
- Improve access to health care for those with unmet health needs.
- Practice relationship-centered care with individuals and families.
- Provide culturally sensitive care to a diverse society.
- Partner with communities in health care decisions.
- Use communication and information technology effectively and appropriately.
- Work in interdisciplinary teams.
- Ensure care that balances individual, professional, systemic, and societal needs.
- Practice leadership.
- Take responsibility for quality of care and health outcomes at all levels.
- Contribute to continuous improvement of the health care system.
- Advocate public policy that promotes and protects the health of the public.
- Continue to learn and help others to learn.

Data from O'Neil, E. (1998) *Recreating health professional practice for a new century.* San Francisco: Pew Health Professions Commission.

and competent with the management of data and information. Opportunities for interdisciplinary interaction and the development of technological competence will be important components of APN programs of the future.

Development of transformational leaders and support for their efforts in leading health care is necessary. Education should emphasize the role APNs have as leaders. Leadership roles will be thrust upon APNs simply because of their unique role and position in health care. Decision-making skills and conflict management are critical skills for all nurses. It does not matter what position an APN has, conflicts must be dealt with. Having knowledge regarding conflict-management techniques is helpful.

All nurses should be aware of the traits of effective leaders and not shirk from serving in a leadership capacity,

Suggestions for Further Learning

- Read the following articles and discuss their application to transformational leadership: Bass, B.M. (1990). From transactional to transformational leadership: Learning to share the vision. *Organizational Dynamics, 18*, 19-31; and Davidhizar, R. (1993). Leading with charisma. *Journal of Advanced Nursing, 18*, 675-679.
- Get the following article and use the Leadership Performance Competence Profile to evaluate your leadership competence and the competence of others, such as your preceptors and fellow classmates: DeSimone, B. (1996). Tranforming curriculum for a nursing leadership course: a collaborative approach. *Journal of Professional Nursing, 12*(2), 111-118.
- Go to the Pew Health Professions Commission website at futurehealth.ucsf.edu/pewcomm.html. Look at the publications related to health professions for the twenty-first century. What are the implications for APNs in those documents? You might also want to look at the one related to physician assistants (PAs) for comparison.
- Read the article: Porter-O'Grady, T. (1999). Quantum leadership: new roles for a new age. *Journal of Nursing Administration, 29*(10), 37-42. Do you agree with his predictions for health care and the implications for APNs? Why or why not?
- Read the editorial: Curtain, L. (1997). How and how not to be a transformational leader. *Nursing Management,*

28(2), 7-8. Do you agree with her position on transformational leaders? Why or why not?
- Obtain the book: Kouzes, J., & Posner, B. (1993). *Credibility: how leaders gain and lose it, why people demand it.* San Francisco: Jossey-Bass Publishers. This book addresses walking the talk, or doing what you say you will do. It offers insights into how APNs can develop credibility and maintain it.
- Another book worth obtaining: Wheatley, M. (1994). *Leadership and the new science: learning about organization from an orderly universe.* San Francisco: Berrett-Koehler Publishers. This book discusses the applicability of quantum physics to our universe. While a challenging read, it may provide some insight into how APNs can use chaos theory to create future health care roles.
- Get the article: Gurka, A. (1995). Transformational leadership: qualities and strategies for the CNS. *Clinical Nurse Specialist, 9*(3), 169-174. This article offers practical strategies on how to personally and professionally transform your leadership qualities and traits.
- Get the book: Rosen, R. (1996). *Leading people: transforming business from the inside out.* New York: Viking Penguin. This book presents the success stories of 36 of the most innovative leaders of our time along with tips for developing leadership skills.

whether it is an informal position or an actual managerial position. As has been mentioned, it is important for APNs to realize their potential as leaders. This can only be accomplished by defining their management or leadership style. Continued learning related to a nurse's own development is important. By the same token, it is important for APNs to promote leadership development in others. All colleagues should have the opportunity to develop to their potential so that the needs of recognition, accomplishment, and sense of belonging are met. The best way to be a part of a radically changing world is to help shape it (Drucker, 1994).

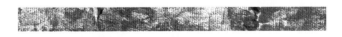

DISCUSSION QUESTIONS

These questions can be used to promote critical thinking and encourage discussion.

1. Discuss the role of the nurse as a knowledge worker in different levels of practice. What can be done to

enhance that role, and how can nursing use that role to its advantage?
2. Discuss leadership characteristics in current employment settings. What characteristics are desired in leaders? Followers?
3. Can the various special interest groups and associations in nursing be brought together for the sole purpose of negotiating for nursing in all settings? Why or why not?
4. How could an APN who sees patients be considered a leader? Describe how an advanced practice leader could be a transformational leader.
5. Draw some organizational charts identifying where an APN might be in various organizations (e.g., in a hospital, ambulatory care practice, independent practice).

REFERENCES/BIBLIOGRAPHY

Allen, D. (1998). How nurses become leaders: perception and beliefs about leadership development. *Journal of Nursing Administration, 28*, 115-120.

Aroian, J. (1990). Assessments of nurse middle managers in patient care settings before and after implementation of the Manager as Developer Model. In B. Henry (Ed.), Research column, *Nursing Administration Quarterly, 16*(1), 81-82.

Aroian, J., Messervey, P., & Crockett, J. (1996a). Developing nurse leaders for today and tomorrow: part one. *Journal of Nursing Administration, 26*(9), 18-26.

Aroian, J., Messervey, P., & Crockett, J. (1996b). Developing nurse leaders for today and tomorrow: part two. *Journal of Nursing Administration, 26*(10), 29-34.

Bass, B. (1985). *Leadership and performance beyond expectations*. New York: Free Press.

Bennis, W. (1989). *On becoming a leader*. Menlo Park, CA: Addison Wesley Publishers.

Bennis, W., & Nanus, B. (1985). *Leaders: the strategies for taking charge*. New York: Harper and Row.

Bernhard, L., & Walsh, M. (1995). *Leadership: the key to the professionalization of nursing* (3rd ed.). St. Louis: Mosby.

Bradford, D., & Cohen, A. (1984). *Managing for excellence: the guide to developing high performance in contemporary organizations*. New York: Wiley and Sons.

Busen, N., & Jones, M. (1995). Leadership development: educating nurse practitioners for the future. *Journal of the American Academy of Nurse Practitioners, 7*(3), 111-117.

Carroll, T., & Adams, B. (1994). The work and selection of first line managers: 1982-1992. *Journal of Nursing Administration, 24*(5), 16-21.

Conger, J. (1992). *Learning to lead: the art of transforming managers into leaders*. San Francisco: Jossey-Bass Publishers.

Curtin, L. (1997). How and how not to be a transformational leader. *Nursing Management, 28*(2), 7-8.

DeSimone, B. (1996). Transforming curriculum for a nursing leadership course: a collaborative approach. *Journal of Professional Nursing, 12*(2), 111-118.

Dienemann, J., & Shaffer, C. (1992). Manager responsibilities in community agencies and hospitals. *Journal of Nursing Administration, 22*(5), 40-45.

Drucker, P. (1994). The age of social transformation. *Atlantic Monthly, 274*(5), 53-80.

Dunham, D., & Fischer, E. (1990). Nurse executive profile of excellence. *Journal of Nursing Administration Quarterly, 15,* 1-8.

Dwyer, D., Schwartz, R., & Fox., M. (1992). Decision-making autonomy in nursing. *Western Journal of Nursing Research, 22*(2), 17-23.

Edwards, P., & Roemer, L. (1996). Are nurse managers ready for the current challenges of healthcare? *Journal of Nursing Administration, 26*(9), 11-17.

Farley, S. (1990). Leadership. In Swansburg, R.C. (1990). *Management and leadership for nurse managers*. Sudbury, MA: Jones and Bartlett Publishers.

Farley, S. (1999). Leadership. In Swansburg, R.C., & Swansburg, R.J. (Eds.), *Introductory management and leadership for nurses* (2nd ed.). Sudbury, MA: Jones and Bartlett Publishers.

Fiedler, F. (1967). *A theory of leadership effectiveness*. New York: McGraw Hill.

Flarey, D. (1996). Reinventing leadership. *Journal of Nursing Administration, 26,* 9-10.

Fullam, C., Lando, A., & Johansen, M. (1998). The triad of empowerment: leadership, environment and professional traits. *Nursing Economics, 16,* 254-257.

Gilbert, J. (1986). *A study of the use of Bradford and Cohen Manager as Developer Model to assess selected staff nurses leadership skills* (Dissertation). Boston: Northeastern University.

Gilbert, M. (1975). Personality profiles and leadership potential of medical surgical and psychiatric nursing graduates. *Nursing Research, 24,* 125-130.

Glynn, P., Arndt, M., Beal, J., & Bennett, N. (1996). The interconnectedness of nurses' lives. *Journal of Nursing Administration, 26*(5), 36-42.

Greenleaf, R. (1991). *The servant as leader.* Indianapolis, IN: The Robert K. Greenleaf Center.

Grohar-Murray, M., & DiCroce, H. (1997). *Leadership and management in nursing*. Stamford, CT: Appleton-Lange.

Grossman, S., & Valiga, T. (2000). *The new leadership challenge*. Philadephia: FA Davis.

Hershey, P., & Blanchard, K. (1988). *Management of organizational behavior* (5th ed.). Englewood Cliffs, NJ: Prentice Hall.

Herzberg, F. (1977). One more time: how do you motivate employees? In L. Carroll, R. Paine, & A. Miner (Eds.), *The management process* (2nd ed.). New York: MacMillan.

Homans, G. (1958). Social behavior and exchange. *American Journal of Sociology, 63*(6), 597-606.

House, R., & Mitchell, T. (1974). Path goal theory of leadership. *Journal of Contemporary Business, 3,* 81-98.

Ingersoll, G., Schultz, A., Hoffart, N., & Ryan, S. (1996). The effect of a professional practice model on staff nurse perception of work groups and nurse leaders. *Journal of Nursing Administration, 26*(5), 52-60.

Jones, L., Soeken, K., & Guberski, T. (1986). Development of an instrument to measure self reported leadership behaviors of nurse practitioners. *Journal of Professional Nursing, 2*(3), 180-185.

Jones, L. Guberski, T., & Soeken, K. (1990). Nurse practitioners: leadership behaviors and organizational climate. *Journal of Professional Nursing, 6*(6), 327-333.

Jones, M., & Clark, D. (1990). Nurse practitioners develop leadership in community problem solving. *Journal of the American Academy of Nurse Practitioners, 2*(4), 160-163.

Klakovich, M. (1994). Connective leadership for the 21st century: a historical perspective and future directions. *Advances in Nursing Science, 16*(4), 42-54.

Krejci, J., & Malin, S. (1997). Impact of leadership development on competencies. *Nursing Ecnomics, 15,* 235-241.

Lewin, K., & Lippitt, R. (1938). An experimental approach to the study of autocracy and democracy: a preliminary note. *Sociometry, 1,* 292-300.

Lipman-Blumer, J. (1992). Connective leadership: female leadership styles in the 21st century workplace. *Sociology Perspective, 35*(1), 183-203.

Marquis, B., & Huston, C. (1996). *Leadership roles and management functions in nursing* (2nd ed.). Philadelphia: J.B. Lippincott.

Marriner-Tomey, A. (1993). *Transformational leadership in nursing*. St. Louis: Mosby.

Marriner-Tomey, A. (2000). *Guide to nursing management and leadership* (6th ed.). St. Louis: Mosby.

Maslow, A. (1970). *Motivation and personality* (2nd ed.). New York: Harper and Row.

McCloskey, J.C., & Grace, H.K. (1997). *Current issues in nursing* (5th ed.). St. Louis: Mosby.

McDaniel, C., & Wolf, G. (1992). Transformational leadership and the nurse executive. *Journal of Nursing Administration Quarterly, 22*(2), 60-65.

McGregor, D. (1960). *The human side of enterprise*. New York: McGraw Hill.

Meighan, M. (1990). The most important characteristics of nursing leaders. *Nursing Administration Quarterly, 15*, 63-69.

Mintzberg, H. (1973). *The nature of managerial work*. New York: Harper and Row.

Mintzberg, H. (1994). Managing as blended care. *Journal of Nursing Administration, 24*, 29-36.

Morrison, R., Jones, L., & Fuller, B. (1997). The relationship between leadership style and empowerment on job satisfaction of nurses. *Journal of Nursing Administration, 27*, 27-34.

Murphy, M., & Deback, V. (1991). Today's nursing leaders creating the vison. *Nursing Administration Quarterly, 16*, 78-80.

O'Neil, E. (1998). *Recreating health professional practice for a new century*. San Francisco: Pew Health Professions Commission. Available online at futurehealth.ucsf.edu/pewcomm.html.

Pike, W. (1997). Entering collegial relationships: the demise of the nurse as victim. In J. McCloskey & H. Grace (Eds), *Current issues in nursing*. St. Louis: Mosby.

Senge, P.M. (1990). *The fifth discipline: the art & practice of the learning organization*. New York: Doubleday Currency.

Shortell, S., & Kaluzny, A. (1994). *Health care management: a text in organization, theory, and behavior* (3rd Ed.). New York: John Wiley and Sons.

Sorrells-Jones, J. (1999). The role of the chief nurse executive in the knowledge intense organization of the future. *Nursing Administration Quarterly, 23*(3), 17-25.

Sorrells-Jones, J., & Weaver, D. (1999a). Knowledge workers and knowledge intense organizations: a promising framework for nursing and healthcare. *Journal of Nursing Administration, 29*(7/8), 12-18.

Sorrells-Jones, J., & Weaver, D. (1999b). Knowledge workers and knowledge intense organizations (part 3): implications for preparing healthcare professionals. *Journal of Nursing Adminstration, 29*(10), 14-21.

Stahl, D. (1998). Leadership in these changing times. *Nursing Management, 29*, 16-18.

Stevens-Barnum, B. (1994, October). Leadership: can it be holistic? *Holistic Nursing*, 9-15.

Sullivan, E., & Decker, P. (1997). *Effective leadership and management in nursing* (4th ed.). Menlo Park, CA: Addison Wesley.

Swansburg, R. (1990). Why nationalize nursing administration? *Journal of Nursing Administration, 20*(6), 8-9, 12-13.

Swansburg, R., & Swansburg, R. (1999). *Introductory management and leadership for nurses* (2nd ed.). Sudbury, MA: Jones and Bartlett.

Taccetta-Chapnick, M. (1996). Tranformational leadership. *Nursing Administration Quarterly, 21*, 60-66.

Tyrrell, R. (1994). Visioning: an important management tool. *Nursing Economics, 12*, 93-95.

Vroom, V., & Yetton, P. (1973). *Leadership and decision making*. Pittsburgh, PA: University of Pittsburgh.

Weaver, D., & Sorrells-Jones, J. (1999). Knowledge workers and knowledge intense organizations, Part 2: designing and managing for productivity. *Journal of Nursing Administration, 29*(9), 19-25.

Wiggens, L. (1997). The conflict between "new nursing" and "scientific management" as perceived by surgical nurses. *Journal of Advanced Nursing, 25*, 1116-1122.

Yoder-Wise, P.S. (1995). *Leading and managing in nursing*. St. Louis: Mosby.

Section III

Health Care Economics and Finance

Margaret M. Anderson & Alice G. Rini

*C*ost containment—these words, or variations of them, have become almost a mantra for health professions at the turn of the millennium. Without cost containment, the health care system, even restructured, may continue to spiral out of control, leading to its ultimate undoing. When one sees only the short-term effects of an economic policy or its effects on a particular group, rather than the long-term effects for all, financial problems are inevitable. To avoid this long-term consequence, advanced practice nurses (APNs) must understand at least the basics of the economics and financing of health care. There will be challenges, in their respective roles as direct care providers, to understand both the bigger picture and the "bottom line" and be able to speak about these with individuals who govern costing, spending, and reimbursing health care dollars. Unit III is not intended to educate APNs for roles as economists or financial planners. Rather, it is designed to provide the foundation in health care economics necessary for an appreciation of how health care is financed and reimbursement is ensured. This foundation is necessary to enable APNs to value fiscally responsible practice and know the way to make such practice possible.

Chapter 10 provides the principles of health economics that serve to explain the current market-driven health care system, as well as discussing both private and governmental influences on consumers and providers within the existing system. Selected concepts of economic theory are presented. The chapter explains how the system works and how economic principles may be applied to the day-to-day clinical realities at practice sites. A historical overview explains the way in which the current system evolved.

Unless patients pay their own health care costs, there is inevitably a third-party payer involved in every health care encounter between an APN and a patient. Chapter 11 details the system for third-party payment, whether from private insurance, Medicare, Medicaid, or some form of managed care. It explores how the social and political events of recent history have shaped health care payment systems and their associated policies. There is considerable coverage of governmental programs that meet the health care needs of children and older adults.

Chapter 12 introduces the budgeting process and its requisites and explains the types of costs that affect both the work of an organization and direct patient care. The important processes of costing-out APN services and analyzing variances are presented. Understanding these concepts of financial planning and budgeting are critical not only to being a fiscally responsible provider, but also to being able to articulate one's financial value to a practice. That fiscal planning must be linked to an organization's mission and practice goals is clearly shown with examples.

An APN without consistent reimbursement for services provided will not survive in practice for very long. Consequently, knowing an APN's rights and responsibilities for billing and reimbursement processes is critical. Chapter 13 presents these aspects of APN practice and provides practical wisdom about how to document effectively for third-party reimbursement, use Current Procedural Terminology (CPT) and International Classification of Diseases (ICD-9) coding effectively, and avoid insurance fraud. The basic requirements necessary for reimbursement are provided, as are numerous suggestions for maximizing reimbursement. The chapter reiterates the importance of APNs knowing the details of practice income in their respective settings to enable rational justification of their specific contributions to the practice.

Chapter 10

Principles of Health Care Economics

Alice G. Rini

The evolving health care environment of the new millennium will demand advanced practice nurses (APNs) who understand the basics of health care economics as a foundation for health care delivery. APNs will need an economic background to interface comfortably with those in fiscal management positions and to appreciate when to seek additional expert guidance in the economic aspects of practice. Certainly there will remain an expectation for all providers to be fiscally accountable for clinical practice.

DEFINITIONS

Several definitions provide a context for understanding the basics of health care economics. The **gross national product** (GNP) is a measure of the total income produced in 1 year through the labor and property supplied by residents of the United States, no matter where the resources are located (Clayton & Geisbrecht, 1997). The **gross domestic product** (GDP) is the market value of all final goods, services, and structures produced in 1 year through labor and property located in the United States, no matter who owns the resources. The conversion to a GDP in 1991 makes the measurement of total output consistent with the World Bank system, though the difference between the GNP and the GDP is generally small. The Bureau of Economic Analysis (BEA) in the United States Department of Commerce issues three estimates of the GDP each quarter; the final one is issued 3 months after a particular quarter ends (Clayton & Geisbrecht, 1997). A **recession** occurs whenever the real GDP declines for two successive quarters. The National Bureau of Economic Research (NBER), a private research institute, makes the determinations.

The **consumer price index** (CPI) is a measure of the average change in prices for a fixed "market basket" of goods and services used by consumers. The Bureau of Labor Statistics (BLS) uses a list of consumer goods and services from a 1982 to 1984 survey as its base period in determining later price changes. The index includes items of consumer use such as food and beverages, housing, clothing, transportation, medical care, and entertainment (Clayton & Geisbrecht, 1997).

Market refers to the area of economic activity in which buyers and sellers come together and the forces of supply and demand affect prices; it is the course of commercial activity by which the exchange of commodities or services is effected. *The Index of Leading Indicators* is a monthly statistical measure that attempts to predict the direction of the economy by measuring such factors as average hours of production, claims for unemployment insurance, orders for plants and equipment, and new housing starts (Clayton & Geisbrecht, 1997).

CRITICAL ISSUES: UNDERSTANDING ECONOMICS FOR HEALTH CARE

If one studies the history of societies in terms of how a society answers questions about management of resources and monetary policy, one finds a variety of strategies used. It is important to note that any policy or system of policies is dependent upon the characteristics of the society itself. What may work in one society will not be successful in another. Therefore it is difficult to transplant one system from a different culture to another merely because it seems to work in a particular place. For instance, in some ancient societies, religious principles were the guide for resource use and distribution. Religious tradition determined the production methods and distribution of goods, and the people accepted this. It is likely that all the members of the society held similar beliefs and values, so this was an acceptable manner of policy strategy. In addition, before the age where most citizens became reasonably educated and sophisticated, central rationalistic planning was the norm. Today, some groups, such as the Kibbutzim, Amish, and other isolationist religious or cultural groups, still rely on cooperative or community principles. However, contemporary societies, even those that are quite homogeneous, rely primarily on a market system of production and distribution. A *market system* is a mechanism for producing, distributing, and allocating resources in a society or group. The market generally is a desirable mechanism for allocating scarce resources because it can lead to a technically cost-effective and efficient system of managing goods and services.

Markets and Prices

Within a market system, goods and services are produced in the least costly manner so that the optimal mix of goods and services are produced and they are distributed in a way that reflects their importance to individuals within the group or society. Price is an important factor in a functioning market system. Prices are a notice to market participants regarding the cost to acquire the goods or services offered.

Most consumers are very conscious of price when they enter the market and shop for everyday necessities. A consumer may choose a store brand of plastic bandages over a national brand if the price for the former seems to provide more value than the latter. However, if consumers have experience with the lower-priced brand and have found it to be of lower quality, they may purchase the national brand, even at the higher cost. If the price for a particular consumer product uses a considerable amount of a person's budget, that consumer may not be able to purchase other things.

Consumers decide how best to spend their resources, purchasing those products that are most important to them and foregoing the less important ones. Prices ensure that resources are used in a productive manner (i.e., taking the opportunity cost into account). *Opportunity cost* may be described as an opportunity (in terms of product or service) for which resources could be used if another choice was made for the expenditure of funds. This can be understood by a simple example. A consumer sees a new mountain bicycle for $500. She has the $500, but she must also pay her college expenses. If she focuses on her long-term goals, she will decide to forego the bicycle to attend college. The college degree may give her a higher earning power so that she may purchase the bicycle if she so desires. The opportunity cost is the bicycle, foregone in favor of the tuition. Consumers make such choices everyday, but these choices seem almost nonexistent in the health care market. Generally, people do not have the opportunity to make choices about health care purchases or do not believe such choices should have to be made.

Markets need some external controls to operate optimally. A well-functioning legal system that can define and adjudicate or mediate claims concerning property rights; enforce contracts; and punish transgressors and fraudulent behavior is necessary. Markets also depend

upon merchants and consumers behaving in certain ways. Also important are consumers who understand the market and can determine the quality and value of goods and services to a reasonable degree or who can use others to provide this information for them. Markets are based on the ability and willingness of consumers to pay for goods or services and an understanding of opportunity cost. When one considers the concept of market prices, the communication and cooperation that such prices permit must also be understood (Lee, 1998b). Consumers often see prices as being too high and a barrier to their ability to obtain what they want. Suppliers see prices as too low. Consumer demand and producer supply determine a price toward which the market tends to go. Prices encourage suppliers to produce the amount that consumers demand. This coordination of action between consumers and suppliers is the result of information that is communicated through market price (Lee, 1998b). Figure 10-1 depicts supply and demand curves that affect the price of any product or service. It should be noted that as supply increases (i.e., more health care providers and more available appointments), demand decreases and prices drop because consumers tend to have all they want; as supply decreases (i.e., fewer health care providers), demand increases and prices go up. The higher the demand is, the higher the price will be. The optimum price is where the lines cross, the point at which suppliers produce as much of a commodity as consumers want or need.

Where there is an interference with the balance of demand and supply, such as price ceilings imposed by a governmental entity, suppliers are likely to produce fewer units of a particular commodity, while consumers may wish to acquire a greater number of those commodities. This is a condition called *shortage*, or the inability of a consumer to obtain a product even though the consumer has the funds to buy it. This is different from a condition of *scarcity*, which Lee (1998b) defines as the inability of

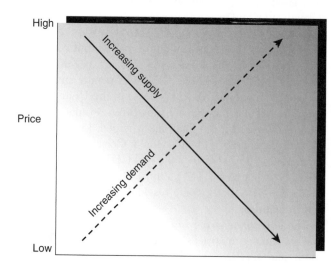

Figure 10-1 Supply and demand curves. Note that as the price of care increases, the number of visits decreases.

consumers to obtain as much as they want of a commodity at zero cost. Shortages are generally eliminated by appropriate prices that have been determined by market communication; shortages, therefore, are created by the government's (or another authority's) restrictions on market prices. There are supporters of price ceilings because it can be demonstrated that they lower the price of a product for consumers. However, prices alone do not account for actual cost, and Lee (1998b) describes how in countries where there are price controls, consumers often spend many hours shopping to find products or stand on long lines to purchase generally inferior materials. There is a cost in terms of time and money, as well as putting up with the poor quality of goods, to the consumers, but it is important to note that the supplier does not receive any more revenues. The higher cost to consumers does not let suppliers know that more of the commodity should be available on the market, so the supplier or manufacturer does not increase production. Some consumers do benefit from price ceilings, but it is mostly those who are politically connected or somehow favored by producers. This does not support a fair and open market, so most consumers are harmed by price ceilings.

Economic Statistics

Economic statistics inform the citizens of a country or of the world how they are doing financially. Statistics also help determine what kinds of action need to be taken to make change or progress. Such decision-making, much as any kind of decision-making, requires accurate and meaningful information and knowledge. Knowledge is the only logical basis for future action (Clayton & Geisbrecht, 1997). The United States generates countless reports and amounts of statistical data, providing different kinds of information addressing everything from local use of electricity to broad-based measures of national spending on agricultural products. The *Statistical Abstract of the United States* provides information and statistical tables on a large variety of topics. It is generally found in the government documents section of public and university libraries. Statistical information that is of broad interest to many citizens is reported on television and radio and in newspapers and magazines. The Dow Jones Industrial Average (DJIA) and the Standard and Poor 500 Index (S&P 500) are reported daily and tend to be of great interest to investors and others who view these indices as evidence of the strength of the stock market and the economy. Additionally the GDP and GNP are of interest to economists and those who see these indices as indicative of changes in the economy of the nation.

As with any statistical information, economic statistics can be abused. The United States and most of the free world countries produce remarkably honest statistics (Clayton & Geisbrecht, 1997). Many private organizations compiling and reporting statistical information also have excellent reputations for reliable data. However, Clayton and Geisbrecht (1997) note that the data emerging from some countries are not trustworthy and are exaggerated or underreported for political and ideological reasons. Such data are not useful and can actually harm the citizens of those countries and their relationships with other countries.

The most common abuse of statistical information is to use it to explain or describe situations for which it was not intended. Other abuses include reporting numbers without an explanation of how they fit with other economic data and discussing statistical data as if they were predictive of certain movements of the overall national economy when they are not. Although not an abuse, it is also important to know that some data are released by an organization before all necessary details are available. This is a problem because the early information affects consumer action, but when the true and complete data become available, people do not pay sufficient attention (Clayton & Geisbrecht, 1997).

Governmental Spending and Taxation

Economic policies at the federal and state levels affect consumers of all kinds of goods and services. According to Hazlitt (1979), economics is both an art and a science. The art of economics requires that one looks at not only the immediate effect of an act or policy, but its long-term effects, as well as the consequences of that policy for all persons and groups in society, not just one. The problem is that immediate effects can readily be seen, but the future is harder to visualize. Something available now, although the result of a poor decision that could be harmful in the long run, often looks better than a hard decision that may be uncomfortable now but best for the future. One should remember the student who chose college expenses over the bicycle. The immediate loss means that she will not be able to take bike trips with her friends or get the exercise she needs by using the bicycle, but the better decision is to achieve the education.

It is understood that everything has a cost; there is never something for nothing. There is always a cost in money, time, effort, and the foregoing of something else. When private citizens and private businesses expend funds it is based on balancing one choice against another. The spending of public funds is different. All government expenditures are made using the proceeds of taxation. People rarely consider the issue, but a government has no money of its own; it has only those funds collected from taxpayers. Governments tax increasingly higher amounts in order to collect enough for it to meet the expenditures it has planned. For every dollar of tax collected, there is one less dollar for consumers to spend as they choose.

One should understand what constitutes appropriate government spending. The United States Constitution addresses the need for the federal and state governments to provide for the defense of the nation; for certain public works such as roads and railways, public buildings, police and fire services; and for the operating costs of these functions. A problem occurs when the government expends funds in ways that bear no relationship to its constitutionally granted powers and responsibilities. When public funds are used to build or produce things that are needed by the public and are not appropriately produced by the private sector, that is a proper use of such funds. Too often, projects are proposed and granted in senatorial and congressional districts as agreements between and among the representatives to federal and state governments. Much legislation is passed by negotiation. Often the represented people believe that government projects that bring jobs to an area are to be desired without understanding the dollar cost and the opportunity costs. Furthermore, when the need for the services the project provided ends, jobs are lost, often after many people have become used to the project and foregone other opportunities. When government spending is creating jobs to produce things that are not necessary to the people, jobs that could have been created in the private sector never come into existence.

The role of government in the economy is to protect property rights and freedom of exchange so that market prices can permit successful commerce. When governments try to influence outcomes or supply certain goods or services, prices lose their ability to convey accurate information about cost and value (Boaz, 1997). A basic principle of economics is that of supply and demand. When better ways of satisfying human needs are discovered or invented, demand for formerly used products or services falls. Resources no longer needed have little or no demand because people want the better product or service. In such situations, there may be a loss of investments or jobs. Still, it is not wise for the government to interfere by attempting to maintain a demand for the product, bar competition, or require that jobs be preserved (Boaz, 1997). One need only think of some products that health care providers have used in the past that are no longer useful. Disposable plastic enema bags, for example, have replaced older ones made of rubber. The disposables provide a significant increase in safety, patient comfort, and efficiency. Glass bottles for intravenous fluids have been replaced by disposables as well, increasing safety and ease of storage. There would have been no sense if some rule had required health care institutions to continue to use outdated products or required manufacturers to continue to employ the people who made them. The Chinese symbol for *crisis* is the same as that for *opportunity*; similarly these economic changes are uncomfortable but provide new opportunities. This does not mean that transition is easy—just that economic and technical progress means change. Although old jobs and products are gone, better jobs generally take their place and make the newer products available; newer products do the same job in a better way. About 100 years

ago, 60% of the workforce was involved in agriculture, domestic service, and jobs related to horse transport. Since then, about two thirds of all jobs existing at that time have disappeared. Today only about 3% of the workforce are in those three occupations (Boaz, 1997).

Scarcity and Shortage

Scarcity could be said to provide opportunities (Lee, 1999). Opportunity cost requires choosing one alternative and foregoing others. It might be said that cost is, therefore, something to avoid. Of course that is impossible to do; few people can choose anything and everything they want. In fact, society is better when each person is required to confront the cost of everything chosen. Consuming services and products without consideration of cost just shifts those costs to others. Any advantage one person might realize is offset by the choices others might make and shift to the first party. Ignoring costs would also mean that consumers lack information and motivation to choose wisely, which results in bad outcomes (Lee, 1999).

Consumers generally cannot purchase goods or services in a free market for less than others are willing to pay or for less than it costs to produce the goods. This is an important feature of the social cooperation that is inherent in market transactions. Without the discipline of considering the opportunity cost of choices, the best use of funds does not occur and the most effective choices are not made (Lee, 1999). Many economic decisions are made outside a market setting in response to political considerations. In such situations, those groups that are politically influential acquire benefits paid for by the general public. Costs are underestimated or justified on the basis that some goods are so important that cost should not matter. Health and illness care is one of those commodities. However, considering the costs of health and illness care is important. To avoid such consideration is essentially claiming that all health and illness care should be provided without regard to any other human needs. That would make sense only if people considered health and illness care as *always* more valuable than anything else, such that all resources should be devoted to it. Economists have asserted that if all the health care desired was provided, it would cost as much as the entire GNP of the country. If a vocal group asserted the importance of another good (such as housing or education) over health care, then people would demand consideration of the other alternatives. Scarcity, and the opportunity costs that result from it, invade the political process despite those who disparage the consideration of cost. Lee (1999) maintains that the imperfection and bias in the political process prevent the opportunity cost of governmental action from being adequately considered.

Shortages occur when there are inadequate supplies of a certain product despite willing buyers, or when the workforce's wage rate is constricted beyond normal market forces (Phelps, 1997). There have been many episodes of a shortage of registered nurses (RNs). During nursing shortages, one might expect market forces to cause the wage rate to increase, eventually attracting more nurses into the workforce, either reentering retirees or more enrollees in nursing programs, but this has not actually been the case. Phelps (1997) describes the monopsony power of hospitals, which are the major employer of nurses (although this is changing), which reflects the power they have in the labor market. *Monopsony power* is present when the power of the market is held by a small number of parties. Boonton and Lane (1985) found that an increase in vacancies in nursing positions actually resulted in lower wages. Historically, as hospitals' total wages to nurses have increased, the cost to manage the payments increased faster than the supply of nurses available. Hospitals then adjusted to hire a manageable level of RNs at the wage they were willing to pay (Box 10-1). However, this situation may be changing. Hospitals and other employers are advertising sign-on bonuses, flexible hours, and other incentives to attract nurses.

Some communities are taking a proactive stance to increase the numbers of nurses for the foreseeable future. For example, Cincinnati, Ohio is launching a major effort to encourage people into health-related fields (especially nursing) and local health care employment by establishing a task force and planning a major event to accomplish their objective of an increase in supply in the health care workforce (Personal communication, Greater Cincinnati Health Council, May 2000).

Market Incentives

Incentives are an important factor in a market economy. Incentives can be used to encourage people to behave in certain desirable ways. Critics may assert that incentives should not be used to get people to do something they should do in any case, but the reality is that incentives motivate desirable action (Lee, 1998a). Incentives can be direct rewards, such as paying health care providers only for patients who remain healthy for a given period of time. However, a direct incentive might not be favorable if it results in a person doing one thing and ignoring another. The incentive to the health care provider in this example above might encourage a practice to limit services for chronically ill persons or older adults, who tend to have more health problems.

Less direct incentives can be established through a set of general rules that allow people to act in an appropriate manner through cooperation. The flow of traffic is a good example. Spontaneous social cooperation permits motorists to allow pedestrians to cross at corners, stop on red traffic lights, and merge into traffic on highways. The incentive, of course, is to move through traffic areas safely and conveniently by accommodating one's behavior to the situation (Boaz, 1997). While some commuters violate the rules of traffic, others avoid difficulties by slowing down, moving out of the way, or sounding a horn to alert an unaware motorist. A market economy is also a good example of how a set of rules creates incentives that promote social cooperation. Prices, profits, and losses are the market incentives that communicate consumer desires to suppliers. The social cooperation in free markets permits prosperity to emerge. The material wealth that is available in countries that embrace market exchange would be lost without the accountability and discipline available only in a market economy (Foundation for Economic Education, 1998). Freedom is often taken for granted, particularly in places where it has always been enjoyed. Like good health, freedom tends to be unappreciated until it is in jeopardy. Short-term advantages are often taken at the risk of long-term loss of health or freedom.

In health care, the incentive to provide quality is based on the desire to market one's product to the health care consumer. Of course, "good quality" is often a subjective determination. The person who consumes a product or service is in the best position to judge quality on the basis of personal perception. However, there are also objective criteria for quality. Care and treatment outcomes, restoration of health, and successful management of chronic illness to an extent that one can be productive, are all measurable outcomes. Incentives to produce this quality arise from the freedom to experiment with modified or new therapies, use a variety of health care practitioners, and attract patients by informing them of these benefits. Real freedom can only survive when it is exercised in ways that are accountable to patients, other professionals, the health care system, and all of society (Foundation for Economic Education, 1998). Freedom without responsibility is an indulgence and will not be long tolerated by the market.

Box 10-1

Mean Annual Wage in the Most Common Health Care Occupations (1998)

Pharmacy technicians and aides	$18,970
Emergency medical technicians	$22,360
Medical technicians	$27,840
Licensed practical nurses (LPNs)	$28,040
Radiological technologists	$34,340
Medical technologists	$38,190
RNs	$43,070
Dental hygienists	$46,570
Pharmacists	$60,090
Physicians and surgeons	$102,020

Data from the Bureau of Labor Statistics (1999). Available online at www.stats.bls.gov.

The marketplace and freedom support each other in society. If there were central ownership or direction of all the means of production, the direction of centralized political authorities would be substituted for the market choices of individual consumers and suppliers. Such decisions would often be made in the presence of deficient information. For example, central planners cannot know local information; consequently, their decisions are imperfect and at times will be ineffective as a result of the knowledge deficit.

Markets, Regulation, and Political Freedom

Hayek (1960) noted that freedom in an open society like the United States is rarely lost in a revolution; it is lost slowly and incrementally over time, without much notice until most of it is gone. Often people do not believe certain restrictions affect them. In comparing current health care systems around the world, critics express concern that the United States is failing because it does not have a centralized, universal health care system. However, states that have enacted centralized, highly regulated health care have experienced negative, unintended consequences. The state of Maryland, for example, enacted an array of regulations on all aspects of health care, purportedly to control cost (Snyder, 1998a). The outcome was cost shifts, an increase in the number of uninsured persons, and the state's Medicaid spending per eligible person being the highest in the country (Snyder, 1998a). Perhaps unrelated to the current cost, but certainly to the regulations, is Maryland's medical record database, a collection of information on all patients' visits to physicians and hospitals. This information is collected without the consent or, in some cases, knowledge of consumers. The databank was intended to provide for central planning related to the health care needs of the population, and legislators and patient advocacy groups from all sides of the political spectrum (who have expressed concern about patient privacy) have been unable to change the law (Snyder, 1998a).

Maryland also has the highest number of mandates for health and medical coverage in the country. Consumers must pay insurance premiums for certain treatments and procedures that legislators believe are medically necessary, whether or not that consumer wants or would ever use them. Such treatments include abortions, chiropractic services, and in vitro fertilization procedures (Snyder, 1998a). Mandates, which are often the result of effective lobbying by special interest groups, tend to significantly increase costs. Furthermore, Maryland imposes caps on premiums and requires guaranteed reissue; this means that insurers may charge only a premium for health care insurance that does not exceed the maximum mandated by the state and that insurers must accept all people willing to pay that premium. Consequently, many insurers have left the state, thereby leaving many Maryland citizens without

insurance or with few choices from which to select. A similar situation occurred in Kentucky, which enacted health care reforms only to find that most insurers could not survive economically with the insurance mandates and premium caps required by the state and so ceased doing business in the state. That left only one insurer for much of the rural population, that being the state system, leaving the consumer with no choice and no competition for quality or service. Many rural people were left with no insurance.

Between 1987 and 1997, health insurance supplanted medical services as the largest component of consumer health care expenditures in every region. The BLS provides important governmental statistical data for those attempting to understand health care finance at their website: stats.bls.gov. For example, BLS data indicate that in the Northeast, the share of health care spending going toward insurance was over 50% in 1997. The proportion of out-of-pocket health care spending on insurance in the Northeast was 32.5% in 1987; in 10 years this share rose to 51%. As a result, the Northeast went from having the smallest share spent on insurance to having the largest. The share of health care spending devoted to medical services in the Northeast fell from 43.9% in 1987 to 28.1% in 1997. There was a somewhat similar pattern of change across the country. In each of the regions, the biggest share of the consumer health care dollar was spent on medical services in 1987 and on health insurance in 1997. For each region, the share devoted to health insurance increased by at least 10% and the share devoted to medical services decreased by at least 10% over the period (Table 10-1).

Effect of Inflation

Inflation is a term used to describe the concept of the increase in the volume of money and credit relative to available goods and services resulting in a continuing rise

Table **10-1**	
Annual Change in Average Consumer Expenditures on Health Care (1990-97)	
YEAR	**PERCENTAGE OF CHANGE**
1990	+5.2%
1991	+5.0%
1992	+5.1%
1993	+8.7%
1994	+1.2%
1995	+1.3%
1996	+2.2%
1997	+4.0%

Data from the Bureau of Labor Statistics (1999). Available online at www.stats.bls.gov.

in the general price level. Inflation is a continuous rise in prices that is sustained by the tendency of wage increases and cost increases to react to each other. Over time, there are persistent patterns in prices and markets. Phelps (1997) identifies three issues that affect inflation in health care—changes in the economy, a demographic shift to an aging society, and an increase in medical knowledge (mostly in the form of technology). Such changes have led to a persistent growth in real medical spending. This growth in spending has induced extensive government regulation and the development of health care insurance plans that have the control of medical costs or spending as their primary goal.

The CPI constructed by the BLS attempts to measure the meaning of prices over time and assist people in understanding inflation. As previously discussed, the CPI is a measure of the average change in prices for a fixed "market basket" of goods and services used by consumers (Clayton & Geisbrecht, 1997). The index includes items of consumer use such as food and beverages, housing, clothing, transportation, medical care, and entertainment. These general categories are further broken down into specific items within the categories so that data are specific enough to be meaningful to individuals using the CPI (Clayton & Geisbrecht, 1997).

Using the CPI to estimate inflation is done by computing the change in the CPI level for any category or item from one period to a later period. It should be understood that the CPI is not the same as a cost-of-living index because it does not account for the changes in consumer buying patterns as consumers adjust to price changes (Clayton & Geisbrecht, 1997). When comparing economic data over time, real meaning can only be derived if the data are adjusted to reveal the real dollar buying power changes from one period to another. According to Phelps (1997), time trends must be deflated with the appropriate measure of inflation to make these data meaningful. The CPI uses a specific year as a base, then either multiplies or divides the base year numbers by the percentage of inflation upward (usually moving forward in time) or downward (usually moving back in time) to obtain an expression of purchasing power over time (Phelps, 1997). For example, if the fee for a particular medical procedure in 1980 was $100, the CPI could demonstrate how inflation would affect the cost of the same procedure in 1999 by knowing the rate of inflation over the past 19 years. The CPI would also reveal how much of the current price was the result of factors other than inflation, but it would not identify those factors.

The CPI is affected by politics. The BLS indicates that the CPI affects the income of Social Security beneficiaries, federal retirees, union members who base their salary demands on changes in the CPI, and the size of the annual adjustments to income tax brackets (Clayton & Geisbrecht, 1997). Questions have been raised about the CPI because the "market basket" categories and items have not been updated since 1984 and may not reflect the consumer behaviors of today. Information on the CPI is available on the BLS website (stats.bls.gov).

IMPLICATIONS FOR MSN EDUCATION AND ADVANCED PRACTICE

The importance of understanding economic influences on health care cannot be underestimated during these times of rapid change. APNs who aspire to leadership roles in the health care system of the future need to understand the effect of private and governmental influence on both consumers and providers. The notion that government entities can solve all the problems of health care needs to be carefully analyzed. Americans have been impelled to believe in the government's inherent responsibility to provide care and economic security to all citizens, but a new realization that resources for health care are finite has begun to reshape this belief. Certainly APNs need to continue to assist with behavior that promotes health and individual responsibility for health, as well as promoting efforts favorable to the health of communities. Additionally, this group will be instrumental in helping consumers better understand how the system works and how to make better choices for their future health. Creating solutions to problems affecting the health of individuals and communities requires the cooperation of both private and public entities. Those with an ability to envision the possibilities that can exist between the two will have a critical voice in shaping a preferred health care future. APNs with a foundation in health care economics and its effects on the health care system and its consumers, both individually and collectively, have a greater capacity to create positive changes toward that future.

APNs, by virtue of their selection of a direct care arena for practice, are less involved in the business and accounting aspects of health care than those in administrative positions. However, they will be more involved in the application of basic principles of care economics to the realities of the clinical situation. Behind the doors of the examination room, the APN needs to manage resources wisely and monitor the effectiveness of clinical decisions with an appreciation for cost-containment. In proposing the essential elements of APN education, the American Association of Colleges of Nursing (1996) suggests that while "a complete background or comprehension of health care economics and accounting is not deemed essential. . .[the APN] graduate must know why and when to seek additional expertise in the area of financing and economics when practicing in, managing, or establishing a health care delivery system of practice." Clearly, graduate education in nursing should include classroom and clinical opportunities to learn the basic principles of health care economics to better understand the health care system and how to influence care in a positive way.

PRIORITIES FOR RESEARCH

Research into the economic issues that affect the health care system should address those issues from the perspective of consumers, institutional and professional providers, and insurers. The health care sector must determine what kinds of care should be produced, what kinds of care are desired or needed by consumers, who should produce the care, how it should be distributed, how it should be paid for, and how to best provide for growth and promote innovation.

In terms of consumers, nurse researchers might want to determine what health services are desired by consumers, whether in the presence of insurance or not. One of the more interesting phenomena of the decade is the interest in and use of so-called *integrative* or *alternative* health care measures, which consumers seem willing to pay for from their own funds. Why will consumers purchase alternative health care while demanding insurers cover traditional medical care? What kinds of providers will patients accept? In what circumstances will they accept, or even prefer, APNs? In what ways, if any, does consumer behavior with regard to seeking health care change with the presence of insurance; the diagnosis of health problems; certain social changes such as marriage or childbearing; or aging? How have prices for care changed over time? Have those prices affected salaries or income for health care providers?

Regarding providers, it would be helpful for research to consider how some of the consumer issues mentioned previously might affect the education of and need for APNs. Of particular interest might be the price of health care and the income of providers. When physician income increases, does the income of APNs in the same types of practice increase correspondingly? An interesting economic issue is protecting against claims of malpractice. Do premiums for liability insurance increase or decrease based on damage awards to clients? An important issue for health care providers is the need to balance income with expenses in managing a practice. How might a practice group with a varied provider skill mix determine how much they need to receive in fees from paying patients, capitation insurers, government payers, and others, and what mix of such payers is needed to pay the office staff; complete the administrative work; and pay the rent, insurance, and other expenses? Without such information, practices will not remain solvent.

Regarding insurers, a study of the different forms of health care insurance could yield important information. What are the similarities and differences among fee-for-service insurers, preferred provider organizations (PPOs), and health maintenance organizations (HMOs) in terms of

bearing financial risk? How are providers paid, and what kinds of providers are paid? What are the incentives for providing and withholding care, and how is care quality affected by any of these factors? What kinds of insurers do providers prefer and why?

Many of these questions may not be difficult to answer given appropriate study methods, yet not much detail is available. However, asking the questions will yield important data about the economics and management of practice. APNs who consider their only concern to be the provision of patient care miss an essential point of managing a practice: the need to balance the economy of care with the desire to do it.

DISCUSSION QUESTIONS

These questions can be used to promote critical thinking and encourage discussion.

1. Discuss the situation described in the section of the chapter on markets and prices in which a college student has to deal with the opportunity cost of purchasing a mountain bicycle or paying college costs. Have you ever had to make such a decision? What did you decide? Why? Explain the concept of opportunity cost in terms of similar decisions.
2. A well-functioning market in any commodity requires certain conditions. Discuss the conditions that are needed, such as the legal system, the behavior of parties in the system, and the balance of supply and demand. What specific conditions are necessary for a well-functioning health care system? Why is a market system an appropriate way to provide health care? How can the present system be adjusted to equate to a market system and still provide for those who are unable to pay for care from their own funds?
3. Compare and contrast the concepts of *shortage* and *scarcity*. Discuss the health care market as it is affected by shortage and scarcity. Be sure to include the health care workforce in your discussion.
4. Discuss how price ceilings may be applied in health care. What would the imposition of such price limits do to the availability of different types of care? Why would you advocate or oppose price ceilings? Justify your position in economic, social, and ethical terms.
5. Review one or more statistical reports or series. Follow one of the reports for several weeks and record the changes you find that may relate to health care or health care markets. Examples might include morbidity or

Suggestions for Further Learning

- Consult the following book: Clayton, G.E., & Geisbrecht, M.G. (1997). *A guide to everyday economic statistics.* Boston: Irwin-McGraw-Hill. This is a great little book that makes economic statistics easy to understand, even if one has little background in economics. It was written by two economists who have as their mission to make such information understandable to the average reader. It also provides links to sites where statistics are available and information on how best to use them.

- Visit the BLS at stats.bls.gov. Their site provides information on the CPI and the PPI, as well as statistical information related to these indices. The site is updated monthly in most cases.

- Visit the Foundation for Economic Education (FEE) at www.fee.org. FEE supports the ideas that sustain a society of free and responsible individuals. The website is full of sound ideas, logical commentary, and a fundamental philosophy of liberty, economic freedom, and individual rights.

- Explore the websites for the following governmental agencies: Department of Health and Human Services, Department of Justice, and Health Care Fraud and Abuse Control Program, as well as examining the *Annual Report for FY 1999.* (2000, January), which is available at www.doj.gov/dag/pubdoc/hipaa99ar21.htm.

- Read the following: Heffley, D., & Miceli, T. (1997, July). *Economics of incentive-based health care plans.* Available online at www.uconn.edu/economics/working/heff_ibhc.pdf. This provides a discussion of medical savings accounts.

- Review the following: American Public Health Association (1997). 125th anniversary retrospective: looking to the future: the nation's health. *The Nation's Health,* 1-7. Discuss the challenges to health care presented by demographic trends, the evolving health delivery system, technological and scientific progress, and the political and economic systems.

- Obtain the following references related to advanced practice nurses in the workforce: Cooper, R., Henderson, T., & Dietrich, C. (1998). Roles of the nonphysician provider clinicians as autonomous providers of patient care. *Journal of the American Medical Association, 280,* 795-802; Cooper, R., Laud, R., & Dietrick, C. (1998). Current and projected workforce of nonphysician clinicians. *Journal of the American Medical Association, 280*(9), 788-794; Grandinetti, D. (1999, February 8). What kind of patient would rather see a nurse practitioner? *Medical Economics.* Available online at www.pdr.net/memag/static.htm?path=docs/020899/article4.html; Lowes, R. (2000, March 20). What do PA, NP, and CNM spell? A revolution in health care. *Medical Economics.* Available online at www.pdr.net/memag/static.htm?path=docs/032000/article1.html; and the many letters discussing the topic in the *Journal of the American Medical Association* issue dated February 10, 1999. What do these articles imply about the supply and demand of APNs and primary care providers (PCPs)? Based on future projections, do you think this will influence salaries, demand, and availability for APNs? What strategies can you identify that would keep the supply side of the equation high for APNs?

mortality rates for a particular health problem. Discuss why such information is useful to APNs and nurses in leadership positions in health care agencies.

6. In small groups, ideally with graduate students or clinicians of varied nursing specialties, answer this question: Where is the health care system headed in the new century? What will that system be like for nurse practitioners (NPs)? Certified nurse midwives (CNMs)? Certified registered nurse anesthetists (CRNAs)? Clinical nurse specialists (CNSs)? Physicians? What will the system be like for patients?

REFERENCES/BIBLIOGRAPHY

Aaron, H. (1994). Thinking straight about medical costs. *Health Affairs, 13*(5), 8-13.

Aday, L.A. (1993). *At risk in America: the health and health care needs of vulnerable populations in the United States.* San Francisco: Jossey-Bass Publishers.

Altman, S.H., & Reinhardt, U.E. (1996). *Strategic choices for a changing health care system.* Chicago: Health Administration Press.

American Association of Colleges of Nursing (1996). *The essentials of master's education for advanced practice nursing.* Washington, DC: American Association of Colleges of Nursing.

American Public Health Association (1997). 125th anniversary retrospective: Looking to the future: The nation's health. *The Nation's Health,* 1-7.

Bayles, P., & Parks-Doyle, J. (Eds.) (1996). *The web of inclusion.* New York: National League for Nursing Press.

Blumberg, L.J., & Nichols, L.M. (1996). First, do no harm: developing health insurance market reform packages. *Health Affairs, 15*(3), 35-54.

Boaz, D. (1997). *Libertarianism: a primer.* New York: The Free Press.

Boonton, L.A., & Lane, J.I., (1985). Hospital market structure and the return to nursing education. *Journal of Human Resources, 20*(2), 184-96

Brecher, C. (1995). The government's role in health care. In A.R. Kovner (Ed.), *Jonas's health care delivery in the United States* (5th ed.) (pp. 322-347). New York: Springer.

Bronow, R.F. (1997). *HMOs—the death of medical ethics.* Available online at www.pwc.org/summer97/ART3.html.

Cassell, E. J. (1996). The two faces of primary care. *The Wilson Quarterly, 20*(2), 28-30.

Clayton, G., & Geisbrecht, M. (1997). *Everyday economic statistics.* Boston, MA: Irwin-McGraw-Hill.

Cooper, R.A. (1994). Seeking a balanced physician workforce for the 21st century. *Journal of the American Medical Association, 272*, 680-687.

Cooper, R., Laud, R., & Dietrick, C. (1998). Current and projected workforce of nonphysician clinicians. *Journal of the American Medical Association, 280*(9), 788-794.

Foreman, S. (1996). Managing the physician workforce: hands off, the market is working. *Health Affairs, 15*(5), 243-249.

Foundation for Economic Education (1998). Markets and freedom. *The Freeman* 48(8). Available online at www.fee.org.

Goldsmith, J. (1996). A different health care world than expected. *Health Affairs, 15*(4), 109-110.

Grandinetti, D. (1999, February 8). What kind of patient would rather see a nurse practitioner? *Medical Economics.* Available online at www.pdr.net/memag/static.htm?path=docs/020899/article4.html.

Gray, S. (1996). *Health of native people of North America.* Landon, MD & London: The Scarecrow Press.

Hayek, F. (1960). *The constitution of liberty.* Chicago: University of Chicago Press

Hazlitt, H. (1979). *Economics in one lesson.* San Francisco: Laissez Faire Books.

Issel, M., & Anderson, R. (1996). Take charge: managing six transformations in health care delivery. *Nursing Economics, 14*(2), 78-85.

Kongstvedt, P.R. (1995). *Essentials of managed health care.* Gaithersburg, MD: Aspen.

Lee, D. (1998a). The power of incentives. *The Freeman.* Irving-on-Hudson, NY: Foundation for Economic Education.

Lee, D. (1998b). Price ceilings cause shortages and higher costs. *The Freeman.* Irving-on-Hudson, NY: Foundation for Economic Education.

Lee, D. (1999). Opportunities and costs. *The Freeman.* Irving-on-Hudson, NY: Foundation for Economic Education.

Lee, P.R., & Estes, C. (Eds.) (1994). *The nation's health* (4th ed.). Boston: Jones & Bartlett.

Liggins, K. (1993). Inappropriate attendance at accident and emergency departments: a literature review. *Journal of Advanced Nursing, 18*(7), 1141-1145.

Lovitky, J.A. (1997). Health care fraud: a growing problem. *Nursing Management, 28*(11), 42, 44-45.

Lowes, R. (2000, March 20). What do PA, NP, and CNM spell? A revolution in health care. *Medical Economics.* Available online at www.pdr.net/memag/static.htm?path=docs/032000/article1.html.

Managed Care Research Reports (1997, April). *Seven trends shaping managed care today.* Bethesda: MD: Health Trends Managed Care Research Reports.

Phelps, C.E. (1997). *Health economics* (2nd ed.). Reading, MA: Addison-Wesley.

Shi, L., & Singh, D.A. (1998). *Delivering health care in America.* Gaithersburg, MD: Aspen Publishers.

Snyder, D. (1998a). Building bureaucracy and invading patient privacy: Maryland's health care regulations. *Backgrounder.* Washington, DC: The Heritage Foundation.

Snyder, D. (1998b). Economic notions: markets and freedom. *The Freeman.* Irving-on-Hudson, NY: Foundation for Economic Education.

Stahl, D.A. (1995). Managed care and subacute care: a partnership of choice. *Nursing Management, 26*(1), 17-19.

Zelman, W.A. (1996). *The changing health care marketplace.* San Francisco: Jossey-Bass Publishers.

Zwanziger, J., & Melnick, G.A. (1996). Can managed care plans control health care costs? *Health Affairs, 15*(2), 185-199.

Chapter 11

Insurers and Other Payers for Health Care

Alice G. Rini

One of the unique aspects of health care in the United States is the complex system of payment for that care. Private and governmental resources are used to pay for care; persons not covered by either are considered uninsured. Over time, public resources to finance health care costs have grown exponentially, while private funding has shrunk proportionately (Wilson & Neuhauser, 1985).

DEFINITIONS

The nomenclature of insurers and other payers is important information for advanced practice nurses (APNs) so that they understand the system better and can help patients and others understand as well. Many of the following terms are expanded upon throughout the chapter, but they are offered here to present a beginning context. First, this chapter deals extensively with information related to **third-party payers**. In the current health care system, private insurance companies and the government are the biggest sources of payment for health care coverage. Because these sources are neither providers nor patients, these groups are called *third-party payers*.

In insurance terms, an **assignment** refers to the agreement by a provider to accept the amount of payment for services established by the payer, usually Medicare or Medicaid. If a provider is not on assignment, the patient is billed for the amount remaining after the insurer has paid. The billing of that leftover sum is known as **balance billing**. Insurance payments may be subject to **copayment**, the portion of charges for health care paid by the patient under the terms of the insurance policy. The portion of health care costs that must be paid by an insured patient, usually an annual limit, before any insurance money is paid is referred to as the **deductible.** These two sums, the copayment and deductible, are sometimes called the patient's *out-of-pocket expenses*.

Insurers generally cover what they have determined to be "customary, prevailing, and reasonable" costs for a particular aspect of health care. Each insurer determines

what those costs are, usually based on a survey of what providers are charging in their local area or state. In insurance terms, **exclusions** are those disorders, health problems, or treatments listed as uncovered (not reimbursable) under the terms of the particular policy. **Preexisting conditions** may be excluded from coverage by insurers or may be covered after a designated waiting interval has passed; these conditions, which may be physical and/or mental in nature, existed before the effective date of insurance coverage. Many insurance contracts also include a provision for **prior approval**, a requirement that the insurer grant permission to a provider before a particular type of care (usually surgery) is provided. This provision is a form of utilization review that controls costs.

Managed care refers to a system that combines health insurance coverage and the actual utilization of services. An **independent practice association (IPA)** is a legal entity that providers in private practice join to enable representation in negotiating managed care contracts (Shi & Singh, 1998). **Health maintenance organizations (HMOs)** are types of managed care organizations (MCOs) that provide comprehensive medical care for a predetermined annual fee. The insurance industry's version of managed care are **preferred provider organizations (PPOs)**. These organizations negotiate contracts with employers to provide health care coverage for their employees at a discounted fee. A PPO may provide a share of the costs of services provided by clinicians not on the preferred provider panel. The HMO generally does not (Shi & Singh, 1998). **Capitation** is a set amount (or flat rate) paid to a provider, usually on a monthly basis, to care for an HMO member. In primary care settings, capitated fees generally range between $5 and $35 per enrollee per month, based on the age and gender of the patient (Buppert, 2000).

Entitlement describes a health program for which certain people are entitled by virtue of some characteristic. Medicare is an example; persons over 65 years of age are generally entitled to Medicare coverage because of contributions they have made through taxes. **Medicare** is a federally funded health insurance program for older adults and certain others who are disabled. **Medicaid** is a health insurance program for the poor that is jointly funded by federal and state money. **Worker's compensation** is a provision for workers, paid by their employers, to compensate for medical costs and lost wages related to an on-the-job injury or work-related illness. It does not cover other illnesses or injuries.

Fee-for-service is reimbursement for health care on the basis of varied factors, such as the number and types of services provided, Current Procedural Terminology (CPT) and International Classification of Diseases (ICD-9) codes, the geographical location of the practice site, and the specific office and training expenses of the provider (Buppert, 2000). **CPT codes** are a uniform coding system developed by the American Medical Association (AMA) and adopted by third-party payers for use in claims submission (Buppert, 2000). **ICD-9 codes** (the ninth revision) classify disease by diagnostic categories, using a six-digit number for each.

Incident to a physician's professional service, sometimes shortened to *incident to services*, is a Medicare term that relates to the regulation stating that reimbursement of a nonphysician provider must be rendered for services that are under a physician's direct personal supervision, when he is present in the office suite and immediately available to provide direction and assistance while service is being provided. The physician must have provided initial services and subsequent services frequently enough to indicate active participation in management of a patient's disease process (Buppert, 2000).

CRITICAL ISSUES: THIRD-PARTY PAYMENT FOR HEALTH CARE

The critical issues about third-party payment for health care are related to understanding the way the varied systems function; eligibility requirements; the way to employ coding, billing, and documenting processes in a way to increase the probability of reimbursement; and measures for being fiscally responsible APNs. Those aspects of third-party reimbursement (as they inform APN practice) are integrated throughout this chapter. Knowledge of isolated processes, however, is inadequate for comprehending how the current reimbursement system evolved and became problematic. A more global perspective is provided here to set a context for comprehension of third-party reimbursement.

Regulation and Insurance Law

Health care insurance does not have a long history. It began with workers' compensation programs in the early 1900s, in the form of cash payments to workers who were injured on the job and replacement of wages lost while

workers were unable to do their jobs. Later, compensation for medical expenses was added. The first insurance against sickness became available in the nineteenth century and was available through employers, fraternal groups, and trade unions. Such insurance originally provided for income during a worker's sickness, but it later added a worker's dependents (Sultz & Young, 1999).

In 1910, workers' compensation programs were initiated in New York (Sultz & Young, 1999), and the programs spread to all states by 1948 (Berkowitz & Berkowitz, 1985). Workers' compensation programs, which operate at the state level, require participation by employers who contribute to an insurance fund that assists employees with expenses incurred from job-related injuries. Employers purchase workers' compensation insurance from commercial insurance companies, and the companies pay legitimate compensation claims. Since both workers compensation and health insurance are employer based, health insurance contracts usually have exclusions for job-related injuries so that duplication of benefits is not an issue.

In 1906, the American Association of Labor Legislation (AALL) had a social reform agenda that included government-sponsored legislation to protect injured workers. The organization also argued for government-sponsored health insurance for the general public. They modeled their proposals after the compulsory sickness insurance that was widely available in Europe (Starr, 1982). The AALL, made up of a small membership of labor leaders, economists, and social scientists, took the position that social reform was best accomplished through government action. Their efforts ultimately failed because of a variety of factors. However, in times of national crisis, there was some softening of this resistance in order to permit a broad-based response to the problem. The Depression was one of those crises, out of which emerged programs such as Social Security. Unfortunately, programs born of crisis or temporary necessity are generally difficult or impossible to extinguish even when circumstances change. The idea of health insurance coupled with Social Security was proposed in 1946 by President Harry Truman, who argued that health care consumed only 4% of the gross national product (GNP) and that the government could afford to provide health care for all classes in the society (Anderson, 1990). Health care now consumes nearly 16% of the gross domestic product (GDP), and many governmental efforts are directed toward reducing the costs of health care. The level of expenditure is high, although government programs provide care for only some groups in the country, not all classes as Truman proposed. Private organizations are also enacting cost-control measures.

State Regulation in the Health Care Industry

States have health policy responsibilities that include regulating the health insurance industry. The state authority arises from a constitutionally granted responsibility for the public's health. Included in this broad mandate are requirements to monitor the environment within the state boundaries, ensure safe workplaces and food service organizations, provide programs and information to prevent injury and promote healthy behavior, and provide certain health services. With regard to health insurance, states are expected to control the content, marketing, and pricing of health insurance products. Legislators, through the McCarran-Ferguson Act (Public Law [PL] 79-15) directed most insurance regulation to the states; however, there is considerable federal legislation that forces the federal government into the insurance regulation process (Longest, 1998). Such federal imposition on state responsibilities tends to make the line between state and federal regulation unclear. The Employee Retirement Income Security Act (ERISA) of 1974 (PL 93-406) preempts state regulation of pensions and self-insured employer health plans. The Consolidated Omnibus Budget Reconciliation Act (COBRA) of 1985 (PL 99-272) provides the opportunity for persons leaving a job to retain existing employer-provided health insurance for up to 18 months if the employee pays the premiums directly. Most recently, the Health Insurance Portability and Accountability Act (HIPAA) of 1996 (PL 104-191) provides guaranteed access to health insurance for employees who work for a company that offers health insurance but then change jobs or become unemployed. It also provides for guaranteed renewability of insurance as long as premiums are paid (Longest, 1998). Of course Medicare and Medicaid, as well as the Veterans Administration health care system, have a significant effect on the regulation of the delivery of health and medical care because all those programs have a considerable array of rules and regulations.

It remains to be seen how state and federal regulation will be able to coexist, particularly with the concerns about managed care and uninsured persons. The federal government is apparently concerned that health care issues are too complex for states to manage. For their part, states want the flexibility to structure systems that will efficiently and effectively serve their citizens (Lipson, 1997). Some of the federal programs that address health care issues were responses to a perceived inability of the states to serve older adults or the poor. The federal role expanded considerably as Medicare and Medicaid grew (in scope and cost) far beyond what had ever been predicted by its early proponents (Liu & Moffit, 1995).

In the 1980s, there was a great effort to return greater control to the states through the use of block grants from the federal government and based on a predetermined formula. One needs to understand that all funds that the federal government has are taxpayer funds paid by individuals and businesses residing in the various states. These tax revenues are then returned to the states after losing some of their bulk in the federal bureaucracy. This money arrives as a block grant, a consolidated dollar amount with which a state endeavors to provide certain

services through use of the grant and also state funds (also paid by taxpayers). States were successful in funding their services in the 1980s primarily because of a healthy economy and the resulting increase in tax revenues. However, the economic downturn in the early 1990s made it difficult to continue to provide services at the level of the previous 10 years. Some states maintained funding by instituting special new taxes such as those on the income of hospitals, physicians, nurses, and other health care providers. In some states, there were lawsuits related to those taxes, and many of the taxes were repealed.

Over the past several years, most states have tried to enact some kind of health care reform in response to rapidly increasing costs. Much of the rising cost is influenced by federal tax policy. When people enter the health care marketplace, they are not experiencing the cost of the care they purchase. For every dollar of health care purchased, the consumer generally pays between 5 and 17 cents. The generous tax subsidy of employer-provided health care insurance tends to encourage overuse of services, while those who are self-insured or who purchase their own insurance do not always have the same benefits (a more detailed discussion of this phenomenon is in the section on medical savings accounts, later in this chapter). Other federal policies affect the ability of states to control their health care expenditures. About one quarter of all Medicaid spending pays for long-term care (LTC). Federal regulations related to approved LTC facilities and accommodations limit states in devising effective, but less costly, alternatives (National Center for Policy Analysis [NCPA] Idea House, 1997). Federal tax policy also affects the value of the subsidy of health care insurance. The value of the subsidy to a low-income family is significantly lower than the value to a middle- or upper-income group.

Federal policy as reflected in the Medicare program is also inefficient. The amount that may be spent by beneficiaries can be excessive. Some of the small fees might be borne by the middle- or upper-income beneficiary. There is no support in terms of tax subsidies for younger people who try to save for future health care expenses or for LTC; in fact, savings and earnings from investments are heavily taxed (NCPA Idea House, 1997). Medicare can leave some older adults uncovered for major illnesses and LTC because the money has been spent on the small, predictable expenses of chronic disease and aging. This means state and local governments must cover the expenses of a serious illness.

Several state health care reform proposals attempt to include people enrolled in health plans that do not fall under state purview. Many of the plans not covered by state insurance regulation have deliberately chosen to select an insurance form that is exempt from such regulation. These employers and other groups have concluded that state regulations tend to increase costs of insuring a given population. Critics argue that state regulation protects insured employees or group members.

It is instructive to analyze the experience of state health policy in states where aggressive regulation has been tried in an attempt to accelerate reform. In a study of the sixteen most aggressive states, all of them had growth in the uninsured population eight times that of the other thirty-four states that did not enact reform or did so only minimally. The citizens who were supposed to be helped by the new state policies were actually hurt by the reforms (Schriver &Arnett, 1998). Many states have since repealed their reform regulations as a result of negative outcomes.

Several factors provided much of the impetus for the increase in state regulation. Rising health care costs increased from 8.9% in 1980 to 13.4% in 1992 and 13.6% in 1996. There was a drop in the percentage of Americans covered by health insurance—from 79.5% in 1980 to 70.5% in 1992—primarily because of increased costs that employers could not afford while still remaining competitive in the global economic environment. As a result, companies that had always provided generous, paid health care insurance for their employees (and often their families) increased the share employees had to pay, limited coverage, and reduced benefits (Schriver & Arnett, 1998). Many younger or lower-income persons declined to pay the higher premiums or lost health care insurance when their employer no longer covered or offered it. Some of the uninsured, therefore, were working people or their dependents (Schriver & Arnett, 1998). Concurrently, more Americans were having their health care expenses paid by Medicare and Medicaid. This situation was a major political issue in the 1992 presidential election. Although national proposals were not successful, the states did make regulatory reforms that were targeted at cost control, increased access, and insurance coverage (Schriver & Arnett, 1998).

The success of the state reforms that were modeled on the universal coverage plan proposed by the Clinton administration has been well researched. Kentucky, Massachusetts, and Washington introduced similar elements that included a strong government bureaucracy, increased regulation, mandates for coverage, defined health care packages, mandatory managed care, and price controls (Cihak, Williams, & Ferrara, 1997). In all three states, the reforms reduced individual choice, increased costs for health insurance, increased the number of uninsured persons, and increased the number of insurers withdrawing from offering its products in those states (Cihak et al, 1997; McCubbin, 1997). Schriver and Arnett (1998) completed a study of the success of state health insurance reforms to determine whether the goals of increased accessibility and decreased numbers of uninsured persons were met. In their review, they provide a description of typical state health policies that relate to insurance market reforms; these include:

1. *Guaranteed issue* provides that any eligible person agreeing to pay a stated premium must be offered an insurance product during a specified enrollment period. Individuals do not have to be offered all of the products of an insurer.

2. Currently covered persons may not be dropped from an insurer's rolls because of high medical expenses in a particular year, which means *guaranteed renewability*. Insurers can make coverage and pricing decisions for a group and can also cancel a whole group policy or leave the state market.

3. Some states imposed limits on noncoverage of preexisting conditions, restricting the waiting time for such conditions to 6 or 12 months. In states without such restrictions, waiting times could be longer or preexisting conditions could be permanently excluded.

4. *Portability of insurance* permits the movement from one job to another without fear of loss of insurance. Persons who maintained continuous coverage are eligible for coverage with a new employer and are exempt from any preexisting condition waiting periods.

5. *Community rating* requires an insurer to charge everyone in the community the same price for health insurance, regardless of risk of illness or current health.

6. The imposition of *mandated benefits* is a system where regulators require coverage for certain treatments and providers. These mandates are costly and force people in the insurance market to accept and pay for coverage they would normally not choose.

The study by Schriver and Arnett (1998) is instructive in revealing the effect of state regulation of health care insurance on the availability and cost of such insurance to the population. This study also provides some conclusions and recommendations for addressing the existing problems.

Private Health Insurance

The first private health insurance policies were directed toward protection from loss of income during an illness through which a person could not work. Soon after such policies were established, some insurers added reimbursement for surgical fees, but most policies continued to be directed toward replacing lost income during periods of illness. These were similar to what are now called *disability insurance policies*. Three factors promoted the establishment of modern health insurance (Shi & Singh, 1998). In the early part of this century, developing technology created better treatments. People responded to the healing nature of health care providers, placed a higher value on health care, and believed they could do something about certain health problems, thereby increasing the demand for care. The health problems of modern society and the expanding industrial environment made it difficult for consumers to predict or plan for health problems, and the cost of care was increasing and unpredictable. These changes led to the emergence of health insurance that initially covered only limited groups, such as industrial employee groups, railroad workers, union members, and some fraternal groups (Shi & Singh, 1998).

Soon hospitals became involved in insurance plans to provide themselves some economic stability (because their philanthropic donations were decreasing). Hospitals became the underwriters of the insurance to prepaid consumers, but the hospitals were not required to maintain a fund to ensure that they would be able to provide payment for hospital services when they were needed. Eventually, the American Hospital Association (AHA) became the coordinating agency, uniting all the hospital plans into what became the Blue Cross network, a not-for-profit corporation. No physician fees were covered. By 1950, almost 60% of the population was covered by Blue Cross. At this point the AMA supported the concept of hospital insurance (Shi & Singh, 1998).

The first health plan for the payment of physician fees was started in California. The California Medical Association endorsed private health insurance to spread the financial risk of paying for serious illnesses throughout the population, ensuring the protection of the public and their own interests. As this voluntary Blue Shield movement gained acceptance across the country, physicians began to underwrite it because they preferred these plans, which kept the control of medical decisions with the physicians. Since there continued to be efforts to establish a national health insurance program, physicians were interested in the voluntary plans expanding throughout the country. Later, commercial insurers began offering health insurance. The wage freezes of World War II promoted the expansion of hospital and medical insurance as part of employee compensation packages; thus private insurance in a variety of forms became the primary manner of providing health services in the United States (Shi & Singh, 1998).

In the years since World War II, health insurance has undergone significant evolution. Private insurance is not monolithic; it includes a variety of forms. More than 90% of people with private health insurance obtain it through the workplace, and nearly 40% of those with workplace-based insurance belong to self-insured programs. The number of self-insured plans varies with the size of the company, and the largest firms (those with 500 or more employees) are most likely to have such plan (Acs, Long, Marquis, & Short, 1996). Self-insured programs are health insurance plans offered by an organization that itself bears the risk of covering the health care expenses of its employees and is not funded by a third party insurer (United States General Accounting Office [GAO], 1997). Employers who provide self-insured plans are not subject to state insurance regulation because of ERISA rules. Although such health plans need not conform to state mandates, most self-insured plans offer similar benefits as those given by other employers who are not self-insured (United States GAO, 1997).

Purchasing commercial health insurance from a third

party is another way of providing health insurance for employees. Large employers (those employing more than 100 persons) are able to do so at an attractive price simply because they bring a balanced risk pool to the market. It is likely that such a group's financial stability would not be adversely affected by high costs from a few of the employees because the large number of employees spreads the risk over the entire employee base (Schriver & Arnett, 1998). It is also likely that because of this spread, no one employee is adversely affected by those few who have high expenses in any single year.

Smaller employers also purchase commercial insurance, but they may not be able to obtain the pricing advantage of larger firms because they are not large enough (or perhaps diverse enough) to have a balanced risk pool of employees. If one or more employees happens to have particularly high medical expenses in any single year, it is likely that premium rates for the entire group would be affected the following year, or their insurance could be cancelled (Schriver & Arnett, 1998). At times, smaller employers have been able to come together in industry groups to gain bargaining power. Some companies can join a local chamber of commerce and receive access to group insurance in combination with a larger number of other companies, thereby better approaching the balanced risk group that is attractive to insurers and results in lower premiums.

Some people do not have access to insurance in any of the ways described above and must purchase individual health insurance. This includes self-employed persons, those who work for employers who do not offer health insurance, unemployed persons, and early retirees not yet eligible for Medicare. In terms of numbers, a projection for 1996 showed there would be approximately 14 million persons with individually purchased insurance (United States GAO, 1995). As might be expected, price is an important consideration for these individuals, who have the same diverse health needs and resources as other working people. Insurance carriers do offer a variety of products, but all have high-risk and cost-sharing features, whether through deductibles or copayments. Those in the individual market pay their entire premium themselves, generally without any of the tax advantages of employees. Self-employed persons may deduct a portion of their insurance costs. In 1998, they were able to deduct 45% of premium costs from their taxable income. This deduction will increase to 100% by 2007 (Schriver & Arnett, 1998). However, not everyone qualifies for the deduction, and 8 years is a long time to wait for a benefit that those who are employed in larger companies have enjoyed for 50 years.

The demand for health insurance arises from an individual's concern about the unpredictable nature of health and illness, specifically the occurrence of serious illness or catastrophic injury. A consumer of health care seeks such care in hope of a cure, or at least an improvement. This response to illness creates a financial risk against which the consumer insures himself or herself via some type of health insurance. In fact, health insurance does not actually insure health; like other forms of insurance, it insures against financial loss related to illness (Phelps, 1997). To seek health or medical care is a rational act when someone is ill. Statistical studies show that as certain factors increase, the use of medical and health services also increases. If all other factors remain constant, the quantity of care increases with: lower prices for care; increased severity of illness; insurance coverage (the level of deductible and/or copayment is also influential); decreased time and effort needed to obtain care; and aging (Phelps, 1997).

Medicare

The Medicare program was established in 1965 as Title XVIII of PL 89-97. For the 50 years before the enactment of Medicare, the idea of government-mandated health plans was rejected (Twight, 1997). However, federal legislators seemed determined to pass such legislation; it was introduced in Congress every year (in some form) until it passed (Friedman, 1995). Much of the proposed legislation during the years from 1934 through 1965 was incremental in nature; it introduced laws piece by piece that would provide for national health insurance. The involvement of the federal government in social legislation actually began in 1934 when President Franklin Roosevelt established the Committee on Economic Security (CES). The CES proposed the idea of Social Security, which included a provision for a health insurance plan. This health care provision was met with such animosity that Roosevelt postponed its inclusion so the passage of Social Security would not be in peril (Corning, 1969; Twight, 1997). A provision in the Social Security bill called for a Social Security Board that would continue to study the health care issue (Chapman & Talmadge, 1970). The Social Security Act was signed into law on August 14, 1935, after which Roosevelt immediately appointed an interdepartmental committee to work on the health insurance issue. Committee recommendations included a program of medical care paid through general taxation or social insurance contributions, as well as federal support for expansion of hospitals, disability insurance, public health services, and programs for the medically needy (Poen, 1979).

Serious legislative efforts for health care were introduced in every session of Congress beginning in 1939. In 1943, the Wagner-Murray-Dingell Bills sought to establish a universal compulsory national health insurance at the federal level. The bill was not successful for many years due to the efforts of the AMA (Friedman, 1995) and vigorous public opposition (as evidenced by a 1942 poll by *Fortune* magazine that revealed that more than three quarters of the American people did not want the federal

government to provide "free" medical care) (Cantril, 1951; Goodman, 1980).

When it was determined that it was unlikely that universal health insurance could be enacted, a plan of incrementalism was proposed. In the 1930s, legislation for the support of public health initiatives and maternal and child health activities was in fact passed. In 1943, during World War II, the Emergency Maternal and Infant Care Act was enacted to provide health care for the families of low-rank servicemen. When Wilbur Mills became chairman of the House Ways and Means Committee, he managed the enactment of the Kerr-Mills Act of 1960, which provided federal funding to help certain states to pay for medical care for low-income residents (Friedman, 1995; Twight, 1997).

Efforts continued in the 1960s during the Kennedy administration, at which time there was a proposal for compulsory health insurance for older adults. There was strong feeling that this group would be the most sympathetic in the eyes of the public. Limiting the proposal to older adults was clearly part of the incrementalism strategy (Cohen & Ball, 1965). In 1962, Kennedy gathered a selected group of senior citizens in Madison Square Garden in New York City, where he called for universal access to health care for the older adult population. The AMA, which had long opposed government-financed health care, responded with strong counter claims 2 days later (in the same place and with an impassioned, televised speech) (Friedman, 1995).

After the death of Kennedy, Lyndon Johnson's administration, aided by a strongly Democratic Congress, was able to push through legislation that provided three things. First, physician services for Social Security beneficiaries would now be paid through a combination of federal funds and copayments by patients. Second, hospital care would be covered through payroll and employer taxes. Third (and added to the main bill as an afterthought), Kerr-Mills coverage of low-income citizens was expanded by attaching the scheme to existing state welfare programs (Friedman, 1995).

Twight (1997) describes a process by which government officials use what she calls *transaction-cost augmentation* to permit passage of legislation that is significantly opposed by the public. Economists describe *transaction costs* as those of negotiating and enforcing exchange agreements and opportunities to obtain relevant information and act upon it. These costs tend to alter the role and scope of government. Costs include obtaining accurate information about exactly what the legislation will do or permit in certain situations, as well as about political agreement and enforcement issues. Twight (1997) describes how a person might have perfect information and yet be deterred from taking political action if the costs of taking political action were increased. Government officials attempt to secure the legislation they want with as little resistance from the public as possible. Whatever actions are needed to build transaction costs, deliberate steps are taken to increase the difficulty of obtaining relevant information about certain legislation by the public and other legislators, so that the scope of governmental authority can be increased without much resistance. Twight (1997) describes how the titles of congressional bills can alter the perceptions of people who understand them literally. Such titles often imply objectives inconsistent with what is really intended. A recent example is the Health Insurance Portability and Accountability Act of 1993. This bill included a provision that jeopardized the privacy of medical records and the ability of physicians and other health care providers to practice their professions. Nevertheless it was possible, even likely, that the general public would not look beyond the words *portability* and *accountability* in a situation where persons who change jobs risk losing their medical insurance. Twight (1997) asserts that Medicare could not have been enacted without the misrepresentation, cost concealment, and deliberate structuring of political transaction costs to overcome the widespread public opposition that lasted for 50 years.

The current Medicare program covers persons 65 years old and older and certain disabled individuals less than 65 years old. People with end-stage renal disease (ESRD) who have permanent kidney failure and need dialysis or a kidney transplant are also eligible for the Medicare program. There are several ways for eligible persons to participate in the program. The Original Medicare Plan is a fee-for-service type plan. Part A is a hospital insurance plan provided with no premium payment. There is, however, a deductible of $768 for each hospital stay, which can last from 1 to 60 days. Beneficiaries stay in a semiprivate room; telephone and television are not covered. Should a hospital stay last more than 60 days, the beneficiary pays $192 per day through the 90th day, and $384 per day through the 150th day. These last 60 days are reserve days that may be used only once in a person's lifetime. Hospital stays that last more than 150 days are charged to the beneficiary because no more Medicare funds are available. Care in a skilled nursing facility (SNF) is also available in the Part A program. After meeting certain preliminary requirements, such as a diagnosis with a serious illness that requires a long rehabilitation period or hospitalization, beneficiaries are eligible for skilled nursing care in a SNF. For the first 20 days, beneficiaries pay no deductible or copayment. Should the stay last for more than 20 days, there is a required payment of $96 per day through the 100th day; beneficiaries pay all skilled care costs after that. Home health care is also available through Medicare Part A. There is no charge to beneficiaries who meet the requirements for the care. If durable medical equipment is needed to provide the care, beneficiaries pay 20% of the Medicare-approved amount for such equipment as wheelchairs, a special bed, oxygen, or mobility

assistive devices. If a Medicare beneficiary is terminally ill, hospice care is available for pain and symptom relief, either in an institutional facility or at home. Beneficiaries pay some of the cost of outpatient drugs and respite care for family caregivers. (It should be noted that all of the preceding dollar amounts were current in 1999 [Health Care Financing Administration (HCFA), 1999].)

In the Original Medicare Plan, there is an option to purchase, for a set premium of $45.50 per month, Part B coverage. Part B provides assistance with the payments for physicians' services; inpatient and outpatient medical/surgical services; physical, occupational, and speech therapy; diagnostic tests; and durable medical equipment (DME). Beneficiaries may see any care provider, whether a primary care provider (PCP), specialist, or nurse practitioner (NP). There is an annual deductible of $100, after which the insurance pays 80% of the approved amount for the service; the beneficiary pays 20%. There is a different plan for mental health care; a 50% copayment is required. With Part B, clinical laboratory tests are covered in full when medically necessary. Under certain conditions, home health care is covered with no copayment except for DME. Outpatient hospital care is also available with a 20% copayment after the initial $100 deductible. (Again, all amounts are current for 1999.) There is also some support through Part B for services such as emergency care, x-rays, eyeglasses after cataract surgery, transplants, and some screening or preventive care (HCFA, 1999). (Table 11-1 explains the preventive care measures and the support provided for them in the Medicare program.) Medicare beneficiaries may only use Part B if they are participating in the Original Medicare Plan (Part A). There are special enrollment periods for Part B if an eligible person failed to join at the time of eligibility for Part A.

There are some health care services for which Medicare will not pay. There is no provision for outpatient prescription drugs (although there is currently activity in Congress to address this), eyeglasses, hearing aids, and routine physical examinations. There is no coverage of emergency care when a beneficiary is outside the United States; home health care and skilled nursing home care if the specified conditions are not met; the first three pints of blood needed in any situation; and the cost of nursing home care that is for personal maintenance only (HCFA, 1999).

If an eligible person participates in the Medicare Part A and Part B programs, he or she may also choose to purchase a supplemental health insurance policy that will cover some of those services not covered in the Original Medicare Plan. These policies provide insurance coverage for Medicare deductibles and copayments, prescription drugs, preventive screening, emergency care outside the United States, and (sometimes) provider charges in excess of Medicare approved amounts. Such policies are generally available through a former employer, union, or fraternal

Table 11-1

Preventive Care Measures and Support in the Medicare Program

PREVENTIVE/SCREENING MEASURE	WHO IS ELIGIBLE	COST
Screening mammogram	Female Medicare beneficiaries 40 years and older	20% of Medicare-approved amount; no deductible
Pap smear and pelvic examination	Female Medicare beneficiaries	No copayment or deductible for Pap smear; 20% of Medicare-approved amount for physician services
Fecal occult blood test (annually)	All Medicare beneficiaries 50 years and older	No copayment or deductible
Flexible sigmoidoscopy (every 4 years)	All Medicare beneficiaries 50 years and older	20% of Medicare-approved amount after Part B deductible
Colonoscopy (every 2 years for those with high risk)	All Medicare beneficiaries	20% of Medicare-approved amount after Part B deductible
Barium enema (instead of sigmoidoscopy or colonoscopy)	All Medicare beneficiaries 50 years and older	20% of Medicare-approved amount after Part B deductible
Diabetic monitoring—glucose monitors, test strips, and self-care training	All Medicare beneficiaries with insulin-dependent or non–insulin-dependent diabetes	20% of Medicare-approved amount after Part B deductible
Bone mass measurement	All Medicare beneficiaries at risk for bone loss	20% of Medicare-approved amount after Part B deductible
Influenza vaccine (once per year)	All Medicare beneficiaries	No copayment or deductible
Pneumococcal vaccination (one time)	All Medicare beneficiaries	No copayment or deductible
Hepatitis B vaccination (if at high or immediate risk of infection)	All Medicare beneficiaries	20% of Medicare-approved amount after Part B deductible

organization, or they can be purchased from a private insurance company. There are ten standardized policy plans that provide for a variety of services for which a person may choose to insure. The plans offer varying levels of service coverage, with premiums that generally reflect the services covered (HCFA, 1999).

Program of All-Inclusive Care of the Elderly

The Program of All-Inclusive Care of the Elderly (PACE) uses Medicare funds (and Medicaid funds for certain eligible persons) to provide outpatient, inpatient, and LTC services. It is available to those persons who have been certified by a state agency as being eligible for nursing home care. The services available through PACE include primary care; restorative therapy; specialty and ancillary medical services; nursing care in homes, day care centers, and nursing homes; transportation to PACE centers; and meals. PACE is interdisciplinary in nature and provides holistic, total care. PACE sites are not available everywhere in the country, and persons who need such care must reside in a service area of a PACE program to be eligible for its service (HCFA, 1999). The goal of PACE programs is to maintain the independence and mobility of the older adults it serves and help them stay in their own homes and communities for as long as possible. Because they work to

coordinate services from a single location, they can provide quality care at low cost.

Other Medicare programs

Some persons who are eligible for Medicare can receive care at a federally qualified health center (FQHC). These include some community health centers (CHCs), tribal health clinics for Native Americans, migrant health clinics, and certain health centers for homeless persons. These centers are found in inner-city and rural areas, as well as on tribal land. Some health care not usually paid for through Medicare is available if a beneficiary uses a FQHC. For example, routine physical examinations, screening and diagnostic tests, and influenza vaccinations are covered. Some deductibles and copayments may also be waived.

Some low-income Medicare beneficiaries may be eligible for Medicaid. Since Medicaid is administered by the states, qualification and benefits vary from state to state.

Medicare abuse and fraud

Any third-party payer for health care can investigate providers for abuse and fraud in billing practices. However, the majority of prosecutions thus far have come from Medicare and Medicaid (Buppert, 2000). The federal government is intent on keeping Medicare solvent, and doing this involves stopping fraud and abuse and requiring that providers adhere to the rules. (This topic is covered extensively in Chapter 13.)

Medicaid

The federal program known as Medicaid was established as Title XIX of the Social Security Act (PL 89-97). These amendments to the Act established a partnership between the federal government and the states to provide health insurance benefits for low-income people. This was a significant economic and political change that involved the federal government in providing and controlling health care more than it had ever been before. As with Medicare, the economic consequences of Medicaid were not adequately predicted, and like Medicare, they have vastly exceeded the initially projected expenditures. No one at the time of passage of the law in 1965, or for the previous years when the premise was being discussed in Congress, considered the effects on demand that such a program would precipitate or the later demand for the increasing availability of health care technology (Phelps, 1997). Since 1989, Medicaid expenditures have increased 112%.

When Medicaid cost increased rapidly in the 1970s, states found that they were forced to spend significantly more than the amount for which they had planned or budgeted. Medicaid was open ended; therefore a state with a cost far more than anticipated could not merely stop paying or deny eligibility. It had to appropriate additional state funds, reduce eligibility or services, reduce provider compensation, or delay payments to providers until the next fiscal year. (This latter strategy likely violates the Medicaid law.) Reducing services tends to increase costs in other areas; for example, reducing drug coverage may increase hospitalization or nursing home admission (Rosenberg, Law, & Rosenbaum, 1997). Unfortunately, states have been denied (by federal regulation) the right to make specific exclusions based on diagnosis, a strategy often used by private insurance. Because of this, states have been forced to cover expensive treatments for a few persons (e.g., organ transplants), while denying more common elements of care to many more persons. Some of the newer managed care programs have alleviated this problem (Rosenberg, Law, & Rosenbaum, 1997). Problems of Medicaid coverage have reached appeals courts, where judges have held that distinctions based on diagnosis or specific illness or condition are inconsistent with the objectives of the Medicaid program and so will not be upheld, but that general coverage limitations, such as the number of physician visits per period, excluding emergencies, are reasonable and consistent with the objectives of the program (*Curtis v. Taylor*, 625 F.2d 645 [5th Cir.1980]).

The Medicaid program is thought to be an important

but unmanageable entity. The complexities of the law make the program difficult to administer, and the move toward managed care for Medicaid recipients has only made the situation more difficult. The only types of managed care entities recognized under federal law are federally qualified or state-licensed HMOs. Reimbursements to hospitals and other institutions tend to be governed by cost considerations. Furthermore, states are still being required to permit freedom in choosing providers, although insured workers in managed care have restricted choices for providers (Rosenberg, Law, & Rosenbaum, 1997). The lag in the trends does not support cost-containment and rational approaches to care in Medicaid.

The Medicaid program serves people who have income below a certain specified amount based on guidelines developed by the state and the federal government. It is administered by the state with federal financial assistance. Medicaid recipients pay no copayments for care under federal law, but they may have certain nominal cost-sharing. Providers, if they participate in Medicaid, must accept all patients who seek care. The earlier Kerr-Mills Act (Title I [1960] of the Social Security Act) established a program that provided health care for low-income older adults, but rather than expand Kerrs-Mill to include all medically indigent persons, the new Medicaid program was developed. Federal law required that Medicaid cover persons and families receiving Aid to Families with Dependent Children (AFDC), as well as other welfare recipients, and that services include hospital and physician care, diagnostic tests, family planning, and LTC in SNFs. Later amendments provided for health screening and assistance to the recipients of Supplemental Security Income (SSI) (Sultz & Young, 1999). According to Phelps (1997), states could also provide care in intermediate care facilities; dental care; prescription medicines; or eyeglasses, for all of which they could charge a copayment.

Medicaid-eligible recipients have low incomes, so it is presumed that they cannot generate the funds to pay for health insurance themselves. The Medicaid program cannot, in managing its care-provision efforts and controlling costs, rely on patient cost-sharing as a mechanism for creating incentives for appropriate use, since it is believed that if costs were imposed, many of the Medicaid population could not afford any care at all. Since Medicaid was originally structured as a combination of welfare assistance and fee-for-service health care, the lack of the cost-control measures in private insurance and a politically precarious funding base has made the program particularly difficult to continue to manage and justify in its current organization (Rosenblatt, Law, & Rosenbaum, 1997).

Eligibility for Medicaid is based on certain income and resource limits. The categories of persons eligible varies by state but, if they meet income and resource limits, generally include those shown in Box 11-1. Limits on

Box **11-1**

Categories of Persons Eligible for Medicaid

- Persons 65 years of age and older
- Blind or permanently disabled persons
- Members of families with dependent children
- Children in foster care homes
- Children under 18 years of age
- Pregnant women
- Persons under 21 years of age residing in psychiatric hospitals
- Qualified Medicare beneficiaries
- Aged, blind, or disabled persons receiving SSI
- Pregnant women with a family income of less than the federal poverty level (may be eligible; resources not considered)
- Persons receiving assistance from the new federal program Temporary Aid to Needy Families (TANF) (replaced the AFDC program, which was repealed by the Balanced Budget Act)

- Institutionalized persons who have 300% of the SSI benefit rate
- Certain older, blind, or disabled persons earning up to 250% of the FPL
- Tuberculosis (TB)-infected persons, with benefits limited to TB related expenses
- Certain persons who have such high medical expenses that those costs reduce their assets to a qualifying level based on the FPL

Sultz and Young (1999) describe the Medicaid program as a transfer payment program from people who are more economically successful (but by no means wealthy) to those who are more needy. Unlike Medicare, which reimburses health care providers through local intermediaries such as other insurers, Medicaid reimburses providers directly. As described previously, each state has its own formulas and policies, as well as variations in benefits.

Between 1980 and 1990 Medicaid expenditures rose 300%. This led to many initiatives at both state and federal levels to control the cost of the program. In 1995, combined federal and state expenditures for Medicaid totaled $159 billion. Despite the use of managed care programs, utilization review, and prospective payments similar to diagnostic-related group (DRG) reimbursement, Medicaid remains the fastest growing component of state budgets (Health Care Industry Analysts, 1996). States have received waivers from the federal government to require Medicaid recipients to enroll in managed care plans and have contracted with HMOs on a fully or partially capitated basis to provide all or most of the benefits. Since this became available, managed care enrollment increased by more than 170% (Health Care Financing Administration, 1997).

The Balanced Budget Act of 1997 projected the intent to reduce Medicaid expenditures by $10.1 billion by 2002. The strategies to accomplish this include reducing payments made to the states for hospital care. It is believed that the greatest effect will be on inner-city hospitals. There will also be increased efforts to fight fraud and abuse. Two of the goals of Medicaid reform are to reach more people with services they need and to expand coverage where possible. One of the areas addressed is health care for children. There is also an effort to introduce managed care to the Medicaid program. Managed Medicaid has its own challenges. Recipients used to accessing the health care system in an unregulated and unrestricted manner will find it difficult to plan for care and accept the controls of a managed care system. Nevertheless, Medicaid managed care enrollments have increased significantly in the last several years. More than 40% of Medicaid recipients are now in managed care programs. States may make managed care enrollment mandatory or voluntary (Sultz & Young, 1999). Managed care systems are beginning to demonstrate that they can reduce inpatient hospital

income and resources are set by the states, using federal guidelines (some mandatory). States are free to expand coverage and may include federally ineligible low-income persons, but they must do it with state funds only (Havighurst, Blumstein, & Brennan, 1998). The limits on resources or assets such as personal property and savings include countable assets such as a house and household materials; clothing and other personal effects; money to provide for a funeral; income-producing property up to a certain amount (generally about $5000 to $6000); an automobile used to get to work or the physician's office; and other equity up to a specified amount, generally under $5000. Income cannot exceed certain limits as well, with the limits based on the number of persons in a family. At least one state provides benefits only if a family of three has an income of less than $3700 or a family of seven has an income of less than $6800. Should income exceed the stated amounts, a person may be eligible if he or she has major medical expenses that would equal or exceed the excess income in a given period. It is not uncommon for persons or families to vary in eligibility from month to month, so qualification is assessed periodically.

States may optionally add other categories of persons to their Medicaid programs and then receive matching federal funds for their health care expenses. However, not every category a state chooses to cover is eligible for matching funds. In addition to coverage for federally mandated categories, states may also cover the following:

- Children in families who earn up to 185% of the federal poverty level (FPL)
- Pregnant women in the same FPL category

days and emergency department use, but it remains to be seen if this can continue.

Care for children in the Medicaid program

Care for uninsured and underinsured children is affected by public policy. Since the federal government's attempt to nationalize health care in 1994, the incrementalism and transaction-cost augmentation that permitted the passage of Medicare and Medicaid and their subsequent expansions and modifications is being used to include health care for children. That this is a political effort is evident from the manner in which health plans were implemented (Lopez, 1998). The effort has been fairly successful; there are more than 900 school-based programs providing some traditional health care, screening, and prevention. In addition, many of the school programs also offer psychological and reproductive counseling to children (Bureau of National Affairs, 1997). This is generally without the permission or knowledge of their parents. States have numbers of school-based health centers varying from 149 centers in New York to a single center each in New Hampshire and Alaska (Making the Grade, 1997.) In 1994, more than $22 million was expended for school-based health clinics, an increase of 140% in 2 years (Bureau of National Affairs, 1997).

State health programs for children

The State Children's Health Program (S-CHIP) is a federal program that expands government health care for children. States may either expand Medicaid or their own insurance plans to provide this care. A small amount of the federal money may be used for direct purchase of care, perhaps through a CHC. Federal guidelines include those children whose families earn up to twice the poverty level. Some legislators are concerned that at that level, some middle-class families will be attracted to it (Shi & Singh, 1998). An aggressive advertising program on television and radio maintains that families can obtain "free" health care coverage for children, whether or not parents are employed. This program is actually somewhat redundant. There are almost five million children who are eligible for Medicaid that do not currently participate in the program, either because their families do not realize the children are eligible or they do not have an immediate need for care (Selden, Banthin, & Cohen, 1998). Often when a child reaches school age and needs assessment and immunization before starting school, families take advantage of the Medicaid program.

Long-term care and Medicaid

One of the provisions of the Medicaid program is coverage of nursing home care or LTC. Many older adults who need LTC, which is not covered by Medicare to any significant extent, expend all of their assets and are eventually unable to fund their continuing nursing home care (Havighurst et al, 1998). LTC in a residential facility costs between $35,000 and $80,000 each year (typical costs from 1998 and 1999) (United States GAO, 1998), and there are many people who cannot fund such expenses; the average nursing home stay is 2½ years (Hollman & Hayes, 1996). Medicaid offers what could be described as universal coverage for residential LTC, but it requires that the ultimate recipient exhaust all his assets to receive the benefit (Havighurst et al, 1998). The aging of the population and changes in family structure have increased the numbers of people needing institutional or home-based LTC. Many of the people who exhaust their funds on LTC are not those who would have been thought of as poor during their working life or retirement. However, one of the features of the Medicaid Long-Term Care Support Program is that it recognizes that older adult couples will not age or experience failing health at the same rate. It is not uncommon for one member of a couple to need LTC and the other to be relatively healthy. For the couple to exhaust their assets to provide LTC for one can leave the person still living at home impoverished, having exhausted all savings on nursing home care for the other. That person may then need public assistance. Medicaid now permits spouses living in the community with a spouse in LTC to avoid impoverishment and still receive Medicaid funds to pay for the LTC. The assets the community-dwelling spouse may retain and the income limits for participants are determined by Congress and imposed upon the states. Before this law, and even now, there has been a problem with families hiding funds, using legal strategies to protect funds from being used for LTC, and permitting the nursing home resident to appear eligible for Medicaid funds earlier than he or she would have otherwise been (Phelps, 1997). This is now considered fraud, and lawyers who attempt to advise their clients to defraud the federal and state governments by hiding or redirecting assets for up to 3 years before applying for Medicaid can be censured or worse by their state bar associations.

Social issues concerning long-term care. A broad social issue is raised when discussing the idea of managing assets and the behavior that results from it. Do families have a responsibility to provide LTC for their older family members? Medicaid rules say that children and other relatives are not so responsible, and that the person in question is responsible for paying for his or her own care for as long as possible. Because society has made provision for intergenerational transfer of assets via a testamentary will or trust, younger generations expect that upon the death of older family members, they will inherit certain assets. However, if there are no assets left because of the cost of LTC, the beneficiary of the will or trust forfeits his inheritance. Economists describe this as de facto, requiring families to pay by relinquishing their right to receive a bequest (Phelps, 1997). This issue may be interpreted in many ways. Although there is never a right to anything until the grantor dies, lifetime behaviors of both grantors and benefactors are very much related to this intergenerational asset transfer. Unfortunately, there is little effort to educate about or encourage the purchase of LTC insurance, which would provide older adults with more choices than those provided by Medicaid. For example, most reputable insurance policies provide for a care recipient to receive care in the home, in an assisted living facility, or in some level of skilled care facility. For a minimally impaired person, this permits a gradual movement to higher levels of care, thereby conserving insurance funds for a longer period because lower levels are less costly.

Many individuals and families pay for much of the cost of LTC out of their pocket. Of people who need LTC, 33% rely on personal savings or financial help from family members to meet their expenses. Without some assistance, 70% of single individuals and 50% of couples are impoverished within 1 year (United States GAO, 1998).

The Health Security Act

While it is not necessarily a part of the current Medicaid program, it is instructive to assess the 1993 Health Security Act proposal by the Clinton administration, which proposed to provide health care for everyone. Although the plan promised more control of access to care by consumers, in reality it demanded a more prominent and prescriptive role for government than was originally contemplated by the advocates of what was termed *managed competition*. When Congress and the public refused to endorse the proposals of the Health Security Act, the bill failed (Havighurst et al, 1998). In a political environment antagonistic to higher taxes and redistributive schemes, the proposers of the Health Security Act tried to manage its passage without revealing the extent of the transfer of funds from workers to others who did not contribute in any way to the program. In the proposal, funds would have been collected by employers and others, pooled in health alliances, and redistributed in ways that would not permit a clear connection between what a person paid in and the value of the health insurance coverage received in return (Havighurst et al, 1998). The drafters of the Health Security Act planned to impose a mandatory payroll tax on employers. Funds so paid were to be sent to private alliances but then used for public purposes, as defined by statute. Critics claimed that the Clinton program would have cost jobs, reduced take-home pay for workers, and rationed beneficial health services to those who thought they were paying for them (Havighurst et al, 1998).

At present, there is an ideological problem of whether the United States can acknowledge that public policy can manage some marginal differences in the level of health care available to individuals in different income categories. The Balanced Budget Act of 1997 does permit higher-income older adults to purchase care in a variety of ways likely to enhance their quality of care. However, at the same time, S-CHIP portends more incrementalism in

government-sponsored health care insurance. Furthermore, although about 75% of employers offer some type of group health insurance, many lower-income and younger workers decline it, possibly to maintain their level of take-home pay or because they do not perceive a need for such insurance.

Managed Care

Managed care is one of the signal events for health care insurance this century (Epstein, 1997). Early forms of managed care were notably found in some fraternal organizations and provided by employers for employees that operated in jobs in remote locations, such as mining and logging. During World War II, shipyard workers in California had a prepaid group practice health plan from Henry J. Kaiser, out of which developed the Kaiser-Permanente Health Plan, which is now an industry leader. The Health Insurance Plan (HIP) in New York was also an early form of HMO. The commonality among such plans was the replacement of a fee-for-service payment system with a prepaid fixed amount to a group of providers who were then responsible for providing all health care to enrollees. HMOs seemed to be able to provide quality care at reasonable cost, and proponents of the concept also considered them useful vehicles for introducing competitive forces into the health care marketplace (Havighurst et al, 1998). The federal government entered the effort in 1973 through the passage of the Health Maintenance Organization Act (42 U.S.C.A. Section 300e; 42 C.F.R. Section 417). It was meant to encourage and subsidize a form of health care delivery more than promote innovative competition. At the same time, states were enacting HMO-enabling legislation that was less restrictive than the federal law. The result was that employers were reluctant to contract with non–federally qualified plans because they believed they would be required to eventually meet the federal requirement (Starr, 1976). Federal regulations, written after the Act was passed, took several years (not an uncommon problem even today). The Health Maintenance Organization Act required the provision of certain contracted health services for a specified periodic payment that was not dependent upon the frequency or kind of services needed or used. State laws that interfered with the formation of federally qualified HMOs were prohibited; such interference might include requirements for medical society approval for licensure, a certain number of physicians on the governing board of the HMO, or financial reserves to prevent insolvency (Havighurst et al, 1998).

In 1976, approximately 10 million people were in managed care health plans. However, the greatest growth in HMO enrollment occurred in the 1980s after the federal subsidies for them had expired, (although many of the regulations continue to be in effect). For example, federal law requires HMOs to use a community rating to determine insurance premiums, with only a few alterations available. By 1995, there were five times as many people enrolled—50 million—and the numbers are expected to increase rapidly as employers, private insurers, and government insurers see cost savings in the programs.

Epstein (1997) describes the move to managed care as a change from a primarily therapeutic relationship with a physician to an interaction that considers primarily financial issues. He describes insurance to protect against the unpredictable and expensive occurrence of injury or illness as the best (if not the only) feasible approach for most people to cope with the risk. However, his premise that insurance also adds complications to the risk equation is true. People who put little or none of their own assets at risk in seeking health care tend to "spend" freely, and physicians and other health care providers, who do not have a stake in the judicious use of limited funds, do not consider the costs relative to the benefits of many aspects of care. In fact, if providers are paid based on the amount of care provided, there is a powerful incentive to provide all available forms of care. Therefore there has been an emergence of cost controls in health care insurance. One of the ways cost control has been instituted is through managed care. Although there has been much criticism of managed care, insurers who offer such products defend them by promoting their advantages. Reducing unnecessary care saves in both money and health risks for patients (Epstein, 1997). Moreover, MCOs are part of the risk equation. In theory, it is in their best interests to maintain the health of the participants in the plan since the more patients who become ill, the greater the expense to care for them. Preventive care, therefore, is the rule rather than the exception. Epstein (1997) describes a paradox in the managed care system. The turnover rate in a managed care network of patients averages about 15%. The higher the turnover rate, the weaker the relationship is between the MCO's efforts to maintain health and the actual patient outcomes. This affects the measured performance of an MCO. Performance is what promotes financial solvency and a reputation that will get that particular MCO additional enrollees.

Iglehart (1992) explains that the defining characteristic of MCOs is the integration of financing and delivery of health care through contracting with selected providers to deliver comprehensive care to a group of enrolled patients in exchange for a periodic predetermined fee. A patient pays a premium to the insurer (or the premium is paid by an employer), and the insurer pays fees to contracted providers. Health care providers are expected to provide all the needed care for their enrollees for the amount of the fees paid, including medical, hospital, and other services. This is typically referred to as a *capitated fee*, a fixed fee for each patient enrolled with that provider.

There are at least three types of MCOs. The HMO has been available since the middle of the twentieth century and is characterized by contracts with health care providers who provide an array of benefits for a fixed fee. PPOs are entities in which employers and insurers contract with providers at reduced rates for the care of an enrollee group. Point-of-service (POS) plans are hybrids. They have the characteristics of both HMOs and PPOs. However, for a higher fee, enrollees are permitted to go outside the provider panel for care (Litman & Robins, 1997).

The goal of managed care is to reduce the cost of health care by changing physicians' practice styles and patient behaviors. To reduce the inappropriate use of specialists and nonparticipating physicians and other providers, PCPs are the main source of all patient care. A referral system is used to regulate the access of patients to more expensive specialty services (Litman & Robins, 1997). PCPs and specialists in the provider panel are actually sharing the financial risk of providing care, so they eventually do change their behavior with regard to indiscriminate use of certain aspects of care.

This does not mean that HMOs are without critics. Bronow (1997), a member of a group called Physicians Who Care (who have a website at pwc.org), is highly critical of managed care. Bronow claims that managed care compromises the ethics of physicians and the care of patients while damaging the trust that existed between them. Other criticisms include the barriers that prevent certain aspects of care, particularly costly care (Bronow, 1997). Bronow does note that HMO contracts are unclear as to exclusions or restrictions on benefits and that patients may not know of such barriers until the HMO denies coverage. Physician contracts often militate against offering certain treatments through penalties for "overtreatment" and bonuses for limiting expenditures. Bronow expresses concern that people are depersonalized by the language that MCOs use to describe them and that participants in managed care do not know or understand contracting arrangements with physicians and other practitioners whose clinical decisions affect patient care. There is an assertion that managed care is good for society because it lowers the cost of health care, and MCOs claim that they need to ration care because resources are scarce and in no way infinite. Bronow also challenges the need to ration care at the same time as physicians and MCO executives are being well rewarded for improving the MCO profits. He does not denigrate profits, but he does question the mechanisms that produce profit not by providing a service that someone wants to buy but through deception and denial. He gives three recommendations for restoring ethics and balance in MCOs: (1) patients should know about the physician contracts and cost-cutting strategies, (2) patients should be informed about the benefits and exclusions in detail, and (3) patients should be provided with all information needed to make fully informed decisions about health care.

A counter argument is that many patients will demand care even if it does not offer them any benefit in terms of longer life or more comfort. Also, particularly desperate patients needing or wanting high-tech or experimental treatments are generally unable to make a dispassionate evaluation of the efficacy of a particular treatment. This is one of the reasons that so-called "gag clauses" were put in MCO contracts, clauses that prohibited panel physicians from offering or informing patients about treatments that would just be denied (Epstein, 1997). Of course such clauses undermine the fiduciary duty that exists between a physician and a patient, such duty arising whenever one person trusts or relies on the integrity and fidelity of another.

Managed care has influenced the entire health system. Such influence is likely to result in pressure on providers to merge into fewer and larger practice and delivery entities. The resulting competition to join managed care groups and retain patient groups will require providers to become more responsive to the price and quality concerns of purchasers, which are employers, the government, and other large purchasing groups, not patients. This is likely to lead to more stringent control of utilization, minimization of staff and managerial positions, standardized treatment for many health problems, and quantification of quality indicators (Litman & Robins, 1997). Managed care has become a powerful player in the health insurance market and affects about one half of all hospitals and three quarters of physicians. Another factor confounding the MCO/HMO emergence is the distinction between for-profit and not-for-profit organizations. In for-profit competitive systems, profit maximization is the driving force. If capitated fees are the payment mechanism, insurers rely on economic self-interest to encourage health care providers to deliver cost-effective care (Miller, 1996.) A positive aspect of the capitated system is the clinical autonomy of the health care providers, who are not restricted by managed care insurers. Of course, such autonomy only exists in reality if the capitation payment is adequate to provide for high-quality patient care and a satisfying income for providers. Despite significant criticism in the popular media, there is little evidence of widespread poor-quality patient care. However, the potential exists for capitation payments to encourage underprovision of care, with the patient as the most vulnerable party in the system (Miller, 1996). Conversely, since capitation payment systems shift the financial risk from the insurer to the provider, there may be a greater incentive for providers to assume insurer function themselves. Then they would not lose the initial profits taken by an insurer after receiving premium payments and before forwarding capitation payments. As for not-for-profit MCOs, they are subject to certain statutory regulations and common laws related to their tax-exempt status, and this favored position carries certain public service obligations.

As hospital mergers and physician group consolidation increase, they may gain some power in the marketplace. Self-insured organizations may also exert power as they bypass insurers to contract directly with providers. The AMA (1994) reports that managerial control of health care

is and will continue to be systematically applied to clinical decisions and treatment plans. A recent ruling by the Office of the Inspector General (OIG) of the Department of Health and Human Services (DHHS) indicates that cost-sharing agreements between hospitals and physicians that have the effect of inducing physicians to reduce or limit care to Medicare or Medicaid recipients violate the Social Security Act (Section 1128A[b][i]). Hospitals and physicians who participate in such arrangements and do not immediately cease to do so are subject to civil penalties of up to $2000 (for both hospital and physician) per Medicare or Medicaid recipient. In the same directive, the OIG indicates that there is sympathy for the need to limit unnecessary use of services, but there can be no regulatory relief for the practice of cost-sharing at this time. There is also some warning that other similar arrangements may violate the Social Security Act (Greenbaum, 1999).

In the past decade, there has been a significant shift by employers and employees, as well as those in Medicare and Medicaid, to MCOs/HMOs and other similar health insurance plans. With this experience, there is also growing acceptance of them. A 300% increase in MCO/HMO enrollees has been reported by the HCFA Office of Managed Care during the past 10 years (Managed Care Research Reports, 1997). The major struggles with this evolution include changed profitability incentives, patient resistance to the reduced choice of providers, hospitals unable to cost-shift from nonpaying patients to paying patients, and the modification of clinical practice based on the need to control costs, continue growth in earnings, manage chronic health conditions, and address changing patient behavior. (The trends affecting managed care are shown in Box 11-2.)

Box 11-2

Trends Affecting Managed Care

- Projected enrollment to exceed 100 million persons
- Increasing numbers of MCOs/HMOs; these may consolidate to reduce competition
- PPO networks increased by more than 50% in the last few years
- Decreased market share of employer-sponsored health care insurance plans held by traditional health care plans (71% in 1988; 26% in 1996)
- Hospitals more likely to have several contracts with PPOs and HMOs
- More than 83% of physicians participate in PPOs and MCOs/HMOs (according to the AMA)
- More pressure to effect continuing health of patients while generating earnings

Data from Managed Care Research Reports (1997, April). *Seven trends shaping managed care today*. Bethesda: MD: Health Trends Managed Care Research Reports.

A patient who is noncompliant with treatment or engages in lifestyle behaviors that mitigate against continued good health is a costly participant in a health care system. Patients who respond to health care provider guidance and information and engage in behaviors designed to maintain and improve health benefit themselves and the other parties in the system.

Medical Savings Accounts

A medical savings account (MSA) is a newer form of health insurance product that has some unique characteristics and is considered to be the most effective reform proposal for controlling the cost of medical and health care while consistently maintaining quality and consumer autonomy. All other cost-control proposals involve shifting more power and control to a third party (either the government or insurance companies) that would limit and ration care to reduce costs.

MSAs are designed to avoid the fundamental cost-control problem. They restore direct incentives to consumers to control costs, which stimulates true market cost-control competition. MSAs permit the ultimate control of health care decisions by consumers. Consumers, not the government or insurance companies, decide whether a procedure or treatment is worth the expense (Goodman & Musgrave, 1992). Rand Corporation studies show that families with a $2500 deductible consume 50% less health care than families with no deductible, with no adverse effects on health (Goodman & Musgrave, 1992).

A MSA works as follows:

1. Regular deposits are made into the MSA by the individual or employer (the funds belong to the insured person).
2. Money can be withdrawn at any time to pay for medical and health care expenses or for insurance premiums.
3. Money not used for such expenses may be rolled over into an individual retirement account (IRA) or a private pension plan after retirement. In any case, the money not used for health care grows, free from taxes on the interest (and the dividends, if invested in dividend-producing equities).

The significant difference with the MSA, compared to traditional insurance or managed care plans, is that the consumer pays for small, initial medical expenses and probably preventive measures, but if they incur high medical costs because of serious illness, those expenses are paid in full by an insurance policy, which is a necessary link attached to the MSA. If money is withdrawn for expenses other than health care, there are penalties and taxes on those amounts. An additional value to a MSA is that expenses paid out of a MSA entail no insurance administrative cost. Tanner (1995) asserts that insurance is a very inefficient way to pay for small or routine health expenses. Significantly more administrative costs are involved in processing a large number of small claims than in processing a few large claims with an equal dollar value. Premiums generally fall as the average claim size increases. With the typical MSA, insurance companies need not be involved in the vast majority of health care transactions, particularly small claims where insurance is least efficient. Therefore the overall cost of health care and the administrative costs for physicians and other health care providers could be significantly reduced (Tanner, 1995).

Under the current third-party insurance system, most health care consumers do not pay directly for their health care. Nearly 95% of hospital bills and more than 80% of physician fees are paid for by private health insurance. Of every dollar used to purchase health care, 76 cents are paid not by a consumer, directly to a provider, but by some third party, which is essentially an invisible expenditure. As a result, consumers have little incentive to question costs and every incentive to demand more services. However, with MSAs, patients pay for much of their care from their accounts or in cash, giving them an incentive to become cost-conscious consumers. Congress has provided only reluctant support of MSAs, permitting a small number to be available and those only to self-employed persons and small businesses with fewer than 50 employees.

When a MSA is chosen, individuals choose a deductible between $1550 and $2300, families a deductible between $3100 and $4600. Total sharing of costs (deductibles, coinsurance, and copayments) is limited to $3000 for individuals and $5500 for families. Individuals may put 65% of their chosen deductible into a tax-free account; families may contribute 75% of their deductible. Only the employer or employee (but not both) may make this contribution in a single year.

Most companies that offer MSAs permit insured persons who accumulate money in the MSA in excess of what is needed to cover the high deductible to invest in a variety of financial vehicles so that the tax-deferred growth of the funds is enhanced. The benefits of the accompanying health insurance policy are available once the deductible is satisfied (American Health Value, 1999).

Under current law, every dollar of health insurance premiums paid by an employee escapes the minimum 28% federal income tax, 15.3% Social Security (Federal Insurance Contributions Act [FICA]) tax, and minimal 6% or larger state and local income tax (depending on location). Thus the government is effectively paying up to half the premium—a generous subsidy that encourages employees to overinsure. At the same time, the federal government discourages individual self-insurance by taxing income that individuals try to save in order to pay their own future medical expenses. By subsidizing third-party insurance and penalizing self-insurance, federal tax law prevents employees and their employers from taking advantage of the opportunities that a MSA option would create. (Box 11-3 shows examples of health care services and health care products that can be purchased using a MSA.)

MSAs will not solve all health care insurance problems.

Box 11-3

Health Care Services and Products That May be Purchased through a Medical Savings Account

Abortion
Acupuncture
Air conditioner (when necessary for relief from an allergy or difficulty breathing)
Alcoholism treatment
Ambulance
Anesthetist
Artificial limbs
Autoette (when used for relief of sickness)
Birth control pills (by prescription)
Blood tests
Braces
Cardiographs
Chiropractor
Christian Science practitioner
Contact lenses
Contraceptive devices
Convalescent home (for medical treatment only)
Crutches
Dental treatment
Dental x-rays
Dentures
Dermatologist
Diagnostic fees
Diathermy
Drug addiction therapy
Drugs (by prescription)
Eyeglasses
Fees paid to a health institute prescribed by a doctor
FICA and FUTA tax paid for medical care service
Fluoridation unit
Guide dog
Gynecologist
Healing services
Hearing aid and batteries
Hospital bills
Hydrotherapy
Insulin treatment
Laboratory tests and x-rays
Lead paint removal
Legal fees (to authorize treatment for a mental illness)

Lodging (away from home for outpatient care)
Metabolism tests
Neurologist
Nursing (including board and meals)
Obstetrician
Operating room costs
Opthalmologist
Optician
Oral surgery
Organ transplant
Orthopedic shoes
Orthopedist
Osteopath
Oxygen and oxygen equipment
Pediatrician
Physiotherapist
Postnatal treatment
Practical nurse for medical services
Premiums for insurance received while on unemployment compensation
Premiums for long-term care insurance
Prenatal care
Prescription medicines
Psychiatrist
Psychoanalyst
Psychotherapy
Radium therapy
Registered nurse
Special school costs for the handicapped
Spinal fluid test
Splints
Sterilization
Surgeon
Telephone or TV equipment to assist the hearing impaired
Therapy equipment
Transportation expenses (to obtain health care)
Ultraviolet ray treatment
Vaccines
Vasectomy
Vitamins
Wheelchair

FUTA, Federal Unemployment Tax Act.

However, they will have a significant effect on reducing health care costs while expanding access to care and preserving consumer choice and the quality of the health care system. Ultimately, only three entities can control health care costs: government, through rationing; insurance companies, through managed care (another form of rationing); or individual consumers (Tanner, 1995). MSAs provide the incentive for individual consumers to make cost-conscious decisions. Tanner (1995) asserts that recent criticisms of MSAs are not accurate; according to him, consumers do indeed have the capacity to be cost conscious while not forgoing necessary or preventive care. He believes that MSAs will reduce costs throughout the health care system, not just on spending below $3000; will not bankrupt the health care system; and are no more regressive than the current health care system. He also believes that any adverse selection problem has been overstated.

IMPLICATIONS FOR MSN EDUCATION AND ADVANCED PRACTICE

This chapter has addressed the various payment systems in the American health care arena and a historical view of how they evolved. This knowledge base is helpful to create an informed citizenship. For APNs, it also provides a knowledge base for the problems with the existing system and the possibilities for the future.

Every day, all APNs deal with patients whose health care costs are being paid by their third-party payers. Questions from those patients abound. Whatever knowledge APNs can share with patients and families to ease the potential struggles they face with health care costs is an advantage. Knowledge is power for patients and families.

APNs may not be in positions that require dealing directly with third-party payers, but most clinical decisions are affected in some way by the cost factors within the system. A fiscally responsible practice is a must.

APNs must know the regulations associated with the various entities and follow them conscientiously. Ignorance offers no protection when one is challenging accusations of abuse or fraud. Knowing the basics of health care financing and economics is an expectation of all Master of Science in Nursing (MSN) graduates (American Association of Colleges of Nursing, 1996). For those being educated for direct care roles, the immediate applicability of these principles to the real world is invaluable. Students may be placed with experts in third-party payment systems within the financial department of their clinical setting to gain experience in handling questions and concerns raised by patients and families. Case studies that deal with older adult patients can ask questions that require application of knowledge about Medicare. Cases that deal with low-income families can require application of knowledge related to Medicaid. As students come to appreciate the politics and ethics in the clinical setting that relate to health care costs, they can be encouraged to debrief in clinical journals or conferences.

In these times of spiraling costs, it is appropriate for students to be evaluated in the clinical setting on the extent to which they practice in a fiscally responsible or cost-conscious manner. Students should learn what things cost and should appreciate, in general, the variance between the cost of a medication, diagnostic test, treatment, or procedure and the amount paid by the third party. As part of their educational program, APN students should be exposed to the essentials of reimbursement. They should learn the appropriate evaluation and management codes and the effective documentation so critical to

optimal payment for services. Knowledge about coding and billing procedures increases the fiscal viability of a practice.

APNs should critically evaluate the systems affecting health care financing. They will have many opportunities to be patient and family advocates, but to be effective in the advocacy role requires knowledge of the system.

Decades of research indicate that APNs, because they provide satisfying quality care at lower costs than some other alternatives, are one answer to the system's problems. APNs can be justifiably proud that this is true. However, they should know the research literature thoroughly and take every possible opportunity to educate the public and other providers of the contributions they can make.

PRIORITIES FOR RESEARCH

Certainly research studies could be done to determine the APN's level of knowledge about third-party reimbursement and the effect of it as seen in the practice setting. It would be interesting to learn what the experience is for the APN who encounters ethical concerns related to health care financing. For example, what was it like for Mary, a certified nurse midwife (CNM), during her encounter with her postpartum patient Ruth? Ruth had a postpartum hemorrhage 7 days after discharge from the hospital due to a retained placental fragment. In collaboration with the obstetrician at her practice, Mary determined that a dilatation and curettage (D&C) would be necessary to resolve the problem. Since Ruth was planning to have a bilateral tubal ligation at 6 weeks postpartum, Mary and Dr. Rolf thought that the tubal ligation could be scheduled earlier without compromising Ruth's safety. Now, with one brief admission to the outpatient surgical center and one administration of anesthesia, both procedures could be done. This would minimize the risk of being anesthetized twice and the amount of time Ruth would be away from her newborn and other children. Her husband would only have to miss work one time, and the money for babysitting would be less. Mary and Dr. Rolf speculated that Ruth would recover more quickly as well. Ruth and her husband found this possibility compelling and were distressed when the insurance company refused to precertify both procedures at one admission. How does this experience affect the APN? How does it affect the patient and her family? How does it affect the nurse-patient relationship?

Other interesting questions for research are related to the care of managed care patients in terms of when to refer to specialists, how an APN determines what medications to prescribe, and what effect the cost of care has on clinical decisions. How does the payment system relate to the number of patient visits and the level of compliance with care regimens? Are the health care outcomes different in different types of health insurance programs? Is patient satisfaction affected?

DISCUSSION QUESTIONS

These questions can be used to promote critical thinking and encourage discussion.

1. Read Schriver and Arnett (1998). They address the issue of state regulation in health care. Analyze why the phenomenon of increased cost and fewer numbers of insured developed.
2. Review the history of the establishment of Medicare. Look particularly at the legislative history in the Congressional hearings and the testimony of the persons who supported and opposed these programs. What kinds of issues were raised in the testimony? Why was this program proposed? What were the objections

to it? What would you have argued at the time? Can you justify or accept the payment of a Medicare tax by middle- and lower-income workers so that wealthy older adults may have their health care for little or no cost? Do you see how it is hard to object to social programs that are presented in a way that makes the objector appear to be uncaring and against good health for a particular group? Discuss these issues in class.
3. Review the various kinds of health care insurance. What combinations of forms are most effective in promoting cost effectiveness, consumer choice, and a coherent health care system? Why?
4. Discuss the concept of incrementalism in legislative enactment. Why is incrementalism an effective strategy for passing laws and programs that would generally be opposed by many citizens? Discuss this theory in terms of several health care programs and laws that have been enacted in the last 50 years.
5. Discuss the idea of Medicaid managed care. How can Medicaid patients be reeducated to conform to the discipline of managed care health plans?

Suggestions for Further Learning

- Consult the HCFA website at www.hcfa.gov. This is a very comprehensive site supported by the federal government that provides information on Medicare, Medicaid, statistics and data, laws and regulations, and links to other government sites. This site has an enormous amount of information, however the reader should be aware that it is somewhat self-serving in terms of explaining and supporting its activities. There are many full text laws and acts.
- Consult the following: Antosz, L.C. (Ed.). (1997). *National Health Directory, Aspen Reference Group.* Gaithersburg, MD: Aspen Publishers. This is a virtual address and telephone book for health related agencies at the federal, state and local levels. Names of officers of federal agencies and health departments of major cities in the United States are available. Even if the people have changed, the addresses and telephone numbers are quite valuable.
- For pediatric specialists, read the following: Lopez, N. (1998). *Are American children being lured into socialized medicine?* Washington, DC: Institute for Health Freedom; Making the Grade (1997). *National survey of state school-based initiatives: school year 1995-96.* Washington, DC: George Washington University; National Governors' Association for Best Practices (1998, May 7). *How states can increase enrollment in the state children's health insurance program* (Issue brief). National Governors' Association Center for Best Practices; and Selden, T.M., Banthin, J.S., & Cohen, J.W. (1998). Medicaid's problem

children: eligible but not enrolled. *Health Affairs 17*(3). This group of articles provides data to assist in analysis of the problems and issues concerning the health care of children.
- For gerontology specialists, read the following: Twight, C. (1997). Medicare's origin: the economics and politics of dependency. *The Cato Journal, 16*(3); Friedman, E. (1995). The compromise and the afterthought: Medicare and Medicaid after 30 years. *Journal of the American Medical Association, 274*(3), 278-282; and Corning, P.A. (1969). *The evolution of Medicare: from idea to law* (Research report no. 29). Washington, DC: US Department of Health, Education, and Welfare Social Security Administration, Office of Research and Statistics, US Government Printing Office.
- Visit the HCFA site at www.hcfa.gov/Medicare. This site's web resources provide much useful information for the analysis of health care opportunities and problems for older adults.
- Read the following: Buppert, C. (2000). *The primary care provider's guide to compensation and quality.* Gaithersburg, MD: Aspen Publishers.
- Visit the Medicare Fraud and Abuse Computer Based Training Course website at www.hcfa.gov.
- Read the following: American College of Physicians–American College of Internal Medicine (1998, February). *Medicare Medical Review: Safeguards and Advice for Internists and Their Staff,* 2-9. Although written for physicians, this is also very relevant for PCPs.

6. Why is it a problem if there is an expansion of government-sponsored health care insurance at the expense of private insurance? How are the current government-sponsored programs affecting the private market? Where might you find this information?

7. One of the major issues of today is how to finance LTC for older adults and disabled populations. What strategies and approaches might be used to address this issue, with the understanding that a tax-supported system cannot be maintained? What are the issues, factors, and concerns that need to be addressed in solving this problem?

8. Review the Health Maintenance Organization Act of 1973. Discuss the positive and negative aspects of managed care. How can the positive aspects be strengthened while minimizing the negative effects? Is there a role for APNs?

REFERENCES/BIBLIOGRAPHY

Acs, G., Long, S.H., Marquis, M.S. & Short, P.F. (1996). Self-insured employer health plans: prevalence, profile, provisions, and premiums. *Health Affairs, 15*(2), 266-279.

American Association of Colleges of Nursing (1996). *The essentials of master's education for advanced practice nursing.* Washington, DC: American Association of Colleges of Nursing.

American Health Value (1999). Information available online at www.americanhealthvalue.com.

American Medical Association (1994). *The future of medical practice* (Order no. OP211594). American Medical Association.

Anderson, O.W. (1990). *Health services as a growth enterprise in the United States since 1875.* Ann Arbor, MI: Health Administration Press

Berkowitz, E., & Berkowitz, M. (1985). Challenges to workers' compensation: an historic analysis in workers' compensation benefits. In Worrall & Appel (Eds.), *Workers' compensation benefits: adequacy, equity, and efficiency.* Books on Demand.

Bronow, R.F. (1997). *HMOs—the death of medical ethics.* Physicians Who Care. Available online at www.pwc.org/summer97/ART3.html.

Buppert, C. (2000). *The primary care provider's guide to compensation and quality.* Gaithersburg, MD: Aspen Publishers.

Bureau of National Affairs (1997). School-based centers gaining attention for providing access for uninsured kids. *Health Care Policy Report, 5*(32).

Cantril, H. (1951). *Public opinion 1935-1946.* Princeton, NJ: Princeton University Press

Chapman, C.B., & Talmadge, J.M. (1970). Historical and political background of federal health care legislation. *Law and Contemporary Social Problems, 35*(2), 334-347

Cihak, R., Williams, B., & Ferrara, P.J. (1997). The rise and repeal of the Washington state health plan: lessons for America's state legislatures. *Backgrounder, 1121/S.* Washington, DC: The Heritage Foundation.

Cohen, W.J., & Ball, R.M. (1965). Social security amendments of 1965: summary and legislative history. *Social Security Bulletin, 28*(9), 3-21

Commonwealth of Pennsylvania House of Representatives (1996). *Findings of fact and report* (pp. 18-19). Committee on Education, Select Subcommittee on Education, Select Subcommittee on House Resolution No. 37.

Corning, P.A. (1969). *The evolution of Medicare: from idea to law* (Research report no. 29). Washington, DC: US Department of Health, Education, and Welfare Social Security Administration, Office of Research and Statistics, US Government Printing Office.

Epstein, R.A. (1997). *Mortal peril: our inalienable right to health care?* Reading, MA: Addison-Wesley

Friedman, E. (1995). The compromise and the afterthought: Medicare and Medicaid after 30 years. *Journal of the American Medical Association, 274*(3), 278-282

General Accounting Office (1998, March 9). *Testimony before the Special Committee on Aging, U.S. Senate.*

Goodman, J.C. (1980). *The regulation of medical care: is the price too high?* (Cato public policy research monograph no. 3). San Francisco: Cato Institute.

Goodman, J. & Musgrave, G.L. (1992). *Patient power.* Washington, DC: Cato Institute.

Greenbaum, Doll, & McDonald (1999). *Kentucky health law letter.* Louisville, KY: Greenbaum, Doll, and McDonald, PLLC.

Havighurst, C. (1970). Health maintenance organizations and the market for health care services. *Law and Contemporary Social Problems, 35*(16).

Havighurst, C.C., Blumstein, J.F., & Brennan, T.A. (1998). *Health care law and policy.* New York, NY: The Foundation Press.

Health Care Financing Administration. *Medicare fraud and abuse computer based training course.* Available online at www.hcfa.gov.

Health Care Financing Administration. *Overview of the Medicare program.* Available online at hcfa/gov/medicare/careover.htm.

Health Care Financing Administration (1997, January 28). *Managed care in Medicare and Medicaid* (Fact sheet). Health Care Financing Administration.

Health Care Industry Analysts (1996). *Comparative performance of U.S. hospitals: the sourcebook.* Baltimore, MD: Health Care Industry Analysts.

Hollman, K.W., & Hayes, R.D. (1996). *Long-term care insurance: planning for independence and security.* Murfreesboro, TN: Business and Economic Research Center, College of Business, Middle Tennessee State University.

Iglehart, J.K. (1992). Health policy report: the American health care system. *New England Journal of Medicine, 327,* 742-747.

Lipson, D.J. (1997). State roles in health care policy: past as prologue. In T.J. Litman & L.S. Robins, *Health politics and policy.* Albany, NY: Delmar Publishers

Litman, T.J., & Robins, L.S. (1997). *Health politics and policy.* Albany, NY: Delmar Publishers

Liu, J.C., & Moffit, R.E. (1995). *A taxpayer's guide to the Medicare crisis.* Washington, DC: The Heritage Foundation.

Longest, B.B. (1998). *Health policymaking in the United States.* Chicago: Health Administration Press

Lopez, N. (1998). *Are American children being lured into socialized medicine?* Washington, DC: Institute for Health Freedom

Making the Grade (1997). *National survey of state school-based initiatives: school year 1995-96.* Washington, DC: George Washington University.

Managed Care Research Reports (1997, April). *Seven trends shaping managed care today.* Bethesda, MD: Health Trends Managed Care Research Reports.

McCubbin, R. (1997). The Kentucky health care experiment: how managed competition clamps down on choice and competition. *Backgrounder, 1119/S,* Washington, DC: The Heritage Foundation.

McMenamin, B. (1996, December). Trojan horse money. *Forbes.*

Miller, F.H. (1996). Health care capitated payment system. *American Journal of Law and Medicine, 22*(2-3). Available online at www.library.usask.ca/ejournals/0099/0098-8588.html.

National Center for Policy Analysis Idea House (1997). Available online at ncpa.org.

National Governors' Association for Best Practices (1998, May 7). *How states can increase enrollment in the state children's health insurance program* (Issue brief). National Governors' Association Center for Best Practices.

Phelps, C.E. (1997). *Health economics* (2nd ed.). Reading, MA: Addison-Wesley.

Poen, M.M. (1979). *Harry S. Truman versus the medical lobby: the genesis of Medicare.* Columbia, MO: University of Missouri Press.

Rapsiler, L.M., & Anderson, E.H. (2000). Understanding the reimbursement process. *The Nurse Practitioner, 25*(5), 36, 43-46, 51-56.

Rosenberg, R.E., Law, S.A., & Rosenbaum, S. (1997). *Law and the American health care system.* Westbury, NY: The Foundation Press.

Scandlen, G. (1999, May 21). Open MSAs to the rest of us. *Cato Commentary.* Available online at www.cato.org.

Schriver, M.L., & Arnett, G.M. (1998). Uninsured rates rise dramatically in states with strictest health insurance regulations. *Backgrounder.* Washington, DC: The Heritage Foundation

Selden, T.M., Banthin, J.S., & Cohen, J.W. (1998) Medicaid's problem children: eligible but not enrolled. *Health Affairs 17*(3).

Shi, L., & Singh, D.A. (1998). *Delivering health care in America.* Gaithersburg, MD: Aspen Publishers.

Starr, P. (1976, Winter) The undelivered health care system. *Public Interest.*

Starr, P. (1982). *The social transformation of American medicine.* Cambridge, MA: Basic Books.

Sultz, H.A., & Young, K.M. (1999). *Health care USA* (2nd ed.). Gaithersburg, MD: Aspen Publishers.

Tanner, M. (1995). Medical savings accounts: answering the critics. *Cato Policy Analysis,* 228. Available online at www.cato.org/pubs/pas/pa228.html.

Twight, C. (1997). Medicare's origin: the economics and politics of dependency. *The Cato Journal, 16*(3). Available online at www.cato.org/.

United States General Accounting Office (1995, June 12). *Health insurance regulation: variation in recent state small employer health insurance reforms* (GAO/HEHS-95-161FS).

United States General Accounting Office (1997, July). *Private health insurance: continued erosion of coverage linked to cost pressures* (GAO/HEHS-97-122).

Wilson, F.A., & Neuhauser, D. (1985). *Health services in the United States* (2nd ed.). Cambridge, MD: Balinger.

Chapter 12

Principles of Fiscal Planning and Budgeting for the Advanced Practice Nurse

Margaret M. Anderson & Cheryl Pope Kish

Financial issues in the health care industry are becoming increasingly important given the current demands for cost containment and efficiency of operation. In a health care context where the demand for balance between quality and cost is unprecedented, the budgeting process is more important than ever. The budget is a powerful management tool. Historically, those in nursing management positions were provided with a budget determined by someone outside nursing, with little (if any) input by those who knew the nursing unit best—the nurses themselves. The situation is very different today; those in nursing leadership positions, including many advanced practice nurses (APNs), have a high degree of control over the budgeting process for their respective units. They receive regular reports from their institution's financial division, which are useful for comparing actual figures with budgeted amounts to identify variances. Nursing managers add a critical voice to identifying and balancing cost and quality.

DEFINITIONS

A **budget** is a blueprint for the efficient use of resources. Marquis and Huston (2000) define it as "a plan that uses numerical data to predict the activities of an organization over a period of time." Most organizations, regardless of size or complexity of operation, have some form of budget that is used as a quantitative representation of the organization's financial goals. According to Marquis and Huston (2000), "Because a budget is at best a prediction, a plan, and not a rule, fiscal planning requires flexibility, ongoing evaluation, and revision."

The **operating budget**, likely familiar to nurse managers, is subdivided into line items and budget codes (account numbers). Money is allocated into each line based on historical data incremented for inflation or justified by the manager. Line items include expendable supplies,

travel, continuing education costs, and office supplies. The costs of utilities and maintenance and repair of equipment are included in the operating budget. This can be a significant expenditure in settings with historical buildings. It is reviewed on both a monthly and a cumulative basis. A **personnel budget** is used to budget labor of all types in the organization; labor usually represents the largest budget expenditure. Items include base salary, productive time (all time worked with patients) and nonworking time (nonproductive or benefit time). Nonproductive time includes the cost of benefits, new employee orientation, employee turnover, sick and holiday time, and education time (Marquis & Huston, 2000). Productive and nonproductive time for staff are closely monitored. The personnel budget is sometimes also called the **labor budget.** Development of a personnel budget requires understanding of the appropriate skill mix for a particular unit and the standard that serves as a basis for staffing that unit. Nursing care hours per patient day are generally calculated as hours per patient day (for general inpatient units), visits per month (for home health units), encounters per day (for primary care clinics), or minutes per day (for operating rooms). Since these figures are static, managers must be flexible in adjusting for staffing patterns that correspond to patient volume (Marquis & Huston, 2000).

Capital budgets include major expenditures for new or replacement equipment and renovations to the organization's physical facilities (i.e., major acquisitions). Each organization has specific criteria for what is considered a capital expense. The criteria often specify the cost and anticipated life expectancy of the item. For example, an organization might define capital expenses as "hard goods with a purchase price greater than $1000 and a useful life of 1 year or more." Capital budgets are often created on a different calendar than the regular budget because the items in this budget reflect long-term commitments. A 5-year capital budget calendar is common, with annual prioritization of available capital funds. The **supplies**

budget is a separate entity in health care organizations because of the amount of supplies necessary for operation; the supplies budget is sometimes subsumed in the operating budget in non–health care organizations. However, having supplies considered within a separate budget allows for better tracking of supply use and for leveraging procurement strength. In terms of purchasing supplies, there really is strength in numbers. An ability to order supplies in bulk quantity translates to better prices.

Several factors about a particular unit are correlated with the benchmarks for major supplies needed on the unit: patient mix, occupancy rate, technology utilization, and procedures common to the unit (Dreisbach, 1994). Obviously the supplies budget is highly responsive to patient volume and services provided. The basic principles are the same if the unit is a primary care setting.

Not unlike a family budget, institutional budgets are divisions of resources—what is available to spend. Knowing this helps one prioritize how to spend available funds. Before the era of managed care, if a unit's spending outpaced income appropriated to the unit, the manager could simply increase charges. Now, to remain viable, an organization must contain costs. It is never prudent to use endowment principles, savings, investments, or loans to supplement day-to-day operations. Therefore, there is a limited pool of money, and APNs and their colleagues must live within those means or be able to clearly justify variances. If one unit overspends its allotment, other units must make up the difference or close the gap by making sacrifices. Primary care practices in several states have been forced into fiscal crisis, even bankruptcy, when expenditures outpaced income. There has been substantial erosion (as much as 30%) in competitive markets in the past 3 years (Aymond, 1999).

It is important to recognize that where an organization places its money is highly indicative of its mission and goals. There should be a clear congruence between the organization's mission and goals and its expenditures.

CRITICAL ISSUES: FISCAL PLANNING AND BUDGETING FOR ADVANCED PRACTICE NURSES

According to Liebler and McConnell (1999), there are five requisites to sound budgeting: (1) a sound organizational structure that lends clarity to the processes of preparing and administering a budget; (2) a consistent, defined budget period; (3) the availability of adequate statistical data; (4) a reporting system that reflects the organizational culture; and (5) uniform account codes that enable meaningful, consistent data. Marriner-Tomey (1996) adds, as a requisite, clear lines of authority and accountability for budgetary programs and non-monetary statistical data

(e.g., average length of stay, percentage of occupancy, number of patient days) useful to planning and controlling the budgetary process.

It is generally accepted that institutional budgetary programs serve the following purposes, regardless of how *institution* is defined: (1) quantifying the mission, policies, and vision of the organization; (2) evaluating fiscal performance and responsibility of leadership and management personnel, both individually and collectively (as an institution); (3) demonstrating cost-containment effectiveness; and (4) raising the universal cost consciousness of the institution and relating cost consciousness to goal attainment (Rowland & Rowland, 1997).

Fiscal Responsibility and Advanced Practice Nurses

For organizations to remain fiscally responsible, it is important to have clear concepts about an organization's direction and the fiscal plans that enable that direction. Administrative tools such as market research, identification of a market niche, and a strategic plan are helpful endeavors to moving an organization forward. The budget records forecasts about income and spending aimed toward the organization's mission and goals.

Financial planning is not a one-time-per-year event but an ongoing process. The budget that guides the financial plan is usually developed for a designated period (usually 1 year). The accounting period encompassed by the budget is the fiscal year (FY); technically the FY may or may not coincide with the calendar year. Historically, health care institutions have used July 1 to June 30 as the FY, which corresponds to the placement of interns and residents for the teaching program. Recently, however, with government encouragement, many health care organizations have adopted the calendar year as the FY (Liebler & McConnell, 1999).

Rowland and Rowland (1997) provide a framework for the budget planning process. Initially, an organization must review and modify organizational goals and objectives for the FY. Because the budget is tied to the organization's mission, that mission must be clear before proceeding with budget preparation. For example, MidSouth Community Health Center has a goal for the upcoming year to become the premiere provider of care to school-aged children, a practice area they envision as a market niche. To realize that goal, they must build marketing and advertising into the budget, looking realistically at what it will cost to be the best in the identified market.

The organization must identify key points of stress, disagreement, agreement, and control. Where are the organization's strengths and weaknesses, financial and otherwise? What is the level of give-and-take between units that will enable necessary compromise? To what extent does crossfunctional awareness exist within the organization? What does one unit know about the work of other units? What are the hot topics that demand attention? Responses to this budgetary step can highlight issues that need resolution.

Next, the organization must evaluate past performance. They must look at the financial history of the organization, then examine the data in light of the existing market for similar services. What is the significance that MidSouth Clinic saw 12,000 patients during the last FY, given the market? Do numbers need to increase for viability? Will the new goal related to school-aged health care help to realize increasing numbers? This budget step demands looking at the whole picture, not wearing blinders related to one's part of the total enterprise.

After evaluating what has been useful or problematic in the past, the organization must identify available resources. This step involves looking carefully at human, physical, and fiscal resources in light of the goals of the organization; it helps determine what additional resources might be needed so that budget figures can reflect those needs. Perhaps in examining the provider mix at MidSouth Clinic, the examiner determines that the addition of significant numbers of school-aged children to the existing patient population necessitates an additional nurse or a staff member with expertise in the developmental aspects of children ages 6 to 12. Those preparing the budget can plan for the advertisement, employment, and education costs accordingly.

Basic budget assumptions need to be stated. Planners must be able to assume what cost increases may occur that will affect the cost of doing business. Some assumptions can be made on the basis of inflation, the consumer price index, and cost-of-living increases for personnel. Perhaps there has been notification that insurance premiums will increase. The cost of renting a building or leasing certain equipment might also increase. Personnel development, including orientation of new staff, may be a significant figure in a given year because of an unusually high staff turnover. Department, division, and unit goals and objectives must be established as subsets of the organization's objectives. Each unit must determine what contribution it makes to the whole organizational effort. If a clinic determines that there is a need to add five examination rooms, each unit must determine what that means to their effort. For example, the properties unit thinks in terms of building costs and equipping the rooms. Housekeeping services consider how the workload and scheduling needs for cleaning can be realized with the five additional rooms. The maintenance department attends to issues in their control, and the utilities department determines to what extent five new rooms will affect heating, cooling, and lighting costs. Costs of extra linen and extra expendable supplies must be considered. Will the addition of five rooms compromise traffic within the clinic? Will new parking be necessary? Will additional staff be necessary? It is amazing to consider how much effect five additional examination rooms can have on an organization.

Clearly, without a team approach in this step of the process, something important may be lost. What if someone forgot to address the question of how linen service would be changed with the addition of the new rooms? This step is a good example of the importance of input of clinical managers in the budget process, as opposed to having the budget developed by financial experts without such input.

With unit objectives in hand, action plans become a necessary component to ensure that objectives can be met. For example, the unit whose role includes provision of linen services may need to do a cost comparison in providing linens in-house versus negotiating with a professional linen service. Someone may need to check with the heating company to determine if the existing system has the capacity to heat the additional space. This phase often requires meetings with outside consultants, such as architects, building inspectors, and various equipment vendors.

Once this groundwork has been laid, the organization must develop operational plans. This phase demands specific details about operating the unit and financing the operation. For example, scheduling for the appropriate provider mix to cover a unit 6 days a week for 10 hours a day, 360 days a year, so that there is always a particular provider mix would be an operation in this phase. This can be very complicated. Perhaps certain staff members only work part-time. For example, Joe can never work Tuesdays because of another commitment. Because of the large Hispanic patient population, a Spanish-speaking interpreter must always be scheduled in-house. Terry is pregnant and doing limited duty at present. Knowing the personnel is imperative in this kind of operation.

Budget recommendations must be examined and modified as necessary. Again, a real-world perspective is imperative. Otherwise, the budget will be too ambitious or too unrealistically low, or a budget will be prepared that is off target for meeting the institution's financial goals. Difficult decisions related to initiatives and funding are made throughout the budget process, and adherence to those decisions is imperative. Otherwise, it becomes time and effort wasted. It is sometimes helpful to revisit the decision-making process as a reminder of the intensity of the experience and the justification for why certain decisions, although painful, were purposefully made.

Once plans are finalized, approval must be obtained and the budget must be implemented. The process for approval of an institutional budget varies according to its governing structure. In some cases, a presentation of the budget is provided to a board of directors for approval. In others, the organization's administrative team makes the approval decision. Once the budget is approved and set, monitoring of income and spending begins. Budget performance data reports are prepared monthly by the finance department and distributed to responsible managers. Managers review budget performance statements and prepare explanations or justifications for variances. A variance indicates that the actual income or amount spent was different (varied) from the figures originally forecast. Some organizations require variance reporting for both positive and negative variances; others require justification only for negative variances. In some cases, the extent to which justification of variance is expected is based on a specific dollar amount or percentage threshold (e.g., it would be impractical for a unit with $100,000 in expenditures per month to work to explain a $10 variance).

The budget may be revised up or down at any time during the FY. As the budget figures are analyzed month by month, it may become evident that an initiative, albeit an important one like the five additional rooms at MidSouth Clinic, cannot progress. If a recession hits, plans for the additional five rooms may be shelved abruptly. Placing an important initiative "on hold" for 2 consecutive years should be an impetus for the organization's administration to reevaluate its need. Should any initiatives be modified, the budget may be revised.

Careful tracking of variances should continue throughout the year. As variances are tracked and interpreted, data is provided that indicate trends and patterns useful for forecasting at the next planning session. In addition to the events in the planning phases of the budget process and the monthly statement review, most institutions have a budget calendar that provides target dates to facilitate planning. In most cases, the planning process for the next FY starts before the current year ends. The preliminary phases of planning, although very time-intensive, must be balanced with regular job responsibilities; daily operations cannot be set aside. It is essential for the individual unit manager or department head to appreciate that an institutional budget must be built in a timely manner; his or her respective unit is one small measure of the entire budget. Consequently, meeting deadlines is crucial to the final product. Decisions made at one level tend to have a domino effect on other units. Any decision affecting spending, hiring, firing, or special programs must be made with a view of the entire organization and a crossfunctional awareness on the part of all managers. Institutional budget preparation without the functional expertise of the clinical representatives is nonproductive. Without the input of real-world experts, the budget loses its richness as a forecasting tool. Building the budget and planning through a team effort not only increases the partnership between financial experts and clinical experts, it tends to increase their mutual accountability to the process and the product. Understanding the budget process within this context helps APNs and nurse managers appreciate that the more detail they provide in variance reporting, the better informed the team will be for making responsible fiscal decisions on behalf of the organization. It is information "from the field" within an organization that allows the chief administrators to have their "finger on the pulse" of the organization.

Finkler (1992) conceptualizes the budget cycle with a circular model (Figure 12-1). This model clearly reflects a continuous venture for those planning, preparing, implementing, and evaluating a budget.

Budget Approaches

Rowland and Rowland (1997) have identified six unique budget approaches useful to business and health care organizations: (1) zero-based, (2) fixed or static, (3) flexible, (4) variable, (5) rolling or moving, and (6) program approaches.

The zero-based budgetary approach assumes that every program must be reviewed at least periodically; there is no automatic continuation or approval without evaluation and justification of continued funding. In this approach, every unit or program begins with a zero balance at every budget period and must justify their request for certain funding, often on the basis of a cost-benefit analysis. For example, a unit might report that it spent $1869 during the last FY by doing flexible sigmoidoscopies that added $4739 after personnel, operating, and supply costs were factored in. The volume of patients enables the unit to be eligible for a cost-savings initiative from a major vendor for the first time; this will lower supply costs for the next FY. The projected patient volume is the same. These facts translate to a forecast of increased revenues for the unit during the next FY. This kind of cost-benefit analysis reveals an advantage of the zero-based budget approach; it forces an examination of cost effectiveness, efficiency, and productivity.

The major disadvantage is that it is a time-consuming approach. Additionally, the frequency with which the budgets must be planned may prohibit adequate time for programs to be successful. For the MidSouth Clinic, there may have been only minimal progress toward the 5-year goal of being the premiere service for the community's school-aged population. In a zero-based budget, one must use caution before closing a program or shelving an initiative prematurely.

A fixed or static budget approach assumes a "fixed annual level of volume activity to arrive at an annual budget total" (Rowland & Rowland, 1997). This approach simply annualizes numbers. The total amount designated for the annual budget is divided by twelve; each month's budget, then, indicates one twelfth of the annual amount. If the annual total is $120,000, the monthly total is $10,000. An advantage of this approach is that it enables an initial budget for a new unit or program when there is no historical data available. Even in situations when historical data is available, though, this approach is used because it is simple and quick.

The major disadvantage of a fixed budget approach is the difficulty of evaluating its effectiveness in relation to actual performance and its failure to allow for normal seasonal or monthly variation. MidSouth Clinic, for

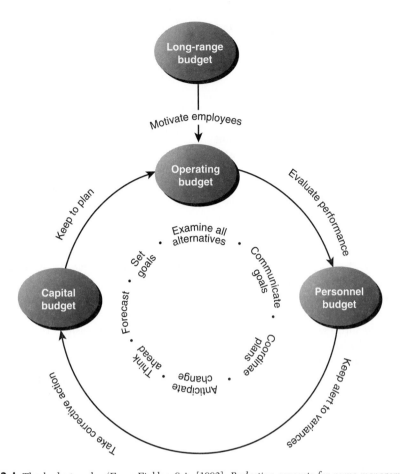

Figure 12-1 The budget cycle. (From Finkler, S.A. [1992]. *Budgeting concepts for nurse managers* [2nd ed.]. Philadelphia: WB Saunders.)

example, has proposed that part of its outreach to a school-aged population will be a preschool immunization program. Based on research that included a visit to a similar program in a nearby state, MidSouth managers predicted a need for $12,000 annually to support the immunization program. In the fixed approach, this would provide $1,000 each month or $10 per patient (with an anticipated volume of 100 patients each month). In reality, the monthly budget reports indicate that 300 immunizations were provided during the peak preschool months of May, June, and July, while the months between September and April showed an immunization rate of 60 or less.

A flexible budget assumes variability in activity that "establishes relevant ranges of volume activity" (Rowland & Rowland, 1997). Its major strength is that it does account for seasonal and monthly variation. The disadvantage is the amount of front-end time it requires. The MidSouth seasonal variances shown above would have been less problematic if a flexible budget had been in place.

The variable budget assumes a formula approach related to volume and activity. This approach is also time-intensive and requires extensive maintenance; to understand the dynamics of activity on a unit may even neces-

sitate construction of a model from which to extrapolate specifics. Variable budgets are generally reserved for huge enterprises, but they may be appropriate for nursing settings because of the variables in nursing-related unit activities. One can imagine the complexity of the variable approach by envisioning coverage of a 30-room operating suite for 24 hours a day, 365 days a year—that coverage accounting for nursing, technical support, and anesthesia services, as well as productive and nonproductive time elements, including "call."

A rolling or moving budget approach assumes the budget to be a management tool in the most dynamic terms; budgeting is ongoing all year, pushing 1 month in advance. The danger is the difficulty of measuring long-term performance. This approach is similar to a family budget that has the family living paycheck to paycheck; it causes a degree of uncertainty and insecurity.

Program budgets are often separate tools in the sense that they include start-up costs for an initial year plus projections into the future, separate from the day-to-day operations budget. This kind of budget is helpful for tracking program success because of its specificity for a given project or program. It can easily be consolidated into the organization's traditional budget at the end of the start-up interval or deleted without affecting the traditional budget unnecessarily.

Types of Costs

APNs need to understand that all costs are not equal. There are five different types of costs, each affecting overall budget expenditures differently: (1) fixed costs, (2) variable costs, (3) sunk costs, (4) direct costs, and (5) indirect costs. These are not mutually exclusive.

Fixed costs occur irrespective of patient volume. They are constant, or fixed, within the budget. Equipment depreciation, base personnel salaries and fringe benefits, and some taxes and loan payments are examples of fixed costs. Variable costs, in contrast, are related to volume. Because they are associated with particular procedures or services, variable costs increase as the numbers of such procedures and services increase. Food, linen, and expendable supplies (e.g., disposable suture sets, dressing materials, medications) are examples of variable costs. Sunk costs are those that, once spent, do not recur and cannot be recovered. Building renovation, advertising, and personnel time expended in planning are examples of sunk costs.

Direct costs are those that have a direct association with a specific unit or department or a particular patient—a cost object. These costs can be traced. Baker and Baker (2000) suggest the following approach to distinguishing direct costs: "As a rule of thumb, if the answer to the following question is 'yes,' then the cost is a direct cost: 'If the operating unit (such as a department) did not exist, would this cost not be in existence?'" A childbirth education class provided by a nurse midwifery service provides an example of direct costs (Box 12-1).

Indirect costs are those costs necessary to support the overall operation and not specific to any one unit, service, or patient. They are often referred to as *overhead costs.* These are shared costs, costs shared with other units; therefore they are sometimes referred to as *joint* or *common costs.* While direct costs are traced to the cost object, indirect costs are allocated to the cost object (Baker & Baker, 2000). In the childbirth education example above, indirect costs would include facility costs and administrative costs. Indirect costs are allocated to the department using them but are direct costs for the department that is their source. For example, housekeepers maintain the cleanliness of the room where the childbirth education classes are taught but that is not their only duty. So, housekeeping services are an indirect cost for the childbirth educators but a direct cost for the housekeeping department because that is where its primary responsibility lies.

Each organization determines how costs are defined and to what departments they are charged. The cost in providing the service or producing the product is determined by adding together all cost types. A modest mark-up is added for profit. In the childbirth class example, the direct and indirect costs would be added with a mark-up of 10% as a profit measure. If the classes were a free service and participants were not billed, the cost minus the mark-up charge is applied to the source department (midwifery services). To further complicate the picture, obstetrical patients, who ultimately profit from the classes, may be charged for the service. In some situations, the cost to the hospital of offering the classes might be hidden within the obstetrical package offered by the hospital. For example, the charge for the hospital's obstetrical package is increased by $200, but the increase is not shown in the patient's itemized hospital bill as childbirth education.

Variance Analysis

Once a budget is prepared, approved, and set and monthly reports become available to track income and spending, the process of variance analysis begins. A variance is the difference between standard and actual prices and quantities (Baker & Baker, 2000). Another way of saying this is that a variance is the difference between the amounts budgeted and the actual amounts. An analysis of these differences is known as *variance analysis.* APNs may be called on to justify variances found in the monthly report. This involves explaining the source of the variance and providing as much supporting evidence as possible. At times, only an educated guess is possible. The information that establishes that educated guess should be provided; the financial managers of the organization do not have access to that information otherwise, and an educated guess is better than wild speculation.

It is important to include in the justification the length of time the variance is expected to continue before baseline is reached once more. Again, supporting rationale is helpful. Perhaps the APN has learned from a colleague at a family practice down the street that they are renovating and will be open limited hours for the next 3 months. This would serve to explain a volume variance in this clinic;

Box 12-1

Childbirth Education Class: Direct Costs

Salary of American Society for Psychoprophylaxis in Obstetrics (ASPO)–certified childbirth educator	$25,000
Duplicating handouts related to childbirth	4100
Registration costs (including postage)	276
Other teaching supplies and models (including maintenance)	500
Total direct costs	$29,876

patients are being temporarily rerouted to the closest practice site.

The variance justification or explanation report also includes any corrective steps implemented or planned to correct, eliminate, or minimize the variance. For example, Zack is an adult nurse practitioner (ANP) who has budget responsibility for the nurse-practitioner (NP)–run clinic where he has worked for 5 years. For the last 2 months, there has been a $78 to $80 variance in telephone services. Zack begins to closely monitor the telephone bills and determines that numerous long-distance calls are being placed after clinic hours. A call to the telephone company pinpoints calls being made to the same three out-of-state numbers. Over time, Zack and his coworkers find that the housekeeper, who works from 7:15 PM until 10:00 PM, is making long-distance calls to his family that are being charged to the clinic. The employee is confronted with this inappropriate behavior and referred to management. The telephone variance, now explained, ends abruptly thereafter.

Costing-Out Nursing Services

Clearly, the cost of an item or service is the amount of money one must pay for it. What is not so apparent is what is included in determining cost. A telling exercise for APNs is taking a particular procedure or service and analyzing every aspect of the cost for that procedure. Too often, one forgets the personnel, equipment, and overhead costs necessary to support a particular procedure or service.

According to Swansburg and Swansburg (1999), the volume of service has the greatest effect on cost. The simple law of supply and demand suggests that the more people who receive a service, the less the cost; conversely, the fewer people who request or obtain a service, the higher the cost. This is related to the economic principle of economies in scale. There are savings in volume.

In health care, many factors other than patient volume affect costs. Length of stay also affects cost, as do seasonal factors. Certain illnesses predominate in one season over another. Both inpatient and outpatient settings know to prepare for an onslaught of respiratory illness at certain times of the year, just as perioperative services know to project for additional elective surgery during school holidays and summer vacations. The patient case mix also influences cost; the cost is higher if the high-volume patients have high-cost, intensive conditions instead of less-intense, low-cost conditions. The ability of the organization to manage high morbidities and mortalities within the patient mix also affects costs.

Regulatory requirements influence costs, whether those are requirements of an internal board or external requirements imposed by agencies of the local, state, and federal government. One need only consider the cost of monitoring an organization's adherence to Occupational Safety and Health Administration (OSHA) or Clinical Laboratory Improvement Amendments (CLIA) recommendations or the costs of secretarial staff to monitor licensure and other credentialing of nursing and medical staff members.

As is true in business enterprises, competition can be an important cost variable in health care. A service for $20.95 at Clinic X may appear more compelling than a similar service, costing $25.95, at a competing clinic 4 miles away. However, this initial advantage may be offset by the convenience of a clinic that is open in the evening, has better parking, or is closer to city transportation lines.

Efficiency of processes and procedures in an organization has the potential to affect costs significantly. Commitment on the part of administration and staff at all levels to cost-containment and elimination of waste can be a huge impetus for cost savings. Systems that reward cost savings can be a plus if the systems clearly delineate cost-containment within quality care as an expectation—not cost-containment at the expense of quality care.

With managed care options in effect, payer demands affect costs today to an extent unprecedented in health care history. Details about managed care and third-party payers were provided in Chapter 11.

The most commonly used methods for determining the cost of hospital nursing services are per diem, or the cost per day of service; costs per diagnosis; costs per relative intensity measures (RIMs); and costs per nursing workload measures specified in patient classification systems (Marriner-Tomey, 1996). In primary care settings, cost accounting is different; some settings use fee schedules. Others use a resource-based relative value scale (RBRVS) (based on relative value units [RVUs]) that allows procedures and costs to be indexed and linked to resources consumed (Shackelford, 1999).

Costing-out nursing services has remarkable benefits, enumerated by Mariner-Tomey (1996) (Box 12-2). Flarey (1990) would add that costing-out of nursing services is beneficial by virtue of establishing a reputation for innovation and responsive leadership.

Costing-out health care services is clearly a complex and, at times, seemingly convoluted process. It is relatively easy to understand how clinicians of the past, by virtue of their educational focus, have been poorly prepared for handling the staggering responsibilities of costing services and programs.

IMPLICATIONS FOR MSN EDUCATION AND ADVANCED PRACTICE

For the first time in nursing's history, professionals must be able to not only understand and manage spiraling costs but also to clearly articulate their financial value to the health care enterprise. No longer can the cost of nursing service be subsumed within the bed-and-board aspect of a

Box **12-2**

Benefits of Costing-Out Nursing Services

- Enables customers to pay for care provided to them.
- Enables an appreciation by customers that direct care has a price and an associated value.
- Allows health care agencies to be compensated for direct care.
- Allows nursing to be envisioned as a revenue-generating and revenue-worthy endeavor, rather than a cost center.
- Enhances the professionalism of nursing associated with the traditional fee-for-service reimbursement process.
- Stimulates productivity in balancing resource use, quality, and cost-containment measures.
- Facilitates cost-accounting systems that improve resource control.

Data from Marriner-Tomey, A. (1996). *Nursing management and leadership.* St. Louis: Mosby.

Box **12-3**

Strategies for Cost-Conscious Nursing Practice

- Understanding what is required to remain financially sound.
- Knowing costs and reimbursement practices.
- Capturing all possible charges in a timely fashion.
- Using time efficiently.
- Discussing the costs of care with patients.
- Meeting patient, rather than provider, needs.
- Evaluating the cost-effectiveness of new technologies.
- Predicting and using nursing resources efficiently.
- Using research to evaluate standard nursing practices.

hospital bill. APNs must have a clear, distinct voice and an informed message about their value to providing a quality alternative at a contained cost. They cannot afford to let others negotiate their place in practice and determine their worth. APNs are well served by a business-wise manner and by having a sense of business discipline. They need to know how to use financial reports and other data sources to quantify their productivity and contribution to the workforce in primary care and other settings. Realistic portrayals of the business of practice are imperative; APNs must understand that, in most settings, the expenditure for overhead is 50%, and that many collaborating physicians require a consulting fee in the novice year of an APN's practice.

An understanding of the financial aspects of health care must be a priority in the education of APNs. Regardless of major, Master's preparation in nursing should include content about the budgeting process and costing-out nursing services and how these are clearly related to the work of advanced practice. Only when costs are known can a cost-benefit analysis answer the question of how beneficial is nursing to the nation's health care. Yoder-Wise (1999) captures the elements of a cost-conscious nursing practice (Box 12-3).

APNs need to understand the financial aspects of health care in order to advocate for reasonable and appropriate patient charges. A position of advocacy demands attention to such moral deliberations as:

- If health care is a business, how much of the cost is a fair representation of the price of doing business?
- Would government control render health care less expensive?

- What evidence exists to lend support for or against governmental control?
- Are the costs currently used to determine the price for services legitimate?

APNs also need to make sure their own "house" is in order in terms of finances. Those graduates who have had to take out loans to finish their MSN program may find that they are quite stressed both emotionally and financially when they graduate. In order to remain financially solvent, it is imperative that APNs apply the same budgetary concepts to their own personal budget. Areas such as retirement, malpractice insurance, vacations, and continuing education activities should be prioritized. Poor fiscal management at home can spill over into all parts of an APN's practice; being fiscally prudent in personal spending reflects a responsible leader who can share his or her wisdom in practice.

PRIORITIES FOR RESEARCH

Studies directed toward methods and programs that lower health care costs are one priority for nursing research. For example, what measures of quality management and redesign have been associated with containing health care costs? What effect on cost is associated with education of the nursing workforce? What are the cost effects of health prevention programs? What evidence exists that regulation versus deregulation of health care by managed care organizations (MCOs) affects costs positively? What are best practice models in other disciplines that can be applied to nursing? What are the best practices in nursing that can be transported from one population to another or one setting to another without sacrificing quality?

It would be interesting to explore the role of each of the APN groups in budget preparation. For example, in what way is the NP involved in budgeting for the practice site?

Does that differ by length of service or specialty area? What role, if any, does the certified registered nurse anesthetist (CRNA), certified nurse midwife (CNM), or clinical nurse specialist (CNS) have in budgeting? If APNs are involved in budgeting, what is the experience like for them? What do they see as advantages of their involvement? Disadvantages? How were they prepared for enacting this budgeting role?

Other research might be devoted to determining what skill mix of care providers is associated with outcomes of quality and cost. What evidence exists that a collective of physicians and NPs (or midwives or anesthetists) is a more advantageous mix than one of all physicians or all APNs? Does the skill mix of the collective influence job satisfaction? Patient satisfaction?

Qualitative studies are needed to determine how APNs have thrived in these turbulent times in health care. How have they been fiscally responsible and responsive?

DISCUSSION QUESTIONS

These questions can be used to promote critical thinking and encourage discussion.

1. Obtain copies of operating statements from various health care organizations. Remove identifying information to protect the interests of the organization or, if no copies are available, use the samples provided in Figure 12-2. In small groups (with each group examining a different operating statement), determine costs, budget priorities, and variances for the month. Speculate on possible justification for variances seen.
2. Within a local health care institution, locate the individual charged with the responsibility for preparing the budget. Invite that individual to speak with the class about the budget preparation process from a financial view.
3. Invite a nursing manager or APN who has a budgeting role to share with the class the "lived experience" of budgeting.

4. In small groups, identify a program or service you would like to see added to a clinic or unit's repertoire. Brainstorm as a group about the costs associated with such an enterprise—fixed and variable costs and direct versus indirect costs.
5. Discuss how an appropriate balance might be found between cost-effective care and quality care.
6. Examine the role of the nurse manager or chief nursing officer in advocacy related to health care costs.
7. Redbud Community Health Center is a federally funded agency with a federal grant accounting for 25% of its current budget. There is a full-time receptionist who answers the telephone 40 hours a week whether or not the clinic is open for patient care; a nurse who works 24 hours a week and is consistently off on Tuesdays; and two part-time family nurse practitioners (FNPs). The NPs are paid $30 an hour. During the first year of operation, the clinic was open as follows: Monday to Friday 1 PM to 5 PM and Thursday 9 AM to noon and 1 PM to 5 PM. After the first 3 months, it was noted that the maximum number of patients seen during the morning hours was three. In response to that data, the clinic was closed in the mornings on Thursday, and hours of operation were reposted as Monday to Friday 1 PM to 5 PM. The receptionist remains on site for the full day, Monday through Friday. Answer the following questions, using the monthly budget reports (see Figure 12-2) for Redbud Community Health Center and Box 12-4 as support:

- What would be involved in adding morning hours on Monday and Wednesday?
- How might you justify the need for a pulse oximeter for Redbud Community Health Center? (Assume the cost of the item as $2400.)
- In this nonprofit agency, how might the staff be awarded a bonus?
- In today's mail, the staff at Redbud Community Health Center received notice that they are about to lose part of their grant funding. Looking at the budget for the center, how would you make the 10% cut demanded by the loss of grant money?

Redbud Community Health Center
MONTHLY FINANCIAL STATEMENTS
FOR 2 MONTHS ENDING MARCH 31, 1999

% of Grant Year   16.67%
Expired

WORK DAYS IN MONTH	20	23	43		

	FEB	MAR	YTD TOTAL	YTD BUDGET	VARIANCE
ENCOUNTERS	257	254	511	332	179
ENCOUNTERS PER DAY	12.85	11.04	11.88	7.71	4.17
RELATIVE VALUE UNITS (RVU'S)	318.08	309.86	627.94	366.83	261.11
RVU'S PER ENCOUNTER	1.24	1.22	1.23	1.11	0.12
REVENUES					
GRANTS AND CONTRACTS	4,570	4,631	9,201	9,261	(60)
MEDICAID	11,462	12,437	23,899	19,939	3,960
MEDICARE	308	246	554	470	84
INSURANCE	1,000	720	1,720	478	1,242
SELF PAY	1,310	1,382	2,692	1,185	1,507
				0	0
TOTAL REVENUE	18,650	19,416	38,066	31,333	6,734
REVENUE PER ENCOUNTER	72.57	76.44	74.49	94.47	(19.98)
EXPENSES					
SALARIES	6,855	8,311	15,166	11,739	3,427
BENEFITS					0
BENEFIT DOLLARS	518	351	869	850	19
F.I.C.A.	521	568	1,089	845	245
TRAVEL			0	33	(33)
SUPPLIES					
MEDICAL	567	2,781	3,348	1,250	2,098
OFFICE	78	34	112	333	(221)
PRINTING	21	63	84	233	(149)
CONTRACTUAL			0	0	0
RENTS/MORTGAGE INTEREST		12	12	800	(788)
EQUIPMENT LEASES		26	26	0	26
UTILITIES	432	217	649	667	(18)
WASTE REMOVAL	42	108	150	133	17
PHONE	496	468	964	1,233	(269)
CONTINUING EDUCATION			0	100	(100)
POSTAGE			0	42	(42)
MAINTENANCE AGREEMENTS		70	70	333	(263)
LIABILITY INSURANCE	31	31	62	83	(21)
LAB AND X-RAY	250	546	796	500	296
PHARMACY			0	67	(67)
REPAIRS AND MAINT.		21	21	417	(396)
DEPRECIATION	136	136	272	500	(228)
PROVIDER TAX			0	25	(25)
FEES AND DUES		200	200	17	183
MARKETING			0	0	0
MISC.			0	83	(83)
TOTAL OPERATING EXPENSES	9,947	13,943	23,890	20,284	3,607
ADMINISTRATIVE OVERHEAD	3,818	3,818	7,636	7,636	0
TOTAL EXPENSES	13,765	17,761	31,526	27,919	3,607
NET INCOME (LOSS)	4,885	1,655	6,540	3,413	3,127
COST PER ENCOUNTER	53.56	69.93	61.69	84.18	(22.48)
DIFFERENCE REVENUE VS. COST	19.01	6.52	12.80	10.29	2.51
COST PER RVU	43.28	57.32	50.21	76.11	(25.90)

A

Figure 12-2 Sample budgets for Redbud Community Health Center. **A,** For 2 months.

Continued

Redbud Community Health Center
MONTHLY FINANCIAL STATEMENTS
FOR 8 MONTHS ENDING SEPTEMBER 30, 1998

% of Grant Year Expired   16.67%

WORK DAYS IN MONTH	FEB	MAR	APRIL	MAY	JUNE	JULY	AUG	SEPT	YTD TOTAL	YTD BUDGET	VARIANCE
	20	22	22	20	22	22	21	21	170	170	
EXPENSES											
SALARIES	4,738	5,816	6,787	5,572	6,161	5,997	5,407	5,867	46,345	49,807	(3,462)
BENEFITS											0
BENEFIT DOLLARS	269	382	518	500	515	509	500	500	3,693	6,000	(2,307)
F.I.C.A.	358	429	496	437	483	467	425	461	3,556	3,717	(162)
TRAVEL		37	18	1	14	11	9	24	114	133	(19)
SUPPLIES											
MEDICAL	428	252	770	887	609	252	263	156	3,617	5,213	(1,596)
OFFICE	18	153	197	0	19	78	108	319	892	533	359
PRINTING	0	47	214	32	0	206	371	80	950	267	683
CONTRACTUAL									0	0	0
RENTS/MORTGAGE INTEREST									0	0	0
EQUIPMENT LEASES							13		13	0	13
UTILITIES	256	210	380	116	101	175	124	253	1,615	3,667	(2,052)
WASTE REMOVAL	0	93	80	42	42	87	46	46	436	533	(97)
PHONE	176	520	525	568	524	599	653	547	4,112	2,133	1,979
CONTINUING EDUCATION	0								0	400	(400)
POSTAGE	0	10	0	5			9		24	333	(310)
MAINTENANCE AGREEMENTS	90	135	250	13	160	203	260	128	1,239	667	573
LIABILITY INSURANCE	30	30	31	31	31	31	31	31	246	267	(21)
LAB AND X-RAY	94	74	325	244	424	78	204	298	1,741	800	941
PHARMACY	0					21			21	267	(246)
REPAIRS AND MAINT.	(34)		805	35	70	1,190	57		2,123	2,333	(210)
DEPRECIATION	250	250	250	250	250	250	250	250	2,000	2,000	0
PROVIDER TAX	92	118		139	136	141	70	55	751	200	551
FEES AND DUES	0			0					0	67	(67)
MARKETING	0								0	0	0
MISC.			34				18	28	80	333	(253)
TOTAL OPERATING EXPENSES	6,765	8,556	11,680	8,872	9,539	10,295	8,817	9,043	73,567	79,671	(6,103)
ADMINISTRATIVE OVERHEAD	2,516	2,516	2,552	2,552	2,552	2,552	2,552	2,552	20,344	20,417	(73)
TOTAL EXPENSES	9,281	11,072	14,232	11,424	12,091	12,847	11,369	11,595	93,912	100,087	(6,176)
NET INCOME (LOSS)	5,438	4,968	1,776	2,990	155	2,218	2,837	2,947	23,328	(1,017)	24,345
COST PER ENCOUNTER	**46.17**	**50.79**	**64.40**	**61.42**	**76.53**	**62.06**	**58.60**	**59.77**	**59.48**	**75.44**	**(15.97)**
DIFFERENCE REVENUE VS. COST	**27.05**	**22.79**	**8.04**	**16.08**	**0.98**	**10.71**	**14.62**	**15.19**	**14.77**	**(0.77)**	**15.54**
COST PER RVU	**42.84**	**45.50**	**55.43**	**51.84**	**63.83**	**51.26**	**43.82**	**51.24**	**50.41**	**68.21**	**(17.80)**

B

Figure 12-2, cont'd Sample budgets for Redbud Community Health Center. **B,** For 8 months.

Box 12-4

Relative Value Units at Redbud Community Health Center

RVUs are a measurement providing weighting of revenue encounters.

For Team A:
Target RVU: 5650
Actual RVU: 5800
RVU over target: 98
Cost/RUV: $45.50
Merit allocation: $1.15

Suggestions for Further Learning

- Locate a web-based personal budget planner. Compare and contrast this process of budget planning with that necessary to budgeting in a health care organization.
- Consult Baker, J. J., & Baker, R.W. (2000). *Health care finance: Basic tools for nonfinancial managers.* Gaithersburg, MD: Aspen Publishers. This is an exceptional text for providing practical information, including case studies and many examples, for those without a financial background.
- Consult Evans, C. (2000). *Financial feasibility studies for healthcare: A practical guide for a changing industry.* New York: McGraw-Hill. This resource includes many aspects of finance as it affects nursing. It also contains employment agreements, operation assessment, a case study, and a disk providing for spreadsheet analysis.
- Spend several hours during a clinical rotation with the individual in the practice site that deals most closely with costing services and assigning charges. Determine how diagnoses (International Classification of Diseases [ICD-9] codes) and procedures affect patient cost.
- Saks (1999) suggests a partnership between a triad of clinicians, finance experts, and information managers. Consult the School of Business about the possibility of a partnership of that sort in discussing financial aspects of health care.

REFERENCES/BIBLIOGRAPHY

Altimer, L.B., & Sanders, J.M. (2000). Financial management—can you make a merger pay off? *Nursing Management, 31*(4), 8.

Angell, M. (1993). The doctor as double agent. *Kennedy Institute for Ethics Journal, 3*(3), 279-286.

Aymond, R. (1999, July-August). Monitoring your practice's financial data: 10 vital signs. *Family Practice Management.* Available online at www.aafp.org/fpm/990700fm/42html.

Baker, J.J., & Baker, R.W. (2000). *Health care finance: basic tools for nonfinancial managers.* Gaithersburg, MD: Aspen Publishers.

Belgeri, M. (1999). The financial report: how it can aid case managers. *Nursing Case Management, 4*(2), 67-70.

Borglum, K. (1997, October). Practical tips to boost your efficiency and cut practice costs. *Family Practice Management,* 86-98.

Brown, B. (1999). Financial management—how to develop a unit personnel budget. *Nursing Management, 30*(6), 34-35.

Bruttomesso, K.A. (1995). Variable hospital accounting practice: are they fair to the nursing department? Selected authors from 1985 update their articles. *Journal of Nursing Administration, 25*(1), 6.

Burner, S., & Waldo, D. (1995). National health expenditure projections: 1994-2005. *Health Care Financing Review, 16*(4), 221-242.

Calmelat, A. (1993). Tips for starting your own nurse practitioner practice. *The Nurse Practitioner, 18*(4), 58, 61,64.

Carruth, A.K., Carruth, P.J., & Noto, E.C. (2000). Financial management: nurse managers flex their budgetary might. *Nursing Management, 31*(2), 16-17.

Corley, M.C., & Satterwhite, B.E. (1993). Forecasting ambulatory clinic workload to facilitate budgeting. *Nursing Economics, 11*(2), 77-81.

Curtin, L. (1996). The bottom line be damned. *Nursing Management, 27*(9), 7-8.

Dreisbach, A.M. (1994). A structured approach to expert financial management: a financial plan for nurse managers. *Nursing Economics, 12*(3), 131-139.

Emmanuel, E.J., & Dubbler, N.N. (1995). Preserving the physician-patient relationship in the era of managed care. *Journal of the American Medical Association, 273*(4), 323-329.

Evans, C. (2000). *Financial feasibility studies for healthcare: a practical guide for a changing industry.* New York: McGraw-Hill.

Finkler, S.A. (1992). *Budgeting concepts for nurse managers* (2nd ed.). Philadelphia: WB Saunders.

Flannary, T.P., & Grace, J.L. (1999). Managing nursing assets: a primer on maximizing investment in people. *Nursing Administration Quarterly, 23*(4), 35-46.

Flarey, D.L. (1990). A methodology for costing nursing service. *Nursing Administration Quarterly, 14,* 41-51.

Foley-Pierce, S., & Luikart, C. (1996). Managed care—will the healthcare needs of rural citizens be met? *Journal of Nursing Administration, 26*(4), 28-32.

Gardner, K., Allhusen, J., Kamm, J., & Tobin, J. (1997). Determining the cost of care through clinical pathways. *Nursing Economics, 15*(4), 213-217.

Gordon, S., & McCall, T. (1996). Helping your patients manage managed care. *Revolution—Journal of Nurse Empowerment, 6*(1), 20-22, 90-92.

Grimaldi, P.L. (1997). Medicare marketing guidelines for managed care. *Nursing Management, 28*(4), 22-23, 25.

Grimaldi, P.L. (1998a). Financial management—managed care glossary: update II. *Nursing Management, 29*(10), 8-11.

Grimaldi, P.L. (1998b). Financial management—two steps to enhance managed care quality. *Nursing Management, 29*(8), 14, 16-17.

Grimaldi, P.L. (1999). Financial management—new managed care glossary. *Nursing Management, 30*(11), 16-17.

Hadley, E.H. (1996). Nursing in the political and economic marketplace: challenges for the 21st century. *Nursing Outlook, 44,* 6-10.

Holman, E.J., & Branstetter, E. (1997). An academic nursing clinic's financial survival. *Nursing Economics, 15*(5), 248-252.

Jones, K.R. (1997). Finance for nurse managers—an introduction to financial statements. *Seminars for Nurse Managers, 5*(4), 162-163.

Jones, K.R. (1998). Finance for nurse managers—operating indicators. *Seminars for Nursing Managers, 6*(3), 104-105.

Jones, K.R. (1999). Finance for nurse managers—The capital budgeting process. Seminars for Nurse Managers, 7(2), 55-56.

Jones, K.R. (2000). Finance for nurse managers—equity financing of capital acquisitions. *Seminars for Nurse Managers, 8*(1), 5-6.

Jost, S.G. (2000). An assessment and intervention strategy for managing staff needs during change. *Journal of Nursing Administration, 30*(1), 34-40.

Kasan, N., & Shkrab, S. (1999). Financial management—how to mobilize an organization with commitment, not cash. *Nursing Management, 30*(12), 16-17, 27.

Keeling. B. (2000). Financial management—how to establish a position and hours budget. *Nursing Management, 31*(3), 26

Kowai, N.S., & Delaney, M. (1996). The economics of a nurse-developed critical pathway. *Nursing Economics, 14*(3), 156-161.

Liebler, J.G., & McConnell, C.R. (1999). *Management principles for health professionals*. Gaithersburg, MD: Aspen Publishers.

Marquis, B.L., & Huston, C.J. (2000). *Leadership roles and management functions in nursing: theory and application* (3rd ed.). Philadelphia: JB Lippincott.

Marriner-Tomey, A. (1996). *Nursing management and leadership* (5th ed.). St. Louis: Mosby.

Parrish, M. (2000, January 24). The California nightmare: is this where managed care is taking us? *Medical Economics.* Available online at www.pdr.net/memag/public.htm?path= dvcs/012400/article5.html.

Pelfrey, S. (1997). Managing financial data. *Seminars for Nurse Managers, 5*(1), 25-30.

Poteet, G.W., Hodges, L.C., & Goodard, N. (1991). Financial responsibilities and preparation of chief nurse executives. *Nursing Economics, 9*(5), 305-309.

Reed, F.M., O'Hara, S., & Schaad, P. (2000). How an employed group redesigned itself to achieve financial viability. *Family Practice Management, 7*(4), 21-25, 65-66.

Rowland, H.S., & Rowland, B.L. (1997). *Nursing administration handbook* (4th ed.). Gaithersburg, MD: Aspen Publishers.

Saks, N.P. (1999). Developing an integrated model for outcomes management. *Advanced Practice Nursing Quarterly, 4*(1), 27-32.

Schmidt, D.Y. (1999). Financial and operational skills for nurse managers. *Nursing Administration Quarterly, 23*(4), 16-28.

Shackelford, J.L. (1999). Group practice management measuring productivity using RBRUS cost accounting. *Healthcare Financial Management, 53*(1), 67-69.

Silva, M.C. (1998, June 10). Financial compensation and ethical issues in health care. *Online Journal of Issues in Nursing.* Available online at www.nursingworld.org/ojin/tpc6_4.htm.

Stuart, M.E., & Weinrich, M. (1998). Beyond managing Medicaid costs: restructuring care. *The Milbank Quarterly, 76*(2), 251-279.

Swansburg, R.C., & Swansburg, R.J. (1999). *Introductory management and leadership for nurses*. Sudbury, MA: Jones & Bartlett.

Wieseke, A., & Bantz, D. (1992). Economic awareness of registered nurses employed in hospitals. *Nursing Economics, 10*(6), 406-412.

Wyad, D.C. (1996). The capitation revolution in health care: implications for the field of nursing. *Nursing Administration Quarterly, 20*(2), 1-12.

Yoder-Wise, P. (1999). *Leading and managing in nursing* (2nd ed.). St. Louis: Mosby.

Zoloth-Dorfman, L., & Rubin, S. (1995). The patient as a commodity: Managed care and the question of ethics. *The Journal of Clinical Ethics, 6,* 339-357.

Zuckerman, H.S., Kaluzny, A.D., & Ricketts, T.C. (1995). Alliances in health care: what we know, what we think we know, and what we should know. *Health Care Management Review, 20,* 54-65.

Chapter 13

Reimbursement for Advanced Practice Nursing

Denise Robinson

Achieving payment for advanced practice nursing (APN) services has been tumultuous over the past 20 years, with progress occurring in small forward steps interspersed with larger steps backward. Traditionally, APNs have been employed by hospitals or physicians in solo or group practices where billing was done by the employer, with reimbursement going to the employer. The APN, in turn, was paid wages by the employer. APNs typically had little or no knowledge of the reimbursement process and their rights within that process. Recently, however, APNs have been acting as primary care providers (PCPs), creating more awareness of their rights and responsibilities in the billing and reimbursement process. With these recent developments, significant changes occurred in the federal laws governing health programs, enabling APNs to be directly reimbursed. This chapter details the status of reimbursement for APNs.

DEFINITIONS

Reimbursement is to pay back someone for services rendered. A similar term is *compensation*, which means to make proper payment. Buppert (1998) defines *reimbursement* as payment for medical services already delivered. Reimbursement is critical to APN practice. If an APN is not reimbursed by their patients' insurers, it is very difficult, if not impossible, to maintain a practice. Many times, a patient with Medicare is seen by an APN in an "incident to" situation. *Incident to* is care provided as a follow-up to the physician's plan of care, and the physician must be an active participant in that care. If "incident to" services are provided by the APN, the physician must be on site and the visit cannot be with a new patient or an old patient with a new problem. *Incident to* means the APN is an employee of the physician, there is direct supervision, and the payment is 100% of the physician's fee. *Provider credentialing* refers to the data that the managed care organization (MCO) obtains to verify that a provider is adequately credentialed (i.e., prepared to care for the organization's

patients). This usually is a fairly long process, sometimes taking from 6 to 9 months to complete.

Collaboration, according to the Health Care Financing Administration (HCFA) guidelines for Medicare reimbursement, must meet the standards for a collaborative process as established by the state in which the APN is practicing. In the absence of state-governing collaborative relationships, collaboration is a process in which APNs have a relationship with one or more physicians to deliver health care services. This collaboration deals with patient care issues outside the usual scope of advanced practice, such as hospitalization of the patient, or patients with more complex illnesses than the APN can handle alone. The collaborative process must be documented. The collaborating physician does not need to be present when the services are provided and does not need to make an independent evaluation of each patient seen by the APN (Federal Register, 1998).

APNs must know how to evaluate and bill for proper reimbursement. In order to bill for services, several codes are required. One code is the *Current Procedural Terminology* **(CPT)**. CPT is nomenclature for the reporting of physician procedures and services under government and private health insurance companies (American Medical Association [AMA], 1998). Each procedure or service is identified with a five-digit code, selected for the procedure or service that most accurately describes the service performed. When necessary, any modifying or extenuating circumstances are added. This is a code developed and copyrighted by the AMA. The billing for the visit is based on the CPT codes identified. Insurance pays based on the CPT code and not necessarily the amount billed. On average, code and time are considered roughly equivalent.

The second code needed is the *International Classification of Diseases (ICD-9)* code (US Department of Health and Human Services [DHHS], 1996). ICD-9 codes are diagnostic codes that classify morbidity and mortality. Diagnostic coding dates back to the seventeenth century in England, and a statistical listing was published in 1948 by the World Health Organization (WHO) to track morbidity and mortality. This listing led the way to the development of the ICD, ninth revision, published in 1977. Clinical modifiers were added, leading to the ICD-9-CM. ICD-10 has been drafted but will not be addressed or adopted until after 2000. ICD-9-CM codes describe the diagnosis, symptom, complaint, condition, or problem. The primary diagnosis is coded first, followed by secondary and other diagnoses. The codes consist of three digits for a limited number of conditions; all others require four or five digits to be as specific as possible. Hill (1999) suggests thinking of the CPT code as describing what one does and the ICD-9 code as describing why one does it. The CPT code is linked with an ICD-9 code to establish the medical necessity of each service or procedure. ICD-9 codes do not include rule-out or suspected conditions. The APN needs to code for what is known to be fact. This also means only coding for a diagnosis that affects the care that the APN gives. If a patient has a fractured arm, the fracture should not be coded if the APN is treating him for diabetes (Box 13-1).

Third-party reimbursement is based on the ***resource-based relative value scale (RBRVS)***. This scale was developed by the HCFA and the AMA in 1988. The RBRVS is determined by provider productivity, malpractice insurance, cost of overhead, staff, equipment, supplies, the geographical costs of various parts of the country, and the payment rate for nonphysician providers. Most third-party payers and physician practices use the RBRVS to establish fees for procedures and services (Rapsilber & Anderson, 2000). In 1994, the term ***relative value unit (RVU)*** was introduced by the HCFA and AMA, along with the *Evaluation and Management Documentation Guidelines*. A RVU refers to a work-relative value unit. Many practices use the RVU as a basis of productivity, awarding bonuses on the number of RVUs obtained in a year.

The HCFA refers to ***fraud*** as "intentional deception or misrepresentation which the individual knows to be false or does not believe to be true, [occurring when] the individual is aware that the deception could result in some unauthorized benefit to him/herself or some other person" (18 U.S.C. §1341, 1343, and 1347). ***Abuse*** is "payment for items or services when there is no legal entitlement to that payment, and [when] the physician has not knowingly and intentionally misrepresented facts to obtain payment (HCFA, 1999). Buppert (2000) defines *false claims* as "those claims that the provider knows or should know will lead to greater payments than appropriate." Many third-party payers are concerned about payments for services not given, but Medicare administrators in particular are on a mission to decrease the costs associated with the program and are investigating more providers and offices with questionable billing practices. In the past, erroneous payments made by Medicare ranged from 7.1% to 11% (Buppert, 2000) costing the U.S. government and taxpayers $12.6 million. Agencies charged with enforcing the law of Medicare are the HCFA, Office of the Inspector General (OIG), Department of Justice, and Medicare carriers. (Table 13-1 describes the role of each agency in Medicare enforcement.)

CRITICAL ISSUES: REIMBURSEMENT FOR ADVANCED PRACTICE NURSES

The earliest record of trying to change reimbursement for nurses is from 1948 (Jennings, 1977). The Social Security Amendments of 1972 (PL 92-603) authorized reimbursement for projects that focused on services for independent providers. This was the beginning of the Physician Extender Reimbursement Study (Morris & Smith, 1976). Most of the proposed amendments for direct reimbursement of APNs (certified psychiatric nurses and certified nurse midwives [CNMs]) by Medicare and Medicaid were introduced by Senator Inouye of Hawaii (Hawkins & Thibodeau, 1993). By 1979, 16 states had authorized payment for nurse midwives under Medicaid and the Civilian Health and Medical Program of Uniformed Services (CHAMPUS) (health care for dependents of the Department of Defense). In 1980, Maryland became the first state to provide for direct reimbursement for nurses and other nonphysician providers through all health insurance (Hawkins & Thibodeau, 1993).

The Rural Health Clinic Services Act of 1977 (PL 95-210) authorized Medicare and Medicaid payment for the services of nurse practitioners (NPs) in qualified rural health clinics. Another important step forward for APN reimbursement took place in 1987. The Federal Employees Health Care Freedom of Choice Act was passed in Congress, mandating third-party reimbursement to nonphysician providers under the Federal Employees Health Benefits Program. Rural clinic reimbursement was en-

---

Box 13-1

Sample of ICD-9 Coding

A female patient comes in with dysuria and increased frequency of urination. A urine dip reveals bacteriuria, and a urine culture is sent. During the visit the patient asks for a refill of her thyroid medication. When checking her chart, the APN notes that a TSH has not been drawn for a while, so that is also drawn. Assuming this patient has Graves disease, the following ICD-9 codes are appropriate: 595.0 for acute cystitis (justifying the urine dip and culture) and 242.00 for hyperthyroidism, linking the TSH to it. The primary reason for the visit is the cystitis (Hill, 1999).

Table 13-1

Role of Agencies in Medicare Enforcement

AGENCY	ROLE
Health Care Financing Administration	Drafts rules governing Medicare; writes rules and regulations that build on statutory law; oversees Medicare carriers.
Office of the Inspector General	Audits and investigates.
Department of Justice	Prosecutes for the government (investigative branch of the Department of Justice is the Federal Bureau of Investigation [FBI]).
Medicare carriers	As private contractors, pay the claims submitted by health care providers (authorized by the HCFA and may refer to the OIG for suspected fraud and abuse cases).

hanced in the Omnibus Budget Reconciliation Act (OBRA) of 1989 for NPs and clinical nurse specialists (CNSs) in rural health clinics, although the payment was made to the employers and not directly to APNs. These regulations stipulated collaboration with a physician for reimbursement. Also in 1989, legislation was passed by Congress to allow Medicare reimbursement for NPs in long-term care (LTC). In 1991, direct reimbursement to APNs was authorized by the Rural Nursing Incentive Act for those NPs and CNSs in rural areas. By 1993, 38 states had passed legislation for some form of reimbursement for APN services (Pearson, 1993); this included reimbursement for Medicaid services as well as from some private insurance carriers.

In the early 1990s, Medicare reimbursement for APNs was limited to those NPs who worked in rural or medically underserved areas, as well as nursing homes. Sections 4511 and 4512 of the Balanced Budget Act of 1997 liberalized Medicare coverage for NPs by removing the restriction of geographical location or practice setting for direct reimbursement for NPs; these changes became effective January 1, 1998. Payment by private insurers is contract specific and varies in each state. While APNs have made many studies of direct reimbursement, many of the same issues remain. It is crucial that APNs recognize where they need to go to remove financial barriers for APN practice. APNs must be included in all reimbursement systems, not just Medicaid and Medicare. They need to work toward direct reimbursement from all third-party payers.

Advanced Practice Nurses as Primary Care Providers

There are a number of issues of importance to APNs relative to reimbursement for services. Perhaps the most critical is the acceptance of APNs as PCPs. In the current climate of managed care, APNs must be recognized as PCPs on insurance panels. If not recognized, they can easily be left out of the running to serve as PCPs, significantly reducing their ability to provide care for patients. It is important for APNs to garner patient support and encourage them to share their voice with insurance companies. APNs must also have working knowledge of state regulations or statues that give APNs the authority to provide care. This knowledge will guide APNs through the legal parameters of practice. It is also crucial that APNs be familiar with Medicaid and Medicare regulations that apply to APN reimbursement. The argument that "I did not know I couldn't bill for that service" is not a defense. When APNs apply for Medicare or Medicaid numbers and sign the application, their signature denotes agreement and adherence to the regulations pertaining to Medicaid and Medicare.

APNs must remember that each payer has its own set of rules for reimbursement. Reimbursement is a high-stakes issue; without steady income, the practice can not survive. Direct reimbursement to APNs is the desired goal; this gives visibility and recognition to APNs as PCPs. APNs need to be recognized by managed care panels as PCPs in order to care for patients. Without this credentialing, APNs will be invisible; patients will not see APNs in the books that list providers.

For example, Rachel provides care in a small office. She decides to take another position in a nearby larger office. The problem is that, in the past, Rachel was not credentialed as a PCP with MegaMCO. She practiced under her collaborating physician's name. Now that she has changed offices, none of her patients can find her. Even if a patient calls MegaMCO, her new office will not be identified because she is "invisible" as a PCP.

In addition, APNs must have an understanding of who the competitors are, how many of them exist, what services are offered, how much they charge, and how much they are paid as a means of comparison. This means that an APN must know how much income he or she is bringing into the practice, as well as his or her overhead costs, as a means of comparison. Unfortunately, in many circumstances, APNs do not know the full details of the practice income and their contribution, because either they do not ask or others are not willing to share that type of information. That leaves APNs without the ability to discuss their competitive niche in the marketplace. APNs need to realize that they may present more of an economic threat to physicians in the future, given the projected increase in nonphysician providers. This may interfere with further advances for increased reimbursement. (Figure 13-1 shows the multiple factors that influence APN reimbursement.)

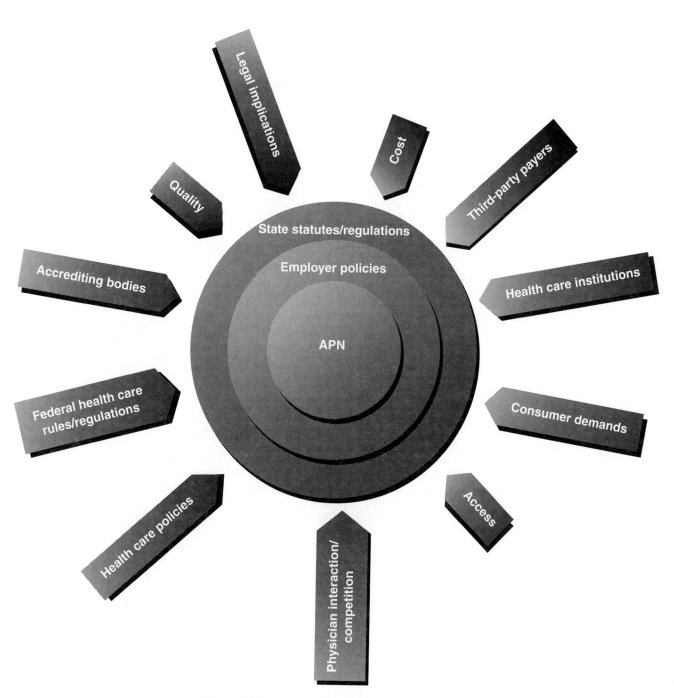

Figure 13-1 Factors that influence APN reimbursement.

Every encounter between a health care provider and patient has a third-party payer (except for those encounters involving patients who pay their own medical bills). Four categories of third-party payers are presented in Table 13-2. Table 13-3 summarizes the current status of reimbursement for APNs by the major third-party payers.

Billing and Reimbursement by Advanced Practice Nurses

Billing for reimbursement from any third-party payers includes documentation of the patient's visit, filing the proper forms, and using the correct diagnostic and procedural codes. The rules and regulations for billing are not simple. APNs must know and follow the rules and use

Table 13-2

Third-Party Payers

PAYER	DEFINITION AND COVERAGE	CRITERIA FOR REIMBURSEMENT
Medicare	Nation's largest health insurance program, Medicare covers 37 million Americans who meet the following criteria: • People 65 years old or older • People who are disabled • People with permanent kidney failure *Benefits:* Hospital insurance (Part A) provides coverage of inpatient hospital services, skilled nursing facilities, home health services, and hospice care. Medical insurance (Part B) (also called supplementary medical insurance) helps pay for the cost of provider services, outpatient hospital services, medical equipment and supplies, and other health services and supplies. Not everyone is covered by Part B because this part requires the payment of a monthly premium.	Two types of arrangements for payment: • MCO; APNs must apply for admission to the provider panel. • Direct billing for patients not enrolled in a MCO; APNs apply as providers. The final rules and revisions to Medicare's physician fee schedule include the following requirements: • Must have an MSN degree (those with current provider numbers are grandfathered in until December 31, 2000). • Must be authorized by the state to practice as an APN and be certified as of January 1, 2001; those applying after January 1, 2003, must have a MSN degree. • Must be a registered professional nurse authorized by the state to practice as a NP in accordance with state laws. • Must be certified by a recognized national certification body. (*Federal Register* [1999, May 12]. 64(91), 25456-25460)
Medicaid	A federal program administered by the states, Medicaid covers people who meet the following criteria: • Mothers and children who qualify on the basis of poverty • Adults who are disabled on a short-term basis (< 1 year) and who qualify on the basis of poverty	Vendor payment program: payment is made directly to providers of service for care given to eligible individuals. • Providers must accept the Medicaid reimbursement level as full payment. • Many states have applied for Medicaid waivers, which allow states to enroll all Medicaid patients in MCOs. • APNs must apply for admission to the group's MCO panels in order to maintain reimbursement.
Managed care organization	This is an insurer that provides health care services and payment for services, usually with some cost-containment provisions. (See Chapter 6 for a detailed discussion of MCOs.). *MCO* is an umbrella term that may include HMOs, provider-sponsored organizations, and physician-hospital organizations.	MCOs can decide if they wish to acknowledge APNs as PCPs. Not all MCOs currently recognize APNs. Some require a cosignature and bill only under the physician's number; others provide no reimbursement for patients seen by APNs.
Indemnity insurance company	This is an insurer that pays for the medical care of its insured but does not deliver health care (Buppert, 1998).	Pay health care providers on a per visit/per procedure basis, usually through a "usual and customary" fee schedule.

the systems to help detect errors. Even though other people actually do the coding, the provider is the one legally responsible for the codes selected and submitted to payers.

Completion of proper forms, using the correct terminology, is critical to get the highest level of reimbursement for which the visit qualifies. The standard billing form is HCFA 1500. The following are required components needed to qualify for reimbursement for a patient visit:

- Face to face contact (in the office, inpatient setting, or patient's home)
- ICD-9 codes
- CPT codes
- Distinction between new and established patients
- Date of service

Table 13-3				
Summary of Reimbursement for Advanced Practice Nurses				
TYPE OF PAYER	**NP**	**CNM**	**CNS**	**CRNA**
Medicare Part B: Paid MCO or fee-for-service. Self-employed NPs receive either 80% of the lesser of either actual charges or 85% of the physician's charge. When a NP is employed by a physician, the NP may receive 100% when subject to "incident to" rules or 85% when the physician is not present. In states with restrictive collaborative requirements, there is no direct reimbursement.	Yes*	Yes (65%)*	Yes*	Yes*
Medicaid: APNs apply as a provider in a state; if through a MCO, they must apply and be admitted to the provider panel of the MCO. Payment is 70% to 100% of the rates set for physicians, with fees controlled by state law.	Pediatric, family, and other specialties (dependent on state)	Yes	Yes	Yes
CHAMPUS	Yes	Yes	Limited to psychiatric CNS	Yes
FEHB (Federal Employee Health Benefit Program)	Yes	Yes	Yes	Yes
Rural health clinics: Per the Rural Health Clinic Services Act of 1977.	Yes	Yes		
Managed care organizations: APNs must apply and be admitted to a MCO provider panel as a PCP. Each MCO negotiates a payment arrangement with each group, practice, or provider on its panel.	?	?	?	?
Indemnity insurers: Payment made on a per visit/per procedure basis. A billing form is submitted to the insurance company. "Usual and customary" fee schedules are used for reimbursement.	?	?	?	?
Self-paying patients: Assumes money is collected at the time of service.	Yes	Yes	Yes	Yes

*Those employed in rural health clinics or federally qualified health centers are ineligible for direct reimbursement.

- Patient-identifying information
- Provider-identifying information

The extent of the history and physical, as well as the medical decision-making, are key components in making a code selection in the evaluation and management services. (Table 13-4 provides a summary of evaluation and management services guidelines.) Also important are counseling, coordination of care, and the nature of the presenting problem. These are considered contributing factors in most encounters and are not required to be present for every patient encounter.

The evaluation and management services codes (CPT 99201-99456) are the most frequently used procedure codes for primary care (Buppert, 1998). The *Evaluation and Management Documentation Guidelines* were developed by the HCFA in 1997 (available online at www.hcfa.gov); these are the criteria by which Medicare audits are conducted. Medical record documentation must support the level of care billed. The most commonly used code for an established patient is 99213. This includes an expanded problem-focused history and physical and a low complexity of medical decision-making. This correlates roughly with a 15-minute patient visit.

The use of a well-designed encounter form (also called a *superbill*) (Figure 13-2) makes it easier to report and bill for services. The form should include the most common ICD-9 and CPT codes. Using a form with the codes already listed increases accuracy in billing. Every claim must include both an ICD-9 and CPT code. Each service or procedure performed must be represented by a diagnosis that would substantiate those services (i.e., thyroid-stimulating hormone [TSH] for the diagnosis of fatigue or hypothyroidism).

Avoiding Insurance Fraud

The best way an APN can avoid an insurance investigation by Medicare or Medicaid is to develop a system by which documentation and billing can be self-audited. This system is called a *compliance program*. Buppert (2000) recommends eight elements that should be included in a compliance program:

- Learning and staying current with the requirements of payers.
- Following the rules in choosing diagnosis and billing codes.
- Following the rules to choose and document visits and procedures.
- Using tools that help decrease the time needed for complete documentation (especially when time is at a premium).
- Conducting periodic audits. (Capko [1998] recommends doing them quarterly, with at least 20 patients per provider.)

- Showing a commitment to detect and correct billing errors.
- Correcting errors when they occur.
- Conducting legal reviews of contracts and operating procedures.

While this compliance program is specific for Medicare, it is very likely to satisfy other third-party payers if it meets Medicare standards.

For example, an audit of a 99214 visit (a level-four visit) should include a minimum of four elements in the history, as well as the status of at least three chronic or inactive conditions; a review of at least two systems, with positives and negatives identified; one item from the past medical, family, or social history (PFSH); and twelve elements within the physical exam. The APN should document at least one of the following: one or more chronic illnesses with mild exacerbation, two or more stable chronic illnesses, an acute illness with systemic symptoms, or an acute complicated injury. Treatment would need to document at least one written prescription drug. Use of a checklist form that identifies these required elements would be helpful to review documentation for a level-four patient.

Dorothy is an example of a 99214 visit. She has uncontrolled hypertension, obesity, and hypercholesterolemia, and she is complaining of swelling of her right leg, with pain. She has a 6-month history of cellulitis in this leg. She states that her shoes are tight (tighter on her right foot). She denies chest pain, shortness of breath (SOB), dyspnea on exertion, and difficulty lying flat. She keeps forgetting to take her medications. Her history, as taken by the APN, is listed in Box 13-2. This visit qualifies for a 99214 visit based on the criteria. More time was spent reviewing medications and ways to remember to take them, but this amount of time was needed to meet the criteria for this level.

Most providers tend to underbill for their services. (According to the Medical Group Management Association (MGMA), approximately 50% to 60% of providers undercode [Jaklevic, 1999].) In some cases, providers are not billing at all for certain billable services. Over a year's time, this can be a significant cost to the practice. Buppert (2000) identifies some specific suggestions that work for enhancing accurate billing and correcting errors (Box 13-3).

The most common level of visit is level three (99213). This visit should include two out of three of the following elements to be accurately considered a level-three visit: expanded problem-focused history, an expanded problem-focused examination, and/or medical decision-making of low complexity. Table 13-5 shows a summary of requirements for the five levels of visit for both new and established patients; Table 13-6 describes the level of risk pertaining to medical decision-making, with examples of presenting problems, diagnostic procedures, and treatment regimens. The highest level of any one of the three aspects determines the overall complexity level for coding.

Table 13-4

Summary of Evaluation and Management Guidelines for Documentation

GUIDELINES	DETAILS
Select the category and subcategory of service. Categories of service are divided broadly. The ones most applicable to APNs are listed at right.	Office visit: • New (no care from anyone in the same specialty/same group in the last 3 years) • Established (received care in the last 3 years) Hospital visit: • Initial hospital care • Subsequent care • Hospital discharge services Home visit: • New patient • Established patient Preventive medicine services: • New patient • Established patient • Individual counseling • Group counseling
Determine the extent of the history obtained.	• HPI: Location, quality, severity, duration, timing, context, modifying factors, associated signs, and symptoms • ROS: Constitutional symptoms and symptoms of the eyes, ear, mouth, nose, throat, and various systems (cardiovascular, respiratory, gastrointestinal, genitourinary, musculoskeletal, integumentary, neurological, endocrine, hematological). Also includes allergic/immunological and psychiatric symptoms • PFSH: Any past history • Problem focused: CC and brief HPI (one to three elements of the HPI) • Expanded problem focused: CC, HPI, and problem-pertinent systems review (of the systems directly related to the problem) • Detailed: CC, extended HPI (four elements), ROS (two to nine systems), and pertinent PFSH (1 history area) • Comprehensive: CC, extended HPI (four elements), ROS (at least ten body systems), and complete PFSH (2 to 3 history areas)
Determine the extent of the examination performed.	• Examination: Head (including face), neck, chest (including breasts/axilla), abdomen, genitalia (including groin and buttocks), back, and each extremity • Organ system: Eyes, ears, nose, mouth, throat; various systems (cardiovascular, respiratory, gastrointestinal, genitourinary, musculoskeletal, endocrine, neurological, psychiatric, hematological, lymphatic, and immunological) • Problem focused: Documentation of one to five elements in one affected body area or organ system (identified by bullet) • Expanded problem focused: Documentation of at least six elements in the affected body area, as well as other symptomatic or related systems (identified by bullet) • Detailed: Should include at least two elements from six organ systems or body areas • Comprehensive: General multisystem examination or complete examination of a specific organ system (at least nine organ systems or body areas)
Determine the complexity of the medical decision-making.	Complexity determined by: • Number of possible diagnoses • Amount or complexity of the diagnostic tests or other information that must be obtained Risk of significant complications, morbidity, and/or mortality: • Straightforward (minimum diagnosis, data, and risk) • Low complexity (limited diagnosis and data; low risk) • Moderate complexity (multiple diagnoses; moderate data and risk) • High complexity (extensive diagnosis and data; high risk)

For new patients seen in the office, all of the required components (history, examination, and medical decision-making) must be met. For established patients seen in the office, two of the required components must be met.

CC, Chief complaint; *HPI,* history of present illness.

Adapted from Health Care Financing Administration (1998). *Evaluation and Management Documentation Guidelines.* Washington, DC: Health Care Financing Administration.

A Office visit est-pat
- 99212 Level 2-est (10 min)
- 99213 Level 3-est (15 min)
- 99214 Level 4-est (20 min)
- 99215 Level 5-est (25 min)
- 99211 Nursing visit Chg/NC

Preventive visit
- 99394 Est patient 12-17
- 99395 Est patient 18-39
- 99396 Est patient 40-64
- 99397 Est patient 65+

Hospital admission
- 99221 Initial visit (30 min.)

B Immunizations
- 90724 Flu vaccine
- 90745 Hep B (11-19) $5
- 90746 Hep B (>19) $5/50
- 90713 IPV
- 90707 MMR
- 90732 Pneumococcal
- 90718 TD (7 yrs or older)
- 90716 Varicella

Injections
- 90782 Therapeutic or diag.
  Sq or im
- 90788 Antibiotic
  Im ___ Chg/NC
- 86580 PPD
- J1055 Depo provera injection

Procedures
- 94640 Aerosol treatment
- 46600 Anoscopy
- 25600 Arthrocentesis major TT
- 92551 Audioscope
- 11730 Avulsion of nail plate
- 16020 Burn 1st, dressing sm
- 53670 Catheterization
- 17100 Destruction of lesion (not of face) 1 or ___
- 57170 Diaphragm fitting
- 69210 Ear irrigation
- 93000 ENG
- 11480 Excision/benign-trunk arms, legs, <5 cm or
- 11420 Excision/benign-scalp neck, hands, feet, genitalia <5 cm or
- 11750 Excision/nail and part of matrix
- 11280 Excision of skin tag

**** Foreign body removal ****
- 69200 Ear
- 65205 Eye
- 38380 Nose
- 10128 Subcutaneous tissue
  Other body part ___
- 90782 Immunizations
- 10050 Incision/drainage cyst
- 20558 Injection tendon/ligament

In house labs
- 82962 Accucheck
- 82270 Hemoccult slide (1-3)
- 85018 Hemoglobin
- 81025 Pregnancy test, urine
- 87210 Slides/smears
- 86580 Strep screen
- 81082 Urine dip
- 81080 Urine dip w/microscopy
- 58300 IUD insertion
- 58301 IUD removal
- 92567 Tympanometry
- 36410 Venipuncture, Phys.
- 36415 Venipuncture, Nurse

LABS M/C bas. lab
- 80049 Basic metab panel
- 85027 CBC
- 85025 CBC w/diff
- 84054 Comp metab panel
- 87068 Cult throat strep
- 87086 Culture urine
- 80051 Electrolyte panel
- 87797 Gen probe
- 82947 Glucose
- 80058 Hepatic func panel
- 83036 HEB AIC
- 80859 Hepatitis panel
- 80861 Lipid panel
- 86309 Mono test
- 88150 Pap smear
- 85618 Pt/INR
- 84132 Potassium
- 80184 Phenobarb level
- 85651 SED rate
- 84702 Serum preg test
- 84436 T-4
- 80198 Theophylline level
- 80091 Thyroid panel
- 84443 TSH by RIA

**** Test Code Description ****
___
___
___
___

C
- 627.0 Abnormal bleeding
- 383.90 Alcoholism
- 477.9 Allergic rhinitis
- 595.3 Allergy unspec
- 626.0 Amenorrhea
- 285.9 Anemia unspec
- 380.0 Anxiety
- 716.9 Arthritis
- 427.31 Artial fib
- 493.90 Asthma
- 724.5 Back pain
- 466.0 Bronchitis acute
- 491.9 Bronchitis chronic
- 414.9 CAD
- 428.0 CHF
- 078.1 Condyloma
- 496 COPD
- 311 Depression
- 250.00 Diabetes non-ins dep
- 250.01 Diabetes ins dep
- 782.3 Edema
- V25.09 Family planning
- V72.3 Gyn exam
- 784.0 Headache
- 307.81 Headache tension
- 346.9 Headache migraine
- V08.0 HIV
- 272.4 Hyperlipidemia
- 401.9 Hypertension (ESS)
- 244.9 Hypothyroidism
- V72.6 Lab exam
- 760.7 Malaise/fatigue
- 382.9 Otitis media
- 462 Pharyngitis
- V70.0 Physical
- 614.9 PID
- V74.1 PPD/TB check
- V22.2 Pregnancy
- 305.1 Tobacco abuse
- V56.3 Suture removal
- 473.9 Sinusitis
- 465.9 URI
- 599.0 UTI
- 616.1 Vaginitis
- 079.99 Viral syndrome

Paid: SP _____ INS Co-pay _____ MC _____ Provider's signature _____
RETURN APPOINTMENT

Figure 13-2 Sample encounter form (superbill) for an adult, established patient. **A,** Evaluation and management CPT codes. **B,** Common CPT procedure codes. **C,** Common conditions with ICD-9 evaluation and management codes.

Box 13-2

Dorothy's History

Medications:	HCTZ 25 mg
	Zestiril 10 mg
	Zocor 10 mg
	KCl 10 mg
	All medications qd
	No known allergies
Social:	No smoking or alcohol
	Lives with her daughter
Examination:	BP 160/108
	P 96
	R 14
	Weight 300 pounds
General:	Well-developed female
Heart:	No lymph adenopathy
	Throat without erythema
	S_1S_2 regular with no murmurs
Lungs:	Clear to auscultation
	Respirations unlabored
Abdominal:	BS+; obese; no hepatosplenomegaly
Ext:	Light edema, left leg
	2t edema left leg; warm to touch
	Erythema present
	Painful to palpation
	Pedal pulse present
Diagnoses:	1. Hypertension (uncontrolled)
	2. Obesity
	3. Hypercholesterolemia
	4. Cellulitis in right leg
Treatment:	Keflex 500 mg bid x 10 days

Box 13-3

Recommendations for Accurate Billing Practices

- Review the CPT manual for the current year.
- Make sure the documentation meets the criteria for the level of visit billed (see www.statcoder.com for a coding program available for palm pilots).
- File all progress notes in the chart.
- Provide a reasonable history and examination, labs, and treatment for each patient.
- Bill for additional services only if they were done.
- Make sure that both ICD-9 and CPT codes are identified for each patient.
- Attend a reimbursement training session once a year; HCFA offers free Medicare training for providers at www.hcfa.gov/medlearn/cbts.htm.
- Note that APN primary provider visits should be coded at least level 2, with most coded level 3.
- Get feedback about coding accuracy from the billing manager.
- Perform self-reviews.

Maximizing Reimbursement

Fee-for-service is still the most common method of reimbursement. Managed care companies negotiate various fees for services performed. It is not unusual that different insurance companies get different fees for the same services. This has had a major effect on the income earned by all PCPs. To keep the same level of income, each PCP needs to see more patients a day, maximize allowable billings, make sure payers pay, negotiate the highest fee agreements possible, and give all employees incentive to bill wisely. For physician practices, there is an incentive to hire nonphysician providers because their salary is less than physicians and the reimbursement rate for their services is the same in many cases.

Methods to maintain the same amount of reimbursement have implications for APNs and other providers. In many cases, APNs will be asked to see more patients each day. This encourages an APN to be as efficient as possible when providing patient care. Soper (1999) recommends a number of ways to manage time wisely when seeing patients. First, all necessary forms should be kept within close reach, either in the examination room or just outside of it. The APN should make sure that necessary equipment is in the room or on his or her person. This might mean keeping a penlight in a pocket, having a percussion hammer in every room, or having the triage person put the needed form with the chart as he or she prepares the patient. References, referral numbers, and patient handouts should be kept in a central location or in each examination room. Using tools that simplify the process

An example of a level-three visit would be a patient such as Aretta, a 45-year-old female with diabetes (type 2) who is being seen for a diabetes follow-up. She has been walking three times a week, watching her diet, and taking her metformin (Glucophage). She denies having any chest pain, open sores, swelling in her legs or hands, or frequent urination. Her examination reveals a well-developed woman who weighs 127 pounds (lbs), has a blood pressure (BP) of 124/68, and a heart rate (HR) of 86. Her physical examination reveals no neurovascular disease (NVD); her lungs are clear to auscultation; and her heart sounds are regular, without murmur. Her extremities are without edema, and a foot examination with monofilament showed sensation being present. The diagnosis is type-2 diabetes mellitus (DM), controlled. The plan is to refill her metformin (six refills) and check her glycosylated hemoglobin (Hgb A1C). Documentation for Aretta would need to include all of these elements to be considered a level-three (99213) visit. A checklist-type form may provide an efficient way to document the review of systems (ROS), examination, and treatment.

Table 13-5

Summary of Requirements for New and Established Patients

LEVEL OF VISIT	HISTORY	EXAMINATION	DIAGNOSIS	TIME (MINUTES)
New Patients				
99201	Problem focus	Problem focus	Straightforward	10
99202	Expanded problem focus	Expanded problem focus	Straightforward	20
99203	Detailed	Detailed	Low complexity	30
99204	Comprehensive	Comprehensive	Moderate complexity	45
99205	Comprehensive	Comprehensive	High complexity	60
Established Patients				
99211	None	None	None	0
99212	Problem focus	Problem focus	Straightforward	10
99213	Expanded problem focus	Expanded problem focus	Low complexity	15
99214	Detailed	Detailed	Moderate complexity	25
99215	Comprehensive	Comprehensive	High complexity	40

Adapted from Health Care Financing Administration (1998). *Evaluation and Management Documentation Guidelines*. Washington, DC: Health Care Financing Administration.

and jog the APN's memory of evaluation and management codes is particularly helpful (Box 13-4).

Another way to be efficient is to dictate or document as soon as possible after each visit. This keeps the information fresh and shortens the time needed to document accurately. Bundling tasks together is also another efficient way to manage time. For example, all the prescription refills can be done once in the morning or once in the afternoon. Using an automated refill request line may save even more time for all staff. While these suggestions will not be priorities in the mind of a new APN graduate, it might be wise to start in an organized fashion; those skills learned early are those that may be the most helpful and long lasting. Any way the APN can increase productivity and generate increased revenue is a powerful negotiator for a salary increase or bonus.

IMPLICATIONS FOR MSN EDUCATION AND ADVANCED PRACTICE

Given the importance of correct billing and documentation, every APN program should address its specifics. While many APN students learn some basics from their preceptors, it is vital to include the basics of coding as one of the "must have" classes. It is also critical for APN students to realize why correct billing and documentation is so important (and likely to become even more important in the next few years).

The implications of prepaid capitation or managed care inventory are a significant and positive development for

APNs. The crucial issue for APNs is being chosen to serve on provider panels so that they can serve as PCPs. APNs are less costly in terms of salary and benefit requirements, so they are an economically attractive option for the roles of PCP and gatekeeper (Fagin, 1992).

It will be critical for all APNs to be aware of and participate in the legislative process; contact with legislators is important so that nursing's views on particular issues are known. Wong (1999) recommends that APNs work together to more effectively influence and affect policy related to patient care.

APNs need to be aware of the six rules related to APN billing of Medicare (Box 13-5). Buppert (2000) recommends that the safest practice is to bill with an APN's own provider number and avoid the use of "incident to." Buppert calculates the difference in revenues using "incident to" and APN provider numbers (based on seeing 20 patients a day, with 25% Medicare patients) to be approximately $6200 per year, a relatively small amount considering the risk involved in following the confusing "incident to" rules.

An APN does not need to have a chart cosigned by the collaborating physician unless state law and/or insurance providers require it. However, APNs can not direct the care of hospitalized patients because federal law requires a physician direct their care. APNs can provide physician services in the hospital but can not be the sole director for care. This same rule applies to ordering home and hospice care and qualifying patients for Social Security disability; this care must be directed by physicians.

Mundinger (1999) demonstrates that APNs are able to compete and be successful in the primary care market. Data reveals that APNs do provide high-quality primary

Table 13-6

Risks, Procedures, and Options

LEVEL OF RISK	PRESENTING PROBLEMS	DIAGNOSTIC PROCEDURES ORDERED	MANAGEMENT OPTIONS SELECTED
Minimal	• One self-limited or minor problem (e.g., cold, insect bite, tinea corporis)	• Laboratory tests requiring venipuncture • Chest x-rays • Electrocardiograph/ electroencephalograph • Urinalysis • Ultrasound • Potassium hydroxide preparation	• Rest • Gargles • Elastic bandages • Superficial dressings
Low	• Two or more self-limited or minor problems • One stable chronic illness (e.g., well-controlled hypertension, non–insulin dependent diabetes mellitus, cataract) • Acute uncomplicated illness or injury (e.g., cystitis, allergic rhinitis, simple sprain)	• Physiological tests not under stress (e.g., pulmonary function tests) • Noncardiovascular imaging studies with contrast (e.g., barium enema) • Superficial needle biopsies • Clinical laboratory tests requiring arterial puncture	• Over-the-counter drugs • Minor surgery with no identified risk factors • Physical therapy • Occupational therapy • Intravenous fluid without additives
Moderate	• One or more chronic illnesses with mild exacerbation, progression, or side effects of treatment • Two or more stable chronic illnesses • Undiagnosed new problem with an uncertain prognosis (e.g., lump in the breast) • Acute illness with systemic symptoms (e.g., pyelonephritis, pneumonitis, colitis) • Acute complicated injury (e.g., head injury with brief loss of consciousness)	• Skin biopsies • Physiological tests under stress (e.g., cardiac stress test, fetal contraction stress test) • Diagnostic endoscopies with no identified risk factors • Deep needle or incisional biopsies • Cardiovascular imaging studies with contrast and no identified risk factors (e.g., arteriograph, cardiac catheterization) • Drawing of fluid from a body cavity (e.g., lumbar puncture, thoracentesis, culdocentesis)	• Minor surgery with identified risk factors • Elective major surgery (open, percutaneous, or endoscopic) with no identified risk factors • Prescription drugs • Therapeutic nuclear medicine • Intravenous fluids with additives • Closed treatment of fracture or dislocation without manipulation
High	• One or more chronic illnesses with severe exacerbation, progression, or side effects of treatment • Acute or chronic illnesses or injuries that pose a threat to life or bodily function (e.g., multiple trauma, acute myocardial infarction, pulmonary embolus, severe respiratory distress, progressive severe rheumatoid arthritis, psychiatric illness with potential threat to self or others, peritonitis, acute renal failure) • Abrupt change in neurological status (e.g., seizure, transient ischemic attack, weakness, sensory loss)	• Cardiovascular imaging studies with contrast and identified risk factors • Cardiac electrophysiological tests • Diagnostic endoscopies with identified risk factors • Discography	• Elective major surgery (open, percutaneous, or endoscopic) with identified risk factors • Emergency major surgery (open, percutaneous, or endoscopic) • Parenteral controlled substances • Drug therapy requiring intensive monitoring for toxicity • Decision not to resuscitate or to deescalate care because of poor prognosis

Data from Health Care Financing Administration (1998). *Evaluation and Management Documentation Guidelines.* Washington, DC: Health Care Financing Administration; and Rapsilber, L., & Anderson, E. (2000). Understanding the reimbursement process. *Nurse Practitioner, 25*(5), 36-56.

Box 13-4

Quick Tips to Identify Needed History, Examination, and Documentation Items

LEVEL 2 (NEW OR ESTABLISHED PATIENT)	LEVEL 3*	LEVEL 4*	LEVEL 5*
• 1 item in history • 1 item in examination • 1 diagnosis and plan	• 2 items in history (1 CC and 1 ROS) • 6 items in examination • 1 new diagnosis, 2 minor diagnoses, or 1 stable chronic condition	• 7 items in history (4 complaints, 2 ROS, and 1 from PFSH) • 12 items in examination • 1 complicated or acute diagnosis, 1 chronic illness with mild flare, or 2 stable chronic conditions • 3 labs or other treatments	• 16 items in history (4 complaints, 10 ROS, and 2 items from PFSH) • 18 items in examination • 1 chronic illness diagnosis with severe flare, or an acute or chronic illness that poses a threat to life or bodily function • 4 labs or other treatments

*Two of three areas must be documented.
Adapted from Health Care Financing Administration (1998). *Evaluation and Management Documentation Guidelines*. Washington, DC: Health Care Financing Administration.

Box 13-5

Rules Pertaining to Medicare Billing for Advanced Practice Nurses

1. APNs can bill for any services for which a physician can bill, in any geographical area and any setting. APNs can perform any services authorized by state law and any services delegated by the physician. Scope of practice, as described in the Balanced Budget Act of 1997, says "APNs may perform such services as the individual is legally authorized to perform in accordance with state law and who meets such training, education, and experience requirements as the Secretary may prescribe in regulations."
2. APNs may not supervise a resident for billing purposes.
3. The use of "incident to" rules requires close attention to the rules.
4. The APN provider number and the group's provider number should be entered on HCFA form 1500.
5. The extent of required physician collaboration is determined by state law.
6. After January 1, 2003, all APNs must possess a Master of Science in Nursing (MSN) degree and be nationally certified. Those who are providers before that date will be "grandfathered" in as long as provider status is maintained (41 U.S.C. § 135x [aa][5]]).

---

care for patients when compared to primary care physicians, and they have been economically successful as well. This group sets a new standard in how APNs might work collaboratively with physicians to better serve patients.

According to O'Nieal (2000), each APN needs to make a commitment to market the APN role to at least one person per week. This may include talking with people in the front office of a practice, neighbors, senior citizen organizations, or public officials. Educating people about the APN role is a job all APNs need to take on. The future of APNs may depend on these interactions.

PRIORITIES FOR RESEARCH

O'Nieal (2000) emphasizes that APN research needs to go beyond the 1985 Office of Technology Assessment to measure effectiveness in health care, cost, and outcomes. Outcomes research can help identify how well APNs do with management of common illnesses, as well as health prevention and promotion; determining the effect of nursing interventions on client response is critical. This research will make a statement regarding how well APNs do in providing primary care. Linking primary care performance to outcomes of care and quality will make

Suggestions for Further Learning

- Locate the following websites for more information related to APN reimbursement:
  - American Academy of Nurse Practitioners (www.aanp.org)
  - American College of Nurse Practitioners (www.nurse.org/acnp)
  - American Nurses Association (www.nursingworld.org/gova/hcfaru/2.htm)
  - Health Care Financing Administration (www.hcfa.gov/medicare/mcarpti.htm)
  - Nurse Practitioner Central legislative section (www.nurse.net/leg)
  - Nurse Practitioner Central Medicare section (www.nurse.net/medicare)
- Review the following articles: Cooper, R., Laud, P., & Dietrich, C. (1998). Current and projected workforce of nonphysician clinicians. *Journal of the American Medical Association,*280(9), 788-794; and Cooper, R., Henderson, T., & Dietrich, C. (1998). Roles of nonphysician clinicians as autonomous providers of patient care. *Journal of the American Medical Association, 280*(9), 795-802. What implications do these articles have for APNs? Do these articles raise the level of competition between physicians and APNs? How might an increase in the numbers of nonphysician providers affect reimbursement? Support your view.
- What are some strategies to achieve savings for a health maintenance organization (HMO), as compared to fee-for-service patients? Review the following article for one suggestion: Flood, A., Fremont, A., Jin, K., Bott, D., Ding, J., & Parker, R. (1998). How do HMOs achieve savings? The effectiveness of one organization's strategies. *Health Service Research, 33*(1), 79-99.
- Go to the MGMA website at www.mgma.com for information related to compliance with HCFA guidelines. What information is available that may help APNs stay in line with HCFA guidelines?
- Examine the following resource: *PMIC CPT coding tool: evaluation and management components.* Available at 1-800-MEDSHOP from Doorstop Medical Consultants. This is a handheld pull-tab tool that simplifies evaluation and management service codes. It also is available online at www.nurse.net/products/billingtools.

APNs much more attractive as PCPs on provider panels. This research has been almost impossible to conduct in the past because many APNs were not credited for their part in the care provided. This was changed with the research published by Mundinger (2000), which verified how well APNs do when compared head to head with physicians.

Research also needs to look at new ways to provide care; for example, how cost effective is a model in which APNs provide health promotion and prevention services as well as basic care, leaving physicians to manage more complex problems? What would the benefits and problems be in such a system? What is the level of patient satisfaction when that type of collaborative care is provided? Long-term results on mortality and morbidity rates when compared to those of other providers would also be important. Overall, APNs need to collect data related to setting, increased access, cost and quality, and long-term outcomes. These data will provide hard evidence by which APN practice can be judged and marketed.

DISCUSSION QUESTIONS

These questions can be used to promote critical thinking and encourage discussion.

1. Using CPT and ICD-9 references, identify the evaluation and management codes that are appropriate for the following encounters:
   - A 5-year-old child having a school physical
   - A 21-year-old woman having a gynecological exam and receiving family planning advice for oral contraceptives
   - A 2-year-old child with otitis media
   - A 67-year-old male having a ½ cm mole removed from his shoulder

   For the situations described, also use the following reference—Healthcare Consultants of America (2000). *2000 physician's fee and coding guide.* Augusta, GA: Healthcare Consultants of America—to identify both Medicare and third-party payer reimbursement amounts.

2. What are the advantages and disadvantages of direct reimbursement? Identify and discuss the remaining barriers to reimbursement. How might APNs address these barriers?

3. What role has consumer demand played in direct reimbursement of APNs?

REFERENCES/BIBLIOGRAPHY

American Association of Colleges of Nursing (1997). *Direct reimbursement for nurse practitioners and clinical nurse specialists.* Available online at www.aacn.nche.edu/government/index.htm.

American College of Nurse Practitioners (1999). *Federal reimbursement for advanced practice nurses*. Available online at www.nurse.org/acnp.facts/reimbur-fed.shtml.

American Medical Association (1998). *Physicians' current procedural terminology: 1999* (4th ed.). Chicago: American Medical Association.

Baldwin, G. (1999, August 2). Attention to detail can be the key to a practice's success. *American Medical News*, 2

Buppert, C. (1998). Reimbursement for nurse practitioner services. *Nurse Practitioner*, 23(1): 67-81.

Buppert, C. (1999). *Nurse practitioner's business and legal guide*. Gaithersburg, MD: Aspen Publishers.

Buppert, D. (2000). *The primary care provider's guide to compensation and quality*. Gaithersburg, MD: Aspen Publishers.

Capko, J. (1998). Use random audits to find payment problems. *Family Practice Medicine*, 6(6). Available online at www.aafp.org/fpm.

Cohen, S., & Juszczak, L. (1997). Promoting the nurse practitioner role in managed care. *Journal of Pediatric Health Care*, 11, 3-11.

Congressional Record (1997). *The Primary Care Practitioner Incentive Act of 1997*. Available online at thomas.loc.com.

Fagin, C. (1992). The cost effectiveness of nursing care. In L. Aiken & C. Fagin (Eds.), *Charting nursing's future: agenda for the 1990s*. Philadelphia: JB Lippincott.

Federal Register (1998, November 2). *Final rule on nurse practitioner, clinical nurse specialist, physician assistant, certified nurse-midwives and Medicare billing* (pp. 58863-58912).

Finefrock, W., & Havens, D. (1997). Coverage and reimbursement issues for nurse practitioners. *Journal of Pediatric Health Care*, 11, 139-143.

Gelman, E. (1999). A reasonable compromise. *Patient Care for the Nurse Practitioner*, 11, 5.

Gelman, E. (2000). Claiming our title as primary care provider. *Patient Care for the Nurse Practitioner*, 1, 4.

Hawkins, J., & Thibodeau, J. (1993). *The advanced practitioner: current practice issues* (3rd ed.). New York: Tiresias Press.

Health Care Financing Administration: *Overview of the Medicare program*. Available online at hcfa/gov/medicare/careover.htm.

Hill, E. (1999). Improve your ICD-9 coding accuracy. *Family Practice Physician*, 6(7/8). Available online at www.aafp.org.

Hoffman, C. (1994). Medicaid payment for non-physician practitioners: an access issue. *Health Affairs (Millwood)*, 13, 140.

Jaklevic, M. (1999, February 8). Practices with best practices. *Modern Healthcare*, 64.

Jennings, C. (1977). Third party reimbursement and the nurse practitioner. *Nurse Practitioner*, 2, 11-13.

Johnson, D. (1999). Coding for nurse practitioners. *American College of Nurse Practitioners Newsletter*. Washington, DC: American College of Nurse Practitioners.

Kongstvedt, P. (1993). Compensation of primary care physicians in open panels. In *The managed health care handbook* (2nd ed.). Gaithersburg, MD: Aspen Publishers

Lindeke, L., & Chesney, M. (1999). Reimbursement realities of advanced nursing practice. *Nursing Outlook*, 47(6), 248-251.

Managed Care: a guide for physicians. (1999). Yardley, PA: Stezzi Communications

McKessy, A., & Saner, R. (1998). Protect your practice with a Medicare and Medicaid compliance program. *Family Practice Management*, 57.

Medicode's 1999 Physician ICD 9 CM. (5th ed.). (1998). Salt Lake City, UT: Medicode Public.

Melby, C. (1998). Physician and nurse reimbursement. *Online Journal of Issues in Nursing*. Available online at www.nursingworld.org/ojin.tpc6/tpc6_3.htm.

Miller, S. (2000). Obtaining a provider number. *Patient Care for the Nurse Practitioner*, 4, 83-85.

Minarik, P. (1993). Legislative and regulatory update: federal reimbursement revisited. *Clinical Nurse Specialist*, 7(2), 102-103.

Mittelstadt, P. (1993). Federal reimbursement of advanced practice nurses' empowers the profession. *Nurse Practitioner*, 18(1), 43-49.

Moore, K. (1998). Billing for NP services: what you need to know. *Family Practice Management*, 5(5), 345-348.

Morris, S., & Smith, D. (1976). *The physician extender reimbursement study: the diffusion of physician extenders* (Working paper No. 1). Washington DC: US Social Security Administration, Office of Research and Statistics.

Mundinger, M. (1999). Can advanced practice nurses succeed in the primary care market? *Nursing Economics*, 17(1): 7-14.

Mundinger, M. (2000). Primary care outcomes in patients treated by nurse practitioners or physicians. *Journal of the American Medical Association*, 293(1), 59-68.

Nurse practitioners: evaluation and management coding. (1997). St. Paul, MN: Medical Learning.

Office of Technology Assessment (1986). *Nurse practitioners, physician assistants, and certified nurse midwives: a policy analysis* (Health technology case study No. 37). Washington, DC: US Government Printing Office.

O'Nieal, M. (2000, May). Recognition, research, reimbursement: ensuring business survival into the 21st century. *ADVANCE for Nurse Practitioners*.

Pearson, L. (1993). 1992-1993 update: how each state stands on legislative issues affecting advanced nursing practice. *Nurse Practitioner*, 18(1), 25.

Rapsilber, L., & Anderson, E. (2000). Understanding the reimbursement process. *Nurse Practitioner*, 25(5), 36-56.

Richmond, T., Thompson, H., Sullivan-Marx, E. (2000). Reimbursement for acute care nurse practitioner services. *American Journal of Critical Care*, 9(1), 52-61.

Romaine-Davis, A. (1997). *Advanced practice nurses: education, roles, trends*. Boston: Jones & Bartlett.

Rustia, J., Bartek, J. (1998). Managed care credentialing of advanced practice nurses. *Nurse Practitioner*, 22(9), 90-103.

Saffriet, B. (1992). Health care dollars and regulatory sense: the role of advanced practice nursing. *Yale Journal on Regulation*, 9(2), 417-487.

Sheehy, C., & McCarthy, M. (1998). *Advanced practice nursing: emphasizing common roles*. Philadelphia: FA Davis.

Silva, M. (1998). Financial compensation and ethical issues in health care. *Online Journal of Issues in Nursing*. Available online at www.nursingworld.org/ojin/tpc6/tpc6_4.htm.

Soper, W. (1999). 13 ways to be more efficient. *Family Practice Management*, 6(4). Available online at www.aafp.org/.

Sullivan, E. (1992). Nurse practitioner and reimbursement: case analyses. *Nursing and Healthcare*, 13, 236-241.

Sullivan-Marx, E. (1998). Medicare reimbursement for advanced practice nurses: in the front door. *Nursing Outlook*, 46(1), 40-41.

Sullivan-Marx, E., & Mullinix, C. (1999). Payment for advanced practice nurses: economic structures and sytems. In M. Mezey & D. McGiven (Eds.), *Nurses, Nurse Practitioners.* (pp. 345-368). New York: Springer.

Synder, M., & Mirr, M. (1995). *Advanced practice nursing.* New York: Springer.

Tower, J. (1999). Medicare reimbursement for nurse practitioners. *Journal of the American Academy of Nurse Practitioners, 11*(7), 289-292.

United States Department of Health and Human Services (1996). *International classification of diseases* (9th ed.). Los Angeles, CA: Practice Management Information Corporation.

Wilken, M. (1995). Nonphysician providers: how regulations affect availability and access to care. *Nursing Policy Forum, 1,* 28-33.

Wong, S. (1999). Health policy: reimbursement to advanced practice nurses through Medicare. *Image, 31*(2), 167-173.

Section IV

Ethical Issues in Health Care

Margaret M. Anderson

Revolutionary changes in health care delivery and finance, combined with advances in technology and science, have created a workplace with many morally perplexing problems for which there are not always clear ethical or legal answers. This is the workplace for which today's advanced practice nurse (APN) is being prepared. Unlike at any other time in nursing's history, today's nursing specialists need a foundation in health care ethics to support their clinical practice because they will be expected to act when ethical problems emerge. Whether they provide primary or acute care in nurse practitioner (NP) roles, provide expertise as clinical nurse specialists (CNSs), manage anesthesia as certified registered nurse anesthetists (CRNAs), or care for childbearing women as certified nurse midwives (CNMs), APNs in their respective roles will encounter virtual strangers and engage those individuals in unique nurse-patient relationships. This connection between two people who are often strangers at the outset is an amazing feat in itself. It is possible, in part, because nurses engage in a process of intentional caring, a patient advocacy based in ethics. This unit clearly reveals advanced practice as a moral endeavor, introduces the ethical foundation that enables this kind of special practice, and lays bare the moral principles that underpin the decision-making process for that practice.

Chapter 14 provides definitions that structure a review of the theoretical dimensions of ethics and examines the major ethical theories, deontology and teleology (utilitarianism), in some detail. Additionally, this chapter introduces the primary ethical principles of beneficence, nonmaleficence, autonomy, justice, veracity, and fidelity, using both clinical and educational examples of each to facilitate understanding. APNs have several resources to enhance their capacity to handle ethical problems in practice. Ethics consultations, written codes of ethics, and ethics committees (including institutional review boards [IRBs] for research) are available to APNs. The chapter exposes the way in which these resources serve APNs in the reality of daily practice.

Nurses face bioethical problems in a unique manner because of their special roles in collaborating with physicians and other providers and their special relationships with patients and families. Chapter 15 examines their unique perspective by defining ethical dilemmas and introducing several decision-making models as approaches to the ethical dilemmas common in contemporary clinical practice. An individual APN's continued maintenance of professional practice amidst ethical problems is a major aspect of the chapter; another is an APN's role in assessing a clinical practice setting for evidence of ethical policies, procedures, and processes.

In Chapter 16, the broad theoretical perspective of ethics/ethical dilemmas is narrowed to the specifics of everyday clinical practice by offering real everyday problems (in case scenarios) for analysis and decision-making. Four case studies—one each for the various types of APNs—are presented and analyzed through decision-making models. Three different decision-making models, introduced in Chapter 15, are used to make decisions about the cases; a series of questions for case analysis is included as well.

Not only must APNs have a foundation in ethics as a basis for their specialty practice, they need knowledge of the law as well. Chapter 17 describes ethics and law as distinct entities and shows how they coexist. A review of intentional torts and the elements of malpractice is included in this chapter. An extensive discussion of risk management for APN practice is also included, with consideration given to systems, interpersonal, and damage-control components of risk management and the appropriateness of liability insurance coverage. Curbside and telephone consultations, so much a part of primary care practice in today's restructured delivery system, are analyzed from the perspective of risk management.

Chapter 14

Foundations for an Ethical Practice

Patricia M. Gray, Margaret M. Anderson, & Cheryl Pope Kish

With continuing advancements in technology and changes in society that include more aged and chronically ill persons; fiscal constraints; and increasingly emotional, often controversial issues such as euthanasia, genetic engineering, and abortion, nurses are bombarded with ethical issues on a daily basis. Nurses may find themselves dealing with internal moral conflicts and conflicts among themselves, patients and their families, physicians and other care providers, and the health care organizations that employ them. Issues related to ethics are pervasive.

Socrates is credited with the emergence of *ethics* as a discipline for study. Ethics is a practical field because it deals with the difference between good and evil and examines issues related to the "good life." The good life is considered to be a life that is lived successfully; it is also one conducted in an ethical fashion—the person who is living a good life is an ethical or good person. Of course, the definitions of *successful* and *ethical* are open to great discussion. Good and evil become synonymous with but are not the same as right and wrong. Socrates, Plato, and Aristotle wrestled with the study of ethics in an effort to define right and wrong, good and evil. Looking back, such study seems almost easy because the times seem easier in comparison to today. However, these philosophers also wrestled with the larger issues—the shades of right and wrong and the constant demands of an ever-changing and evolving civilization (Husted & Husted, 1995). Socrates lost his life for questioning the beliefs of others and forcing them to question their own beliefs. Self-examination is not a pleasant practice, especially when one must look at long-held beliefs with no apparent basis other than having been learned during one's life. Socrates is famous for his method of examination. He would ask a question and then question the answer until the responder was down to his or her basic beliefs and concepts. It is impossible to understand and know one's ethics without considerable self-examination of the origin of one's beliefs. Understanding of one's beliefs and ordering of those beliefs are essential to ethical decision-making.

The field of *bioethics* is only about 30 years old; until 1970, it was a part of ethics in general. However, this subset of ethics has exploded into its own as a result of changes in medical technology and a realization that health care resources are indeed finite. The capacity of contemporary medicine to affect even the most fundamental aspects of life—birth, death, and human suffering—is astonishing. As technology and medical treatment continue to advance and resource allocation affects patients' access to and potential quality of care, the need for constant examination of beliefs and ethics will continue. With the sweeping changes in the health care system, individuals must be prepared to examine and accommodate their respective belief systems accordingly. For today's advanced practice nurse (APN), this involves examining, clarifying, and possibly reframing the professional value system for new role expectations.

DEFINITIONS

Professional nurses have an obligation to help and sustain their patients and support their colleagues as they face difficult moral and ethical choices in the clinical arena. To do justice to this role, it is important to understand the related terms.

Values are the enduring attitudes and beliefs, developed through life experience, which serve to influence one's behavior. According to the classic work of Raths, Harmin, and Simon (1978), one's beliefs or values are chosen freely after consideration of many possibilities; are important (even cherished) to the person; and are so much a part of the person that they are acted on consistently, both privately and publicly. To some extent, others can tell what values a person holds dear by seeing how he or she spends time, energy, and money. Herein lies the idea of "putting your money where your mouth is." Because values shape the consistency of one's behavior, others begin to associate certain values with an individual over time. For example, they may learn from observing Nancy's office behavior that she values neatness and care for the property of others. By noting Steve's daily agenda and the way he sometimes schedules his last appointment early, others begin to appreciate that, while Steve has a strong work ethic, he loves fatherhood and values leisure time with his family. *Values clarification* refers to the process of examining one's set of values and the way in which they shape behavior. Self-discovery comes when values clarification leads to ranking one's values or understanding the priority of one over another. Values are learned through the process of socialization as individuals observe others and gain life experience within the context of their social and cultural circumstances. As the saying goes, "Children learn what they live." For example, the child who lives in a home where racial bigotry and hatred are the norm can easily learn those values unless exposure to different circumstances, perhaps in school, leads to alternative values. As another example, individuals in different cultures learn how to react to pain in public situations by modeling themselves on family members or friends in that cultural group. The implications that such values hold for a practicing nurse are fairly obvious.

Because values are incorporated into a person's character, they affect both the personal and the professional life. Nurses cannot put on or take off the values they have learned like a lab coat, donning them in the clinical setting and leaving them behind once off duty. For nurses, clarification of values promotes self-awareness and offers insight into why they act as they do. Such insights are not always easy, but they are necessary for making choices about what values to keep and what values need modification.

Bandman and Bandman (1995) indicate that values clarification is a three-stage process. The first stage involves making an initial value choice from the alternatives, examining the alternatives, and ranking the alternatives. Stage two involves reflection on these values to find those worth honoring. In stage three, an individual determines how to achieve the particular value. **Values inquiry** refers to the process of examining social issues and the values that affect choices related to them (King, 1984). Nursing students learn the values and inherent social issues of their intended profession from the first day they step onto campus; they learn in the classroom, in clinical settings, and by and through the socialization process for nursing. (Attaining a professional value set is part of the professional socialization process described in Chapter 19.) The student gains a professional identity in this process; the same is true for an individual who returns to school to be educated as an APN—now this individual gains a professional identity for specialty practice. According to King (1984), until individuals gain a self-identity, they perform on the basis of external values, values reflecting what they have witnessed in others and not what they have found in themselves. However, with a professional identity and the esteem to match, one can rely on the new value set to guide decisions and actions.

When students at either the generalist or specialist level of nursing education examine nursing's heritage, they learn the values and traditions that have shaped the profession, the most central being unconditional regard for the worth and dignity of humans. Florence Nightingale's personal "call to service" reflected these values at a time when nursing was looked on as a service provided by the lowest members of society (Craven & Hirnle, 2000).

Morals are those personal standards or principles that guide an individual's sense of what is right and wrong, what one should do in certain situations and how one should treat others. Morals are often associated with the conscience, which guides behavioral choices and causes one to feel guilty when behavior deviates from what is believed to be right. Morals are learned. An individual's value set determines his or her morality, albeit often unconsciously. APNs practice within a moral context. Every day, APNs face choices in clinical practice that challenge their fundamental values. They can be guided in their choices by the *Standards of Clinical Nursing Practice* (American Nurses Association [ANA], 1998) and by the ethical codes of conduct prescribed by the ANA (1985) and the International Council of Nurses (2000). **Ethics** is that branch of philosophy that deals with morality and moral reasoning—the rules and principles that determine which human actions are right and which are wrong (Zerwekh & Claborn, 1997). **Bioethics** concerns what is right or wrong in relation to human life and the life and death decisions one faces. Euthanasia, advanced directives, assisted reproduction, and abortion are concerns in the arena of bioethics, as are issues related to the quality of life. **Clinical ethics** is a practical discipline that offers a structured approach useful for making ethical decisions in clinical practice (Jonsen, Siegler, & Winslade, 1998). Clinical ethics relies upon the "conviction that, even when perplexity is great and emotions run high," its framework can enable clinicians and patients, working together, to construct a correct decision. According to these authors, ethical features are part of every patient encounter. It is only when there is disagreement between providers and patients, or when the choices challenge a person's values, that problems or ethical dilemmas arise.

Ethical dilemmas are those problems that force decisions between alternatives that are equally undesirable. The fundamental principles of right and wrong may appear to be in conflict; this places the decision-maker "between a rock and a hard place," which is never an easy place to be.

CRITICAL ISSUES: APPLYING ETHICS TO PRACTICE

Before one can understand how ethical dilemmas arise, much less get resolved, it is helpful to have an understanding of how ethics are derived, the relationship between ethics and values, and the ethical theories prevalent today. Bandman & Bandman (1995) identify key differences between scientific theory and ethical theory. Scientific theory explains and describes whether a phenomenon is true or false. In contrast, ethical theory "aims to justify human action [and] may be right or wrong but not regarded as true or false, and presents obligations or ought statements" (Bandman & Bandman, 1995). Ethical theories employ moral principles and fact-based premises to justify action, and they tend to be more prescriptive; ethical theories may include principles to guide action. For example, the Ten Commandments are the generally accepted guide to Judeo-Christian ethics (Bandman & Bandman, 1995).

There are two broad ethical approaches to decision-making that are generally accepted: teleology and deontology. A third, situational theory, merges the other two but is not considered normative in the same way as the others because it lacks the definition to influence decision-making (Zerwekh & Claborn, 1997).

Teleology, also called *utilitarianism*, derives from humanistic origins and is often associated with nineteenth century philosopher John Stuart Mill. In utilitarian terms, useful outcomes are good. Human reason is the basis of authority, not some absolute revealed by God. Because the focus is on outcomes or results, the actions chosen are always driven by the potential results. This approach tends to protect the interests of the majority, sometimes at the expense of the individual (Zerwekh & Claborn, 1997).

The concept of determinism is a beginning point in utilitarian theory. *Determinism* means "every human action is a response to a prior action" (Husted & Husted, 1995). The original action comes from outside the current actor. Deciding and choosing are only illusions that the determinist holds. The belief is that one acts to seek pleasure and avoid pain and can not choose to act otherwise. Pleasure is therefore good and pain is evil. The greater good is what is best for more than one, but the pleasure of one is equal to the pleasure of every other. Therefore the greater good is the goal of every ethical agent, and people should act to obtain that greater good. This theory directs humans "to look at the results of an action in making moral judgements" (Husted & Husted, 1995). Utilitarianism is a single principle theory, and the theory is consequential. One can consider the benefits and detriments of potential actions and, hopefully, reach some balance of good over evil. That which causes good outcomes is believed to be a good action. Simplistically, this ethical approach "is sometimes interpreted as 'the end justifies the means'" (Zerwekh & Claborn, 1997).

Deontology has a Judeo-Christian origin, often associated with eighteenth century philosopher Immanuel Kant. The concepts of right and wrong are at the center of this ethical approach, and right and wrong are based on absolute moral obligations revealed by God. Also, "right or wrong is based on [the] duty and obligation to act, not on the consequences of one's actions" (Zerwekh & Claborn, 1997). The deontologist is committed to universalizability. This means "when one makes a moral judgement in a given situation, one will make the same judgment in any similar situation" (Davis, Aroskar, Liaschenko, & Drought 1997). Deontology assumes that rules justify decisions and actions. Simplistically, people have rules to go by, and the

decisions they make are right when they follow those rules. Of course, there are times when the rules are in conflict with one another. Obligations are primary and have no exceptions. For example, the deontological belief that all life is worthy of respect obligates against abortion and euthanasia, irrespective of the circumstances. In deontology, because truthfulness is an obligation, lying is always wrong, even when one knows that the truth will cause pain.

The *situational approach* to ethical decision-making is often credited to Episcopal theologian Joseph Fletcher, who appealed for love to be the only norm. Within this approach, there are no steadfast rules or absolute prescriptions for behavior. Instead, the merits of each situation determine what decision best respects the individuals involved. Risks and benefits of each action are considered for the unique situation; consequently, decisions made in one situation are not generalizable to other situations. Although this approach seems arbitrary, it probably accounts for the way most people make day-to-day decisions (Zerwekh & Claborn, 1997). An individual taking a situational approach might be opposed to abortion in general but support it in cases of rape or incest.

Moral and Ethical Principles

Regardless of the worldview of ethics being used, certain principles are common: autonomy, beneficence, nonmaleficence, respect, justice, fidelity, and veracity. While some of these principles are more cogent to one theory than another, ethicists concur that all are relevant to ethical decisions.

Autonomy, or self-determination, implies the freedom to choose and make decisions for oneself without external interference. The presupposition exists that the individual has the intellectual capacity to make the decision and has been informed of the consequences in cases where they were not obvious. For example, Mr. London, a 54-year-old fisherman, has a right to refuse a coronary bypass procedure, but that decision should be made only after he is informed about what nonsurgical treatments are available and how the results compare to the anticipated surgical results. The health care team must be sure that Mr. London was not under the influence of sedatives at the time he changed his mind about the surgery and should feel comfortable that he is not being pressured in his decision. At times, the principle of autonomy is challenged because the individual's decision infringes on the rights of another person. For example, Mrs. Tanner refuses a blood transfusion because she is a Jehovah's Witness, and receiving blood products is not acceptable in her religion. As a rational adult, once informed, she can refuse the blood, even though her life might be in jeopardy as a result. However, the scenario becomes complicated (and the principle may be challenged) if Mrs. Tanner is pregnant and her decision also jeopardizes her unborn child.

The principle of beneficence implies doing good or

doing as little harm as possible under the circumstances, or making sure that the good outweighs the harm. Davis et al (1997) relate this concept to infant immunizations. The pain and discomfort, both at the injection site and systemically for a couple of days, are worth the ultimate measure of good derived from disease prevention on a long-term basis.

Related closely to beneficence is the ethical principle of nonmaleficence—the obligation to avoid doing harm, either intentionally or unintentionally. Zerwehk and Claborn (1997) relate this principle to a situation where a nurse is asked to float to an unfamiliar hospital unit where part of the assignment is administration of medications. The nurse might consider refusing the assignment out of concern that her unfamiliarity with the medications might contribute to errors that would compromise patient safety.

The principle of respect for persons not only supports personal autonomy, it also relates to the interconnectedness and relatedness of humans. This principle recognizes that respect for the individual also affects those who are around or interact with that individual. When interpreted broadly, this principle means that each individual is equal to all other individuals, and that each individual is unique. Therefore individuals deserve respect for their own purposes, privacy, and nature. Interference by others requires quite special circumstances (Davis et al, 1997). In keeping with this idea, the role of the nurse as advocate is purposive and directed to the patient's goals. The patient has the right and duty to make decisions regarding care and, in accord with the principle of autonomy, the health professional is required to respect, accept, and even support those decisions (Davis et al, 1997). This is an expectation even in cases where the patient's decision does not agree with what the nurse or other members of the health care team would have wanted, and this is particularly difficult when the patient's choice is something that will ultimately cause him or her harm.

The principle of justice implies fair treatment—not making treatment decisions, including allocation of resources, on the basis of age, gender, socioeconomic status, religion, ethnic group, sexual orientation, and other such variables. There is currently no consensus about the concept of justice as it relates to either health care or society, but the principle is often used to justify the distribution of goods and services (distributive justice). Justice has some interesting implications for health care. It implies that health care is a right (an implied right that has become a political issue) and that fairness is a doctrine for employment as well as the distribution of care. For example, can employers force nurses to work overtime with additional compensation, and can staffing be so short that one patient dies of a preventable condition while the nurse is busy with a critical patient at the other end of the hall? Is there justice in the distribution of the nurses' skills, or would more nurses or nurses with different types of skills have prevented the preventable death? Assuming

nurses are professionals, should they expect compensation for overtime work, or is this a function of the profession?

Philosopher John Rawls proposes a creative view of "justice as fairness." According to Rawls (1971), when making ethical decisions, rational people choose an alternative that supports the most disadvantaged because they are perceived as less able to advocate for themselves. Two principles reflect the essence of his theory: (1) each individual is to have an equal right to the most extensive basic liberty compatible with a similar liberty for others, and (2) social and financial inequities should be arranged so that they are reasonably to everyone's advantage and attached to positions and offices open to all individuals. Silva (1998) suggests that this means inequities are morally justifiable so long as they are fair. An individual or corporation can have advantages if these advantages can benefit the least fortunate members of society.

The restructuring of health care witnessed in the last decade has profoundly affected not only the delivery systems, but also health care financing. The market-driven system has elicited criticism from patients and providers and forced a renewed interest in the ethical principle of justice. As managed care evolves, APNs will be challenged to attend to the many ethical issues it raises. Beauchamp and Childress (1994) suggest that health care professionals consider allocation of resources according to these factors: (1) to each person an equal share, (2) to each according to need, (3) to each according to effort, (4) to each according to contribution, (5) to each according to merit, and (6) to each according to free-market exchanges. Silva (1998) adds that allocation of resources should also be to each according to moral relevance. Allocation of resources should never be capricious or based on irrelevant characteristics such as race, economic circumstances, or gender.

Loewry and Loewry (1998) suggest that, given the current health care environment, physicians' roles have been distorted; they have been forced to attend to more of the financial aspects of illness, becoming fiscal officers. They explore the inherent difficulty in simultaneous attempts to be both patient advocates and resource stewards. For APNs in primary care settings, the same might be said. Certainly APNs are being asked to see more patients and limit their time with patients in an effort to be more cost effective.

The principle of fidelity refers to the duty to be faithful to commitments, keep promises, and maintain privacy and confidentiality (Zerwekh & Claborn, 1997). To whom the nurse owes fidelity can complicate what would seem an otherwise straightforward principle. For example, is the APN's obligation for fidelity to the patient, family, physician, clinic, or profession? What if these are at odds? Mary, an acute care nurse practitioner (NP), promised Mr. Tolen that she would share the results of his colonoscopy with him, tell him "if cancer is there." While Mr. Tolen is recovering from his sedation and before his test results are

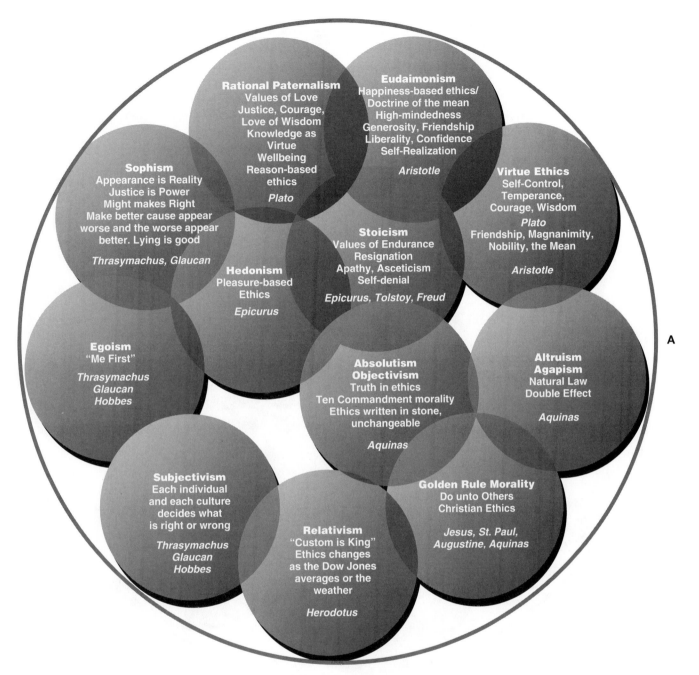

Figure 14-1 A, Traditional theories of ethics. (From Bandman, E.L., & Bandman, B. [1995]. *Nursing ethics through the life span* [3rd ed.]. Upper Saddle River, NJ: Prentice-Hall.)   *Continued*

known, Mr. Tolen's adult children disclose to Mary that they do not wish for him to know if he has cancer. They seem genuinely worried about the effects of that prognosis; they suspect he would "just curl up and die now without even trying therapy of any sort." Mary's collaborative physician agrees. To whom does Mary owe an obligation for fidelity?

Veracity is an ethical principle that specifies a duty to tell the truth. The principle of veracity is an issue in the example of fidelity given above. Is something less than the total truth justified when the truth will cause anxiety or emotional pain? Veracity also relates to actions like documenting accurately and honestly, not attempting to minimize or cover up an error, and reporting research findings accurately and fully.

No worldview of ethics addresses the issues that arise in nursing situations on a daily basis. They each provide different perspectives from which to examine ethical issues, and each perspective has strengths and weaknesses. There is considerable overlap (as indicated in Figure 14-1), and it is immediately apparent that no one theory has been confirmed through research as *the* ethical theory.

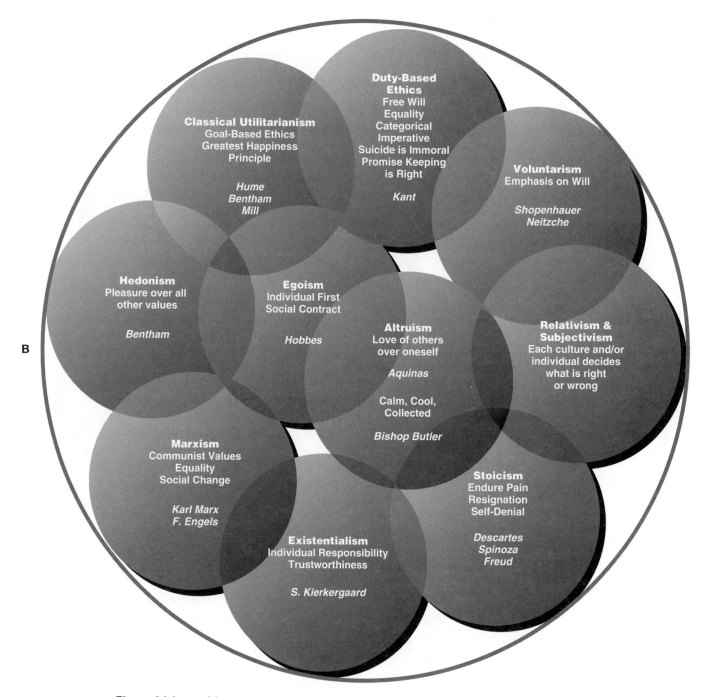

Figure 14-1, cont'd B, Modern theories of morality. (From Bandman, E.L., & Bandman, B. [1995]. *Nursing ethics through the life span* [3rd ed.]. Upper Saddle River, NJ: Prentice-Hall.)   *Continued*

The Ethic of Caring

Recently, nurse ethicists have proposed that an ethic of caring would serve the needs of the profession well. Hartman (1998) believes that caring is so perfectly intertwined with ethical principles that "together they provide a perfect circle of ethical justification." She continues, "Nurses' call to care is a moral imperative to enter into a relationship with individuals, families, groups, and communities. It is an obligation to take the ethical high road, so to speak, and put patients before convenience and to

remember that without patients needing care there would be no profession of nursing."

Caring has its roots in the altruistic theory developed by the medieval Christian philosopher St. Thomas Aquinas (Bandman & Bandman, 1995). *Care* is a concept compatible with the principle of beneficence—the commitment to do good and avoid doing harm. Begany (1994) found that "caring" was the most common adjective selected to describe a typical nurse, which is certainly a positive commentary on the profession. Accusing a nurse of "not

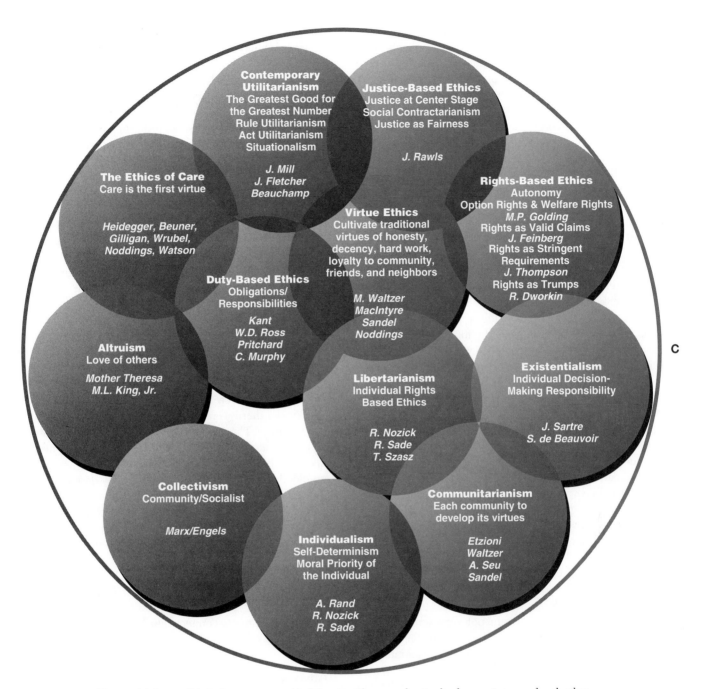

Figure 14-1, cont'd C, Contemporary ethical theories. These may be visualized as moving around each other.

caring" is quite an insult. The concept of caring as described by Benner and Wrubel (1989) means that "persons, events, projects and things matter to people." Caring is an interactive, dynamic concept that includes involvement. Benner and Wrubel (1989) believe that caring is a response to stress—helping people in distress to cope. Nurses care for others in a distressed state by helping them cope with the recovery of health or with the failure to recover.

The theoretical underpinnings of caring are found in feminist theory. Carol Gilligan (1982) and Nell Noddings

(1984) both assert that women have a softer, less aggressive approach to ethics than men (i.e., a caring approach), and that the rule-driven, justice approach to ethics espoused by others is more compelling to men. Women are attracted to virtues of love, caring, nurturing and sympathy. Gilligan (1982) writes that women develop "an 'ethic of care' whose underlying logic is a psychological logic of relationships, which contrasts with the (generally male) formal logic of fairness that informs the justice approach." Noddings (1986) believes that "caring lies at the very heart of morality and gives it stability."

In nursing, caring is a central concept that actually provides the legitimate base of the profession. During the current shortage of nurses, one of the complaints most often heard from nurses is that they do not have enough time to care for their patients, or that there is such heavy assignment that patients are not getting the necessary care. When new nursing students are asked why they entered nursing, the most common answer is to "help and care for people." The individual nurse looks at caring as the role necessary to return a patient to health, provide a meaningful life, or provide a peaceful death. At the very core of the caring ethic lies the nurse-patient relationship and the responsibility it entails. According to Steckler (1998), a nurse's ethical decisions are made within the context of an implicit agreement between patient and nurse. Wilmont (1998) would agree; he argues for a contractarian perspective on ethics and sees the nurse-patient relationship as grounding for such concepts as accountability, rights, and duty. The nurse's commitments are clearly identifiable and highly explicit in the agreement. The two people, nurse and patient, mutually agree (to an extent) what the relationship will entail. Each finds it meaningful, and it is likely that each will be changed to some extent by it.

In 1992, Hartman conducted a study of the values guiding the practice of professional nurses using 100 Bachelor's-degree prepared medical-surgical nurses as her research sample. She asked, "What is a good thing a nurse like yourself can do? What is a bad thing that a nurse like yourself can do?" The most dominant theme of the "good thing I can do" was caring. The "bad thing I can do" related to a lack of caring or to actual harmful actions (e.g., being prejudiced, providing poor care, harming a patient, ignoring negligence.) In her article *Revisiting the Call to Care: An Ethical Perspective* (1998), Hartman reports on her study and reflects that it showed commitment to the bioethical principles of autonomy, fidelity, beneficence, veracity, and freedom; she notes that (surprisingly) confidentiality and privacy were not represented in the responses. A vital condition for establishing the kind of nurse-patient agreement that encourages collaboration in times of ethical crisis is trust. Veracity, confidentiality, and privacy are critical to that level of trust; no firm relationship can develop without them. "It might be questioned whether or not privileged information can exist within the complex environment of the prevailing health care delivery system" (Hartman, 1998). Hartman questions whether the health care team's need to know supercedes patient privacy, especially in situations of interdisciplinary care.

The intentional act of caring by the professional nurse transcends place; intentional caring happens in homeless shelters, intensive care units, prison infirmaries, and even at accident sites along a busy interstate where a nurse-volunteer has stopped to give aid. In other words, it happens virtually anywhere. As Manthey comments in an interview about timeless nursing values and all the places nursing takes place (Manthey, Wolf, Carlson, Salmon, & Moccia, 2000), "It's always about the nurse and the patient. Despite technology, materialism, finances, managed care, and everything else, it still has to be about a nurse and a patient."

Ann, a women's health NP and sexual assault nurse examiner, tells her story as evidence of the "anywhere" about which Manthey spoke. Ann took her completed doctoral dissertation to a small print shop in her hometown and left it for several days while copies were made for members of her dissertation committee. Her research dealt with immediate care of the rape victim and included a detailed clinical simulation she developed as the independent variable for the study. The simulation was a case involving a college student raped by a stranger; the clinical details of the nurse-patient encounter were graphic, as were the trauma diagrams in the "chart." There was also a transcribed telephone crisis call between the simulated victim and the APN/sexual assault advocate. When Ann returned to collect her copies near closing time, the female clerk was alone in the shop. While putting the newly printed pages into boxes for Ann, the clerk commented, "I hope you don't mind that I read some of your paper." Ann said that it was okay; this was not a real patient that needed her privacy protected, but a "paper patient" Ann had created. The clerk responded, "I wish I had known there were nurses like your nurse—the nurse in your story." Then she began to cry and disclosed that she was raped at age 16 and never told anyone until this day because she was afraid and ashamed. Slowly, the story unfolded. After a time, she locked the shop door and asked Ann to come in the back and have tea while she continued to share her story. In that print shop, over chipped mugs of tea, Ann performed victim counseling, 26 years after the rape. Ann would have to agree with a statement attributed to Zane Robinson Wolf in an interview on the timeless values of nursing (Manthey et al, 2000). Wolf, who presides over the International Association of Human Caring, stated, "Caring takes place during single moments as nurses and patients connect. During such encounters lie the rewards of nursing."

Advocacy as a Component of Intentional Caring

Recently, the nursing profession has determined that one of its necessary roles in the nurse-patient relationship is one of advocacy. An advocate is one who pleads the cause of another. The values and ethical framework adopted by the individual nurse have a tremendous effect on how the role of patient advocate is implemented. Major components of the advocacy role are the provision of information and support of the patient's rights. This presupposes that the patient is willing to have the information provided; that the nurse either knows or has access to the information needed by the patient; and that the nurse has the capacity to frame the information in words understandable to the patient and the other people significant to his or her decision-making process.

The support component of advocacy refers to objective support and not taking over the decision oneself; it implies that a nurse show neither approval nor disapproval for the decision. The nurse must show acceptance and respect for the decision, whatever it is, even if it does not conform to the nurse's personal belief or to the decision the nurse would have made. In a way, advocates must place their own morals or values "on hold" for the sake of the patient's views. This can be a challenge. Even if nurses do not verbally disagree with or try to dissuade the patient from a particular decision, they must realize that nonverbal messages can have a powerful effect. When there is conflict between the values of a nurse and patient, the principle of advocacy demands that the nurse find another advocate for the patient. For example, Vivian is a clinical nurse specialist (CNS) who is morally opposed to abortion in any circumstance. Although she would never tell a patient how she personally feels about abortion or encourage a patient not to have an abortion, she realizes that her facial expressions might give away her beliefs, unfairly influencing a patient's decision. Therefore Vivian says to her patient, who has hinted that she is considering abortion, "It sounds as if you might want to discuss the abortion option further. Susan, one of my colleagues, has considerable experience working with women who are considering abortion. Why don't I get her to come in so the two of you may explore that option." Vivian then asks Susan, another CNS, to work with the patient, agreeing to take on some of Susan's work to offset her additional assignment.

Donahue (1985) reiterates that patients and peers must be allowed to have their own values, which they will use to direct their courses of action, or to "dispose" of those values in certain situations without external pressure or coercion. Sam, a nurse anesthetist, is working in a pain management center when Gloria, one of his coworkers, comes in for help with her incapacitating chronic pain. Several times in the operating room, Gloria, a scrub technician, has made disparaging remarks about pain clinics. She has often been quite verbal about people "who claim disability and get someone to let them quit work and draw a government check." However, as an advocate for Gloria, Sam allows her to receive care at this "pain clinic," never mentioning the past discussions. Sam has, in effect, allowed Gloria to "dispose" of her values about chronic pain sufferers in order to meet her own needs. The example of Sam and Gloria emphasizes that advocacy goes beyond information and support to taking action on the behalf of others. It also exemplifies the notion of contractarian ethics about which Wilmont (1998) wrote. As a result of this nurse-patient relationship, both parties will likely change to some extent.

Advocacy is sometimes risky. Some actions on the part of nurses and in the name of advocacy conflict with the loyalty institutions expect from their employees. Sometimes a job may even be jeopardized by an advocate's actions. The ultimate question may become, "For what am I willing to sacrifice my position at this institution?" The following case, relating to a potential loss of a clinical placement site, serves as an example of this principle. Haley is a family nurse practitioner (FNP) student setting up a clinical site for a women's health course. Working from the list of potential preceptors provided by the course coordinator, Haley has become desperate to find a legitimate spot that meets her own learning needs, her part-time work schedule, her family's needs, and her desire not to commute long distances on clinical days. Although she is a good student and presents herself well in negotiations with prospective preceptors, there is considerable competition for clinical spots. Her dialogue with this new physician in the community seems positive, despite his not having served as a preceptor before. The physician agrees to the preceptorship in principle, but he asks that Haley leave the preceptor orientation materials and her clinical objectives with him. She is to return in 4 days to pick up the signed agreements. The physician phones Haley 2 days later and says that when he noticed a clinical objective relating to advocacy, he decided he should call her. The physician emphasizes that this is a "Christian practice staffed by people, including himself, opposed to abortion." He informs Haley that he will not tolerate discussion about abortions in his practice, irrespective of the circumstances. If that is agreed, he will welcome her as a clinical student. Haley has serious concerns that this expectation will compromise her work with pregnant women. She says, "I would never suggest an abortion to someone, but I would like to be able to help any woman with an unwanted pregnancy explore all the available options. At the very least, I would want to answer her questions." Haley's decision in this matter can be a risky one for her.

In this scenario, Haley has to answer the questions Padgett (1998) suggests will become ever more common in corporate settings and in case management. To whom is the nurse advocate accountable? To what standard? What tradeoffs are options? Who or what is the prime focus of obligation and duty?

Can an APN be both advocate and gatekeeper of the health care purse? Chafey, Rhea, Shannon, and Spencer (1998) used interviews of 17 hospital and community nurses in an effort to discover whether and in what ways the nurses exercised advocacy as part of their practice. The respondents identified supporting, teaching, and informing as part of nursing advocacy; they also suggested that qualities of empathy, assertiveness, self-confidence, and connection were conducive to advocacy. Personal fatigue, fear, frustration, patient acuity, domineering people, financial imperatives, and time constraints were listed as impediments to being a patient advocate. As a result of this study, the authors conclude that advocacy is a critical, perhaps unique dimension of professional nursing, the nature of which is changing in the existing health care system.

Ethical Dilemmas

That nurses confront moral and ethical problems frequently in practice does not diminish the potential uncertainty and angst they feel at such times. Feelings of powerlessness are common because, as is described in the very definition of ethical dilemmas, the decisions made must come from equally unsatisfactory alternatives (Erlen & Frost, 1991). Discussing the commonness of ethical dilemmas in contemporary practice, one perinatal CNS remarked, "It would be unlikely in these times for a week to go by on any busy clinical unit without some moral dilemma arising—without some level of concern or distress about the right choices to make."

Davis et al (1997) describe three features of ethical dilemmas: (1) conflicting values, obligations, loyalties, interests and needs are involved; (2) ethical principles or values are at issue; and (3) the feelings and values of the stakeholders in the situation will be affected, despite the ultimate decision made. After a decision has been made to resolve an ethical dilemma, there can be no legitimate argument as to the inherent rightness or wrongness of the decision. Second-guessing the decision is pointless; the case cannot be redone. However, a review of the process and the resolution may be cathartic and engender further values clarification that can ease the burden of future decision-making. (Details about the process of ethical decision-making are provided in Chapter 15.)

In the midst of ethical dilemmas, nurses often find their greatest support coming from coworkers, from fellow nurses. Those who work from a different ethical perspective, such as physicians and administrators, are likely to be perceived as less supportive. Some clinical settings have established informal support forums for difficult clinical situations "after the fact," much like the notion of a "screaming room" for those who deal with difficult diagnoses in practice day-after-day. Nurses are wise to affirm each other in the moments and hours after ethical dilemmas have been resolved as a means of empowerment. It is also important to know about other more formal mechanisms for assistance during or immediately after ethical dilemmas that might exist within an institution.

On occasion, an ethical dilemma is further complicated by conflicts between providers who work from different models. Grundstein-Amado (1992) finds that nurses place the highest fundamental value on a caring perspective (i.e., the nursing model), while physicians' value the scientific perspective (i.e., the disease/cure or medical model). This difference in professional orientation and approach may place nurses, as patient advocates, in conflict with colleagues in social work, pharmacy, occupational therapy, physical therapy, and dietetics. An example reveals this variance in approach. Julie, a 45-year-old divorced woman who has breast cancer, is receiving outpatient chemotherapy. She desperately wants her children, ages 4, 6, and 8, who are on school vacation, to remain with her in this setting, even though she has some difficulty caring for them. While the CNS wants to honor this request, the social worker believes that the children would be better served by staying with their father.

Some of the ethical dilemmas faced in today's clinical settings relate to the fact that health care is now considered big business, and the goals of big business and health care can be at odds. Mohr and Mahon (1996) warn professional nurses about what they label "dirty hands situations." In such situations, "one agent is morally forced by someone else's immorality to do what is, or otherwise would be, wrong." They give the example of what greed has done to the tobacco industry; out of greed came (apparent) lies and coverups that have produced "dirty hands" for many in the industry. Mohr and Mahon advise nurses to be cautious about the "dirty hands" phenomenon in light of what is occurring in health care. Although the principles of efficiency, competition, and profit-making are not unethical when prudently applied, they become problematic when the corporate culture ceases to be morally responsible to its employees and clients. A lack of moral responsibility in health care organizations can lead to abuses, such as charging for services never rendered, unwillingness to pay for legitimate insurance claims, and financially penalizing consumers who use out-of-system providers or who exceed capitation prepayments.

Ethics Committees, Ethical Consultations, and Institutional Review Boards

The Joint Commission on the Accreditation of Healthcare Organizations (JCAHO) mandates that a health care organization have mechanisms in place to address ethical issues in providing care. These mechanisms may include an established ethics committee, a formalized ethics forum, or ethics consultation provided by a staff ethicist or one outside of the institution (JCAHO, 1996). Today, most hospitals and other health care organizations have ethics committees that were formed to deal with the complex issues facing heath care providers. Ethics committees are often interdisciplinary, an advantage because answers to ethical dilemmas come from a variety of disciplines. Ethics committees may be composed of community members (possibly former patients or family members), physicians, nurses, other health professionals, clergy, ethicists, and legal representatives. Members of the agency's administrative staff are also often members, although their inclusion has sometimes been questioned.

Expecting the executive staff to implement decisions without a voice in them places the executives in an untenable position—possibly carrying out decisions with which they are uncomfortable or that are contrary to the agency's mission or policies. The ethics committee typically reviews cases, makes policies, educates staff, and acts as mediators in ethical conflicts. In some cases they may meet to make the actual collective decision about how to resolve an ethical conflict. As part of the formal hospital structure, the ethics committee is expected to conform to the rules and protocols of the agency.

Jonsen et al (1998) maintain that an ethics committee requires the following:

- Endorsement and support by administration, medical staff, and nursing staff, including sufficient resources to work effectively. The committee's placement within the institution's organizational chart should be clear, showing designated lines of reporting.
- Respect by peers. The committee members should be individuals who are willing to meet regularly and keep confidential records of their deliberations, in accord with relevant laws.
- An educational function for informing staff about the existence, role, and processes involved in the work of the committee, including how to contact them.
- Opportunities for bioethics education of members and prospective members.
- A systematic method for review of cases.

An example of the way in which an ethics committee works is shown in the following scenario, an actual case with fictitious names. Baby Boy Navarez was born prematurely (22 weeks gestation) at an inner-city major medical center. The baby's single, 17-year-old mother Juanita and her mother Rutha were told during the premature labor that the baby would likely not survive because of his level of immaturity. Throughout labor, the perinatal staff and the grief team provided care and grief support for Juanita and Rutha. Juanita saw her son briefly in the birthing room, expecting (because of what she has been told by everyone on the perinatal/neonatal team) that she would have photographs taken of her son and spend private time with him later; during the hours of labor, she and her mother saw evidence that the staff honors such commitments (fidelity). Juanita and her mother understood that the baby's prognosis was poor, and because they were given truthful information in terms clear to them (veracity) about the options for care, they decided (autonomy) for the "care and comfort" option. Everyone involved perceived care and comfort as more humane than "heroic" measures, such as invasive and painful procedures, especially given understanding of the quality of life expected for such a premature infant (beneficence/nonmaleficence). However, despite all of this, a neonatology resident on weekend call made a unilateral decision to place the baby on life support, irrespective of the team's collective concerns about this decision.

When the attending neonatologist returned from his weekend off, he was met by the nurse manager and neonatal nurse practitioner (NNP), who were both upset. They explained what happened and shared their frustration. He also heard of the mother's confusion and despair, made worse when another resident told her that she would probably have to make a decision to remove the baby from life support. The neonatologist then learned that, despite

life support, the baby's condition was deteriorating. After speaking to all the people involved, the neonatologist asked that the Committee for Clinical Ethics be impaneled to recommend some resolution to this complex dilemma. The committee carefully reviewed the facts; interviewed the staff members directly involved in the baby's care; and spoke with Juanita and her mother (through the aid of an interpreter) to learn their wishes in the matter. Committee members also sought the recommendation of the attending physician. After lengthy, careful deliberation and advice from the legal representative of the committee, the informed opinion was offered: discontinuation of life support was appropriate. The life support disconnected, Juanita, with Mrs. Navarez and the NNP at her side, held her dying son.

APNs are often invited to serve on ethics committees because of their knowledge of the clinical domain; leadership ability; foundation in bioethics; ability to think critically and analyze complex phenomena; and articulate a professional position, even in the face of disagreement. As a committee member, the APN is expected to become familiar with the literature and research methods of bioethics and share informed opinions about the issues with the group (Jonsen et al, 1998).

In general, important moral decisions are and should be made together by an APN and his or her patient. The decisions with which clinicians are faced in today's health care arena, however, are so complex that ethics consultation can be of inestimable value. At times, an ethical consultant is on an institution's staff or on a retainer. The process for accessing the assistance of that individual should be clear to the professional staff. Ethical consultation is modeled on the familiar practice of patient consultation. The consulting individual, who has special education in bioethics, is available to clinicians, and sometimes to patients and their families, to review the case and provide informed, prudent counsel related to it (Jonsen et al, 1998).

The ethics demanded of research are associated with a special type of ethics committee: the Institutional Review Board (IRB) (sometimes referred to as the Human Subjects Committee). This collective must consist of more than five individuals, one of whom is not a researcher, that have no personal or family affiliation with the institution sponsoring the committee (e.g., hospital, university). To further eliminate potential bias, both men and women must be on the committee, and they cannot be members of the same profession (Polit & Hungler, 1995).

The role of the IRB is to review research proposals to ensure that the rights of humans, as research subjects, are being protected. To do that, the group ensures that the benefit of the research outweighs the risks involved to the subjects, and that the essential provisions of informed consent have been diligently followed. An IRB has the choice to approve the research being conducted as proposed; suggest specific modifications to ensure humans are protected; or disapprove of the research. Based on the

Rights of Human Research Subjects Ensured by an Institutional Review Board

1. The right to self-determination (autonomy). This refers to subjects' control of their own destiny with respect to the research study and the freedom to determine for themselves, without external pressure from the researcher, their level of participation in the study.
2. The right to privacy.
3. The right to anonymity or confidentiality. This refers to the assurance that subjects' individual responses can not be linked in any way to them unless they approve.
4. The right to fair treatment (justice). This refers to subjects being given what they were promised or owed as a result of their participation in the study.
5. The right to protection from discomfort or harm (beneficence).

Adapted from Polit, D., & Hungler, B.P. (1995). *Nursing research: principles and methods* (6th ed.). Philadelphia: JB Lippincott.

American Nurses Association Code for Nurses

1. The nurse provides services with respect for human dignity and the uniqueness of the patient unrestricted by considerations of social or economic status, personal attributes, or the nature of health problems.
2. The nurse safeguards the patient's right to privacy by judiciously protecting information of a confidential nature.
3. The nurse acts to safeguard the patient and the public when health care and safety are affected by the incompetent, unethical, or illegal practice of any person.
4. The nurse assumes responsibility and accountability for individual nursing judgments and actions.
5. The nurse maintains competence in nursing.
6. The nurse exercises informed judgment and uses individual competence and qualifications as criteria in seeking consultation, accepting responsibilities, and delegating nursing activities to others.
7. The nurse participates in activities that contribute to the development of the profession's body of knowledge.
8. The nurse participates in the profession's efforts to implement and improve standards of nursing.
9. The nurse participates in the profession's effort to establish and maintain conditions of employment conductive to high-quality nursing care.
10. The nurse participates in the profession's effort to protect the public from misinformation and misrepresentation and to maintain the integrity of nursing.
11. The nurse collaborates with members of the health professions and other citizens in promoting community and national efforts to meet the health needs of the public.

From American Nurses Foundation & American Nurses Association (1985). *Code for nurses with interpretive statements*. Washington, DC: American Nurses Publishing.

nature of the study, the decision is made for full review (the entire panel is convened to review the study because of the risk element) or expedited review (only the chairperson or designee conducts the review because the study's risk to humans is minimal). Alternately, the research may be exempt from review in cases where there is no apparent risk involved. For example, a study would be exempt if it involved only retrospective reviews of charts or test results. In deciding which of the three alternatives is appropriate, the IRB follows federal guidelines. (Box 14-1 summarizes the human rights required for protection of human research subjects; the ethical principles involved are the same as for direct care of patients.)

Ethical Codes

Nursing professionals have adopted codes to assist in guiding their moral practice obligations and responses to ethical dilemmas. A code of ethics is "a formal statement of a group's ideals and values. It is a set of ethical principles that is shared by members of the group, reflects their moral judgment over time, and serves as a standard for professional actions"(Kozier, Erb, Blais, & Wilkinson, 1998). The first ethical code for nursing was provided in 1950 by the ANA; it was last updated in 1985 (Box 14-2). The American Nurses Association (ANA) also published standards of professional performance for APNs (Box 14-3). The *International Code of Ethics for Nurses* was initiated in 1953 and last revised in 2000 (Box 14-4).

Kozier et al (1998) list the following purposes for a nursing code of ethics: (1) informing the public about minimum professional standards and professional conduct, (2) signifying the profession's commitment to the public, (3) outlining the major ethical considerations of the profession, (4) providing general guidelines for professional behavior, and (5) guiding professionals in self-regulation. Standards of clinical nursing practice, established by the professional nursing organizations for their specialty populations, also serve to guide ethical practice by APNs. The ANA developed a generic set of professional standards to guide all of nursing practice. In 1996, the ANA published *Scope and Standards of Advanced Practice Registered Nursing*. This document says the following about ethical expectations for those in APN practice: "The advanced practice registered nurse makes ethical decisions and takes ethical actions . . . acknowledges the client's rights of self-determination, truthful disclosure, privacy, and confidentiality and respects the client's dignity [and]

Box 14-3

American Nurses Association Standards
of Professional Performance

Standard V: Ethics
The advanced practice registered nurse integrates ethical
principles and norms in all areas of practice.
Measurement criteria
1. The advanced practice registered nurse maintains a
   therapeutic and professional relationship and discusses
   the delineation of roles and parameters of the relationship with the patient.
2. The advanced practice registered nurse informs the
   patient of the risks, benefits, and outcomes of health
   care regimens.
3. The advanced practice registered nurse contributes to
   resolving the ethical problems or dilemmas of individuals or systems.

From American Nurses Association (1996). *Scope and standards of
advanced practice registered nursing.* Washington, DC: American Nurses
Association.

cultural beliefs. She or he serves as an advocate for the
client and is obligated to demonstrate non-judgmental
and non-discriminatory behaviors that are sensitive to
client diversity . . . [he or she also] works to facilitate client
decision-making, promote ethical practice environments,
and protect professional integrity" (ANA, 1996). When
specialty organizations publish standards for the professional practice of their constituency, they are usually more
detailed and specific.

IMPLICATIONS FOR MSN EDUCATION AND ADVANCED PRACTICE

The American Association of Colleges of Nursing (AACN),
in its *The Essentials of College and University Education
for Professional Nursing* (AACN, 1996a), identified seven
core values as essential to the practice of nursing: altruism,
equality, esthetics, freedom, human dignity, justice, and
truth. Weis, Schank, Eddy, and Elfrink (1993) conducted a
study to determine whether these seven core values were
reflected in the program objectives of baccalaureate
programs. Using a cross-sectional survey of both public
and private programs accredited by the National League
for Nursing Accrediting Commission, stratified according
to geographical locale and program type, the researchers
analyzed professional nursing behaviors reflecting the
seven core values in program objectives. Five values—
altruism (caring), equality, freedom, human dignity, and

justice—were found in the majority of programs, while
truth and esthetics were found in a minority of programs.
These findings seem to indicate that values permeate
professional nursing education at the generalist level. The
implication, then, is that APN education can build on this
foundation as values are reexamined in preparation for a
new place in the health care system as specialists.

Husted and Husted (1998) believe the nurse's ethical
obligations are formulated within the context of the
nurse-patient relationship. Since the nature of the nurse-
patient relationship changes with specialization, it seems
likely that one's ethical duty, as an APN, is reformulated as
the new role evolves. According to Husted and Husted
(1998) the nurse's ethical self develops in stages. They
frame that notion in the stages of Benner's justly celebrated
theory "novice to expert." With regard to ethics, the APN
is likely never a true novice again; however, there may be
some self-recognition that a renewed sense of ethical
accountability is developing with each clinical encounter.
Gaining clarity about one's philosophical and ethical base
for advanced practice is facilitated by case analysis followed
by reflection on the experience, either verbally or in
writing.

There are three distinct levels of ethical inquiry: descriptive ethics, normative ethics, and metaethics. Descriptive ethics explores ethical theory as a basis for finding
answers to moral and ethical questions. Normative ethics
attempts to answer questions about what decision would be
right or wrong in a particular situation. Metaethics refers to
analysis of the meaning of terms associated with the study
of ethics (Cameron & Shaffer, 1992). In an APN program,
students are ideally exposed to all three levels of inquiry.
When a student group debates the virtue of utilitarianism
versus deontology as an approach to a particular dilemma,
they are engaging in descriptive ethics. While analyzing the
case of a patient who is "dumped" from one emergency
room to another because of his lack of insurance, students
are involved in normative ethics inquiry. Students engage
in metaethics when they debate the question of what it
means to be faithful.

In educating APNs to be ethically competent, it is
imperative that educators structure learning opportunities
based on real-world experiences. The ability of students to
think critically about ethical issues and to handle ethical
situations skillfully and sensitively is essential to a liberal
education for most professional disciplines today. Interdisciplinary study of ethics is of inestimable value for APN
students because they will learn that the answers to such
dilemmas come from multiple perspectives. Some programs have a separate course in philosophy or ethics; more
often, the topic of ethics is integrated throughout the
curriculum and applied in clinical settings and through
case analysis in the classroom.

Using case studies helps students practice a structured
analytical approach to a reasoned decision outside of the
"noise" of the real world. Not only does this approach

Box 14-4

International Council of Nurses Code of Ethics for Nurses

An international code of ethics for nurses was first adopted by the International Council of Nurses (ICN) in 1953. It has been revised and reaffirmed at various times since, most recently with this review and revision completed in 2000.

Preamble

Nurses have four fundamental responsibilities: to promote health, to prevent illness, to restore health, and to alleviate suffering. The need for nursing is universal.

Inherent in nursing is respect for human rights, including the right to life, to dignity, and to be treated with respect. Nursing care is unrestricted by considerations of age, color, creed, culture, disability or illness, gender, nationality, politics, race, or social status.

Nurses render health services to the individual, the family, and the community and coordinate their services with those of related groups.

The Code

The Code of Ethics for Nurses has four principal elements that outline the standards of ethical conduct.

Elements of the code

1. *Nurses and people*

The nurse's primary professional responsibility is to people requiring nursing care.

In providing care, the nurse promotes an environment in which the human rights, values, customs, and spiritual beliefs of the individual, family, and community are respected.

The nurse ensures that the individual receives sufficient information on which to base consent for care and related treatment.

The nurse holds in confidence personal information and uses judgement in sharing this information.

The nurse shares with society the responsibility for initiating and supporting action to meet the health and social needs of the public, in particular those of vulnerable populations.

The nurse also shares responsibility to sustain and protect the natural environment from depletion, pollution, degradation, and destruction.

2. *Nurses and practice*

The nurse carries personal responsibility and accountability for nursing practice and for maintaining competence by continual learning.

The nurse maintains a standard of personal health such that the ability to provide care is not compromised.

The nurse uses judgement regarding individual competence when accepting and delegating responsibility.

The nurse at all times maintains standards of personal conduct that reflect well on the profession and enhance public confidence.

The nurse, in providing care, ensures that use of technology and scientific advances are compatible with the safety, dignity, and rights of people.

3. *Nurses and the profession*

The nurse assumes the major role in determining and implementing acceptable standards of clinical nursing practice, management, research, and education.

The nurse is active in developing a core of research-based professional knowledge.

The nurse, acting through the professional organization, participates in creating and maintaining equitable social and economic working conditions in nursing.

4. *Nurses and coworkers*

The nurse sustains a cooperative relationship with coworkers in nursing and other fields.

The nurse takes appropriate action to safeguard individuals when their care is endangered by a coworker or any other person.

From International Council of Nurses (2000). *ICN code for nurses: ethical concepts applied to nursing.* Geneva, Switzerland: Imprimeries Populaires.

---

enhance the students' knowledge of ethical theory, it increases their ability to publicly articulate difficult positions with confidence. Over time, students become more tolerant of resolutions different from their own and come to appreciate the pervasiveness of ethical problems in practice (Vallentyne & Accordino 1998). They learn that this system of case analysis can be counted on in the future. Debates (especially when a person argues a position to which he or she is morally opposed), values clarification exercises, and roleplaying can also be used effectively in examining ethical issues. Several strategies increase the effectiveness of roleplaying while decreasing student anxiety: debriefing after roleplaying, using fictitious names for participants, and ensuring that the content of the role being played is the focus, not the acting ability of the participants.

As the ability to use research in practice and to formulate researchable problems are expectations of the graduate of a Master's program, students must learn about the ethical dimensions of research, including the often troubling historical basis for a concern with ethics in empirical studies. The concept of informed consent deserves considerable attention, as do the elements of research design that ensure protection of human subjects. As students learn the process of research critique, they may be asked to apply the principles to a critique of both quantitative and qualitative studies relevant to APN practice. Knowledge of the work of the IRB in full, expedited, and exempt reviews of study proposals is of value to understanding the research subrole of APN practice.

"Educators are moral agents helping to form other

moral agents" (Steckler, 1998). In the same way that nursing faculty models caring behavior by the way they treat students, patients, and colleagues, they model ethical behaviors. The principles of ethics are no less applicable to educational settings than to practice settings. For example, a professor shows a value for autonomy by treating students as adults who are responsible for their own learning and by serving as a facilitator of learning, not a "sage on the stage, but a guide on the side." When educators allow students the freedom of selecting their own clinical sites and preceptors and developing personal learning objectives, they are giving students autonomy.

The principle of beneficence is shown by educators through being a good role model; preparing students for the reality of clinical practice and the subroles of their particular specialty; and ensuring that students are safe practitioners with the necessary knowledge base, values, and technical skills for the practice of advanced "nursing" (not "semi-medicine"). Beneficent faculty give students a voice in the program and monitor their progress closely, giving objective constructive feedback. To ensure credibility and a reality-based approach, a beneficent educator likely engages in faculty practice and teaches students how to work within and help change the existing delivery system. A beneficent educator wants students to succeed and exit their formal education with a commitment to lifelong learning; such an educator puts mechanisms in place to that end.

The principle of fidelity is evidenced in a curriculum designed and implemented as is promised by the marketing campaign and the university recruiter. When faculty return phone calls, adhere to scheduled office hours, and protect students' privacy and confidentiality, they are engaging in behaviors consistent with fidelity. "If fidelity can be viewed as the glue that holds the nurse-patient relationship together in the moral sense, it certainly can be viewed as the glue that holds together the relationship between a learner and an educator" (Steckler, 1998). Examples of the principle of veracity include providing honest information about program expectations, costs, and required travel; conducting candid clinical evaluations; reporting certification and job placement rates; and adhering to published deadlines and policies. The ethical principle of justice is demonstrated when faculty are fair and nondiscriminatory in the way they treat students and in their allocation of program resources.

In her work with children with disabilities, Savage (1998) introduces a common attitude held by most physicians and nurses—*humanism*, a term attributed to Ehrenfeld (1978). Humanism is the belief that all problems are solvable given enough resources and technology. Health professionals tend to feel a sense of personal failure when a patient does not get well. One must learn, though, that it is unnecessary to use all the resources at one's command to keep everyone alive. The patient and family may decide that death is preferable to a life without

quality. Introducing APN students to the concept of humanism can be of inestimable value to them as direct providers and supportive colleagues. For example, Chris, a pediatric nurse practitioner (PNP) student, worked all semester with Joey and his family as they first awaited Joey's kidney transplant and then went through the surgery. Chris was at the hospital when Joey died as a result of organ rejection. The nurses on the unit were frustrated and dispirited; the physician with whom Chris had worked came into the nursing station after walking Joey's parents to the exit and threw a chart across the room, not at Chris but in her general direction. Instead of getting angry, Chris picked up the chart and handed it to the physician, saying, "It hurts like heck, doesn't it?" This simple phrase seemed to empower the physician and the nurses, who overheard Chris's question, to speak about Joey and their feelings of loss and failure. Such support works both ways; on another occasion, it may be Chris who has a poor outcome and needs to understand the emotions associated with humanism.

Nurses and nursing are well served when professionals in practice clarify the core concept of caring within the context of the nurse-patient relationship. There must be an appreciation that the competitive, money-driven medical system is likely here to stay; conflicts with ethical principles will abound, but the tenets of an ethical practice must remain inviolate. Nurses must put their patients first and not allow the aims of the business of health care to replace humanistic values (Larkin, 1999). APNs will discover that it is not easy to be morally accountable; every ethical dilemma is intertwined with ambiguity. As never before, APNs need to realize that caring, moral principles, and ethical ideals meet at the center of the nurse-patient relationship. "Nursing is a behavioral manifestation of the nurse's value system" (Fowler & Levine-Ariff, 1987). APNs must examine their value system, engage in values clarification, and embrace a philosophy of practice guided by ethical tenets. When they can bring that to the health care arena, APNs are positioned for a preferred future as providers, with the potential to influence equity in health care and ethical treatment of patients. In this era of managed care, there is a perpetual focus on the bottom line. For APNs, an appropriate bottom line would be this one by Weston (1997): "Ethics asks us to resist close-heartedness, to keep the heart open."

PRIORITIES FOR RESEARCH

Empirical study of ethical issues with professional nurses is limited; research related to APNs is virtually nonexistent. Consequently, well-designed studies would be welcome in helping the profession understand how APNs respond to protracted dilemmas; the nature of their ethical reasoning; and whether their position partly within the medical domain affects the kinds of ethical problems they face. For example, in what ways do physicians and APNs approach ethical dilemmas similarly? Differently? Does a particular corporate culture affect the types of dilemmas faced by APNs or the approaches used for resolution? To what extent are employers involved in solving ethical conflicts among staff? What is the lived experience of APNs who serve as members of an ethics committee?

Descriptive study might determine approaches being used to teach ethics in graduate programs, as well as determining student and faculty perception of their effectiveness. Can a "thinking out loud" approach be used by an APN experienced in moral reasoning to help a novice learn a structured approach? Do APNs educated through a nursing model solve moral problems differently than those who were educated through a medical model?

Penticuff and Walden (2000) examined the relative contributions of practice environments and personal characteristics on the willingness of perinatal nurses to be engaged in resolving ethical dilemmas. A correlational design and multiple regression was used to analyze the responses of 127 nurses in high-risk obstetrical and neonatal intensive care settings. Nurses who perceived a higher degree of influence in the practice environment and had higher levels of concern about ethical aspects of clinical situations were more likely to become involved in dilemma resolution activities. The level of nursing education was not found to be a significant factor. Might this result be different if a replication were conducted for APN-level nurses? Would this study design be appropriate for examining the contributions of the primary care environment in a capitated system?

Interested in the way in which nurses reason through ethical dilemmas to clarify "real versus assumed profes-

sional reasoning," McAlpine, Krisjanson, and Poroch (1997) developed and tested an ethical reasoning tool (ERT). With this tool, respondents first analyze a case study. Researchers are then able to outline exemplar behaviors for the eight components of ethical thinking: recognition of ethical issues, use of an ethical framework, use of personal values, use of professional values, perception of the role of the nurse, perception of therapeutic nurse-patient relationship, communication patterns, and potential action. The theoretical base for this study indicates that "ethical thought lies along a continuum of cognitive progression from a narrow and self-serving perspective to a potential reflective and pluralistic perspective." Cognitive progression appears to be based on a variety of personal and contextual factors, including the professional mindset. These researchers believe the ERT holds promise for measuring professional responses to ethical dilemmas and evaluating the effectiveness of ethics education in a trustworthy way. Replication of this study with students in APN programs would be both interesting and informative.

DISCUSSION QUESTIONS

These questions can be used to promote critical thinking and encourage discussion.

1. In a small group format, discuss which of the ethical principles discussed in this chapter is most significant, offering a rationale for each choice. Examine the extent

---

Suggestions for Further Learning

- Husted and Husted (1998) suggest that "very few skills on the part of nurses have a greater ethical importance than skill at encouraging communication from the dying." With that idea in mind, read Ott, B. (1998). Physician-assisted suicide and older patient's perceived duty to die. *Advanced Practice Nursing Quarterly, 4*(2), 65-70. Discuss your reaction to the comment and the article in a peer group.
- Consult your particular specialty group for information about standards of practice.
- Consult the following websites for additional information on professional ethics:
  - National Institutes of Health (www.nih.gov/sigs/bioethics)
  - National Reference Center for Bioethics (Georgetown University) (www.georgetown.edu/research/nrcbl/)
  - Hastings Center (www.cpn.org/sections/affiliates/hastings_center.html)

- Nursing Ethics Network (infoeagle.bc.edu)
- Ethics Health Science Library Loyola University (this site has multiple links) (www.meddean.luc.edu/libraryofethics.html)
- The Center for Ethics and Human Rights (American Nurses Association) (www.nursingworld.org/ethics/)
- Read the following: Gordon, S. (1997). *Life support: three nurses on the front lines.* Boston: Little Brown. It provides insights about the professional scope of practice and the ethical dilemmas experienced in the cases of the three nurses.
- Also read: Tate, E.D., & Pranzatelli, M.R. (1999). *Unforgettable faces: through the eyes of a nurse practitioner.* Jacksonville, FL: Atheneum.
- Consult a current research text for criteria that distinguish among *full review, expedited review,* and *exempt review.* Also review the history of health care research to better appreciate the heritage that provides the basis for ethical research.

to which the views of the group reflect those in the interviews with nursing leaders in the following: Manthey, M., Wolf, Z.R., Carlson, K., Salmon, M., & Moccia, P. (2000). Nursing values: a look back, a view forward. *Creative Nursing, 6*(1), 5-11.

2. Bring up current dilemmas encountered in practice or in books of case studies. Debate or discuss the issues, taking a stance opposite of what you normally would.

3. Speculate on the response of deontology, teleology, and situational ethics to the following topics, consulting a reference as necessary:

   - Gay and lesbian couples who wish to be parents
   - People who wish to donate their organs for profit
   - Couples on Medicaid who require in vitro fertilization to achieve a pregnancy
   - Impaired nurses
   - Female circumcision.

4. Write your personal philosophy of advanced practice.
5. Read about caring theory and write your personal ethic of caring.
6. Discuss your own experiences with humanism.
7. According to several authors, the health care delivery system itself can compromise moral reasoning by a nurse. Chambliss (1997) refers to a nurse giving up to the "rhythm" of the institution. Explore the meaning of that idea with a group of peers.
8. Respond to Chafey's (1996) comment that the ethic of caring can not provide nurses with the power necessary to effect change.
9. Husted and Husted (1998) suggest that one's ethical self develops in stages in much the same way that Benner (1984) conceptualizes professionals developing from novice to expert. How have you seen your own ethical stance change in stages?

REFERENCES/BIBLIOGRAPHY

American Association of Colleges of Nursing (1996a). *The essentials of college and university education for professional nursing.* Washington, DC: American Association of Colleges of Nursing.

American Association of Colleges of Nursing (1996b). *The essentials of Master's education for advanced practice nurses.* Washington, DC: American Association of Colleges of Nursing.

American Nurses Association (1985). *Code for nurses with interpretive statements.* Kansas City: American Nurses Association.

American Nurses Association (1998). *Standards of clinical nursing practice.* Washington, DC: American Nurses Association.

American Nurses Association (1996). *Scope and standards of advanced practice registered nursing.* Washington, DC: American Nurses Association.

Bandman, E. L. & Bandman, B. (1995). *Nursing ethics: through the life span* (3rd ed.). Norwalk, CT: Appleton & Lange.

Barnett, T. (1993). Are there employment risks to unethical decisions? *Nursing Forum, 28,* 17-21.

Beauchamp, T.L., & Childress, J.F. (1994). *Principles of biomedical ethics* (4th ed.). New York: Oxford University Press.

Begany, T. (1994). Your image is brighter than ever. *RN, 57*(10), 28-35.

Benner, P., & Wrubel, J. (1989). *Primacy of caring.* Menlo Park, CA: Addison-Wesley.

Berger, M.C., Severson, A., & Chvatel, R. (1991). Ethical issues in nursing. *Western Journal of Nursing Research, 13*(4), 514-521.

Bishop, A.H., & Scudder, J.R. (1996). *Nursing ethics: therapeutic caring presence.* Boston: Jones & Bartlett.

Cameron, M.E., & Schaffer, M.A. (1992). Tell me the right answer: a model for teaching nursing ethics. *Journal of Nursing Education, 3*(8), 377-380.

Cassells, J., & Redman, B. (1989). Preparing students to be moral agents in clinical nursing practice. *Nursing Clinics of North America, 24,* 463-473.

Cassidy, V.R., & Oddi, L. F. (1991). Professional autonomy and ethical decision making among graduate and undergraduate nursing majors: a replication. *Journal of Nursing Education, 30*(4), 149-151.

Chafey, K. (1996). Caring is not enough: ethical paradigms for community-based care. *Nursing and Health Care, 17*(1), 10-16.

Chafey, K., Rhea, M., Shannon, A.M., & Spencer, S. (1998). Characterizations of advocacy by practicing nurses. *Journal of Professional Nursing, 14*(1), 45-52.

Chambliss, D.F. (1997). *Beyond caring: hospitals, nurses, and the social organization.* Chicago: University of Chicago Press.

Corley, M.C., & Selig, P.M. (1992). Nurse moral reasoning using the Nurse Dilemma Test. *Western Journal of Nursing Research, 14,* 380-388.

Craven, R.F., & Hirnle, C.J. (2000). *Fundamentals of nursing: human health and function.* Philadelphia: JB Lippincott.

Davis, A.J., Aroskar, M.A., Liaschenko, J., & Drought, T.S. (1997). *Ethical dilemmas and nursing practice* (4th ed.). Stamford, CT: Appleton & Lange.

deCasterle, B.D., & Janssen, P.J. (1996). The relationship between education and ethical behavior of nursing students. *Western Journal of Nursing Research, 18*(3), 330-351.

Donahue, M. (1985). Viewpoints: euthanasia: an ethical uncertainty. In J.C. McCloskey & H.K. Grace (Eds.), *Current issues in nursing* (2nd ed.). Cambridge, MA: Blackwell.

Ehrenfeld, D. (1978). *The arrogance of humanism.* New York: Oxford University Press.

Erlen, J.A., & Frost, B. (1991). Nurses' perceptions of powerlessness in influencing ethical decisions. *Western Journal of Nursing Research, 13*(3), 397-407.

Feutz-Harter, S.A. (1991). Ethics committees: a resource for patient care decision-making. *Journal of Nursing Administration, 21*(40), 1, 2,44.

Fowler, M., & Levine-Ariff, J. (1987). *Ethics at the bedside.* Philadelphia: JB Lippincott.

Gilligan, C. (1989). *In a different voice.* Cambridge, MA: Harvard University Press.

Gordon, S. (1997). *Life support: three nurses on the front lines.* Boston: Little Brown.

Gordon, S., & Fagin, C.M. (1996). Preserving the moral high ground. *American Journal of Nursing, 96*(3), 31-32.

Grundstein-Amado, R.J. (1992). Differences in ethical decision-making processes among nurses and doctors. *Journal of Advanced Nursing, 17*(2), 129-137.

Hadley, E.H. (1996). Nursing in the political and economic marketplace: challenges for the 21st century. *Nursing Outlook, 44*, 6-10.

Hartman, R.L. (1998). Revisiting the call to care: an ethical perspective. *Advanced Practice Nursing Quarterly, 4*(2), 14-18.

Heitman, L.K., & Robinson, R.E.S. (1997). Developing nursing ethics roundtables. *American Journal of Nursing, 97*(1), 36-38.

Hewa, S., & Hetherington, W. (1990). Specialists without spirit: crisis in the nursing profession. *Journal of Medical Ethics, 16*, 179-184.

Hosford, B. (1986). *Bioethics committees.* Rockville, MD: Aspen Publishers.

Husted, G. L., & Husted, J. H. (1995). *Ethical decision making in nursing* (2nd ed.). St. Louis: Mosby.

Husted, G.L., & Husted, J.H. (1998a). New perspectives on bioethical decision-making. *Advanced Practice Nursing Quarterly, 4*(2), v.

Husted, G.L., & Husted, J.H. (1998b). Strength of character through the ethics of nursing. *Advanced Practice Nursing Quarterly, 3*(4), 23-25.

Husted, G.L., & Husted, J.H. (1998c). With the ethical agreement: where are you now? *Advanced Practice Nursing Quarterly, 4*(2), 34-35.

International Council of Nurses (2000). *ICN code for nurses: ethical concepts applied to nursing.* Geneva, Switzerland: Imprimeries Populaires.

Jecker, N.S. (1994). Managed competition and managed care: what are the ethical issues? *Clinics in Geriatric Medicine, 10*, 527-539.

Joint Commission on Accreditation of Healthcare Organizations (1996). *Accreditation manual for hospitals.* Chicago: Joint Commission on Accreditation of Healthcare Organizations.

Jones, R., & Beck, S. (1996). *Decision making in nursing.* Albany: Delmar Publishers.

Jonsen, A.R., Siegler, M., & Winslade, W.J. (1998). *Clinical ethics* (4th ed.). New York: McGraw-Hill.

Kelly, C. (1998). Investing or discounting self: are moral decisions shaped by conditions in the workplace? *Advanced Practice Nursing Quarterly, 4*(2), 8-13.

King, E. (1984). *Effective education in nursing.* Rockville, MD: Aspen Publishers.

Kohne, M.F. (1980). The nurse as advocate. *American Journal of Nursing, 80*(11), 2038-2040.

Korniewicz, D.M., & Palmer, M.H. (1997). The preferred future for nursing. *Nursing Outlook, 45*, 108-113.

Kozier, B., Erb, G., Blais, K., & Wilkinson, J.M. (1998). *Fundamentals of nursing: concepts, processes, and practice* (5th ed.). Menlo Park, CA: Addison-Wesley.

Larkin, G.L. (1999). Ethical issues of managed care. *Emergency Medicine Clinics of North America, 17*(2), 397-415.

Liaschenko, J. (1998). Moral evaluation and concepts of health and health promotion. *Advanced Practice Nursing Quarterly, 4*(2), 71-77.

Loewry, E.H., & Loewry, L.S. (1998). Ethics and managed care: reconstructing a system and refashioning a society. *Archives of Internal Medicine, 158*(22), 2419-2422.

Loewry, E.H., & Loewry, R.A. (1999). Editor's correspondence—ethics and managed care can coexist with a free market. *Archives of Internal Medicine, 159*(12). Available online at archinte.ama-assn.org/issues/v159n12/full/ilt0628-6.html.

Manthey, M., Wolf, Z.R., Carlson, K., Salmon, M.E., & Moccia, P. (2000). Nursing values: looking back, a view forward. *Creative Nursing, 6*(1), 5-11.

McAlpine, H., Kristjanson, L., & Poroch, D. (1997). Development and testing of the ethical reasoning tool (ERT): an instrument to measure the ethical reasoning of nurses. *Journal of Advanced Nursing, 25*, 1151-1161.

Mohr, W.K., & Mahon, M.M. (1996). Dirty hands: the underside of market place health care. *Advances in Nursing Science, 19*(1), 28-37.

Noddings, N. (1984). *Caring: a feminist approach to ethics and moral education.* Berkeley, CA: University of California Press.

Noddings, N. (1982). Doubts about radical proposals on caring. In N. Burbules (Ed.), *Philosophy of education.* Normal, IL: Illinois state University.

Ott, B.B. (1998). Physician-assisted suicide and older patients' perceived duty to die. *Advanced Practice Nursing Quarterly, 4*(2), 65-70.

Padgett, S.M. (1998). Dilemmas of caring in a corporate context: a critique of nursing case management. *Advanced Practice Nursing Quarterly, 4*(1), 1-12.

Penticuff, J.H., & Walden, M. (2000). Influence of practice environment and nurse characteristics on perinatal nurses' responses to ethical dilemmas. *Nursing Research, 49*(2), 64-71.

Polit, D., & Hungler, B.P. (1995). *Nursing research: principles and methods* (6th ed.). Philadelphia: JB Lippincott.

Porter-O'Grady,T. (1998). Ethics in health care: are nurses at the table? *Advanced Practice Nursing Quarterly, 4*(2), 83-84.

Raths, L., Harmin, M., & Simon, S. (1978). *Values and teaching.* Columbus, OH: Merrill.

Rawls, J. (1971). *A theory of justice.* Cambridge, MD: Harvard University Press.

Saarman, L., Freitas, L., Rapps, J., & Riegel, B. (1992). The relationship of education to critical thinking ability and values among nurses: socialization into professional nursing. *Journal of Professional Nursing, 8*(1), 26-34.

Savage, T.A. (1998). Children with severe and profound disabilities and the issue of social justice. *Advanced Practice Nursing Quarterly, 4*(2), 53-58.

Silva, M.C. (1997). Ethics of consumer rights in managed care. *Nursing Connections, 10*(2), 24-26.

Silva, M.C. (1998, June 10). Financial compensation and ethical issues in health care. *Online Journal of Issues in Nursing.* Available online at www.nursingworld.org/ojin/tpc6_4.htm.

Sofaer, B. (1995). Enhancing humanistic skills: an experiential approach to learning about ethical issues in health care. *Journal of Medical Ethics, 21*(1), 31-35.

Steckler, J. (1998). Examination of ethical practice in nursing continuing education using the Husted model. *Advanced Practice Nursing Quarterly, 4*(2), 59-64.

Tate, E.D., & Pranzatelli, M.R. (1999). *Unforgettable faces: through the eyes of a nurse practitioner.* Jacksonville, FL: Atheneum.

Vallentyne, P., & Accordino, J. (1998). Teaching critical thinking about ethical issues across the curriculum. *Liberal Education, 84*(2), 46-51.

Weis, D., Schank, M.J., Eddy, D., & Elfrink, V. (1993). Professional values in baccalaureate nursing education. *Journal of Professional Nursing, 9,* 336-342.

Weston, A. (1997). *A practical companion to ethics.* New York: Oxford University Press.

Wilmont, S. (1998). Nursing by agreement: a contractarian perspective on nursing ethics. *Advanced Practice Nursing Quarterly, 4*(2), 1-7.

Winland-Brown, J.E. (1998). Death, denial, and defeat: older patients and advance directives. *Advanced Practice Nursing Quarterly, 4*(2), 36-40.

Wynia, M.K. (1999, November-December). Performance measures for ethics quality. *Effective Clinical Practice.* Available online at www.acponline.org/journal/ecp/novdec99/wynia.htm.

Zerwekh, J., & Clabon, J.C. (1997). *Nursing today—transition and trends* (2nd ed.). Philadelphia: WB Saunders.

Zoloth-Dorfman, L., & Rubin, S. (1995). The patient as commodity: managed care and the question of ethics. *The Journal of Clinical Ethics, 6,* 339-357.

Chapter 15

Decision-Making for an Ethical Practice

Margaret M. Anderson & Cheryl Pope Kish

Advances in medicine, science, and technology have combined to make moral reasoning and ethical decision-making more necessary (and infinitely more complex) in today's health care setting. Scientific advances such as genetic engineering and cell regeneration, unheard of a decade ago, are now part of everyday specialty practice. The most intimate issues surrounding the way individuals are born and die force ethical thinking to a degree not felt at any other time in history. Compounding the situation is the fiscal reality in health care of attempting to accomplish more with less resources. The decisions being thrust on patients and families, as well as advanced practice nurses (APNs), require thoughtful analysis to determine the ethical or moral thing to do. As nursing specialists and leaders, APNs will be expected not only to practice ethically but also to facilitate ethical inquiry among staff and enable decision-making for patients. Veath and Fry (1995) suggest that nurses face bioethical problems in a unique manner because they stand in special role relationships with patients, families, physicians, and other members of the health care team.

The preceding chapter provided a foundation to inform ethical practice and examined the nature and derivation of ethical dilemmas. In this chapter, several approaches to resolution of ethical dilemmas are considered within the larger context of clinical practice. Additionally, the chapter addresses the manner in which APNs can affect the mission and ethics of the organizations in which they work.

There are many models for analysis and resolution of ethical problems; indeed, several are examined in this chapter, and two that appear to have special relevance to the role of APNs are examined closely. The profound clinical problems inherent in nursing can seem overwhelming. This is especially true when shortages of staff or lack of structural support exist. Emotions run high. Using decision-making models to frame close examination of the issues at such times decreases the chances of errors based on personal bias or strong paternalism (Thompson & Thompson, 1990). In the past, ethical decisions were made in private between a patient and a health care professional. Today, decisions that affect vulnerable populations are often a topic of public scrutiny and the focus of public debate (Raines, 1993).

DEFINITIONS

Although ethical dilemmas were defined in the previous chapter, it is helpful to review the definition in juxtaposition to information about using ethical decision-making models to resolve such dilemmas. **Ethical dilemmas** "occur when there are at least two compelling defensible alternatives or when two or more clear moral principles apply but support mutually inconsistent courses of action," and the balance is not between "what can be done and what one wishes could be done, but among two or more morally right but inconsistent alternatives" (Raines, 1993). Davis, Aroskar, Liaschenko, and Drought (1998) propose three characteristics of ethical dilemmas: (1) value conflicts exist, (2) ethical principles or values are at risk, and (3) the values and feelings of all stakeholders in the decision are implicated.

Ethical decision-making models, for purposes of this chapter, refer to approaches or frameworks used purposefully by APNs to guide ethical reflection and analysis of case situations in the clinical setting; they use moral reasoning to affect decisions about the most ethical course of action. Using ethical decision-making models in situations of uncertainty presupposes the capacity to critically think and problem-solve and the obligation to adhere to the code of conduct expected in professional nursing. Additionally, to use the models effectively requires a basic understanding of ethical theory and the inherent principles of autonomy, beneficence/nonmaleficence, justice, privacy, fidelity, and veracity.

Paternalism refers to governing decisions made, by others, in a fatherly manner. For clinical ethics, this implies enacting a role that views the professional as one with authority over patients, a "father knows best" attitude. This approach is obviously in conflict with the ethical principle of autonomy.

CRITICAL ISSUES: ETHICAL DECISION-MAKING IN ADVANCED PRACTICE NURSING

Several general decision-making models have been proposed within professional relationships. In the *priestly model*, decisions are made for individuals, with limited patient input and little regard for the patient's desires, feelings, and level of expertise. The *engineering model* involves decision-making on the basis of facts presented, without regard for personal ethical codes. The caregiver makes the decision; the patient is expected to accept it without question. In some cases, the patient may not even know the facts. Paternalism is a feature of these models because the caregiver decides what the patient needs.

The *contractual model* presupposes an agreement between two or more people. This may be a superior-subordinate relationship, or the situation may be more egalitarian in nature, like a nurse-patient relationship. In this model, the morals and needs of both people are considered in a decision made through compromise. The *collegial model* also has applicability to nursing decisions. By mutual discussion of needs and sharing of feelings, decision-makers reach consensus. This approach minimizes conflict and is helpful to team building in decision-making (Marriner-Tomey, 1996).

Ethical Decision-Making Framework

Davis et al (1998) developed a complex but thorough decision-making framework. Box 15-1 contains the elements in their decision-making model. The elements focus on several things: the character of the decision-maker, the ethical theory or principles at risk in the situation, and the relationship between caregiver and patient. No decision made in the midst of an ethical dilemma is without potential flaws or without at least a modicum of self-doubt, frustration, or even despair. For this reason, having structural supports or peer networks in place can be of inestimable value. A certified nurse midwife (CNM) voiced colleague support in these terms, "Without the others [midwives] watching out for the 'blahs' and 'blues' that come with ethical practice decisions, it would be easy to stay angry or lose spirit over time. When we can share [the experiences] we don't get so discouraged."

Husted and Husted (1995) also offer a model for ethical decision-making. Their model (shown in Figure

---

Box **15-1**

Elements to Assist in Discussion, Analysis, and Development of Ethical Decisions

1. Review the overall situation to identify what is going on.
2. Identify significant facts about the patient, including his or her medical and social history, his or her decision-making capacity, and the existence of any advanced directive for treatment.
3. Identify the parties or stakeholders involved in the situation or affected by the decisions that are made.
4. Identify relevant legal data.
5. Identify specific conflicts of ethical principles or values.
6. Identify possible choices, their intent, and the probable consequences to the welfare of the patient as the primary concerns.
7. Identify practical constraints (e.g., legal, organizational, political, and economic constraints).
8. Recommend actions that are determined to be ethically supportable, recognizing that the possible choices often have both positive and negative aspects.
9. Take action if you are the decision-maker and the person to implement the decision that is made.
10. Review and evaluate the situation after action is taken to determine what was learned that will be helpful in resolution of similar situations in patient care and related policy development.

Data from Davis, A.J., Aroskar, M.A., Liaschenko, J., & Drought, T.S. (1997). *Ethical dilemmas and nursing practice* (4th ed.). Upper Saddle River, NJ: Prentice-Hall.

15-1) is a contractual model for decision-making within the context of a nurse-patient relationship based on six bioethical standards. The standards are autonomy (patient's unique nature), freedom, veracity (objectivity), privacy (presumption of self-ownership), beneficence, and fidelity (faithfulness to the relationship agreement). Violation of any of these standards makes the relationship suspect and therefore compromises ethical decision-making.

Before APNs can make ethical decisions, they must understand the way in which decisions are made. Although there are numerous approaches to decision-making, the familiar steps of the nursing process can serve well for making informed choices. Jones and Beck (1996) identify a decision-making approach that contains the familiar nursing process steps:

1. Determine the problem and carefully assess the situation as extensively as possible. Data-gathering in this initial step presupposes examining multiple perspectives of the problem.

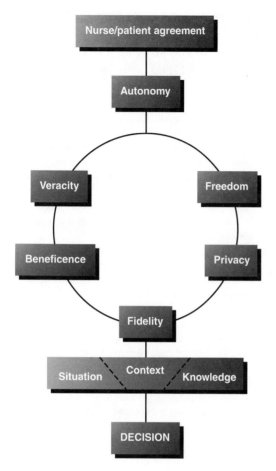

Figure 15-1 Bioethical decision making model. (From Husted, G.K., & Husted, J.H. [1995]. *Ethical decision making in nursing.* St. Louis: Mosby.)

2. Analyze the data for common components and differences that will precede examination of potential solutions (as many as can be generated).
3. Select the optimal solution after examining the advantages and disadvantages of each option identified in step 2.
4. Implement the selected option or decision.
5. Evaluate the effect of the decision on the individuals involved to determine the extent to which the decision worked. If a determination is made that the decision was ineffective in solving the problem, collect data to justify why the option failed to work. At this point, subject the new problem (the one unresponsive to the selected strategy) to the decision-making process and start the cycle again.

Ethical Decision-Making Process

Dozens of decisions are made every day. Even with inconsequential personal decisions such as what to wear or what time to have dinner, the decision-making process

is used, albeit not as obviously as for more significant decisions. At times, the best choice might well be one chosen from several equally unsatisfactory options. Such is the nature of an ethical dilemma. For example, Mr. Giles, a man with recently diagnosed prostate cancer, may be asked to decide to do nothing in response to his cancer, to have radiation seeds implanted in the gland, or to have surgery. None of these options is a guaranteed cure; indeed, all may contain a level of discomfort, the potential for unpleasant results, and even permanent effects like impotence. The APN might have a role in helping Mr. Giles examine the options, with as much information as possible made available to him in understandable terms. The nurse could refer questions beyond the APN scope of practice to the appropriate provider to ensure that the patient has an additional perspective. Furthermore, there might be the option of asking a patient who has experienced one of the available treatment options to talk with Mr. Giles and his family. The effect of the potential consequences on the individuals involved obviously has a great effect on the final decision. As is always the case, the decision may be rendered quickly, or it may require considerable time and data. The profundity of the effect determines the extent of the data needed, how many other people are consulted, and the amount of time needed for a decision.

Working with Mr. Giles and patients like him requires particularly close and continuing contact to appreciate his perspective. The potential for conflict exists when respect for an autonomous patient's freedom and an APN's interest in doing good (beneficence) are juxtaposed (Dormire, 1993). A patient's stance demands objective support from the APN that lends comfort; it does not warrant the APN taking over the decision or influencing it by showing approval or disapproval to the way the patient is leaning. Ultimately, this kind of clinical encounter demands that the APN enable the patient's decision. Such enablement involves "that communicative process whereby situational participants are provided with the understanding, the means, opportunities, power or authority, already intrinsic to their situation, to effect change by their decisions" (Zaner, 1988).

What separates ethical decisions from other kinds of decisions is that moral principles are the focus of the resolution. This is not to imply that routine decisions are not made by ethical people or based on principles of ethics; however, in those decisions ethical principles are not at risk of being violated. In other words, if a clinical decision does not involve an at-risk ethical principle, it may be a routine decision made by (hopefully) ethical professionals, but not an ethical decision.

Ethical decisions are ones that hold the highest ethical principle as inviolate. For example, Diane is a nurse practitioner (NP) at a public clinic. Jimmy, age 7, and his mother, Mrs. Lutz, have come in for Jimmy's school

PRACTICE Model for Resolution of Essential Ethical Issues by Advanced Practice Nurses

Patient	What facts about the patient are available from a holistic patient assessment?
Relationships	What connections exist with significant others (e.g., family, friends, other social support persons)? What role, if any, should they have in the decision?
Advocacy	Does the patient have the capacity to make the decision? What information is needed to enable that? In situations where the patient is not able to make an autonomous decision, who is the appropriate substitute in the decision process (e.g., parent, adult child, legal authority, advanced directive)?
Conflicts	What conflicts exit in the case? Are there conflicts between stakeholders? Between ethical principles?
Treatment	What treatment options are available? What details are available about each and about the extent to which they might be successful? What is likely to happen without treatment?
Interests	What are the interests of the various stakeholders in the situation? Has there been a previous expression of interest, such as an advanced directive or living will? What are the motives attached to the interests expressed? Is the motive advocacy or some hidden agenda?
Consequences	What are the short-term and long-term consequences of each choice being considered?
Ethical Principles	Which ethical principles are at stake in the decision?

Data from Perlin, T.M. (1992). *Clinical medical ethics: cases in practice.* Boston: Little Brown.

physical examination. As Diane is questioning Jimmy about school, his dietary likes and dislikes, and his relationships with peers (common questions appropriate for school-aged children), Mrs. Lutz tells her not to ask Jimmy those questions. She says her son is here for a physical examination and that the NP does not need the additional information. She further tells Jimmy not to answer these questions. At this point, Diane faces an ethical dilemma. Who is her patient—Jimmy or his mother? In advocating for Jimmy, will she make his mother angry? Since Mrs. Lutz is a custodial parent and Jimmy is a minor, should Diane comply with the mother's request to limit the visit to the physical assessment only? Will doing so compromise the integrity of data collection? If the NP decides, in analysis of the case, that Jimmy is her patient, is his autonomy violated by not being able to answer questions? Is there a potential harm to his health status (nonmaleficence) if the mother limits Diane's data collection? What should be done? If she continues asking questions despite the mother's request, the mother may leave the clinic setting with Jimmy before his examination is complete, thereby complicating his pre-school assessment. If she refrains from asking the questions, Jimmy may not be getting the care he deserves; potential health problems might be missed. There is obviously no best answer. The decision must be made on the basis of determining which ethical principle has priority.

Obviously, information is important to the NP's decision. Have the Lutzes been to the clinic in the past? If so, what has been their reason for coming? Is Jimmy generally a healthy child without developmental delays? Or does he have chronic problems? Is the mother's behavior today an anomaly, or is this typical? Diane must make a decision based on her assessment of the facts, then implement that decision, fully appreciating the possible consequences. Covey (1991) advises that an NP in this situation must ask herself the following regarding her decision: (1) Is the decision right, as opposed to the most popular or the expected decision?; and (2) can I live with myself, defending the decision to the face looking out from the mirror every day?

Models for Resolving Ethical Dilemmas

Perlin (1992) proposed the PRACTICE model for resolving ethical dilemmas in medical practice. Because so much of advanced practice overlaps the medical domain, this model has relevance for the ethical decision-making of APNs as well. Box 15-2 provides an overview of Perlin's model, modified for use by APNs.

When one examines a patient scenario using the PRACTICE model (or any other model), attention to the consequences of the decision should include quality of life as well as quantity of life. Menzel (1990) suggests that decision-makers may need to distinguish quality-of-life issues from sanctity-of-life issues. "Sanctity of life is sometimes associated with the idea that human life is so valuable that it must be preserved at all costs, under any conditions, for as long as possible." Ott (1998) maintains that concern about being a burden to family and friends serves as a critical determinant of how many patients decide about treatment options.

According to Ernst (1996), quality of life before the illness, as well as that expected with and without treatment, should be considered. Will pain be relieved? Function restored? Will improvement be effected quickly and easily, or is the situation more time intensive, even hopeless? Sometimes, "quality life" is less easily defined. For example, is it defined by mobility to perform the activities of daily living without dependence on others? Or perhaps by continued mental acuity or ability to socially interact. The cost of treatment is a priority for some. For example, Mrs. Winslow wants to have a legacy for her grandchildren. She is a widow who is trying to decide whether she should undergo prolonged treatment for metastatic cancer. She discloses to the oncologist clinical nurse specialist (CNS), "I lost my husband Willard 2 years ago, and life has been so painful since then. He supported me through the mastectomy, and I nursed him through kidney failure. We had planned on leaving money for our grandchildren, but Willard's illness took a large part of the money. I understand this treatment the doctor is talking about will take most of the remainder. There's no guarantee it will work, and I am in so much pain—do you understand that I might rather just leave my money for 'my babies' and go on to be with my Willard?"

Jonsen, Siegler, and Winslade (1998) appreciate the difficulty of organizing a decision-making framework around ethical principles. They offer this rationale for the clinical framework: "Moral rules and principles are best appreciated in the specific context of the actual circumstances of a case." Furthermore. these authors (a professor of ethics, a physician, and an attorney/ethicist) developed an organizing device with a better "fit" to making quick decisions in clinical situations. Their model for thinking about the complexities of ethical problems includes four topics: (1) medical indications, (2) patient preferences, (3) quality of life, and (4) content of problems (Box 15-3). This case analysis approach to clinical ethics has particular relevance for APNs who have a primary care focus in their clinical practice. Accustomed to analyzing and presenting cases to formulate a diagnosis and management plan, APNs will find the topics familiar and constant. With experience, they will note the moral or ethical equivalents in the case scenarios. It should be noted that the order of the questions in the model does not correspond with their relative importance.

The category for medical indications in this clinical ethics model includes the typical information gained in a clinical discussion. Answers to questions in this section relate facts that prompt a diagnosis and treatment plan; the ethical discussion of the case can then go beyond facts to the purposes and goals of treatment. "Indications refer to the relation between the pathophysiology presented by the patient and the diagnostic and therapeutic interventions that are 'indicated', that is, appropriate to evaluate and treat the problem." To assess the ethical aspects of a clinical case, the potential benefits of treatment are an important first consideration.

According to Jonsen et al (1998), "In all medical treatment, the preferences of the patient, based on the patient's own values and personal assessment of benefits and burdens are ethically relevant. In every clinical case, the questions must be raised: 'What are the patient's goals? What does the patient want?'" APNs should ensure that a patient's free choice is not being constrained, but such assurance presupposes information necessary to informed consent. In cases where a patient is mentally incapacitated at the time a decision is necessary, the APN must question "Who, then, has authority to make the decision for the patient?"

The patient preferences category includes advanced planning done by patients concerned that when crucial decisions about health care are demanded they will lack the capacity to make such decisions. Advanced planning includes formalized advanced directives, less formal living wills, and durable powers of attorney for health care. Most people agree, at least in principle, that humans should have a right to express their preferences about termination of life support in a legally valid document. "Although the legality of advanced planning has been formalized by legislation and upheld by courts, medical practice has been slow to respond to the preferences of terminally ill patients for less aggressive end-of-life care" (Jonsen et al, 1998). Although the APN is not involved in implementing advanced planning documents, an understanding of their processes, procedures, and emotional effect on patients and families is critical. It may well be an APN who ends up assuming the role of supporting family members in decision-making related to do not resuscitate orders.

Illness and injury are associated with a threat to one's actual or potential quality of life, depending on the extent of the symptoms experienced. The extent of the threat perceived is relative. For example, one may assume that, for the concert pianist, the pain and decreased mobility of rheumatoid arthritis likely threatens quality of life differently than it does for a corporate officer in a bank. A female neurosurgeon who is losing her visual acuity might perceive that threat differently than a female homemaker. An APN can only speculate on these assumptions; however, accurate assessment of patient perceptions is critical to decision-making. Quality of life evaluations are subjective, reflecting the personal views of the person making the judgment, and agreement is difficult at best. Jonsen et al (1998) suggest that broad, if not universal, agreement might be made on the following descriptions:

- *Restricted quality of life:* An objective description of a situation wherein a person suffers severe physical or mental health such that his functional capacity departs from the norm. Clearly, evaluations by an observer and by one living with the deficits may differ. Mr. Franklin,

Box 15-3

Clinical Case Approach to Ethical Decisions

Medical Indications

1. What is the patient's medical problem? History? Diagnosis? Prognosis?
2. Is problem acute or chronic? Critical? Emergent? Reversible?
3. What are goals of treatment?
4. What are the probabilities of success?
5. What are plans in case of therapeutic failure?
6. In sum, how can this patient be benefited by care, and how can harm be avoided?

Quality of Life

1. What are the prospects, with or without treatment, for a return to the patient's normal life?
2. Are there biases that might prejudice the provider's evaluation of the patient's quality of life?
3. What physical, mental, and social deficits is the patient likely to experience if treatment succeeds?
4. Is the patient's present or future condition such that he or she might judge continued life as undesirable?
5. Is there any plan and rationale to forgo treatment?
6. What plans exist for comfort and palliative care?

Patient Preferences

1. What has the patient expressed about preferences for treatment?
2. Has the patient been informed of benefits and risks? Has the patient understood and given consent?
3. Is the patient mentally competent? What evidence exists of incapacity?
4. Has the patient expressed previous preferences?
5. If the patient is incapacitated, who is the appropriate surrogate decision-maker? Is the surrogate using appropriate standards?
6. Is the patient unwilling or unable to cooperate with medical treatment? If so, why?
7. In sum, is the patient's right to choose being respected to the extent possible in ethics and law?

Contextual Features

1. Are there family issues that might influence treatment decisions?
2. Are there provider issues that might influence treatment decisions?
3. Are there financial and economic factors?
4. Are there religious and cultural factors?
5. Is there any justification to breach confidentiality?
6. Are there problems of allocation of resources?
7. What are the legal implications of treatment decisions?
8. Is clinical research or teaching involved?
9. Are any provider or institutional conflict of interests involved?

Data from Jonsen, A.R., Siegler, M., & Winslade, W.J. (1998). *Clinical ethics: a practical approach to ethical dilemmas in clinical medicine* (4th ed). New York: McGraw-Hill.

a cardiac patient with significant disability, may consider his life a good one; observers may judge otherwise.

- *Minimal quality of life:* An objective description of a situation wherein an individual's general physical condition has deteriorated to a point that his ability to communicate and have relationships with others is severely restricted and includes pain and discomfort. An example would be Mrs. Rafferty, an aging woman struggling with severe Alzheimer's disease.
- *Quality of life below minimal:* An objective description of a situation wherein a patient suffers extreme physical debilitation and irreversible loss of sensory and intellectual activity. The ability for human interaction or relationships is severely limited or lost completely. Mr. Jones, a patient involved in an automobile accident that rendered him brain dead, would be an example.

"The object of all medical intervention is to restore, maintain, or improve quality of life" (Jonsen et al, 1998). Therefore all medical situations necessitate raising the issue of quality of life and the meaning it has for a particular individual. Issues of life quality must be considered cautiously because there is room for bias. An APN should remember that persons seem to evaluate quality of life differently when imagining a situation, as opposed to when they are actually experiencing the situation. For example, Mr. Pope, on learning of his early renal failure, verbalized that he would never agree to dialysis, that he would rather die than be dependent on a machine. Over time, however, he agreed to dialysis, almost apologetically. "I have decided I was wrong in the beginning. Don't misunderstand—I'm prepared to die. I know there is a Heaven, and I'm going there one day. But I'm not ready to leave my daughter and my grandson. My work is not done in this world."

Patient care during an illness or injury does not exist in a vacuum; the case unfolds within a context with psychosocial, legal, economic, and institutional circumstances. As clinical experts in holistic care, APNs are accustomed to addressing the multiple dimensions of health and illness. Both patients and APNs live in the context of a social system that requires responsibilities and duties outside the nurse-patient relationship. Many values affect the relationship between these individuals: goals and obligations of each, laws, institutional policies, economic concerns, religious beliefs, professional standards, and (sometimes) teaching and research issues. Changes in health care delivery systems and financing in particular have created conflicts of interest for those who must be both providers of care and gatekeepers for the system (with its utilization and cost constraints). The social burden is often perceived as being imposed at the expense of benefits to particular patients. Therefore it is imperative that the core value of caring is evident in interactions between APNs and patients. "Caring presence affirms the humanity of both nurse and patient and accords each the respect due a human being. It comforts and supports those cared for as they face suffering, treatment, and possible death, and at the same time it inspires and enlightens the caregiver" (Zaner, 1993).

Several models have been advanced thus far for analysis and resolution of ethical dilemmas. Many others are available in the ethics literature. APNs are advised to select a model that is a comfortable fit for their professional practice and to use it in situations calling for moral reasoning. With experience, such a model becomes integrated into the professional self; its use then becomes second-nature. At times, merging the best features of several approaches into an eclectic model can work best for a particular professional. (Several case studies, related to APN roles, that can be used in practicing the various ethical decision-making models are provided in Chapter 16.)

Ensuring Ethical Practice Settings

Ethical practice is the individual APN's effort to practice in his or her respective area of advanced practice while being true to professional values. As health care organizations merge, close, and change ownership and profit status, it is difficult to keep up not only with their ownership status but also their mission and philosophy. Certainly restructuring in the health care delivery system has had profound effects on the delivery methods and financing of care; it has also changed the nature of a market-driven workforce. Jobs have changed or been lost; a number of unlicensed assistant personnel have been added, shifting responsibility and accountability from professional nurses; and there is a sense in many of job insecurity. Complicating those changes is a severe nursing shortage. Hadley (1996) suggests that "nurses need to prepare for the inevitable dislocation that will occur as a result of hospital downsizing and other dramatic changes in health services." Ethical issues arise when there are changes in the way care is financed and incentives are provided (Silva, 1998).

Loewy and Loewy (1998) suggest that health care professionals perceive themselves in one of three basic ways: (1) as individuals in a system over which they have no control, making individual ethical choices in an attempt to comply with or circumvent the system; (2) as members of a collective who, through action and solidarity, might reshape the system and thus the way ethical situations are handled; and (3) as a combination of both of these—as individuals attempting to do their best in the given context, working collectively toward constructive change. However, all professionals place themselves within the context of the system of care and their respective employing institution, so they must carefully assess the ethical perspective of that workplace. The system often determines both one's options and one's moral and ethical choices. "One cannot practice truly ethically within the context of an unethical or corrupt health care system" (Loewy & Loewy, 1998).

Whether one agrees that managed care is the panacea for health care, it is obvious that it has reshaped the provider-patient relationship adversely, or at least has the potential to. There are now imposed time limitations for clinical encounters, thus inhibiting the dialogue between providers and patients. Patients appear less secure in the health care system, and there is considerable uncertainty about the motives prompting some health care decisions. Wynia (1999) cites the results of a 2-year study by the Kaiser Foundation, showing public concern for the communal ethical norms of health care, one example of which is the limitations on care for vulnerable populations. Wynia further explores the responses of the American Medical Association's (AMA's) Institute of Ethics to the public concerns, specifically the initiation of a program (E-Force) to discern and develop sets of ethics performance standards against which practices can judge themselves. APNs would be well served to continually self-assess the ethical perspectives of the corporate culture of their own practice sites, perhaps considering how to formalize that evaluation by using performance measures suggested by the E-Force program.

As both a condition of initial employment and with the substantive changes in the practice setting, APNs need to know that the mission of their organization remains within the individual professional framework they embrace. APNs are in a position to affect the mission and ethics of the organizations with which they are associated by virtue of their leadership roles and to enjoy input into policy and organizational decisions.

Ethics in Organizations

The ethics of an organization are reflected in their mission statement or philosophy (if they have one) and in the policies that govern the organization. These may be implied rather than explicitly stated, but loyalty to the ethical stance of the organization is still expected. Swansburg and Swansburg (1999) believe that business or organizational ethics aid employees and practice providers in making decisions before an ethical dilemma arises. Although most businesses do not have written policies on ethics and ethical practice, it would actually be a good idea to write down an organizational code of ethics and have employees review and commit to it at regular intervals. This would promote ethical practice and enable employees and employers to hold each other accountable for ethical behavior, reinforcing each other's commitment to an ethical stance. Health care organizations, community organizations, and physicians' offices should base their existence on values supporting the basic ethical principles of autonomy, beneficence, justice, privacy, veracity, and fidelity. These universal principles promote both individual and common good. The ethical code of a practice site or organization is the standard against which policies and actions are measured. If a written code is unavailable, a decision-making model (like those explored in this chapter) can be substituted. A nurse's relationship with the patient is a social contract entered into by both partners willingly and voluntarily, and both expect ethical behavior from the other. For help with this, *The International Code of Ethics for Nurses* is always appropriate for guiding nurse-patient relationships and actions and decisions of an organization. Ethical practice stems from these core values.

No matter what an APN's practice site is, it is important that he or she accept the values of the employing organization. However, when the nature of the practice agency changes over time, commitment may waiver. Perhaps the core values have shifted and are no longer comparable to the APN's personal value set. In cases where personal and organization values are no longer compatible, change must occur. Either the APN must find ways to modify the organization's stance so it is supportable or he or she must find work elsewhere. Jerry, a geriatric nurse practitioner (GNP), provides a good example. When Jerry was first employed by Elder Care Community Clinic, he was impressed by the autonomy and justice accorded the older adults in his care. However, 2 years later the clinic merged with another geriatric clinic in the community to increase the patient base. The new clinic used a paternalism care model that became the reality in Jerry's clinic setting. He could not support this ethic of practice because he valued the older adult's right to self-determination in health care; he could not be satisfied making decisions for his patients. He spoke candidly with the physicians and other providers in the clinic and learned that most were satisfied with the new approach to care and not likely to change. Jerry gave the situation considerable thought and decided that to be true to his personal mission of care, he must tender his resignation.

The amount of autonomy permitted in a practice setting is a good measure of an organization's respect for the nurse-patient relationship. Accountability for practice not only refers to the accuracy and currency of assessment and treatment and the responsibility and realism shown in decision-making, it also means that APNs should ensure that an ethical stance pervades the practice and its policies.

Values clarification can be a valuable exercise not only for an individual but also for an organization. Assessment of an organization's value stance includes questions such as:

1. How does the practice site develop policies? Is there an effort to articulate a mission and clarify the ethics of the organization?
2. Are employees involved in developing an ethical code? Are they asked to review it at intervals and commit to it?
3. Do the actual policies and practices in the organization reflect a commitment to the ethical code or principles of ethics?
4. Is the *International Code of Ethics for Nurses* used as a basis for practice in the organization? Is there evidence of respect for professional and accountable practice at the organization?
5. How are ethical dilemmas resolved? How are conflicts handled?
6. What is the APN's role in resolving ethical dilemmas?
7. What policies demonstrate respect for the individual's ethical code?
8. Is an ethicist available for consultation?
9. What support is available during and after ethical dilemmas?

Congruence between Practice Environment and Personal Ethics

During the search for employment, an APN is well served by examining the ethical stance reflected in the corporate culture of the clinical sites being considered. The questions listed in the previous section are useful in that kind of assessment. Accepting a position in an institution whose ethics are incompatible with one's own can only lead to frustration and unease. Even when there is congruence between an APN's value set and that of an institution, there is likely to be a period of adjustment. Many APNs find it impossible to replicate the patient-centered models of their educational experience in the real practice world (Lurie, 1981).

Corley and Raines (1993b) propose a model for assessing "goodness of fit" between the ethics of a practice environment and one's personal perspective. The model, which can be used both prospectively and retrospectively, includes these features: (1) role orientation and role modeling by administrators, (2) institutional support of education, (3) ethically responsive guidelines, (4) procedures for addressing ethical or unethical practice, (5) individual counseling or debriefing after ethical dilemmas are resolved, (6) adequate staffing, (7) practices that reflect value for the worth of staff to the organization, and (8) in-place systems that clearly show value for autonomy, trust, and communication. Corley and Raines (1993a) later added other components: (1) codes as guides for practice, (2) a philosophy that promotes ethical decisions and decreases the risk of making them, (3) inclusion of ethics rounds, (4) representation on ethics committees, (5) stability of staff, (6) encouragement of clinical expertise and credibility of nurses, and (7) support to change protocols, a suggestion attributed to Penicuff (1989).

Jameton (1993) explores the very real moral distress sometimes associated with a nurse's moral responsibility. Moral distress can occur when the nurse feels morally responsible but fails to act, not out of irresponsibility or lack of motivation, but due to institutional constraints or colleague opposition. These scenarios are remembered even years later as "failures" by some nurses who regret their inaction but felt powerless to act at the time of the incident. For example, Terry tells a story about her own powerlessness with respect to Baby M, an encounter that happened 32 years ago at the beginning of her nursing career. Now a doctorally prepared CNM teaching in an academic program, Terry recounts the delivery of Baby M at a small community hospital where she was "the nurse" for labor and delivery on the 3 PM to 11 PM shift. Baby M was delivered at term by a family physician. As was the custom at the time, the mother was sedated and the father was in the waiting room. The baby required basic resuscitation, which Terry tried to provide. When it became evident that her resuscitative efforts were ineffective, Terry informed the physician, who was, at the time, repairing the episiotomy. Terry acknowledged candidly that she needed assistance and wanted to telephone for someone more experienced; in this case, the hospital's anesthesiologist. The physician stopped stitching and came to evaluate the baby. After a cursory evaluation, he pronounced that nothing could be done and that Terry should not only stop attempting to resuscitate the baby but not call anyone. Terry made several more attempts to convince the physician to let her call someone to assist the baby, but he always said no. "The baby is gone—nothing more can be done." As a novice, Terry thought she had been wrong. In later years, she realized instead that the physician was wrong in his approach. "I wish I had known more about advanced resuscitation. Sometimes I think about that little girl—she would be almost 33 years old today. If only I had known how to help her or been more courageous! I should have just walked out to the telephone and paged anesthesia, regardless of what the physician said. I should have been a better nurse, a better advocate." When reminded that she had helped and advocated for thousands of patients since that event in her first year of practice, Terry smiled tentatively and said, "Yeah, but not that night!"

Wilkinson (1987-1988) defines this kind of moral distress as "psychological disequilibrium and [a] negative feeling state experienced when a person makes a moral decision but does not follow through by performing the moral behavior indicated by that decision." Although inaction seems to be a more prevalent cause of moral distress, taking action amid obstacles and opposition can also contribute. Anger, guilt, frustration, depression, and physical symptoms like headache, gastrointestinal upset, and palpitations have been associated with moral distress (Jameton, 1993; Wilkinson, 1987-88). In a look at how a limited pool of critical care nursing staff affects moral distress, Fowler (1989) speculated that the phenomenon of moral distress is a contributory factor in burnout.

IMPLICATIONS FOR MSN EDUCATION AND ADVANCED PRACTICE

To provide ethical care in today's health system one must be informed about basic rights, ethical principles, and philosophies; be able to apply conceptual models as a way of thinking about ethical dilemmas; and have opportunities to explore and resolve ethical dilemmas (Dormire, 1993). Educational programs must ensure inclusion of these elements in the curricula. Not only should students have the necessary philosophical foundation to inform their specialty practice, they must also have practice opportunities in clinical settings. Educators cannot assume that graduate students have had adequate exposure to ethical philosophies and clinical experience with models in their basic nursing education. Furthermore, irrespective of knowledge base, the moral perplexity associated with APN roles in practice is very different, as are the expectations for individuals within those roles.

APN programs have an advantage when faculty members bring credible examples from their own practice for consideration by student groups. Inclusion of ethical features of every case analysis can be helpful, as can practice with multiple models until one declares "goodness of fit." Students should be helped to appreciate that there are no right or wrong answers in ethical dilemmas, that they can feel comfortable sharing their candid beliefs within a setting that promotes freedom to do so. As Veath and Fry (1995) remind readers, "Each question has several plausible answers, which have been developed over two thousand years of Western thought." Not all cases for ethical analysis should be clinical cases; APNs face ethical dilemmas in their nonclinical roles as well. Consequently, cases for practice should include those pertinent to education, research, and management roles as well as direct care roles.

APNs need to appreciate the extent to which they can shape the ethical mission of a practice setting and to understand how to evaluate settings for evidence of an ethic congruent with their own. Opportunities to reflect on the ethical dimensions of clinical practice in a clinical journal can be helpful not only as a cathartic activity but as a component of experiential learning. Understanding how the health care system itself affects ethics can also be an asset, as can knowing the common sources of value compromise.

According to Veath and Fry (1995), nurses face bioethical problems uniquely because they share special role relationships with patients, families, physicians and other members of the health care team. No doubt this statement is universally accepted as truth by APNs. Therefore, it is essential that APNs individually and collectively have a practice informed by bioethical theory and clinically applicable models and guided by a professional value system appropriate to their roles. As Fowler (1977) suggests, "A set of values serves to orient a person in a complex world . . . without values, a person's judgment and actions would be whimsical, disorderly."

PRIORITIES FOR RESEARCH

The existing research related to ethical practice in the APN population is limited. Many questions need to be addressed by either quantitative or qualitative research approaches or through triangulation studies.

Eddy, Elfrink, Weis, and Schank (1994) conducted a study with baccalaureate nursing students and their faculty that would provide for an interesting replication with graduate students and faculty. These researchers developed a professional nursing behaviors instrument based on the values identified in the American Association of Colleges of Nursing's (1996) *Essentials of Baccalaureate Education for Professional Nursing*; these values are altruism, integrity, autonomy, human dignity, equality, individual freedom, and justice. Interested in determining if senior nursing students and nursing faculty had different perceptions of the importance of values on the profession, the researchers sought responses from 10 public and 16 private National League for Nursing Accrediting Commission (NLNAC)–accredited baccalaureate programs. They found that faculty perceived values as significantly more important to the profession than did students.

Another study of professional values was conducted by Weis and Schank (2000). Theirs was methodological research involving development and testing of an instrument to measure professional values: the Nursing Professional Values Scale (NPVS), a 44-item norm-referenced instrument with a Likert-type format based on the ANA's *International Code of Ethics for Nurses*. The authors reviewed the literature from 1970 to the present, noting 18 studies measuring professional values from which few generalizations could be drawn because of the diversity of instrumentation and of the value indicators under study. The caregiving factor accounted for 31.4% of the variance in professional values, confirming the importance ascribed to the caregiving role. Activism accounted for 10.1% of the variance. Based on factor analysis, the authors suggest that other values, such as accountability, freedom, integrity, trust, safety, and knowledge, should be retained for future research with the instrument. Initial testing of the NPVS showed high reliability and validity. The researchers believe that the instrument is promising as a "preintervention or screening instrument, a postintervention tool for programs targeting development of professional nursing values, and for assessment of professional nursing values over time."

Kelly's (1998) exploratory study of how nurses make ethical decisions and the factors they perceive as helping or hindering moral choices, also has relevance for APNs. In this study, 26 experienced Australian nurses with advanced degrees kept diaries for 7 to 10 working days during 1 month, noting any practice-related situation that presented an inherent moral problem. Two central constructs were found to explain ethical decision-making: (1) investing the self to act on the problem, and (2) discounting the self in not acting on the problem. Investing included several subprocesses: (1) reflecting, which involved taking time to think through the possible decision, often under pressure for an immediate answer; (2) personalizing, the second most common approach, which included relating to the problem from a highly personal level; and (3) transcending, which involved visualizing the problem in a broader context, with clarity about ownership of the problem and the potential resolution in light of existing time and resources. Those who invested themselves were likely to use assertive techniques such as fact-finding, identification of resources, exploration of other options, risk-taking, and verbal or written communication for follow-up. These nurses learned to take pride in small victories and recognize that resolution of moral problems might occur in stages. Conversely, nurses discounting themselves involved: (1) reacting, which is described as rushing about in their concern, urging others to act, or grumbling, with only later reflection; (2) distancing, which is described as vacillating in their lack of knowledge and fearing; and (3) limiting, which involved engaging in avoidance behavior (common with moral distress), conforming to the status quo position, and playing doctor-nurse games instead of confronting issues directly. Action in response to moral problems was more likely when patient safety was threatened, the problem was a highly visible one, and the patient or significant other was aware of the problem. Action was also associated with ideal timing in the clinical day; a nurse's number of years of experience in the setting; and whether the problem fell within the clinical expertise of the nurse respondent.

It would be interesting to replicate this Australian study with APNs in the United States to determine if responses to moral problems would be similar. Perhaps the research population could include all four types of APNs to determine similarities and differences in response between NPs,

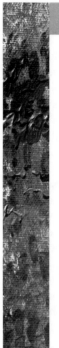

Suggestions for Further Learning

- Consult the following journal article: Wynia, M.K. (1999, November-December). Performance measures for ethics quality. *Effective Clinical Practice*, 1-8. Available online at www.acponline.org/journal/ecp/novdec99/wynia.htm. Pay particular attention to the appendix, which includes examples of measurement questions for assessing ethical behaviors. Critique the questions and speculate on others that could be included in the list.
- Interview a currently practicing APN to discuss his or her perception of ethical practice in health care today. If possible, debrief in a peer group where others have interviewed APNs in a different specialty.
- Read Zaner, R. (1993). *Troubled voices: stories of ethics and illness.* Cleveland, OH: Pilgrim Press.
- Consult the following websites for additional information on ethical decision-making and ethical practice:
  - The Kennedy Institute of Ethics (Georgetown University) (www.georgetown.edu/research/kie)

- Bioethics Links2Go (www.links2go.com/topic/Bioethics)
- Bioethics Links on the Web (www.mcw.edu)
- The Journal of Clinical Ethics (www.clinicalethics.com/)
- Review *21 Competencies for the 21st Century* from the Pew Health Professions Commission. Note that the first two items in the competency list pertain to ethics. Available online at futurehealth.ucsf.edu/pewcomm/competen.html.
- Consult the Kaiser Foundation (1998). *Survey of Americans' views on the consumer protection debate.* Available online at www.kff.org/archive/health_policy.
- Read Shilts, R. (1988). *And the band played on: politics, people, and the AIDS epidemic.* New York: Penguin Books. In a small group, discuss the ethical issues in this book.
- Consult Jonsen, A.R., Siegler, M., & Winslade, W.J. (1998). *Clinical ethics* (4th ed.). New York: McGraw-Hill. It provides detailed examples of the authors' clinical model for decision-making.

CNMs, certified registered nurse anesthetists (CRNAs), and CNSs. How would the moral problems be alike or dissimilar? Would the nature of the setting be an important variable? What other demographic factors might be correlated?

It would also be helpful to further explore the lived experience of moral disequilibrium and distress for APNs. What helps? What exacerbates the experience of discomfort? What are the most common ethical issues facing APNs? Are they similar across specialties? What guides decision-making in morally perplexing situations? Which models have been perceived as most helpful? What measures are most helpful in preparing APN students for those kinds of experiences? In terms of ethical practice environments, what is the corporate culture experienced by APNs? What questions are useful in assessing the prospective corporate culture? What is the experience of those who either attempt to reshape the practice environment or who choose to leave an environment incongruous with their practice values? These are just a few of the myriad researchable questions worthy of attention in contemporary practice.

DISCUSSION QUESTIONS

These questions can be used to promote critical thinking and encourage discussion.

1. Identify an ethical dilemma from your clinical practice, or select one from the literature. Employ one of the decision-making models in this chapter as a guide for analysis of the dilemma and for suggesting resolution. Evaluate the "goodness of fit" of the particular model for that activity. Consider working in a group where the same dilemma is analyzed with a different model from the chapter. Afterward, consider the advantages and disadvantages of each model.

2. In a group setting, use the work of Raines and Corley (1993b) as a framework for determining questions suitable for assessment of a clinical practice environment. Use the finished list to evaluate a clinical practice site, documenting your findings. Bring the written documentation back to the group for discussion. Brainstorm measures for improving the clinical site as an ethical environment.

3. Keep a clinical diary or journal for a minimum of 1 week. Write about any encounter that involves a moral problem. Include not only the factual information but also a description of the feelings the experience evoked.

4. Review your professional history for moral situations that have elicited moral distress for yourself or those with whom you have worked. Discuss this in a small group, being certain to protect the confidentiality of those involved.

5. In a small-group setting, explore the way in which you perceive the tidal wave of changes in health care delivery and health care financing to have affected the ethical stance of professionals in practice.

6. Write your personal philosophy of nursing and outline your practice ethics.

7. Select some ethical issue of particular relevance to the professional practice of APNs. Stage a debate in which individuals argue the position opposite their personal belief. This process encourages examination of self-beliefs. Examples include: right to abortion vs. right for fetal tissue for transplantation; cost of health care vs. right to health care; and right to privacy vs. right to know for the insurance industry.

8. Define quality of life. React to the categories suggested by Jonsen et al (1998) in this chapter.

9. Answer this question: How does the system of financial compensation in the health care system of the United States generate ethical issues and affect the ethical values of nursing?

REFERENCES/BIBLIOGRAPHY

American Association of Colleges of Nursing (1996). *The essentials of baccalaureate education for professional nursing.* Washington, DC: American Association of Colleges of Nursing.

Bandman, E.L., & Bandman, B. (1995). *Nursing ethics through the life span* (3rd ed.). Norwalk, CT: Appleton & Lange.

Barnett, T. (1993). Are there employment risks for unethical decisions? *Nursing Forum, 20,* 17-21.

Bartholome, W.G. (1992). A revolution in understanding: how ethics has transformed health care decision making. *Quarterly Review Bulletin, 18*(1), 6-11.

Broom, C. (1990). Conflict resolution strategies for ethical dilemmas: when ethical dilemmas evolve to conflict. *Dimensions of Critical Care Nursing, 10*(6), 354-363.

Corley, M.C., & Raines, D.A. (1993a). Environments that support ethical nursing practice. *AWHONN's Clinical Issues in Perinatal and Women's Health Nursing, 4*(4), 611-619.

Corley, M.C., & Raines, D. (1993b). An ethical practice environment as a caring environment. *Nursing Administration Quarterly, 17,* 68-74.

Covey, S. (1991). *Principle-centered leadership.* New York: Simon & Schuster.

Czerwinski, B. (1990). An autopsy of an ethical dilemma. *Journal of Nursing Administration, 20,* 25-29.

Davis, A.J., Aroskar, M.A., Liaschenko, J., & Drought, T.S. (1998). *Ethical dilemmas and nursing practice* (4th ed.). Upper Saddle River, NJ: Prentice-Hall.

Dormire, S.L. (1993). Ethical models: facilitating clinical practice. *AWHONN's Clinical Issues in Perinatal and Women's Health Nursing, 4*(4), 526-532.

Eddy, D.M., Elfrink, V., Weis, D., & Schank, M.J. (1994). Importance of professional nursing values. *Journal of Nursing Education, 33*(6), 257-262.

Erlen, J., & Frost, B. (1991). Nurses' perceptions of powerlessness in influencing ethical decisions. *Western Journal of Nursing Research, 13,* 397-407.

Erlen, J., & Sereika, S.M. (1997). Critical care nurses: ethical decision-making and stress. *Journal of Advanced Nursing, 26*(5), 953-961.

Ernst, E. (1996). The ethics of complementary medicine. *Journal of Medical Ethics, 22,* 197-198.

Fowler, J. (1977). The problem of values in futures research. *Futures, 9,* 303-313.

Fowler, M.D.M. (1989). Moral distress and the shortage of critical care nurses. *Heart & Lung, 18,* 314-315.

Garrett, T.M., Baillie, H.W., & Garrett, R.M. (1998). *Health care ethics: principles and problems* (3rd ed.). Upper Saddle River, NJ: Prentice Hall.

Gordon, S., & Fagin, C.M. (1996). Presenting the moral high ground. *American Journal of Nursing, 96*(3), 31-32.

Hadley, E.H. (1996). Nursing in the political and economic marketplace: challenges for the 21st century. *Nursing Outlook, 44,* 6-10.

Heitman, L.K., & Robinson, R.E.S. (1997). Developing a nursing ethics roundtable. *American Journal of Nursing, 97*(1), 36-38.

Husted, G.K., & Husted, J.H. (1995). *Ethical decision making in nursing* (2nd ed.). St. Louis: Mosby.

Jameton, A. (1993). Dilemmas of moral distress: moral responsibility and nursing practice. *AWHONN's Clinical Issues in Perinatal and Women's Health Nursing, 4*(4), 542-551.

Jecker, N.S. (1994). Managed competition and managed care: what are the ethical issues? *Clinics in Geriatric Medicine, 10,* 527-539.

Jones, R., & Beck, S. (1996). *Decision making in nursing.* Albany, NY: Delmar Publishers.

Jonsen, A.R., Siegler, M., & Winslade, W.J. (1998). *Clinical ethics: a practice approach to ethical decisions in clinical medicine* (4th ed.). New York: McGraw-Hill.

Kelly, C. (1998). Investing or discounting self: are moral decisions shaped by conditions in the workplace? *Advanced Practice Nursing Quarterly, 4*(2), 8-13.

Kenney, J.W. (1996). *Philosophical and theoretical perspectives for advanced nursing practice.* Sudbury, MA: Jones & Bartlett.

Loewy, E.H., & Loewy, R.S. (1998). Ethics and managed care: reconstructing a system and refashioning a society. *Archives of Internal Medicine, 158*(22). Available online at archinte. ama.assn.org/issues/v158n22/full/ied80612.htm.

Ludwick, R., & Sedlack, C.A. (1998). Ethical issues and critical thinking: students' stories. *Nursing Connections, 11*(3), 12-18.

Lurie, E. (1981). Nurse practitioners: issues in professional socialization. *Journal of Health and Social Behavior, 22,* 31-48.

Lutzen, K. (1997). Nursing ethics into the next millennium: a context-sensitive approach for nursing ethics. *Nursing Ethics, 4*(3), 218-226.

Marriner-Tomey, A. (1996). *Nursing management and leadership* (5th ed.). St. Louis: Mosby.

McCloskey, J.C., & Grace, H.K. (1997). *Current issues in nursing* (5th ed.). St. Louis: Mosby.

Menzel, P.T. (1990). *Strong medicine—the ethical rationing of health care.* New York: Oxford University Press.

Omery, A. (1989). Values, moral reasoning, and ethics. *Nursing Clinics of North America 23,* 499-507.

Ott, B.B. (1998). Physician-assisted suicide and older patients' perceived duty to die. *Advanced Practice Nursing Quarterly, 4*(2), 65-70.

Padgett, S.M. (1998). Dilemmas of caring in a corporate context: a critique of nursing case management. *Advances in Nursing Science, 20*(4), 1-12.

Pearlman, R.A., Cain, K.C., Patrick, D.L., Applebaum-Maizel, M., Starks, H.E., Jecker, N.S., & Uhlmann, R.F. (1993). Insights pertaining to patient assessment of states worse than death. *Journal of Clinical Ethics, 41*(1), 33-41.

Penicuff, J.H. (1989). Infant suffering and nurse advocacy in neonatal intensive care. *Nursing Clinics of North America, 24,* 987-997.

Perlin, T.M. (1992). *Clinical medical ethics: cases in practice.* Boston: Little and Brown.

Raines, D. (1993). Ethical reflection and resolution. *AWHONN's Clinical Issues in Perinatal and Women's Health Nursing, 4*(4), 641-647.

Raines, D.A. (1997). From covenant to contract: how managed care is changing provider patient relations. *AWHONN Lifelines, 1*(4), 41-45.

Raines, D.A. (1993). Values: a guiding force. *AWHONN's Clinical Issues in Perinatal and Women's Health Nursing, 4*(4), 533-541.

Silva, M.C. (1998, June 10). Financial compensation and ethical issues in health care. *Online Journal of Issues in Nursing.* Available online at www.nursingworld.org/ojin/tpc6/tpc6_4htm.

Swansburg, R.C., & Swansburg, R.J. (1999). *Introductory management and leadership for nurses.* (2nd ed.). Sudbury, MA: Jones & Bartlett.

Thompson, J., & Thompson, H. (1990). Values: directional signals for life choices. *Neonatal Network, 8,* 83-84.

Veath, R.M., & Fry, S.T. (1995). *Case studies in nursing ethics.* Boston, MA: Jones & Bartlett.

Viens, D.C. (1994). Moral dilemmas experienced by nurse practitioners. *Nursing Forum, 5*(4), 209-214.

Viens, D.C. (1995). The moral reasoning of nurse practitioners. *Journal of the American Academy of Nurse Practitioners, 7*(6), 277-285.

Weis, D., & Schank, M.J. (2000). An instrument to measure professional nursing values. *Journal of Nursing Scholarship, 32*(2), 201-204.

Wilkinson, J.A. (1987-1988). Moral distress in nursing practice: experience and effect. *Nursing Forum, 23,* 16-29.

Williams, A.M. (1998). The delivery of quality nursing care: a grounded theory study of the nurse's perspective. *Journal of Advanced Nursing, 27,* 808-816.

Winslow, B.J., & Winslow, G.R. (1991). Integrity and compromise in nursing ethics. *The Journal of Medicine and Philosophy, 16,* 307-323.

Wurzbach, M.E. (1998). Managed care: moral conflicts for primary health care nurses. *Nursing Outlook, 46*(2), 62-66.

Wynia, M.K. (1999, November-December). Performance measures for ethics quality. *Effective Clinical Practice,* 1-8. Available online at www.acponline.org/journal/ecp/novdec99/wynia.htm.

Zaner, R. (1993). *Troubled voices: stories of ethics and illness.* Cleveland, OH: Pilgrim Press.

Zaner, R. (1998). *Ethics and the clinical encounter.* Englewood Cliffs, NJ: Prentice-Hall.

Chapter 16

Case Studies for Ethical Analysis

Cheryl Pope Kish

Each person brings to the study of advanced practice a set of personal values that have frequently been accepted without critical reflection, unless such reflection is forced by educators. Nursing education for advanced practice nurse (APN) roles generally reintroduces theoretical frameworks for ethics learned in basic nursing education, pronounces principles that should direct actions, and forces values clarification. There is a very real reluctance at times to avoid the arduous study of one's self-assumptions about morality, "but only the intellectually naive will deny that professional codes are built on presupposed theoretical principles" (Schultz, 1993).

At the turn of the millennium, it is not clear if the ethical dilemmas to be faced by APNs will be different than those faced by nurses in general. A decade ago, Omery (1990) found that the top five ethical dilemmas for nurses were do not resuscitate orders, quality of life issues, organ transplants, dealing with difficult patients, and beneficence issues. In 1991, Berger, Severson, and Chvatal learned that 71% of their respondents felt inadequate staffing was a pressing ethical issue. Other issues included prolonging life with heroic measures, inappropriate resource allocation, inappropriate discussion of patients, and irresponsible actions of colleagues. Today, new ethical issues have surfaced; these are as varied as genetic engineering, care of very-low birth weight neonates, use of unlicensed assistive personnel, fetal tissue harvesting and use, reproductive choices, physician-assisted suicide, and the nursing shortage. With the mapping of human deoxyribonucleic acid (DNA), questions abound about how this knowledge will affect both medical treatment and insurance coverage. With spiraling costs, questions are being raised about allocation of resources and rationing of selected aspects of care. As primary care providers (PCPs) are pushed to see more patients in less time to reduce costs, there is added pressure to cut the "talking and teaching time" with patients. Quality of life issues continue to present dilemmas, as do shortages of staff. Whistle-blowing, more common in society than ever, is occurring among health care professionals who, as patient advocates, bring evidence of negligent clinical acts and health care fraud to the attention of authorities. With declining funding of health care research, there has regrettably been data tampering by researchers hoping to compete for those dollars. Furthermore, technocentric problems will continue as technical capabilities increase. Now, since nursing has always attended to issues related to human suffering, nurses' actions are not likely to change; however, as can be seen, ethical dilemmas will continue to be a prominent part of clinical practice; APNs need education and experience for handling them.

This chapter presents case studies that offer opportunities for reflection and for examining the kinds of realistic dilemmas APNs face in clinical practice. Four cases, one for each kind of APN, are analyzed; three different decision-making models are used in the analysis.

DEFINITIONS

To provide patient care within an ethical framework, APNs need an ethical framework for determining what ought to be done; knowledge of the basic human rights, patient rights, and ethical principles; a conceptual model to structure their thinking about ethical dilemmas; and opportunities to explore and resolve clinical dilemmas in realistic situations. Without this level of foundation for ethical practice, one can be emotionally paralyzed when confronted by an ethical dilemma. Chapters 14 and 15 introduced the theoretical foundation for ethical study and ethical problem-solving and provided definitions to that end. Those two chapters also established the principles of beneficence, nonmaleficence, autonomy, justice, fidelity, and veracity as compelling principles appropriate to guide APNs' decisions. Still, it is important to redefine selected terms here as a context for case analysis.

An ***ethical theory*** is a general view of ethics that provides a coherent set of principles and claims that help objectify clinical decisions about ethical dilemmas (Schultz, 1993). ***Ethical dilemmas*** are problems that arise in clinical situations because people, attempting to make decisions guided by their value set, weigh differently the competing moral principles under consideration. In ethical dilemmas, no choice exists that preserves both of the competing values. Either decision is morally defensible because either is guided by an ethical principle, but neither is ideal. For example, allowing autonomy for a terminally ill person might clash with one caregiver's view of saving life at any cost. Each clinical predicament is unique and based on the individual attributes of those involved as patients, families, and caregivers; the situational context; and the consequences of any decision. Ethical dilemmas, then, are resolvable but not solvable (Raines, 1993).

Case studies are short scenarios that present the basic information necessary to make a decision about some situation confronted in practice. Case analysis gives students opportunities to engage in what Wright (1987) and Steele (2000) refer to as "doing ethics." Veatch and Fry (1995), experienced in developing case studies for both medical and nursing education, suggest that one cannot approach a case in the abstract: "It is the real-life, flesh and blood cases that raise fundamental ethical questions." These allow one to lay bare the principles derived from an ethical framework. This is an unequaled practicum: students can be present vicariously in the patient encounter, and there is a possibility for an eventful decision-making experience; however, the experience is within an atmosphere where values can be safely tested and group wisdom

can be used as students analyze the dilemma, reach consensus, and analyze the implications of that decision.

The strength of case studies is likely in their ability to provoke critical thinking. According to Fuszard (1995), the case study also "permits development of professional synergy, because students learn to work together with professionals of other disciplines for increased problem-solving and decision-making acumen." Wright (1987) offers two limitations of case studies: they are artificial and as such, there is a danger that the case will be trivialized. It is true that nothing on paper can capture the richness of an actual patient encounter; however, case studies can be made less artificial by developing them out of real-world situations. In examining a case study, some participants tend to suggest that more information is a prerequisite to resolving a case. This can be overcome by the specific assignment: part of the analysis activity can be to suggest what additional data is needed to enable a more informed decision. Wright (1987) also offers this caveat: participants may be tempted to elicit legal questions from the cases. This should be discouraged because one cannot assume that what is legal is ethical or that what is ethical is legal. Furthermore, as Wright suggests, "Philosophy [ethics] recognizes the fallibility of the human endeavor, while law tends to immortalize these failings through decisions which serve as precedent and are thus frequently difficult to overturn." Conversely, "The doing of ethics is seen as a recursive activity, a process that is never really complete but always making progress."

CRITICAL ISSUES: RESOLVING ETHICAL DILEMMAS IN ADVANCED PRACTICE

Ethics does not involve recitation of one's moral viewpoint. It involves applying one's theoretical views of ethics into a rational and careful process of thought about how best to handle a realistic situation. Sometimes this can be accomplished by answering key questions about the situation (Box 16-1). Other times, one may approach the case with what Wright (1987) refers to as a situation assessment procedure (Box 16-2). Often, a clinical decision-making model like the PRACTICE model suggested by Perlin (1992), the clinical ethics model proposed by Jonsen, Siegler, and Winslade (1998), or the model proposed by Davis, Aroskar, Liaschenko, and Drought (1997) (all detailed in Chapter 15) can be used to analyze a dilemma. At other times, one might wish to merge the best features of several models. The main objective is to engage in a rational enterprise for an ethical judgment that shows balance between the spontaneous emotions inherent in facing difficult situations and a carefully reasoned approach to a decision (Ruggerio, 1984).

The following case scenarios have been derived from the actual experiences of APNs; all names have been

---

Box 16-1

Questions that Enable Good Ethical Decision-Making

1. What do I know about the situation? What do I need to know that I do not know at this point?
2. What is my purpose in this situation? Am I the person who has the right to make this decision?
3. What are the ethical concerns inherent in this situation?
4. What organizational policies and professional guidelines should be considered?
5. Should others who have a different perspective and diverse ideas be included in the decision-making process?
6. Who are the stakeholders affected by the ultimate decision (whatever it is)? What is their motivation? Which motivation is legitimate?
7. What if the roles were reversed? How would I feel in the shoes of the person in the situation?
8. What are the possible consequences of the action in the short term? In the long term?
9. What alternatives exist that have the potential to maximize response and minimize harm?
10. Can I clearly and fully justify my thinking and decision to colleagues, stakeholders, and the public if need be?

Note: The Poynter Institute is an educational program for journalists and teachers of journalism. That these questions are valid for APN practice validates Wright's (1987) contention that, "Ethical problems are problems of persons who just happen to be professionals." In other words, personal issues are raised in a professional context.
Modified from Steele, B. (Director, The Poynter Institue). *Doing ethics: ask good questions to make good ethical decisions* (Handout). Available online at www.poynter.org.

changed, and all case situations have been somewhat modified. In some cases, composites have been used. These actions have all been taken to protect the privacy of those involved. Consequently, any resemblance to public cases is entirely coincidental. As will be seen, ethical dilemmas occur not only in the daily work of direct care but also in nonclinical roles such as leadership, research, and education.

The Family Nurse Practitioner and the Williams Family: Disagreement over Treating a Viral Illness

Ned and Carol Williams and their children, Jim (age 17) and Josh (age 8), leave their home in the southeastern United States for a skiing adventure in the Rockies. They have been saving for and anticipating this trip for an entire year. During the last few hours of the drive, Josh begins to complain of a headache and sore throat. He is irritable and has no appetite. By the time the family arrives at their motel, Josh feels feverish and says his neck is sore. So the Williams locate a community clinic, where Beverly, an experienced family nurse practitioner (FNP), sees Josh.

Over the past 2 weeks, Beverly and her partners have seen dozens of patients with symptoms similar to those experienced by Josh and have successfully treated this presumed viral illness symptomatically. After a careful history and physical, Beverly decides that Josh has a viral upper-respiratory illness and informs Mr. and Mrs. Williams, suggesting ibuprofen, rest, increased fluids, warm saline gargles, and a decongestant as treatment. She is careful to explain the difference between viral and bacterial illness and how management is different.

Both parents are concerned about this diagnosis and management plan. They mention that Josh has always received antibiotics for similar symptoms in the past. The antibiotics have always worked rapidly, and they cannot understand why a pediatrician uses antibiotics and the FNP plans a different treatment. Mrs. Williams is particularly vocal. She is obviously upset about her son's illness and about how uncomfortable Josh is. She also talks about how it will affect their vacation. All their plans will be ruined. She is legitimately upset about being so far from home with a sick child, and she also mentions all the money that will be wasted "because none of us will be able to enjoy the trip." "We certainly can't go skiing now, can we? If you would just give him the penicillin shot like Dr. Howard [their pediatrician] does, he'd be better by tomorrow." Mr. Williams begins to button Josh's jacket and says, "Come on, son. Let's go find a doctor who will do something for you." *If you were in Beverly's position, what would you do?*

Application of the PRACTICE model in this case reveals the following:

- *Patient*—Josh Williams is an 8-year-old child who looks and feels ill. He is in generally good health and has

---

Data from Wright, R.A. (1987). *Human values in health care: the practice of ethics.* New York: McGraw-Hill.

met all developmental milestones on time. At present, Josh has symptoms indicative of a viral respiratory illness and finds himself in an unfamiliar health care environment. He is likely disappointed that he might not get to ski on this vacation and may be concerned about his parents' obvious displeasure with the lady who is taking care of him. He is irritable during the visit and frequently says, "I wanna ski. I wanna go to the motel."

- *Relationships*—Mr. and Mrs. Williams, Josh's parents, are present in the clinic with him and anxious that he is ill. Additionally, they are worried about how his illness will affect their vacation. Their motives seem reasonable. As parents, they feel responsible for their child's health care and in an unfamiliar environment may be uncertain about the credentials and reputation of this provider. Their pediatric experience has been with a physician; they may not be familiar with the FNP role or its comparability to a physician provider. They may wonder how they will manage a sick child and a teen in a motel environment or on a return trip home. They may be concerned that Jim, the other son, will also become ill. During Josh's examination, Jim remained in the clinic waiting room; he had wanted to stay at the motel to watch a movie, but his parents refused. He has already begun to worry about how his brother being sick will affect the vacation.

- *Advocacy*—Because Josh is a minor, he cannot make decisions for himself, so his parents are the preferred decision-makers. Parental autonomy is almost universally accepted in pediatric health care. The minor child cannot give consent, and a child as young as Josh cannot have a meaningful discussion about treatment options.

- *Conflicts*—Beverly has a conflict about ordering an antibiotic for this child as the parents have requested. She knows that antibiotics are not indicated for a presumed viral illness. The antibiotic will likely do little, if any, harm in the short term. However, unnecessary antibiotics can contribute to antibiotic resistance, complicating any future infection for Josh. To order the antibiotic, Beverly cannot be true to what she understands as the appropriate treatment.

- *Treatment versus nontreatment options*—Beverly believes that medically she is better able to make decisions about treatment than these parents are. Over several weeks of treating this illness in her setting, she has witnessed numerous children with similar symptoms respond favorably to symptomatic treatment. At the same time, she understands the plight of a family in an unfamiliar setting with a sick child. Ordering an antibiotic is a simple enough action, and although it will likely not make Josh feel better, it will not make him worse.

- *Interests of various parties*—Beverly may tell the family she will not order the antibiotic. Beverly wants to help Josh (beneficence), and she certainly does not want to cause him harm (nonmaleficence). She knows that the

antibiotic will affect the cost of treatment for the family and that it likely will not help Josh; more likely, the viral illness needs to "run its course." If she does not give in to the parent's request, they will likely leave the setting. They are interested in obtaining a particular type of care for their child. It is growing late in the evening and they are in a town unfamiliar to them; they may not be able to find a pediatrician at this hour.

- *Consequences*—This family is likely to have negative feelings about this health care experience and possibly about nurse practitioners (NPs) as providers if Beverly does not order the medication they want. Beverly may wonder if the Williams' word-of-mouth complaint in the community could affect her practice negatively. Beverly may wonder what the decision of her collaborative physician would be if he were on site. If he randomly selects this particular chart for review, what will be his response to Beverly's present treatment plan? What if she orders antibiotics?

- *Ethical principles at stake*—The principles at stake are autonomy, beneficence, and nonmaleficence.

The Clinical Nurse Specialist and the Research Dilemma

Kate is a student clinical nurse specialist (CNS) in mental health nursing. She is completing her Master's thesis, a qualitative study related to the experience of adult daughters who lose both parents to death within a 1-year interval. She needs at least two more interviews to meet the requirement set by her thesis advisor. Kate is flying out of state to a work-related seminar. During the flight, the person next to her begins a conversation with Kate, disclosing how she is returning home after burying her father. "My mother died 10 months ago," she says, "and I think Daddy just died of a broken heart. They had been together 52 years and raised four children." During the 2-hour flight, the woman talks at length about what this experience has been like for her. She seems to feel comfortable with Kate, who has identified herself only as a nurse. She has not mentioned her research. Indeed, the woman appears to find the discussion therapeutic and tells Kate, when the plane lands, " I should pay you for counseling. Talking to you has done me a world of good."

Reflecting on the conversation later, Kate realizes that the woman described every theme she has identified in her study. Moreover, in several cases, she used words highly descriptive of the theme, words that would add considerable meaning to the study if they were included. Kate briefly considers using this unknown woman as a research subject, but hesitates because she neither disclosed the study nor gained any kind of consent from the woman. Kate vacillates briefly, but she begins to think more seriously about including the woman in her study when graduation draws near and she still lacks the necessary research subjects. *What should Kate do in this situation?*

Although this is not a clinical scenario, the PRACTICE model may provide some direction for appropriate action on Kate's part:

- *Patient*—Not a patient in the strict sense of the word, Kate's companion on her airline flight is a would-be research participant, albeit one unaware of that status. If Kate should include her in the study, Kate owes her a duty as an ethical researcher.
- *Relationships*—There is no information about the woman on the airplane other than about her parental losses in the last 10 months. She was traveling alone and never even mentioned her name to Kate.
- *Advocacy*—The woman has a right to know if she is being included as a research participant and a right to an opportunity to learn enough about the conditions of the study to provide her informed consent. Perhaps if she had known about the study, she would have agreed to participate, but perhaps not. She might well have been less candid if she thought Kate would be putting her comments in writing. As a researcher, Kate has an obligation to meet the conditions of informed consent. There is no one to advocate for this woman if Kate decides to include her in the study without permission.
- *Conflicts*—Because the woman in this scenario is completely unaware of the circumstances, there is no conflict for her. The only conflict is for Kate: what should she do? She feels pressured to complete her thesis; a timely graduation depends on that. She is having difficulty finding two more participants. Kate is also seeing redundancy in her interviews and believes her professor is being overly demanding. Furthermore, the woman on the plane will never know her comments are being included in the study. As Kate tells herself, "That woman's words will absolutely give voice to all the themes. Her words would be perfect." Can what the woman does not know possibly hurt her?
- *Treatment versus nontreatment options*—In this case, the treatment/nontreatment issue does not relate to medical treatment but to inclusion in a research study without having given one's permission. It is straightforward; either Kate will include the woman as a participant or not. The woman will have no say in the decision. If she decides to include the woman in the study, Kate will have an additional ethical conflict over whether to explain this inclusion as a procedural variance or omit the facts altogether.
- *Interests of various parties*—The woman disclosed aspects of a painful personal experience during their time together; clearly, the loss of two parents in less than a year is an emotional situation. The woman felt comfortable being candid with Kate, who was a good listener. She actually felt comforted in sharing her experience and was unaware of any other component of their encounter. On the other hand, Kate's initial motivation no longer exists. The conversation is over; now Kate is interested in using these "perfect words" to realize her requirements for the thesis. She wants to complete her degree requirements and sees this as a possible way to do so. Kate tells herself that the comfort she provided during that 2 hours is a fair exchange for using the woman's case in her study. Moreover, there is no risk to the woman or the profession, and possibly other individuals will benefit from the information shared when Kate publishes her study.
- *Consequences*—For the woman, there are likely no consequences, regardless of Kate's decision. For Kate, graduation might be delayed if she does not include the woman's responses. However, this choice may contribute to a greater sense of pride in the ultimate accomplishment. The consequences of the opposite choice likely depend on how Kate's self-perception is affected by the decision and whether the facts of the decision become public.
- *Ethical principles at stake*—Autonomy, veracity, and fidelity are the major ethical principles in conflict in this dilemma.

The Certified Registered Nurse Anesthetist and the Surgeon: at Odds over Protocol

Bill is a certified registered nurse anesthetist (CRNA) in his second year of practice at a large teaching hospital. Today he is giving general anesthesia for an abdominal surgical procedure. The patient, Ben, is a police officer injured in a motorcycle accident. The supervising anesthesiologist is Dr. Ann Fleming, who is circulating between three rooms and has just gone next door to help another nurse anesthetist with a problem situation.

Shortly after Dr. Fleming leaves the room, the surgeon tells Bill to give Ben two units of whole blood. Bill recognizes that the patient fails to meet the objective criteria for a blood transfusion according to the written nurse anesthesia protocol. Bill informs the surgeon, who asks loudly, "And just where did you go to medical school?" He again demands that a blood transfusion be started, saying that it is his decision, not Bill's. He even accuses Bill of careless disregard for the patient's well-being. *What should Bill do in this situation?*

For this case, the clinical ethics model proposed by Jonsen et al (1998) will guide analysis:

1. **Medical indications:**

- *Patient's medical problem/history/diagnosis/prognosis*— The patient is a 37-year-old policeman who prior to this motorcycle accident was in good health. He is undergoing an exploratory laparotomy, which has been ongoing for approximately 30 minutes when the surgeon demands the blood transfusion. Objective parameters, baseline labs, vital signs, blood loss, fluid replacement status, and urinary output by catheter fail to indicate a need for blood at this time. A recheck of arterial blood gases, a hematocrit, and pulse oxygen readings validate those parameters. Additionally, this is a healthy, well-conditioned male whose prognosis is good. He has no chronic conditions and leads a healthy lifestyle.

- *Problem: acute/chronic/critical/emergent/reversible*—This is an acute problem related to an accidental injury. The patient had been in the emergency room for approximately 1 hour before the surgery. His only other injuries were scrapes and bruises and a laceration of the right knee requiring 20 sutures. The decision for surgery was made on the basis of signs suggestive of an acute abdominal condition and an inconclusive ultrasonography. His preoperative status was good.
- *Goals of treatment*—The exploratory laparotomy is intended to identify the causative problem and allow timely surgical intervention.
- *Probabilities of success*—Given the status of the patient preoperatively, there is every indication that the surgery will be effective. A full recovery is expected.
- *Plans in case of therapeutic failure*—There is no reason to doubt that surgery will be successful in this situation. It is an appropriate remedy for diagnosing and treating an acute abdominal condition related to accidental injury.
- *Benefits of medical and nursing care*—This is a complicated question because the medical and nursing care in this scenario are at odds. The physician is ordering a blood transfusion, but the APN has determined that the patient does not meet the criteria for blood transfusion at this time.

2. **Quality of life:**

- *Prospects with or without treatment for return to normal life*—The surgeon does not provide a rationale for his demand for a blood transfusion. As he is operating within a sterile field, his knowledge of objective parameters would seem to be somewhat less than that of the CRNA, whose role it is to monitor the patient's health status during surgery. The CRNA has attended closely to objective findings and compared these to the written protocol in making his decision that blood is not warranted.
- *Biases that might prejudice the provider's evaluation of quality of life*—None are evident.
- *Present or future conditions such that continued life might be judged undesirable by the patient*—None are evident.
- *Plan or rationale to forego treatment*–None has been made.
- *Plans for comfort and palliative care*—None have been prepared, with the exception of usual postoperative comfort measures. Full recovery is expected.

3. **Patient preferences:**

- *Patient's expressed preference regarding treatment*—The informed consent, which the patient signed, did mention blood transfusions as an option for treatment. Although the patient signed the consent form, he requested that blood be withheld unless absolutely necessary.
- *Patient informed of risks and benefits*—The surgeon did not go into detail about the need for blood transfusions. He did respond to the patient's request by saying he doubted blood would be necessary and would use blood "only as a last resort."
- *Patient's competence to give consent*—Although the patient is under the influence of general anesthesia at the time of the incident, he was alert, nonsedated, and fully capable of giving informed consent preoperatively.
- *Surrogate if incapacitated*—This is not applicable.
- *Unwilling or unable to cooperate*—This is not applicable.
- *Patient's right to choose being respected to extent possible*—Although the CRNA's primary motivation is not related to the patient's preference not to have a blood transfusion, this is a factor.

4. **Contextual features:**

- *Family issues possibly influencing treatment*—None are known.
- *Provider issues influencing treatment decisions*—The surgeon in this case is experienced; he has been in general surgery practice for 11 years and enjoys a good reputation. There is no rationale given for why he believes the patient needs blood at this point in the surgery. Therefore it is difficult to know what factors might be influencing his treatment request. Bill is new to the CRNA role but is capable and conscientious. He is following hospital protocol and seems not to have any other motivation for failing to honor the surgeon's request immediately. Dr. Fleming, the supervising anesthesiologist, is in the surgical suite but not in the room at the time of the surgeon's request.
- *Financial and economic factors*—Although there is a charge for blood transfusions at this hospital, cost is an insignificant factor in this case. The cost of the blood transfusion would be borne by third-party payers.
- *Religious and cultural factors*—The patient is not a member of a particular organized religious group; consequently, this is not a factor. He is not a member of an ethnic or racial group that prohibits blood transfusions.
- *Justification to breach confidentiality*—This is not applicable.
- *Problems of allocation of resources*—There are none.
- *Legal implications of treatment decisions*—The patient is owed a duty by the nurse anesthetist. If his care fails to meet the standard of practice and he sustains damages as a result, there would be legal implications. At present, it appears that the CRNA is attempting to meet the standard of practice by following acceptable written protocols. He is working under the supervision of a licensed anesthesiologist who is meeting the legal

requirement of covering nurse anesthetists by being present in the surgical suite.

- *Clinical research or teaching involved*—None is involved.
- *Provider or institutional conflict of interest*—Clearly there is conflict between the two providers. It is unknown if they have worked together before or if there has been a problem in the past.

The Certified Nurse Midwife and the Patient Who Does Not Want an Abortion

Shanna is a 16-year-old girl who comes to the nurse-midwifery clinic for a follow-up visit on Tuesday afternoon. On the preceding Saturday, Shanna had been brought to the clinic by her mother, who asked for a prescription for birth control pills for Shanna. At that time, Shanna was found to have a positive pregnancy test. The pelvic examination revealed a uterus approximately 14 weeks in size. At that point, Shanna and her mother were informed and asked to come back to the clinic for follow-up because full prenatal examinations are not done on Saturdays at the clinic.

Today Shanna is scheduled to see Jo, an experienced certified nurse midwife (CNM). When Jo enters the examination room, she finds both Shanna and her mother. A quick interview reveals that the mother is determined that Shanna have an abortion. She says to the midwife, "She is at the top of her class and has a scholarship for track; this girl is an Olympic hopeful. She can't just let all that go. Plus, I'm a single mom with two other daughters, and I don't get help from their father. If she has this baby, that'll be on me too—she can't take care of a baby. I have to work, and I can barely make ends meet feeding three folks, let alone a baby. A baby! What was she thinking?" Jo notices that throughout this tirade, Shanna is sitting quietly, staring straight ahead without facial expression.

Jo asks the mother to wait outside while she talks to Shanna. At this time, she learns that Shanna does not want an abortion; she believes abortion is wrong. She acknowledges that the baby's father is no longer "in the picture" and that her mother is "right about it being too soon for me to have a baby." Still, she would prefer to have the baby and place it for adoption than have an abortion. *What should Jo do in this situation?*

The elements for ethical decisions suggested by Davis et al (1997) will be used to analyze this ethical dilemma:

- *Overall situation*—There is a disagreement between the patient and her mother about how this unexpected, recently diagnosed pregnancy will be managed. There is a readily apparent lack of communication between the two. This disagreement has apparently been escalating for the 4 days since the pregnancy was diagnosed.

- *Significant facts*—Shanna is a 16-year-old primigravida in good health, approximately 14 weeks pregnant. She is a junior in high school and has recently broken up with her boyfriend of 1 year. He is the father of this baby but wants no part of the decision about what to do. Shanna lives with her mother and two sisters, (14 and 12 years old). Since her mother does shift work, Shanna has responsibility for caring for her younger sisters at times; she does not mind the role, except that they frequently argue. She is a runner on the track team and has won numerous medals. She has been offered scholarships in track by four different universities and realizes that her continued education might be compromised by this pregnancy. She says that since the clinic visit on Saturday, her mother has been upset, shouting and crying. With tears in her eyes, Shanna says, "I have really disappointed a lot of people." She says her mother refuses to listen to her. Her mother has consulted an abortion clinic and has started trying to borrow the money for an abortion, assuming that Shanna will agree to have the procedure. Physical examination shows a tall, extremely slender girl who appears to be her stated age. The findings of the examination are entirely normal and confirm pregnancy.

- *Stakeholders involved*—Stakeholders include Shanna and her mother; Shanna's sisters; and Shanna's grandmother, who is actively involved in the situation. The father of the baby knows about the pregnancy, but he has a new girlfriend and has said this is Shanna's decision. Whatever she decides is fine with him; he has no money to help with an abortion or with prenatal care.

- *Relevant legal data*—Although Shanna is only 16 and lives with her mother, the law says she has the right to make decisions related to pregnancy. Shanna is the patient; the CNM owes a legal duty to her, not her mother.

- *Specific ethical conflict*—The conflict is between Shanna's right to choose (autonomy) not to undergo an abortion and her mother's wishes that the pregnancy not continue.

- *Possible choices, intents, and consequences*—The possible actions in this situation are provided in Table 16-1.

- *Practical constraints*—There is no abortion clinic in the community; if abortion is the ultimate decision, arrangements will be necessary. Finding the necessary funds will also be a problem. If the alternate decision is made, Shanna will need to be scheduled for prenatal visits after school. Since pregnant students are not allowed to attend the school in which she is currently enrolled, arrangements will need to be made for transfer to a different school. Shanna's health care coverage is paid by Medicaid, but a pregnancy and new baby will seriously tax the limited financial resources of this family. Shanna will be eligible for WIC foods.

- *Recommended action*—On the basis of the outlined facts, *what should you do?*

Table 16-1

Possible Choices, Intents, and Consequences

CHOICES	LIKELY CONSEQUENCES
Inform the mother of Shanna's desire not to have an abortion. Provide information about how forcing someone into an unwanted abortion has been shown to increase emotional problems postabortion.	The mother may or may not change her opinion as a result of this action.
Advise Shanna to listen carefully to her mother's concerns about continuing the pregnancy and how this will likely affect her future and that of her family.	This action may compromise the nurse-patient relationship and decrease Shanna's trust in the midwife, who will be an important member of the childbirth team if Shanna does continue her pregnancy.
Refer Shanna to an abortion clinic for assessment.	Although this may be an appropriate action later, resolution of the conflict between Shanna and her mother must be given priority.
Refer Shanna and her mother to a social worker for counseling and encourage them to use this resource to see each other's point of view. Schedule a follow-up visit with the prenatal clinic after the social work visit.	Since the patient is in the late first trimester of pregnancy, the decision to abort must be made soon. If the opposite decision is made, prenatal care should continue to create an optimal outcome for mother and baby. With the help of an informed and neutral professional, Shanna and her mother can consider the situation less emotionally and hopefully come to some resolution. Additionally, irrespective of the ultimate decision, the social worker will be able to provide anticipatory guidance and practical support.

IMPLICATIONS FOR MSN EDUCATION AND ADVANCED PRACTICE

Case studies like the four given here can be used as a basis for individual reflection or group discussion and decision-making, or they may be used as an interactive learning activity. They can also be used as a stimulus for roleplaying, with individuals playing the parts of the stakeholders in the situation.

APN educators who also practice can bring real-world examples into the classroom using the case-study format. Students can share cases from their own clinical practice experiences for discussion. Students often need support as decision-makers in ethical dilemmas. They need help in appreciating that such cases, by virtue of being dilemmas, have no one right answer. Tolerating ambiguity and working in "shades of gray" can sometimes be difficult, especially for novices.

A systematic approach to ethical problems, such as those used here, enables a more rational thinking process and ensures that a decision is informed and reasoned, not emotional. APNs may wish to try several approaches before deciding which serves their practice most effectively. Having a copy of the various professional codes that guide practice can facilitate case analysis.

PRIORITIES FOR RESEARCH

Priorities for research relevant to ethical decision-making are offered throughout this unit. It is enough here to suggest that the case study makes a valuable addition to research as a medium for studying the decision-making processes of APNs in situations calling for moral or ethical reasoning. It would be interesting to compare decisions made with the various decision models. One might also determine whether decisions made by individual APNs vary considerably from those made collectively by APNs in a group exercise. Finally, in generic cases, how do decisions compare when made by different types of APNs? For example, in the case related to the graduate student's completion of a thesis, does the decision made by the CNS student differ from one made by an NP, CNM, or CRNA? If it does, what factors contribute to that different decision? To what extent does the specialist use professional codes to guide role-related decision-making?

DISCUSSION QUESTIONS

These questions can be used to promote critical thinking and encourage discussion.

Chart
16-1

Case Studies

The Woman who Could Not Pay

Julie is a FNP working for a group of physicians in private practice in a small community. She is at her desk doing paperwork when an aide approaches her about a woman who is in the otherwise empty waiting room, hoping to be seen. She says the woman is "dirty and smells bad." "She is toting a canvas bag full of her belongings and says she has no money, but she looks sick and hopes someone will help her. She says she's lived under the Richmond Street Bridge since losing her job. She says it hurts to 'pass her water,' and when she used the gas station bathroom an hour ago, there was blood in the toilet. What should I do?" Julie knows that the other providers have left for the day and that the decision is hers. *What should Julie do?*

The Clinical Nurse Practitioner and the Camper with a Do Not Resuscitate Order

Carol, a pediatric nurse practitioner (PNP), volunteers in a camp for developmentally and physically challenged children every summer. This year, she has agreed to precept baccalaureate students doing several days of their pediatric clinical experience at the camp. One day when she enters the camp infirmary to check on the students, she meets one of the camp nurses exiting the building and saying, "I'm not going back in there. I can't stand this." When Carol enters the waiting room, the two nursing students are sitting on a sofa talking quietly and looking anxious. The volunteer physician is seated at a desk reading. Carol asks about the location of the 8-year-old girl who was admitted for observation because of respiratory difficulty. The students point to a closed door. Carol knows that the child has both developmental delays and a serious heart defect; she also has a do not resuscitate order on her chart. The little girl has had great fun at camp, but in the last 24 hours she has had difficulty breathing. Carol enters the room to find the child lying supine and struggling to breathe. Carol motions for the students; with their help, Carol intervenes to ease the child's breathing efforts. Then she learns that the physician has put the child in the room and told everyone not to go in. The students report being afraid to disobey his order; the nurse is the one who has left the building. *How should Carol handle this dilemma?*

The Nurse Practitioner Student who Wants to Precept Classmates

Christy is a certificate-prepared women's health NP enrolled in a Master of Science in Nursing (MSN) program, where she is learning the FNP role. Based on Christy's certification and experience in women's health, she is exempt from the women's health course. One of her classmates in the program, now taking that course, asks that Christy be her preceptor at the clinical site where Christy works full time. It is a choice setting, and Christy is an experienced preceptor who enjoys a reputation in the community as "one of the best." Christy asks a faculty member if she can be a preceptor for this classmate. *How should the faculty member respond and why?*

The Nurse Anesthetist and the Boss's Wife

Sam is a CRNA in practice with an anesthesiologist, Dr. Roth, in a small community. They are the only providers offering anesthesia at the local hospital. Sam is the first nurse anesthetist in the community. Until 6 months ago, Dr. Roth had another anesthesiologist in the partnership, but that person left for a practice site 40 miles away. Sam feels very fortunate to have the position and has liked the work until recently, when Dr. Roth's wife began to "help out" in the practice by keeping financial records. Shortly thereafter, Mrs. Roth began to comment about how much more money her husband could make if he did not have a partner. She complains about the cost of a seminar Sam hopes to attend and about the cost of his malpractice policy, which is paid as part of his contract. Mrs. Roth also makes disparaging remarks about the former anesthesiologist, making Sam very uncomfortable. Sam is told by an operating room nurse that the other doctor "left because Mrs. Roth made him miserable." None of these incidents occurs when Dr. Roth is present. *What should Sam do in this situation?*

The Student who Knew too Much . . . about a Boyfriend

Polly, a CNM student who desires more practice with microscopy and sexually transmitted disease (STD) diagnosis and management, arranges for a clinical experience at the STD clinic. At the clinic, Polly sees the record of a young man being treated for gonorrhea and chlamydia. She recognizes this person as a boyfriend of one her classmates in the program. Polly knows her fellow student believes she is in a mutually monogamous sexual relationship. *What should Polly do?*

The Nurse Practitioner and the Paternalistic Physician

Janis is an adult nurse practitioner (ANP) in private practice with two physicians. Her new patient, Linda, has been previously seen by one of the physicians but has asked to be scheduled with Janis this time. She is seeking reliable contraception and provides her history. Linda had a copper intrauterine device (IUD) inserted by the physician, for which she paid an $800 charge on the installment plan (and she was grateful for that provision). During her first annual examination after the IUD placement, however, Linda mentioned to the doctor that she was having heavier menstrual periods with the IUD in place than she had before. At that point, the physician said, "Well, you don't need it then," and removed the IUD without her permission. Linda begins to weep. "It was so hard to come by that money. I had to save from the grocery budget and from doing part-time mending at night. That much money for 1 year of birth control. How could he do that [remove the IUD] without asking me? Now I still need birth control because we don't want another baby right now and Joe refuses to use condoms." Janis meets Linda's request for contraception. *What else should Janis do about this dilemma?*

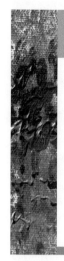

Suggestions for Further Learning

- Read the following: Zaner, R. (1993). *Troubled voices: stories of ethics and illness.* Cleveland. OH: Pilgrim Press.
- Visit the Northern Arizona University website (www.nauonline.nau.edu) to participate in the ethical case studies there.
- Consider additional cases in the following sources: Perlin, T.M. (1992). *Clinical medical ethics: cases in practice.* Boston: Little Brown; and Veatch, R.M., & Fry, S.T. (1995). *Case studies in nursing ethics.* Boston: Jones & Bartlett.

1. Revisit the four case studies in this chapter using the questions provided in Boxes 16-1 and 16-2. Which did you find most helpful in case analysis and resolution? What did you perceive as the advantages and disadvantages of each approach?
2. Review the case studies in the chapter that do not represent your particular area of specialization. Have you encountered any similar issues in your clinical practice?
3. Apply one of the decision-making models or series of questions to the following case studies in Chart 16-1.

REFERENCES/BIBLIOGRAPHY

Astrom, G., Jansson, L., Norberg, A., & Hallberg, I.R. (1993). Experienced nurses' narratives of their being in ethically difficult care situations: the problem to act in accordance with one's ethical reasoning and feelings. *Cancer Nursing, 16*(3).

Bailey, M.A. (1992). Developing case studies. *Nurse Educator, 17*(5), 10-14.

Beauchamp, T.L., & Childress, J.F. (Eds.). (1993). *Principles of biomedical ethics* (2nd ed.). New York: Oxford University Press.

Berger, M.C., Severson, A., & Chvatal, R. (1991). Ethical issues in nursing. *Western Journal of Nursing Research, 13*(4), 514-521.

Broom, C. (1990). Conflict resolution strategies for ethical dilemmas: when ethical dilemmas evolve to conflict. *Dimensions of Critical Care Nursing, 10*(6), 354-363.

Coope, C. (1996). Does teaching by cases mislead us about ethical morality? *Journal of Medical Ethics, 22*(1), 46-52.

Czerwinski, B. (1990). An autopsy of an ethical dilemma. *Journal of Nursing Administration, 20,* 25-29.

Davis, A.J., Aroskar, M.A., Liashencko, J., & Drought, T.S. (1997). *Ethical dilemmas and nursing practice* (4th ed.). Stamford, CT: Appleton & Lange.

Fry, S.T. (1986). Moral values and ethical decisions in a constrained economic environment. *Nursing Economics, 4,* 160-164.

Fuszard, B. (1995). *Innovative teaching strategies in nursing* (2nd ed.). Gaithersburg, MD: Aspen Publishers.

Garrett, T.M., Baillie, H.W., & Garrett, R.M. (1998). *Health care ethics: principles and problems* (3rd ed.). Upper Saddle River, NJ: Prentice Hall.

Haddad, A.M. (1993). Problematic ethical experiences: stories from nursing practice. *Bioethical Forum, 9,* 5-10.

Hawley, D.J., & Jeffers, J.M. (1992). Scientific misconduct as a dilemma for nursing. *Image: Journal of Nursing Scholarship, 24,* 51-55.

Heitman, L.K., & Robinson, R.E.S. (1997). Developing a nursing ethics roundtable. *American Journal of Nursing, 97*(1), 36-38.

Henkelman, W.J. (1991). Analyzing ethical dilemmas. *Journal of Nursing Administration, 21*(1), 6.

Holland, S. (1999). Teaching nursing ethics by case studies: a personal perspective. *Nursing Ethics: An International Journal for Health Care Professionals, 6*(5), 434-436.

Jecker, N.S. (1994). Managed competition and managed care: what are the ethical issues? *Clinics in Geriatric Medicine, 10,* 527-539.

Jonsen, A.R., Siegler, M., & Winslade, W.J. (1998). *Clinical ethics: a practical approach to ethical decisions in clinical medicine* (4th ed.). New York: McGraw-Hill.

Ludwick, R., & Sedlack, C.A. (1998). Ethical issues and critical thinking: students' stories. *Nursing Connections, 11*(3), 12-18.

Lutzen, K. (1997). Nursing ethics into the next millennium: a context-sensitive approach for nursing ethics. *Nursing Ethics, 4*(3), 218-226.

McGuire, D.C. (1978). *The moral choice.* New York: Doubleday and Company.

Omery, A. (1990). Ethical issues. In S.L. Smith (Ed.), *Tissue and organ transplantation: implications for professional nursing practice* (pp. 103-116). St. Louis: Mosby.

Perlin, T.M. (1992). *Clinical medical ethics: cases in practice.* Boston: Little Brown.

Raines, D.A. (1993). Ethical reflection and resolution. *AWHONN's Clinical Issues in Perinatal and Women's Health Nursing, 4*(4), 641-647.

Ruggerio, V. (1984). *Beyond feelings: a guide to critical thinking* (2nd ed.). Palo Alto, CA: Mayfield.

Ryan-Wenger, N.A., & Lee, J.E.M. (1997). The clinical reasoning case study: a powerful tool. *Journal of Nursing Education, 22*(5), 66-70.

Schultz, R.C. (1993). Ethical principles and theories. *AWHONN's Clinical Issues in Perinatal and Women's Health Nursing, 4*(4), 507-525.

Steele, B. *Doing ethics: ask good questions to make ethical decisions* (Handout). Available online at www.poynter.org.

Swenson, M.M., & Sims, S.L. (2000). Toward a narrative-centered curriculum for nurse practitioners. *Journal of Nursing Education, 39*(3), 109-115.

Uustal, D.B. (1990). Enhancing your ethical reasoning. *Critical Care Nursing Clinics of North America, 2*(3), 437-442.

Veatch, R.M., & Fry, S.T. (1995). *Case studies in nursing ethics.* Boston: Jones & Bartlett.

Viens, D.C. (1994). Moral dilemmas experienced by nurse practitioners. *Nurse Practitioner Forum, 5*(4), 209-214.

Winslow, B.J., & Winslow, G.R. (1991). Integrity and compromise in nursing ethics. *The Journal of Medicine and Philosophy, 16,* 307-323.

Wright, R.A. (1987). *Human values in health care.* New York: McGraw Hill.

Wurzbach, M.E. (1998). Managed care: moral conflicts for primary health care nurses. *Nursing Outlook, 46*(12), 62-66.

Zaner, R. (1993). *Troubled voices: stories of ethics and illness.* Cleveland, OH: Pilgrim Press.

Chapter 17

Health Care Ethics and Law

Alice G. Rini

An understanding of ethics and law and how they affect the contemporary health care arena is important to advanced practice nurses (APNs). Nursing exists as a moral enterprise in a time when science and technology outpace ethics and law, and ethics and the law are changing in response to the revolutionary changes in health care. One must stay informed to make moral, legally prudent decisions. With advanced practice comes a role with greater autonomy and potentially greater risk, and with this new role, for the first time, one may become accountable not only for one's personal practice but also for managing general risks in a practice setting.

DEFINITIONS

Although the reader has been introduced to the concept of ethics throughout this section of the text, additional definitions are provided here to serve both as a review and to offer a slightly different perspective. Now concepts related to law are interspersed. This ethical-legal context is an important one because many problems in health care have both a moral component and a legal one; moreover, resolutions to problems sometimes require that a professional's practice be informed by both law and ethics.

Ethics is the branch of philosophy that deals with the nature of and justification for the principles that guide conduct. *Normative ethics* is the ethics of everyday life and the substantive moral problems inherent therein. *Bioethics* deals with issues of life, health, patient-caregiver relationships, and other substantive applied ethical concerns (Ahronheim, Moreno, & Zuckerman, 1996). *Health care ethics* is a branch of bioethics. (Figure 17-1 describes the organization of ethics as it leads to its application in health care and nursing situations.) Health care and nursing ethics are applications of bioethics, which deals with ethical decision-making related to practice and research. Application of ethical values requires interpretation by individuals based on their belief system and understanding of rights and values.

Law refers to constitutions (both state and federal), written or codified laws promulgated by state and federal

legislatures, and the decisions of judges in courts. There are also numerous rules, regulations, and ordinances that contribute to the body of law within a jurisdiction. APNs will be most influenced by the parts of law dealing with intentional torts and professional negligence/malpractice.

Morality relates to principles of right or wrong. It involves conforming to a standard of what is considered right and good; it also refers to the established ideals of human conduct.

As mentioned, normative ethics is a type of ethics that involves everyday questions and dilemmas requiring a choice of action and a conflict of rights and obligations. Normative ethics serves as a guide for action (Guido, 1997). *Deontological ethical theory* refers to a particular worldview of ethics that involves norms and rules based on the duty of one human being to another and respect for obligations arising from one's role. *Situational ethics* refers to an ethical approach in which decision-making is based on the characteristics of the individuals in the situation, their relationship, and the conditions of the environment at the time of the encounter. *Teleological ethical theory,* the other major worldview of ethics (along with deontological ethical theory), relates to the consequences of actions. According to this ethical approach, the end justifies the means. Often referred to as *utilitarianism*, it calls for the greatest good for the greatest number of people, good generally being interpreted as happiness or well-being.

Autonomy refers to one of the principles of importance in ethical decision-making; some would call this the most important principle. Autonomy, or *self-determination,* arises from the ideal of persons as moral agents who have the right of sovereignty over themselves. In biomedical ethics, the principle of self-determination, the notion that a competent adult (one of sound mind) has the right to determine whether or not any health care will be accepted, is highly influential in clinical practice (Ahronheim et al, 1996). Autonomy and self-determination are supported in law (*Natanson v. Kline* 350 P.2d 1093 [Kansas 1960]; *Canterbury v. Spence*, 464 F.2d 772 [DC Cir.] *cert. denied*, 409 US 1064, 1972).

An *intentional tort* is a civil wrong intentionally committed by a defendant who specifically desires the

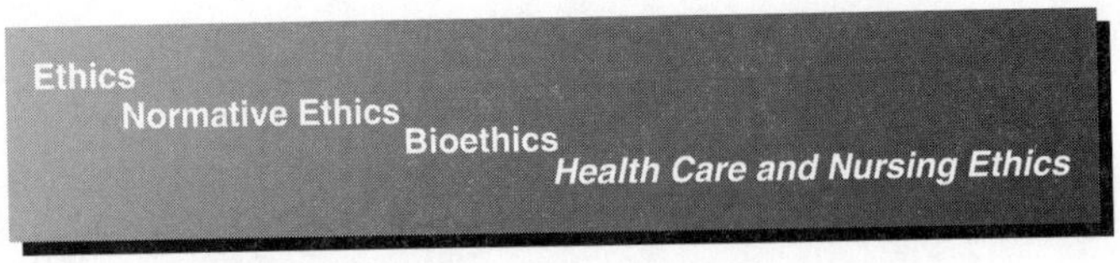

Figure 17-1 The organization of ethics as applicable to advanced practice nursing.

result or knows with substantial certainty that a particular result will occur. Examples include *battery* (harmful or offensive touching), *assault* (putting a person in reasonable apprehension of an immediate harmful or offensive contact, although no contact need actually occur), and *trespass to personal property* (interference with personal property that denies access by the property owner and causes damage to the property). Other intentional torts are *defamation of character* (harming someone's reputation by means of the written word [*libel*] or spoken word [*slander*]), *invasion of privacy* (disclosing confidential information to an inappropriate third party), and *false imprisonment* (unjustified retention of a person without consent). The intentional tort of *fraud* has special significance for APNs who bill patients for services. Fraud is the "willful, purposeful misrepresentation of self as an act that may cause harm to a person or property" (Craven & Hirnle, 2000). APNs who bill for care that has not actually been given may be committing fraud.

Negligence refers to conduct that falls below a reasonable standard of care. Negligence consists of several elements, all of which are essential to establish, or refute, a negligence action. These elements are:

• *Duty*—This is the legally recognized relationship between parties that establishes some accountability by one of the parties to the other.
• *Standard of care*—This is the health care practitioner's (defendant's) required level of expected conduct, generally established by custom, law, a professional organization's statements, or expert witnesses.
• *Breach of duty*—This is the defendant's failure to meet the standard of care.
• *Causation*—An injured party's damage must have a connection to the defendant's breach of duty, and there must be no policy reason to relieve the defendant of liability.
• *Damages*—The plaintiff must have suffered an injury that can be compensated, such as physical harm, mental or emotional harm, or financial loss (Diamond, Levine, & Madden, 1996).

In situations where an APN is being sued for professional negligence, all of these elements must be proven by the plaintiff (the patient alleging that an event of malpractice has occurred).

CRITICAL ISSUES: HEALTH CARE ETHICS AND LAW

Health care ethics encompasses the rules of conduct and practice norms established by professional health care (e.g., the *Code of Ethics* [American Nurses Association, 1985]), as well as the array of ethical problems, dilemmas, and questions that arise in clinical practice. (Many such problems have been discussed in Chapters 14, 15, and 16.)

Health care ethics, while always an important issue, has emerged recently as a major force in the relationships between health care providers and their patients. Although Hippocrates addressed medical ethics, the face and practice of ethics has changed considerably in the twentieth century (Ahronheim et al, 1996). Science and technology have given health care practitioners an unprecedented ability to affect the course of illnesses and provide patients fairly reliable means to prevent, or at least minimize, disease. Some of the interventions have increased the risk of other problems such as reactions to drugs, side effects of treatments, and pain and suffering from highly invasive but possibly life-saving treatments (Ahronheim et al, 1996). Health care interventions have also provided unknown benefits, such as "cures" for cancer and heart disease and the opportunity to transplant organs and tissue to prolong life. These benefits and risks have changed the relationship between providers and recipients of care. The patient, at least in Western society, is more knowledgeable about health, illness, and the workings of his or her own body than ever before; he or she is not a passive recipient but one who demands information about and participation in treatment decisions. Furthermore, there is a greater array of types of health care providers today, far more than just traditional physicians. Some of these new clinicians, such as APNs, emulate long-established and well-accepted norms. Others enact roles practiced in so-called "primitive" societies but contemplated by more modern societies only a quarter of a century ago; these roles include healing touch therapists, art and music therapy practitioners, and herbalists.

There is a need for ethical practice by all health care workers. For those professionals who supervise ancillary or unlicensed workers, there may also be some responsibility for the ethical behavior of those workers. It cannot be overlooked that sometimes the cultural and socioeconomic differences between professionals and ancillary workers mean that their values and behaviors also differ. Professionals need to set appropriate standards, but they must also be open to the ideas and concerns of other workers so that the patient is well served. Professionals must also be aware that although there are ethical obligations, many such obligations have been codified into law. There are now legal requirements that dictate and mandate relationships between licensed health care providers and others who assist in the process.

Ethics and Law as Distinct and Coextensive Entities

Ethics and the law may operate separately, coextensively, or while partially overlapping (Kjervik, 1990). In a coextensive relationship, the law and ethics are able to deal with similar subject matter. One can call upon the law to address some ethical issues, and ethics can guide the development and interpretation of law. Although some laws are clearly based on ethical principles, there are many instances where there is little support in the law for ethical questions. Additionally, there are laws that appear to defy ethical principles. Kjervik (1990) asserts that a purely coextensive relationship between law and ethics is an ideal rather than a reality. However, one might argue that the law of informed consent (i.e., the requirement in most states that patients receive all the information about a proposed treatment, including the expected outcome, the alternatives, and the risks before beginning such treatment) has a coextensive relationship with ethics. The ethical part is the recognition of human autonomy, liberty, and the idea of self-ownership. The law supports both autonomy and self-ownership by requiring informed consent before treatment, and where the law is not followed, it allows the opportunity for a patient to seek redress for damages related to the lack of informed consent.

If the law and ethics are seen as completely separate, there is no support for either principle by the other. Should existing law conflict with someone's morality, civil disobedience to protest that law may be morally required (Brent, 1997). If the law and ethics are completely distinct from each other, one could not use the legal system to resolve situations of an ethical nature, nor would ethics influence the development of law. This is the opposite of coextensiveness, likely exists only in limited circumstances, and probably does not exist in health care.

Law and ethics may also overlap, either by having areas where matters are influenced by both concepts or by the notion that the law is actually imbedded in ethics (Kjervik, 1990). The previous example of informed consent may also be explained in terms of an overlap of law and ethics, or as one imbedded in the other. Some laws address only social regulation, however, and do not necessarily consider moral values. Furthermore, moral values vary by culture and often age or generation. Even autonomy and liberty, very

important in the Western culture, are not necessarily the most important moral concepts in cultures where community and harmony are more valued. There is support for the notion that the law often follows ethics; in other words, laws are generally not enacted until there is a relatively clear picture of the ethical trends in the community. The people's attitudes alone, however, cannot be the controlling factor because judging what is morally correct or incorrect on such relativism is not appropriate for important matters. An example of the problem of moral relativism is arguing for the correctness of slavery based on its being approved by most persons in the society. The enslavement of humans is morally wrong, whether society approves of it or not.

Another example is infanticide. In the case of a physically defective infant, there are societies that consider it not only morally correct but also a duty to terminate the child's life (Arras & Rhoden, 1989). However, in most of the Western world, terminating the child's life would be considered murder. An affirmative, intentional act that results in the death of another is not legal. This tends to raise the argument about some forms of abortion; that is, termination of the life of an infant is legal, if not moral, on the day *before* its birth but not on the day *of* its birth. Critics of abortion law assert that there is little difference between the fetus at term and the newborn, and for some ethicists, this also does not make sense, but it is the situation one faces under the current law.

Law and Morality

It is difficult for the law to represent the diversity of moral positions held by members of a population. Many laws that use ethical language in their codification are actually inconsistent with the moral values of those who are bound by them. What happens in such situations is a continued agitation against implementation of the law. There is no requirement that the law specifically reflect the values of any majority or minority position. However, there is an expectation that the rights of all individuals be respected and not violated by the passage of certain laws. Because Americans tend to be individualistic, the general attitude is that people can choose to take advantage of a particular law or not. The right to be left alone is a rather important concept inherent in the Constitution through so-called *negative rights*, typically exemplified by the "Congress shall make no law" prefix in the Bill of Rights, the first ten amendments to the Constitution. An example of a law that exemplifies the problem of the law's potential conflict with ethical and moral values is the "right" to terminate a pregnancy, arising from the U.S. Supreme Court case *Roe v. Wade* (410 U.S. 113 [1973], modified several times in ensuing years). *Roe v. Wade* dealt with a Texas law that prohibited procuring an abortion. It was challenged by a woman who claimed that she was being discriminated against, based on her personal liberty rights under the

Fourteenth Amendment to the Constitution. The Court found that there was an inherent right of privacy in the Constitution that permits a woman to choose abortion. The conflicting rights of the fetus were addressed by declaring that the fetus was not yet a person and therefore not entitled to constitutional protection. This view of the fetus was, and is, protested by those who believe that a fetus is a person at the time of conception, because they consider it to be at that time, or very soon after, that ensoulment occurs. This religious belief is quite strong and continues to drive efforts to overturn the law, which prohibits states from enacting laws that unreasonably interfere with access to safe abortions.

Law and Human Autonomy

Another important example of conflict between law and ethics is with the notion of human autonomy. The quest for autonomy in health care decisions has yielded laws governing informed consent, generally at the state level and created either through legislation or court decisions; and self-determination, exemplified by the Patient Self-Determination Act (PSDA) of 1991. The health care community and the courts continue to struggle with both concepts, and there are many lawsuits that demand interpretation of these laws in a variety of situations. The conflict and the subsequent legal decisions affect the power and independence of patients, health care providers, and others who are part of the system.

There is conflict in the law as well as in ethics. If one accepts Kjervik's (1990) position on the interrelationship between law and ethics, these conflicts are often related. The issues surrounding end-of-life care reflect such dilemmas. While people search for a morally correct answer, it may be that health care providers and others must recognize that people do not know what is right or wrong in certain situations. One view is that an individual's feelings or decisions should be followed, but this can be as difficult to rationalize as the argument to follow societal attitudes (discussed previously in regard to relativism). One's feelings, while relevant because they reflect personal taste, can not determine moral correctness. When attempting to solve ethical dilemmas, one does not look only within the self, but toward the available external and objective alternatives and their implications, to make a determination (Arras & Rhoden, 1989).

An example of an ethical dilemma that illustrates this concept is the decision to provide certain kinds of end-of-life care. Can a health care provider provide medication and other comfort measures that may also have the effect of shortening the life of a patient? Two issues are in question. The first issue is the autonomy of the patient to choose to be free of pain during his final days or hours. The second is the requirement that the health care provider do no harm. No matter what choice is made in such a situation,

some moral principle may be violated. Which is the lesser "wrong" (if either is)?

Principle of Double Effect

It is not uncommon for both ethical and legal dilemmas to arise in the course of caring for patients. Particularly at times of crisis, the intended outcome of a treatment or therapeutic action may also bring about unintended consequences. This is the principle of *double effect*, a notion derived from Catholic theology. It describes how in certain circumstances, more than one outcome or effect may result from the actions of an individual, including a health care provider. Theology interprets that the morality of an action is determined by the intended outcome, even if there is a second, unintended outcome that would be legally or morally wrong (if it had been the true intention) (Ahronheim et al, 1996). The principle of double effect can be at work in an end-of-life care situation. If a health care provider intends to reduce pain, suffering, and fear in a terminally ill person, and yet knows that the medication to achieve that effect will also have the effect of shortening the person's life by some measure, the morality and legality of the action is decided on the basis of the original intent. If a provider is to do no harm and respect patient self-determination (and there are laws to support self-determination), there must be a way to justify the double effect dilemma. Arras and Rhoden (1989) quote one authoritative source, Gerald Kelly, who suggests that the principle of double effect can be justified if the harm done is not the means of producing the good effect. In the example above, the shortening of lifespan is not the means of reducing pain; one does not kill a patient to cure his or her pain. Kelly also asserts that the harm must not be directly intended and that there must be some positive reason for taking action in spite of the harmful outcome. It can be ascertained that providers do not intend to shorten a patient's life; therefore the respect for self-determination and pain relief are adequately positive reasons for action.

Law and the Health Care Provider

Laws affecting the decisions of health care providers affect APNs in a variety of ways. Administrative laws, promulgated by state and federal agencies, are regulations that govern practice, use of treatments and medicines, and payment schemes. Administrative law deals with licensure issues at the state level. Professional boards such as state boards of nursing address the quality of educational programs that prepare practitioners; determine if certification is to be required for advanced practice; establish testing for licensure; monitor continued competence through continuing education requirements; and investigate and discipline inadequate practitioners.

Civil law deals with private differences between people where redress for damages is sought. Nurses, including APNs, may be sued by patients who believe they have not been treated appropriately and have suffered damage because of it. Generally, an injured patient must prove that the nurse or other provider provided treatment or care that fell below an accepted standard and that because of that substandard care, the patient experienced some loss, damage, or injury. The loss or damage may be physical, mental/emotional, or financial. These claims are called *negligence claims*. Nurses may also be sued under other legal theories such as intentional torts (e.g., battery, assault, invasion of privacy, defamation of character, false imprisonment, fraud). Liability insurance generally protects a nurse from financial loss if he or she is sued; however, if the provider's acts are done with malice or other inappropriate intent, insurers often exclude such actions from protection.

Criminal law deals with violations of law that are deemed to interfere with important societal interests. Recently, there have been criminal actions against health care providers for acts that heretofore had been addressed in civil court through a negligence or civil tort theory. However, several cases were brought against nurses by the state because prosecutors believed that the actions of the nurses were so egregious as to exceed normal negligence and become criminal acts. This change in the law and in the manner that malpractice is addressed is of concern. Liability insurance is not likely to defend a nurse in a criminal action.

Liability Insurance for the Advanced Practice Nurse

Not uncommonly, when a malpractice lawsuit is filed, it names a list of individuals at a practice site, some of whom had no involvement with the incident in question. Those names are dropped off the list at a later time. The attorney for the patient looks for the maximal amount of damages on behalf of the patient bringing the suit—the so-called "deep pocket" effect. Since liability insurance coverage gives an APN "deeper pockets"—access to more money in damages for the person alleging malpractice—some believe that malpractice insurance coverage increases a professional's vulnerability (Pearson & Birkholz, 1995). (Box 17-1 lists some important questions for those seeking professional liability coverage.)

Having one's own personal insurance coverage, however, can be advantageous. It often provides coverage for circumstances outside the job setting and can help protect the APN's interests when such interests are in conflict with the interests of the employing agency. For example, ABC Anesthesia Group, because it is better served by settling a malpractice case out of court, does so, even though it would be advantageous to Jake, one of the nurse anesthetists involved in the malpractice case, to have a "day

---

Box 17-1

Questions to Ask when Considering Malpractice Coverage

1. What type policy is this? Is it claims-made or occurrence-based?
2. What kind of policy do I need, given my specialty area of practice? What are the inherent risks in my practice area?
3. What actions are included in the coverage? Does it cover me 24-hours-a-day, irrespective of setting?
4. What injuries are covered?
5. Who is covered?
6. What exclusions does the policy contain?
7. What is the dollar amount per incident? Per year?
8. What are my rights in choosing my own legal counsel?
9. What are my rights in consenting to settlement or trial?
10. What is the cost of the policy? Does membership in a particular nursing organization provide a discounted cost?

Data from Stock, C. (1997, Spring). Malpractice insurance: what you should know. *Contemporary Nurse Practitioner*, 30-32.

---

in court." If Jake has individual insurance coverage, he can proceed with what better protects his individual interests and not be impelled to follow the group's decision.

APNs who are to be covered by a group liability policy are advised to review the policy carefully to determine if they are individually named as persons covered by the policy and protected appropriately for the roles they undertake. It is important to discern the extent of coverage in dollars and be certain that coverage includes professional tasks performed outside the clinic walls. Generally, insurance coverage cites a dollar amount per occurrence and an aggregate limit (total amount paid in a policy year). For example, Jake, the nurse anesthetist, notes that his policy specifies $1 million/$3 million coverage. This means the insurer will pay $1 million for any incident of malpractice in the policy year, but no more than $3 million in that policy year no matter how many incidents occur.

There are two distinct types of professional liability policies: claims-made policies and occurrence-based policies. The coverage of the two can differ substantially. If one is insured by a claims-made policy (the more restrictive of the two types), coverage exists for claims made against the policyholder during the period in which the policy is in effect and reported to the insurance company during the policy period. "The policy is enforced unless there is a specific provision to the contrary, even if the events or occurrence that gave rise to the claim took place outside the effective period of the insurance policy" (Anderson & Gold, 1996). Vivian, for example, was a certified nurse midwife (CNM) named in a malpractice case filed in August 1999. Unfortunately, Vivian was not conscientious about paying her insurance premium on time; coverage lapsed 6 months earlier. Because hers was a claims-made policy, Vivian lacked financial protection for the incident; she was covered only for incidents that occurred while her policy was in effect. Professionals who wish to extend the coverage on claims-made policies to protect their interests can buy "tail" coverage for that purpose. Jill chose this option. She had malpractice coverage with one company for 15 years as a registered nurse (RN). When she became a nurse practitioner (NP), Jill's coverage by the same insurer would have been prohibitive in cost, even though she had never been sued. Therefore she sought and purchased coverage from a new company, one with better rates for NPs. To ensure she would still be protected by her old policy should a malpractice suit be filed for some incident unknown to her at the time, Jill purchased "tail" coverage for the old policy. An individual preparing to let a claims-made policy lapse for any reason, including retirement, would be wise to investigate tail coverage.

An occurrence-based policy provides coverage for any claim against the policyholder so long as the wrongful act or error that gave rise to the claim occurred during the time the policy was in effect. This means that the individual is covered for the incident even if the claim is filed after the policy expires (Anderson & Gold, 1996).

Risk Management for the Advanced Practice Nurse

APNs, especially those whose roles involve diagnosing and prescribing, need to know about risk management for their respective practices. Formally, risk management is an approach or program that includes precautionary measures intended to prevent problems that place patients, individual providers, or a practice site at risk. This approach to practice involves three components: system precautions, interpersonal precautions, and damage control. System precautions are efforts directed at the design of policies, procedures, and processes that enable safety checks and balances, like "tickler" files that ensure follow-up of abnormal diagnostic tests or a documentation system that includes notes about telephone advice given to a patient. Interpersonal precautions include all the intangibles inherent in good patient-provider relationships, including the general milieu of the office environment and personnel. Damage control includes those processes put in place after an untoward event that continue until the problem is resolved or some settlement occurs (Starr, 2000).

Effective risk management is informed by an appreciation on the part of health care providers of what potential problems exist and how best to prevent or minimize the risk of those problems. This demands some foreseeability on the part of providers—to foresee, for example, that without a way to track the results of diagnostic tests,

abnormal findings might be lost and patients harmed as a result. An APN must be able to foresee that a patient who has a complaint that is not addressed in a timely manner or one who does not have appropriate follow-up for an abnormal Pap smear because of a lack of timely notification are more likely to sue. The APN must also foresee that the potential exists for any chart to be subjected to legal scrutiny; thus, good documentation always serves well as a risk-management strategy.

System components

According to Preston (1998), failure to follow up referrals and abnormal findings on diagnostic tests is among the top reasons health care providers are sued for malpractice. These incidents represent "system failures" that can be minimized by strategies that "flag" laboratory results, referral summaries, and the like to ensure that these are not lost in the system but receive appropriate and timely review, including notification of the patient of the results and necessary follow-up. It also would include follow-up of problems at subsequent visits. Appropriate risk management strategies to that end include:

- Tickler file systems or logs to remind an APN that the results of diagnostic tests are back and ready for their review and action decisions.
- Policies requiring review and the initials of the reviewer on all diagnostic test results and all information provided by professionals to whom patients have been referred.
- Clear procedures that specify the way in which patients will be notified of abnormal test results (e.g., by the NP within 24 hours) and normal diagnostic findings (e.g., by telephone call or letter sent by the office nurse within 24 hours).
- Processes that include having abnormal x-ray or laboratory results telephoned or faxed to the clinic as soon as available (which serves as an additional prompt).
- Summary notes or problem lists indicating that a particular test was ordered or a particular problem was discovered on a specific date so that follow-up can be ensured. For example, if the NP finds a skin rash on a patient at an office visit, whether the rash is treatable or not, there should be some system to remind that NP or another to follow up on the skin rash and document accordingly. Is the rash the same? Better? Worse? If there has been minimal or no improvement, what is the treatment plan at this visit? According to Cummings (1996), "Failure to show the 'apparent resolution' might suggest the problem was being ignored."
- Careful documentation of attempts to follow up with patients by telephone or mail (several attempts should be made in cases where a patient could be harmed by not receiving follow-up information).
- Systems that alert an APN of a patient who "no shows" an appointment. The APN can review the chart and determine if the patient's status is such that a telephone

call or printed reminder is necessary. In situations where the patient's health is clearly compromised by missing an appointment (e.g., a pregnant woman with pregnancy-induced hypertension), follow-up is obviously in order.

- Documentation of all care provided to patients by telephone.
- Expectations that patients admitted to the hospital by a consultant will be visited or telephoned by someone in the practice.

Interpersonal components

All that APNs do to ensure good will within the nurse-patient relationship can be considered an interpersonal aspect of risk management, even though that is not its motivation. In general, patients who are satisfied with care, even in the event of poor outcomes, are less likely to resort to legal action; those who have been treated impersonally or whose concerns or complaints have not been handled to their satisfaction are more likely to sue. Happy patients rarely sue; unhappy patients often do. Even if malpractice is not ultimately proven, the legal process can be costly in terms of time, money, and emotional distress, and the reputation of a professional can be adversely affected.

Effective communication is an essential part of interpersonal risk management. Is there a positive atmosphere in the setting? Are patients treated with dignity and warmth? Are their questions answered? Is anticipatory guidance provided? Do telephone calls receive prompt responses? Are the practice's policies and procedures clearly outlined in writing or in a printed brochure? Do staff members really listen to patients with a sympathetic ear? Positive answers to these questions demonstrate good interpersonal risk management. However, despite the best intentions on the part of APNs and office staff, occasional patient complaints arise.

Starr (2000) recommends that patient concerns and complaints be taken seriously and handled quickly and at the highest level possible without disrupting the work of the office or clinic. It is appropriate to thank patients for sharing their concerns, thereby allowing one not only to remedy patient problems (if possible) but also to improve practice in general. Careful attention to the problem and a show of appreciation to the patient for letting one know about it can go a long way in making the patient feel better in the situation. The patient and provider can explore ways in which the situation can be made right; many such options exist, including decreasing or writing off the cost for a particular service. Starr (2000) recommends asking the patient, "What would make this right for you?" and then proceeding accordingly if possible. Starr says, "It may be the last chance you have to do some effective risk management on this particular patient before he or she consults a lawyer." Of course, the interpersonal gains that come with problem resolution for patients can also lend positively to their word of mouth endorsement of the practice to others.

Damage control components

There is clearly an element of damage control in attending to patients' grievances in a timely, appropriate manner as previously outlined. Sometimes there is no remedy and the patient will seek redress through the legal system. In such cases, everyone involved should participate in a retrospective evaluation of what went wrong and what strategies can be used to prevent the same or similar problems in the future. The willingness and capacity to learn from one's mistakes is of inestimable value.

Diagnostic interviews, physical examinations, and prescription of medications, all within the purview of APNs, fall within the top five areas for malpractice claims; diagnostic errors and failure to treat are the major sources of lawsuits filed against primary care providers (PCPs) (Preston, 1998; Buppert, 2000). According to Pearson and Birkholz (1995), APNs are at low risk for malpractice allegations. One supporting example is revealed by a review of data from the National Practitioner Data Bank, established in 1990 in response to the Health Quality Improvement Act of 1986; this data indicates that NPs are rarely sued.

APNs should, of course, practice within their defined scope of practice according to the law and carefully follow the standard of care in their actions and interactions. It is when care falls below the standard and a patient with whom one has a relationship is harmed as a result that questions of professional negligence arise. In the event that there has been an incident of that nature, the APN should file a report with the insurer and seek legal counsel according to the terms of the policy agreement. Other actions should be taken to minimize the effects as soon as possible. There should be no attempt at cover-up of the facts and no alteration of documents; this will only make the situation worse. The APN should not communicate with the person alleging malpractice or talk about the situation with others; the legal counsel is the appropriate source of advice in this situation.

Legal Aspects of Curbside and Telephone Consultations

APNs, especially those who are PCPs, may find two contexts for practice uniquely challenging: telephone consultations and consultations provided out of the office setting. Starr (1999) refers to the latter as "curbside consultations" although they may occur anywhere in nonclinical, often social situations. Although most nurses, beginning as early as nursing school, have had neighbors and friends ask for free professional advice, this becomes almost the norm for those in primary care practices. On occasion, it is one's own patient who happens to ask for advice or a prescription outside the practice's walls; at other times, it is a nonpatient who happens to learn one is a PCP and seeks advice or a prescription. Either way, curbside consultation is not without legal risk. If the person seeking advice is a patient, a duty is owed and the APN will be held to the standard of care for that type of problem. In this case, it is important that when the provider returns to the office or clinic, a note be made in the patient's chart about the problem and its resolution.

Even if the person is not a patient, once the APN offers advice, a nurse-patient relationship exists and a duty is owed that the standard of care be followed. This is true whether or not the provider intends to charge the person for the "curbside" service. The problems inherent in consultations provided outside the office setting are fairly obvious: history is often inadequate, even vague; any physical assessment is cursory, at best; there is generally no examination equipment available; privacy is rarely ensured; and follow-up is problematic, often impossible. Diagnosis and treatment are made, at best, on limited clues provided by the individual. The wise APN attends carefully to this kind of situation and proceeds cautiously. The APN can often convince the person to come to the office for a visit by reminding him or her that the problem under review deserves more time and attention than is available outside the office (Starr, 1999).

Today, some form of telephone triage is becoming the norm in most primary care practice sites. *Telenursing*, the name often given to providing any measure of nursing care over the telephone, is also on the increase, so most, if not all, APNs will experience its effect. There should be clearly written policies that govern telephone triage in a practice site. Policies should cover, at the very least, how emergencies are to be handled, how nonpatient callers are to be advised, who will handle which sorts of problems, and how messages will be gathered and relayed (Johnson, Schmitt, and Wasson, 1995).

Certainly, patients need to be aware that they have access to the APN by telephone and that every call will elicit a response, whether taken promptly or returned in a timely manner. This assurance is at the heart of the patient-nurse relationship (Johnson et al, 1995). A polite, calm, and concerned demeanor is appropriate in situations involving telephone triage, whether in an after-hours program or during office hours. It is legally prudent for the telephone call to elicit prompt action by the qualified professional and that the problem, advice given, and any other aspects of management be documented. Many practices have telephone logs or special forms for this purpose. One must remember that telephone message sheets are rarely subpoenaed, while patient records are; it is therefore imperative that notes related to the telephone triage find their way to the chart (Buppert, 2000). Having the chart at hand for review before attempting telephone triage can be of immeasurable value not only to the process of the call but also to the patient outcome.

Furthermore, having the chart at hand facilitates timely documentation.

Stock (1997) offers this caveat about the efficient and effective use of the telephone in care, "There is no duty to provide a particular service to a stranger—a non patient caller, for example; however, once you attempt to help the stranger, you are required to meet and exercise reasonable care." Charges of negligence are associated with bad outcomes, especially as they relate to hanging up prematurely; disconnecting the caller, albeit inadvertently, and not reconnecting; and prolonged waiting (usually interpreted as more than 2 to 3 minutes). Strategies to minimize the probability of those occurrences are recommended (Stock, 1997).

IMPLICATIONS FOR MSN EDUCATION AND ADVANCED PRACTICE

Managing one's practice while maintaining compliance with the law and adhering to ethical principles takes some effort. APNs must be willing to engage in serious discussion about the ethical questions that arise in practice. They must be familiar with ethical theories as ordered sets of standards so as to evaluate their application to practice. Only a careful examination of one's own values and the values of one's professional colleagues yields meaningful and useful answers to moral questions.

Nurses must also be familiar with trends in the laws of negligence and torts. The law is always changing, and it varies in interpretation from place to place and time to time. The autonomy of APNs puts them at greater risk than those nurses who work in more stable, controlled environments. The knowledge requirements are greater, and courts will hold nurses, as well as other health care practitioners, to the standards accepted by national organizations. As APNs seek to establish themselves in a variety of practice settings and as legitimate health care providers, professional organizations set the standards quite high. Nurses need to be aware of those standards and always adhere to them, for these are the evidence that any court will use to evaluate a nurse's actions.

The varied dimensions of ethics and law as they relate to APNs should be a focus of educational programs. Opportunities to explore theories and principles of ethics and law in the classroom and to apply them in the realities of the clinical setting are imperative. Educators cannot afford to assume that graduate nursing students who have been in generalist practices have the necessary knowledge base to provide ethical and legally prudent care. Students must clearly understand the elements of malpractice and the ways in which risk management can be used to advantage in their practices.

Nurses have learned, almost from the first day of their first nursing course, the importance of documentation in a patient's chart—the legal account of the care. They can cite the critical principle that, "If it wasn't charted, it wasn't done." Educators need to appreciate, however, that knowing how to chart effectively as a generalist does not automatically demonstrate adequacy of charting in specialty situations. Moreover, many will be recording—not writing—notes for the first time. Consequently, time spent in a review of documentation principles is rarely time wasted. Critiques of charting that include constructive feedback from preceptors and faculty can be important to APNs learning to use SOAP charting (subjective, objective, assessment, plan) in a primary care or specialty practice. Some faculty have students critique each other's notes (minus the patient's identity) and raise questions to clarify points or suggest additions; this approach is an example of the reminder to "write every note as if it will be read by a jury of your peers."

The concept of risk management is an important one to APN practice. Students and practicing APNs should continue to investigate the best practices for ideas that can be integrated into their systems of care. For example, they can explore the ways in which various clinical sites "flag" lab data or referral notes to ensure follow-up and the approaches used to notify a patient of abnormal test results. Dealing with dissatisfied or complaining patients can be challenging. Roleplaying that offers students opportunities to practice this skill in nonjudgmental, safe settings can be very helpful.

PRIORITIES FOR RESEARCH

Research in nursing related to health care ethics and law, perhaps unlike other clinically based study, should include both patient and practitioner perspectives. The following ideas are possible directions for research in nursing ethics and law.

Patient Perspective

Patients have concerns about coping with health care situations, and these raise ethical issues. It is known from the efforts of citizens that people want to participate in health care decisions that affect them and their families. The law of informed consent and the opportunity to establish advanced directives are just two examples of such participation. Research related to the extent of patient use of these opportunities to control, to some degree, the health care situation may yield interesting information regarding patient interest in these matters. Questions might include: What do patients expect in terms of information about procedures and treatments proposed by health care providers? What information do patients de-

mand before consenting to treatment proposed by health care providers? How often do patients refuse treatment when they are unclear on or do not understand fully the purpose of a treatment or the problems associated with it? Why do patients refuse treatment?

Another interesting avenue for research is the decision-making processes that patients and families use to decide about treatments and procedures. Do they value autonomy and exercise it? Do they rely exclusively upon the direction or advice of the health care provider? Or do they use some combination of these? It is important for APNs to be aware of these forces so as to determine how to support patients in their decision-making while being consistent with the law and ethical practice.

Practitioner Perspective

The attitudes and practices of APNs are valuable elements to understand. It is well established that nurses' attitudes affect their practice decisions, so knowledge of their attitudes could provide direction for educators regarding issues to address in classroom work and for practicing nurses themselves to assist in understanding their own motivations.

Wurzbach's (1996) study of the effect of nurses' certainty about their moral values when caring for patients at the end of their lives provides an interesting example. The study found that nurses who were morally certain about their values concerning the provision of futile tube feedings to dying patients were more likely to believe such feeding was inappropriate and that its use violated the dignity of patients. One might study the effect on practice of moral certainty versus uncertainty, or whether educational programs that permitted nurses to clarify their values about particular ethical dilemmas changed the nurses' practice.

Another useful avenue might be to determine what resources nurses use to assist in solving ethical dilemmas or obtain information about legal practice. This would provide information about how to direct nurses to appropriate information and sources of assistance in these areas so that they do not feel alone or abandoned in such efforts.

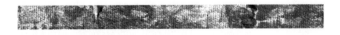

DISCUSSION QUESTIONS

These questions can be used to promote critical thinking and encourage discussion.

1. Patient autonomy is a fundamental principle in approaching patient care. However, many patients are not

always assertive in demanding their right to autonomous decision-making. How would you manage a patient who waived all rights to his or her own decision-making and simply indicated a desire for the provider to say what to do? Are there legal perils inherent in such a situation?

2. Suppose you are an APN working in long-term care (LTC), managing and monitoring the care of many residents. One particular resident has made her wishes if she should become terminally ill very clear, both verbally (to anyone who would listen) and in writing. Then she experiences a major stroke and is neither conscious nor able to eat or drink independently. Her advanced directive requests the withholding of artificially provided food; it asks for fluids only to the extent of minimizing any discomfort associated with dehydration. However, the nurses and nursing assistants caring for the resident demand that you order tube feedings. What is the best way to handle the staff? What should you do for the resident? Why did you make those decisions? Are there other people who should be involved in the decisions? Who and why?

3. A 62-year-old severely retarded man, living in an institution for the developmentally disabled, is diagnosed with acute myelogenous leukemia (AML). Treatment is usually chemotherapy, but his prognosis is poor with or without treatment. He has no known family, and his living expenses are paid with public funds. Although he does not speak, this man has developed a friendly relationship with you, the NP for the institution. Once in the past when he was sick and required treatment that caused discomfort, he screamed and tossed on the floor during even minor discomfort and then became less friendly for several days; it was clear that he did not understand the treatment and considered it an attack by someone he previously trusted. Now, at a staff meeting, his potential chemotherapy treatment is discussed. What would you recommend? Since this man has never had decisional capacity, how, if at all, is his autonomy protected? Can someone so disabled have the ability to participate in treatment decisions? What interest might the state have in his care since they are paying for it? Who or what is the appropriate party to make health care decisions for such patients? Is there legal or ethical

---

Suggestions for Further Learning

- Read Ahronheim, J.C., Moreno, J., & Zuckerman, C., (1996). *Ethics in clinical practice.* Boston: Little, Brown, and Company. This reference provides an overview of ethical theory as it applies to clinical practice in health care situations. It addresses ethical issues across the lifespan. It also includes several case studies, with extensive analysis of each question or issue that arises in clinical practice. Written by a physician, a philosopher, and an attorney, this source is a good one for examining the relationships of ethics, law, and clinical practice realities.

- Review Diamond, J.L., Levine, L.C., & Madden, M. S. (1996). *Understanding torts.* New York: Matthew Bender. This small treatise on the law of torts refers to civil wrongs for which the law provides redress. It can be used as a comprehensive reference and is clearly written to help explain the law and torts in the light of ethical theory. Although written primarily for law students, it may be easily read by any graduate student.

- Read Goodman, J.G., & Musgrave, G.L. (1992). *Patient power: solving America's health care crisis.* Washington, DC: The Cato Institute. This is a study of rights and autonomy in health care, addressing the issues from the perspective of the health care consumer. It argues that none of the health care systems currently in place support patient choice and patient-based decision-making. It offers some possible solutions and is excellent reading for APNs who see themselves as patient advocates.

- Obtain a copy of several malpractice insurance policies. Read them for evidence of answers to the questions presented in Box 17-1.

- Read Johnson, B.E., Schmitt, B.D., & Wasson, J.H. (1995, June 15). Taming the telephone. *Patient Care,* 136-156. This is an exceptional reference with implications for APNs. It includes development of sensible, noncumbersome policy, including telephone triage and patient education, which is both legally and medically prudent.

- Consult Buppert, C. (2000). *The primary care provider's guide to compensation and quality.* Gaithersburg, MD: Aspen Publishers. It contains additional ideas about documentation and other aspects of risk management.

- Consult Cotterell, Mitchell, and Fifer at 1-800-221-4904 (151 Williams Street, New York, NY 10038) regarding *The Nurse Practitioner Risk Management Procedure Guide.* This excellent manual, which has a selling price of $4.95, is provided by these insurers and the American International Group.

- Consult the following websites for additional information about the legal aspects of nursing:
  - USLaw.com (www.uslaw.com)
  - National Practitioner Data Bank (www.npdb.com/)
  - Nurses Protection News (www.npg.com/npg/cases. htm) (this site has malpractice case scenarios for 1998, 1999, and 2000 listed week by week).
- American Society for Healthcare Risk Management of the American Hospital Association (aslm.org/asp/home/home.asp)

support for your answer? Where would you find it? What is the significance of the poor prognosis in your decision-making?

4. As a women's health NP working in a practice group, you often encounter women with unwanted pregnancies. However, you are opposed to abortion under any circumstances. A 32-year-old patient presents with a first trimester pregnancy and a breast mass. Her family history reveals an aunt and grandmother on her father's side with premenopausal breast cancer, both of whom were treated and are still living. The physician has suggested that the patient terminate the pregnancy and aggressively treat the cancer. The patient wants to wait until the baby can be delivered and then commence treatment, but her husband wants her to treat her cancer immediately and considers the baby a secondary issue. How would you work with this family? How can you balance the interests of the pregnant woman with the interests of the fetus? Should that be an issue in the first trimester? Does the father/husband have any rights in the situation? Consult the following cases for guidance: *Roe v. Wade*, 410 U.S. 113 (1973); *Planned Parenthood v. Danforth*, 428 U.S. 52 (1976); and *Planned Parenthood v. Casey*, 112 S.Ct. 2791 (1992).

5. Locate a malpractice attorney or paralegal in your area. Invite that person to class to discuss malpractice law.

REFERENCES/BIBLIOGRAPHY

Ahronheim, J C., Moreno, J., & Zuckerman, C. (1996). *Ethics in clinical practice*. Boston and New York: Little, Brown, and Company.

American Nurses Association (1985). *Code for nurses with interpretive statements*. Kansas City, MO: American Nurses Association.

Anderson, E.R., & Gold, J. (1996). Medical malpractice insurance: are you covered? *Advanced Practice Nursing Sourcebook*, 15-17.

Applebaum, P.S., Ledzt, C.W., & Meisel, A. (1997). *Informed consent: legal theory and clinical practice*. New York: Oxford University Press.

Arras & Rhoden (1989). In Furrow, B.R., Johnson, S.H., Jost, T.S., & Schwartz, R.L. (Eds.). (1991). *Bioethics: health care law and ethics*. St. Paul, MN: West Publishing.

Bergman, J. (1999). Legislative developments: California enacts nurse-to-patient ratio law. *Journal of Law, Medicine, and Ethics, 27*(4), 387-395.

Birkholz, G. (1995). Malpractice data from the National Practitioner Data Bank. *The Nurse Practitioner, 20*(3), 32-35.

Brent, N. (1997). *Nurses and the law*. Philadelphia: WB Saunders.

Broom, C. (1990). Conflict resolution strategies for ethical dilemmas: when ethical dilemmas evolve to conflict. *Dimensions of Critical Care, 10*(6), 354-363.

Buppert, C. (1996). Nurse practitioner private practice: three legal pitfalls to avoid. *Nurse Practitioner, 21*(4), 32-37.

Buppert, C. (2000). *The primary care providers' guide to compensation and quality*. Gaithersburg, MD: Aspen Publishers.

Cavico, F.J., & Cavico, N.M. (1995). The nursing profession in the 1990s: negligence and malpractice liability. *Cleveland State Law Review, 43*, 557-626.

Craven, R.F., & Hirnle, C.J. (2000). *Fundamentals of nursing: human health and function* (3rd ed.). New York: JB Lippincott.

Cummings, C. (1996, July). Strategies in documentation. *ADVANCE for Nurse Practitioners*, 15.

Cummings, C.M. (1997, May). The basic issues in risk management. *ADVANCE for Nurse Practitioners*, 15.

Dennis, B.P. (2000). The origin and nature of informed consent: experiences among vulnerable groups. *Journal of Professional Nursing, 15*(5), 281-287.

Diamond, J. L., Levine, L.C., & Madden, M. S. (1996). *Understanding torts*. New York: Matthew Bender.

Ely, J.W., Dawson, J.D., Young, P.R., Doebbeling, B.N., Goerdt, C.J., Elder, N.C., & Olick, R.S. (1999). Malpractice claims against family physicians—are the best doctors sued more? *The Journal of Family Practice, 48*(1), 23-29.

Eskreis-Nelson, T. (1999). Preparing for deposition. *Journal of Nursing Law, 6*(1), 7-16.

Faherty, B. (1998). Medical malpractice and adverse actions against nurses: five years of information from the National Databank. *Journal of Nursing Law, 5*(1), 17-25.

Guido, G.W. (1997). *Legal issues in nursing* (2nd ed.). Stamford, CT: Appleton and Lange.

Hall, J.K. (1996). *Nursing ethics and law*. Philadelphia: WB Saunders.

Johnson, B.E., Schmitt, B.D., & Wasson, J.H. (1995, June 15). Taming the telephone. *Patient Care*, 136-156.

Johnson, L. (1999). Legislative regulatory update. The advanced practice nurse: change the practice law: what did we learn? *Clinical Nurse Specialist, 13*(5), 243-247.

Kjervick, D. (1990). Legal and ethical issues: the connection between law and ethics. *Journal of Professional Nursing, 6*, 138.

LaDuke, S.D. (1999). When the blaming stops: lessons in risk management. *Journal of Nursing Law, 6*(2), 23-32.

Lutzen, K. (1997). Nursing ethics into the next millennium: a context sensitive approach for nursing ethics. *Nursing Ethics, 4*(3), 218-226.

McKessey, A., & Saner, R.J. (1998, July-August). Protect your practice with a Medicare and Medicaid compliance program. *Family Practice Management*, 57.

Morrison, C.A. (1999, February). A malpractice primer for NPs. *ADVANCE for Nurse Practitioners*, 23.

Pearson, L. (2000). Annual legislative update: how each state stands on legislative issues affecting advanced nursing practice. *The Nurse Practitioner, 25*(1), 16-68.

Pearson, L., & Birkholz, G. (1995). Report on the 1994 readership survey on NP experiences with malpractice issues. *The Nurse Practitioner, 20*(3), 18-30.

Preston, S.H. (1998, August 24). Malpractice danger zones. *Medical Economics*, 106.

Rich, B.A. (1998). Advanced directives: the next generation. *Journal of Legal Medicine, 19*, 63-97.

Sheehan, J.P. (2000). Legal checkpoints: defeating malpractice risk: part I. *Nursing Management, 31*(4), 12.

Starr, D.A. (1998, January). Legal consult: tips for everyday clinical practice. Suit-proofing your medical records. *The Clinical Advisor,* 81.

Starr, D.A. (1998, March). Legal consult: tips for everyday practice. Watch out for those laboratory results. *The Clinical Advisor,* 77.

Starr, D.A. (1998, July-August). Legal consult: tips for everyday clinical practice. Altering the chart. *The Clinical Advisor,* 76.

Starr, D.A. (1999, February). Legal consult: tips for everyday clinical practice. The curbside consultation. *The Clinical Advisor,* 77.

Starr, D.A. (1999, July-August). Legal consult: tips for everyday clinical practice. Referrals and consultations. *The Clinical Advisor,* 80.

Starr, D.A. (1999, September). Legal consult: tips for everyday clinical practice. Handling patient complaints. *The Clinical Advisor,* 80.

Starr, D.A. (2000, May). Legal consult: tips for everyday clinical practice. Is your practice at risk? *The Clinical Advisor,* 106.

Stock, C.M. (1997, Spring). Malpractice insurance: what you should know. *Contemporary Nurse Practitioner,* 30-32.

Stock, C. M. (1997, Summer). Malpractice dangers in telephone nursing: how you can avoid them. *Contemporary Nurse Practitioner,* 31-32.

Trott, M.C. (1998). Legal issues for nurse managers. *Nurse Manager,* 29(6), 38-41.

Wetli, C.V. (1995, July). Answering the call to court. *ADVANCE for Nurse Practitioners,* 49-50.

Wurzbach, M.E. (1996). Long-term care nurses' ethical convictions about tube feeding. *Western Journal of Nursing Research,* 18(1), 63-76.

Section V — Professional Role Development

Cheryl Pope Kish

A strong cadre of advanced practice nurses (APNs) are on the scene in the contemporary health care arena, connecting with patients and meeting health care priorities in a manner unparalleled in nursing's history. Throughout history, practice has evolved in response to need. Now the shift in the locus and character of the health care delivery system has created amazing potential for APNs to align their talents with the public's need for health care. These specialized professionals—clinical nurse specialists (CNSs), certified nurse midwives (CNMs), certified registered nurse anesthetists (CRNAs), and nurse practitioners (NPs)—have a proud history. In addition, growing empirical evidence concludes that their work and their singular commitment to quality care have produced cost-effective, positive health outcomes and health care encounters satisfying to patients. APNs have a bright future.

So, who are these professionals, and what is their role? APNs concentrate their efforts in a specialty area of professional nursing practice. They have a knowledge base with depth and breadth to inform clinical ethical decision-making and a skill mix to enable technical competence. They have the education and experience to form the interdisciplinary relationships necessary for successful collaboration and the unique connections necessary for successful partnerships with patients. While their regulation comes from state and federal laws and their sense of accountability comes from national standards, their heritage comes from nursing. They are first and always *nurses*.

Four APN roles are currently recognized; others may emerge in response to changes in health care delivery. The CRNA provides perioperative services related to the administration of anesthesia, including induction, maintenance, emergence, and recovery; management of acute and chronic pain; and clinical support of respiratory care and emergency resuscitation. The CNM manages the antepartum, intrapartum, and postpartum experiences of childbearing women, provides primary care to their newborns, and provides well-woman gynecological care. NPs provide primary health care and specialized health services to individuals, families, groups, and communities. CNSs develop research-based care guidelines and work to prevent and resolve non–disease-based symptoms, functional problems, and risk behaviors. This section provides a longitudinal view of all of these APNs along the continuum of role development: envisioning a career trajectory, enacting a role, and ultimately evaluating its effectiveness. This section also provides unifying information to help APNs better understand their roles.

Chapter 18 examines the subroles related to the ultimate mission of APNs: expert clinician, educator, collaborator, researcher, and leader. This chapter focuses on emphasizing the nurse in the varied APN roles.

Today, as throughout recorded history, work roles occupy nearly one half of one's adult life. Chapter 19 is devoted to describing the development of the work roles of the APN—the role socialization process. The education that enables role acquisition is evaluated.

APNs are in a position to invest in the future of the profession one individual at a time by serving as preceptors or mentors for others. Chapter 20 is concerned with the way in which preceptors and mentors influence role attainment. Suggestions are provided for selecting an ideal preceptor or mentor; choosing or creating a clinical site conducive for optimal learning; and capitalizing on a mentorship. The phases of preceptorship and the inherent expectations for both individuals in this special pairing are examined in detail.

Chapter 21 elaborates on how to market oneself for the prospective role of APN and how to promote the role once it is attained. This chapter examines the 4 *P*s of marketing the APN role: product, price, place, and promotion. Guidelines for preparing a resume or curriculum vitae and a list of marketing strategies are included.

Too often, APNs lack the business savvy to negotiate an employment agreement or collaborative practice arrangement that contributes to their maximal potential, protects them legally, and ensures appropriate compensation and benefits. Chapter 22 stresses the importance of a written contract, discusses what to include in a contract, and teaches how to calculate an appropriate compensation package. Strategies useful before, during, and after an interview to increase the probability of being employed are also a focus of the chapter. A sample practice agreement is included.

The focus of Chapter 23 is how to write a business plan for a revenue generating or not-for-profit venture. A sample business plan is included. Details in this chapter are helpful to APN entrepreneurs.

Chapter 24 presents a comprehensive view of Benner's "novice to expert" theory as it relates to role attainment of APNs. Attention is given to the way in which expertness develops.

Finally, Chapter 25 continues to elaborate on role development, addressing the specifics of role-performance evaluation. The CIPP and Waltz evaluation models are detailed, as are the processes of self-evaluation, peer evaluation, and chart audit evaluation. Additionally, both external and internal outcome evaluation measures are examined, and a case study is used to integrate the evaluation models.

Chapter 18

Roles of the Advanced Practice Nurse

Janet L. Andrews

Advanced practice nurse (APN) roles have evolved over the past 30 to 40 years in response to the demand for affordable, high-quality health care. Nursing stepped up to the demand by filling the void with highly educated nurses who deliver quality health care in acute and primary care settings within today's managed-care environment. In the past, nurses were allowed to practice as APNs if they had attended post-associate degree or diploma training through a certificate program. Recently, there has been discussion about whether "certificate" APNs (as they are known) should be allowed to receive third party reimbursement. In most states, certificate APNs have been "grandfathered" so that they may continue to practice; however, the issue of reimbursement is still being debated. Presently, APNs are required to obtain graduate degrees, and in many states they pass a certification examination in order to practice. Thus APNs must now have a minimum of a Master's degree for entry into practice, with all the education, practical experience, and skills that implies.

CRITICAL ISSUES: DEFINING THE MAJOR ROLES OF THE ADVANCED PRACTICE NURSE

APNs practice in a variety of specialty areas, but they usually choose one of four routes to advanced practice: (1) nurse practitioner (NP), (2) clinical nurse specialist (CNS), (3) certified nurse midwife (CNM), or (4) certified registered nurse anesthetist (CRNA). APNs must assume multiple roles within the health care system in their effort to provide primary and acute care for patients. Although the multiple roles provide richness for practice, performing them presents challenges.

Generally, APNs assume five major roles: (1) expert, (2) educator, (3) collaborator, (4) leader, and (5) researcher. As will become evident in this chapter, an APN may perform these roles simultaneously at any given time or may perform a variety of roles throughout any given day. Although these roles may overlap and thus are circular in nature (Figure 18-1), they are presented separately in this chapter for the sake of clarity of discussion.

Expert

Nursing as a profession is rooted in practice. Because they are able to focus on an area of specialty, APNs are experts in a defined area of knowledge and become expert clinicians in their field. In its definition of a CNS, the American Nursing Association (ANA) (1986) describes specialty practice in nursing as "the diagnosis and treatment of actual or potential health problems within a specialized area of nursing." This definition is particularly compelling for APNs because it retains the flavor of nursing more than medically focused interpretations. Indeed, an APN is prepared to diagnose and treat patients' health problems. Clinical decision-making, both independent and collaborative, is one the hallmarks of advanced clinical practice in nursing. As students, APNs branch out into specialty areas and study complex issues in depth; however, all APNs have a common base from which to begin—nursing. Therefore they not only communicate holistically with patients, they also communicate with each other using a common base of knowledge and understanding.

APNs are clinical experts in their respective fields. Research supporting this fact has recently been widely disseminated (Mundinger, 2000). Gift (1998) describes the expert clinician as the APN who "manages the care of patients with complex needs, instructs other nurses about the care of these patients, and is responsible for the quality of patient care." An APN is neither a physician extender nor a physician substitute (Ford, 1999). Although both physicians and nurses collect similar data, the difference lies in what they do with it (Ford, 1999). APNs have the advantage of bringing knowledge and expertise from the unique perspective of nursing to the advanced practice arena. Advanced assessment knowledge builds on the basic

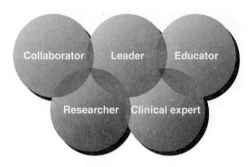

Figure 18-1 The roles of the advanced practice nurse are circular and overlap.

skills and information that APNs gain during undergraduate education. Building on an already established base of assessment skills, the APN becomes an expert at patient assessment. In addition, nursing's perspective of holistic care and their understanding that each patient is an individual with unique needs and concerns allows the APN to approach each patient with an open mind and a willingness to accomplish patient assessment from the patient's perspective. In a strictly medically focused examination, the health-related concerns of a patient may go undetected; not so with the expert holistic assessment of the APN. Hirschberg (1998) described an APN's skilled assessment as automatic and accompanied by an ability to "provide a truly focused and caring presence within a short period of time." APNs are experts in listening to patients and interpreting subjective information that patients may have difficulty putting into words. They are able to view the world through a patient's eyes. Beddoe (1999) called this the "reachable moment." Although she acknowledged that this level of understanding does not occur with every patient encounter, she described it as one of the benefits of the APN-patient relationship. Patients will tell nurses things that they will not share with anyone else (Gordon, 1997). Virtually every nurse has experienced a patient encounter in which the root of a patient's health problem turns out to be an emotional situation. For example, a middle-aged woman presents with hypertension but is also dealing with a complicated family situation involving a full-time job, troubled grandchildren in the home, and a disabled husband who is dying of brain cancer. APNs are experts in uncovering etiologies that only a holistic assessment can reveal.

The depth of knowledge in a specialty area allows the APN to actively influence patient outcomes through diagnosis, treatment, and follow-up. The additional knowledge and skill obtained in graduate education (following the practice experience gained as a baccalaureate nurse) allows APNs to build on basic knowledge and skill and begin to diagnose and treat. APN education entails numerous hours of both didactic and clinical course work, including pathophysiology and pharmacology, to prepare graduates to be clinical experts. The right to diagnose and treat is recognized through the prescriptive authority and reimbursement granted by most state governments or the federal government. APNs are also experts at analyzing and interpreting findings and clinical decision-making. Thus an APN is able to analyze large volumes of data and arrive at conclusions concerning diagnosis, treatment, and individualized patient needs. If the patient's condition lies outside the boundaries of APN care, the APN recognizes this situation and institutes consultation, referral, and follow-up.

Because of their clinical expertise, APNs are actively involved in developing and revising the protocols and clinical guidelines under which they practice; they do not have to wait for the hospital administration to recognize a need for change or a medical director to institute a new direction for care. As new diagnostic tools or treatments become available, APNs can propose the most effective and cost-efficient methods for their practices. They can identify problems, visualize and formulate answers, identify possibilities, and influence others (Forbes, 1997). Often, APNs serve as the voice for the nurses with whom they work and can present proposals for new equipment or procedures to improve patient care at all levels

The APN's clinical specialty expertise opens up doors of opportunity. APNs contribute significantly to cost-effective, quality health care for hospitals, clinics, and private practice (Aiken, Lake, Semaan, Lehman, O'Hare, Cole, Dunbar, & Frank, 1993; Cronenwett, 1995). Many APNs are discovering that not only is their expertise valuable within an institution or clinic, it is marketable as well. Advanced practice entrepreneurs are opening independent practices in community settings, performing health education, testing, and screenings for high-risk groups such as diabetics, human immunodeficiency virus (HIV)–positive patients, and patients with sickle cell anemia. Other APNs are contracting out their expert assessment skills, performing admission physical assessments for drug and alcohol rehabilitation centers or correctional facilities. Still others are contracting as forensic nurses performing post-rape examinations in emergency settings. APN expertise can be particularly valuable in the courtroom when an expert witness is needed in a legal case. Contracting for this service provides a valuable policing of APN practice and can be a learning experience for the practitioner as well. Nurse midwives are opening and managing freestanding birth centers in response to the demand by women for less paternalistic health care (Spitzer, 1995). CNSs are moving from inside hospital walls out into community settings (Nokes, 2000), while NPs are moving into hospitals in the acute care arena. Although this "blurring of roles" has raised the flag of concern about regulation and education (Cronenwett, 1995), as the tracks and specialties for APNs become more clearly defined, such crossovers will become more common without breaching the practice boundaries of any advanced practice specialties. The development of entrepreneurial nurses in all health care settings is a process of growth for nursing as a profession.

Educator

Education is integral to advanced practice. Educational responsibilities range from individual patient education to education of families, peers, and the public, with a commitment to personal lifelong education. With every patient encounter, the APN educates individual patients and/or their families. Often education is aimed at prevention of illness or complications from illness and the promotion of wellness. Patient education not only includes information about injuries or illness, including assessments, treatment, medications, and follow-up, it includes information about how to avoid future illnesses and improve overall health. Providing health promotion information is central to APNs, but providing information about avoiding future complications from a current illness is crucial as well. For example, teaching a woman with gestational diabetes how to control her blood sugar is critical to the nurse midwife. However, teaching her what to do if her blood glucose reading is high is equally important because complications from hyperglycemia may be avoided if the woman is armed with knowledge. Research shows that although physicians ask pregnant patients if they smoke, they tend not to counsel them about stopping (Mullen, Pollak, Titus, Sockrider, & Moy 1998; Thornedike, 1998). In contrast, most nurse midwives report that they counsel women about smoking cessation during pregnancy (Murphy, 1996). Thus one of the major goals of APNs is educating patients to become well and stay well. Medical care is directed toward detecting and treating disease or illness—that is, a curing focus. APNs are experts at patient and family teaching—a caring focus. Both physicians and APNs are great detectives; they are just looking for different things.

Often an APN can develop written educational materials to be used by the majority of the patients seen in the unit or practice. Knowing the individual patient and family's educational level, ethnicity, cognitive ability, socioeconomic status, emotional and psychological state, and level of wellness or illness gives the APN the advantage when planning and developing educational materials. Education can empower patients and their families to reach and maintain optimal wellness. Often patients are too anxious to remember instructions that were given to them at discharge or during an office visit. Fear of the unknown can lead many patients to avoid following instructions that seem unfamiliar or difficult, and often these patients may be labeled "noncompliant." Many complications can be avoided if patients are willing and able to follow instructions. Written materials sent home with the patient and family can serve to reinforce and clarify verbal instructions and improve compliance, but only if the written materials can be read and understood by the patient and family. If the patient speaks and reads only Spanish, instructions written in English will do no good.

Sometimes an APN has to be creative when developing materials. For example, a CNS encountered a family who were all legally blind. She explained the complicated instructions for medical care of the aging father at discharge and realized the family was distracted during her explanation by phones ringing and numerous interruptions by staff. She returned to her office, quickly tape-recorded the instructions, and took the tape back to the patient and family. The family could then listen to the instructions again at a time when they could absorb and use the information. The same technique could be used for patients who cannot read. The point is the APN is in a position of having the freedom, power, and knowledge to develop educational materials for patients based on their individual needs.

APNs also educate their peers and colleagues. APNs have extensive knowledge about disease processes, assessment, health promotion, and disease prevention. In addition, they understand how to interpret and use the results of research studies to improve patient care. A willingness to share knowledge and information not only establishes good relationships with staff, it fosters the provision of high-quality care to patients. Education is empowering; there is no limit to knowledge, and sharing information can improve the staff's understanding of a clinical case, a new technique, a medication, or a new piece of equipment. For instance, when a NP explained to a registered nurse (RN) in a clinic how to read and interpret a Pap smear report, the RN was able to follow up with patients and teach them much more effectively when they had questions about their Pap results. Once the RN understood the meaning and implications of each type of report, the importance of follow-up and the fact that the nurse could have a part in the patient outcome became a reality. The nurse felt empowered, and she empowered patients by passing the knowledge along, reinforcing the NP's' initial patient teaching. As knowledge is freely shared, it is passed along in a "domino effect" to improve patient care. This type of education can be accomplished informally as opportunities arise, or it can be formally offered through classes for staff. Either way, the outcome of disseminating knowledge is improved patient care.

Because they are experts in their fields of clinical practice, APNs are called upon to organize and participate in formal education programs. APNs have a commitment to lifelong learning, realized through attending conferences, workshops, and seminars while continuously keeping abreast of the latest research results, legislative issues, and practice innovations by reading numerous journals and flyers and accessing the Internet every week. Knowing other experts in the field can be as important as being an expert in the field. Networking is a particularly important part of continuing education for APNs; when the need for an expert opinion or presentation arises, the APN has a pool of professionals on whom to call. The route to networking is ongoing communication with other professionals throughout the country and reading the most current literature. Two heads are always better than one when accomplishing any large task. such as organizing a conference. There are distinct advantages to working with another APN to develop a conference for professionals. The organizational responsibilities and program planning are easier when their contacts and knowledge are brought together. Many APN programs are incorporating professional conference planning, professional presentations, and community presentations into the curricula as a way to introduce graduate students to the process and rewards of such endeavors.

Another component of being an educator is teaching others about the role of the APN. There is still much confusion among physicians, other health professionals, and the public about what an APN is and what a nurse in advanced practice does, confusion over the fact that the focus of nursing is different from that of medicine. APNs still practice nursing, and their expertise is not meant to replace or "extend" medicine. It is designed to fill a void in health care delivery to which nursing, by its very philosophy and practice, is an excellent fit. For example, the NP role was developed to fill an identified gap in primary care, a gap which physicians were reluctant to fill (Brush & Capezuti, 1996). The boundaries between medicine and nursing may have been blurred by the evolution of APNs, but the realms of practice remain distinct. Every day, APNs model their practice of nursing to peers, physicians, staff, students, and patients; this is one of the most effective ways of educating others about the role. Physicians (who have opportunities to work closely with APNs), consult specialists, and collaborating professionals can observe APNs as they perform their roles. The advantages of such firsthand observations are readily discerned. As physicians work with APNs they have an opportunity to become familiar with the clinical expertise, critical thinking, patient education ability, and knowledge that APNs demonstrate.

APNs are frequently called upon to serve as preceptors for APN students. As preceptors for graduate students, APNs can influence individual students' experiences and practice, and they can influence the profession as a whole. They not only have the opportunity to model their role for students but also an opportunity to further develop their role and shape the very future of advanced practice. Professional preceptorship can have a profound influence on both the student and the APN. It is a true partnership in learning. Often the preceptor is challenged by the student to explain a procedure or the rationale behind a particular test or treatment. In turn, the student is challenged by the preceptor to explain an assessment, a pathophysiology, a treatment, or the choice of a particular clinical path or topic for a conference. Commitment and excitement about challenges is contagious; both the preceptor and the student learn from each other and can experience a renewed sense of enthusiasm about their role when knowledge is shared.

Collaborator

Collaboration is part of the role of the APN. No one can know everything. The APN may collaborate in a practice relationship with a physician or with an interdisciplinary team. APNs have often informally consulted with other health care professionals when faced with complex patient situations and dilemmas. However, collaboration can take place in a more formal context involving joint practice or contractual obligations. *Collaboration* is defined as working together to meet complex patient needs. Although this definition seems straightforward, successful collaboration is not easily accomplished. Merely signing a contract or an agreement to collaborate does not guarantee that the partnership will work as it is designed to work (Stapleton, 1998). Although on the surface it appears that collaborative efforts should mean less work because of shared responsibility, collaboration actually requires concerted effort on the part of all involved.

The advantage to collaborative practice is that the patient benefits from the expertise, knowledge and practice of two practitioners. Collaboration is often a process that has to be learned through practice; physicians and APNs approach patients from different perspectives and have different ways of looking at the same problem. This can lead to miscommunication unless a concerted effort is made to understand each other's perspectives and communicate effectively (Stapleton, 1998). Both the APN and physician in collaborative practice must have open communication, a willingness to express opinions freely, and an appreciation for the other's expertise and unique practice patterns. This open system of collaboration requires continuous effort on the part of both people. They must recognize how their differing patterns of practice complement each other, how the gaps in one's practice are filled by the other. They must have an appreciation and respect for each other that is evident to patients, staff, and other health professionals.

Nurse midwives have established successful collaborative practices with physicians that can serve as examples for all health professionals desiring to collaborate (Stapleton, 1998). The physicians respect the expertise of the nurse midwives and value their contributions to the practice. In a society that has traditionally relegated nurses to positions of subservience to physicians, this demonstration of respect may elicit criticism and opposition from others who are not involved in cooperative interdisciplinary relationships. Thus collaborators in practice must educate through communicating and being role models. APNs and physicians in collaborative practice must be committed to the philosophy and goals of collaboration and willing to endure criticism for the sake of the improved quality of patient care afforded by such practice.

In today's system of managed care, more than ever before, APNs find the need to collaborate with a wide variety of other health professionals, such as physicians, dietitians, social workers, physical therapists, and mental health professionals. According to Keleher (1998) collaboration of many individuals that integrates their knowledge directly affects the quality of health care. The APN serves as a facilitator of interdisciplinary teams and is often called upon to serve as case manager (Holt, 1997). All disciplines must participate willingly, and all parties involved must understand and value each participant's expertise and contribution to the case. In a profession such as medicine, which values independence and competition, such valuing is difficult, but not impossible (Stapleton, 1998). Open communication and negotiation assist all members to arrive at creative solutions to patient problems. Often the patient or patient's family can be included on the team, contributing to decision-making. Thus collaboration in case management is an equal partnership without hierarchical relationships (Keleher, 1998). Within the health care system, the health care team must be supportive of each other, demonstrating respect for each other's roles in and opinions about patient care. In this form of collaboration, with patient care team involvement, the team has a vested and ongoing interest in patient outcomes. The multidisciplinary team involvement in the case management system allows coordination of care, improved quality of patient care, efficient use of resources, and control of costs. CNSs have taken the lead in assuming the responsibility for case management. The holistic focus of nursing ensures that the APN is uniquely qualified to lead an interdisciplinary team as case manager.

Collaboration for the APN may also take the form of consultation. A patient's care may be so complex that staff nurses require assistance from an APN to interpret assessments, work with complicated equipment, or implement a new experimental protocol. APNs may also be called upon as consultants to assist with specific projects or program planning. As experts in a specialty area of care, APNs have the depth of knowledge to develop programs and carry out projects efficiently and well. APNs can develop a network of APNs with specific areas of expert knowledge and expertise so that at any one time, they can call an expert for consultation. Of course, the process is reciprocal, and APNs who request consultation would be expected to serve as consultants for others when the need arises. This provides an efficient way of dividing and sharing valuable resources while ensuring high-quality programs and projects. Consultants move in and out of

situations, and their assistance is required only for a limited period, but the value of consultation lies in tapping into the expertise of individuals when needed.

Researcher

A variety of research activities can be incorporated into nursing. At different times during an APN's career, research may assume a different priority. Nursing at all levels is both a science and an art. In general, quantitative research supports the science, and qualitative research supports the art. Both types are needed to maintain the balance of science and art. The APN uses research results to improve patient care and outcomes, conducts research to document quality of care and cost-effectiveness, and facilitates the research of others.

Nurses in advanced practice are in an ideal position to use results of research studies to improve patient care. During graduate education, APNs critique research studies and learn to discriminate quality research from poor research. Because of this experience, APNs are in a position to sort the reams of information to better plan patient care. A natural sense of curiosity is invaluable to an APN in asking the questions about patient care and outcomes from which research studies are derived. How many times have nurses wondered why one patient fares better than another with the same disease process or treatment? Solutions to problems in clinical situations can improve patient outcomes by "decreasing complications, facilitating timely discharges, assisting in multidisciplinary effort, preventing re-admissions, and promoting comfort, patient and family coping, and patient satisfaction" (Chase, Johnson, Laffoon, Jacobs, & Johnson, 1996). APNs can share their clinical questions with expert researchers and thus form a partnership in research projects. Research partnerships are developed for the sharing of expertise between the APN, who is an expert at clinical questions, and the expert researcher, who is familiar and comfortable with the research process (Alvarez, 1998). This can be a powerful partnership with the potential to further the knowledge base for nursing (Goldberg & Moch, 1998). The immediate goal is improved patient care.

Leader

APNs are leaders in practice and in the profession of nursing. They have the ability and power to bring about change and influence others. Whether practicing in primary care or the acute care arena, APNs teach and empower other health care providers. The APN's leadership abilities are evident in each previously mentioned role: expert, educator, collaborator, and researcher. The role of leader includes political activism. Today's health care world is characterized by constant and consistent change. Many of these changes are political in nature and

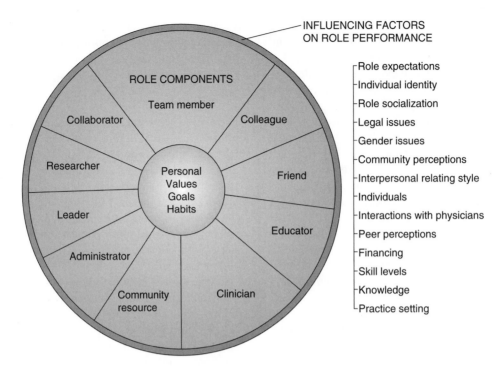

INFLUENCING FACTORS
ON ROLE PERFORMANCE

ROLE COMPONENTS

Team member

Collaborator

Colleague

Researcher

Personal
Values
Goals
Habits

Friend

Leader

Educator

Administrator

Community
resource

Clinician

- Role expectations
- Individual identity
- Role socialization
- Legal issues
- Gender issues
- Community perceptions
- Interpersonal relating style
- Individuals
- Interactions with physicians
- Peer perceptions
- Financing
- Skill levels
- Knowledge
- Practice setting

Figure 18-2 Role performance components for the advanced practice nurse. (Redrawn from Mackey, T. [1993]. *The nurse practitioner role: issues and education* [Paper presented at SREB regional conference]. Atlanta, GA: Southern Council on Collegiate Education for Nursing.)

ultimately affect APN practice. Staying current with relevant legislation affecting practice is vital to survival and growth. This does not mean that APNs must lobby on a daily basis or be constantly present at the capital, but it does mean they should stay current on the literature concerning practice legislation. APNs must be willing to express viewpoints to legislators when practice issues come up for a vote.

Today, APNs are becoming more involved in planning health care policy at a national level (Sharp, 1999). Nurses are experts at working with vulnerable populations. Surgeon General David Satcher outlined the national health agenda for America's immediate future, and he included disease prevention and patient education as priorities. Satcher says that putting more disease prevention into the health care system requires leadership (Buppert, 1999). And who better to meet this political agenda than APNs—experts in both health promotion and disease prevention? APNs need to make themselves known as the answer to this national health challenge, and the avenue for this is political activism. Belonging to professional organizations and supporting the lobbying efforts of those organizations will go far to promote the growth of nursing.

The role of the APN is being developed globally. Although the United States was the first country to demonstrate a need for APNs, countries such as Australia and the United Kingdom are beginning to develop the role. How the role develops in America not only has implications for America, it has implications for the world. As the role evolves and changes, it is important for APNs to stay true to nursing. Everyone goes into nursing to be nurses. If nurses do not practice nursing, they lose their collective voice in the health care system and the political arena. The pressures for acute care APNs to defer to the medical model may become intense. It is important, even imperative, that nurses remember that to be different is not to be inferior. To remain a nurse and to practice nursing is a reward in itself.

PRIORITIES FOR RESEARCH

There is still a need for research concerning patient outcomes experienced with APN care. APNs need to validate what they do as valuable and show that it is cost effective and contributes to the quality of patient care. Qualitative research regarding patient satisfaction with APN care is an area to explore. There is little information from patients, in the patients' words, about their perceptions of and experiences with APN care. One topic of interest for research may be the differences between the care provided by acute care APNs and primary care APNs. Another topic may be an exploration of the differences between the care delivered by certificate-prepared APNs and Master's-prepared APNs.

Suggestions for Further Learning

- Read the following references related to APN roles: Abraham, T., & Fallon, P.J. (1997). Caring for the community: development of the advanced practice nurse role. *Clinical Nurse Specialist, 11*(5), 224-230; Buchanan, L. (1996). The acute care nurse practitioner in collaborative practice. *Journal of the American Academy of Nurse Practitioners, 8*(1), 13-20; Decker, B. Reproductive health care: a case for uniform prescriptive privileges. *Journal of Nurse-Midwifery, 43*(6), 403-405; Hamrick, A.B., Lindebak, S.,Worley, D., & Jaubert, S. (1998). Outcomes associated with advanced nursing practice prescriptive

authority. *Journal of the American Academy of Nurse Practitioners, 10*(3), 113-118; and Mundinger, M.O. (2000). Primary care outcomes in patients treated by nurse practitioners and physicians: a randomized trial. *Journal of the American Medical Association, 283*(1).
- Consult the websites for the traditional APN groups:
  - Clinical nurse specialists (www.nacns.org)
  - Nurse practitioners (www.aanp.org)
  - Certified nurse midwives (acnm.org)
  - Certified registered nurse anesthetists (www.aana.com/information/)

IMPLICATIONS FOR MSN EDUCATION AND ADVANCED PRACTICE

While reading this chapter, the graduate student in nursing may feel that pursuing the role of the APN is an overwhelming proposal. However, one needs to bear in mind that at any particular time, an APN may only be performing one role. Thus, as an APN's career advances, he or she may spend more time in the educator role, in the researcher role, or in collaboration. No one can perform all the roles at the same time all of the time. APNs develop into experts over time. When entering practice, the APN needs to find a practice site that allows professional growth and development, as well as the time needed to grow and develop. Graduate education should also include opportunities to learn all aspects of the APN role.

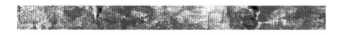

DISCUSSION QUESTIONS

These questions can be used to promote critical thinking and encourage discussion.

1. Interview several APNs about their respective roles. What have their biggest challenges been? What have been the biggest barriers they have faced? What do they find the most rewarding? How do they handle the demands of their careers? How have they become politically involved? What are the most critical issues they feel APNs are facing today? How do they enact the various roles of the APN (expert, leader, educator, collaborator, and researcher)?

2. Join a listserve of APNs in your specialty area, and join the discussion about the varied roles of the APN.
3. Look at Figure 18-2. How does this model align with Figure 18-1? How are they alike? How are they different? Would an APN using the model in Figure 18-2 have a different role than an APN using the model in Figure 18-1? Why or why not?

REFERENCES/BIBLIOGRAPHY

Aiken, L.H., Lake, E.T., Semaan, S, Lehman, H.P., O'Hare, P.A., Cole, C.S., Dunbar, D., & Frank, I. (1993). Nurse practitioner managed care for persons with HIV infections. *Image: Journal of Nursing Scholarship, 25*(3), 172-177.

Alvarez, C.A. (1998). Research collaboration: harder than it should be, better for nursing. *Clinical Nurse Specialist, 12*(6), 250.

American Nurses Association (1986). *The role of the clinical nurse specialist*. Kansas City: American Nurses Association.

Beddoe, S.S. (1999). Reachable moment. *Image: Journal of Nursing Scholarship 13*(3), 248.

Brush, B. & Capezuti, E.A. (1996). Revisiting "a nurse for all settings": the nurse practitioner movement 1965-1995. *Journal of the American Academy of Nurse Practitioner, 5*(1), 5-10.

Buppert, C. (1999). Satcher spells out national health agenda: Surgeon general sets sights on prevention. *Clinician News, 3*(2), 1, 8-9, 22.

Chase, L.K., Johnson, S.K., Laffoon, T.A., Jacobs, R.S., & Johnson, M.E. (1996). CNS role: an experience in re-titling and role clarification. *Clinical Nurse Specialist, 10*(1), 41-45.

Cronenwett, L.R. (1995). Molding the future of advanced practice nursing. *Nursing Outlook, 43*(3), 112-118.

Forbes, K.E. (1997). Leader and teacher. *Clinical Nurse Specialist, 11*(2), 76.

Ford, L. (1999). Editor's memo: the acute care nurse practitioner. *The Nurse Practitioner, 24*(11), 21, 25-26.

Gift, A.G. (1998). The advanced practice nurse as clinical expert. *Clinical Nurse Specialist, 12*(2), 85.

Goldberg, N.J., & Moch, S.D. (1998). An advanced practice nurse-nurse researcher collaborative model. *Clinical Nurse Specialist, 12*(6), 251-255.

Gordon, S. (1997). *Life support: three nurses on the front lines.* New York: Back Bay.

Hirschberg, S. (1998). A rose by any other name. *Clinical Nurse Specialist, 12*(6), 211.

Hoke, K.M. (2000). Exploring the clinical nurse specialist role in an AIDS community-based organization. *Clinical Nurse Specialist, 14*(1), 8-11.

Holt, F.M. (1998). Do we need a report card for interdisciplinary collaboration? *Clinical Nurse Specialist, 11*(3), 133.

Keleher, K.C. (1998). Collaborative practice: characteristics, barriers, benefits, and implications for midwifery. *Journal of Nurse Midwifery, 43*(1), 8-11.

Mackey, T. (1993). *The nurse practitioner role: issues and education* (Paper Presented at SREB regional conference). Atlanta, GA: Southern Council on Collegiate Education for Nursing.

Mullen, P.D., Pollak, K.I., Titus, J.P., Sockrider, M.M., & Moy, J.G. (1998). Prenatal smoking cessation counseling by Texas obstetricians. *Birth, 25*(1), 25-31.

Mundinger, M. O., (2000). Primary care outcomes in patients treated by nurse practitioners and physicians: a randomized trial. *Journal of the American Medical Association, 283*(1), 59-68.

Murphy, P.A. (1996). Primary care for women: health assessment, health promotion, and disease prevention services. *Journal of Nurse Midwifery, 41*, 83-91.

Nokes, K.M. (2000). Exploring the clinical nurse specialist role in an AIDS community-based organization. *Clinical Nurse Specialist, 14*(1), 8-11.

Sharp, N. (1999). Wanted: nurse leaders to craft health policy. *Nurse Practitioner, 24*(10), 85-89.

Spitzer, M.C. (1995). Birth centers: Economy, safety, and empowerment. *Journal of Nurse Midwifery, 40*(4), 371-375.

Stapleton, S.R. (1998). Team-building: making collaborative practice work. *Journal of Nurse Midwifery, 43*(1), 12-18.

Thornedike, A.N., Rigotte, N.A., Stafford, R.X., & Singer, D.E. (1998). National patterns in the treatment of smokers by physicians. *Journal of the American Medical Association, 279*, 604-608.

Chapter 19

Role Acquisition

Carol Ormond & Cheryl Pope Kish

The health care system evolving for the new millennium demands graduate education that prepares a professional who has strong critical thinking and decision-making skills informed by ethics, theory, research, and practical wisdom; who can communicate effectively; who understands the organization and financing of contemporary health care; who knows how health policy is formulated and influenced; who has a global awareness that enables culturally sensitive health care; who has built a foundation to promote health, prevent illness, and maintain functional status for patients across the health-illness continuum; and who is committed to lifelong learning. For the nursing professional who intends to provide direct care of individuals, families, aggregates, or communities, there will be an additional focus on preparing for a practice role informed by advanced knowledge and clinical skills.

Currently, four direct care practice roles are recognized in advanced practice: clinical nurse specialist (CNS), certified registered nurse anesthetist (CRNA), certified nurse midwife (CNM), and nurse practitioner (NP). This chapter examines the manner in which one acquires practice roles.

DEFINITIONS

To understand the way in which one acquires an advanced practice nurse (APN) role, it is helpful to review selected definitions and conceptualizations associated with role theory.

A *role* is defined as "the culturally defined rules for proper behavior that are associated with every status (social category) one occupies. Roles may be thought of as collections of rights and responsibilities" (Tischler, 1999). The term *role* has its roots in the theater and was used there to describe a part played by an actor in a drama. However, it has come to refer to the predictable behaviors in which one engages as an expectation of a particular circumstance, of a particular "part being played" in the world. For example, over time, patients come to expect that professional nurses will behave in a certain way while providing care to them or their family members. A certain amount of predictability about this likely behavior lends security to individuals seeking such care.

The *role set* is the collective set of roles associated with a particular status; the behaviors within a role set depend on a particular social context (Tischler, 1999). The role set one assumes depends on whom that individual is interacting with at a particular point in time. For example, the role set of a graduate nursing student may be displayed quite differently in a seminar setting while interacting with student peers and faculty than in a clinical site with an ill toddler and his parents.

Socialization can be considered the process of acquiring knowledge, skills, and values associated with membership in a particular group, society, or culture; it occurs over a lifetime (Marquis & Huston, 2000). So, the process through which one learns an occupation and its inherent values, ethics, and responsibilities and acquires the associated role set can be called socialization (Kozier, Erb, & Blais, 1991).

Resocialization is the process of redefining one's role identity by reshaping or changing a role set. When nurses return to graduate school to prepare for advanced practice roles, they hold fast to parts of their former nursing identity—that professional self they initially acquired as a nursing role set—but they connect it to new conceptualizations, and their sense of nursing is forever altered as a result of the new education.

Resocialization is not an easy or smooth process for APNs. This role transition demands broadening the scope of nursing while expanding somewhat into medicine and acquiring parts of the medical role set. "By expanding into medicine, [APNs] will need, more than ever before, to increase consciousness of what nursing is all about. The values of nursing must not get lost in the dominant medical culture. If they do, [APNs] justly risk the epithet of junior doctor[s]" (Bates, 1990).

Role stress is a "social structural condition in which role obligations are vague, irritating, difficult, conflicting, or impossible to meet" (Hardy & Conway, 1978). *Role strain*, a subjective sense of distress when exposed to role stress, is inherent in all major role transitions. The identity crisis aspect of role strain may actually facilitate role acquisition by motivating one to self-evaluate and attempt to narrow the perceived gaps in knowledge and skill needed for practice.

Role ambiguity refers to a lack of clarity about expectations or responsibilities associated with a role or its subroles. Role ambiguity is common for APN students and new graduates. Not the least reason for such ambiguity is that APN roles continue to evolve depending on the clinical focus or practice setting. For example, CNSs, who have traditionally functioned as inpatient experts, have begun to practice in community sites, while many NPs have begun to practice in hospital settings. Blurring of the lines between primary care providers (PCPs) and physicians also contributes to role ambiguity.

CRITICAL ISSUES: THEORIES ON ADVANCED PRACTICE NURSING ROLE ACQUISITION

The process of acquiring the advanced practice role is not easy; growth is irregular and sometimes painful. Brookfield's (1993) comments about acquiring the ability to think critically are particularly descriptive of the process of role acquisition. The emerging APN's role is acquired through "incremental fluctuation" where the overall direction moves forward. As APNs develop in their new role, they refine their ability to see alternative perspectives on familiar situations and become more confident with challenging assumptions and tolerating ambiguity.

Role socialization of the APN involves acquiring a set of values, a knowledge base, technical skills, and the decision-making ability to inform the direct patient care one provides to individuals, families, aggregates, or communities as part of the APN role. Role socialization begins within the graduate classroom and is cumulative, continuing in clinical settings where the classroom theories and national standards of care are applied.

In both classes and clinical settings an individual learns and tests competence and develops an appreciation that this role is associated with a need for perpetual learning. Here, too, the APN internalizes the professional identity and develops what Styles (1982) calls the "professional soul." Several models have been developed to substantiate the way in which APNs acquire the role and to identify the domains and competencies that represent the APN role.

Domains of Practice and Levels of Competency

Benner (1984) used an interpretive approach to examine the knowledge imbedded in clinical practice and identified five levels of competency (Box 19-1). (Benner's conceptualization of the "novice to expert" model of role acquisition is described in Chapter 24.) Additionally, Benner identified seven domains of nursing practice with the potential to describe the clinical judgment process of expert nurses in acute care settings (Figure 19-1).

Interested in determining clinical role expectations for

Box **19-1**

Benner's Five Levels of Competency

Novice
Advanced beginner
Competent
Proficient
Expert

Data from Benner, P. (1984). *From novice to expert*. Menlo Park, CA: Addison Wesley.

CNSs and NPs, Fenton (1985) and Brykczynski (1989) modeled their research after Benner's classic interpretative approach. An interpretative research approach is a qualitative design, "a situation, contextual, or narrative research method for understanding the knowledge and meanings in everyday (naturalistic) settings" (Fenton & Brykczynski, 1993).

Fenton (1985) analyzed 242 clinical situations, using interviews and participant observations of 30 CNSs in varied acute care settings. All seven domains, previously identified by Benner, were evident in the acute care practice of the CNS research participants. However, numerous examples of how CNSs provided both formal and informal expert guidance to other providers led to a new domain of practice with supporting competencies: "consulting role of the nurse." Although similar studies related to the domains of practice for CNMs or CRNAs have not been forthcoming, one could speculate that commonalities exist because their roles are enacted primarily in acute care settings.

The Brykczynski (1989) study involved analysis of participant observations and interviews for a total of 199 clinical scenarios provided by 22 NPs engaged in ambulatory care practices. Not surprisingly, their involvement in primary care as opposed to acute care justified inclusion of a new domain: "management of patient health/illness status in ambulatory care settings." As is evident from Figure 19-1, this new domain consolidated and replaced two of Benner's original domains more typical of acute care practice settings, specifically "diagnostic and monitoring function" and "administering and monitoring therapeutic interventions and regimens." A list of competencies associated with the new domain was also added for the NP group. Otherwise, the study validated that the remaining five of Benner's original seven domains were applicable for NP practice. Although there was little support in the study for the domain related to "effective management of rapidly changing situations" as typical of NP practice, Brynczynski retained it in the listing because many practitioners do now work in urgent care settings.

The domains and competencies of expert practice identified by these classic researchers are appropriate to

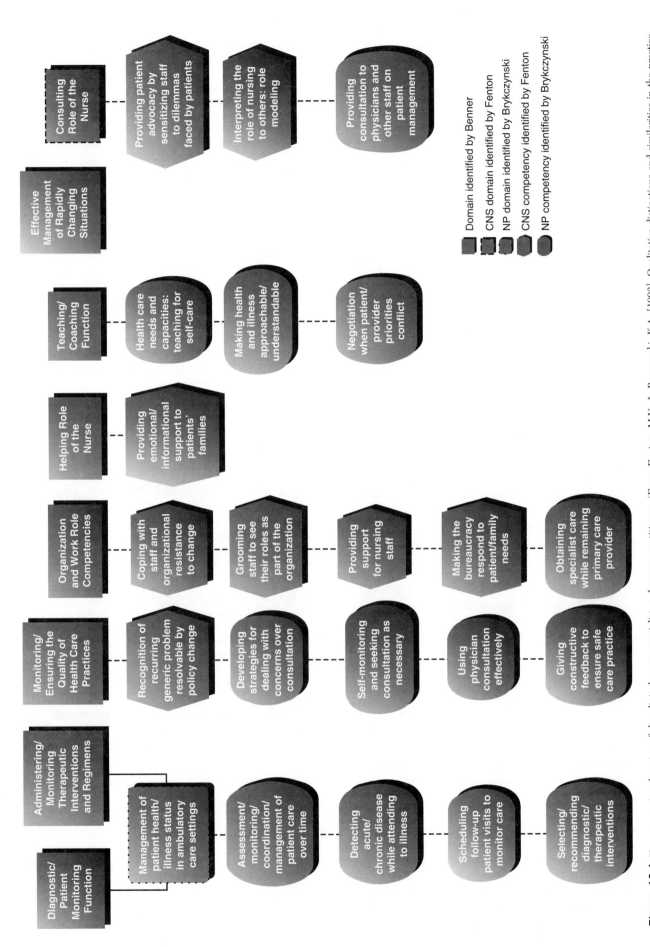

Figure 19-1 Expert practice domains of the clinical nurse specialist and nurse practitioner. (From Fenton, M.V., & Bryczynski, K.A. [1993]. Qualitative distinctions and similarities in the practice of clinical nurse specialists and nurse practitioners. *Journal of Professional Nursing, 9*[6], 317.)

Consulting Role of the Nurse

Effective Management of Rapidly Changing Situations

Teaching/ Coaching Function

Helping Role of the Nurse

Organization and Work Role Competencies

Monitoring/ Ensuring the Quality of Health Care Practices

Administering/ Monitoring Therapeutic Interventions and Regimens

Diagnostic/ Patient Monitoring Function

Providing patient advocacy by sensitizing staff to dilemmas faced by patients

Interpreting the role of nursing to others: role modeling

Providing consultation to physicians and other staff on patient management

Health care needs and capacities: teaching for self-care

Making health and illness approachable/ understandable

Negotiation when patient/ provider priorities conflict

Providing emotional/ informational support to patients' families

Coping with staff and organizational resistance to change

Grooming staff to see their roles as part of the organization

Providing support for nursing staff

Making the bureaucracy respond to patient/family needs

Obtaining specialist care while remaining primary care provider

Recognition of recurring generic problem resolvable by policy change

Developing strategies for dealing with concerns over consultation

Self-monitoring and seeking consultation as necessary

Using physician consultation effectively

Giving constructive feedback to ensure safe care practice

Management of patient health/ illness status in ambulatory care settings

Assessment/ monitoring/ coordination/ management of patient care over time

Detecting acute/ chronic disease while attending to illness

Scheduling follow-up patient visits to monitor care

Selecting/ recommending diagnostic/ therapeutic interventions

Domain identified by Benner

CNS domain identified by Fenton

NP domain identified by Brykczynski

CNS competency identified by Fenton

NP competency identified by Brykczynski

guide curriculum development in APN education and to structure both courses and instructional strategies to enable realization of expert potential. Further, they can serve as criteria against which professional clinical competency may be evaluated. Indeed, the national curriculum model proposed by the National Organization of Nurse Practitioner Faculties (NONPF) (1995) and supported by the agencies that accredit nursing education is consistent with the domains and competencies.

Formal Educational Programs

In 1994, the board of directors of the American Association of Colleges of Nursing (AACN) established a taskforce, which focused on inclusion and consensus-building processes, to develop a proposal of the essential elements of Master's education for APN roles. This group conceptualized a curriculum inclusive of three components: nursing core content that is essential for all graduates of Master's programs, irrespective of their clinical or functional focus; APN core content that directs advanced patient care; and specialty content defined by specialty organizations as appropriate for enacting direct care roles. A particular institution offering the Master's degree in nursing can use these elements as a framework to customize according to its unique mission and needs, geographical area, and student population (AACN, 1996) (Box 19-2).

The graduate program that educates APNs should build on the generalist base of baccalaureate education, which includes courses in the liberal arts and sciences as well as didactic learning and practice in the art and science of nursing. The graduate curriculum expands the knowledge, skill, and value base in scope, breadth, and depth. Graduates are prepared to use clinical judgment and decision-making, interpersonal, and technical skills as they apply theory to clinical practice in an area of nursing specialization. There must be a commitment to preparing learners for the lifelong learning demanded for a preferred competitive future.

Additional guidance for development of curricula to educate APNs for roles in a changing health care arena can be found in *Recreating Health Professional Practice for a New Century* (O'Neil & Pew Health Professions Commission, 1998). The standards of practice for APNs can also serve as guides for educating APNs and helping them fully understand the depth and scope of the role for which they are preparing and the accountability of that role to the public. According to the *Scope and Standards of Advanced Practice Registered Nursing* (American Nurses Association [ANA], 1996), "Standards are authoritative statements by which the nursing profession describes the responsibilities for which its members are accountable. Consequently, standards reflect the values and priorities of the profession." Written standards of care can be obtained from the specialty organizations supporting APNs or the ANA. In addition to serving as guides for curriculum, these written statements are invaluable in writing a job description or

designing a performance evaluation instrument against which one will be evaluated annually.

Continuing Education and Lifelong Learning

An indisputable fact for anyone engaged in a contemporary health care provider role is that the knowledge and technology required for practice will continue to expand exponentially. For that reason, remaining current in practice requires a commitment to and capacity for lifelong learning (Box 19-3). The predominant source of learning after graduation is the clinical practice itself and the workplace-related learning associated with encountering new situations and an increasingly diverse patient population. A more formal means of continuing education is also essential if one is to have a credible current practice and remain certified as an APN. In some states, continuing education units (CEUs) are specified as a requirement for relicensure as well.

APNs are best served by planning their continuing professional education to ensure a broad perspective with

---

Box 19-2

Outline of Essential Curriculum Elements for Advanced Practice Nursing Programs

Graduate Core Content (for All Master's Degree Students)
Research
Health Care Policy
Organization of the Health Care Delivery System
Health Care Financing
Ethics
Professional Role Development
Theoretical Foundations of Nursing Practice
Human Diversity and Social Issues
Health Promotion and Disease Prevention

APN Core Content (for All APN Students)
Advanced Health/Physical Assessment
Advanced Physiology and Pathophysiology
Advanced Pharmacology

Specialty Content
Content specific for specialization as a:
   CNS
   CRNA
   CNM
   ACNP
   Primary care NP

From American Association of Colleges of Nursing (1996). *The essentials of Master's education for advanced practice nursing.* Washington, DC: American Association of Colleges of Nursing.

balance between formal courses and self-directed learning that relates to the different subroles of their practice. Continuing education should focus not only on the direct-care role of advanced practice but also include topics such as research, health policy, advocacy, and business management. Formal continuing education courses, skill workshops, and seminars have an advantage of networking as a means for learning; however, self-directed continuing education can be invaluable in terms of convenience and expense. Membership in professional organizations often provides a cost-saving avenue to continuing education through formal courses, journal subscriptions, newsletters, and prepackaged content units. Today, CEU offerings are associated with particular articles in professional journals and with audiocassette packages. The *Nurse Practitioner Informer* offers a combination of audiocassettes, newsletters, and a website (www.npinformer.com) for self-study, with an option for earning CEUs. Additionally, there are ever-expanding resources on the Internet. Websites such as *MDConsult* (www.mdconsult.com) and *Nurse Practitioner Student Journal* (www.npeducation.com/~npsj/index.html) can be invaluable to continuing education; indeed, website addresses are becoming a common feature on course syllabi, and learning guides in many APN programs serve as an enduring resource for practice.

In many communities, APNs have initiated journal clubs and other groups for continued learning; in some of these, physician assistants (PAs) have been included in the collective. Pharmaceutical and medical supply companies are rich sources of continuing education access for such groups. These companies are often willing to arrange onsite speakers or teleconferences that include information about their products or services as part of the instruction.

Experiential Learning Theory

How does one gain the cognitive, affective, and psychomotor competencies associated with an APN role? How does one learn to be a CNM, CRNA, CNS, or NP? People learn, or at least prefer to learn, in a particular way. They acquire, process, and master information using a preferred learning style. Although several learning style theories have been posited, the work of Kolb (1984) has particular significance for APNs.

Kolb (1984) advanced a phenomenological concept of experiential learning—learning that occurs as a result of active engagement in a real-world, lived experience. For an APN student, this translates to a patient encounter in an actual clinical setting or an encounter that is contrived through media, such as a case study, simulation, or role-play. According to this theory, even if two students could be exposed to the exact same learning activity, their learning experience would be different because learning occurs uniquely and is internal to the learner, depending on how personal meaning is constructed from the experience. Faculty, then, can never plan learning *experiences*; those occur within the learner. Faculty can only plan *activities* from which one may learn.

According to Kolb's theory, four sequential stages must be completed as part of a learning cycle for experiential learning to occur: concrete experience, reflective observation, abstract conceptualization, and active experimentation (Figure 19-2). The prospective learner may enter the cycle at any of the four stages, generally progressing clockwise through the sequence. However, a learner generally selects an entry point that corresponds to his or her preferred learning style. Once the learner has progressed through the process and gained new knowledge,

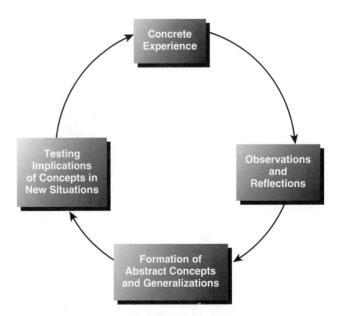

Figure 19-2 Experiential learning cycle. (From Cooper, C. [Ed.]. [1975]. *Theories of group process.* New York: John Wiley and Sons Limited.)

the cycle starts anew. Experiential learning occurs whether the assignment is one involving total patient care or some isolated task, such as a prenatal history and physical examination. Because safety is an overarching concern in nursing, the learner must have basic knowledge before the experiential learning opportunity. The concepts related to experiential learning are relevant for formal education as well as lifelong learning.

In the concrete experience stage, the learner either executes a planned task based on specified objectives or encounters some spontaneous opportunity to perform with guidance. Here the learner tends to interpret the problems encountered in a personal way, relying more on feelings than a logical approach to resolutions. Opportunities to "shadow" an experienced APN for a time in a new clinical setting can be effective for this learning process, as can opportunities to review, practice, and discuss the expectations before performance of the objectives.

The reflective observation stage is marked by examining a situation from multiple perspectives, using intuitive and empathetic thinking to come to terms with the problem situation and the actions taken. Clinical journals and post-encounter conferences with a preceptor are appropriate strategies for reflection.

The abstract conceptualization stage involves logical thinking and a systematic, reasoned approach that is based on thoughtful planning. Here learners begin to build theories. A valuable approach in this part of the learning

cycle is having the learner "think out loud" as he or she makes clinical decisions.

Finally, the active experimentation stage is characterized by highly organized, goal-directed "doing" with the intent of solving a problem or otherwise obtaining results. Unlike the "doing" in concrete experience, this is more systematic and rational in nature. Varying the approaches with different patients works well in this stage. Here learners appreciate that theory is guiding their practice and being tested. This realization leads back to the concrete experience stage of the cycle (Dunn & Campbell, 1985).

Dunn and Campbell (1985) suggest that experiential learning, when used fully, provides for professional socialization and limits reality shock during transition from the idealized world with its espoused theories to the real world with its practice theory or theory-in-use. This practice theory evolves over time as learners experience encounters in varied settings and gain assurance that theory can indeed guide practice in the real world. "Each nursing encounter should add dimension to the practitioners' individualized theory of practice" (Dunn & Campbell, 1985). (Figure 19-3 shows how the experiential learning cycle is central to developing professional effectiveness in nursing.)

Raschick, Maypole, and Day (1998) maintain that students who prefer inductive versus deductive reasoning might selectively enter the learning cycle at different points. Consider how Carol and Kim, two classmates in a

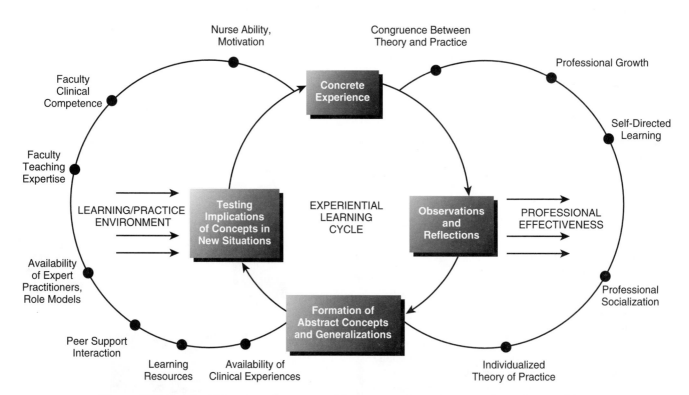

Figure 19-3 Experiential learning cycle as a central feature in professional nursing role socialization. (From Dunn, D., & Campbell, J. [1985]. *Developing professional effectiveness in nursing.* Upper Saddle River, NJ: Prentice-Hall.)

NP program, approach the cycle of learning differently based on this idea. Enrolled in an advanced assessment course, the two students are assigned to a women's clinic where they are each scheduled to perform breast examinations and teach self-examination techniques to two women patients. Carol, the more inductive thinker of the two, enters the examination room and carries out the assigned assessment, teaching, and appropriate documentation; comes out of the room; and takes a few minutes to reflect on her experience. In reviewing, she realizes that she forgot to put a rolled towel under the patient's shoulder during the breast examination. Also, because the woman was African-American, Carol wishes she had used a dark-skinned breast model instead of the one she chose. After a quick chart review of the second patient, Carol makes a plan for her examination approach, then enters the room and begins the examination.

In contrast, deductive thinker Kim notes that her first assigned patient's history indicates breast augmentation surgery. Kim considers how she will modify the procedure for breast examination given this circumstance. She asks the preceptor to demonstrate the appropriate modified technique on the breast model. Then Kim enters the room and performs the examination, using the preplanned creative approach. Afterwards, Kim pauses to reflect on how she did, how the patient responded to her approach, and what she will do differently next time. She makes a mental note to read more about this topic before the next clinical session, then moves on to the second examination.

Kolb (1984) believed that true experiential learning could not occur without reflection. Reflection can occur during or immediately after a patient encounter (as in the examples just given) or after the student has exited the clinical setting. Clinical logs, diaries, and journals, which provide an opportunity for learners to reflect on their experiences, are popular and effective measures for ensuring reflective observation as a part of the learning cycle. Written reflection not only serves to increase the probability that learning occurs by helping one see connections between theory and practice, it can also be a valuable medium for catharsis. The process of written reflection is enhanced when there is a purposeful link with the learning objectives and when guidance is given for the content and structure. Reflective writing may need to be nongraded; otherwise the writer may be hesitant to be candid. Emotive entries are acceptable, as are responses to questions such as: What did I learn? How will I use this? How did I perform? Students might also be asked to use the "thinking out loud" method on paper for exploring their clinical reasoning, reflecting on the context of practice, or reacting to some event or encounter. For example, a CRNA student wrote emotionally about her discomfort in the sociopolitical environment of the operating room when there was an argument at the table about whether blood should be administered to a patient whose religion forbade blood products. The student used reflection in this clinical log to explore the ethics of the scenario as well as her distress when it appeared that a decision contrary to her ethical position was about to be made.

Although there is universal support for actual patient care encounters to enable experiential learning for APN students, clinical reasoning can be learned experientially even in classroom settings. Case studies, simulations, and roleplaying are all experiential learning methods. Faculty using these methods should ensure that the full learning cycle is possible, and debriefing at the conclusion of these methods can provide for reflective observation.

Kolb (1984) further conceptualized four styles of adult learning: accommodator, diverger, assimilator, and converger, each combining two of the processes in the cycle of learning (Figure 19-4). Learning style is an acquired trait, somewhat stable over time, which is determined by heredity, past experience, and the demands of a particular situation. According to Highfield (1988), learning style determines the way an individual masters content and skill and how that person reacts to and interacts with the learning environment. Kolb designed a learning style inventory (LSI) in the mid-1970s and revised it in 1986 in response to criticism of its psychometrical properties. The revised LSI employs 12 sentence-completion items, such as "When I learn . . . " and "I learn best from . . . " Scoring determines one's preferred learning style. The instrument reflects the basic tenets of Kolb's theory and has considerable face validity; hence, it is used for diagnostic purposes by many disciplines. However, Kolb suggests that it is as well suited as a stimulus for thinking and talking about how learning occurs (Atkinson, 1991).

Knowing one's preferred learning style can aid in planning optimal learning. Instructional methods can be selected or designed to coincide with the predominant learning styles of the student group in an attempt to increase motivation and academic success. The value of this matching of teaching and learning styles, however, has not been consistently validated by research. Perhaps it is just as valuable to support learners as they attempt to learn with less familiar styles, thereby increasing their learning repertoire. Regardless of which instructional approach one favors, it is important to recognize the characteristics associated with particular learning styles and their relevance to clinical learning. Students should appreciate that learning styles are different and none is superior to the others. All humans likely use all styles to some extent; however, approximately 25% of the population falls into each of the four predominant styles (Kolb, 1994).

When the accommodator style predominates, learning occurs through concrete experience and active experimentation. This style is people oriented and involves a hands-on approach. Accommodators tend to address problems intuitively or by trial and error; they like timely feedback. These learners like novel situations and dislike repetition. According to Alspach (1995), their learning orientation is emotional and intuitive, and they benefit most from structured situations that need management. Appropriate teaching methods for this group include skills laboratories, computer-assisted instruction, case studies, and supervised clinicals.

Divergers rely heavily on concrete experience and reflective observation to learn. Also people oriented, these learners examine problems and alternative solutions from multiple perspectives, gaining insights from watching others and becoming personally involved in problem-solving. The orientation to learning is emotional and imaginative (Alspach, 1995). Persons in the social sciences and service occupations are often divergers. Effective teaching methods include brainstorming, group discussions, small group work, roleplaying, seminars, and drawing on past experiences (Alspach, 1995).

Assimilators have a theoretical orientation and prefer abstract thinking to interpersonal exchanges. These more passive learners value theory over practice, excel at organization, approach problems logically and with inductive techniques, and may need help in the application of theory. Alspach (1995) suggests lectures (with time for reflection and integration), self-instruction, reading, computer-assisted instruction, and independent study as appropriate teaching methods. Many scientists, researchers, and academicians have this predominant learning style.

Convergers prefer deductive reasoning for problem-solving; appreciate structure, factual information, and concrete answers to questions; and have a good understanding of practice. Technical skill and precision are important to these learners, more so than interpersonal skills. They tend to be uncomfortable with ambiguity and somewhat unemotional. Their orientation to learning is analytical and pragmatic. Effective teaching methods include hands-on experiences; return demonstrations; lectures followed by practice and questions; workshops; and simulations (Alspach, 1995). Engineers and computer technicians commonly share this predominant learning style. (Figure 19-4 shows Kolb's learning styles along the two experiential learning continua: active-reflective and concrete-abstract.)

Developmental Phases in Role Acquisition

Hamric and Taylor (1989) examined role development in CNSs and identified four major developmental phases: orientation, frustration, implementation, and integration. However, their schema for understanding role acquisition actually has relevance for all APNs. During the orientation phase, individuals are excited about the opportunity to experience a new challenge, that of enrolling in graduate school and studying to be a CNS, CRNA, CNM, or NP. Concurrently, they experience anxiety secondary to the uncertainty they face. Questions abound: Am I smart enough to do this? What sacrifices will I have to make in my work situation and personal life? Will I fit in? Am I capable of learning all I need in order to practice in this role? Do I remember how to write research papers? Will I succeed? If not, how will I ever go back to work and face my coworkers, some of whom said I was a fool to try this? The orientation phase resurfaces after graduation when one faces employment in the new role. Again, enthusiasm and anxiety are blended, and again, questions borne of facing the unknown arise.

In the frustration phase, feelings of inadequacy abound, and discouragement looms large. The very real challenges of graduate education become evident, as does the realization of reclaiming the place of a novice despite years of expert clinical practice as a nurse. Additionally, the ambiguities inherent in clinical practice become discomforting. An APN student, having described the excitement of going to her first class in the post–Master's program an hour early because she could not wait any longer to start a new life, recounts the frustration of this phase. "I purchased my pathophysiology course syllabus and textbook the day before class my first semester and looked over it that night in the dorm. Everything seemed new . . . a whole new language. It had been many years since A&P [Anatomy and Physiology]. I had to laugh when I picked up my coffee mug and saw the logo—'Toto, I don't think we're in Kansas anymore.' Cause that's exactly how I was feeling at the moment." Hamric and Taylor (1989) advise that frustration appears in other phases as well. This second phase recurs with the first job after graduation.

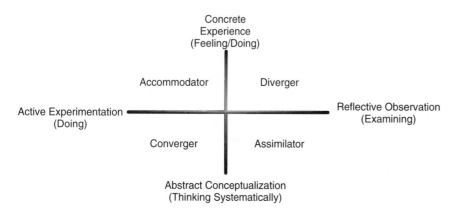

Figure 19-4 The experiential learning continua and predominant learning styles. (From Raschick, M., Maypole, D.E., & Day, P. [1998, December]. Improving field education through Kolb learning theory. *Journal of Social Work Education.*)

The implementation phase finds the APN student thoroughly immersed in the role. There has been enough learning and repetition to enhance confidence and competence. Feedback from persons in the reference group has occurred and helped to shape behavior positively. The individual feels more balanced as role expectations are realigned. One CNM student decided after weeks of discomfort suturing episiotomies to ask that the labor and delivery (L&D) nurse position the patients differently for episiotomy repair. She commented, "I finally realized that I should make this easier on myself. Most new mothers were willing to be in stirrups briefly for the repair—they had their babies in the position of choice. I had to find the best way for me to do a good job and not take forever." Some of what were once perceived as subroles by student APNs move upwards on the priority list and get enacted in this stage. For example, change theory may be used by a CNS student as a basis for a time and motion study to negotiate for a different patient transport system.

Integration, the final phase of role acquisition, occurs after the other phases are completed. Although individuals in this phase respect the experts around them, they are gaining confidence in themselves and seeking opportunities for continued development of the role.

Transition to the First Year of Practice

Kramer's classic work (1974) has relevance for role socialization of APNs. Kramer discovered that reality shock could be minimized by associating novices with real-world role incumbents already socialized in the professional roles. This lends further support for planned clinical experiences with preceptors as part of the learning process in APN programs. Using realistic clinical scenarios for discussing role acquisition can also be helpful. Edmunds (1982) believes that APNs face a type of reality shock because of the following mistaken assumptions about the role: (1) it will be easy; (2) the role will be valued, sought after, and well rewarded; (3) independent practice will be possible; (4) upward mobility will be possible; and (5) the new role will offer an escape from some of nursing's problems. For example, the experience of working with a NP in a community health center (CHC) or rural health center is dramatically different than being one of many care providers in a large private physician's office. Exposure to both settings would provide novices with a means to make comparisons and know what obstacles might be ahead in clinical practice. The practical experience also helps students appreciate that their new role is neither easy nor clearcut.

Brown and Olshansky (1998) developed a research-based model for explaining a NP's first year transition into practice, and although their study dealt solely with NPs, their transition theory would likely also predict the initial year of practice for other types of APNs. This nonlinear process entails four stages and several substages

(Figure 19-5). Stage one involves laying the foundation and includes time spent recuperating from school; negotiating the bureaucracy related to licensure and certification; looking for a job; and worrying about the credentialing process and the job search. Individuals in this stage experience a type of limbo, with concurrent waiting and business. "Without realizing it, they were busy doing both the external work of becoming legitimate and the internal work of establishing and incorporating the new legitimacy into their identity" (Brown & Olshansky, 1998).

The study defined stage two as launching—beginning a "first" position and continuing for at least 3 months. Individuals in this stage feel catapulted into the uncomfortable position of a new NP, progressing backward in expertise from being an expert in the RN role. "Feeling real" is a theme of this stage, referring to the beginning internalization of new role expectations and NPs feeling as if they have earned the legitimacy accorded to them by colleagues and patients. Another theme, "getting through the day," involves the slowness and heavy reliance on resources for guidance in the expediency of making clinical decisions without hurting patients. "Battling time,"

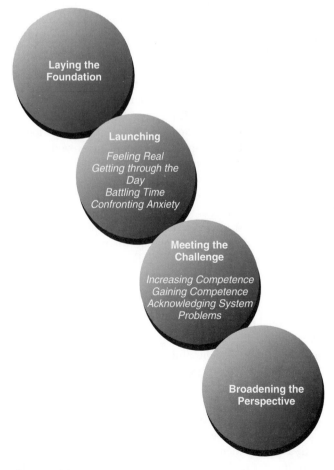

Figure 19-5 Brown and Olshansky's model for transition into the first year of practice. (From Brown, M.A., & Olshansky, E. [1998]. Becoming a primary practitioner: challenges of the initial year of practice. *The Nurse Practitioner, 23*[7], 75-104.)

theme three, focuses on a sense of burdening the practice by being slow and asking so many questions; negative sanctions related to time management are particularly difficult. A final theme, "confronting anxiety" and managing it while presenting an outward appearance of confidence and competence, is an exhausting demand of the early weeks of new practice.

In stage three, meeting the challenge, more realistic role expectations become apparent. "Increasing competence," "gaining competence," and "acknowledging system problems" were themes identified by participants at this stage.

The final stage, broadening the perspective, finds participants developing savvy in their role, affirming their progress based on feedback from the reference group, and seeking opportunities for developing more complex skills.

Challenges to Role Socialization

Transition to a new professional role is not without potential problems. Role ambiguity is a common phenomenon among both APN students and new graduates. The extent and timing of role ambiguity for this group was a surprise to Fenton and Brynkczynski (1993), who discovered that role ambiguity was more prevalent in CNSs after graduation. At the time of the study, a CNS was expected to enact the following professional roles: expert clinician, educator, change agent, researcher, and consultant. These multiple role components were not always well defined in the job setting, contributing to a sense of ambiguity. With the increase in managed care, many CNSs were moved to positions as outcome managers and away from patients' bedsides, thereby complicating the picture even more. Further ambiguity was created by a lack of public understanding of the CNS role and a lack of consensus about what the role could mean to an organization and individual patients.

The CNS student is likely to experience less role ambiguity than students preparing for roles that overlap with medicine, like NPS, CNMs, and CRNAs, while enrolled in an educational program but more ambiguity than such students after graduation. Their clinical exposure is not much different than it has been during previous educational periods; they still work primarily with nursing staff and administration doing advanced nursing. To fully appreciate this, it is helpful to remember that unlike the NP role, the CNS role was created for nursing reasons: a need to decrease depersonalization and fragmentation of care, thereby increasing quality. For the NPs in the Fenton and Brykczynski (1993) study, role ambiguity was greatest during their graduate education as they were struggling with a type of identity crisis in being exposed to that part of primary care that overlaps medical practice. These NPs often responded to the central question—"Am I nurse or physician?"—with an overemphasis on medical diagnosis and prescription to the detriment of holistic nursing.

As they gained knowledge, skill, and self-assurance, they were able to reclaim the holistic approach unique to nursing. Usually by graduation, the full extent of the identity crisis was over and the new graduates knew that they were, without question, APNs. Whether this same situation occurs with CRNA and CNM students has not been addressed empirically; however, since these roles involve some degree of diagnosing and prescribing, one may speculate that similarities in identity do exist.

The National Association of Clinical Nurse Specialists (NACNS), initiated in 1995 to provide role development for CNSs, has published CNS competencies and unique practice-related outcomes that will hopefully better clarify the CNS role and minimize role ambiguity. The *Statement on Clinical Nurse Specialist Practice and Education* (1998) reconceptualizes the role of the CNS around three spheres of influence, representing all the pertinent stakeholders of CNS services: patients, nursing personnel, and organizations or networks. It preempts the former traditional roles of the CNS.

Another role-related phenomenon that causes discomfort in role acquisition is a type of role reversal that is almost universal for NPs and may exist for other APNs as well. This phenomenon might well be called "expert to novice" role reversal. APN students enrolled in clinical courses in their graduate program have often assumed the level of competent, proficient, even expert providers in their work as nurses. Now, with resocialization, they are novices once more. This realization produces the incremental fluctuation about which Brookfield (1993) wrote, and it can be difficult and painful. The highly competent clinicians surveyed in the study by Roberts, Tabloski, and Bova (1997) disclosed anxiety similar to that of beginning nursing students, a desire to shadow the preceptor for extended periods, and feelings of incompetence. They reported forgetting to obtain the usual data for patient histories, an inability to recall even the simplest facts, and a feeling of awkwardness with patients.

One NP student described this role reversal phenomenon as "roller coaster-like . . . one day feeling up . . . pretty confident . . . then next week (in clinical) crashing down the hill, feeling stupid, discouraged, ready to quit. In my job, I have been auscultating fetal heart rates for 15 years; now I often couldn't even locate them. I would come out of the exam room and give the case presentation to my preceptor and she would ask a simple question, like 'is anybody else sick at home?' that I had not even thought about. I should have thought about that—I know about contagion and food borne illnesses." She continues, "I would question if I should do this . . . be a NP . . . after all, I have a good job . . . well paying. Why am I putting myself through this?" This student and others like her struggle with the notion of "expert to novice" role reversal. The ego of the adult learner is fragile, and it is difficult to feel as if one is going backward with regard to skill, to look like a beginner, sometimes inadequate, when one has been an expert. For APN students to have members of their reference group—peers, faculty, and preceptors—validate this singleness of emotion and doubt helps them realize that this is a common, yet transient phenomenon and find the renewed confidence to go forward in role socialization. This role discomfort occurs with traditional Master's degree students and those in post-Master's programs, even doctorally-prepared students returning for APN credentials (Margolis & Sneed, 1999).

The research of Roberts, Tabloski, and Bova (1997) relates to another potentially problematic role transition. Using an ethnographical approach involving 6 years of observation and journal review for 100 students, these researchers noted that role confusion, a decreased sense of confidence, and anger were experienced by students when they realized that faculty and preceptors lacked all the answers in clinical situations. However, over time and with an increasing sense of professional identity in their roles, these individuals tolerated ambiguity more comfortably and began to appreciate that even competent providers do not know everything. The study also established three distinctive types of student groups. One group had worked in positions with similarities to the NP role for which they were being educated and had learned to be autonomous and accountable. This group had the most successful transition to the role. A second group consisted of students with critical care nursing backgrounds in which experts were in control; this group had a difficult transition to primary care practice, where patients have more control and providers are partners in their care. Students in the third group seemed capable and confident on the surface and rarely verbalized discomfort. However, the reference group (faculty and preceptors) perceived these individuals as less than fully engaged in the program and found that progression for them was difficult and uncertain.

Three students, Richard, Laura, and Betsy, enrolled in a family nurse practitioner (FNP) program serve as examples of the distinctive groups about which Roberts et al (1997) wrote. Richard had worked full time in the intensive care unit (ICU) of a large tertiary care center for 7 years. Now enrolled in graduate school, he cut his work hours to 24 hours a week to accommodate evening classes and 1 day each week as a clinical learner. Accustomed to the fast-paced ICU setting with its multiple technologies and myriad specialists, Richard became frustrated in the primary care clinic where he was a student. He felt limited by a lack of technology and wanted to schedule unnecessary tests because he could not imagine deriving a diagnosis without them. He had frequent frustrations with "noncompliant patients" and with teaching and anticipatory guidance, not always a first priority for his critically ill patients on the job. Notes in Richard's clinical log mentioned the difficulty he was having exchanging the bedside excitement of the "post–open-heart surgery patient" or "the man with major trauma" for the daily "sameness" of sinusitis and sexually transmitted diseases (STDs). At other times, his frustration could not be put into words; he was just unhappy and considering dropping out of the program.

Richard's classmate Betsy had worked for 12 years in a public health department of a rural county. There she had an expanded role and worked under state protocols. She performed complete physical assessments, including Pap smears and STD screening, every day and saw between 15 and 20 patients per day, patients representing every age and diverse ethnic groups. The pace of primary care was a comfortable one, and she was accustomed to making decisions without the benefit of other providers nearby. She clearly knew her strengths and limitations. Seeing patients day-after-day with similar diagnoses was not boring to Betsy, who viewed them all as unique. Her clinical logs addressed this comfort level and the excitement she felt about learning more about new drugs not on the cost-effective formulary at the health department and about expanding her diagnostic abilities. She was delighted that she was able to use information from her class on respiratory illnesses to affect the health care of many people in her county with tuberculosis.

Laura had worked as a staff nurse on an adult health unit of a community hospital since earning her baccalaureate degree 6 years ago. For the last 2 years, she had been involved in infection control and staff education, moving further from patients' bedsides. After lengthy deliberation between a degree in nursing administration and the FNP program, Laura chose the latter. She then made mostly *B*s in the core courses. In her first primary care clinical course, Laura sometimes seemed hesitant in her case presentations in the clinical seminar. She did not appear to be progressing as quickly as her classmates but said things were going well in clinical and that she was learning a lot. Clinical logs were not particularly revealing. Three weeks into the semester, when the faculty first visited Laura's clinical site, a problem was immediately obvious. Laura was performing a thorough history and physical and exiting the examination room to provide the preceptor with a case presentation. Instead of offering a tentative diagnosis, discussing rule-outs, and suggesting a tentative management plan, however, Laura was doing little more than accompanying the physician as he saw the patients, made all of the clinical decisions, and provided patient teaching. Laura seemed genuinely surprised when the faculty mentioned that she is not performing in the expected student role, even though written objectives and class discussions have clearly outlined the expectations. The physician disclosed privately that Laura had seemed reluctant to perform any differently. She rarely asked questions; instead, she looked up information in the numerous texts she carted to clinical in her backpack and responded to his questions correctly, albeit without confidence. He mentioned that Laura "seems to lack the same degree of passion for this kind of work" that he had seen in other students from the program. The faculty member was concerned about Laura's ability to finish the course successfully without major changes in her clinical performance and planned to confer with Laura.

A final potential problem related to APN role acquisition is one concerning a lack of value for and use of the nontechnical subroles of APN practice: teacher, researcher, change agent, leader/manager, evaluator, and user of nursing theory (Stanford, 1987; Hupcey, 1990, 1994; Scott, 1999). Scott (1999) found that CNSs spent a surprising amount of time in the technical direct care and administrative roles and the least amount of time in the research role. Stanford's (1997) study showed that NPs were not practicing in more than the technical direct care role.

Hupcey (1990) examined 13 adult nurse practitioner (ANP) programs for evidence that students were being socialized for roles common to the Master's-prepared APN—roles beyond direct patient care. Less than half of the participants engaged in the teacher or leader subroles. (*Teacher* in this study referred to the preceptor role, not patient teaching.) The importance placed on the technical and medical roles was significantly higher than that for all Master of Science in Nursing (MSN) role behaviors, with the role of researcher being considered the least valuable. These findings were irrespective of personal or program characteristics. There was modest indication that opportunities to practice MSN role behaviors in clinical settings as a student increased the probability that they would be perceived as valuable.

In 1994, Hupcey replicated the study with practicing NPs, again looking for actual use and perceived importance of the MSN role behaviors. Respondents included 49 MSN-prepared and 31 non–MSN-prepared practitioners representing several practice specialties. The results of the second study were essentially the same—the technical/medical role behaviors were considered significantly more important and practiced to a greater extent. That role behaviors related to direct care of patients are favored and used more in practice by NPs is not surprising; what must be of particular concern, however, is that other role behaviors are valued and practiced so little. While empirical study has been limited thus far to only two of the four APN groups, one can easily speculate that similar findings would exist in the CRNA and CNM populations.

IMPLICATIONS FOR MSN EDUCATION AND ADVANCED PRACTICE

No nursing program preparing APNs can teach all of the possible nursing knowledge or prepare individuals for every eventuality of clinical practice. Consequently, programs must prepare students to think critically; use scientific inquiry and know how to access informational resources; and communicate effectively. APN educational programs must ensure the quality and relevance of their respective curricula.

Role socialization is a complex phenomenon that deserves faculty support. Inviting a panel of graduates of an APN program to describe their personal experiences with the role transition can be helpful in preparing students for the challenges they face. In enacting their role in the clinical setting, students are exposed to both positive and negative experiences. An opportunity for debriefing one-on-one, in student group settings, in a virtual discussion group, or via a clinical log is of inestimable value. Students should be encouraged to incorporate the positive behaviors they witness into their own practice repertoire and to identify strategies for resolving problem performances. Students must understand that they have a choice about how to conduct their own personal practice.

When faculty and students fully understand role theory, they can capitalize on strategies that enhance role socialization. Faculty and preceptors are encouraged to speak candidly about the challenges and rewards they have experienced in acquiring and practicing the roles of advanced practice, including the MSN role behaviors. For faculty to give voice to their own stories of "expert to novice" role reversal helps students appreciate how common and transient the phenomenon is. Students often gain surprising comfort from the anecdotes of faculty and preceptors they revere as clinical experts. To learn that a professor, exemplary physician, or APN preceptor once felt incompetent in the role may give hope to a student in the midst of a role identity or role reversal crisis.

There is undeniable empirical support for the worth of clinical practice as an agent for role socialization. Chances to practice MSN role behaviors in actual or contrived clinical settings may increase their value to students. Appreciating these facts makes selection of practice sites for clinical placements and preceptors critical. Planning didactic learning activities that have fidelity to actual practice capitalizes on experiential learning theory and extends the options for diagnostic reasoning and decision-making. For example, participating in a case study or managing a simulated (paper) patient can be used as a concrete experience in advance of encountering a similar situation in the real world. Making a wrong diagnosis or prescribing an inappropriate antibiotic for a paper patient in a case analysis or simulation promotes rich and meaningful learning without doing harm. Performing a pelvic examination on a paid instructional model capable of providing feedback can not only significantly lessen anxiety but also serve as effective role rehearsal for patient examinations.

It is imperative that APN programs prepare students to be leaders and innovators in health care, create a vision of the future, and embrace lifelong learning as a way of attaining that vision. Changes in the health care system may necessitate changing or expanding the present role of APNs as certainly as the knowledge explosion, technology, and sweeping changes in reimbursement and cost containment have affected the last decade. APNs look ahead at a future where the human genome experience is expected to revolutionize health care, innovative group practice arrangements and hospital and nursing home affiliations will change care demands, alternative medicine will continue to affect care, and nursing entrepreneurship will thrive.

It is understandable that students focus closely on those areas of practice they will face on national certification examinations and behind the closed doors of a patient's examination room. After all, they must be safe practitioners, and there is a lot to learn; moreover, the primary focus of the MSN program is appropriately on the clinical role. (AACN, 1996). However, the fact that many graduate students and practicing APNs view nontechnical subjects, such as research and health care economics, as less important should concern APN program faculty and administrators. This concern presents an immediate challenge to APN education (Table 19-1).

The engagement theory of program quality (Conrad, Haworth, & Miller, 1993; Haworth & Conrad, 1996) can serve as a helpful framework for nursing faculty and administrators of programs educating APNs. This theory, which is empirically based, identifies attributes suggestive of program quality in Master's education, based on student learning outcomes. The attributes include: (1) diverse and engaged learners, (2) collegial stakeholders and participatory culture, (3) practices that extend theory to practice, (4) interactive teaching and learning where students and faculty are co-learners, and (5) adequate support resources for faculty, students, and the infrastructure.

Designing and implementing stable and credible programs for the preferred future of APN practice will be accomplished amidst continued change in health care. Those who know the practice arena best—those in practice, whether they be faculty who practice or advisory panels of APNs in practice—should be given a strong voice in this endeavor. It is worth remembering that those who prepare one best for a role are those who know the workplace.

PRIORITIES FOR RESEARCH

Much of the recent research related to APN roles has addressed NPs only. Similar studies should address other types of advanced practice. The new conceptualization of the CNS role should serve well to guide research related to that APN group. Replication of the Brown and Olshansky (1998) study of role acquisition in the initial practice year with CRNAs, CNMs, CNSs, and acute care NPs would not only be fascinating, it would guide preparation for role taking. A study comparing role socialization and how it develops in Master's-degree APNs versus those completing post-Master's specialization would be of value.

It would also be worthwhile to study measures for ensuring that APNs claim the roles associated with graduate nursing core content, particularly the role of researcher. Initially, one might need to address students and graduates in some qualitative method, examining what they perceive as happening in this regard and what meaning they associate with it.

Priorities for research in role acquisition also include studies devoted to developing and testing measures for assisting nurses to better understand their role. Can the process of role acquisition be improved? Are there innovative educational methods that will enable students to make the role transition faster or more comfortably? Are certain methods associated with internalizing values and ethics in role development? What is the best way to prepare students to incorporate the nursing standards in the "daily" of their practices? What program variables, if any, are associated with role socialization?

Research might be updated using an LSI. Laschinger and Boss (1984) discovered that both incoming and enrolled undergraduate nursing students preferred concrete strategies. A decade later, the work of Cavanaugh, Hogan, and Ramgopel (1995) led to similar conclusions: for 54% of baccalaureate nursing students, concrete learning styles predominate, irrespective of age or gender. These studies, if replicated with a graduate student population, would be advantageous in guiding instructional design. Raschick, Maypole, and Day (1998) found that when student social workers' preferred learning styles matched those of their field supervisors, students had a more positive experience. Using their findings, the researchers developed an orientation for field supervisors that capitalized on knowing preferred styles and matching similar dyads for field experiences. Would a similarly designed study with APN students and their preceptors yield similar results? Is clinical learning enhanced when preceptors know more about planning and implementing Kolb's cycle of learning because they have been trained to use the student's predominant learning style effectively?

DISCUSSION QUESTIONS

These questions can be used to promote critical thinking and encourage discussion.

1. Write a job description for one of the APN roles of CRNA, CNS, CNM, or NP using the *Scope and Standards of Advanced Practice Registered Nursing* (American Nurses Association, 1996) as a guide. Review and discuss the job descriptions with a group of

Table 19-1

Strategies/Objectives to Facilitate Nontechnical/Medical MSN Role Behaviors of Advanced Practice Nursing Students*

ROLE EXPECTATION	STRATEGIES/OBJECTIVES
Teacher (refers to participation in the instruction of students, not patients)	In group format, discuss preceptor behaviors that group members have found lessen anxiety and facilitate learning in the clinical setting versus those behaviors that they have found ineffective. What similarities and differences have group members seen in physician and APN preceptors? Between male and female preceptors?
	Identify your preferred learning style and the way in which you learn best experientially. Using case scenarios of students who have different predominant styles, have group members offer suggestions for how best to teach those individuals.
	With a group of peers, practice using a style of learning opposite your preferred style to learn some simple non-nursing subject (e.g., cooking a particular dish, playing a game). Reflect afterward on how what you each gained could be used in teaching students in a clinical setting.
Leader/manager	Shadow the office manager in a clinic for several hours and reflect on that leadership and management role.
	Write a job description for a licensed practical nurse (LPN) or RN who might be employed as a clinical assistant after graduation.
	Read about leadership styles. Write a brief paper about your personal leadership style and the rationale for your choice.
	Work with those in other disciplines to suggest a management approach for a certain clinical situation that capitalizes on the strengths of each discipline.
	In a group and using a case study that calls for generation of a management plan inclusive of pharmacological and nonpharmacological interventions, investigate the cost of each strategy in the plan; generate a cost comparison; and specify how the patient and family can access the resources (e.g., drugs, equipment, supplies) needed to implement the plan. Ensure that one group member investigates the extent of typical third-party payment for each strategy (including private, Medicare, and Medicaid funding).
	Attend a legislative session or board meeting at the local or state level. Afterward, reflect on the experience and how you might affect decisions made by that particular agency through political activism or advocacy processes.
	Write a letter to a senator or congressman related to some aspect of health policy.
Change agent	Identify an aggregate of the population that could benefit from health promotion (e.g., inner city fireman in need of dietary changes). Using change theory, generate a plan for assessing the need, designing an approach for behavioral change, and implementing and evaluating the change. If possible, carry out the project, which has the additional benefit of service learning.
	Identify some aspect in the clinical setting that needs modification. Generate a plan for effecting change. This might involve a patient, personnel, or organizational problem.
User of nursing theory	Select a nursing theory that has "goodness of fit" for your own clinical practice. Write a brief paper about how you applied that theory on a given day.
	Write a brief philosophy of practice. In a group setting, discuss the similarities and differences of the group's philosophies of practice. Considering your assigned clinical setting this semester, how does this philosophy match what you perceive as the philosophy of other staff members and your preceptor?
	Write a one-paragraph mission statement for your own practice or your graduate education.
	In a group format, discuss what theories of nursing relate best to your particular area of advanced practice. Speculate on which theory or theories might best relate to some other APN role.
	In addition to the medical diagnoses for each patient, generate a list of relevant nursing diagnoses.

*Note that these are examples only. This is not meant to represent an inclusive list.

Continued

Table 19-1

Strategies/Objectives to Facilitate Nontechnical/Medical MSN Role Behaviors of Advanced Practice Nursing Students—cont'd

ROLE EXPECTATION	STRATEGIES/OBJECTIVES
Researcher	Select a quantitative research study with implications for your practice. Critique the study. Propose replication of the study.
	Select a qualitative research study with implications for your practice or role as an APN. Critique the study. Propose replication of the study.
	Select a policy, procedure, or protocol from practice. Find empirical support to: (1) retain it without change, (2) modify it (include how it will be modified), or (3) discard it completely. Provide a rationale for your decision.
	As part of your clinical log, keep a list of all the researchable questions that come to mind during the course of the semester or all the times you find yourself asking "what if?" or "I wonder if . . . "
	Select an intervention you prescribed in the clinical setting this week. Offer empirical support for that choice.
	Complete a research project or thesis.
	Conduct a literature review of a topic of interest to your clinical practice or role acquisition. Write a state-of-the-science paper.
Evaluator	Using a faculty-provided case study or simulation on management of a specific problem and a group format, generate a plan for evaluating patient response to the planned interventions.
	Perform a self-evaluation using the clinical objectives for the course.
	In a group format, address the following questions: Who has a right to evaluate an APN's role performance? On what criteria should performance be based? What kinds of instruments might be used or designed to measure the criteria?

Suggestions for Further Learning

- "APNs must include research as part of their role to ensure excellence in practice and achieve definition and validation of the APN role." Respond to this statement. Is it valid or not? Support your answer with a rationale. Also, read the following article and use it to develop a research plan for a clinical project in your practice setting: Dumas, M.A., Shurpin, K., & Gallo, K. (1995). Getting started in clinical research. *Journal of the American Academy of Nurse Practitioners, 7*(12), 591-596.
- Consult the following article concerning the initial year in practice for an excellent list of "comforting thoughts for the first year": Brown, M.A., & Olshansky, E. (1998). Becoming a primary nurse practitioner: challenges of the initial year of practice. *The Nurse Practitioner, 23*(7), 46, 52-66.
- Further investigate the respective roles of APNs by consulting the websites for their professional organizations:
  - American College of Nurse Midwives (www.acnm.org/)
  - National Association of Clinical Nurse Specialists (www.nacns.org)
  - American Association of Nurse Anesthetists (www.aana.com/)
  - American Association of Nurse Practitioners (www.aanp.org)
  - American Nurses Association (www.ana.org)

APNs, providing criticism and clarifying misunderstandings and uncertainties about the respective roles.
2. Review the standards carefully and answer the following questions about using them in clinical practice: Why are the standards important to practice? What examples from practice indicate that the standards are being employed? What legal significance do the standards have for advanced practice?
3. Discuss the following questions in writing or as a group: What values have you seen in the behaviors of your

clinical preceptors? What values do you attempt to convey to patients and others during your residency experiences or clinical practice? What value, if any, do you embrace so strongly that you would quit a job in order to not compromise that value?

4. In a group venue, differentiate the roles of the registered nurse (RN) and the APN. Discuss changes required in self-concept and professional identity when role change occurs from RN to APN. Discuss the attitudes and interactions you have witnessed or personally experienced between RNs and APNs. Examine ways in which the relationships between the two groups can be enhanced.

5. Speculate on the reasons why CNSs appear to experience more role ambiguity after graduation than other APNs.

6. Using the three student types identified by Roberts et al (1997), determine which type best describes you. Compare your socialization process as an APN student with that of someone in one of the other two groups. Do the findings by Roberts et al apply to you and your classmates?

7. Consult Mauksch (1990). Mauksch states that in order to achieve excellence in advanced practice, nursing must address "low self-esteem, which was a significant occupational characteristic of the nursing collective." Was this valid in 1990? What about in 2000? Support your answer with a rationale.

REFERENCES/BIBLIOGRAPHY

Alspach, J. (1995). *The educational process in nursing staff development*. St. Louis: Mosby.

American Association of Colleges of Nursing. (1996). *The essentials of Master's education for advanced practice nursing*. Washington, DC: American Association of Colleges of Nursing.

American Nurses Association (1996). *Scope and standards of advanced practice registered nursing*. Washington, DC: American Nurses Association.

Atkinson, G. (1991). Kolb's learning style inventory: a practitioner's perspective. *Measurement and Evaluation in Counseling, 23*(4), 149-162.

Bass, M., Rabbett, P., & Siskind, M. (1993). Novice CNS and role acquisition. *Clinical Nurse Specialist, 7*(3), 148-152.

Bates, B. (1990). Twelve paradoxes: a message for nurse practitioners. *Journal of the American Academy of Nurse Practitioners, 2*(4), 136-139.

Bellack, J.P., Graber, D.R., O'Neil, E.H., Musham, C., & Lancaster, C. (1999). Curriculum trends in nurse practitioner programs: current and ideal. *Journal of Professional Nursing, 15*(1), 15-27.

Benner, P. (1984). *From novice to expert*. Menlo Park, CA: Addison-Wesley.

Benner, P., Tanner, C., & Chesla, C. (1992). From beginner to expert: gaining a differentiated clinical world in critical care nursing. *Advances in Nursing Science, 11*(3), 13-28.

Brody, C.M. (1994). Collaborative learning: fostering dialogue across the professions. In C.M. Brody & J. Wallace (Eds.). *Ethical and social issues in professional education* (pp. 49-66). Albany, NY: State University of New York Press.

Brookfield, D. (1993). On impostership, cultural suicide, and other dangers: how nurses learn critical thinking. *Journal of Continuing Education in Nursing, 24*, 197-207.

Brown, M.A., & Olshansky, E. (1998). Becoming a primary nurse practitioner: challenges of the initial year of practice. *The Nurse Practitioner, 23*(7), 46, 52-66.

Brykczynski, K.A. (1989). An interpretive study describing the clinical judgment of nurse practitioners. *Scholarly Inquiry for Nursing Practice: An International Journal, 3*(2), 75-104.

Cavanaugh, S.J., Hogan, K., & Ramgopal, T. (1995). The assessment of student nurses' learning styles using the Kolb Learning Styles Inventory. *Nurse Education Today, 15*, 177-183.

Christensen, M.G., Lee, C.A.B., & Bugg, P.W. (1979). Professional development of nurse practitioners as function of need motivation, learning style, and locus of control. *Nursing Research, 23*, 51-56.

Conrad, C.F., Haworth, J.G., & Miller, K.A. (1993). A silent success: Master's education in the United States. Baltimore, MD: Johns Hopkins University Press.

Curriculum guidelines and regulatory criteria for family nurse practitioners seeking prescriptive authority to manage pharmacotherapeutics in primary care. (1998). Washington, DC: Department of Health & Human Services Health Resources and Services Administration, Agency for Health Care Policy and Research.

Dewar, B.J., & Walker, E. (1999). Experiential learning: issues for supervision. *Journal of Advanced Nursing, 30*(6), 1459-1467.

Diers, D. (1985). Preparation of practitioners, clinical specialists, and clinicians. *Journal of Professional Nursing, 1*(1), 41-47.

Dunn, D., & Campbell, J. (1985). *Developing professional effectiveness in nursing*. Upper Saddle River, NJ: Prentice-Hall.

Edmunds, M. (1982, September). NPs face different reality shock. *Nurse Practitioner*, 64, 68.

Elkema, R.C., & Knutson, M. (1983). Basic principles for new role development: a ten-year experience. *Journal of Long Term Care Administration, 11*, 10-14.

Fenton, M.V. (1985). Identifying competencies of clinical nurse specialists. *Journal of Nursing Administration, 15*(12), 31-37.

Fenton, M.V., & Brykczynski, K.A. (1993). Qualitative distinctions and similarities in the practice of clinical nurse specialists and nurse practitioners. *Journal of Professional Nursing, 9*(6), 313-326.

Frik, S.M., & Pollack, S.E. (1993). Preparation for advanced nursing practice. *Nursing & Health Care, 14*(4), 190-195.

Hamric, A.B., & Spross, J.A. (1989). *The clinical nurse specialist in theory and practice* (2nd ed.). Philadelphia: WB Saunders.

Hamric, A.B., & Taylor, J.W. (1989). Role development of the CNS. In A.B. Hamric & J.A. Spross (Eds.), *The clinical nurse specialist in theory and practice* (pp. 41-82) (2nd ed.). Philadelphia: WB Saunders.

Hardy, M. E., & Conway, M.E. (1978). *Role theory: perspectives for health professionals* (2nd ed.). New York: Appleton-Century-Crofts.

Haworth, J., & Conrad, C. (1996). Refocusing quality assessment on student learning. *New Directions for Institutional Research, 92*, 45-60.

Highfield, M.E. (1988). Learning styles. *Nurse Educator, 13*(6), 30- 37.

Hinshaw, A.S. (1982). Socialization and re-socialization for professional nursing practice. In E.C. Hein & M.F. Nicholson (Eds.), *Contemporary leadership behavior: selected readings* (pp. 17-39). Boston: Little, Brown.

Hupcey, J.E. (1990). The socialization process of master's level nurse practitioner students. *Journal of Nursing Education, 29*(5), 196-201.

Hupcey, J.E. (1994). Graduate education for nurse practitioners: are advanced degrees needed for practice. *Journal of Professional Nursing, 10*(6), 350-356.

Kitchie, S. (1997). Determinants of learning. In S.B. Bastable (Ed.), *Nurse as educator: principles of teaching and learning* (pp. 55-89). Boston: Jones & Bartlett.

Klaich, K. (1990). Transition in professional identity of nurses enrolled in graduate educational programs. *Holistic Nursing, 4*(3), 17-24.

Kolb, D.A. (1984). *Experiential learning: experience as the source of learning and development.* New York: Prentice Hall.

Kozier, B., Erb, G., & Blais, K. (1992). *Concepts and issues in nursing practice* (2nd ed.). Reading, MA: Addison-Wesley.

Kramer, M. (1974). *Reality shock: why nurses leave nursing.* St. Louis: Mosby.

Laschinger, H.K., & Boss, M.W. (1984). Learning styles of nursing students and career choices. *Journal of Advanced Nursing, 9*, 375-380.

Margolis, F., & Sneed, M. (1999). From expert to novice: doctorally prepared nursing faculty retooling for the future. *Nurse Educator, 24*(1), 9-11.

Marquis, B., & Huston, C. (2000). *Leadership roles and management functions in nursing.* Philadelphia: JB Lippincott.

Mauksch, I. (1990). Nursing practice evolves into excellence. *Nurse Practitioner Forum, 1*(3), 175-179.

Merritt, S. (1983). Learning style preferences of baccalaureate nursing students. *Nursing Research, 32*(6), 367-372.

Mundinger, M. (2000). Primary care outcomes in patients treated by nurse practitioners and physicians: a randomized trial. *Journal of the American Medical Association, 283.*

National Association of Clinical Nurse Specialists (1998). *Statement on clinical nurse specialist practice and educa-* *tion.* Glenview, IL: National Association of Clinical Nurse Specialists.

National Organization of Nurse Practitioner Faculties (1995). *Curriculum guidelines and program standards for nurse practitioner education.* Washington, DC: National Organization of Nurse Practitioner Faculties.

O'Neil, E.H., & Pew Health Professions Commission (1998). *Recreating health professional practice for a new century.* San Francisco: Pew Health Professions Commission, Pew Charitable Trust Foundation.

Page, N.E., & Arena, D.M. (1991). Practical strategies for CNS role implementation. *Clinical Nurse Specialist, 5*(1), 38-43.

Papai, P., Bourbonnais, F.F., & Chevrier, J. (1999). Transcultural reflection on clinical teaching using an experiential teaching-learning model. *Journal of Continuing Education in Nursing, 30*(6), 260-266.

Pew Health Professions Commission (1998). *Recreating health professional practice for a new century: the fourth report of the Pew Health Professions Commission.* San Francisco: University of California at San Francisco.

Raschick, M., Maypole, D.E., & Day, P. (1998). Improving field education through Kolb learning theory. *Journal of Social Work Education, 34*(1), 31-43.

Roberts, S., Tabloski, P., & Bova, C. (1997). Epigenesis of the nurse practitioner role revisited. *Journal of Nursing Education, 36*(2), 67-73.

Russell, J., & Hezel, L. (1999). Role analysis of the advanced practice nurse using the Neuman health care systems model as a framework. *Clinical Nurse Specialist, 8*(4), 215-220.

Scott, R.A. (1999). A description of the roles, activities, and skills of clinical nurse specialists in the United States. *Clinical Nurse Specialist, 13*(4), 183-190.

Shugars, D.A., O'Neil, E.H., & Bader, J.D. (Eds.). (1991). *Healthy America: practitioners for 2005: an agenda for action for U.S. health professional schools.* Durham, North Carolina: Pew Health Professions Comission.

Stanford, D. (1987). Nurse practitioner research: issues in practice and theory. *Nurse Practitioner, 12*(1), 64-75.

Styles, M. (1982). *On nursing—toward a new endowment.* St. Louis: Mosby.

Tischler, H.L. (1999). *Introduction to sociology* (6th ed.). Fort Worth, TX: Harcourt Brace.

Chapter 20

Role Attainment: Preceptors and Mentors

Cheryl Pope Kish

The nursing profession recognizes clinical experiences as an invaluable measure for socialization for new practice roles. In the clinical arena, the prospective advanced practice nurse (APN) working within a holistic framework undertakes a deliberately planned sequence of actions and interactions to meet the particular needs of patients and to facilitate clinical learning objectives. The knowledge, skills, and values of APNs, learned in the university classroom, can be applied in a clinical site containing all the uncertainty and "noise" one faces in the daily activities of advanced nursing practice in the real world. In this setting, supported by a seasoned, expert clinician, a student APN can learn more about handling ambiguity amidst the multiple variables that exist. By being in juxtaposition with providers from other disciplines, one learns that differing approaches can be used for similar problems. To take advantage of the inestimable value the clinical setting brings to APN education, most academic programs use preceptorships, negotiating for veteran clinicians who work in practice settings to lend their time and expertise as preceptors.

Having a seasoned expert to offer guidance, support, and empowerment once the formal education is past can be of incalculable value as well. Mentorships are effective for that purpose. While the literature has focused primarily on mentors in educational or leadership roles, there is no reason that APNs can not engage in a mentoring relationship to their personal and professional advantage.

DEFINITIONS

Preceptorships and mentorships enjoy some similarities: both are measures appropriate for role development and role rehearsal and work from a vision of quality care. Preceptorships tend to be more short term, while a mentoring relationship persists over time, possibly a lifetime. Both involve a relationship with some degree of mutuality; a preceptorship tends to be more contractual in nature, while mentoring tends toward an informal agreement.

A *preceptorship* is a clinical teaching model that involves a consistent one-on-one relationship between an experienced practitioner and a student enrolled in an educational program with a practice component. The intent of the encounters between the practitioner and student is for increasing the probability that learning and role socialization will occur. This model provides for oversight and support by a member of the academic faculty before, during, and after the practitioner-student encounters to facilitate a positive educational outcome.

Preceptorships got their start in the 1960s with undergraduate educators who determined a need for additional reality-based clinical learning opportunities to prepare prospective nurses for the inherent stress of the real world to prevent the "reality shock" so evident in that era. When it was not feasible for faculty to oversee such learning experiences, which extended over all shifts, expert nurses were identified onsite who were willing to engage students in opportunities to "be the nurse" under their watchful eyes. Preceptors were helpful as "guides on the side," and the experiences were generally rated positively by students and preceptors. This model continues to be used extensively for undergraduate nursing education. Holly (1992) believes that preceptorships serve the following purposes:

1. Enhancing skill performances in situations of uncertainty, unpredictability, and stress (*Skill* refers not just to technical skills but also cognitive skills such as decision-making)
2. Promoting comfort and confidence in performance for the novice
3. Enabling application of nursing theory to practice
4. Facilitating understanding of the organization in which practice occurs
5. Increasing leadership ability

Bahrych (1999) would add that preceptorships serve as a "means of passing on the values and unspoken truths" of the profession.

Mentorship is defined as a form of socialization for a

professional role that involves an "intense long-term relationship between a novice and a recognized expert in a given discipline"(Hawkins & Thibodeau, 1996). This relationship, which is dynamic and noncompetitive, is instrumental in fostering the career of many novices, enabling a protégé to reach his or her full potential. At times, mentorship may also serve to rejuvenate the career of a seasoned professional. The term *mentor* derives from Greek mythology; Athena, the goddess of wisdom, disguised herself as a man, Mentor, in order to serve as protector, guide, and advisor to Telemachus, whose father Odysseus was fighting the Trojan War. Today, a mentor is "involved with the mentee in a cognitive and an affective relationship of trust, preference, and mutuality" (Hawkins & Thibodeau, 1996).

CRITICAL ISSUES: BENEFITS OF PRECEPTOR AND MENTOR RELATIONSHIPS

Preceptors

Being a preceptor is a time-consuming, labor-intensive activity. First, preceptors must balance the priority of patient care, for which they remain ultimately responsible, with the student's learning needs. At times, these are at odds, contributing to possible role conflict. For example, an excellent learning opportunity may become apparent, but the patient or family may feel uncomfortable with a student provider, albeit one that is well supervised. In other cases, a patient may proclaim loudly, "I am paying to see a doctor. I won't see some green student." This juggling act—having one more person (the student) whose needs must be met in the hectic clinic environment—can be stressful. Second, there is rarely financial compensation for preceptors, although rewards are given in some programs—certificates, journal subscriptions, books, items with a particular university's logo (e.g., coffee mugs, pens), access to university events and facilities, tuition reductions or continuing education courses, adjunct positions, and/or opportunities for collaborative publishing with faculty.

Satisfaction for the preceptor comes from the pleasure of witnessing professional development in his or her student; stimulation of the intellectual exchange that challenges preceptors to "stay on their toes"; and the assurance that the profession will lay claim to the best and brightest. For the preceptor who is an alumna of a university, preceptorship lends an opportunity to give something back. Precepting can increase job satisfaction by allowing the experienced practitioner to learn new things and granting him or her status, admiration, and respect (O'Mara, 1997). In clinical agencies with career ladder programs in place, being a preceptor can assist in advancement.

Preceptorships are beneficial to both the educational enterprise and the quality of patient care. Additionally, they can play a powerful role in recruitment. The staff has opportunities to preview student performance, and students, because their familiarity with the agency increases over time, require shorter orientation intervals upon employment.

Sloand, Feroli, Bearss, and Beecher (1998) suggest that being a good preceptor requires: (1) thorough understanding of the multifaceted APN role, (2) willingness to assume responsibility for student learning, (3) knowledge of the strengths and limitations of the site, and (4) skill in clinical instruction. These requirements ideally blend exemplary clinical performance and wise time management with the qualities of being a good teacher, gracious host or hostess, and caring professional.

Mentors

While one may be assigned a preceptor for the purposes of learning a new role, one "finds" a mentor (Olson, 2000). Mentorships are extraordinary relationships formed when chemistry exists and the people involved experience a special bond that progresses over time, contributing most to the career of the junior member of the pair. Virtually any aspect of one's career quest can be an aspect of such a mentorship. "In a mentorship, the personal and professional are beautifully and messily compounded and intermixed" (Barnum, 1997).

While the power base in a mentorship is unequal, both individuals have the potential to gain from the experience. Barnum (1997) believes that there is "not enough money in the world to reimburse a mentor" for the selfless acts undertaken in behalf of the protégé. Many of the satisfactions of the mentoring role are similar to those for the preceptor—mainly the excitement of being a generative professional.

Fuszard and Taylor (1995) identify behaviors of a mentor, based on *The Seasons of a Man's Life* (1978) by Levinson, Darrow, Klein, and McKee; these include:

1. Promoting intellectual development and teaching new skills
2. Guiding acquisition of the values, customs, and resources of the profession
3. Serving as an exemplar and role model
4. Offering wise counsel and moral support during times of crisis
5. Fostering a student's development by believing in him or her
6. Supporting and facilitating life's goals and dreams
7. Advising

IMPLICATIONS FOR MSN EDUCATION AND ADVANCED PRACTICE

Gray (1983) describes three phases of a preceptorship, comparable to the development of therapeutic relationships with patients: orientation, working phase, and termination. Gray's stages serve as an excellent organizing framework for exploring preceptorships. (Box 20-1 identifies the myriad tasks involved in each stage.)

Orientation Phase

During the orientation phase, the foundation on which a student's learning will develop is established. Strategic planning occurs among faculty, preceptor, and student; curriculum materials that inform the preceptorship are shared; mutual expectations are examined; and a climate of trust, inclusive of a sense of mutual approachability, is created. The collaboration started in this first phase must continue throughout the relationship; otherwise, it is doomed to fail.

One of the most important tasks of the orientation phase involves site selection. In most programs, this is done well in advance of the experience; many sites have lists of acceptable preceptors from whom students may select. Other programs allow students to identify preceptors with whom they wish to work, who are geographically closer to their residence, or who are located in a community in which the student ultimately hopes to be employed. There are benefits to self-directed, actively involved adult learners selecting their own preceptors: they can identify someone with whom they feel comfortable in what can otherwise be an inherently stressful setting, and they can select a setting of particular interest, such as a clinic seeing all indigent patients or a unit with a particular patient population. The disadvantages of selecting one's own preceptor are that familiarity may contribute to an atmosphere too relaxed for optimal learning and effective evaluation, as well as the possibility of selecting someone incongruous with program objectives. Moreover, in these times of increased enrollments and competition for clinical sites, locating a preceptor can be particularly stressful for a novice. No matter how a preceptor is identified, the faculty must select preceptors based on identified program standards (Miller, 2000).

Even when students identify potential preceptors, the faculty has responsibility to assess the sites and preceptors before negotiating a contract or placing a student. A selected clinical site for the preceptorship should include the following:

- Professionals with appropriate credentials (e.g., licenses, certifications).
- Flexibility to allow additional time for student learning, onsite visits, and evaluation by faculty.
- A philosophical perspective on advanced practice and holistic primary care (or another specialty) that is congruent with that of the nursing program.
- A variety of patients in sufficient numbers to allow attainment of objectives. A range of other types of learning experience (e.g., nursing home visits, hospital rounds) can also be a plus.
- Current protocols or clinical guidelines in place.
- Knowledge among staff about community resources for referral.
- Accessibility of patient records for student use.
- Staff willing to collaborate with faculty, student, and preceptor in the learning process.
- Access to consultation as needed.
- Resources available for student use (e.g., reference materials, policies).
- Space for private conferences, patient panels, storage of belongings, safe parking, and accessible dining (when prolonged hours are involved).

Students are well advised to negotiate preceptorships with both APNs and physicians while in school. Doing so enhances the appreciation that there are different approaches to similar problems and that the medical and nursing models are, in fact, different. Physician preceptors often have particular strengths in pathophysiology and pharmacology, and they often share invaluable clues about physical assessment and patient management. NP preceptors help students absorb the new identity associated with the APN model and those dimensions that distinguish APN practice.

Working Phase

The working phase includes those patient-care encounters, designated at the outset, that have as their purpose the student's attainment of the clinical objectives. This is the longest of the three phases, often running over a full semester. Onsite visits by faculty are a critical part of the working phase. Preceptors have a vital role in helping students discover the knowledge embedded in a clinical practice itself and learn to work within the infrastructure of a particular setting, with its inherent rules, customs, culture, and politics. Within a one-on-one preceptorship, learners observe and experience the reality of practice in a secure environment, with the preceptor adjusting the teaching as determined by the learner's needs (Shah & Politroni, 1992). To accomplish this, preceptors find themselves coaching, teaching, questioning, encouraging, reassuring, motivating, and correcting. Through it all, hopefully they share their passion for the role with their students.

Preceptors are expected to develop an environment

Box 20-1

Overview of Each Phase of Preceptorship

Orientation Phase

The faculty identify a clinical site.

The faculty identify a qualified preceptor with:

- Academic credentials desired by the program and a current license to practice
- Experience in the role (18 to 24 months minimum)
- Experience at the site to be used (1 year minimum)
- A willingness to serve in the role
- Unquestioned clinical expertise
- A practice philosophy congruent with that of the academic program
- A passion for the role

The faculty negotiate a contract or letter of agreement for use of the clinical site and the preceptor's involvement, as dictated by the university, state regulation, and/or the clinical agency.

The preceptor, student, and faculty mutually delineate expectations.

The faculty:

- Share information with the preceptor about the student's ability, level in the program, and credentials (e.g., proof of registered nurse [RN] license, liability insurance, health and immunization status, cardiopulmonary resuscitation [CPR] training).
- Review course objectives with the preceptor.
- Provide curriculum materials as needed to facilitate the preceptor's understanding of the academic program (e.g., description of courses, philosophy).
- Ensure a match of the student and preceptor to the extent possible before the experience begins.
- Negotiate to meet with the preceptor on a regular basis, either in person or by telephone or e-mail; to be accessible at other times by telephone or beeper; and to make onsite visits for the purpose of talking with the preceptor and student and evaluating student performance.

The student:

- Agrees to candid self-appraisal and identification of learning needs.
- Appreciates the importance of reliance on the professional wisdom of the preceptor and the need to assert learning needs to capitalize on that wisdom.
- Agrees to prepare for each clinical experience.
- Agrees to write learning objectives for each experience.
- Agrees to ongoing self-evaluation during the experience.
- Provides a resume or curriculum vitae (CV) as required by the agency or preceptor before beginning the experience.

The preceptor:

- Orients the student to the agency.
- Develops an environment conducive to learning.
- Identifies ways for the student to meet clinical objectives.
- Guides the actions of the student.
- Provides feedback on student clinical performance.
- Maintains communication with the faculty, attending meetings as negotiated.

- Provides the faculty with data for a final evaluation of the student's performance.

Working Phase

The preceptor, student, and faculty collaborate to facilitate learning experiences based on clinical objectives. Prerequisite skill and student entry behavior are starting points in patient selection.

The patient, preceptor, and student prioritize safety throughout each encounter.

The student is given opportunities for role rehearsal in each of the aspects of the multifaceted role of the APN.

The student is provided a mixed patient population to ensure cultural, age, and gender diversity, as well as varied diagnoses.

Based on observation of the student's performance, the preceptor modifies the learning environment as needed to increase the probability of student learning.

Termination Phase

Appraisal of each phase of the preceptorship by the preceptor, student, and faculty occurs, which enables evaluation of the overall learning experience.

Summary meetings occur.

A determination is made about the extent to which the student was able to attain expected competencies in collaboration with the preceptor. Examples of appropriate competencies for an advanced student include:

- Performing complete histories and physical examinations in a manner appropriate to patients' problems.
- Differentiating normal variations and abnormal findings based on examination, history, and diagnostic test results.
- Developing a working diagnosis, differential diagnoses, or a problem list.
- Developing a preliminary plan of care.
- Presenting a concise, accurate, and organized review of a patient and preliminary management plan to enable the preceptor and student to jointly critique and revise a final plan for implementation.
- Considering the cost implications of the management plan under consideration.
- Providing anticipatory patient guidance and education for managing identified health problems and promoting health.
- Recognizing when to refer patients to another health care provider.
- Documenting in the patient's record, using agency procedure, those elements of the clinical encounter necessary to continuity of care, third-party reimbursement, and a legally prudent record.
- Demonstrating relationships with patients, family, staff, and others that exemplify professionalism, appreciation of the worth and dignity of individuals, caring, and unconditional positive regard.

conducive to student learning. Some universities offer inservice programs for prospective preceptors that teach them how best to accomplish this, including content about working with adult learners and varied teaching approaches. Written information can be provided to preceptors that explains the basic elements of a conducive learning environment; these include:

- An available examination space to allow students to proceed at a "learning" pace without disrupting patient flow within the agency
- Opportunities to perform histories and physical examinations, propose necessary diagnostic tests or formulate a list for consideration, propose a tentative management plan for critique by the preceptor, and document encounters either in the patient record or on a worksheet for preceptor review
- Availability of the preceptor to hear a student's case presentation, then to see and/or reexamine the patient with the student (as necessary) to provide a critique of the student's assessment findings and proposed plan of care
- Opportunities for students to observe or participate in the care of a patient (with the patient's permission) who, in the opinion of the preceptor, has a demonstrable pathology or some other factor of educational interest
- Opportunities to perform technical procedures consistent with the student's learning objectives while under the supervision of the preceptor
- Appreciation by all involved that learners are in the setting to function as health care provider students, working at a slower pace and requiring more consultation than an experienced provider

Because students entering APN programs are often experts in the area of their pre–graduate school practice, they often come into the preceptorship with a peculiar mix of confidence and insecurity. To return to novice status in a new nursing role is predictably hard for all involved (Sloand et al, 1998).

Students can be embarrassed by their limitations. There is a certain vulnerability described by most APNs. Some days go well; other days, they can't seem to do anything right. In these situations, it is valuable for preceptors to reach within their memories for what it was like to be a novice at performing new, complex skills and share those memories with students (Manley, 1997). For students to know that they are "on target," progressing as expected, and not alone in their sense of insecurity and vulnerability offers both reassurance and hope (Sloand et al, 1998).

The real world is not always a supportive learning environment. Clinical sites are unpredictable and can sometimes border on chaos. Students can encounter situations that threaten their self-esteem and individuals who are judgmental, nonsupportive, and closed to questions. Preceptors can intervene by helping students examine and reflect on a particular occurrence and proposing solutions.

At times, preceptors have to intervene more directly to ensure that student learning is not compromised.

In their qualitative study of teaching styles of expert preceptors—both physicians and NPs—Davis, Sawin, and Dunn (1993) discovered that regardless of the level of student, all preceptors tend to manipulate the learning environment to minimize student stress. Role-modeling was also used by all participants. Two distinct preceptor styles/teaching philosophies, depending on the level of the student, emerged from this study: immersion style (where experiences are "sink or swim" or "all at once") versus incremental structure style (which gradually adds responsibility).

In the three videotapes titled *Partnerships in Clinical Teaching* (1994) and based on the research of Davis et al (1993), the immersion and incremental structure styles are evident. Preceptors describe their initial work alongside novice students, sometimes allowing students to shadow or observe them for a time to become familiar with what is expected in a particular practice. Pre- and post-observation conferences are widely used. In many cases the preceptor reviews a student's history of a patient or redoes portions of a patient's physical examination to ensure that nothing was missed. Gradually students take over more hands-on care. Extra time is built in for beginning students, who tend to take longer for patient encounters and need additional time to think about what they are doing. The major goal for beginning students is a more strongly focused assessment. Preceptors in the video reported leaving advanced students more on their own, letting them set the pace of patient encounters; in these cases, preceptors found themselves serving more in a consultant role. Post-visit critiques were commonly used. The goal for advanced students was stronger time management. Preceptors tended to buffer stresses as much as possible for both beginning and advanced students.

A study by Snyder, Modly, Hancock, and Hekelman (1998) revealed that physician and APN faculty have different teaching styles in preceptorships. In general, physicians tend to give information or direction, seek information and comprehension, encourage questions, and substantiate findings. APN preceptors use some of those techniques, but they are more likely to use caring or nurturing behaviors than physicians, such as listening to student concerns and giving positive feedback. It is not uncommon to hear from those who have had physician preceptors that the medical education model tends to be slightly more confrontational.

Termination Phase

Preceptors oversee student performance with a watchful eye. A preceptor needs to be able to keep apprised of all student activities and be watchful for potential errors or missed data (Sloand et al, 1998). Although faculty retain the final evaluation of students, one of the important roles of the preceptor that overlaps the working and termination stages is providing corrective feedback. Ideal feedback from preceptors is:

- Offered in private, with respect for confidentiality.
- Clearly communicated so there is no room for misinterpretation.
- Provided fairly soon after the incident in question (if possible).
- Based on observable behavior that can be modified on the basis of feedback.
- Explicit and concrete and, if possible, inclusive of information about the consequence of the specific performance on outcomes for the patient and the functioning of the clinical team.
- Inclusive of both positive and negative behaviors observed over time.

It can be helpful to have students perform self-critiques and explore what they might change in similar situations. However, students are usually well aware of any deficient performance; indeed, they are often too critical and profit from some balance from their preceptors.

Preceptors generally have considerable input into the final evaluation of students. Data for these evaluations is objective-based and focused on the multidimensional roles of the APN: interviewing and data collection; diagnostic skills; management approaches and their basis in sound rationale; functioning amidst a culturally diverse clientele; and functioning as a team player. Those role aspects that particularly distinguish APN practice—teaching, anticipatory guidance, counseling, and providing health promotion—should receive consideration. Professional behavior and work ethic issues are also commonly addressed.

During the evaluation phase, there is typically an end-of-preceptorship meeting, with opportunities for summary of experience by those involved. Preceptors may be given some acknowledgment or reward for their willingness to serve. Students are frequently asked to complete evaluations of their preceptors' effectiveness, which are shared with the preceptors at some point. (Figure 20-1

Name of preceptor:_____

Course:_____ Semester:_____ Clinical setting:_____

Name of evaluator (optional): _____

Instructions: Rate your clinical preceptor on each item below, giving the highest scores for unusually effective performances. Place the number that most nearly expresses your view in the blank space before each statement. Provide comments as desired as evidence for your choice.

Highest			Average				Lowest	Not applicable
7	6	5	4	3	2	1	0	NA

_____ 1. Provided orientation to the agency, staff, and essential policies and procedures.
_____ 2. Selected patients for me that provided opportunities to meet course and personal learning objectives.
_____ 3. Assisted me in new or unfamiliar situations without taking over.
_____ 4. Provided me with helpful and timely feedback.
_____ 5. Provided a non-threatening atmosphere where I could learn comfortably.
_____ 6. Answered questions freely.
_____ 7. Expressed willingness to help me learn.
_____ 8. Offered encouragement.
_____ 9. Served as an appropriate role model of advanced practice.
_____ 10. Behaved in a supportive and enthusiastic manner.
_____ 11. Made me aware of my professional accountability.
_____ 12. Identified additional resources to enhance my learning.
_____ 13. Assisted me in learning the multifaceted role of advanced practice nurse.

To offer your clinical preceptor an additional view of his or her performance, please share your comments about the following:

1. Would you recommend this preceptor to your peers or future students of this program? Please explain.

2. What actions by this preceptor do you believe can be described as exemplary?

3. What specific suggestions would you make concerning how this preceptor might improve his or her performance in this role?

Figure 20-1 Sample instrument for student evaluation of a clinical preceptor's effectiveness.

shows an example of such an evaluation.) Both faculty and student evaluate the clinical site for future use.

Finally, just as an APN learns the clinical role from a more experienced professional, graduates can continue their professional growth by being mentored by a master. Novice APNs would be wise to identify a mentor, even if it is one accessible only by telephone or e-mail. A mentoring relationship does not have to be an all-encompassing one. New Master of Science in Nursing (MSN) graduates frequently comment that they feel very isolated in the early days of practice because they no longer have the peer group in class with whom they can network and share confidences. Hayes (1998) believes that the mentoring model might be especially effective for full socialization of APNs—the series of short-term assigned relationships between students and preceptors may not be adequate because the practitioner role is so multifaceted.

Although mentors are sometimes assigned when a new employee joins an agency, they tend to work more effectively if they are simply allowed to begin mentoring when "something clicks" between the mentor and protégé. Some time is spent in initiating the relationship and mutually identifying the role for the mentor. The working phase of the mentoring relationship is typically long lasting and the power inequality may be slightly more evident. In later stages, the relationship becomes more collegial. Tigges (1998), in a survey of 150 executives from the nation's top 1000 largest companies, discovered that 50% of executives believe having a mentor is very important; another 44% believe it is somewhat important. The greatest benefits were seen as having a confidant and advisor; being introduced to contacts; and being given encouragement, which boosted morale. Roche (1979), Vance (1992), and Allen, Russell, and Maetzke (1997) find that those who are mentored are more likely to serve as mentors themselves. Some mentors and protégés stay in touch over time, occasionally for a lifetime.

PRIORITIES FOR RESEARCH

Most of the early research on mentoring has been conducted within the context of organizational settings; the business and educational literature is filled with such studies. However, in the last decade, health care researchers have turned their attention to preceptorships and mentorships as worthy areas of study. Caine (1989) developed and tested an instrument for judging the mentor role; it is the Quality of Mentoring Tool (QMT), developed for the purpose of exploring the relationship between mentoring and job satisfaction. The QMT consists of specific mentor qualities—model, envisioner, energizer, investor, supporter, standard-prodder, teacher, coach, feedback-giver, eye-opener, door-opener, idea-bouncer, problem-solver, career counselor, and challenger—scored on a five-point Likert scale. The total score for the QMT is a sum of the values for each quality; the higher the score, the

greater the quality of the mentoring relationship. Caine found that 83% of the clinical nurse specialist (CNS) sample in the study engaged in a mentoring relationship; moreover, there was a significant relationship with having done so and subsequent job satisfaction. Cuesta and Bloom (1998) conducted a direct replication of Caine's work, using newly certified nurse midwives (CNMs) as their study population. Fewer (65%) of the midwives had been mentored; however, there was a significant, albeit low, correlation between stated job satisfaction and the quality of the mentoring relationship. Of the CNMs, 81% (compared to Caine's 83%) reported job satisfaction; however, the relationship between mentoring and job satisfaction was not found to be statistically significant. Additional replication of these studies with other types of APNs, like certified registered nurse anesthetists (CRNAs) and NPs, would prove interesting. Research designed to match preceptor-student or mentor-protégé pairings might explore these relationships more fully, possibly identifying incentives and disincentives for engaging in them. It would be interesting to compare matched pairs of APNs against APN-physician pairings; to examine gender variances; and to correlate self-selection versus assigned preceptorships. Capitalizing on Hagerty's (1996) notion that the more ambitious individual is more likely to seek a mentor, one could design a study with ambition as a variable.

Wing (1998) describes an 80-hour business preceptorship within a NP program designed to facilitate the prospective clinician's competence in business operations, which are now so critical in health care practice. Research to determine if this kind of preceptorship results in better preparedness for using coding systems and understanding reimbursement would be of value. Does a preceptorship with a business manager result in a higher proficiency level with International Classification of Diseases (ICD-9) coding? A better understanding of the business of primary practice? The capacity to develop a funded business plan for a CNS-managed education program for diabetic patients?

Hayes (1998) studied the self-efficacy of NP students based on their clinical preceptorship experience, which she called "mentoring." She found a modest correlation between student perceptions of mentoring behaviors and the confidence with which they faced undertaking the APN role. (Interestingly, this study used Caine's 1989 QMT in addition to several other instruments.) Students who self-selected their mentors had higher confidence scores. Time in the clinical practicum itself and the preceptors' actual years of experience in the APN role were also predictive of positive mentoring outcomes.

Hayes (1999) also used qualitative methodology to explore NP preceptor–student relationships and the meaning of the relationships to students, including "mentoring" (positive) or "nonmentoring" (negative) preceptor behaviors. Positive behaviors include such actions as giving case studies or references to enhance learning, celebrating

Suggestions for Further Learning

- Read the following resource, which includes an excellent series of guided questions for facilitating clinical decision-making in a relatively brief interval: Neher, J.O., Gordon, K.C., Meyer, M., & Stevens, N (1992). A five step "microskills" model of clinical teaching. *Journal of the American Board of Family Practice, 5*(4), 419-424. This resource refers to educating family practice physician residents in an ambulatory care setting. To what extent can it be applied to preceptors working with APN students? What, if anything, would need modification?
- Interview an APN who has served as a preceptor about the experience. What were the challenges? The rewards? What advice would he or she offer to someone considering the preceptor role?
- There is a possibility that differences in communication between genders affect preceptor-student relationships when one member is female and the other is male. Consider your own experience. For further insights, read Tannen, D. (1990). *You just don't understand: women and men in conversation.* New York: Ballantine Books.
- Find a compelling study on mentorships in business or educational literature. Draft a proposal for replicating the study in an APN context.
- Consult the following: How to be a great mentor. (1999, February 15). *Newsweek, 133*(7). This special issue was designed by Kaplan Educational Centers and the National Mentoring Partnership.

- Generate a strategy for either seeking a mentor or becoming one. To inform your strategic planning, read Biehl, B. (1997). *Mentoring: confidence in finding a mentor and becoming one.* Nashville, TN: Broadman-Holman.
- To learn more about how to be an effective preceptor, consult Case, B. (1999). *Advanced practice nurse preceptor workbook.* Chicago: Marcella Neihoff School of Nursing, Loyola University. This resource is available from the publisher for $27.00 (cost of the book and shipping). Contact Marcella Neihoff School of Nursing, Loyola University (Attention Meg Gulani), 6525 N. Sheridan Road, Chicago, IL 60626-5385; phone (708) 216-3542; email mgulani@luc.edu. This is an excellent 98-page, spiral-bound workbook with over 50 pages of appendices devoted to information and activities related to preceptorships for APNs.
- To learn more about how to be an effective mentor, consult one or more of the following:
  - Mentoring Made Easy (www.eeo.nsw.giv.au)
  - The Medical College of Wisconsin Faculty Mentoring Program (www.mcw.edu/edserv/facdev/mentor.htm)
  - Masterplanning Group International (PO Box 952499, Lake Mary, FL 32795-2499; phone (800) 969-1976; website: master-planning.com [this is a business devoted to information, brochures, books, and tapes about mentoring])

student successes, being open to questions, and modeling patient care without taking over. Negative behaviors include being unwelcoming, not letting go, being impatient in the learning situation, and being competitive with the student. Students in the study perceived that the mentoring preceptor was indispensable to them in preparing for the APN role. Since studies like those of Hayes use the terms *preceptor* and *mentor* interchangeably, readers of research in this topic area are well served to attend closely to the operational definitions being used.

A priority for additional research is on facilitative and hindering preceptor and mentor behaviors for others in advanced practice and the effects of these relationships not just on novice members of the dyad but also on the more seasoned clinicians, preceptors, or mentors. It will be helpful to have empirical studies that investigate how preceptorships and/or mentorships can enable the nonclinical roles of APNs, such as consultant and researcher.

DISCUSSION QUESTIONS

These questions can be used to promote critical thinking and encourage discussion.

1. Reflect on your own experiences of being precepted. What behaviors by your preceptors facilitated your learning? What behaviors or approaches were less effective? Have you had experience with a preceptor who used immersion style? Incremental style? Which was more comfortable for you as a learner? Which approach will you hope to emulate as a future preceptor?
2. Compare and contrast the styles of physician and APN preceptors with whom you have worked. Discuss with peers their experiences with APN versus physician preceptors.
3. Reflect on the individuals who have served as role models in your graduate education and career thus far. What characteristics of these individuals made them compelling role models? Could any of these individuals qualify as mentors? Why or why not?

REFERENCES/BIBLIOGRAPHY

Allen, T.D., Russell, J.E.A., & Maetzke, S.B. (1997). Formal peer mentoring: factors related to protégés' satisfaction and willingness to mentor others. *Group & Organization Management, 22*(4), 488-507.

Bahrych, S. (1999). Mentoring. *Clinician Reviews, 9*(10), 23-27.

Barnum, B.S. (1997). Precepting, not mentoring or teaching: vive la difference. In J.P. Flynn (Ed.), *The role of the preceptor* (pp. 1-13). New York: Springer.

Beihl, B. (1997). *Mentoring: confidence in finding a mentor and becoming one.* Nashville, TN: Broadman-Holman.

Belcher, A.E. (1997). Mentorships. In J.P. Flynn (Ed.), *The role of the preceptor* (pp. 119-137). New York: Springer.

Bodman, E.J. & Weintraub, J. (2000, March). Essential to the profession's future: clinical preceptors. *ADVANCE for Nurse Practitioners,* 58, 60, 62.

Caine R.M. (1989). *A comparative survey of mentoring and job satisfaction: perceptions of clinical nurse specialists* (Unpublished doctoral dissertation # 8918736 [50] 05A, 36). Pepperdine University Dissertation Abstracts International.

Case, B. (1999). *Advanced practice nurse preceptor workbook.* Chicago: Marcella Neihoff School of Nursing, Loyola University.

Corcoran, S., Narayan, S., & Moreland, H. (1988). "Thinking aloud" as a strategy to improve clinical decision making. *Heart & Lung, 17*(8), 463-468.

Cuesta, C.W., & Bloom, K.C. (1998). Mentoring and job satisfaction: perceptions of certified nurse midwives. *Journal of Nurse Midwifery, 43*(2), 111-116.

Davis, M.S., Sawin, K.J., & Dunn, M. (1993). Teaching strategies used by expert nurse practitioner preceptors: a qualitative study. *Journal of the American Academy of Nurse Practitioners, 5*(1), 27-33.

DeLong, T.H., & Bechtel, G.A.(1999). Enhancing the relationship between nursing faculty and clinical preceptors. *Journal for Nurses in Staff Development, 15*(4), 148-151.

Flynn, J.P. (Ed). (1997). *The role of the preceptor.* New York: Springer.

Fuszard, B., & Taylor, L.J. (1995). Mentorship. In B. Fuszard (Ed.), *Innovative teaching strategies in nursing* (pp. 200-207) (2nd ed.). Gaithersburg, MD: Aspen Publishers.

Gibson, S.E., & Hauri, C. (2000). The pleasure of your company: attitudes and opinions of preceptors toward nurse practitioner preceptees. *Journal of the American Academy of Nurse Practitioners, 12*(9), 360-363.

Gray, A.P. (1983). How to utilize a preceptor. In S. Stewart & J.M. Haberlin (Eds.), *Preceptorship in nursing education.* Rockville, MD: Aspen Publishers.

Hagerty, B. (1996). A second look at mentors. *Nursing Outlook, 34*(1), 16-24.

Hagopian, G.A., Ferszt, G.G., Jacobs, L.A., & McCorkle, R. (1992). Preparing clinical preceptors to teach master's level students in oncology nursing. *Journal of Professional Nursing, 8*(5), 295-300.

Hawkins, J.W., & Thibodeau, J.A. (1996). *The advanced practice nurse—current issues.* New York: Tiresias.

Hayes, E. (1999). Athena found or lost: the precepting experiences of mentored and non-mentored nurse practitioner students. *Journal of the American Academy of Nurse Practitioners, 11*(8), 335-342.

Hayes, E. (1998). Mentorship and self-efficacy for advanced nursing practice: a philosophical approach for nurse practitioner preceptors. *Journal of the American Academy of Nurse Practitioners, 10*(2), 53-57.

Hayes, E.F. (1998). Mentoring and nurse practitioner student self-efficacy. *Western Journal of Nursing Research, 20*(5), 521-535.

Holly, C.M. (1992). A program design for preceptor training. *Nursing Connections, 5*(1), 49-59.

Kersbergen, A.L., & Hrobsky, P.E. (1996). Use of clinical maps in precepted clinical experiences. *Nursing Educator, 21*(6), 19-22.

Lambert, V.A., McDonough, J.E.M., Pond, E.F., & Billue, J.S. (1995). Preceptorial experience. In B. Fuszard. *Innovative teaching strategies in nursing* (pp. 190-199) (2nd ed.). Gaithersburg, MD: Aspen Publishers.

Levinson, D., Darrow, C., Klein, M., & McKee, B. (1978). *The seasons of a man's life.* New York: Ballantine.

Manley, M.J. (1997). Adult learning concepts important to precepting. In J.P. Flynn (Ed.), *The role of the preceptor* (pp. 15-46). New York: Springer.

Miller, S.K. (2000). Should students find their own preceptors? *Patient Care for the Nurse Practitioner, 3*(1), 72.

Olson, K. (2000). Time spent in a mentor's garden: sowing the seeds of promise and future in nursing. *AWHONN Lifelines, 3*(6), 10.

O'Mara, A.M. (1997). A model preceptor program for student nurses. In J.P. Flynn (Ed.), *The role of the preceptor* (pp. 47-74). New York: Springer.

O'Mara, A., & Welton, R. (1995). Rewarding staff nurse preceptors. *Journal of Nursing Administration, 25,* 64-67.

Partnerships in Clinical Teaching (1994). *So you're considering being a preceptor; Strengths for beginning students;* and *Strategies for advanced students* (Series of three videotapes). Richmond, VA: Virginia Commonwealth University School of Nursing.

Poison, C.J. (1993). *Teaching about adult students* (Idea paper # 29). Kansas City, KS: Kansas State University Department of Continuing Education, Center for Faculty Evaluation & Development.

Roche, G.R. (1979). Much ado about mentors. *Harvard Business Review, 57*(1), 14-28.

Shah, H., & Politroni, C. (1992). Preceptorship of CNS students: an exploratory study. *Clinical Nurse Specialist, 6*(1), 41-46.

Sloand, E.D., Feroli, K., Bearss, N., & Beecher, J. (1998). Preparing the next generation: precepting nurse practitioner students. *Journal of the American Academy of Nurse Practitioners, 10*(2), 65-69.

Snyder, C.W., Modly, D., Hancock, L., & Hekelman, F.P. (1998). Comparison of teaching behaviors used by nurse practitioner and physician faculty teaching primary care. *Journal of the American Academy of Nurse Practitioners, 10*(1), 23-28.

Stokes, L. (1998). Teaching in the clinical setting. In Billings, D.M., & Halstead, J.A. (Eds.), *Teaching in nursing: a guide for faculty* (pp. 281-297). Philadelphia: WB Saunders.

Tigges, L. (1998). Mentoring is more than a trend. *Women in Business, 50*(3), 24-25.

Vance, C. (1992). The mentor connection. *Journal of Nursing Administration, 12*(4), 7-13.

Wing, D.M. (1998). The business management preceptorship within the nurse practitioner program. *Journal of Professional Nursing, 14*(3), 150-156.

Yoder, L.H. (1990). Mentoring: a concept analysis. *Nursing Administration Quarterly, 15*(1), 9-19.

Chapter 21

Marketing the Advanced Practice Nursing Role

Cheryl Pope Kish

Advanced practice nurses (APNs) have been on the professional scene in the United States for many years, during which they have gained a reputation, empirically justified, as providers of cost-effective, quality care that is productive and satisfying to patients. Thanks to segments on "60 Minutes" and articles in *The Washington Post* and *The Wall Street Journal*, the advanced practice role is entering the cultural mainstream (Edmunds, 1999). Yet in many practice sites (indeed, in entire communities), patients and office staff, even physicians, are asking, "What exactly is an APN, and why should we hire one?" The first APN employed by a practice site has the unenviable task of explaining the unfamiliar role to physicians, staff, and patients and making a convincing argument in favor of employment. Brown and Olshansky (1998), in their examination of nurse practitioners' (NPs') initial practice years, discovered that pressure to present oneself as a positive role model was one of the challenges for the NP. The first-year practice experience is no doubt similar for other types of APNs.

When responding to a notice advertising for an APN, the presupposition exists that the staff will be informed about the role and that the environment will be "APN friendly." If the advertisement does not specify the type of provider sought or the prospective job candidate is making a "cold call," there is less certainty about the milieu. It does appear that the increased visibility of the advanced practice role has been met with increasing animosity and tension within parts of the medical community (Edmunds, 1999). Giordano (1994) refers to the backlash against NP success as "friendly fire." This negative response appears to derive from concerns about the propagation of the NP role, incursion into physicians' practice territory, requests for inclusion of NPs on health maintenance organization (HMO) primary care panels, and economic competition for primary care roles. As Buppert (1999) suggests, "What primary care is is not particularly controversial. Who practices primary care is somewhat controversial. Who receives reimbursement for primary care is very contro-

versial." The implication is that conflict may extend to other APN roles.

Ford and Kish (1998) determined that many physicians still remain uninformed and, outside one-to-one experiences with NPs, are more inclined to base perceptions on the negative rhetoric of some of their physician counterparts. Physicians in the study who had direct experience with NPs mostly rated them favorably. Aquilino, Damiano, Willard, Momary, and Levy (1999) had similar findings in their study comparing perceptions of physicians who had experience with NPs and those who lacked such experience. The former group had more positive perceptions of NPs, perceptions borne of actual joint experiences.

Hopefully, in the educational programs preparing APNs, opportunities exist for interpreting the role to various audiences and articulating the worth of the role to a practice site and its community of patients, even in less-welcoming environments. Certainly, at the time of negotiating an initial contract, it is critical to appreciate the richness of the role; how it can be actualized in practice; how to articulate it to multiple audiences, both lay and professional; and the ways in which the role can be promoted or marketed, both initially and over time. An ability to deal with "friendly fire" is a definite plus.

DEFINITIONS

Those in the health care profession often have difficulty with the notion of promoting their practices and the idea of "selling" themselves and their profession. They believe it somehow counters the provision of health care services and seems unprofessional, even unethical. APNs, like other providers of care, have not been socialized to compete and may find the idea of business plans and marketing offensive. In this era of competitive care, however, it is no longer possible for APNs to resist the idea of marketing or promoting their roles.

Promotion refers to the process of telling prospective consumers, customers, or patients about a particular service that one is capable of providing. It involves marketing oneself as a recognized expert provider who produces positive outcomes and engaging in those measures that contribute to an image or reputation that attracts referrals and recommendations for that service (Lachman, 1996). Finnigan (1996) believes that "in developing a new business, what the person must count on most is the use of self."

Marketing is defined as determining the needs and desires of prospective consumers and then designing services, products, or programs to meet those needs (Zwelling, 1993; Lachman, 1996). It is more than buying and selling. It involves finding a "niche" for unique and distinguished professional services where there is an unquestionable need or minimal competition, then setting out to see those services realized in an actual practice setting (Gallagher, 1996), or finding out what patients do not want and designing the practice accordingly (Baum & Henkel, 2000).

According to Baum and Henkel (2000), effective marketing is less about creating a flashy public relations campaign and more about "taking extraordinary care of the patients you already have." They state that marketing is simply making the community aware of the APNs' services and areas of expertise while remaining within the perimeters of ethical and professional behavior.

CRITICAL ISSUES: MARKETING THE ADVANCED PRACTICE NURSING ROLE

Experts in the world of business talk about the 4 *Ps* of marketing: product, price, place, and promotion. All are relevant to APNs and each is discussed here; *product* is placed first, because without the product, APNs and the other 3 *Ps* would be unnecessary.

Product

For the APN, human service is the product. When one hears the word *physician*, an immediate set of skills, abilities, and values comes to mind because the role is a familiar one. That does not yet happen for the title *advanced practice nurse*, so clearly articulating what the role entails is critical, whether one is addressing a prospective employer, a parent whose child is ill, a mentally ill adult, a laboring woman, or a family in a preoperative reception area. It is important that others understand that an APN is first a registered nurse (RN) who maintains all the knowledge, skills and benefits from clinical experience in the RN role. However, there has been additional education to enable an advanced level or practice in a specialty area; there has not been a divorce from nursing.

What makes the APN role unique is the overlap between the domains of medicine and nursing. One can appreciate the distinction by visualizing a Venn diagram (taken from mathematics), with medical practice as one full circle, nursing practice as another full circle, and the overlapping area as APN practice (Figure 21-1). Based on their basic nursing education, APNs can practice *all* of nursing, and based on advanced education, they can practice some aspects from the traditional domain of medicine. The scope of practice in both is legislated by their respective state's Nurse Practice Act. The Office of Technology Assessment (1986) determined that NPs can complete 80% of a physician's primary care measures without consultation, freeing the physician's time for more complex and remunerative tasks. How this translates to the roles of certified registered nurse anesthetist (CRNA) and certified nurse midwife (CNM) has not been determined. The clinical nurse specialist (CNS) role, by virtue of being more amorphous and generally outside the primary care arena, is not affected by this statistic in the same way. That is a huge 80%, however, because that 80% represents the source of much of the conflict between APNs and physicians.

It is critical that APNs retain their commitment to their nursing roots. The APN role is unique, and it is imperative that an APN retain an identity as a nurse rather than shifting to a disease-focused model. Sprague-McRae (1996) notes that the risk of shifting to the medical model is greater when an organization views the APN only as a "physician extender." This author also argues that appreciation of the differences between the APN role and the physician's role and recognition of the value of the APN are necessary for optimal role attainment.

The prospective APN needs to present convincing evidence of professional competence likely to make significant contributions to a particular practice site, either now or in the future. The resume or curriculum vitae (CV) is an important marketing tool because it provides a professional snapshot that can give one a competitive edge. This marketing tool helps one secure an interview and tests

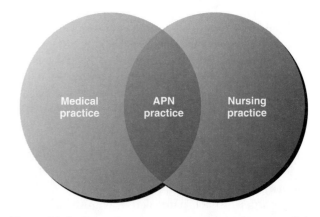

Figure 21-1 Advanced practice nursing is uniquely positioned between the overlapping domains of medical practice and nursing practice.

marketability as a provider. Although the terms *resume* and *curriculum vitae* are often used interchangeably, they refer to different types of documents. The CV is traditionally used for positions in academic or research settings. It tends to be longer because academic credentials, research, publications, professional presentations, and professional associations are included; these accomplishments are of importance in academic circles.

Resumes are used for positions outside academia; therefore, this choice is appropriate for a position in the clinical marketplace. Straka (1996) defines the resume as a "logical, straightforward process for the purpose of showing your knowledge, skills, accomplishments, and other pertinent qualifications." Hinck (1997) describes it as a "running list of professional accomplishments." The resume is important whether one is personally investigating a position or using the services of a professional recruiter as one's marketing agent. (Box 21-1 provides a list of what is typically included in a resume or CV.)

Box 21-1

What to Include in a Resume or Curriculum Vitae

Contact Data
Identify ways in which one can be contacted (e.g., address, telephone, e-mail, fax). Place this information in the center of the page.

Education
List educational experiences in reverse chronological order, with the most recent first. High school is not listed unless it represents the highest level of education. List the institutions attended, their locations, the dates they were attended, and the degrees conferred. A grade point average (GPA) from one's university education should be included only if it is greater than 3.75 on a 4.0 scale.

Clinical Experiences/Positions
List the dates, positions and titles, organizations, and locations, with the current one first. If the duties of a position are not immediately evident or are particularly relevant to the job sought, list them briefly. Jobs held before one's nursing career may be included if they are related to the job sought. If one has held multiple roles within an organization, list them in reverse chronological order with the position and chief responsibility given for each.

Honors/Awards
Describe each award if this is not immediately evident from its title (e.g., Mary Vinney Hickey Award for Outstanding Academic Performance).

Licenses/Certifications
Identify the issuing state, the date issued, and the expiration date (license number is not necessary).

Identify your APN certification number, the issuing agency, the date issued, and the expiration date.

List special short courses that ended with presentation of certificates (e.g., advanced or basic cardiac life support, pediatric advanced life support).

Publications
Underline or bold your name for multi-author papers to make it stand out. Place publications in American Psychological Association (APA) format. If you have more than one publication in a given year, place them alphabetically. Do not include those written for a job (e.g., newsletters, policies). Place service on editorial or review panels here.

Research/Grants
Identify the name of any study, and for ones with multiple researchers, bold or underline your name. Include your MSN thesis or research project here. If projects were funded, list the source and amount of funds.

Memberships in Professional Organizations
Identify full names of organizations and list any offices held. Organizations attended as a student-professional may be listed.

Presentations
List names of presentation, audiences, places, and dates. Do not include those presentations required to meet course or job requirements.

Community Service/Volunteer Efforts
List dates, agencies, and services provided. This includes only those service activities for which no pay was earned.

Military Service
List dates of service and branch of service.

Language Ability
Refers to any language other than English that you are able to speak or to write well enough for basic communication or a focused patient history. Levels usually include native, basic, intermediate, and fluent.

Continuing Education Offerings Attended
List the dates, names of conferences, and locations. Place here any other career-related study (e.g., computer courses, any non–degree-level university study done for enrichment). Do not include courses unrelated to your career.

Objectives
Include only if one is a specific match to the position offered or is requested in instructions for a particular position.

Unless the prospective employer has already met the APN, the resume is the only information available before the interview. Consequently, this document and the accompanying cover letter are critical. Every word of a CV or resume sends a message (Meador, 1999). It must be able to capture the attention of the prospective employer and be compelling enough in 20 to 30 seconds to justify an interview. It must clearly indicate a match between the particular job and the candidate's strengths, talents, interests, and potential. If an individual is responding to a written advertisement for a position, all instructions in the ad should be carefully followed to ensure that the resume is not discarded before being seen by the prospective employer.

A well-structured resume implies that the candidate can think logically and organize well (Meador, 1999). Particular attention should be given to grammar and spelling because errors in either can imply carelessness in practice. Sloppiness in preparing the document translates in the mind of the reader to sloppiness in clinical practice. In addition, one can not count entirely on a computer's spelling and grammar checks; items pertinent to a clinical setting may not be in the computer bank. The extra time of having the resume proofread by another person is well worth it (Box 21-2).

There are many opportunities for use of the resume or CV beyond job searches. For example, many universities require a file copy of the CV for each clinician precepting their students. Selection panels and conference planners often request a copy from each presenter on the program. A copy must often accompany any research abstract submitted, and some journals require them with submission of a manuscript; they are also required with submission of grants. A current resume may also be needed for moving up the job ladder; it often provides evidence to justify promotion or advancement.

In some job searches, the prospective employer receives 200 or more inquiries or resumes for each position advertised. To be compelling enough to open the door to future communications between employer and candidate, the cover letter should be short and dynamic, introducing the candidate and showing how the candidate's strengths and skills match the practice's needs (Harbert, 1994). The letter is the candidate's "voice," providing an invaluable opportunity to say why the particular job is of interest. Harbert (1994) suggests that a cover letter have four main, but concise, paragraphs: (1) an introduction of the applicant and how he or she learned of the position, (2) a few sentences about how the candidate's strengths match the position, (3) a summary of academic and experiential background pertinent to the position, and (4) a statement of the desire for an interview or meeting. According to Harbert (1994), it is helpful to include the date one is available to start work and information about how to access oneself by telephone, voice-mail, or e-mail, even though

---

Box 21-2

Guidelines for Preparing a Resume or Curriculum Vitae

- Locate the name of the individual who will make the ultimate decision. Direct the cover letter and resume or CV to that particular person.
- Limit the document to three pages or less. It needs to be readable in less than 2 minutes (Straka, 1996). If the document must be longer because of a lengthy or illustrious career, place the most important factors first.
- Use highlighting and spacing between sections and as margins to your advantage. This "white space" rests the eyes and makes reading easier. Highlight with different fonts or bold print, and always use 10-point font or larger and common fonts such as Times New Roman.
- Avoid gimmicks like bright colored paper, drawings, or artistic fonts. Do not aim for creativity in this document (Bensing, 2000).
- Be honest and avoid padding and redundancy.
- Write in an active voice. (e.g., "screened for STDs "instead of "was given the opportunity for STD screening").
- Do not say that references will be provided on request; this is assumed by the reader (Straka, 1996).
- Keep the document current by keeping it on disk. Update it every 6 months or so with major changes.
- Print on 8½ x 11 size, 20# bond quality paper in a white or ivory stock color.
- Use black or royal blue ink only.
- Do not Xerox the document; each copy should appear to be an original.
- Do not scrimp on the quality of the paper and printing for the final document.
- Mail the document in an 8½ x 11 inch envelope; this looks more professional and lessens the chance of it being misplaced (Bensing, 2000).
- When updating (as described previously), document the last update in the right lower corner (Hinck, 1997).

---

this information may duplicate portions of the resume. There should also be a sentence or notice that a resume is enclosed. The letter should always be customized; form letters are not acceptable for attracting attention or demonstrating creativity or initiative. (Figure 21-2 shows a sample cover letter.)

The APN may choose to rely on a professional recruiter or headhunter to assist in the job search. This option is especially valuable when one is relocating because the recruiter can "cast a nationwide net that includes as many potential employers as possible" (Feicher, 1997). Because recruiters who work with APNs are in the business of negotiating employment, they are familiar with market demographics, salary potential, and the level of support for nonphysician providers in a particular geographical setting.

March 25, 2000

Dr. Bruce Pennington
Middle Georgia Anesthesia Associates
590 First Street Extension Suite 245-D
Macon, Georgia 31218

Dear Dr. Pennington:
I am responding to your advertisement for a certified registered nurse anesthetist from The Atlanta Journal and Constitution (Sunday, March 20th edition). I am a CRNA with 3 years of clinical practice experience with an anesthesia group in Louisville, Kentucky. My wife has just completed her graduate degree in church music at the seminary here, and we hope to move back to Georgia, nearer to our respective extended families.

As you see from my resume, which is enclosed, I received a Master of Science in Nursing degree with specialization in nursing anesthesia from Frances Payne Bolton School of Nursing, Case Western Reserve University in Cleveland, Ohio. I continue to enjoy all aspects of the nurse anesthetist role. Because I had worked in a pain management setting before graduate school, however, I completed an additional rotation in pain management in graduate school in my final practicum experience. I understand that you and your colleagues are hoping to expand your pain management practice and believe that I have the academic preparation and clinical experience to be an asset in that kind of effort.

I can be reached at 502-555-1000 (home) or 502-555-8888 (pager), or by e-mail at emdcc@sbs.edu if you wish to discuss my qualifications or schedule an opportunity for us to meet in person.

Sincerely,

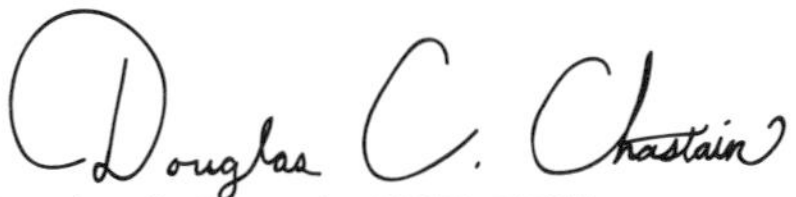

Douglas C. Chastain

Douglas C. Chastain, MSN, CRNA
2121 Landrum Avenue
Apt. 1307
Louisville, KY 40216

Figure 21-2 Sample cover letter.

Recruiters can screen job options for evidence of compatibility with the goals and job specifications of candidates, saving them significant time and energy. A recruiter also has the experience, contacts, and ability to "prep" the candidate for the interview and provide a negotiating edge. Recruiters are paid by the employer who hires the APN, never by the job candidate (Feicher, 1997).

Within practice sites and communities where physician assistants (PAs) are providers, one of the most frequent questions is "What is the difference between a PA and an APN?" This comparison is most likely between the PA and NP and the PA anesthetist and CRNA. Obviously, APNs need accurate information and a carefully worded answer to promote a positive image of APNs without seeming, in any way, disparaging of the other role. The same advice serves well in differentiating the practice of physicians and NPs. In primary care settings and anesthesia practices, the job descriptions of the two types of nonphysician providers are remarkably similar. Because of the similarities of roles and the problems inherent in being a nonphysician provider in times of conflict, many APN groups have joined with PAs for support and continuing education; having this additional alliance can be a great benefit politically as well. (Table 21-1 shows a comparison of the APN and PA roles.)

The talking points most compelling to prospective employers are those related to quality, service, cost, and patient satisfaction. There has been significant anecdotal and empirical support over many years that APNs are highly qualified, perform 80% of primary care at a level equal to physicians, provide care satisfying to patients, and save costs. These findings are sustained whether the researcher was a nurse or a physician. NPs have distinguished themselves with respect to: (1) less cost despite more time with patients (Brown & Grimes, 1993), (2) more thorough history-taking (Moody, Smith, & Glenn, 1999), (3) a more participatory and egalitarian approach (Grandinetti, 1999), and (4) more teaching and counseling (Hankins, Shaw, Cruess, Lawrence, & Harris (1996). Research points and citations on the ability of APNs to provide quality care for less cost, available from the professional organizations, can serve as convincing evidence of the worth of the APN role. APNs are wise to stay current with the literature and research related to their respective role, continually adding to the list of talking points helpful for marketing and image-making. Once in practice, APNs should tell everyone in the community about the role they fill in their practices. They should provide patients with clear and compelling evidence about what distinguishes the APN role and differentiates it from the physician provider in regard to scope, philosophy, and authority. For example, this type of comment would be of value for some APNs, "While the physician cares for those

Table **21-1**

Comparison of Physician Assistants and Advanced Practice Nurses

FACTOR FOR COMPARISON	PHYSICIAN ASSISTANT	ADVANCED PRACTICE NURSE
Licensure	Has no license for practice; practices under the license of a supervising or collaborating physician	Has a license to practice as a RN/APN issued by a board of nursing in the state of practice
Model for practice	Medical model	Holistic nursing model
Education	PA program for 108 weeks; may have a baccalaureate or Master's degree	Master of Science in Nursing (MSN) degree in nursing required*
Certification	Takes a national examination; recertifies through an examination every 6 years and 100 hours of continuing education units (CEUs) every 2 years	National certification examination required for practice in 29 states, with variable recertification intervals and CEU requirements
Supervisory status	Functions under the supervision of a physician	Can function independently or collaboratively with a physician (status determined by a state's Nurse Practice Act)

*The MSN requirement began in 1999. NPs educated in a certificate program will be "grandfathered in" to practice in accordance with state law.

in the practice who are extremely ill or does procedures for which I am not trained, I'll have time to sit down with you and listen to your concerns. I'll teach you how to stay well or manage your illness, and I'll answer all of your questions."

An APN can not be all things to all people and must determine through critical self-analysis what particular talents and interests can be marketed and who represents the target market for those abilities. Who is the competition? Where are the gaps in service? What can be done to fill these gaps? For example, a CNM or women's health NP might decide to market childbirth education classes in the community. An adult NP might become a certified diabetes educator. A CNS in mental health nursing may offer a group session for those concerned about retirement stress or be a part of a crisis service. These kinds of subspecializations can offer a competitive advantage in the clinical marketplace. An ability to be a futurist can also be important in determining a possible marketing niche. What will be the health care needs in the future? Where do potential markets lie? With growing numbers of elderly women, a market niche might be a menopausal support group or educational program in osteoporosis prevention. As male baby boomers age, male health, with a focus on lowering cancer risk, might be particularly compelling. Appreciating the trend toward a more culturally diverse clientele might encourage learning a second language. Some providers believe that writing personal mission statements can provide direction to understanding what their mission will be. These mission statements, borne out of introspection and candid self-review, have the capacity

to provide strategic direction for the distinctive practice one wishes to have. Furthermore, it can show how the provider's philosophy and practice values are comparable to the institutional goals of the practice. In some practices, the mission statement is printed on all written patient materials.

When an APN joins a practice, it is valuable to release information for press coverage introducing the newest "partner"; list the new provider's name on the office door, letterhead, and prescription pads (in states where APNs have prescriptive authority), as well as in the yellow pages; and display posters, flyers, or brochures about the APN. The APN can capitalize on event marketing too. *Event marketing* refers to using a major event or occasion as a publicity tool (Gallagher, 1996). For example, an APN could write articles or public service announcements on the following topics: during February, heart disease; for Memorial Day, sun safety and skin cancer prevention; in July, heat stroke; and at Halloween, safe trick or treating.

Volunteering in the community can also be a means for introducing oneself and one's role. For example, a volunteer shift in a homeless shelter or school not only exposes an APN to a patient population in need but also to professionals with whom interdisciplinary collaboration is possible.

Written materials, including some colorful glossy brochures, can be obtained from professional organizations serving APNs and some state boards of nursing; these can be used outright or modified and personalized for a particular practice setting. These can be of value in promoting the role; many new APNs place brochures in clinic reception areas for that purpose and display them at health fairs and other events.

Price

Like never before in health care, cost sensitivity is a realistic demand in the marketplace. APNs promoting the benefits of their services are well advised to meet patient needs while being cost efficient and to promote patient awareness of this cost advantage. The APN is well served by having a system for tracking numbers of patients seen; numbers added to the practice; and revenues generated for the practice as a means of demonstrating cost savings. Physicians also need to be educated about costs pertinent to hiring APNs. According to McGrath (1990), the overall financial savings resulting from employing a NP instead of a physician were 24%. According to Fitzgerald, Jones, Lazar, McHugh, and Wang (1995), in a capitated environment, an employer hiring a NP can increase the numbers of patients in a cost-effective, care-effective range for approximately half the cost of a physician partner; some NPs can earn five times their cost. Similar findings are a likely expectation for other types of APNs as well. It should be noted that cost savings are often less tangible, involving such things as more leisure time for the partners and more time for their professional development.

Place

APNs may have little choice about where their services will be provided. A hiring office or clinic is already in existence and the APN assumes a space in that site, or a practice is affiliated with a particular hospital or birthing center and the CNM or CRNA simply gains privileges there. Knowing that a competitive edge in practice goes to those sites that are convenient may encourage APNs to explore options that focus on convenience. For example, would an afternoon clinic or occasional Saturday meet the needs of working patients? Is access through the office quick and easy? What is the waiting time to see the provider? If delays are inevitable, does someone advise those waiting? Are there materials or programs that can provide health education during the wait? APNs should look at the practice setting from the door inward and determine what messages patients are receiving from the environment and the systems in place. Tracking a typical patient from his or her scheduling of an appointment through final billing can be particularly valuable (Baum & Henkel, 2000). Are directions easy to follow? Is the office or clinic clearly marked? Is the process for signing in clear? Is the reception area comfortable or cluttered? Are the reading materials varied and current? Is the temperature and noise level comfortable? Is it called a *waiting room* (which has a negative connotation [Baum & Henkel, 2000]), and if so,

can that be changed? Is the patient's privacy compromised by questions by the receptionist or the requirements of placing personal information, including a chief complaint, on the sign-in sheet? Can those in the reception area overhear confidential information during staff exchanges or telephone calls? Is the reception area child friendly? Teen friendly? Gender friendly? Are examination rooms warm enough for undressing? Are stirrups padded? Is there reading material in examination rooms in case of provider delay? Are billing questions handled sensitively?

If or when services or special programs are extended outside the office or clinic, an APN may be able to capitalize on the niche or place. For example, can a health fair be located in an area with ample parking and access for patients who have physical challenges? Can a support group for grieving parents meet at times when both mothers and fathers can attend, and can it be located away from the maternity or childbirth education class entrances?

Promotion

Promoting the advanced practice role has been discussed throughout this chapter as it relates to initiating a practice; however, promoting one's advanced practice is an ongoing enterprise (Box 21-3). APNs promote their practice and a positive image of their role by providing exemplary care. The best advertisement of such excellence in practice is word-of-mouth endorsement from satisfied patients. One may wish to seek permission from patients to have their positive testimonials used on brochures or websites.

Gallagher (1996) refers to any efforts made after a patient's visit to increase the probability of "repeat business" as *aftermarketing*. Examples of aftermarketing include follow-up telephone calls or cards to patients and thank-you notes for referrals.

Baum and Henkel (2000) advise, "Remember, when a person or practice fails, some people call it fate. More often it is bad marketing discovered far too late." Evaluating patient satisfaction is worth the effort in determining how improvements can be made. The American Medical Association (AMA) suggests surveying 20% of patients annually (to a maximum of 200 patients) (Baum & Henkel, 2000). Sellers (1989) further suggests that keeping a customer one already has costs about one fifth of what it costs to acquire a new one. The practice of an APN is likely no different. Surveying can occur one patient at a time or with onsite or virtual focus groups. Written surveys that take no more than 3 to 5 minutes can be sent with a self-addressed stamped envelope to facilitate return, and a suggestion box with cards that say "What can I do to make your visits with me more pleasant or comfortable?" can work effectively and is inexpensive. Baum and Henkel (2000) advise providers that "not only do your patients need an annual check-up, so does your practice," no matter how the evaluation is done.

Box **21-3**

Measures for Marketing Useful to Advanced Practice Nurses

- Negotiate your own panel of patients, gaining a quick reputation for consulting when problems occur that need a different level of provider.
- Display diplomas, certifications, honors, and awards in your office.
- Become listed as an expert source on the speaker's bureau and prepare several health-related topics for use with quick notice.
- Write a health-related column or article for the local newspaper.
- Develop a practice newsletter that includes both information and consumer tips.
- Develop a website and put consumer tips on the site.
- Offer to serve on advisory boards or panels.
- Volunteer for health fairs or other health-related events.
- Send a note to all first-time patients thanking them for choosing you as a provider and welcoming them to your practice. Do not include anything about money in this mailing (Baum & Henkel, 2000).
- Communicate with nursing programs in the area. Send a CV and ask to be placed on the mailing list for events and as a prospective preceptor.
- Use business cards to enhance professional image.
- Sponsor an open house in your early days with a new practice.
- Cultivate media support in the area. If acceptable to your patients and employer, invite the media to photograph you in action.
- If possible, have your name mentioned by the receptionist who handles phone calls.
- Consult the business and management sections of local bookstores for resources on service and client satisfaction, then integrate these ideas into practice.
- Send a thank-you note to all providers who refer patients to you.

- Join a professional organization to gain a voice in policy development that ensures that the APN role is not compromised by other groups.
- Consider sending health-related "stuffers" with bills from the practice (Baum & Henkel, 2000).
- Jot selected personal information about clients inside the chart to facilitate a brief chat when entering the examination room. When cards have been received for special occasions or as a thank you, place them in the chart as a reminder to comment on them at the patient's next visit. To hurry into the chief complaint without a few minutes of chatting to show a personal interest in a patient as a "complete person" fails to lessen his or her anxiety and misses a "precious moment" for the provider (Baum & Henkel, 2000).
- Appreciate that sound time management contributes to promotion of a positive image:
  - Keep interruptions of patient encounters to a minimum or eliminate them entirely.
  - Dictate in real time.
  - Build an extra 15 to 30 minutes into your day for "catching up."
  - Have a designated callback time to prevent patients from waiting long times by the phone for your call.
  - Place the pharmacy telephone number on the chart rather than having to look it up at each visit (Baum & Henkel, 2000).
- Design information sheets with cost comparisons for frequently prescribed medications that show popular pharmacy prices in the community.
- Use follow-up telephone calls when possible.
- Connect with other APNs in the community for external alliances, professional development, collaboration on projects, and a singleness of promoting a collective positive image.

Nurses have long appreciated that it is the little things one does for patients that make the biggest difference. APNs, then, are in a unique position to put this into daily practice. This is an example of marketing and role promotion at its best. As Finnigan (1996) says, "Image is not generated by the person's latest monumental act, but rather by the accumulation of all the little things said and done over time. Focus on results, but remember the little things." APN practice today can rarely compete on price alone. The wise, caring APN can learn a lot from the business world, from companies like Nordstrom and Federal Express who have a reputation for attention to detail that distinguishes them from their competitors. Little things pay off in big ways.

IMPLICATIONS FOR MSN EDUCATION AND ADVANCED PRACTICE

APN and entrepreneur Mimi Secor suggests that individuals can succeed as APNs because they "do the usual unusually well or do the unusual" (Bramble, 1991). Promotion of either or both would require consideration of product, price, place, and promotion and an unwavering commitment not to lose the nursing part of the process of advanced practice. A positive image borne of a strategic promotion plan would serve both individual APNs and the profession well. Educators of APNs must make concerted efforts to see that the nursing domain continues to get a proper focus, even as students take selected tasks from the medical domain. Basing practice on nursing theory, using nursing diagnoses as well as medical diagnoses, and identifying what is medical management versus what is nursing management can all be helpful to that end.

APN education should include information about successful marketing of the role. Students need to know how their respective role evolved, how it is enacted in the existing health care arena, and what the preferred future of the role is likely to entail. Familiarity with research that indicates the effectiveness of APNs in promoting quality care and containing health care costs is important; it will be the results of such research (in part) that can be used to promote the advanced practice role. Students need to be given opportunities in roleplaying experiences and clinical settings to interpret their respective advanced practice roles to many audiences, including patients and prospective employers. Roleplaying scenarios can be developed to allow students to practice articulating their position not only to those prospective employers favorable to the APN role during a job interview but also to those who need convincing.

APNs promote their practice by the professional manner of their speech, behavior, and dress and by maintaining passion and enthusiasm for their work. These aspects of clinical practice need to be part of the education and evaluation of student APNs. Some programs invite recent graduates to return and discuss their experiences in various aspects of marketing. Others ask marketing experts to offer tips about clothing and makeup suitable for interviews or invite headhunters to prepare students for the kinds of questions they are likely to be asked by interviewers.

Ensuring a preferred future for APNs demands practitioners who are actively involved in their respective professional organizations and remain politically active. APNs must stay informed about local, regional, and national legislation and join forces to see that role-supportive legislation is enacted. A professional network that includes the collective efforts of all types of APNs can be a powerful force.

PRIORITIES FOR RESEARCH

APNs would be well served by research devoted to answering questions about what professional behaviors are correlated with successful recruitment and retention of patients and what marketing strategies are most efficient and effective for gaining and maintaining a practice.

An APN may wish to engage in an evaluation study based on patient survey data. What kinds of factors do patients prefer? Are these cost efficient? What kind of reception area is most comfortable and capable of reducing

anxiety? Does it help (as Baum and Henkel [2000] suggest) to provide healthy drinks or coupons for designer coffee if the provider is very late, or to provide puzzles and unusual reading materials, bulletin boards, collections, aquariums, or portable CD or tape players with headphones in the reception area? In fact, is there a relationship between renaming the room *reception area* as opposed to *waiting room*?

A study might be designed to determine the relationship of health knowledge and compliance with treatment and the provision of health-related materials in the reception area or special patient education room. Study comparing different methods for patient teaching and matching specific teaching styles with learning styles might also be of value.

It would be interesting to determine if follow-up telephone calls in certain situations are associated with more positive patient outcomes or fewer calls from the patients themselves. Baum and Henkel (2000) recommend telephone follow-up in these situations: (1) when one has prescribed a difficult procedure, (2) after an outpatient procedure, (3) after hospital discharge, (4) when a patient seemed concerned about difficult diagnostic studies ahead, (5) when new medications have been ordered for a chronic problem, and (6) with a new diagnosis. Does using telephone calls as an anticipatory or primary prevention measure for anticipated problems actually prevent complications? Lessen patient anxiety? Affect patient retention in a practice?

Another study might address the question, "Is there less stated anxiety in patients whose APNs spend a few minutes in casual conversation when compared with those who go directly to a discussion of the chief complaint?"

Novice APNs, especially those in the final part of graduate education, would profit from a study addressing the most impressive components of a resume or cover letter for prospective employers.

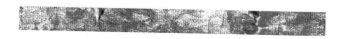

DISCUSSION QUESTIONS

These questions can be used to promote critical thinking and encourage discussion.

1. Draft a brochure or press release to introduce the public to a CRNA, CNM, CNS, and/or NP.
2. Prepare a resume or CV and cover letter for a job search.
3. Write a mission statement or personal philosophy for your particular APN specialty.

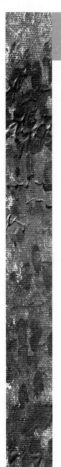

Suggestions for Further Learning

- Read Baum, N., & Henkel, G. (2000). *Marketing your clinical practice ethically, effectively, and enthusiastically.* Gaithersburg, MD: Aspen Publishers. This source provides additional examples of strategies that can be integrated into your practice as an APN.
- Refer to Goitein, M. (1990). Waiting patiently. *New England Journal of Medicine, 323*(9), 604-608. This provides information useful to APNs planning a practice.
- Check out the business section of local bookstores for resources related to customer satisfaction and service that can be employed by APNs. Start with these selections: Berry, L.L. (1998). *Discovering the soul of service.* New York: Free Press; Frieberg, K., & Frieberg, J. (1996). *NUTS! Southwest airlines' crazy recipe for personal success.* Austin, TX: Bard Press; and Spector, R., & McCarthy, P.D. (1995). *The Nordstrom way.* New York: Wiley.
- Consult the appropriate professional organization for your APN specialty for additional information useful in promoting your role.
- Consult the current update of legislation and how it affects APNs, published annually by *The Nurse Practitioner* journal, for more information about APN practice in your state.

4. Draft answers or structure a roleplaying scenario related to the following questions:
   - You have been asked by a faculty member of an associate degree or baccalaureate nursing program to visit his professional issues class to present a 20 to 30 minute presentation on your type of advanced practice. The goal of the session is to introduce students to the APN role. What would you include in this presentation?
   - You realize that your office's receptionist will decide, in part, what patients you are assigned. How will you prepare him or her to select those within your scope of practice?
   - You are in a very busy practice where you have about 15 minutes per patient encounter. Few of the patients have experience with an APN, and questions abound. How do you handle this?

REFERENCES/BIBLIOGRAPHY

Aquilino, M.L., Damiano, P.C., Willard, J.C., Momary, E.T., & Levy, B.T. (1999). Primary care physician perceptions of the nurse practitioner in the 1990s. *Archives of Family Medicine, 8,* 224-227.

Bates, B. (1990). Twelve paradoxes: a message for nurse practitioners. *Journal of the American Academy of Nurse Practitioners, 2*(4), 136-139.

Baum, N., & Henkel, G. (2000). *Marketing your clinical practice ethically, effectively, and economically.* Gaithersburg, MD: Aspen Publishers.

Bensing, K. (2000, September 20). Resume writing for new graduates: your ticket to a successful career. *ADVANCE for Nurses,* 31.

Bramble, K. (1991). Spotlight on nurse practitioner practice—Mimi Secor: nurse practitioner entrepreneur. *Nurse Practitioner Forum, 2*(3), 142-143.

Brown, M.A., & Olshansky, E. (1998). Becoming a primary care nurse practitioner: challenges of the initial year of practice. *The Nurse Practitioner, 23*(7), 46-66.

Brown, S.A., & Grimes, M.E. (1993). *Nurse practitioners and certified nurse midwives: a meta-analysis of studies of the nurse in primary care roles.* Washington, DC: American Nurses Publishing.

Buppert, C. (1999). *Nurse practitioner's business practice and legal guide.* Gaithersburg, MD: Aspen Publishers.

Burgess, S.E., & Misener, T.R. (1997). The professional portfolio: an advanced practice nurse job search marketing tool. *Clinical Excellence for Nurse Practitioners, 1*(7), 468-471.

Burke, C.E., & Bair, J.P. (1996). Marketing the role: formulating, articulating, and negotiating advanced practice nursing positions. In Sheehy & McCarthy (Eds.), *Advanced practice nursing: emphasizing common roles* (pp. 192-216). New York: FA Davis.

Dill, P.Z. (1991). Marketing the nursing practice of obstetrics. *Journal of Obstetric, Gynecologic, and Neonatal Nursing, 20*(4), 328-332.

Edmunds, M.W. (1999). NP News—increasing professional tension limits NP opportunities. *The Nurse Practitioner, 24*(5), 101-104.

Feicher, J.D. (1997). Professional recruiters—simplifying your job search. *Clinical Reviews, 7*(5), 194-200.

Finnigan, S. (1996). Getting started in business: from fantasy to reality. *Advanced Practice Nursing Quarterly, 2*(1), 1-8.

Fitzgerald, M.A., Jones, E., Lazar, B., McHugh, M., & Wang, C. (1995, January 15). The midlevel provider: colleague or competitor? *Patient Care,* 20-37.

Flanagan, L. (1998, June). Family physicians and nurse practitioners: a perfect team. *American Family Physician.* Available online at www.aafp.org.

Ford, V., & Kish, C.P. (1998). Family physicians perceptions of nurse practitioners and physician assistants in a family practice setting. *Journal of the American Academy of Nurse Practitioners, 10*(4), 167-171.

Gallagher, S.M. (1996). Promoting the nurse practitioner by using a marketing approach. *The Nurse Practitioner, 21*(3), 30-40.

Gardner, K.L., & Weinrauch, D. (1988). Marketing strategies for nurse entrepreneurs. *The Nurse Practitioner, 13*(5), 46-49.

Giordano, B.P. (1994). Watch out for "friendly fire" from our medical allies. *AORN Journal, 50*(2), 360-366.

Goitein, M. (1990). Waiting patiently. *New England Journal of Medicine, 323*(9), 604-608.

Grandinetti, D. (1999, February 8). Midlevel providers: making their mark in doctor's offices. *Medical Economics,* 141-156.

Grandinetti, D. (1999, February 8). What kind of patient would rather see a nurse practitioner? *Medical Economics,* 156-158.

Hankins, G.D.V., Shaw, S.B., Cruess, D.F., Lawrence, H.C., & Harris, C.D. (1996). Patient satisfaction with collaborative practice. *Obstetrics and Gynecology, 88*(6), 1011-1015.

Harbert, K.R. (1994). Developing the curriculum vitae/resume. *The Clinician's Reference Guide,* 10-14.

Herrick, T. (1998, November-December). MDs put Pas/NPs under microscope: docs scrutinize how NPCs influence supply and demand. *Clinical News,* 1-9.

Hinck. S.M. (1997). A curriculum vitae that gives you a competitive edge. *Clinical Nurse Specialist, 11*(4), 174-177.

Huch, M.H. (1992). Nurse practitioners and physician assistants: are they the same? *Nursing Scientific Quarterly, 5*(2), 52-53.

Lachman, V.D. (1996). Positioning your business in the marketplace. *Advanced Practice Nursing Quarterly, 2*(1), 27-32.

Longworth, J.C.D., & Di Nardo, E.D. (1995). Marketing your services. In M. Snyder & M.P. Mirr (Eds.), *Advanced nursing: a guide to professional development* (pp. 241-252). New York: Springer.

Maragopoulos, D. (1998). Synchronized rowing. *Clinician Reviews, 8*(3), 33-39.

McGrath, S. (1990). The cost effectiveness of nurse practitioners. The Nurse Practitioner, 15(7), 40-42.

Meador, J.A. (1999). Writing an effective curriculum vita or resume. Available online at www.pracnurse.com/article/feature/f105.htm.

Miller, S.K. (2000, March). Get ready for the next round of opposition. *Patient Care for the Nurse Practitioner,* 94.

Moody, N.B., Smith, P.L., & Glenn, L.L. (1999). Client characteristics and practice patterns of nurse practitioners and physicians. *The Nurse Practitioner, 24*(3), 94-103.

Office of Technology Assessment (1986). *Nurse practitioners, physician's assistants, and certified nurse midwives: a policy analysis* (Health technology case study no. 37). Washington, DC: U.S. Government Printing Office.

Pearson, L.J. (2000). Annual legislative update—how each state stands on legislative issues affecting advanced nursing practice. *The Nurse Practitioner, 25*(1), 16-68.

Peters, S. (1999, March). Making an impression. *ADVANCE for Nurse Practitioners,* 75-76.

Sellers, P. (1989, March 3). Getting customers to love you. *Fortune,* 38-39.

Smithing, R.T., & Wiley, M.D. (1990). Marketing and management—marketing techniques in person. *Journal of the American Academy of Nurse Practitioners, 2*(2), 88-89.

Sprague-McRae, J.M. (1996). The advanced practice nurse and physician relationship: considerations for practice. *Advanced Practice Nursing Quarterly, 2*(1), 33-40.

Straka, D.A. (1996). Are you your resume? *Advanced Practice Nursing Quarterly, 2*(1), 75-77.

Ward, R. (1998, October). Public relations for advanced practice nurses. *AWHONN Lifelines,* 48.

Zwelling, E. (1993, Spring). Marketing your childbirth education practice. *Childbirth Instruction,* 20-23, 37.

Chapter 22

Contract Negotiation

Alice B. Loper

As clinicians, nurses are rarely expected to have business savvy. Historically, there has been little opportunity for them to negotiate employment contracts. Rather, it was enough to know what to expect and how to handle oneself during an interview with either the director of nursing or the human resources department. Salary scales and benefit packages were generally preset, and registered nurses (RNs) tended to earn the same compensation and agree to the same basic job description upon employment. Any differential salary rates were not so much negotiated as assigned—a few dollars more for a baccalaureate degree, a night shift, a highly technical assignment, or specialty certification. An offer was made and either accepted or declined on its merit; negotiation was not an option. For some advanced practice nurses (APNs) today, parts of the contractual process remain essentially the same, with the exception that more opportunity may exist for verbalizing what value one expects to add to an agency by practicing there. However, for other APNs, the capacity to negotiate an employment contract or a collaborative practice agreement is now required.

DEFINITIONS

As APNs gain more opportunities for negotiation in the contract process, it is imperative that a few key concepts are defined. An *employment contract* is a legally binding written agreement between an employer and a prospective employee that delineates the terms and conditions of the working relationship and serves to protect the interests of both (Buppert, 1999).

A *collaborative practice agreement* is a written document that specifies the way in which an APN and physician agree to work together for the good of their mutual patients, taking into account their respective scopes of professional practice (Sebas, 1994). According to Pearson (2000), collaborative practice agreements are required in nearly half of all states. They may be part of the employment contract or a separate legal entity. In some cases, the collaborative practice statement must be approved by the state's board of nursing in advance of employment.

CRITICAL ISSUES: NEGOTIATING A CONTRACT

To some APNs, negotiating for salary and fringe benefits seems contradictory to the legacy of service long associated with professional nursing practice. This mind set must change as APNs come to clearly appreciate that health care is now an art, a science, and a business. In a competitive market, without the capacity to negotiate, one is at a distinct disadvantage.

Even in states where written employment agreements are not legislated, prudence dictates that the contract or collaborative practice agreement be written. Bourne (1996) suggests that if the employer does not take the initiative to get the agreement written, the APN should volunteer to draft a document that represents their mutual decisions about the terms of the practice. The employment contract may contain any item mutually acceptable to both prospective employer and employee; a typical contract specifies the scope of services expected, the compensation and fringe benefits to be paid for those services, the nature of the relationship between the parties, the rights and responsibilities of each, and the way in which the conditions of the agreement can be modified or dissolved.

Many contracts between physicians and APNs also contain a clause that relates to competition in the event the agreement is terminated. The non-compete clause is referred to as a *restrictive covenant*. Employers wish to avoid a situation where a popular APN who has built a large patient following leaves a practice and has that patient group follow him or her to the new practice. A restrictive covenant—"a promise not to compete"—is a way to avoid this (Buppert, 1999). In general, the restrictive clause specifies not practicing within a prescribed geographical region for a particular period. For example, the contract may specify that the individual not practice within a 30-mile radius of practice "X" for a period of 5 years. To be upheld legally, this agreement must be reasonable in balancing the business interests of the employer with the needs of the employee, and the restriction can not compromise the ultimate health care of the public by limiting access to providers unnecessarily. Buppert (1999) advises APNs to seriously consider "the circumstances of the job offer, the severity of the restriction, the potential hardship imposed by the covenant, the availability of health care providers in the area, and the availability of other practice opportunities."

Looking at Potential Contracts: Points of Consideration

Contracts typically describe the scope of services to be provided by an APN. Obviously, there should be a clear match between this job description and the APN's legal scope of practice as outlined in the respective state's Nurse Practice Act. Under no circumstances should one sign a contract where any concern exists about incongruency between job expectations and the law; it is the APN's responsibility to seek clarification, if needed, from the state board of nursing. Both clinical and nonclinical expectations in the job should be identified. For example, will the employee be expected to make rounds in hospitals, nursing homes, or prisons? Is there an expectation that the APN will train staff, maintain a website, lead a support group, or maintain Occupational Safety and Health Administration (OSHA) documents? If so, this should be clearly delineated.

The contract provides details about the exact time commitments of the prospective position so that there are no surprises after employment. For example, is the APN agreeing to a 40-hour per week job with overtime paid separately? Will there be 8-hour days, or will the APN continue to see patients until the reception room is empty? Is "call" an expectation? Is coverage of evening or weekend clinics expected? Are clinical rounds part of the regular workday, or are they expected to commence before or after hours in a clinic? Will there be required meetings in the evenings?

The typical contract is in effect for 1 year and renegotiable. This is an advantageous arrangement because it allows APNs to use data from the first year of practice to demonstrate the way in which the practice has been positively affected by their work. Moreover, data showing the exact numbers of patients seen, the revenue generated and costs saved, the need for less physician consultation than in the novice year, the increased public visibility of the practice, and the patients' satisfaction can all be used to justify requests for additional compensation and other benefits for a second year. Annual renewal of contracts continues to be an advantage throughout an APN's years of practice.

There should be some discussion of how the contract can be altered or terminated by either party. Buppert (1999) suggests that a contract that can be terminated without cause, even with adequate notice, fails to lend job security. This arrangement, however, may be necessary when an APN cannot commit to a full year of employment. In such cases, the contract will specify that a 30-day notice of termination is required or, in lieu of notice, that the APN be given 30 days' pay. Many contracts have a termination "with cause" statement. Events that are considered legitimate justification or "causes" for termination typically include conviction for a felony, loss of one's license to practice, and gross negligence that compromises the safety of patients or staff (Buppert, 1999).

Types of Compensation

What compensation one is to receive for services rendered should be clearly identified in the employment agreement. APNs are well served to know the salary range for similar positions (locally, regionally, and nationally) to enable wise negotiation of salary and fringe benefits. Compensation for an APN is generally believed to be approximately half what a physician partner would cost a practice. Burnett and Martin (1999) report that it takes a minimum of generated revenue of two to three times a nurse practitioner's (NP's) salary to support employment. Similar numbers have not been cited for other advanced practice roles but may be similar. Salaries tend to be variable by specialization, higher for those with more experience, and determined by supply and demand.

The most common method for compensating an APN is a straight salary or a percentage of the revenue generated by the APN. APNs in primary care are often paid on the basis of fee-for-service, on the basis of the agency's fee schedule, or (in the case of managed care) at a designated amount per member per month. The collection rate must be calculated and deducted from that amount. Buppert (1999) suggests that a collection rate of 90% is good; however, in many practices, the rate is less. Overhead costs must also be deducted. A practice's overhead costs are highly variable, depending on whether it is a solo or multiple-partner practice; whether the furnishings are fancy or functional; and the number and credentials of the support staff. Overhead costs include everything needed to keep the doors open, from staff salaries and expendable supplies to window washing, microscope maintenance, and snow removal. Burnett and Martin (1999) propose $111,000 per year as a minimum amount and cite a mean of 3.2 support staff for every provider. The APN may be expected to deduct 20% to 40% for a share of overhead costs. In some practices, a consultation fee is charged against the compensation of the APN; this fee generally declines year by year as the APN gains autonomy and needs to consult with the physicians less for help with clinical decisions. It is not uncommon for the consultation fee to be 10% to 15% of the net income the APN brings to the practice (Buppert, 1999).

How does all this translate to determining compensation? Suppose a salary is being based on fee-for-service. If the APN provider sees 18 patients per day, 5.5 days per week, for 48 weeks (deducting 4 weeks for vacation, continuing education, and illness), that would be 99 patients per week or 4752 patients per year. With an average fee of $35 per patient, this accounts for $166,320. In a practice with a 90% collection rate, this means $149,688. Deducting 15% for consultation and 40% for overhead, the amount becomes $82,328.40.

In a capitated practice, there is a 100% collection fee for the enrolled patients at a predetermined amount per month. If the APN has 1000 patients, at $10 each per month, this accounts for $120,000 per year from which overhead and a consultation fee are deducted.

Contrary to popular opinion, the compensation package is not generally predetermined; rather it is determined by an informed negotiation process. It is easy to see, in the presence of such numbers, why APNs are often pushed to increase their patient volume. It is not uncommon for the novice to negotiate for a lighter patient load initially, even if that translates to a lower salary. Given these numbers, it is also obvious how helpful conscientious records can be to support a clinician's request for a salary adjustment, bonus, or other incentive.

Bonuses and incentives are generally calculated on the basis of the numbers of patients seen in the allotted time or the numbers of patients who schedule appointments repeatedly with the APN. They may also be contingent on new skills acquired, excellent performance, or some other added value provided to the practice. Bourne (1996) mentions 3% to 10% of the gross collections on patients examined as a possible incentive. Bonuses or incentives are generally mentioned last during salary negotiation and, according to Bourne (1996), are usually a compromise to attempt to equalize what is perceived by the prospective employee as an otherwise imbalanced compensation package.

Fringe benefits

Fringe benefits, also explicitly detailed in an employment agreement, can add a minimum of 25% to 30% in worth to one's salary (Mackey, 1996). The benefits one prefers may vary significantly over the course of a career. For example, an APN may be willing to receive fewer benefits in exchange for working closer to home but expect more to compensate for a grueling commute. Flexible hours might be more important to a clinician with young children, whereas additional dollars might be preferred by another to enable purchase of a new home or to offset the costs of daycare. Someone with health insurance coverage through a spouse's job might negotiate for additional financial support of continuing education because the practice is saving money by not having to match monthly insurance dollars. Although vacation, holidays, retirement, and insurance coverage are relatively standard employment benefits, what can be considered a fringe benefit is highly variable depending on the nature of the job. Box 22-1 reveals some fringe benefits successfully negotiated by APNs. A prudent APN is reasonable in negotiating a benefit package and willing to work toward a win-win compromise for both parties.

APNs often feel more secure if their employment agreement includes explicit statements about the status of their liability coverage in the position. Some APNs have been advised by prospective employers that the general malpractice policy for the practice covered all providers, only to discover later that the language of the policy was not as

---

Box 22-1

Examples of Fringe Benefits in Advanced Practice Nursing Employment Contracts

Health insurance (e.g., medical, dental, optical, maternity)	Repayment of college loans
Life insurance	Dues for membership in professional organizations
Disability insurance	Fees for license renewal
Retirement	Fees for recertification
Malpractice insurance	Incentives and bonuses
Continuing education (including paid time off and tuition)	Profit sharing
Sick leave	Marketing/advertising
Vacation	Fees related to clinical privileging, certification, and license renewal
Paid holidays	Free or discounted health care (for self and dependents)
Overtime pay	Family/maternity leave
Uniforms and scrubs (including the costs of purchase and maintenance)	Partnership
Car telephone (when considerable travel is required to cover practice obligations)	Journal subscriptions and books for in-office reference
Pager	Prescription drug card
Cafeteria meals in the hospital	Paid relocation for accepting position

clear on coverage as they had hoped. A careful review of a practice's policy is worth the effort. To be certain of coverage in an APN role, one might request to select the insurance carrier and have premiums paid as part of the contract. APNs are often eligible for lower premiums as a benefit of membership in a professional organization. Occurrence-based insurance is generally considered the best for APNs because it provides tail coverage, meaning that all claims made against the individual provider are covered, regardless of when they occurred. Claims-made policies, because they do not provide tail coverage, cease to be effective for an individual who leaves a practice or changes insurance carriers. An APN should seek at least a $1 million per incident/$3 million per year amount of coverage; in specialty areas that are highly litigious, he or she may wish for a $3 million per incident/$5 million per year coverage option. Since malpractice is a business expense, many prospective employers are willing to offer it as a fringe benefit. This may also be the case for costs associated with renewal of licensure to practice and renewal of certification.

APNs may wish to have a statement in the agreement about performance evaluation—specifically when it will be done and by whom. It is critical that performance be evaluated by someone, such as another APN or physician, who can judge the clinical performance of the provider, rather than an office manager who evaluates nonclinical staff as a part of a job requirement. Ideally, the clause related to performance evaluation will specify that an APN be given a copy of the performance evaluation instrument in advance of the evaluation.

Additional Items in the Employment Agreement

The APN may seek to have other items inserted into the employment agreement. Virtually anything that is fair and reasonable and would increase the sense of job security can be added so long as the addition is mutually agreeable with the employer. For example, if APNs want legal assurance concerning expectations of patient volume or whether they will have their own nurse or other support personnel assigned to them, this would be an appropriate detail for the written contract. Then, if the obligation is not honored by the employer and problems arise as a result, there is some legal recourse. (The sample contract in Figure 22-1 provides additional ideas about legitimate additions to an employment agreement.) Bourne (1996) has this caveat for APNs pursuing contract agreements: employers generally want to treat them fairly; however, there are usually clauses that are surprises to both parties at the end of negotiations.

In states where collaborative practice agreements are required, additional attention is given in the written agreement to defining the roles of the APN and collaborating physician clearly and explaining the nature of the relationship within an organizational structure. Additional details of the role boundaries of each would be an

expectation of this document, as would how certain clinical issues should be handled when the collaborating physician is onsite versus not onsite. Sebas (1994) suggests clarifying such clinical issues as triaging patient assignments, charting procedures, working from protocols, requesting diagnostic tests or consultations, prescribing medicines, admitting patients to hospitals, requesting referrals, and handling emergencies. APNs in those states with a legal requirement for collaborative practice agreements may wish to seek guidance from the state's board of nursing for preparation of a suitable document. Developing such a detailed agreement forces careful negotiation of the prospective duties of the providers involved and serves as an excellent opportunity for each to appreciate the synergism inherent in a collaborative practice—that what each provider brings to the table makes practice outcomes different and better than any one provider could accomplish alone. "Collaboration assumes that interfacing partners are strong enough and secure enough to hear the other's feelings or opinions without being shaken within themselves" (Kyle, 1995). Negotiating to work within this kind of practice requires professional maturity and a keen sense of trust.

Preparing for Successful Negotiation

Whether one is considering an employment contract or collaborative practice agreement, the key to successful negotiation is conscientious preparation. When an APN is preparing to enter the job market, one of the first things to do is to create a professional portfolio (Hawkins & Thibodeu, 1996). The portfolio is a collection of documents relevant to professional development: a resume or curriculum vitae (CV), a copy of one's license(s) to practice within the APN role, a copy of one's certification notice, and documentation of malpractice coverage. Some employers also request documentation of immunization status and certification for performing either basic or advanced cardiac life support, depending on the position sought. An APN may wish to include documentation of special awards, honors, or accomplishments; previous clinical evaluations; a written personal philosophy or mission statement about the APN role; an overview of the theoretical basis for advanced practice; and any other documents believed to showcase ability or give a competitive edge toward employment. Sending the portfolio in advance serves to provide more time for the prospective employer to peruse the contents. Having this kind of information in advance of a formal meeting between the two parties has the potential to enhance the interview process.

It is also helpful for APNs to learn as much as possible about potential practice sites before the formal meeting. What is the general reputation of the practice in the community? Are the providers known for ethical behaviors? Do they have a reputation for supporting APNs? Have they employed APNs? If so, how has that worked

Employment Agreement between
Central City Health Systems
and
Carol Jean Cusack
Pediatric Nurse Practitioner

Carol Jean Cusack, hereinafter referred to as "PNP," agrees to employment and duties of pediatric nurse practitioner at Central City Health Systems, hereinafter referred to as CCHS. The clinical practice of the named practitioner will be limited to the primary care of and minor urgent treatment of children patients of CCHS, seen within the context of the family care philosophy espoused by CCHS, in a collaborative relationship with W. Harvey Doe, MD, FAAP and Mary Beth Jones, MD.

Schedule: PNP accepts employment for 40 hours per week scheduled Monday through Friday 9:30 AM to 5 PM at the CCHS practice site. PNP will be expected to make AM hospital rounds in the newborn nursery at Central City Hospital, said rounds to include education of parents of newborns born in the last 24 hours to patients of the CCHS practice. This obligation at Central City Hospital will occur before the 9:30 AM hour. This schedule may be modified with mutual agreement by both parties. In situations where the final patient has not been seen by 5 PM on any given day, PNP may agree to stay overtime (not to exceed a total of 48 hours per week) for an additional payment of $35.00 per hour. There are no weekend work or call hours required during this contract period.

Salary: The base salary shall be $55,880.00 annually, payable in equal increments of 1/24 on the first and third Thursdays of each month. Adjustments to this salary base will be made at the minimum of 5% annually, coinciding with the initial date of employment. CCHS will pay an additional $5.00 per patient in excess of 5000 patients at the end of the calendar year, the payment being made as a bonus check on December 20. All other adjustments in salary, except as outlined above, will be negotiated at the end of the annual performance evaluation and will commence with the first paycheck of the following month.

Other Employment Benefits:

Health Insurance—PNP agrees to participate in the medical and dental options of Monmart Health Insurance Plan at the rate of $23.42 per pay period, to be matched equally by CCHS. Details of health insurance coverage will be described in a separate contract with Monmart Health Insurance Plan.

Retirement—CCHS agrees to contribute $150.00 per month toward PNP's retirement plan beginning after the first 90 days of employment by CCHS, so long as the retirement plan in effect conforms to the guidelines of the U.S. Internal Revenue Service.

Paid Leave—CCHS agrees to pay 8 days salary for leave due to illness and an additional 2 days salary for "unspecified" leave annually. If all 10 days are not used by December 31, CCHS agrees to compensate PNP in dollars or time off at the discretion of PNP. Any dollar amount will be paid in the first paycheck of January.

Paid Holidays—CCHS agrees to pay for the following holidays when the practice is closed: January 1, Martin Luther King Day, July 4, Labor Day, Thanksgiving Day, the day after Thanksgiving, Christmas Eve, and Christmas Day. CCHS further agrees to pay for a holiday on PNP's birthday each year.

Vacation—CCHS agrees to paid time off for PNP for vacation 10 days annually (2 work weeks) after the first 6 months of employment. After 2 years, paid vacation will increase to 15 days and after 4 years, paid vacation will increase to 20 days per year. Paid vacation will not increase thereafter.

Continuing Education—CCHS agrees to 5 days paid time off for PNP's participation in continuing education courses and will pay a maximum of $1500.00 annually for tuition. Other expenses related to continuing education will be the obligation of PNP.

Malpractice Insurance—CCHS will pay for an occurrence-based insurance policy in the amount of $3 million per occurrence, $5 million total claims per year. Insurance carrier may be chosen by PNP. The total amount of said policy will be paid on the day this contract commences and annually thereafter for the duration of employment. It is the obligation of PNP to submit necessary documentation for said payment to office manager in advance of the due date each year.

Professional Licensure and Recertification—CCHS agrees to pay the fees associated with renewal of the RN license every 2 years in accordance with Board of Nursing policy and renewal of PNP certification as designated by the certifying organization, not to exceed a maximum of $350.00 in a 3-year period. PNP is obligated to provide documentation to enable such payments in advance of the due date.

Loan Repayment—In lieu of a first year bonus, except as otherwise specified in this agreement, CCHS agrees to repay the educational loan of $2680.60 in PNP's name at First National Bank. The full amount is due on the day after the 90-day probationary period for PNP ends.

Contractual Agreement:
A probationary period shall extend from the day this agreement commences to 90 days thereafter, during which time either party may terminate this agreement with a 72-hour notice; thereafter, a 30-day written notice of such termination shall be required by either party. CCHS reserves the right to compensate PNP for 3 days' salary in lieu of 72-hour notice or with 1 months' salary in lieu of the 30-day written agreement.

PNP will receive a written performance evaluation from the collaborating physicians at the end of the probationary period, 6 months thereafter, and annually or as otherwise requested by either party. PNP will receive a copy of the criteria for performance evaluation in advance of such evaluation.

This employment agreement renews itself automatically on a monthly basis until either party serves notice to terminate in accord with procedures designated in this agreement, or employment of PNP may be terminated with cause with a 24-hour notice in the event of conviction of a felony, loss of license to practice as an APN, or gross negligence that compromises the safety of CCHS patients or staff.

_____   _____
                                                     Date
Signature of PNP

_____   _____
                                                     Date
Signature of CEO of CCHS

Figure 22-1 Sample advanced practice nurse contract.

out? If the practice site is a hospital, how are APNs being used? For example, are the clinical nurse specialists (CNSs) being employed for traditional roles or are they being forced into case management or administrative roles? Are the APNs situated within the division of nursing or within medicine? Does there appear to be congruence between the prospective practice and the APN? What is the salary range for APNs in similar practice sites in the community? Do they compare favorably with regional and national figures? What is the mix of providers in the practice, and what age groups and genders are represented? In a group practice, who is the "power center?"

Burnett and Martin (1999) realize that some information helpful to the negotiation process will not be easily accessible to the APN seeking employment. They suggest asking the following questions at the initial meeting to enable more informed negotiation: What is the most frequently billed Current Procedural Terminology (CPT) code? What is the collection rate for the practice? What percentage of the provider's generated income is generally applied to overhead costs? How much consultation cost can be expected in the initial year of practice and later? What will be the patient mix for me? Will the patient load consist solely of those with a historically low payment rate? Before the interview, the APN is also well advised to spend some time in honest reflection, considering the following questions: How many patients can I reasonably see during a day? How many times a day will I likely need to consult with the physician or some other authority about a patient before making a decision? What salary is fair and reasonable, given my current ability in the role? What is most important to me as I anticipate negotiating a fringe benefit package? Where am I willing to compromise, and what must I have from the deal? What is so critical in the negotiations that I will walk away rather than compromise? Asserting one's legitimate needs rather than adapting an attitude of servitude is not a stance that comes easily, so practicing negotiation in front of a mirror or on videotape (for later review) or roleplaying with a peer can be helpful. Putting together and practicing a list of "talking points" from the literature and research about APNs and their potential contributions to outcomes, cost savings, and patient satisfaction is worth the time and effort. This is especially important if the prospective employer is not totally familiar with the role.

Some APNs negotiate for an opportunity to come into the setting for a few days without pay to observe the nature of the practice setting. This allows an individual to become acquainted with the staff and the management system and to learn more about the physical layout of the unit. How many examination rooms are there? How many offices? Will there be an office for a newly employed APN? Does a policy manual exist? Is there an orientation plan? Are there signed protocols or clinical guidelines (if required by the state)?

A few years ago, a dandruff shampoo was associated with an ad campaign with the slogan: "You never get a second chance to make a first impression." This is a powerful idea, not just for shampoo, but also for anticipating a job interview. It is critical to be well prepared and to demonstrate a professional image. Appropriate attire includes a business suit or similar apparel, with conservative makeup and hairstyle and minimal jewelry; it is appropriate to dress for the position one desires, not the position one already holds. One should be prompt (ideally 15 minutes early) for the appointment and remember that office staff—the group one is hoping to work with—begin to form an impression from the first moment of the encounter. An APN who is less than warm and courteous to office staff will not receive their quick endorsement for the job. Greeting the interviewer with a firm handshake and eye contact reflects a positive image. It is important to remember that all nonverbal clues can convey an image of power or powerlessness (Vogel & Jackson, 1992).

It is not uncommon for the APN to be invited to a lunch or dinner meeting with prospective employers. This can be advantageous because it places the parties on neutral turf and can be more relaxing than an office setting. The prudent APN will select a medium-priced meal and decline alcohol. (If the prospective employer orders and drinks wine with the meal, one glass is usually acceptable for the candidate.) Selecting an entree with which one is familiar and comfortable tends to lessen anxiety. For example, eating spaghetti or buttered lobster in public in a silk dress may create considerable anxiety, and nothing is more embarrassing than a poorly handled escargot flying across the room.

Burnett and Martin (1999) identify the 3 As of business basics as availability, affability, and ability, in that order of priority. The APN's capacity at those three aspects of the business of health care will hopefully come across at the interview. This is the time to propose the way in which one can add value to a practice, not the time to be timid or overly modest. The more specifically one can address this the better. For example, a certified nurse midwife (CNM) who speaks Spanish fluently might say, "Dr. Swanson, I understand that 17% of your obstetrical clients are Hispanic. I believe that my ability to speak the language will be a real asset to your practice." Being able to cite such specific information about a practice reveals that the APN has done homework in preparation for the meeting and provides an excellent example of initiative and interest on his or her part.

Throughout the meeting, as questions are asked and answered and details of the anticipated position are forthcoming, the APN will wish to display enthusiasm for the role and appear self-confident in the ability to perform. It is important to use this time to clarify all terms of the agreement being proposed and to listen carefully. Some interviewers ask candidates to verbalize a philosophy that guides advanced practice or to answer hypothetical questions, often of a clinical nature. In these cases, an APN is advised to pause to organize thoughts before providing an answer and to remember the legal scope of practice in answering the question. A certified registered nurse anesthetist (CRNA) relating his personal interview experience with an anxiety-provoking and controversial hypothetical question recommends this kind of answer: " I would follow policy and practice norms and would make it my priority to discern what those were before a situation of this sort arose." Common questions asked at professional interviews for APNs include these: What qualities do you have that you believe will lead to success? What do you think is your greatest strength and your greatest limitation? What were your previous jobs, and why did you leave? Why did you choose us as a prospective place of employment? What can you do for us that would make hiring you a good decision?

Hawkins and Thibodeu (1996) recommend that one wait until near the end of the interview to discuss salary, thereby capitalizing on the opportunity to learn more about the nature of the work first. If the prospective employer raises a question earlier about what salary would be required, the APN might delay until a firm job offer is made by a comment such as, "I'm certain you'll pay a wage that is fair. I'd like to learn more about your expectations before discussing salary." Once the position and salary offer are made, no matter how impressive, the APN should be silent, perhaps counting to 30, before accepting. If the offer is not competitive, it can be countered with a researched response.

Having decided in advance what fringe benefits are essential will make this part of the discussion more productive. Frequently, the benefit package is an area on which compromise can be made to achieve more balanced compensation. It is wise to appreciate that the relationship between the two parties will extend into the future if the position is offered and accepted. An otherwise collegial relationship can be adversely affected by an attitude of inflexibility and unwillingness to compromise at the time of contract negotiation. Behaviors that appear greedy or connote a lack of team spirit can lose the job for even the most talented candidate.

APNs are advised to accept offers made, but not the jobs, at the initial meeting. If a written contract is presented, it should not be signed on the spot. Instead, one should ask for time for an objective, critical, and unemotional review. This delay provides time for closer examination of the offer and for having an attorney review the document to ascertain that the best interests of the APN have been served by the agreement. Buppert (1999) and Ryan and Ryan (1999) agree that the value of attorney review of an employment contract is worth the usual $100 to $200 charge. Even though a request is made for time to consider the offer and have an attorney review the contract, arrangements can be made at the time of the interview for closing the deal.

Regardless of the outcome of the interview, it is appropriate to follow-up with a letter of appreciation for the time invested on behalf of the candidate. Asking for a business card at the interview facilitates correct titles and spelling and ensures an accurate address. Even if an APN has no intention of accepting the position, it is never wise to "burn bridges" by being less than the consummate professional.

An APN may wish to consult a professional recruiter to facilitate job placement. This approach is particularly compelling for those who are relocating to an unfamiliar practice area. Working with a professional recruiter decreases the stress, time, and energy directed toward a job search. Because of their knowledge of and access to multiple locations across the country, recruiters can increase one's ultimate marketability. Additionally, because of their considerable networks, they are knowledgeable about compensation issues and job demands. Recruiters are also paid by the potential employer, not the APN; however, if an APN terminates a contract prematurely, repayment of the cost may be required.

IMPLICATIONS FOR MSN EDUCATION AND ADVANCED PRACTICE

While a written practice agreement or employment contract may seem cumbersome and confusing, it offers some sense of job security and protection. Knowing how to negotiate a contract is a critical skill for APNs. Ideally, one will have opportunities to learn these skills during graduate education. Audiotaping or videotaping oneself in practice sessions can enhance the art of skillful contract negotiation. Seeking guidance from experienced APNs is also of inestimable value in preparing to negotiate. The importance of conscientious preparation for this venture can not be overestimated.

One of the most powerful benefits of contract negotiation is that it forces a discussion between the APN and prospective employer about the anticipated relationship and the complementarity of their respective roles. An appreciation that together they can accomplish more than either one alone can be quite powerful.

Obviously the employer wishes to hire someone who represents the best match for the job requirements. "With the cost of hiring and orienting each new employee ranging from $3000 to $5000, an interviewer must make a point to scrutinize candidates from both a recruitment and a retention perspective" (Vogel & Jackson, 1992). With so much at stake in a short interview, it is imperative that prospective APNs be prepared to make a positive impression.

According to Sprague-McRae (1996), three factors ultimately affect the professional interaction possible between APNs and physicians: the conditions of employment, the physician's perceptions and understanding of the APN role, and the physician's subsequent commitment to role preservation. Confusion and misperceptions do still exist, despite the lengthy history of advanced practice. APNs and APN educators have an obligation to continue to clearly articulate their role at every opportunity to affect collaborative practice possibilities.

PRIORITIES FOR RESEARCH

Campbell. Mauksch, Neikirk, and Hosokawa (1990) studied collaborative practices between NPs and physicians and discovered that 54% of those surveyed believed that a practice agreement had been negotiated; in reality, only 31% of such agreements existed. Another interesting discrepancy was identified in the study: 76% of the physician respondents felt they had final decision-making authority in the practice; only 47% of the NPs held the same perception. In a similar study, Moser and Armer (2000) examined characteristics and factors influential in successful collaborative practices among NPs and physi-

cians. They found that 31% of NPs and 74% of physicians perceived that the physician partners had final authority for decision-making. It would be interesting to replicate this study with other APNs.

Descriptive research should be designed to explore characteristics associated with satisfactory contract negotiation experiences among APNs. It would be fascinating to compare the findings from APNs with those of their employing physicians to determine the level of congruency. Research might also address the relationship between job satisfaction and retention and a particular type of collaborative practice agreement.

Arslanian-Engoren (1995) used a phenomenological approach to examine the experiences of four CNSs in collaborative relationships with physicians. It was the researcher's intent to learn what served as the essential component of collaboration needed by the CNS for facilitating enactment of the clinical expert role. Five themes emerged in the study: the need for mutual trust and respect, the importance of maintenance of a nursing perspective, establishment of a collegial relationship, definition of a practice role, and a positive life experience

---

Chart 22-1

Case Study: The Value of a Written Contract

Megan was eager to begin working as a FNP after completing her program and passing the certification examination. During one of her clinical rotations as a student, two physicians approached her about a job in their office in Megan's community. Megan was thrilled with the opportunity. The physicians, Dr. Moore and Dr. Champ, had been in family practice together for over 10 years and owned their own office. The practice was busy, with new patients being added weekly. Megan knew both physicians and respected their work.

Megan met with the two physicians late one afternoon to discuss a possible job opportunity. She explained her role as a FNP and discussed her clinical experiences during her education. The physicians seemed impressed with Megan and her potential contribution to their practice. They offered her a job in their office, working Monday through Friday, 8:30 AM to 5:00 PM. The physicians did not see the need for Megan to make rounds in the hospital nor take calls, but they did suggest she apply for hospital privileges in case she needed them in the future. She was told she would be added to their group health insurance policy and given 2 weeks paid vacation and six paid holidays per year. The deal was sealed with handshakes, but no written contract was drafted.

During the first few months at work, Megan was happy with her job. She enjoyed the patients and felt she relieved some of the physicians' workload. Both physicians were complimentary of her work, and the patients she saw seemed

pleased with their care. In talking with former classmates, Megan began to realize that she should have negotiated for additional benefits such as paid malpractice insurance and some type of retirement benefits or profit-sharing. Megan was also working overtime several hours a week with no additional pay. This caused a hardship because she was often late in picking up her daughter from daycare and had to pay an extra fee.

Six months into the job, Dr. Herbert Moore died suddenly from a heart attack. The entire staff was shocked and upset, but according to Dr. Champ, "the show must go on." Megan felt obligated to do her part and share the additional patient load. In addition, Dr. Champ asked her to begin making rounds at the hospital, beginning at 7:30 AM. Megan complied, but this again created a daycare hardship and an extra expense. Megan received no additional pay or other compensation for the additional work.

Three months after Dr. Moore's death, Dr. Champ informed Megan that he was adding two new physicians to the practice and would not need her anymore. He told her he was getting older and just could not keep up the current pace. He indicated that bringing in two physicians would be very costly for the practice, and he could not afford to keep her on the payroll too. Dr. Champ gave Megan 2 weeks notice. Megan was shocked and devastated. She had lost her job in less than a year and was suddenly without income or insurance. She had no leads on a new job in her small community.

(enjoying the work and the relationship). Although these research respondents did not see the collaboration as necessarily easy, they were resolute in their commitment to it. Advanced education, clinical preparation, an ability to understand the overall health system, and professional maturity were credited as components necessary for an evolving collaboration. Using similar methodology, one might address the lived experiences of other types of APNs in collaborative relationships and determine how a flat structure, rather than a hierarchy, is maintained. Is the evolution of and components needed for collaborative physician-APN relationships different for APNs whose roles are less amorphous than those of CNSs?

Finally, it would be helpful to learn, through descriptive research, what items have been requested in fringe benefit packages. Having examples of what other APNs have received could guide novices in the negotiation process.

Suggestions for Further Learning

- Consult a bank or other investment group for details on retirement plans.
- Consult your state's board of nursing for regulations about collaborative practice agreements and details about preparation. For specific information on how to contact your state board, contact the National Council of State Boards at www.ncsbn.org.
- Refer to the following websites for information on the legal aspects of contracts and other business advice: www.freeadvice.com and www.profnet.co.uklawyer/#services
- Contact a business supply store for contract forms and computer software (such as Quicken Lawyer). Determine if either of these things could facilitate contract negotiation for the APN.
- Consult the following references for additional details on negotiating contracts and collaborative practice agreements: Bourne, H. (1996). *A great deal: compensation for nurse practitioners and physician assistants*. Areta, CA: Western Practitioner Resources; Buppert, C. (1999). *Nurse practitioner's business and legal guide*. Gaithersburg, MD: Aspen Publishers; and Woomer, S. (1993). Negotiating an employment contract. *The Clinician's Reference Guide 1994, 4*(Suppl 1), 21-28.
- Read Straka, D. (1996). Resume preparation—are you your resume? *Advanced Practice Quarterly, 2*(1), 76-77.

DISCUSSION QUESTIONS

These questions can be used to promote critical thinking and encourage discussion.

1. Read the case study in Chart 22-1. Could a similar scenario affect the CNS, CNM, or CRNA? Why or why not? What can be learned from Megan's case? Discuss these questions.
2. Write a resume and begin to collect other documents for a portfolio.
3. Draft a realistic contract agreement or collaborative practice statement.
4. Answer the following question: Why should an employer want me for a job?
5. Draft a position statement that addresses how you plan to meet the business basics of availability, affability, and ability in your practice.
6. Ask other APNs about their experiences in contract negotiation.

REFERENCES/BIBLIOGRAPHY

Arslanian-Engoren, C. (1995). Lived experiences of CNSs who collaborate with physicians: a phenomenological study. *Clinical Nurse Specialist, 9*(2), 68-73.

Bourne, H. (1996). *A great deal: compensation for nurse practitioners and physician assistants*. Areta, CA: Western Practitioner Resources.

Buppert, C. (1998). Justifying nurse practitioner existence: hard facts to figure. *The Nurse Practitioner, 20*(8). 43-48.

Buppert, C. (1999). *Nurse practitioner's business and legal guide*. Gaithersburg, MD: Aspen Publishers.

Burnett, B.L., & Martin, S. (1999, July 16-20). *The nuts and bolts of building your own practice* (Tape no. 31). American Association of Nurse Practitioners 14th Annual National Conference. Atlanta, GA: American Association of Nurse Practitioners.

Campbell, J.D., Mauksch, H.O., Neikirk, H.J., & Hosokawa, M.C. (1990). Collaborative practice and provider styles of delivering health care. *Social Science and Medicine, 30*, 1359-1365.

Hamric, A.B., & Spross, J.A. (Eds.). (1989). *The clinical nurse specialist in theory and practice* (2nd ed.). Philadelphia: WB Saunders.

Hawkins, J., & Thibodeu, J. (1996). *The advanced practice nurse: current issues* (4th ed.). New York: Tiresias.

Henry, P. (1995). The nurse practitioner's guide to practice agreements. *Nurse Practitioner Forum, 6*(1), 4-5.

Kyle, M. (1995). Collaboration. In M. Snyder & M.P. Mirr (Eds.), *Advanced practice nursing: a guide for professional development* (pp. 169-182). New York: Springer.

Leccese, C. (1998, January). Who's making what—and where. *ADVANCE for Nurse Practitioners*, 31-35.

Mackey, T. (1996, June). Compensation for nurse practitioners. *ADVANCE for Nurse Practitioners,* 47-48.

Mackey, T. & Chandler, H. (1996). Choosing a practice: key issues to consider. *Nurse Practitioner, 21*(12), 87-89.

Miller, S.K. (2000, February). Negotiating your salary. *Patient Care for the Nurse Practitioner,* 72.

Moser, S.S., & Armer, J.M. (2000). An inside view—NP/MD perception of collaborative practice. *Nursing and Health Care Perspectives, 2*(1), 29-33.

Pearson, L.J. (2000). Annual legislative update—how each state stands on legislative issues affecting advanced practice. *The Nurse Practitioner, 25*(1), 16-68.

Peters, S. (2000, February). Get what you're worth. *ADVANCE for Nurse Practitioners,* 21.

Ryan, M., & Ryan, T. (1999, July 16-20). *Understanding contracts and development of successful negotiation skills for nurse practitioners* (Tape no. 87). American Association of Nurse Practitioners 14th Annual National Conference. Atlanta, GA: American Association of Nurse Practitioners.

Sebas, M. (1994). Developing a collaborative practice agreement for the primary care setting. *Nurse Practitioner, 19*(3), 49-51.

Sprague-McRae, J. (1996). The advanced practice nurse and physician relationship: considerations for practice. *Advanced Practice Nursing Quarterly, 2*(1), 33-40.

Straka, D. (1996). Resume preparation—are you your resume? *Advanced Practice Quarterly, 2*(1), 76-77.

Vogel, D., & Jackson, P. (1992). The interview: reflections from the recruiter's side of the desk. *Healthcare Trends and Transitions, 3*(4), 24-26,40.

Woomer, S. (1993). Negotiating an employment contract. *The Clinician's Reference Guide 1994, 4*(Suppl 1), 21-28.

Chapter 23

The Business Plan

Margaret R. Murphy

Nursing has been defined as an art and a science, but in these days of managed care, it must also consider itself a business. Costs of services are monitored carefully at every site, and nursing must educate patients about the value of their services. Advanced practice nurses (APNs) are in the exciting and unique situation of being a fairly new entity in the health care market, providing services either as sole proprietors who own their own practices, consultants, or entrepreneurs who seek new opportunities in existing systems. Because the transition into the advanced practice role is difficult in the first year, many APNs choose to look into business opportunities after establishing themselves in their roles and reevaluating their goals. The definition of those goals is the groundwork for the development of a business plan.

Often, nurses do not see themselves as business people, undervaluing the extensive management and organizational experience gained early in the nursing career. These are valuable skills in the business world. To any new entrepreneur, the task of developing a business plan can be daunting and formidable; however, with the wealth of resources available, the task should not be a roadblock on the path to a successful business opportunity. The job of writing a business plan serves as a vehicle to define who and what an APN is in a way no other theoretical definition can, and it functions as the blueprint for a career in a new and evolving role.

One of the most important steps before initiation of the business plan is an APN's development of a written personal mission statement. Sheehy and McCarthy (1998) say that "this statement will explain who you are." The process of creating a personal mission requires intensive introspection that usually begins in the student role. Before embarking on a business venture, APNs must be sure they are willing to devote the time, energy, and financial and personal resources into operating a business as well as providing service. They must be able to clearly define what they do and why their service is necessary.

In the United States alone, there are approximately one billion new businesses started each year; only 20% of these are viable after 5 years (Haag, 1997). Careful planning is a key aspect to the success of any new venture. A sound, written business plan is the introduction to a world of encouragement, finances, and success. There are numerous guides and worksheets available in software packages, books, journals, and on the Internet to assist APNs in developing business plans.

DEFINITIONS

The **business plan** is an organized, written snapshot of what a business is, what that business does, and what that business plans to do over time. Business plans are often used to elicit capital funds from banks or investors; therefore they must be succinct in describing how the business will make money and repay financing. An APN may choose not to use a business plan to seek a loan for venture capital; they may use it to prove to a prospective employer or contractor that he or she can generate a salary, benefits, and a profit while enhancing a new or existing practice. A plan requires a studied view of the business, market, and goals and may need to be initiated at least 6 months before beginning a new business (Haag, 1997).

CRITICAL ISSUES: CREATING A BUSINESS PLAN FOR ADVANCED PRACTICE NURSING

The business plan serves as a written map to guide the developer through the planning process and management decisions for a business venture. It is a mechanism for analyzing the existing market and placing one's planned venture within that context. Because it is framed in the language of investors, the business plan can project the viability of a venture before any financial commitment is made. A main purpose, however, is to garner financial support from prospective investors or other conventional financial sources. According to Goodspeed, (1985), development of a business plan forces an objective, critical, and unemotional examination of the business proposition.

All business plans must have certain elements (Chart 23-1). The suggested total pages for content should be no

Chart 23-1

Sample Business Plan

Ann has been a CNS in perinatal nursing for some time, employed for the last 2 years in a tertiary care center in a metropolitan area. Ann enjoys her fairly traditional CNS role. Ann's Master's thesis related to perinatal grief and loss, an interest she developed over time. After graduation, she enrolled in several continuing education courses on the topic, including a week-long session devoted to becoming a certified grief counselor and coordinator that was sponsored by Resolve Through Sharing (now RTS Bereavement Services). Subsequently, Ann helped to initiate a successful RTS service at her medical center, and she continues to be instrumental in its day-to-day work. Lately, Ann has experienced a growing concern that the couples, albeit effectively supported while in the inpatient setting, are being sent home to cope with the most devastating experience of a lifetime (the death of a baby) without continued support from the health care community. Hypothesizing that a perinatal support group would be of inestimable value to these couples, Ann approaches the nursing and medical administrators of the hospital's perinatal services. There is administrative support for the proposition, and Ann is advised to develop a written proposal (business plan) for presentation to the hospital's foundation for "seed money." The group agrees with Ann's request that this be a counseling group marketed for the entire community and not affiliated directly with their medical center. Although Ann recognizes that this decision affects the long-term financial support for the effort, she believes the plan is a philosophical imperative.

Appreciating that the ideal support group is egalitarian in nature and that collaboration enhances the planning process, Ann convinces her fellow CNS Frances to be a professional partner in this enterprise. These two APNs mutually develop the following business plan. (Note: Appendices are not included here, but they would include CVs of the principals involved, details of the budget, and a copy of the letters and announcements mentioned in the marketing section.)

**A Business Plan for a Not-For-Profit Venture
Presented to the
Central State Medical Center Foundation
by Ann Logue, RNC, MSN, CNS,
and Frances Holden, RN, MSN, CNS
for Seed Funding for
Central City Parent Support Group**

Executive Summary
Last year in this city, 151 childbearing couples were discharged from a hospital without their baby because of a stillbirth, early pregnancy loss, or newborn death. These individuals went home to face one of the most devastating of personal tragedies without continuity of care from the health professional community. With a support group in place, this would not have been the case. Healthy grief resolution might have been

facilitated and complicated grief quickly identified and referred for appropriate therapy. This will be a group that belongs to the community. It has no direct hospital affiliation but does enjoy the support of all three hospitals in the city.

The Central City Parent Support Group proposes to serve local couples and their peers in the counties contiguous to Montgomery by providing a professionally led, mutual self-help support group that meets monthly but allows ongoing access to the group network via telephone. The meeting place on the St. Mary's Medical Center campus has been donated. The APNs who will serve as co-leaders are volunteering their time and expertise, as are other members of the professional team. All team members have academic and experiential preparation appropriate to meet the mission of the proposed support group—to provide continuity of planned grief intervention for couples experiencing perinatal loss, with the ultimate goal of healthy grief resolution.

Financial assistance in the form of "seed money" is being requested from the Community Service Account of the Foundation of Central State Medical Center for a total 3-year amount of $2357.50, all of which will be devoted to either a lending library for group members or to marketing the enterprise. The first year's projected budget is $1857.50, which would have been an investment of $12.30 for each of the 151 couples who suffered perinatal losses in Montgomery last year.

The addition of this postvention (post-event intervention) service will add a primary prevention measure that has the potential to affect the mental health of hundreds of childbearing families annually and to make subsequent childbearing emotionally easier.

The Business and the Market
The Central City Parent Support Group is a professionally led, voluntary, confidential, mutual self-help group without cost, composed of couples and their significant others who have experienced a perinatal loss. *Perinatal loss* refers to a loss associated with stillbirth, miscarriage, other early pregnancy losses (e.g., ectopic pregnancy, elective medical termination), or newborn death. This is not a therapy group. Group members who need therapeutic intervention beyond the scope of the group's co-leaders will be referred to appropriate providers for such intervention.

There is no other support group of this type in this city of 619,000 or in its contiguous counties. There is one Compassionate Friends group in the city that serves the needs of parents grieving the loss of a child of any age. However, perinatal loss has some unique components, and its grief-counseling model is different than those for other losses. The Central City Parent Support Group will meet the unique needs of a particular population not being addressed by the existing group.

Courtesy of Cheryl Pope Kish.

Continued

Chart
23-1

Sample Business Plan—cont'd

The Business and the Market—cont'd

National statistics on perinatal loss indicate that the stillbirth rate is 1.2%, early known pregnancy loss is 20% or greater, and the newborn death rate is 1.6%. Those statistics in Central City translate into the following numbers:

Perinatal Loss Statistics for Central City: 1996-1998*

TYPES OF LOSS	1996	1997	1998
Stillbirths	24	21	27
Early pregnancy loss at less than 20 weeks gestation	96	107	116
Newborn deaths	9	6	8

*Does not reflect losses in situations without hospital admission. Data provided by hospital liaison personnel.

This data represents 634 total losses; when both members of the childbearing couple are considered, this accounts for 1268 parents experiencing perinatal loss in the last 3 years. These data do not begin to reflect grandparents or others who might profit from grief support, nor do they represent losses that occur without a requisite hospital admission or those that occurred in contiguous counties within commuting distance of a support group. If, as empirical study suggests, 10% of affected individuals attend a support group, the numbers show the value of a perinatal grief group in the city.

As an open self-help group, couples can enter at any point in their grief experience and stay for as long as needed. Consequently, the group will continue to evolve over time. As they begin to heal, the couples in the group will serve as a self-help network to other couples and as panel members for training health care professionals and medical and nursing students to better understand perinatal loss and grief resolution.

Objectives

The purpose of the Central City Parent Support Group is to provide continuity of planned grief intervention for couples experiencing perinatal loss, with the ultimate goal of healthy grief resolution. To that end, the objectives are as follows:

1. Provide emotional support while creating a context for learning about how to cope with the profound grief associated with perinatal loss.
2. Enable individuals who have experienced perinatal loss to come together in a safe, nonjudgmental, and confidential forum for the purpose of sharing their mutual concerns.
3. Provide an atmosphere where group members can develop sensitivity to the needs and feelings of others and come to recognize the universality of emotion, even as they are being supported in gaining insight into their own loss.

After the initial 6 months, the effectiveness of the group method as a postvention strategy for grief resolution will be monitored by member survey. This data and the numbers of participants will be documented and shared with obstetrical services at the area hospitals. Data will be presented only in aggregate form to protect individual confidentiality of group members. Annual evaluation will commence on the 1-year anniversary date of the group's formation.

In the second year and thereafter, nursing and medical students will be allowed to observe the group with permission of the participants and a vow of confidentiality. No more than two students will be allowed to attend any session. Student requests for experience in the group will be managed by Ann Logue.

Management

Group co-leaders

- Ann Logue, RN, MSN, CNS: Holds a Master's degree in nursing with specialization in perinatal nursing and is nationally certified as a CNS and a perinatal grief counselor and coordinator; has 14 years of clinical experience in hospital and community settings with obstetrical patients and families and currently works as a clinical specialist in the perinatal services division of Central State Medical Center; has served as a consultant on varied aspects of obstetrical care, authored two articles, presented at numerous professional conferences, and served as a clinical faculty member for both nursing and medical students; MSN thesis topic dealt with *The Lived Experience of Losing a First-Born Child*; has had graduate-level coursework in group dynamics.
- Frances Holden, RN, MSN, CNS: Holds a Master's degree in nursing with specialization in mental health/psychiatric nursing and is nationally certified in that area of specialization; has 17 years of clinical experience with populations experiencing emotional crises and mental illness; currently employed as a certified CNS at Central State Medical Center where she is the mental health liaison nurse for the hospital; has served as a clinical faculty member for both medical and nursing students, authored several manuscripts related to emotional crisis and mental health, and served as consultant and presenter on related topics; has also taught courses in group dynamics and led support groups over her years of clinical practice; also brings personal perspective to her role as group leader, having experienced a perinatal loss herself.

Referral team

In the event that group members need intervention beyond the scope of professional practice of the APN co-leaders of the support group, the following individuals have agreed to accept referrals. Compensation for services will be negotiated with individuals who need ongoing intervention with these health professionals, but a one-time referral visit will be at no cost. All have also agreed to serve as consultants to the group and to provide-30 minute didactic sessions on occasion to the group.

- John Lacosse, MD: Psychiatrist with 31 years of clinical experience; currently serves as chief of Mental Health Services, Central State Medical Center.
- Susan Gill, MSW: Licensed social worker assigned to the Maternity Pavilion at St. Mary's Medical Center; has 6 years of clinical practice experience, with a focus in social work interventions for childbearing families.

Chart
23-1

Sample Business Plan—cont'd

- Patty Mitcheli, MD, FACOG: Board-certified OB/GYN with 8 years of clinical practice; holds associate professor rank in the medical school at Central State University and has a private practice in the city with privileges at all hospitals serving obstetrical patients.

Other personnel

- John Paul Sorbin, CPA: Group volunteer; will provide annual review of financial records of the group.
- Lydia Chastain, RNC, BSN, OB/GYN nurse manager, St. Mary's Medical Center: Group volunteer; will serve as hospital liaison with the support group.
- Betty Lou Jones, RN, OB/GYN nurse manager, Langley Community Hospital: Group volunteer; will serve as hospital liaison with the support group.
- Geraldine Wentworth, RNC, MSN, patient care coordinator of Perinatal Services, Central State Medical Center: Group volunteer; will serve as hospital liaison with the support group.

Service Description

When the mysteries of birth and death coincide in the case of perinatal loss, couples are forced to shift quickly from preparing for a normal, happy childbirth to dealing with the life-shattering loss of a baby. All three hospitals in the city—St. Mary's Medical Center, Langley Community Hospital, and Central State Medical Center—have effective inpatient grief support programs in place and based on national standards of care. Even smaller hospitals in the contiguous counties have similar programs, thanks to the perinatal outreach efforts of Central State Medical Center. However, at present, there is no continuation of planned intervention for these couples—no planned follow-up with health care providers until the medical checkup after miscarriage or childbirth at an interval of 4 to 6 weeks. Sending grieving couples home after perinatal loss without postvention negates what we know empirically to be true: that their journey of grief is just beginning. Moreover, research indicates that for some this journey will last up to 24 months.

When a couple experiences such a loss, emotional healing comes not from forgetting, but from remembering. A grief support group will facilitate the kind of remembering that enables healing and serves as a measure of primary prevention of mental health problems. This co-led self-help group will provide a monthly forum for couples to connect with professionals capable of facilitating grief resolution and with others who share the singleness of perinatal grief. The leaders will bring a practical wisdom borne of advanced education and their collective clinical experience to promote healthy coping with loss.

The group leaders will use the caring model, which involves caring without obligating others to reciprocate; nurturing; and personally committing to be present in the group setting and at other times by telephone. They will assume responsibility for

helping couples gain the usual benefits of a grief support group: (1) instillation of hope that they can heal; (2) recognition that certain emotions are universally experienced by grieving couples; (3) information about how to adjust to loss, cope with holidays and other events, help family members cope, and plan for another pregnancy; (4) problem-solving related to grief and loss; (5) cohesion associated with a newly evolving network of peers; (6) expression of emotions in a cathartic way; and (7) examination of existential questions about life and loss.

Market Analysis

The market for the Central City Support Group is patients of childbearing age and their family members in a six-county area who have sustained a perinatal loss and seek the services of a self-help group as a way of resolving their grief. The one support group in this area, Compassionate Friends, has as its mission serving patients who have lost children of any age. It is not perceived to be a direct competitive service because it does not deal exclusively with the unique needs inherent in situations of perinatal loss.

Marketing Strategy

The support group will meet monthly on the third Tuesday evening of the month, from 7:30 PM until 9:00 PM in the Women's Center reception room of Building C at St. Mary's Medical Center. This space, provided free of charge, is a comfortable, homelike reception area designated for women awaiting non–pregnancy-related diagnostic tests. It is not used in the evenings. The location is distant enough from the obstetrical service and Lamaze classrooms that patients will not encounter painful reminders while going to and from meetings. There is free adjacent parking in a well-lighted lot. Restrooms, public telephones, and snack machines are located nearby.

Prospective group members will learn about the group in the following ways:

1. Printed notices will be provided in the packet of materials given to couples experiencing perinatal loss in all hospitals in the city and all those served by the perinatal outreach program of Central State Medical Center. Verbal referrals will be made by hospital staff members working with these couples.
2. A reminder of the group meeting will be printed monthly in the Support Group section of the *Montgomery Telegraph and News.*
3. Co-leaders will be interviewed about the group 2 weeks before the first meeting on the television program "Mornings with Dell" on WGIX.
4. Notices about the support group will be sent to all obstetricians in the city and the five surrounding counties, along with a professional letter from the co-leaders asking for referrals.

Continued

Chart 23-1

Sample Business Plan—cont'd

Marketing Strategy—cont'd

5. Notices about the support group will be sent to all mortuaries in the city and five surrounding counties, along with a professional letter asking that notices be provided to appropriate patients.
6. Notices about the support group will be sent to all outpatient surgical centers in the area where patients experiencing early pregnancy loss might receive care.
7. Co-leaders will provide 1-day sensitivity training sessions and participate in week-long training sessions annually for health professionals who care for this patient population. Written announcements about the group will be included in conference materials.
8. The support group will be listed with the national RTS Bereavement Services office at LaCrosse Lutheran Hospital, Gundersen Clinic Ltd., LaCrosse, Wisconsin, as a potential referral site.
9. The support group will be mentioned in all written public-service materials related to perinatal or obstetrical services at the city's three hospitals that provide such care.

Financial Projections

There is no charge for participation in the support group; co-leaders are volunteering their time, as are other professionals. The meeting space is being provided without cost.

The financial needs for the first year reflect the purchase of books, pamphlets, and teaching audiotapes and videotapes for a lending library and storage for these library resources. Multiple copies of some of the items will be purchased. Other first-year needs include letterhead stationery and envelopes, note cards, and business cards. Financial needs during the second and third years will be upkeep of the lending library and replacement of the expendable supplies noted above ($250.00 per year). Funds are being requested in the following amounts from the Foundation of Central State Medical Center's Community Service Account. Funds will be maintained in the First National Bank of Montgomery.

Budget: Year One

ITEM	COST
Multiple copies of books and pamphlets for lending library	$1400.00
Lockable wooden bookcase for storage of lending library materials (to be housed in Women's Center reception area)	150.00
When a Baby Dies video	150.00
Stationery with letterhead (250 sheets)	32.50
Envelopes with logo (250)	44.00
Business cards (100)	18.50
Teaching kits on facilitating healing	62.50
TOTAL	$1857.50

Summary

The Central City Parent Support Group is a voluntary, self-help group led by APNs with specialization in caring for this patient population. This is a group that belongs to the community; it does not have a hospital affiliation as such, but it does enjoy support from all hospitals in the city. The group will meet on a monthly basis in a donated space conducive to the group's purpose; group membership will be free. The primary mission of the group is helping couples experiencing the life-shattering experience of perinatal loss to resolve their grief in healthy ways. A secondary mission is to provide expertise and a forum for teaching prospective health care professionals about the unique dimensions of this kind of loss and how to intervene to facilitate healthy grief resolution. The requested funds are being devoted to marketing the group and providing a lending library for members on topics related to perinatal grief and coping.

---

more than 15 to 35, and the appendix should not exceed the number of pages of the plan. Some experts suggest that any plan less than 10 pages long may be viewed as inadequate. However, others argue that if no loan is sought, a shorter version is appropriate (Haag, 1997).

Executive Summary

This element may be the only component a prospective investor needs to view before a tentative decision is made. Its purpose is to present a well-organized, concise narrative of the business' description, major players, proposed financial needs and projections, and place in the market.

These first few pages set the tone of success for the plan, so it is imperative that the executive summary be complete and convincing. It should be limited to 1 to 2 pages, and it is typically the last part of the plan to be written. The executive summary functions much like a research abstract; it contains the salient points of the presentation and helps the reader know if the fuller contents are worth reading.

The Business and the Market

This section introduces the business and describes the effect of current markets on the business. This places the proposed business within the context of the world in which it will be competing. A description of the background and history of the given industry, including how the business originated and developed, should be detailed. If an APN is developing an adjunct practice for an existing one, the history of the original practice and the background of the principal providers and managers becomes the focus of this segment.

With a new business, the form of the business must be chosen. There are four forms of business: sole proprietorship, partnership, corporation, and limited liability company (Buppert, 1999.) In a sole proprietorship, the owner is the business. Assets and liabilities are the owner's, and taxes are filed on that individual's return. In a partnership, two or more people share assets, liabilities, decision-making, and responsibilities for management of the business and provision of services. The partnership files taxes, with distributions reflected on each individual partner's income tax return. Laws affecting partnerships vary from state to state. The corporation is a legally separate business from the owner, even if the owner is the only stockholder, officer, and director. The corporation files a separate tax return on profits, and the distribution of profits is reported on stockholders' tax returns. State and federal laws require specific paperwork for corporations, again with regulations varying from state to state. The limited liability company is a combination of the partnership and corporation forms. The members are accountable for assets and losses, as in the partnership, but they may have only a limited accountability for liabilities, as with the corporation.

Current conditions within the industry that affect the business (e.g., effect of managed care, population trends, significant numbers of particular diseases that require additional services in the area) should be explained in this section of the plan. Finally, the last part of this section should include any future projections for growth, development of new services, potential new markets, and new competitors, if such information is available.

Business Objectives

The APN needs to define short- and long-term business goals and identify what the business and owners will accomplish in the next 5 years. Steiger (1996) refers to this component of business planning as a *vision*. "Determining a vision is essential in setting the direction of the practice and for evaluating progress." Objectives could be growth in volume of services, addition of personnel and equipment, attainment of additional education and training, and financial outcomes.

Management

Key management personnel are described in this section, with emphasis on their talents, skills, and years of experience in both patient and business areas. This includes

consultants (e.g., lawyers, accountants, collaborating providers and researchers). Resumes and curriculum vitae (CVs) of these key personnel should be attached.

Product/Service Description

This may be the most difficult section for an APN to complete because nurses are not accustomed to objectifying the myriad of tasks the role can entail. This section must concisely describe what the APN offers. All services should be illustrated, including who will use the service, how it will be provided, how much of the service can be offered, and what makes it unique. Emphasis on this unique product or service is the key to the success of the venture. With so many providers in overlapping and similar roles, a lender or administrative supporter wants to know what makes a new service different and better than existing services, what gives it a competitive edge or market niche. Technology and innovative products are imperative in many fields and may serve as an adjunctive service, but the APN's approach to practice may be the unique indicator that will ensure success. It is the portrayal of this approach that will be the foundation of the marketing strategy. Analyzing data on Internet marketing, Scott Kurnit of MiningCo.com says, "Technology will never replace smart people who care." It is the wise APN who can translate this advice into the business plan.

Also in this section, any products that may be sold along with services should be described with manufacturer's information and pricing. If drawings, charts, or pictures are helpful descriptors, these can be included in the appendix. Websites are exceptional forums for this information and a worthy investment for a new business.

Market Analysis

In this section, an APN proves to the potential lender and others that knowledge of the market can result in a successful business. Therefore the APN must be able to define who the market is in detail. Who are the potential patients individuals, families, aggregates, businesses, or organizations? Where are these patients, and what are their characteristics (e.g., age, financial resources, health problems)? What are the trends in the potential market? For example, if the APN is targeting a specific group, does this group exhibit an increased risk for a problem for which the APN will provide a service?

The market analysis must also address the competition, which the APN should be able to easily identify. Having already described the product or service, the APN now must be able to compare the strengths and weaknesses of the proposed product or business against those of the competition. This section must be comprehensive, allowing no room for investors to question why a potential competitor was omitted, thus suggesting inadequate preparation.

Marketing Strategy

The marketing strategy is the overall plan for advertisement of the product or service. Since the product has been discussed earlier, the other *P*s of marketing—price, place, and promotion—should be addressed in this part of the plan.

First, the price of the product or service must be established and the method of calculation reported. Since long-term profitability has to be appraised during development of the financial analysis, evaluation of the price and structure of price changes should be assessed within the context of the entire financial plan.

Second, where is this service or product going to be offered (the place)? Is this a home-based business or clinic, or will the service be delivered to patients? The accessibility of the business to patients should be described, including details about the size of the facility and its proximity to parking or transportation. If there is a special significance to the location of the business, such as optimal exposure to traffic patterns or proximity to other facilities, it should be emphasized. Another consideration should be the hours and days of the week the business will operate.

Finally, how will the patient learn about the service (the promotion)? What strategies will promote this service over the competition? Will patients find it easier to make an appointment? Are payment arrangements clear and straightforward? Does the business accept insurance reimbursement? Will the APN be a member of managed care organizations (MCOs) and specified on the provider list, separate from a physician collaborator? Would a website reach the target market? Can potential or existing patients correspond via e-mail or the Internet with the APN? Who makes the health care decisions? Women handle 75% of family finances and control 80% of purchase decisions—does that translate into health care decision-making as well (Pack, 1999)?

If the APN is collaborating with existing businesses and the new service will be included in the company's marketing plan, the new marketing strategy is described in this section. If any written advertisements have been developed, samples can be appended, including website addresses.

Financial Projections

If a business is already in existence, at least 3 years of balance sheets and income statements should be provided. For new businesses, plans for the use of startup money are listed in this section. Financial projections for 1-year, 3-year, and 5-year income and expenses must be made. Other important components of this section are the break-even analysis and projections for cash flow that demonstrate how the business will generate cash for future endeavors. Consultation with accountants or use of worksheets in software packages and business planning books lead new business owners step by step through the process of developing these documents.

Conclusions and Summary

The final narrative section of the business plan must summarize all the previous components of the plan, with a concluding statement about how the business will be a profitable success. The strength of this summary lies in how effectively the business planner can state how the business will meet its goals.

Appendix

The length of the appendix is dictated by the complexity of the plan. The things included in this section should be corporate agreements, resumes of owners and key personnel, and tax returns of the principals and the business (if already in existence). Items also appended are credit reports for the business and owners, licenses from regulatory agencies, and tax numbers. Photos, charts, and samples of products, services, and marketing tools should be added. Other components may be letters of intent, patient lists, and competitor lists.

IMPLICATIONS FOR MSN EDUCATION AND ADVANCED PRACTICE

Because one of the key components of development of the business plan is description of the product, an important element in the educational process is encouraging students to continually evaluate and postulate their role development and definition.

As more programs graduate more APNs, individuals are becoming more creative in developing positions to meet the needs of communities. The process of business planning incorporates the concepts of market evaluation and supply and demand, and schools must respond by training APNs not only for practice but also for seeking out market niches.

An APN may wish to propose a special project to enhance patient care that is not a traditional business. For example, the clinical nurse specialist (CNS) in a diabetic clinic might wish to offer cooking classes to supplement her patient's ability to plan and prepare appropriate meals. Finding gaps in service such as this one and filling those gaps is part of the uniqueness of the holistic practice of the APN. Although this venture may not be perceived as a business, especially if there is no venture capital being requested, it deserves the same kind of detailed planning. Perhaps it is this kind of enterprise, rather than a money-making venture, that will be the focus of many APNs. With some exceptions, the planning process and the written document necessary to gain administrative and financial support will be similar.

Throughout their graduate education, APNs are ideally encouraged to think creatively about the potential gaps

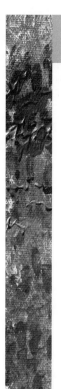

in health care that might be remedied by an APN business enterprise. It is helpful when faculty can role model such endeavors, as have two faculty, Cheryl Giefer and Ellen Carson, from Pittsburg University in Pittsburg, Kansas; they designed and implemented WorkWell, Inc.— Industrial Nursing Service. This business provides health screening, work-related physical examinations, drug screening, injury prevention and ergonomics, safety education, and immunizations in a small community where no such services had previously existed. Not only has this part-time, evening business met a critical need in this industrial community, it has also been profitable for the individuals involved and has provided a model of a tremendous spirit of entrepreneurship for CNS and family nurse practitioner (FNP) students.

PRIORITIES FOR RESEARCH

Much of the advance practice research of the 1970s and 1980s focused on consumer satisfaction and productivity of the role, but there is little research on advanced practice outcomes on patient health status; cost savings and cost analysis of APNs in the current health care system; and projections for opportunities in the new millennium. With emphasis on outcomes research and evidence-based practice, many research opportunities arise related to expanding roles, creative and innovative endeavors, and implementation of evidence-based practice guidelines by APNs.

As APNs become business leaders in the health care industry, evaluation of the success of these businesses and the usefulness of developed business plans in advanced practice models will be valuable information for future entrepreneurs. Qualitative studies might be designed to examine the lived experience of designing a business and seeing it implemented and evaluated.

DISCUSSION QUESTIONS

These questions can be used to promote critical thinking and encourage discussion.

1. Describe your "dream job" in near-complete detail (e.g., types and numbers of patients, location, hours, color of the walls, style of the furnishings). How can you make this dream job come true?
2. Develop a business plan for a potential position or an existing position that would fill an existing gap in health care services.

REFERENCES/BIBLIOGRAPHY

Batstone, D., & Waz, W. (1999, April). Mine Fields. *Business 2.0,* 82-86.

Buppert, C. (1999). *Nurse practitioner's business practice & legal guide.* Gaithersburg, MD: Aspen Publishers.

Calmelat, A. (1993). Tips for starting your own nurse practitioner practice. *Nurse Practitioner, 18*(4), 58-68.

Crow, G. (1996). The business of planning your practice: success is no accident. *Advanced Practice Nursing Quarterly, 2*(1), 58-61.

Finnigan, S. (1996). Getting started in business: from fantasy to reality. *Advanced Practice Nursing Quarterly, 2*(1), 1-8.

Gardner, K.L., & Weinrauch, D. (1988). Marketing strategies for nurse entrepreneurs. *Nurse Practitioner, 13*(5), 46, 48-49.

Goodspeed, S.M. (1985). How to write a business plan for a new venture. *Health Care Strategic Management,* 11-14.

Grimes, B.G. (1997). Developing a business plan for your legal nurse consulting practice. *Journal of Nursing Law, 4*(4), 7-13.

Haag, A.G. (1997). Writing a successful business plan. *AAOHN Journal, 45*(1), 25-34.

Johnson, J.E. (1988). *The nurse executive's business plan manual.* Rockville, MD: Aspen Publishers.

Johnson, J.E., Sparks, D.G., & Humphreys, C. (1988). Writing a winning business plan. *Journal of Nursing Administration, 8*(10), 15-19.

Lachman, V.D. (1996). Positioning your business in the market place. *Advanced Practice Nursing Quarterly, 2*(1), 27-32.

Manthey, M., & Avery, M. (1996). Remembering the nurse in the business of advanced practice. *Advanced Practice Nursing Quarterly, 2*(1), 49-54.

Pack, E. (1999, June). She's gotta have it. *Business 2.0,* 145.

Prucka, L. (1995). *Developing a business plan.* Midland, TX: The University of Texas of the Permian Basin Small Business Development Center.

Sheehy, C. M., & McCarthy, M.C. (1998). *Advanced practice nursing: emphasizing common roles.* Philadelphia: FA Davis.

Steiger, N., Hagenstad, R., & Anderson, A. (1996). Budget development and implementation for the APN in independent practice. *Advanced Practice Nursing Quarterly,* 2(1), 41-48.

Turini, N.N. (1995). Business plans: an effective tool for making decisions. *Nursing Leadership Forum,* 1(4), 116-121.

Vogel, C., & Doleysh, N. (1988). *Entrepreneuring—a nurse's guide to starting a business.* New York: National League for Nursing.

Chapter 24

Role Attainment: Novice to Expert

Pamela C. Levi

Continuing competency is a career-long concern, both for a nurse in his or her own practice and for those individuals who the nurse mentors or supervises. Skill and knowledge are expected to increase and progress throughout a practitioner's career. However, it is sometimes difficult to " know what you don't know," to maintain a realistic awareness of individual weaknesses and gaps in knowledge. Several useful models exist to help in assessing and planning for continuing professional growth. Perhaps the best known model involves the work done by Dreyfuss and Dreyfuss (1986) and significantly applied to nursing by Benner (1984).

In studying how expertness is developed and manifested, Dreyfuss and Dreyfuss (1986) worked with airline pilots and chess players. A continuum of "novice to expert" resulted, which is a useful method of conceptualizing how practitioners at differing points in their career acquire skills and exhibit understanding of processes. Benner then researched how this model of skill acquisition and clinical decision-making is manifested in expert nurses. From this work on how individuals acquire and process information related to clinical decision-making, strategies for teaching and learning for the various levels were suggested.

CRITICAL ISSUES: BENNER'S MODEL OF SKILL ACQUISITION

It is important to understand that, in the Benner model, acquisition of skill and the use of the terminology "skilled practice" do not refer to psychomotor skills or other enabling skills that could be demonstrated in a simulated laboratory setting. Instead, the model uses these terms to mean the applied skill of nursing in actual clinical situations. The model is a situational model and not a trait or talent model; this means that in different situations, the same advanced practice nurse (APN) could find himself or herself in different categories. Five levels of skill acquisition are described: novice, advanced beginner, competent, proficient, and expert.

Novice

Novices are new to a role and have little experience in the situations in which they are expected to perform. Individuals on this level are operating from essentially context-free rules. This tends to make their performance inflexible and unsuccessful because of their inability to prioritize and adapt the "rules" to different situations. Novices are not only students of academic programs but may also be nurses with years of clinical practice who make significant changes in their practice areas. Novices want to do a good job, but they evaluate their performance by how well they follow the rules. After only a short time in practice, the sheer numbers of rules can overwhelm individuals and impair their ability to listen and respond appropriately in complex situations.

All "new" APNs are novices; however, many new APNs are also expert nurses. This influences how quickly a novice APN progresses through the levels described by Benner. Expert nurses transfer knowledge and skills (e.g., communication skills, teaching skills, conflict management techniques) from one type of practice to the new advanced role. Knowing whether a nurse is a novice nurse in advanced practice or a "true" novice nurse affects learning experiences and expectations for performance. However, movement from novice to more advanced levels is not solely dependent on years of practice. Progression toward acquisition of expertise is also dependent on factors such as individual intelligence, motivation, career goals, quality of supervision received, and the quality of mentoring.

The descriptors of a novice APN include the following: slow in pace, taking much time with each patient (a patient may get aggravated over the length of the visit); consults with a physician or other APN on almost every patient; sees in "black and white" and is unable to analyze "gray" areas or read between the lines; and misses many diagnostic clues patients give. The novice APN often gives multiple diagnoses in fear of missing something and is understandably insecure about treatment options. The novice APN also over-orders diagnostic tests and feels the need to evaluate every problem the patient has, in spite of the specific reason given for the patient's visit. The novice is often overwhelmed by large amounts of patient information and is unable to prioritize.

Confronting and managing anxiety is an exhausting component of the first months of practice (Brown & Olshansky, 1998). Commonly, novice nurses in advanced practice remark on their experiences of being overwhelmed, feeling "stupid," and "forgetting" skills they had mastered in previous roles. This regression in functioning is particularly stressful for experienced nurses. Novice APNs are not ready to serve as preceptors, and some APNs may not move from this level or continue in the role. The novice APN does not "earn her keep" in most settings. However, this is a "natural" starting point for all APNs and such behavior should be expected in the beginning year of practice. Novice APNs who are completely self-assured should be a source of concern for any supervisor!

Advanced Beginner

Advanced beginners are individuals who have coped with enough real-life situations that recurring components or themes are being noted. Benner refers to these components as *aspects*. Aspects are defined as global characteristics that can be identified only by previous experience, are different from the procedural lists of things to be accomplished, and are used most often by beginners. Novices and advanced beginners tend to take in very little of the overall situation, often not focusing on the most significant aspects of a situation. Similar to the novice, the advanced beginner tries to address all problems that a patient has, but he or she is better able to focus on the reason for that day's visit and prioritize other problems. The advanced beginner requires less consultation time but continues to consult on a regular basis (appropriately), and he or she begins to take less time with each patient. The advanced beginner may overwhelm the patient with information and education in an attempt to "fix" the patient.

The advanced beginner works well in slower-paced settings where the same type of patients are usually seen (e.g., ones with similar diagnoses and receiving similar treatments). The advanced beginner is usually not willing or able to serve as a preceptor for students. Generally this level of practitioner does well with wellness and preventative treatment issues and education. It often takes 1 year of experience to reach this level of practice.

Competent

Competent APNs are often nurses who have been in a relatively stable job position for 2 to 3 years. These individuals tend to see their actions in terms of long-term outcomes and goals for patients. Competent practitioners are able to determine which aspects of the presenting situation should be considered and which can safely be ignored. There is a sense of being able to cope with most situations that arise in the practice setting.

Competent APNs are able to focus on a patient's chief complaint without feeling an obligation to address all of the patient's problems in one visit. (The relevance of other conditions that affect the safety and effectiveness of treatment are noted.) A competent APN has developed good diagnostic skills and is comfortable with assessment, diagnosis, and plan development. Little consultation time is required, and this individual functions at a productive level, being able to see larger numbers of patients each day. In a practice where patients are seen repeatedly, he or she knows the patients and their likely responses, including what they may or may not be willing to do in response to a particular treatment plan. The competent nurse is able to accept such responses and treat on that basis (i.e., he or she has learned that most people do not do all the right things just because they know they should or because they are told to do them.)

Competent APNs may not recognize their own limitations and fail to refer when it is indicated because they are quickly building self-confidence from successful experience. This level nurse practitioner (NP) may enjoy being a preceptor for students and being in a challenging work environment. APNs often reach this level in the 2 to 3 years that Benner suggests is average for individuals to become competent.

Proficient

Proficiency is the transition from competent to expert (Benner, Tanner, & Chesla, 1996). A proficient APN perceives situations as a whole and works with more speed and flexibility than a competent nurse. These APNs have learned, from experience, what typical events to expect in a given situation and are aware when deviations from normal are present. "Maxims" and long-term goals of patients guide the performances of proficient practitioners. In treating patients, a proficient APN considers less options and focuses correctly on the relevant area of the problem; this reflects acquisition of nuances in practice (maxims). Proficient nurses may feel that the theory underlying their practice is "useless" and express their devaluing of the educational process. Benner states this level can be reached in 3 to 5 years in non–advanced practice roles, particularly if an individual works with similar patient groups. While this appears to also be a useful benchmark for advanced practice roles, continuing research specific to the APN role is needed.

Proficient APNs are able to quickly derive a diagnosis, and they order fewer and more pertinent tests. They may function in a true "medical model" mode, seeing large numbers of patients and treating the essentials safely and efficiently, but with less time spent on activities such as detailed heath education. Proficient APNs generally make good decisions quickly and may question why they did not go to medical school. They may ask, "Who has time for nursing theory at this pace?" Proficient APN practitioners work well in a fast-paced, varied practice with challenging cases; they can become bored by the "same old" routine. Proficient APN practitioners do well in acute care "hospitalist" type roles. While they can make good preceptors for less-skilled individuals, they may have a tendency to be negative towards their educational process and the theory component of practice.

Expert

Expert practitioners have an "intuitive" grasp of many situations and quickly identify and treat the accurate area of the problem with limited consideration of a larger range of options. Not all practitioners achieve this level of functioning. It is very difficult to capture all the steps in the process of highly skilled human performance, and expert nurses often have difficulty explaining actions and decisions on a step-by-step basis. The basis for the "intuitive" knowledge is particularly difficult to describe because it is the result of a continual integration of experience and knowledge. Experience, in this context, does not mean the passing of time; it is the ongoing refinement of understandings, perceptions, and theory through many actual encounters with patients. The nuances labeled "intuitive" result from the perfected skills of observation, data interpretation, and validation certain practitioners display in practice. While experts may experience difficulty in describing rationale, they describe the outcomes achieved and the goals established for patients with clarity (Sheehy, McCarthy, Walsh, & Bernhard, 1998).

Expert APNs perform a wide variety of functions and activities well. They possess the skills of proficient APNs and have the added skills of "knowing" when something is not right and "sensing" when more exists in a situation than is obvious. This level of APN is highly skilled in knowing how and when to ask key questions and elicit pertinent data. Experts tend to use many cues and labels that are more abstract in their categorization. Experts are often "insiders," describing a situation as if they are a part of a patient's story (Itano, 1991). Experts tend to take pleasure in teaching others and may be catalyst mentors for competent or proficient practitioners. Experts exhibit behaviors that are directed at improving practice and adding to the scientific base of practice.

Developing the Advanced Practice Nursing Role

A formal, step-by-step model of decision-making in advanced practice, one that lays bare the complete explanation of a decision, would be very attractive if it were possible to accomplish. Beyond the novice level, however, the complexity in thinking and information-processing

by the human brain is beyond the current understandings of science. In those areas where skill can be objectively assessed (e.g., flying an airplane, playing chess, driving a car), the similarity-based, situational understanding used by an experienced human being leads to better performance than does the formal approach of context-free rules used most often by novices and advanced beginners. The point at which an APN has integrated sufficient experience in a particular area to outperform a "formal rules" model is not clear; the decision to trust one's own knowledge and skill is an individual one and related to one's sense of self-preparedness.

What should the nurse in advanced practice do in a situation of equally attractive alternatives? The generally suggested advice is to seek further information and the advice of trusted peers. Often in advanced practice, situations present without obvious resolutions. Sharing of expertise and a mutual and cultivated system of colleague support is important to the development of all levels of APNs. Continual, deliberate attention to evaluation of one's own learning and knowledge acquisition is also critical for nurses in advanced practice to move through the stages of skill acquisition described by Dreyfuss and Dreyfuss (1980) and Benner (1984).

In evaluating progression through the stages, special attention should be given the initial employment opportunity. Novice APNs, whose initial work environments are hostile, experience escalated self-doubts and delays in building confidence and competence. The drain in time and energy needed to deal with coworkers unsupportive of the APN role delays the progression of novice APNs significantly (Brown & Olshanky, 1998).

PRIORITIES FOR RESEARCH

The three major changes that occur as proficiency levels advance are changes in paradigm, perception, and level of engagement (Sheehy et al, 1998). Research studies are needed in the resource and strategy combinations most beneficial to facilitate the progression of APNs through these changes. Benchmarks for self-evaluation and peer evaluation should be refined in terms of clinically significant outcomes. Whether the Benner model or other models (such as the one proposed by Muscari and Kasar [1997]) are used, career planning and development can be facilitated by studies that increase understanding of how APNs progress in their acquisition of skills and understanding. Brykczynski (1989) defined *clinical wisdom* as a global integration of the body of knowledge that develops when theoretical concepts and practical understanding are refined with actual experience. The process of acquiring clinical wisdom is a complex one, and an understanding of differences in the acquisition of skills specific to the development of APN roles requires specifically targeted studies.

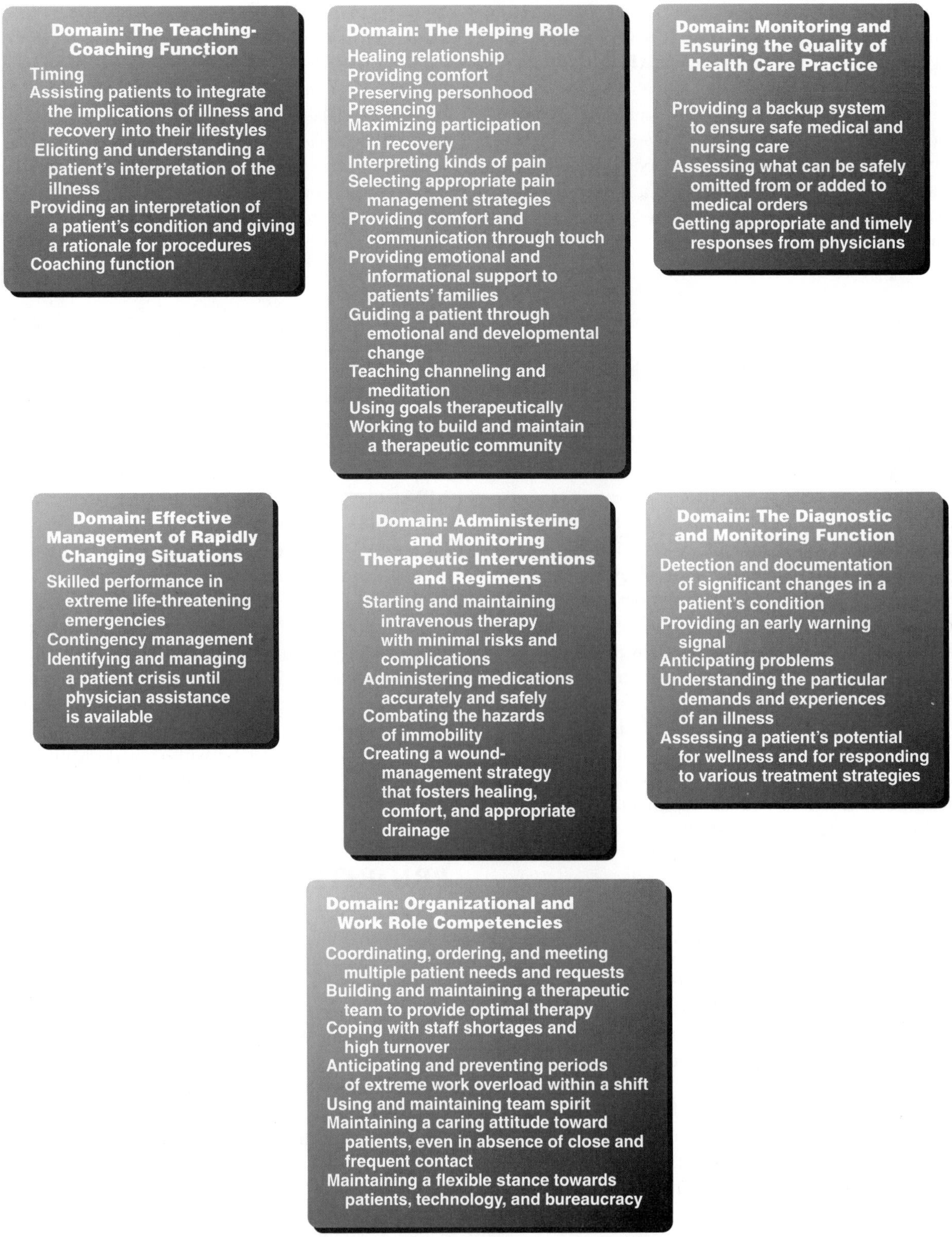

Domain: The Teaching-Coaching Function

Timing
Assisting patients to integrate the implications of illness and recovery into their lifestyles
Eliciting and understanding a patient's interpretation of the illness
Providing an interpretation of a patient's condition and giving a rationale for procedures
Coaching function

Domain: The Helping Role

Healing relationship
Providing comfort
Preserving personhood
Presencing
Maximizing participation in recovery
Interpreting kinds of pain
Selecting appropriate pain management strategies
Providing comfort and communication through touch
Providing emotional and informational support to patients' families
Guiding a patient through emotional and developmental change
Teaching channeling and meditation
Using goals therapeutically
Working to build and maintain a therapeutic community

Domain: Monitoring and Ensuring the Quality of Health Care Practice

Providing a backup system to ensure safe medical and nursing care
Assessing what can be safely omitted from or added to medical orders
Getting appropriate and timely responses from physicians

Domain: Effective Management of Rapidly Changing Situations

Skilled performance in extreme life-threatening emergencies
Contingency management
Identifying and managing a patient crisis until physician assistance is available

Domain: Administering and Monitoring Therapeutic Interventions and Regimens

Starting and maintaining intravenous therapy with minimal risks and complications
Administering medications accurately and safely
Combating the hazards of immobility
Creating a wound-management strategy that fosters healing, comfort, and appropriate drainage

Domain: The Diagnostic and Monitoring Function

Detection and documentation of significant changes in a patient's condition
Providing an early warning signal
Anticipating problems
Understanding the particular demands and experiences of an illness
Assessing a patient's potential for wellness and for responding to various treatment strategies

Domain: Organizational and Work Role Competencies

Coordinating, ordering, and meeting multiple patient needs and requests
Building and maintaining a therapeutic team to provide optimal therapy
Coping with staff shortages and high turnover
Anticipating and preventing periods of extreme work overload within a shift
Using and maintaining team spirit
Maintaining a caring attitude toward patients, even in absence of close and frequent contact
Maintaining a flexible stance towards patients, technology, and bureaucracy

Figure 24-1 Benner's domains and competencies for nursing practice. (From Benner, P [1984]. *From novice to expert.* Upper Saddle River, NJ: Prentice-Hall.)

In designing studies, Benner's (1984) seven domains of nursing practice may be a useful construct (Figure 24-1). Benner defines a *domain* as a cluster of competencies. The seven she identifies are: effective management of rapidly changing situations, administering and monitoring therapeutic interventions, the helping role, diagnosis and monitoring, teaching-coaching, monitoring and ensuring quality, and organizational and work-role competencies. Acquisition of skill in each of these domains does not occur simultaneously. Studies aimed at more fully understanding the acquisition of "clinical wisdom" could be designed using these seven conceptual categories.

IMPLICATIONS FOR MSN EDUCATION AND ADVANCED PRACTICE

Practice models can serve a variety of purposes, including giving direction to educational programs and providing direction for theory development (Styles, 1996). One of the most useful components of the "novice to expert" model is the acknowledgment that at these various stages of skill acquisition, different strategies are indicated for optimal learning. Benner (1994) notes that competent, proficient, and expert practitioners may find the strategies used to help novices and advanced beginners cumbersome and unnecessarily redundant. Novices and advanced beginners need support and guidance in aspect recognition, while competent nurses have mastered more routine clinical situations but benefit from decision-making exercises and simulations that give practice in managing less common and more complex situations. Proficient nurses have already achieved comfort with many differing patient situations, so one strategy for their further education is to use complex case studies. Using patient situations from a proficient nurse's practice that he or she felt did not result in a desired outcome is one source of such case studies.

Expert clinicians benefit from reflection on situations they have found challenging and in systematic documentation of their performances. This analysis contributes to the generation of researchable clinical problems and aids in an understanding of problem-solving in complex and ambiguous clinical situations. Experts can provide consultation, and their own learning can benefit as they validate their understanding with other experts.

Since career-long learning and the continued development of the scientific basis for practice are role expectations for nurses in advanced practice, practice models are appropriate for initial programs and for programs delivered to more advanced practitioners. New students benefit from knowing about practice models in establishing realistic goals for their early years of practice, while also using practice models as benchmarks for themselves.

Suggestions for Further Learning

- Interview APNs in other specialties and peers in your area. Explore with them their perceptions of how they have progressed through the stages of novice to expert. What factors in practice facilitated or inhibited their progression?
- Keep a journal during your first year of clinical practice to follow your progression through the challenges of the first year. Compare the trends from your journal with those cited in Brown, M., & Olshansky, E. (1998). Becoming a primary care nurse practitioner: challenges of the initial year of practice. *The Nurse Practitioner, 23*(7), 46-66.

DISCUSSION QUESTIONS

These questions can be used to promote critical thinking and encourage discussion.

1. Discuss situations in practice you consider to have been good learning experiences. What made the experiences good ones? How could you engineer similar learning experiences for yourself or a colleague?
2. Evaluate how you like to learn and identify learning situations where you are uncomfortable. Articulate your answers to a colleague.
3. Everyone is a novice at one time or another. How can the legitimization of novices and their safe initiation into advanced practice be accomplished?
4. Continued competency is defined in various ways. Define what an APN can do to assess self-competency.
5. Evaluate your current level of functioning using Benner's model. Identify three strategies that would assist you in moving to the next level of the model.

REFERENCES/BIBLIOGRAPHY

Benner. P. (1984). *From novice to expert*. Upper Saddle River, NJ: Prentice-Hall.

Benner, P. (1994). The role of articulation in understanding practice and experience as sources of knowledge in clinical nursing. In Tully, J. (Ed.), *Philosophy in an age of pluralism: the philosophy of Charles Taylor in question*. New York: Cambridge University Press.

Benner, P. (1998). *Expertise in nursing practice: caring, clinical judgment and ethics*. New York: Springer.

Benner, P. (1999). Claiming the wisdom and worth of clinical practice. *Nursing and Health Care Perspective, 20*(6): 312-319.

Benner, P., Hooper-Kyriakidis, P.L., & Stannard, D. (1998). *Clinical wisdom and interventions in critical care: a thinking-in-action approach*. Philadelphia: WB Saunders.

Benner, P., Tanner, C., & Chelsla, C. (1996). *Expertise in nursing practice*. New York: Springer.

Benner, P., & Wrubel, J. (1988). *The primacy of caring: stress and coping in health and illness*. Menlo Park, CA: Addison-Wesley.

Brown, M., & Olshansky, E. (1998). Becoming a primary care nurse practitioner: challenges of the initial year of practice. *The Nurse Practitioner, 23*(7), 46-66.

Brykczynski, K. (1989). An interpretive study describing the clinical judgment of nurse practitioners. *Scholarly Inquiry for Nursing Practice: An International Journal, 3*(2), 75-103.

Dreyfus, H., & Dreyfus, S. (1986). *Mind over machine: the power of human intuition and expertise in the era of the computer*. New York: Free Press.

Itano, J. (1991). The organization of clinical knowledge in novice and expert nurses (No. PUZ9215018). *Dissertation Abstracts International*.

McGregor, R. (1991). *Expert practice and career progression in selected clinical nurse specialists* (No. PUZ9214586). Virginia Polytechnic University.

Muscari, M., & Kasar, J. (1997). Professional behaviors in nurse practitioners. *The Nurse Practitioner, 22*(6), 199-208.

Rubin, J. (1996). Impediments to the development of clinical knowledge and ethical judgment in critical care nursing. In P. Benner, C. Tanner, & C. Chesla (Eds.), *Expertise in nursing practice: caring, clinical judgement and ethics* (pp. 170-192). New York: Springer.

Sheehy, C., McCarthy, M., Walsh, M., & Bernhard, L. (1998). Selected theories and models for advanced practice nursing, In C. Sheehy & M. McCarthy (Eds.), *Advanced practice nursing: emphasizing common roles* (pp. 89-113). Philadelphia: FA Davis.

Styles, M. (1996). Conceptualizations of advanced practice nursing practice. In A.B. Hamric, J. Spross, & C. Hanson (Eds.), *Advanced nursing practice: an integrative approach*. Philadelphia: WB Saunders.

Tanner, C., Benner, P., Chesla, C., & Gordon, S. (1993). The phenomenology of knowing a patient. *Image, 25*(4), 273-280.

Taylor, C. (1994): Philosophical reflections on caring practices. In S. Phillips & P. Benner (Eds.), *The crisis of care: affirming and restoring caring practices in the helping professions* (pp. 174-187). Washington DC: Georgetown University Press.

Chapter 25

Role Performance Evaluation

Cheryl Pope Kish

Within the contemporary health care arena, there is a demand for extracting maximal benefit from each dollar and for accountability to improve access, promote quality, increase optimal outcomes, and contain costs. At the same time, health care providers are grappling with a paradigm shift to a service orientation. In a marketplace fraught with competition, there is a new demand for a competitive edge that exemplary customer/patient service can give. To meet today's demands, it is imperative to evaluate provider performance and the way in which it affects service, cost, and health outcomes. Because advanced practice nurses (APNs) are still pioneering this level of care in some communities and clinical enterprises, the potential exists for the performance of individuals to reflect either positively or negatively on APNs in general. Increasingly important, performance evaluation is a means by which APNs can demonstrate their unique value to a practice setting and show that they are, in fact, making an obvious difference. In this last decade, the concept of outcome-managed care has presented an unparalleled avenue for APNs to determine exactly and comprehensively in what ways their work affects the lives of patients, families, aggregates and communities as *nurses*—not "mini-doctors" (Galvan, 1999).

In a manner unlike at any other time in history, there is a different level of outcome surveillance being imposed from sources external to clinical practice. The National Committee on Quality Assurance (NCQA), a nonprofit consumer-oriented organization that accredits health plans and reports data on quality, collects data on selected measures of health outcomes according to the Health Plan Employer Data and Information Set (HEDIS). According to the NCQA website, HEDIS is designed to focus on significant concerns to public health and now measures health care aspects of the leading causes of premature death in the United States: cardiovascular disease, cancer, asthma, pneumonia, influenza, and diabetes, which collectively account for 1.6 million deaths annually. HEDIS details are updated annually, with additional expectations of more providers being added to the list. APNs in primary care who engage in evaluation of outcomes at the practice level are positioned well as more external evaluation is imposed. This is because they can use their evaluation findings to modify areas that will yield improvements in practice and have data sets to substantiate the reasons for and results of such improvements (Buppert, 2000).

APNs will have a "voice" in many performance evaluations within the clinical area, not just their own. They will likely have occasion to evaluate peers, staff, and students and to negotiate employment contracts that clearly delineate the evaluation system in place; they may suggest modifications if needed. For these reasons, these advanced clinicians need an understanding of the methods of evaluation.

DEFINITIONS

Evaluation is the process of delineating, obtaining, and providing useful information for judging decision alternatives (Stufflebeam, 1971). The word itself, *evaluation*, indicates placing value. *Measurement* is the process of assigning a rating based on data collected from reliable evaluation instruments that can serve decision-makers. Data may be quantitative, qualitative, or mixed. *Quantitative data* refers to facts and claims represented by numbers from rating scales, checklists, and audits, while *qualitative data* describes facts and interpretations presented in narrative rather than numerical form and subjected to careful scrutiny to ensure supportable interpretation. A combination of the two adds credence to the evaluation results. *Formative evaluation* occurs at some time during performance when feedback has the potential to alter behavior. Formative evaluation can occur with a nod across an examination table or a comment at the end of a clinical day or week, so long as there is still opportunity to improve before a final decision is made. *Summative evaluation* is conducted at the conclusion of a particular performance and serves as a summary of behaviors on which decisions may be made about the effectiveness or efficiency of performance, retention of knowledge, rewards (e.g., salary adjustment, bonuses), or ways to improve the outcomes of care.

Evaluation, as a type of applied research, may be either norm-referenced or criterion-referenced. In norm-referenced evaluation, performance is compared between one individual and others, contributing to a bell-shaped curve with outliers at the extremes of exemplary and poor performance and the majority of scores clustered around the mean, which indicates average performance. When a criterion-based evaluation is used, performance is compared to a standard or criterion, such as expectations in the job description or the professional standards of care (hopefully both).

CRITICAL ISSUES: EXPLORING MODELS OF PERFORMANCE EVALUATION

Systematic evaluation has as its intended end the judgment of one's adequacy to perform the tasks, fulfill the role expectations, and exercise the requirements associated with a particular role. The bedrock purpose of performance evaluation for APNs is the improvement of clinical practice; all other ends are collateral to that purpose. Performance evaluation is time consuming and potentially burdens an already busy practice. Consequently, there must be commitment to the process, irrespective of the model in use.

Performance evaluation represents only a sample of the cognitive abilities, skills, and values inherent in the "daily" of APN practice. Ideally, the evaluation is representative of what occurs within the privacy of the closed-door examination room or at a patient's bedside. Evaluation should be impartial and fair, with meticulous data collection and indisputable evidence—not rumor, invective, or praise that lacks support. A valid evaluation is one that represents reality. In a reliable evaluation, a performance is seen in the same way by a variety of sources. Stufflebeam (1971) maintains that evaluation is not just to prove, but to improve. Performance evaluation, then, is predicated on the notion that every professional is capable of improving performance and willing to make the effort to do so.

Most of the models for evaluation were developed in educational settings and were designed to structure program evaluation. If one uses the definition of "program" as any on-going activity designed to produce specific changes in behavior of individuals exposed to it (Waltz, Chambers, & Hechenberger, 1989), it has relevance to advanced practice nursing. Certainly, the APN's role performance produces changes in the health care of patients and in the health care system itself.

Two evaluation models from education are particularly compelling for performance evaluation in advanced practice: Stake's Countenance Model (1973) and Stufflebeam's CIPP Model (1971, 1980, 1983). Although these approaches to evaluation were proposed several decades ago, they remain useful for contemporary practice.

In the Countenance Model, two chief operations, description and judgment, are based on a formal inquiry

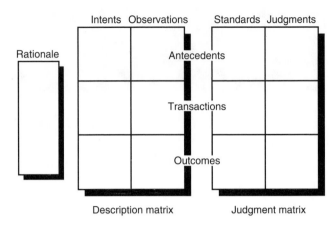

Figure 25-1 Stake's Countenance Model, which depicts the statements and data required for evaluation. (From Popham, W.J. [1975]. *Educational evaluation.* Upper Saddle River, NJ: Prentice-Hall.)

process (Figure 25-1). Stake designed an evaluation matrix with the potential for finding contingencies between three factors: antecedents; processes; and outcomes and congruence between the intent (performance goals) and observations of what actually occurred. Antecedents are those characteristics of the individual and practice setting in existence before encounters with patients; they include such factors as the practitioner's knowledge, skill mix, credentials, motivation, and resourcefulness and the resources at the practitioner's command for affecting patient care. Transactions are the actual processes of caregiving, teaching, supporting, and providing anticipatory guidance that occur during countless encounters with patients. Outcomes are the effects or results that are short- or long-term consequences of care provided by an APN. Stake's model is sometimes called *patient-centered* because of the value with which he views stakeholders' input into the evaluation process. Patient surveys that address perceptions of their care by an APN fit well into this model.

Stufflebeam's decision-oriented evaluation, or CIPP model, is intended to be employed proactively (formatively) to improve performance and retroactively to judge performance, for the specific purpose of decision-making (Figure 25-2). Four types of evaluation—context, input, process, and product—are included. In the language of role performance of the APN, context evaluation determines unmet needs and problems in the context of the practice and provides a rationale for specific practice goals.

Input evaluation provides details about what resources are available and how they should be used on behalf of patients. (Cost-benefit analyses are sometimes a focus here.) The key to process evaluation is to judge the efficiency and effectiveness of the processes of care, identifying exemplars and deficiencies. Product evaluation involves measuring and interpreting the extent to which goals were attained. The CIPP model is a cyclic process that seems familiar because it is very much like the nursing process (Galvan, 1999). To fully appreciate this point, an APN has only to examine each step fully.

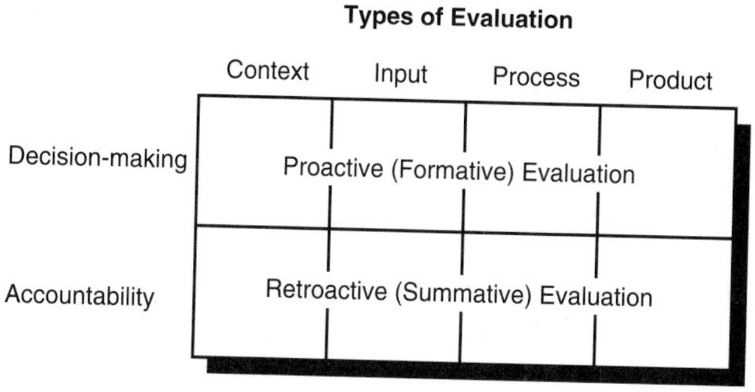

Types of Evaluation

	Context	Input	Process	Product
Decision-making	Proactive (Formative) Evaluation			
Accountability	Retroactive (Summative) Evaluation			

Figure 25-2 Stufflebeam's framework for relating the CIPP model to the formative and summative roles of evaluation. (From Popham, W.J. [1975]. *Educational evaluation.* Upper Saddle River, NJ: Prentice-Hall).

Context Evaluation

The context evaluation stage begins when a problem arises or a need for change becomes obvious to either those within a health care setting or to external constituencies like accrediting agencies, consumer groups, or individual patients (and now the NCQA). The problem is examined carefully through needs-assessment surveys. What are the needs of those involved? What are the features of the health care environment—the strengths and limitations of the human, physical, and financial resources? What services already exist? Are they being utilized efficiently and effectively? Are they being marketed to those who would most profit from them? Are there resources in the community (e.g., programs, services, providers) to whom referrals may be made? What might be done to solve the identified problem or meet the need? The endpoint of context evaluation is identification of priorities for action (Stufflebeam, 1983).

A need for context evaluation became evident at Central City Health Services, a primary care clinic, when a team of APNs noted that the numbers of diabetic patients in the practice had increased precipitously. Moving quickly to assess the context of the situation, the APNs, in collaboration with physicians and staff, designed and implemented a series of surveys. Through patient interviews, written surveys, random chart audits, careful attention to utilization of space, and a time-use study, the team discovered a patient knowledge deficit about diabetes self-management that was not being met by the clinic's existing services. On the basis of these findings, a contemplative team decision was made that these priorities for action existed:

1. A need for space and educational materials devoted to better educating diabetic patients about the disease and self-management
2. A need for better documentation to facilitate consistency for evaluation of outcomes for diabetic patients

3. A need for an increased knowledge base of key providers related to educating diabetic patients, both individually and collectively, about the disease and self-management
4. A need for an approach to empower diabetic patients in self-management

As Galvan (1999) suggests, data collection does not end in the context phase of the process. As in the nursing process, assessment continues throughout other stages of evaluation; however, at this stage, a diagnosis of a problem or need has been derived from the data. At Central City Health Systems, the diagnosis was this: self-management of diabetes mellitus in partnership with health care providers does not exist in this setting to the extent that it should, and there is a limited educational enterprise to inform and empower patients for a patient-provider partnership that will result in better health. The key question for the team was, "If we better educate and empower our diabetic patients for self-management, will their health outcomes improve?" Because the staff believed that the answer was a resounding "yes," starting input evaluation was justified.

Input Evaluation

With the list of priorities in hand and an ongoing commitment to evaluation, the next evaluative steps begin to guide the choice of a specific strategy for intervention. In this stage, evaluators seek guidance from "authorities" to inform their decisions about changes in policy, procedures, and practices. Authorities may be theoretical or empirical literature; unpublished research findings; written standards of practice; protocols; organizations; and experienced clinicians, managers, and other professionals. Guidance may also come from additional chart audits, patient surveys, onsite research, and consultation with other providers who have attempted to resolve similar problems. This stage of evaluation ends with the selection of a specific plan to resolve the existing problem. Evaluators consider alternative possibilities and choose the most sound, reasonable, cost-effective plan that has the greatest probability of success for the particular setting (Stufflebeam, 1983).

At Central City Health Systems, input evaluation involved the following actions by APNs, physicians, and staff:

1. Contacting the American Diabetes Association, consumer groups, and drug company representatives for patient education materials (e.g., printed, audiotapes, videotapes, computer-assisted materials)
2. Consulting a local architect about renovating unused office space for a patient education library
3. Carefully reviewing the standards of care related to diabetes management
4. Inviting a certified diabetes educator from the local medical center to a dinner meeting to gain his input

5. Designing a chart form to facilitate better documentation of various aspects of self-management and patient teaching and learning
6. Reviewing continuing education brochures and college catalogs for seminars and courses related to teaching and empowering diabetic patients for partnered self-management
7. Locating free foot-check filaments for each patient from the National Primary Care Clearinghouse
8. Planning for a cost-accountable educational program

Process Evaluation

The devised plan having now been implemented, process evaluation involves judging its implementation via predetermined feedback mechanisms. Careful documentation is important because accurate records reward success and encourage and inform others who wish to implement similar strategies (Stufflebeam, 1983).

At Central City Health Systems, the interventions being evaluated included the following:

1. Conversion of an unused clinic room for patient education, with shelves for books, tapes, brochures, and a VCR for patient and family use during clinic visits
2. Support of the practice's clinical nurse specialist (CNS) through release time and funding as she obtained credentials as a certified diabetic educator
3. Provision of tuition and 4 hours per week of release time for the adult nurse practitioner (NP) to enroll in a group dynamics course at the local college with the intent of joining the CNS in co-leading a support/education group for diabetic patients in the practice
4. Pilot-testing the new chart form, which documents outcome measures associated with well-controlled diabetes (e.g., self–blood glucose monitoring [SBGM], glycosylated hemoglobin [Hgb A1C], daily foot inspection, yearly eye examination), and checklist indicating educational efforts
5. Ensuring that each diabetic receives a foot filament and instructions for its use

Product Evaluation

In the product evaluation part of the overall evaluation, desired outcomes are measured through supporting evidence. Results are used to make decisions about continuing, revisiting, or terminating an intervention and/or the need for additional measures. Each previous step of the evaluation is reviewed, and a recycling process is possible. Results of the intervention are documented (Stufflebeam, 1983). In the Central City experience, outcomes associated with the support group, presence of a certified diabetes educator on staff, new tools and expectations for documentation of patient care, and educational efforts were measured.

In the nursing process, assessment determines a patient's status upon entering the nurse-patient relationship; evaluation determines the difference the nursing interventions have made in a patient's status. At this point, the stage is set for assessment to begin again because the context is different than it was at the beginning of the relationship. The same is true for CIPP evaluation; product evaluation ends with patients or systems existing in a different context than where they began, meaning that context evaluation is justified once more. (Table 25-1 indicates some key questions addressed in each step of CIPP evaluation.)

Although education's evaluation models are obviously useful for nursing, as seen in the Central City example, knowledge of a nursing-specific model adds a helpful dimension to an APN's evaluation repertoire. As early as 1989, Waltz, a name synonymous with evaluation in nursing, wrote "The imperative is clear: nurses must be accountable not only for quality care, but also for providing important audiences with evidence that nursing *does* make a difference" (Waltz, Chambers, & Hechenberger, 1989).

The components of the Waltz evaluation model, framed in the context of APN practice, are as follows:

- *Inputs*—Knowledge, skills, values, aspirations, purposes, and philosophies of APNs as providers; characteristics of participants in each encounter between patients and APNs; human, time, financial, and physical resources available to the health care enterprise
- *Processes*—Procedures, policies, and philosophies; actions and interactions in behalf of a patient, whether it

Table 25-1

Questions Asked at Each Stage of CIPP Evaluation

Context evaluation	Where are we with respect to "X"?
	Where do we need to be?
	What are the priorities to get us there?
Input evaluation	How do we get where we need to be?
	Who or what can help us?
Process evaluation	What evidence exists that this plan is working to get us where we hope to be?
Product evaluation	Did we end up where we hoped to be with respect to "X"?
	What worked? What did not work?
	What should change? How?
	What should stay the same?
	What is the context of problem "X" now?

is an individual, family, aggregate, community, or entire society; approaches by those who administer practice and provide care

- *Outcomes*—Results of actions to affect health on the part of APNs, framed in a way to allow decision-making by internal or external stakeholders of the practice

Waltz (1989) advises the use of a master plan for systematic evaluation, with specificity necessary to decision-makers. This master plan should specify the following aspects of evaluation, irrespective of the model used:

- *Who*—What individual or group is charged with oversight of each aspect of the evaluation process and assumes ultimate accountability? Who will amass the data? Who will report findings?
- *What*—What individual or group will need to use the data to make decisions? What components of practice will be addressed (e.g., access, quality, cost, patient satisfaction or perception)? What population will be considered?
- *Why*—What is the purpose of the evaluation? Is it formative? Summative? For what decision? Performance appraisal? Policy or procedure change? Management decision? Purchase decision? Is the evaluation proactive or reactive to some particular problem?
- *How*—What data sources and instruments are to be used in data collection? What evidence exists that these instruments are reliable, valid, trustworthy, and credible for that purpose? Are the instruments sensitive enough to capture even small levels of progress toward a particular goal or outcome?
- *When*—What is the timeline for evaluation? What is a reasonable measurement point for showing progress toward the goal? When will specific data be collected (e.g., at every patient visit, monthly, annually)?

The fundamental components of accountability and comprehensive management of quality health care are addressed by Juran (1993) in the idea of total quality management (TQM), a type of evaluation system that assumes every process can be improved. The TQM model advises structure, process, outcome evaluation, and the inclusion of criteria or standards in the evaluative process; for the first time, it also includes third-party payment and the percentage of reimbursable cases as an issue for consideration. Although the definition of *structure evaluation* was not significantly changed from other models, now process and outcome evaluation address issues of productivity; changes in health status, morbidity and mortality; cost-effectiveness; patient satisfaction; and practitioner job satisfaction. Quality management demands measurement and ideally captures the "voices" of stakeholders in the practice. Appropriate measures to that end include chart audits, peer review, patient surveys and interviews, and self-evaluation. This model can demon-

strate the uniqueness each level provider brings to the processes and outcomes of care, and it is particularly valuable for APNs, who are still pioneers in some communities.

Hamric (1989) delineated a model for patient care evaluation by CNSs based on the notion of quality improvement. In the Hamric model, outcome evaluation has prominence because improved outcomes are the reason for advanced practice. While the traditional outcomes of access, quality, and cost are assessed, Hamric suggests that outcome evaluation also reflect the end results of the relationships between APNs and patients.

IMPLICATIONS FOR MSN EDUCATION AND ADVANCED PRACTICE

Regardless of the model used to structure evaluation, certain guidelines are useful to the process. An APN may need to negotiate an evaluation system that follows these guidelines as a point of employment.

1. As in educational settings, there is a time for learning and a time for evaluation; the person being evaluated needs to know which is which.
2. Predetermined criteria are used unless special circumstances indicate that additions should be made.
3. Results of an evaluation are shared in a timely manner; delays in feedback weaken the evaluation system. Confidentiality is ensured. Results are stored in a personnel file with the guarantee of privacy.
4. Any criterion of evaluation that rates as "unsatisfactory" or "needs improvement" is supported by a narrative rationale, and either the written statement or a discussion with the evaluator leads to suggestions for correcting any deficient areas of performance.
5. With evaluation comes a commitment to help one improve identified weaknesses as well as ongoing professional development.
6. Criteria used for evaluation are directly and clearly related to effective and efficient job performance and issues of cost, quality, access, and patient satisfaction. Standards against which one is judged should reflect the mission statement of the practice and the job description of the clinician, as well as support the *Scope and Standards of Advanced Practice Registered Nursing* (American Nurses Association [ANA], 1996).
7. Procedures for evaluation are mutually agreed upon by both the APN and the employer. There are opportunities for the individual to have an ongoing "voice" in the evaluation process.
8. Multiple sources of data are used for evaluation, and the APN's performance is judged not on an isolated event but on trends of behavior. An exception exists in cases

where patient safety and other areas with legal implications are a concern.

9. Evaluation of role performance for this level of provider should be conducted by an employer, not an office manager who would not understand the intricacies of advanced nursing.

Novice APNs often report to former faculty that one of the frustrations of their initial employment is a lack of feedback concerning performance in the role. At school, timely feedback comes in many forms (e.g., examinations; verbal and written faculty feedback on papers, projects, and clinical performance), and there is an inevitable comparison of self with classmates. Without feedback, the early days of "feeling one's way" in a new role can be a time of insecurity. Not surprisingly, a new APN latches onto every positive patient comment as a way to gauge progress, and he or she commonly reviews a day's clinical performance in his or her mind. Subjective feelings of increasing mastery constitute early role identification. It is helpful, though, to initiate early dialogue with others in the practice to gauge role performance from their perspective. In most settings, the initial formal evaluation occurs after 6 months at the earliest.

Typically, evaluations occur annually after that. Goal-setting is often an annual activity coinciding with evaluation and may accompany a self-evaluation (sometimes called an *annual report*). It is important to demonstrate early and often those ways in which one has had a positive effect or provided a competitive advantage for the practice. Have the numbers of patients increased? Have additional clinic hours outside the traditional schedule been added? Have the physicians or other partners had more opportunities for time off or professional development? Have positive outcomes been noted in target patient groups? Are patients referring friends and family members to the practice because of excellent care? Has education to the community at large increased through the APN's outreach services? Have other settings been added? Are patients being seen who would otherwise not receive care (e.g., the poor, minorities, homeless, the disenfranchised)?

The APN may wish to compile an evaluation portfolio containing multiple sources of data showing evidence of role performance. Several common data sources include self-evaluation; peer evaluation; patient surveys; a list of the numbers and classifications of patients seen; data about the percentage of reimbursement; and chart audits. Cards and letters from patients affirming good care can also be added to the portfolio, as can performance checklists or rating scales that allow for quantifiable data. Most nursing research texts have sections on designing such instruments.

Self-Evaluation

Reviewing one's clinical performance for purposes of self-evaluation is an essential task in quality improve-

ment and professional accountability. Hopefully, a newly employed APN gained experience in self-evaluation in his or her Master's program. Too often, a novice tends to produce a long list of deficiencies. It is human nature to focus on areas of inadequacy and remember in detail those times of feeling unprepared, to grieve over the number of times questions were asked or guidance was sought in areas one "should have known." However, it is important to review performance candidly, identifying both strengths and limitations as well as areas needing continued development. A strategic plan for addressing any deficiencies is also appropriate.

Each role should be addressed in the evaluation, and input, process, and outcomes should receive attention. This is not a time for modesty, which may lend a false sense of security and imply that no decision is needed. To create a criterion-based evaluation, an APN can use criteria from the job description or reflect on the *Scope and Standards of Advanced Practice Registered Nursing* (ANA, 1996). Data related to how many patients have been seen and how much revenue has been generated for the practice can be addressed in the self-evaluation, as can committee service, special projects, supervision of staff, and student preceptorships, which are all evidence of productivity.

Peer Evaluation

Peer evaluation refers to a system by which an experienced peer makes judgments about the effectiveness and efficiency of an APN's care of patients as measured against an *a priori* standard. The primary reason for a peer evaluation system is improvement of patient care. Komelasky, Bridges, Golas, Pence, and Woodard (1997), in discussing a peer review system in their health maintenance organization (HMO), suggest that peer review can be used to: (1) ensure uniformity of practice standards, thus promoting continuity of care; (2) provide standard evaluation for practitioners by the administration and supervising physicians; (3) enable self-regulation of the APN group; (4) provide positive validation of a practitioners' practice; (5) encourage continued learning through peer coaching; and (6) develop computer templates for common diagnoses that can serve as a research base. Sheahan and Simpson (1999) add these benefits of peer evaluation: (1) enabling proactive risk management, (2) encouraging professional interaction and positive validation for practice, and (3) maximizing internal regulation of practice, minimizing external control. Peer review is an important feature of professionalism and continuous quality improvement. It is helpful when both an APN's strengths and his or her limitations are identified by a peer evaluator. However, Barrett-Barrick (1993) warns against a seesaw approach that lists weaknesses and strengths side-by-side to allegedly show balance.

Peer review can be threatening. For that reason, in some settings, peer evaluation is for formative purposes

Criteria	#	#	#	#	#	Comments
S: HPI — seven critical variables documented appropriate to chief complaint						
Allergies listed/response described						
Current drug history documented						
Significant PMH documented						
Significant FH documented						
Diagnostic tests ordered: Appropriate to presenting problem? Most cost-effective?						
O: Focused physical examination appropriate to presenting problem						
A: Appropriate brief list of differentials R/O and identified definitive diagnosis						
P: Medications ordered: Appropriate to diagnosis? Most cost-effective?						
Follow-up instructions documented						
Health promotion suggestions documented						
Patient education documented						
Consultation and/or referral documented						

Diagnosis appropriate? _____ Suggestions for the future: _____

_____

Management approach effective? _____ Suggestions for the future: _____

_____

Documentation comprehensive and legally-prudent? _____ Suggestions for the future: _____

_____

Protocol or national guidelines followed? _____ If no, consultation sought to justify deviations? _____

Overall rating:	Excellent		Very Good		Good		Needs Improvement		Unsatisfactory
	7	6	5		4	3	2	1	0

Signature of Evaluator: _____ Date _____

Figure 25-3 Sample chart audit instrument. *FH,* Family history; *HPI,* history of present illness; *PMH,* past medical history; *R/O,* rule out.

only. The element of friendship can color the value of a peer evaluation; to offset this, a criterion-based checklist is helpful, as are ratings from several peers. Another APN is best able to evaluate the discrete aspects of performance related to patients and adherence to standards. Furthermore, a colleague is in a unique position to spot limitations and aid in their correction. It is helpful to have a meeting between an APN and his or her peer evaluator up front to enable a discussion about particular behaviors on which the individual being evaluated desires feedback. For example, a certified registered nurse anesthetist (CRNA) may wish to have feedback on some aspect of intubation technique or a particular way of communicating with a preoperative patient to support relaxation. A certified nurse midwife (CNM) may ask for feedback on managing women who are experiencing back labor secondary to persistent posterior position of the fetal head. Sheahan and Simpson (1999) believe peer evaluation is made less threatening when APNs have input into developing the measurement instrument and assurances of confidentiality and of corrective measures being addressed privately. These aspects of role performance evaluation may be discussed during the preevaluation meeting as well.

Chart Audits

Charts for a review may be selected at random or may focus on a particular patient population, target diagnosis, or age group (particularly valuable in a child health setting). While a chart audit does not capture all that occurred behind the closed doors of the examination room, by following SOAP format (subjective, objective, assessment, plan), it can demonstrate adherence to standards, precision of diagnosis, attention to health promotion, and effectiveness of the management approach. It can show evidence that targeted behaviors (e.g., violence assessment, "quit smoking" information) are part of every patient's plan of care. The chart audit may be documented by a checklist or quantified in a rating scale. A section for comments is particularly helpful. (Figure 25-3 shows a sample chart audit instrument.)

Patient Satisfaction Reports

In a practice setting with a patient-centered culture, patient satisfaction can be a valuable measure of a practitioner's successful performance. In fact, according to Reidy (1997), in 75% of jobs in the United States, performance is measured by how well customers perceive service and not by products. Baker (1996) reminds NPs that the first 60 seconds of an encounter with a patient is critical to service success. This is also likely true for other types of APNs. While a satisfied patient will tell three to four others about the experience, each dissatisfied patient will tell 10 to 15 others (maybe more) (Reidy, 1997). Word-of-mouth is a

wonderful advertisement; therefore patient satisfaction is sacred. It cannot, however, be the sole measure of performance because of the inherent subjectivity involved.

Most health care providers likely believe that the care they provide is of good quality and satisfying to patients. According to Buppert (2000), there are some indicators that reality, when measured, does not match this perception. "Today it will not be enough to *think* you provide outstanding services and quality medical care. You must take the time to measure quality, outcomes, and patient satisfaction" (Baum & Henkel, 2000).

Patient satisfaction can be evaluated with surveys as simple as anonymous index cards with the question "How am I doing?" written on them, with more elaborate surveys, or with onsite or virtual focus groups, suggestion boxes, and advisory panels. Some evidence of patient satisfaction (e.g., cards, letters, referrals), though not solicited, can be extremely valuable evidence for an evaluator. If a patient perceives the front office staff as cold and impersonal, the wait too long, and the NP hurried, he or she comes away from the encounter with a negative impression that may not have been warranted. For the patient, perception is all there is (Bell & Zemke, 1992). Evaluation instruments should be designed with the constructs of patient satisfaction in mind. (Box 25-1 shows some common aspects of care associated with patient satisfaction.)

Box 25-1

Constructs for Evaluating Patient Satisfaction

- Access at a convenient time, which is not always the conventional times for clinic appointments
- Reasonable wait to be seen, with an apology for unexpected delays; resources available during waits
- Time with the clinician without feeling unduly rushed
- A feeling of welcome, made through smiles, the use of names, eye contact, shaking hands, sitting at the provider's level, and formal introductions if new to each other
- Active listening
- Minimal distractions and interruptions during the visit
- Unconditional acceptance and positive regard
- Recollection of facts about a patient's health and about the patient as a person
- Sacredness of confidentiality
- Follow-up cards or telephone calls
- Using complaints as an opportunity to improve instead of getting defensive
- Comfortable examination rooms
- A tangible "something" to take home (e.g., booklet, medication samples)

Considering Outcomes in Advanced Practice Nursing Evaluation

"Today's consumer is interested in obtaining the highest quality and most easily accessed care with the least amount of time and money invested" (Galvan 1999). For that reason, outcome evaluation must be a part of the systematic plan for ensuring quality care. Buppert (2000) categorizes outcomes as those related to medicine, service, and cost. In Buppert's opinion, medical outcomes include complication rates, improvement in functional status, and attainment of therapeutic goals associated with prescribed treatment measures. To evaluate service outcomes, one must collect data about patient satisfaction, the promptness of attention to abnormal examination findings, and timely responsiveness to telephone calls from patients and families. Patients expect cost outcomes to reveal reasonable and justifiable charges for treatment of illnesses and preventive care; decreasing costs associated with hospitalization, should hospitalization not be preventable; and minimization of emergency room charges.

Outcome evaluation is not new to nursing; it has always been part of the nursing process. For the APN, however, outcomes are a direct measure of accountability because they are linked to particular interventions. Demonstrating a direct link between APN action and outcomes is complicated by the fact that much of care is collaborative in nature and because of the increased savvy of consumers. For example, was it the CNM who positively affected an anemic pregnant patient's diet, or was it a comment by the physician or clinic nurse? Was it a library book on nutrition in pregnancy the patient read? Furthermore, lifestyle variables occurring between the intervention and the outcome often confound the evaluation picture (Gavin, 1999). For example, a NP ordered oral Prandin 30 minutes before each meal, and this was added to the diabetic's other medications. However, the patient failed to have the prescription filled for a week because of an important business trip. He was concerned about the uncertainty of blood glucose changes because self-monitoring would be difficult and mealtimes would be uncertain.

For APNs working in primary care settings, some guidance in outcomes criteria comes from national

---

Table 25-2

Use of HEDIS for Benchmarking in a Primary Care Practice

OUTCOME MEASURE	BENCHMARKS AGAINST WHICH PRIMARY CARE IS EVALUATED
Adolescent immunization status	Second MMR vaccine, third hepatitis B vaccine, and tetanus booster by the age of 13
Antidepressant drug management	Antidepressants prescribed for patients diagnosed with major depression
Smoking cessation counseling	Antismoking advice for patients who smoke
Beta-blocker treatment	Beta blockers (unless contraindicated) after discharge from the hospital following a MI or other acute CV event
Breast cancer screening	Mammograms every 2 years for women between the ages of 52 and 69
Cholesterol screening	LDL cholesterol screening for patients who have had an acute CV event in the past year
Childhood immunizations	Four DPT vaccines, three polio vaccines, one MMR vaccine, one varicella vaccine, two H-influenza type B vaccines, and two hepatitis vaccines by the age of 2
Eye examination for diabetics	Yearly eye examination for diabetic patients
Follow-up of mental health hospitalizations	Outpatient visit with a mental health provider within 30 days of hospital discharge for patients with a diagnosis of schizophrenic or manic depressive illness
Prenatal care in the first trimester	Prenatal visit with a NP, PA, CNM, or physician 176 to 280 days before EDC
High blood pressure	BP remains less than 140/90
Asthma	Appropriate therapy for long-term control for patients with chronic asthma
Chlamydia screening	Screening of sexually active women between the ages of 15 and 25
Cervical cancer screening	Pap smears obtained on time

BP, Blood pressure; *CV*, cardiovascular; *DPT*, diphtheria-pertussis-tetanus; *EDC*, estimated date of confinement; *LDL*, low-density lipoprotein; *MI*, myocardial infarction; *MMR*, measles-mumps-rubella; *PA*, physician assistant.
Data from Buppert, C. (2000). Measuring outcomes in primary care practice. *The Nurse Practitioner*, 25(1), 88-98; and the National Committee on Quality Assurance (www.ncqa.org).

Chart 25-1

Case Study: Performance Evaluation

Claire Kent was a FNP employed with Dr. Perrin Whiteside and his son, Dr. Joe Whiteside. She had been employed with them since graduation from a Master of Science in Nursing (MSN) program and national certification in 1997. Claire's practice site was in a small community. She and Dr. Perrin saw primarily adult patients because Dr. Joe was a pediatrician and saw all the children. In fact, Claire accepted the position for exactly that reason. Claire, who had a special interest in working with patients with diabetes mellitus, asked for a group of diabetic women as a target population for 1 year, hoping to see positive outcomes based on interventions she initiated. Based on the success of her MSN research, which included a support group for women with diabetes, Claire started a support group at the practice last year. She planned to document the outcomes for her target group of patients as part of her annual evaluation, which was planned for the anniversary date of her employment. She hoped the outcome data, in print, would give her the confidence to request an outcome-based bonus. Claire's first year annual evaluation went well but dealt primarily with skill development and efficiency because those were the areas on which she focused as a novice.

This year, Claire has been collecting exact data about her patient volume, both onsite, in the emergency room, and in the nursing home, in addition to the outcome data from her project group. She also has data from her charts (audited at random) and, as an afterthought, decides to Xerox and attach copies of cards and letters from patients and referring providers as evidence of satisfaction with her work.

A friend in graduate school recently shared information about the Waltz Evaluation Model, which Claire decides to use to organize her evaluation this year. Her plan is to write an annual report, using her job description to list criteria on which she wishes to be evaluated. The physicians are in agreement with this approach. They have been extremely pleased with Claire's performance this year and think her contributions to the practice have been remarkable for someone so new to the role.

Following the Waltz Evaluation Model handout from her friend, Claire decides that information about her qualifications and the steps she has taken to improve them fits well under a section she labels "Input Evaluation." The portions of her job description related to implementing her role she places under "Process Evaluation." Evidence related to her patients' health status seems more obvious; this becomes part of her "Outcomes Evaluation." Although she has all the patient data on a matrix, she decides to aggregate the data for her evaluation; if the physicians want to see the raw data, she will have it available. She also compiles a mean from the chart audit scores and reports it. (Figure 25-3 shows the form Claire used for her chart audits.)

Claire begins writing a narrative annual report and, midway through, finds it cumbersome, deciding to prepare a table instead. She divides the table into three sections: Input Evaluation, Process Evaluation, and Outcomes Evaluation. She takes the performance criteria from her job description and places them on the left of her table. Using her updated resume, she pulls out examples that correspond with each criterion. She also transfers the data she has summarized about her diabetic patients to the appropriate evidence column. (Table 25-3 shows Claire's completed evaluation, based on the Waltz Evaluation Model.)

---

standards and from attention to HEDIS criteria. (Table 25-2 shows the way in which HEDIS can be used to benchmark for evaluation in primary care settings.) For APNs who practice in secondary and tertiary care settings, it may be even more difficult to determine in what way their being involved in a particular patient's care affects health care outcomes (Snyder & Mirr, 1995). Certain outcomes may be evaluated by randomly assigning patients who require difficult interventions to different types of providers who can provide these services (Galvin, 1999).

All systematic evaluation is labor intensive; however, outcomes evaluation can be especially so. Evaluators identify a target problem on which to focus; familiarize themselves with standards against which benchmarks may be set; and locate or design instruments with validity, reliability, and trustworthiness for data collection. Charts are audited for baseline data, and a procedure is set for selection of patients for the study group; then a particular,

carefully planned intervention is initiated. Following predetermined measurement points, data are collected and analyzed. Results are used to make decisions about continuing the intervention unchanged or after revision or testing another intervention in its place. "Persons intent on the bottom line will be intensely intolerant" of what they perceive as nonproductive periods during evaluation (Galvan, 1999).

Evaluation of the role performance of an APN begins with a job description that clearly delineates role expectations within the recognized scope of practice. An ideal system includes data collected through the multiple lenses of self-evaluation, peer review, supervisor review, chart audit, and assessment of outcomes (Chart 25-1). Table 25-3 shows a sample performance evaluation for a family nurse practitioner (FNP) that addresses input, process, and outcome variables using Waltz's 1989 model.

Table 25-3	

Sample Performance Evaluation

ROLE EXPECTATIONS FOR JOB PERFORMANCE	EVIDENCE
Input Evaluation Has sound knowledge base for making clinical decisions with families in a primary care setting Maintains current legal authority to practice in Georgia Maintains continued professional development to support knowledge and skill base for practice	• MSN/FNP major, The University of Texas: 1997 • GPA 3.8 on 4.0 scale • FNP Certification: AANP, 1997 • APN License: Georgia Board of Nursing, 1997 Continuing education (1997-98): • Pharmacotherapeutic Update for APNs • Reimbursement Issues for the APN & PA • Women's Health Care in the New Millennium, First National NANPRH Conference
Process Evaluation Provides primary care to adult patients Provides education and support to meet aggregate health needs Participates in research or other scholarly activities	• Managed 2317 adult patients in office setting • On call in ER 400 hours, managing approximately 15 patients every 8 hours (n = 750) • Made "sick call" rounds in nursing home with Dr. Whiteside (n = approximately 200 patients) • Chart audit results: 50 charts at random, with a mean score of 5.88 • Authored four health-related briefs for local newspaper • Presented health-related speeches at the B&PW Club, Senior Citizens Group, and local diabetes chapter • Presented original research (MSN thesis): *The Relationship between Support Group Membership and Compliance in Adult Women with Type 2 Diabetes* at Sigma Theta Tau Research Day at GSU • Professional memberships: Sigma Theta Tau, International and AANP
Outcomes Evaluation Promotes optimal health outcomes in patients (target group [1997-1998] = diabetic women)	Attached for review: • Eight referral notices for diabetic teaching • Four letters from patients • Two thank-you cards from families • Results of patient satisfaction surveys Diabetic women in target group (n = 31) • Mean Hgb A1C: < 7.5% (target < 7%) • Mean annual eye exam: 20 (target 100%) • Mean weight loss: 18.9 pounds • One hospital admission • 6 of 11 quit smoking (target 100%) • No patient had lower extremity ulcers • 29 of 31 had Pap smears (target 100%) • 30 of 31 had mammogram (target 100%)

PRIORITIES FOR RESEARCH

In their descriptive survey related to performance evaluation of APNs, Gregg and Bloom (1999) discovered that 56.9% of their sample of 654 APNs received formal annual evaluations, with 75.9% evaluated by physicians and only 17.5% by peers. The evaluation parameters most fre-quently used for evaluation were appropriateness of care, patient satisfaction, patient volume, and patient outcomes (e.g., clinical endpoints, compliance, complications, functional status). Further study on performance evaluation is warranted.

Many NPs report feeling pressured to see more patients and express concern that the intangibles that make their

Suggestions for Further Learning:

- For information on applying the nurse practitioner rating form in performance evaluation, read the following: Courtney, R., & Rice, C. (1997). Investigation of nurse practitioner-patient interactions: using the nurse practitioner rating form. *The Nurse Practitioner, 22*(2), 46-65; and Prescott, P.A., Jacox, A., Collar, M., & Goodwin, L. (1981). The nurse practitioner rating form—Part I: conceptual development and potential uses. *Nursing Research, 30*(4), 223-227.
- For additional information on evaluating productivity, read Kearnes, D.R. (1992). A productivity tool to evaluate NP practice: monitoring clinical time spent in reimbursable patient-related activities. *The Nurse Practitioner, 17*(4), 50-55.
- For learning more about TQM, contact The Juran Institute at 11 River Road, PO Box 811, Wilton, CT 06897-0811; phone (203) 834-1700; website at www.juran.com.
- For more information on "customer" patient service, read Bell, C., & Zemke, R. (1992). *Managing knock*

your socks off service. New York: American Management Association. Also, consult the management and business section of your local bookstores or library for other sources on customer satisfaction and service that might be applicable to health care.
- For ideas about job descriptions and criteria for performance evaluation, see Smith, M.A. (1996). Job descriptions for primary care nurse practitioners. *The Nurse Practitioner, 21*(5), 160-163.
- For more information about the NCQA and HEDIS, consult the following: Buppert, C. (1999). HEDIS for the primary care provider: getting an "A" on the managed care report card. *Nurse Practitioner, 24*(1), 84-99; and the National Committee on Quality Assurance at www.ncqa.org.
- For information on using focus groups for evaluation, see Baum, N., & Henkel, G. (2000). *Marketing your clinical practice ethically, effectively, economically.* Gaithersburg, MD: Aspen Publishers.

advanced nursing practice unique will suffer as a consequence of having to see more patients during a clinic day. As patient volume increases, research designed to address job satisfaction and patient satisfaction and perceptions of APN care would be advantageous. It is imperative, too, that research focus on what patients perceive as satisfying dimensions of care rather than what providers perceive as appropriate measures of patient satisfaction.

Outcome evaluation must stay focused on the unique care provided by APNs. APNs in primary care settings are well served to audit outcomes guided by HEDIS criteria. All APNs should insist that performance appraisal be driven by their job descriptions and standards of advanced practice and focus on health, cost, access, and satisfaction specific to their practice arenas.

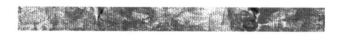

DISCUSSION QUESTIONS

These questions can be used to promote critical thinking and encourage discussion.

1. Answer this set of questions related to your practice as an APN student or provider: Who are your patients or "customers"? What perception of their encounters with

you do you want them to have? How can you contribute to that perception?
2. Respond to the following self-evaluation questions: What activities should I incorporate in my practice that I am currently not doing? What are my practice strengths? What things should I try to improve in my practice? How can I best accomplish this in a timely way?
3. According to Geary Rummier, President of the Rummier-Bache Group, "You can take great people, highly trained and motivated, and put them in a lousy system and the system will win every time" (Bell & Zemke, 1992). With that in mind, reflect on the system in which you practice. In what ways, if any, is the system "winning"? How can this be remedied? Where do you fit into the remedy?

REFERENCES/BIBLIOGRAPHY

American Nurses Association (1996). *Scope and standards of advanced practice registered nursing.* Washington, DC: American Nurses Association.

Baker, S.K. (1996, January). Making yourself memorable to your patients. *ADVANCE for Nurse Practitioners,* 54.

Barrett-Barrick, C. (1993). Promoting the use of program evaluation findings. *Nurse Educator, 18*(11), 10-12.

Baum, N., & Henkel, G. (2000). *Marketing your clinical practice ethically, effectively, economically.* Gaithersburg, MD: Aspen Publishers.

Bell, C.R., & Zemke, R. (1992). *Managing knock your socks off service*. New York: American Management Association.

Bensing, K. (2000, February 7). Career planning: preparing your annual report. *ADVANCE for Nurses*, 24.

Buppert, C. (1999). HEDIS for the primary care provider: getting an "A" on the managed care report card. *Nurse Practitioner, 24*(1), 84-99.

Buppert, C. (2000). Measuring outcomes in primary care practice. *The Nurse Practitioner, 25*(1), 88-98.

Case, B. (1999). *Advanced practice nurse preceptor workbook*. Chicago: Niehoff School of Nursing, Loyola University.

Galvan, T.J. (1999). Identifying outcomes. *Nurse Practitioner Forum, 10*(4), 185-190.

Girouard, S.A. (1996). Evaluating advanced nursing practice. In A.M. Hamric, J.A. Spross, & C.M. Hanson (Eds.), *Advanced nursing practice: an integrative approach* (pp. 569-600). Philadelphia: WB Saunders.

Gregg, A.C., & Bloom, K.C. (1999). Performance evaluation and patient outcomes monitored by nurse practitioners and certified nurse midwives in Florida. *Clinical Excellence for Nurse Practitioners, 3*(5), 279-285.

Hamric, A.R. (1989). A model for CNS evaluation. In A.B. Hamric & J.A. Spross (Eds.), *The clinical nurse specialist in theory and practice* (2nd ed.) (pp. 83-104). Philadelphia: WB Saunders.

Harris, M.R., & Warren, J.J. (1995). Patient outcomes: assessment issues for the CNS. *Clinical Nurse Specialist, 9*(2), 82-86.

Houston, S., & Luquire, R. (1997). Advanced practice nurse as outcome manager. *Advanced Practice Nursing Quarterly, 3*(2), 1-9.

Ingersoll, G.L. (1997). Evaluation of the advanced practice nurse role in acute and specialty care. *Critical Care Nursing Clinics of North America, 7*(1), 25-33.

Juran Institute (1993). *Quality improvement in health care*. Wilton, CT: Juran Institute.

Kennedy-Malone, L.M. (1996). Evaluation strategies for CNSs: application of an evaluation model. *Clinical Nurse Specialist, 10*(14), 195-198.

Komelasky, A.L., Bridges, C., Golas, G., Pence, D., & Woodard, I. (1997, April). Developing a peer review system. *ADVANCE for Nurse Practitioners*, 73-76.

McAlpine, L.A. (1997). Process and outcome measures for the multidisciplinary collaborative projects of a critical care CNS. *Clinical Nurse Specialist, 11*(3), 134-138.

Nugent, K.E., & Lambert, V.A. (1997). Evaluating the performance of the APN. *The Nurse Practitioner, 22*(2), 190-198.

Reidy, P. (1997, February). Who has the right to say "good job"? *Lifelines*, 46.

Sheahan, S., & Simpson, C. (1999, July 16-20). *Nurse practitioner peer review: development, process, and outcome*. American Association of Nurse Practitioners 14th Annual National Conference. Atlanta, GA: American Association of Nurse Practitioners.

Smith, M.A. (1996). Job description for primary care nurse practitioners. *Nurse Practitioner, 21*(5), 160-163.

Snyder, M., & Mirr, M.P. (Eds.). (1995). *Advanced practice nursing: a guide to professional development*. New York: Springer.

Stake, R. (1973). The countenance of educational evaluation (Handout for EDS 964: Educational Evaluation Course, The University of Georgia, Summer 1986). Adapted from B. Worthen & J. Sanders (Eds.), *Educational evaluation: theory and practice*. Belmont, CA: Walsworth Press.

Stufflebeam, D. (1971). *Educational evaluation and decision making*. Ithaca, NY: Peacock Publications.

Stufflebeam, D. (1980). The relevance of the CIPP evaluation model for educational accountability. *Journal of Research and Development, 5*(1), 19-25.

Stufflebeam, D. (1983). The CIPP for program evaluation. In G. Madaus & M. Scriven (Eds.), *Evaluation models: view points on education and human services evaluation*. Boston: Kluvner and Nijhoff.

Waltz, C.F., Chambers, S.B., & Hechenberger, N.B. (1989). *Strategic planning, marketing, and evaluation for nursing education and nursing service* (No. 15-2282). New York: National League for Nursing.

Section VI

Theoretical Foundations of Nursing Practice

Anne M. Dollins & Louise M. Niemer

As advanced practice curricula have evolved, many programs have had to limit the length of the program. In spite of this, graduate students have had to master much new content, primarily in the areas of medical diagnosis and treatment. Baumann (1998) believes that these advanced practice programs (especially nurse practitioner [NP] programs) have lost substantive nursing content. However, most advanced practice nurses (APNs) see themselves differently than physicians, and nursing content is an integral part of this difference. Education about holism, prevention, families, communities, caring, and a view of a patient as an essential component of health is vital to emphasize the differences between APNs and physicians. Nursing has a unique body of knowledge that can serve to guide APNs. Nursing theory, according to Baumann (1998), allows APNs to "structure ideas and interpret information in a way different from the strict biomedical model. It also means being able to consider two views of information, looking at provocative questions and new practice approaches." Baumann argues that using a theory such as the Human Becoming Theory, which prioritizes a person's values and beliefs, provides a way for APNs to be "present" to the full range of human experiences. The American Association of Colleges of Nursing (1996) identifies theoretical foundations of nursing practice as a core concept for advanced practice. This means graduates should be prepared to critique, evaluate, and use both nursing and non-nursing theory within their practices. The use of theory enables APNs to provide care that focuses on the whole range of a person's health and illness experience and leads to holistic care.

This section provides a capsulated view of nursing and non-nursing theory, including how to evaluate it, how to use it, and how to apply selected theories to advanced practice.

Chapter 26 examines the nature of nursing theory and nursing. The basics of nursing theory, definitions of concepts inherent in nursing theory, and how nursing theory developed are all discussed within this chapter.

Evaluation of nursing theory is presented in Chapter 27. This chapter briefly presents a number of evaluation frameworks with which to critique theory. Parse's (1987) framework is used to evaluate Roger's Science of Unitary Human Beings.

Ways in which nursing can use nursing theory are discussed in Chapter 28. Nursing theory is nothing more than an academic exercise unless it is used in practice. This chapter focuses on the application of theory to practice.

The relationships of nursing theory, practice, and research are presented in Chapter 29. The use of conceptual-theoretical-empirical systems of nursing knowledge is examined as a means for APNs to apply nursing theory and research to practice.

In Chapter 30, selected grand range theories are discussed. Roy's Adaptation Model, Orem's Concepts of Practice, Neuman's Systems Model, Paterson and Zderad's Humanistic Nursing, and Newman's Health as Expanding Consciousness are included.

Finally, selected midrange nursing and non-nursing theories are presented in Chapter 31. Kolcaba's Theory of Comfort, Erickson's Modeling and Role Modeling, and Mishel's Theory of Uncertainty are discussed. Non-nursing theories, including Rogers' Diffusion of Innovation Theory, are also highlighted.

REFERENCES/BIBLIOGRAPHY

American Association of Colleges of Nursing (1996). *The essentials of Master's education for advanced practice nursing.* Washington, DC: American Association of Colleges of Nursing.

Baumann, S. (1998). Nursing: the missing ingredient in nurse practitioner education. *Nursing Science Quarterly, 11*(3), 89-90.

DeVit-Dabbs, A. (1994). Theory-based nursing practice: for our patients' sake. *Clinical Nurse Specialist, 8*(4), 214, 220.

Parse, R. (1987). *Nursing science.* Philadelphia: WB Saunders.

Chapter 26

Nursing Theory and Advanced Practice

Anne M. Dollins & Louise M. Niemer

Theory represents a discipline's effort to imbue phenomena of concern with meaning that is unique to that discipline's worldview. This meaning allows for an understanding of those phenomena and contributes to the greater purpose of explanation and prediction of future related events; it ultimately allows the discipline to prescribe a course of action that will bring about a desired result. A discipline's efforts in the realm of theory culminate in the development of an integrated larger body of knowledge that underpins and directs the activities of the discipline. This chapter reviews nursing's theoretical heritage and discusses the function of theory and its significance through examination of critical issues and implications for Master of Science in Nursing (MSN) education, practice, and research.

DEFINITIONS

Paradigm reflects the predominant system of philosophy, science, and theory acknowledged by the discipline. The prevailing paradigm makes the phenomena of interest apparent to the discipline and subsequently influences the discipline's research and practice activities. Paradigm is also referred to as *worldview* in some literary contexts. A *philosophy* is constituted by fundamental beliefs about the nature of phenomena. Philosophical beliefs are derived from opinion; because they are not empirically based, they are untestable (Keck, 1998). The prevailing philosophy of the discipline and theorist shapes what subject matter is viewed as appropriate for attention and influences the focus of its theory.

A *phenomenon* is an object, event, or property that constitutes subject matter of unique concern to a discipline. A phenomenon is identified empirically rather than intuitively and can be the subject of scientific investigation (Keck, 1998). A *concept* is intended to represent an abstract idea or term that symbolizes a phenomenon and creates mental images of the phenomenon being described (Fawcett & Downs, 1992). Concepts are the foundations for theory. A *construct* is similar to a concept in that it, too, is an abstraction. However, a construct is not just an abstraction. A construct consists of more than one abstract idea or term and symbolizes the association or interaction of two or more concepts. Patient satisfaction is an example of a construct; the two concepts are patient and satisfaction. This construct conveys a mental image of the phenomenon that either of the concepts individually fail to achieve. Concepts and constructs are used to generate statements that propose a relationship between or among concepts. This type of statement is called a *proposition*. For example, "Restlessness increases as pain increases" is a propositional statement. Concepts and constructs are also constitutive of *models*. A model is a concrete representation of conceptual and theoretical abstractions. Models are devised to enhance understanding of ideas that cannot be directly observed or visualized and are therefore difficult to grasp (Holder & Chitty, 1997). Models may be represented symbolically through language, though most are commonly communicated graphically.

Concepts, constructs and propositions come together to constitute theory. A *theory* is a set of propositions that are logically connected to provide a systematic view of phenomena in order to describe, explain, predict, or prescribe the phenomena. A *science* is a unified body of knowledge derived from theory that is concerned with a specific focus of interest. The science of a discipline includes the skills and methodologies needed to provide this knowledge (Keck, 1998).

CRITICAL ISSUES: SIGNIFICANCE OF NURSING THEORY FOR ADVANCED PRACTICE NURSES

There are a number of issues critical to the topic of theory that will influence the direction and level of autonomy that distinguishes advanced practice nursing. These issues include:

1. Reluctance of advanced practice nurses (APNs) to recognize the significance of nursing theory
2. Lack of conceptual clarity as to what constitutes advanced nursing
3. Negative consequences of nursing's history
4. The interface between theory for nursing and theory for advanced nursing

Each of these issues is discussed in this chapter.

Reluctance to Recognize the Significance of Nursing Theory

The first critical issue related to theory is the reluctance of APNs to recognize the significance of nursing theory. This reluctance is evidenced within the APN practice community, APN educators, and APN students. A limited presence of explicit references to nursing theory in APN literature is but one part of the evidence that supports this perception of reluctance. A review of APN program curricula reveals the existence of APN programs that do not require a nursing theory course at the Master's level. In evaluating one APN program, student comments reflected this reluctance. Students commented that their preference lay in learning medical theory over nursing theory (Personal communication, D. Robinson, May 8, 2000). What do APNs need to know about APN theory?

In 1996 the American Association of Colleges of Nursing (AACN) recommended that APNs should be prepared at the Master's level. APN program graduates earn a Master's degree in the science of nursing. Thus it is not unreasonable to expect that they have content in their curricula to help them achieve a level of knowledge greater than that of the baccalaureate graduate. APN program graduates should possess knowledge about the origins, characteristics, and classification of theory to understand the significance of theory for a practice discipline.

Origin of theory

Because theorizing is a creative endeavor to systematically describe phenomena in a logical and plausible fashion, it will necessarily reflect the perspectives and values of its creator. Thus nursing theory represents phenomena of unique interest to nursing in a manner that is congruent with the philosophy and goals of the discipline. When APNs borrow or utilize theories from other disciplines, they must be cognizant of the values and beliefs that characterize the discipline that are embedded within the theory. Theories of business and economics, for instance, may have applicability to aspects of health care, but indiscriminate utilization of these theories without evaluation of the underpinning assumptions may prove counterproductive. Similarly, when APNs employ medical theory, they must be mindful of the philosophical stance and goals of medicine. One may tend to assume that objectives of the disciplines are synonymous. However, although a similarity between medicine and nursing may exist by virtue of both being related to health, medicine has as its goal the diagnosis and cure of disease, whereas nursing's goal is the diagnosis and treatment of human responses to actual or potential health problems (American Nurses Association, 1995).

APNs frequently avoid associating themselves with theory and often claim that it is too ethereal for practical purposes. However, it is not uncommon to overhear nurses in situations where an explanation of a particular event is lacking or unknown to exclaim "It is my theory that . . . " or "I have a theory. . . . " In these situations, nurses are doing precisely what they claim to avoid—theorizing. By seeking to understand a phenomenon by placing it in a context that accounts for elements associated with the phenomenon, theory serves to explain similar phenomena in the future. Informal theorizing provides the opportunity for a nurse to comprehend the course and sequence of similar future events and possibly provide a basis for action.

The following scenario helps to illustrate a process of informal theorizing in practice. An APN who specializes in cardiology notices when preparing patients for certain procedures that almost all of the patients remind family members where important papers and belongings are in case these may be needed. This is a first step in the conceptualization process for the nurse—recognizing the phenomenon. At this point, the APN surmises that the patients think that somehow the procedure will affect their memory. This is a second step of the conceptualization process—positing an explanation for the phenomenon. The nurse shares these observations and ideas with nursing colleagues. During the discussion, other nurses identify that they too have recognized similar patterns of behavior. However, another APN hypothesizes that this behavior is derived from patient concerns that they will not survive, or perhaps complications might arise that will preclude them from taking care of routine activities in their usual manner. This activity represents a third element of conceptualizing—seeking alternative explanations for the phenomenon. They discuss the issue further and come to a conclusion that the phenomenon occurring is best explained by the idea that patients feel vulnerable and that there is the potential for untoward events. This last stage of conceptualizing is the derivation of a simple explanatory theory; with further formalized development at the descriptive and explanatory level, it could be subject to testing and ultimately evolve into a predictive microtheory for preoperative nursing care.

Though seemingly unsophisticated, this process represents theoretical activity that APNs (and other health care practitioners) routinely utilize. This level of theorizing has inherent value in that it emerges from practice. The advantages of this "grass roots" approach of making sense out of practice, questioning current practice and beliefs, and thinking critically increases the meaning attached to the work of APNs. It engenders theory that is rooted in nursing. The disadvantage of this activity is the failure to disseminate the theory for further professional debate and discourse, testing and refinement, and evaluation for correspondence with other related theory. In short, unless it is subjected to formal theoretical development, it ultimately fails to contribute to the continued growth and evolution of a recognized body of unique nursing knowledge. Furthermore, if the theory is erroneous and is applied to practice without the benefit of further development, negative patient outcomes may occur.

Role of theory in a practice discipline

A theory is a general explanation used to "explain, predict, control, and understand commonly occurring events" (Holder & Chitty, 1997) and is of unique interest to a discipline. Theory organizes and classifies events into a logical, conceptual whole that allows a practitioner to recognize, understand, and manage the phenomenon at hand. For example, a theory of pain would encompass notions of causation and response. Thus a well-defined theory of pain would enable a nurse to recognize predictors and indicators of pain. A theory of pain management would further facilitate a systematic approach to intervening to achieve goals relative to preventing or minimizing pain.

Characteristics of theory

Theory functions to provide an internally consistent framework for a discipline's activities in light of its goals. The utility of a theory is a function of its ability to consistently guide activities of the discipline congruent with the goals of the discipline. The demonstrated utility of a theory enhances it value to the discipline because it provides a reliable basis for understanding, explaining, and predicting phenomena of interest and concern to the discipline. Continued use and testing of the theory, plus understanding of its ongoing relevance to society, influence its refinement and expansion.

If a theory is readily applicable to a discipline, it will be utilized and refined. Such theories possess certain characteristics. Evaluation of theory for practice is discussed in Chapter 27. However, for further clarification of theory, it is useful to present these characteristics here as well. Torres (1990) provides the following characteristics that enhance the utility of a theory.

1. Theories interrelate concepts in such a way as to create new and more useful ways of looking at a particular phenomenon.
2. Theories must be logical in nature.
3. Theories must be relatively simple, yet generalizable.
4. Theories can be the basis for hypotheses that can be tested.
5. Theories contribute to and assist in increasing the general body of knowledge within the discipline through the research implemented to validate them.
6. Theories must be consistent with other validated theories, laws, and principles, but they will leave unanswered questions that need to be investigated.

Stress theory provides an example that can help to illuminate these characteristics. Stress theory has been widely embraced by health care disciplines as a highly relevant and usable theory. A proposition of stress theory postulates that an individual's success in coping with a stressful event favorably influences his or her response to subsequent similar stressors (Lazarus & Folkman, 1984). When this proposition is applied to patient care situations, it follows that previous experience of successfully coping with a stressful event would enhance coping and diminish stress. Thus the provision of practice scenarios with anticipatory guidelines provides patients with the opportunity to practice successful coping strategies, so that when an actual event occurs, the patient can employ the skills gleaned from the practice activity.

Theories regarding childbirth education, preoperative teaching, developmental anticipatory guidance, and the like have become routine interventions that employ these basic constructs from stress theory to create a different way of understanding phenomena. Stress theory provides a logical and simple (yet generalizable) basis for activities to enhance coping and reduce stress. Hypotheses can be derived from the theory for testing that will enhance the general body of knowledge of the discipline and guide practitioners in improving their practices. Stress theory is conceptually consistent with other validated theories, such as the uncertainty in illness theory (Mishel, 1988) and the health belief model (Rosenstock, 1966). However, when used in conjunction with these theories, new questions for further investigation arise.

Over time, a discipline's prevailing philosophy evolves in response to social change, and a corresponding change in theoretical perspectives will occur. For instance, before World War II, nurses assumed patients would comply with care directives, and patients assumed a passive role in their own health care. However, subsequent to the consumer movement of the 1970s, society's views and expectations of the health care system shifted, as did nursing's. Nurses became more consumer focused, and the involvement of patients in decisions regarding their own care became valued and expected. Corresponding theories of autonomy, interpersonal relations, and mutuality surfaced in response to this paradigm shift. Thus a discipline's theoretical base is not static. Rather, it is dynamic and responsive to phenomena both inside and outside its realm.

Levels of theory

Dickoff, James, and Wiedenbach (1968) propose four levels of theory, with each lower level being a necessary prerequisite for the next. At the most basic level, *descriptive theory* entails the naming of concepts. This activity is often overlooked in the theorizing process. However, if the purpose of a theory is to place ideas into a conceptualized whole, then the development, defining, and naming of those ideas is an essential theoretical activity. Descriptive theory provides an operative frame of reference for concepts and constructs. Returning to the example of pain, without a clear conceptual understanding of pain, it could be difficult to differentiate it from discomfort or even emotional distress.

Once individual concepts are isolated and defined, the second level of theory connects related concepts in an explanatory fashion. *Explanatory theory* examines the correlations and associations between and among concepts. Grimacing and increased pulse and respiratory rates may be identified as correlates of pain. However, heightened pulse and respiratory rates in the absence of a behavioral component (e.g., grimacing) may have a different clinical significance. Thus explanatory theory explores and confirms the relationships among the concepts of the theory and ensures the conceptualization of ideas necessary for prediction.

Predictive theory, the third level, enables the prediction of events when certain situational factors exist. Whereas explanatory theory relates concepts, predictive theory relates situations and represents the classic theory of causal laws. Simply stated, predictive theory enables one to identify that a defined condition or set of circumstances (situation A) will predictably result in a related situation (situation B) (Dickoff et al, 1968). Pain theory does operate at the predictive level. According to this theory, pain (situation A) interferes with cognitive functioning (situation B).

The fourth and most complex level of theory is *prescriptive theory*. Predictive theory roughly states that if situation A occurs, it will produce situation B. However, prescriptive theory acknowledges that the results brought about by a situation are desirable and prescribes actions to facilitate these. Criteria for a prescriptive theory include: (1) a desirable goal for the activity, (2) prescriptions for activity that will achieve the goal, and (3) conceptual awareness of the relationship between the goal and activities and the context in which they occur. (Dickoff et al, 1968). Pain management theory also represents a prescriptive theory. It asserts that by maintaining a specified level of narcotic analgesia (situation A, or the activity), pain will remain at a minimal level and be prevented from escalating (situation B, or the desired goal). Conceptual awareness of contextual elements that affect prescription include, though are not limited to, such factors as who must delegate the activity (the physician), who may implement the activity (the nurse), safe levels for administration of the narcotic, institutional protocols, and so forth.

Scope of theory

Theories differ in their level of scope. The scope of a theory reflects: (1) the range of phenomena to which the theory relates, or (2) a theory's level of abstraction (Chinn & Kramer, 1991). Theories may be very broad in their range of phenomena of interest and try to portray the larger picture, or they may be very limited in their focus. While theories are classified according to their level of scope, one should keep in mind that categorization of scope is relative (Chinn & Kramer, 1991). Starting from theory with the broadest scope and moving to the most limited, the different classifications include metatheory, grand theory, midrange theory, and microtheory.

Metatheory is oriented towards philosophical and methodological issues of theory development. This orientation focuses on concerns related to the nature of theories. Metatheory asks questions about knowledge and about the broader issues within a discipline. It examines questions such as: What type or types of theory is or are needed by a discipline? What are appropriate criteria for the analysis and evaluation of theory? What is the nature of theory? (Powers & Knapp, 1990; Chinn & Kramer, 1991; Walker & Avant, 1995)

A *grand theory*, or *broad-range theory*, has within its focus a wide range of phenomena. Its goal is to explain the totality of events related to a discipline. Theoretical formulations within a grand theory are general. In nursing a grand theory would attempt to explain the mission and goals of nursing care (Jacox, 1974; Meleis, 1997). Examples of grand theories include Orem's Self-Care Deficit Theory of Nursing, Rogers' Science of Unitary Human Being, and King's Theory of Goal Attainment (Marriner-Tomey & Alligood, 1998).

Compared to grand theory, a *midrange theory* is more limited in scope and level of abstraction. However, the focus of midrange phenomena and concepts can be relevant to all nursing specialties and applicable to a number of nursing care situations. A midrange theory seeks to provide answers to specific nursing questions (Jacox, 1974; Meleis, 1997; Marriner-Tomey & Alligood, 1998). This level of theory may be derived either from earlier nursing theories or from disciplines related to nursing. A midrange theory is based on specific practice concepts and is characteristically more concrete than a grand theory. Examples of midrange theories include Peplau's Interpersonal Relations Theory, Leininger's Cultural Care Theory, and Parse's Human Becoming Theory.

Microtheory is also known as *practice theory*, *empirical generalization*, or *partial theory*. The range of microtheory is more limited and prescribed than that of midrange theory. The goal of microtheory is to provide a nurse with specific desired patient goals and precise practice directives (Walker & Avant, 1995; Fitzpatrick & Whall, 1996). An example of a microtheory would be the physiology of pain phenomena.

Conceptual Clarity of the Advanced Practice Role

The second critical issue related to theory is the lack of clarity regarding the conceptual and operational meaning of the term *advanced practice nursing*. Other terms that have been used include *expert nurse, expert practice, advanced practitioner*, and *clinical nurse specialist* (CNS). No precise, universally accepted definition of *advanced practice nursing* exists within the nursing literature (Salussolia, 1997; Brown, 1998). (This deficit is not meant to deny the existence of legal definitions of advanced nursing in state nurse practice acts, but these definitions vary from state to state.)

It is proposed that part of this problem originates from nursing's search for professional identity and its efforts to extricate itself from the imperatives of medicine. In a sense, APN is the proverbial "white elephant" that encumbers this objective. For some in nursing it appears that the elements that constitute advanced practice are the elements of medicine. This aspect is not easily acknowledged, not without cost to the identity of the profession. The idea that nursing knowledge does not provide adequate depth and scope to support a level of advanced practice is demeaning to the self-image of the profession and reinforces the supremacy of medicine (even given the current call for multidisciplinary views and frameworks).

The cost of denying that medical theory is the foundation for advanced practice would be equivalent to admitting to the absence of theoretical grounding for advanced practice. If the profession continues to integrate medicine into the APN's role but does not attend to its own theoretical development, it will negatively affect the future of autonomous practice. This failure will result in the development of role competencies and subsequent curricula that are not consistent with the discipline. As a result of this, the profession will be following instead of determining its own future.

Negative Consequences from Nursing's History

Throughout history, class and gender have influenced nursing's roles. Nursing emerged from women's traditional caretaking roles in the family and community (Ehrenreich & English, 1973). Care for the sick and indigent was provided by women healers, and in many Western cultures nuns assumed this responsibility. Society's misfits and undesirables (women prisoners and prostitutes who had no formal preparation in the care of the ill and dying) were also left with the undesirable task of caring for diseased

and dying people. While science and the humanities became valued and legitimized within universities, the knowledge of healers who were women or from lower socioeconomic classes was suppressed, devalued, and not formally developed. While science differentiated into discreet bodies of knowledge such as biology, chemistry, physics, and astronomy, the work of women healers and caretakers continued without formalized knowledge about ways to provide care.

Traditional healing focused on caring and comforting the ill and dying. Women healers effectively used herbs and treatments but had no recognized theoretical basis for their use. Health was at that time equated with the absence of disease. As science advanced the notion of cause and effect, it could focus on problems related to curing. However, science was privy to acceptance in university settings, and only men were granted admission to university institutions. Hence, the theory of cure developed into the science of healing and was claimed by men under the auspice of medical science.

Concurrently, the realm of care was historically relegated to women and thus received limited recognition as having a scientific basis for practice. Furthermore, the concept of care was diminished because it was women who provided it (Reverby, 1987). Subsequently, tasks became more rigidly divided along lines of gender. Men functioned under the auspice of science to cure, and women employed less-formalized theory embedded in their traditions and customs of care. Societal gender role expectations of the time reinforced the appropriateness of these roles, thus strengthening the division between care and cure.

Science was developed and refined, and as the ability to cure became a scientific reality, it also became a profitable possibility. Men had the advantage on both of these horizons and were able to dominate health care with little effort. In contrast, women's education lacked formal theorizing and was restricted to learning domestic and aesthetic crafts that would enhance their desirability as wives and mothers. Women did not find ready acceptance in university settings until the latter twentieth century. Even then, their presence was tolerated, and they were expected to pursue traditional female roles such as nursing and education.

In 1859, Florence Nightingale was the first to conceptualize nursing's work into a theoretical framework. The application of a formalized framework to nursing practice was the first attempt to value and systematize the work of nursing. An element of this effort included the use of processes associated with research to validate the work of nursing (Pfettscher, de Graff, Marriner-Tomey, Mossman, Slebodnik, 1998). Nightingale recognized the negative perceptions held by society of the current providers of "nursing care" and sought to alleviate these perceptions. She purposely sought to fill the ranks of nursing with women of sound character and good moral standing who would accept and value altruism. Importantly, she also advocated for the formal preparation of women so as to groom them to apprehend the situation of patient care within a systematic framework of practice.

The first formalized educational approaches to nursing in the United States occurred in the late 1800s. These schools operated under the auspices of hospitals and were controlled by physicians and hospital administrators. Curricula reflected biomedical theory and emphasized nursing work relative to this, thus supporting the activities and status of physicians. They also perpetuated the existing gender-based hierarchy. To establish an environment that recognized the unique work of nurses, nurses needed to achieve professional autonomy.

For nursing to gain professional autonomy, it was necessary to create a unique theoretical basis for practice. This was the impetus to provide nursing education in university settings, away from control of the interests of hospitals and the dominance of physicians. At first, universities were reluctant to accept nursing as a valid academic discipline, but the first baccalaureate program was founded in 1909 at the University of Minnesota (Nichols, 1997).

Unfortunately, nursing was not able to easily free itself from the influence of medical theory and the role expectations imposed by society (Reverby, 1987). Because the theoretical development of the discipline had been thwarted, it had no clearly defined theoretical basis for practice. No organized framework existed that clearly delineated the elements that defined and constituted nursing. Hence, nursing continued to struggle for professional autonomy in the shadow of medicine.

By the 1950s it became clear that nurses needed to develop their own theoretical perspectives. Significant events followed. The journal *Nursing Research* began publication in 1955, and multiple theories of nursing emerged. Columbia University's Teachers' College undertook the formidable task of determining curricula appropriate to baccalaureate nursing education. The classical theoretical works of Abdellah, Hall, Henderson, King, Peplau, Rogers, and Wiedenbach emerged from this effort (Meleis, 1997).

Nightingale's initial attempts to theoretically ground nursing during the mid-1800s reached fruition 100 years later with the work of nursing theorists at Columbia. This latter work provided momentum that has continued to shape the theoretical development of nursing. In the 1960s, federal grants were awarded to nurses to pursue doctoral degrees in basic sciences. In 1964, Dorothy Johnson asserted that nurses must be educated to take on the role of scholar and to value research and theory development. By the next year, the American Nurses Association issued a position paper asserting that the most important goal for the profession was the development of theory (Meleis, 1997).

Over the intervening years, nursing theorists have successfully endeavored to develop nursing theory that holds relevance for practice and research. In the 1990s, nursing theorists and APNs examined existing nursing theory to identify its relevance for the practice. One such example is Nelson-Marten, Hecomovich and Pangle's (1998) attempt to demonstrate the applicability of Watson's Theory of Caring to advanced practice. In contrast, Brown (1998) proposes that advanced practice lacks a comprehensive conceptual framework and seeks to develop a framework that will address this perceived shortcoming.

Nursing theorists and APNs are asking questions relating to the APN's role (Salussolia, 1997; Komnenich, 1998). Questions that examine and challenge the relation of APNs to physician assistants (PAs), other nurses, physicians and the health care system are also being asked (Christman, 1998; Bellack, Graber, O'Neil, Musham and Lancaster, 1999). The theoretical basis for curricula in APN programs is being examined (Salussolia, 1997; Bellack et al, 1999). Each of these concerns has theoretical implications for advanced nursing.

As discussed, nursing's history gives witness to the historical practice of assigning healing activities based upon gender and class. Women took on caring activities, which later became formalized as nursing. Men took on curing activities, subsequently formalized into the discipline of medicine.

Genderfication was also responsible for women being denied access to institutions of higher learning. This exclusion has long influenced women's relationships with those who have had the advantage of this privilege. Medicine, with its longer access to universities and traditional male membership, has reaped the benefits of social and scholarly recognition. Nursing's acquiescent relationship with medicine is strongly influenced by this history.

As with other groups whose heritage includes a history of oppression, nursing has experienced a relationship with medicine that at times is characterized by extreme tension. This gender and class history and resulting tension is partially responsible for nursing's reluctance to appropriately frame the integration of medicine into a nursing role. This confusion causes nursing to both identify with medicine and denigrate the identity of nursing bound into this role.

Interfacing Theory for Nursing and Theory for Advanced Practice

The final critical issue is derived from the relationship of theory for nursing and theory for advanced nursing. Are existing nursing theories adequate to ground the practice of APNs? Nelson-Marten et al (1998) believe that current nursing theory can serve as the framework for APNs. As previously mentioned, they describe the applicability of Watson's Theory of Caring for advanced practice as a case in point. Conversely, Brown (1998) argues that APNs need a theoretical framework specific to advanced practice roles. She believes that such a framework would: (1) assist in the recognition of ideas that have contemporary currency, (2) specify plans to facilitate the purposeful planning of a preferred future for advanced practice, (3) specify broad concepts that may be employed to provide a description and explanation of advanced practice, (4) identify relationships among concepts recommended or studied in the research literature, (5) explicitly define concepts and integrate them into a consistent theoretical structure, and 6) make clear the theoretical assumptions upon which the framework is developed. Brown's framework includes four major concepts: environments, role legitimacy, advanced practice nursing, and outcomes. From these concepts Brown derives 17 more specific concepts to ground the framework.

PRIORITIES FOR RESEARCH

The questions remain: Which is the best long-term path for APNs and nursing in general in terms of theoretical growth? Should advanced practice only acknowledge its nursing history and orientation in its use of theory? Is it possible that an intermediate theoretical stance between the directives advocated by Nelson-Marten et al (1998) and Brown (1998) would be more fruitful and beneficial in the long term for both nursing and advanced nursing? Perhaps APNs should embrace nursing theory and search for specific concepts or domains to add to the framework of advanced practice? Or (as Brown recommends) would it be most advantageous for advanced practice to derive a new theoretical framework? Consideration in this regard could heal the gendered history of nursing with a theoretical blending of caring and curing (uniting the roles as they originally existed) to provide a more holistic framework of health care. Other questions that need to be answered are: How do APNs read nursing theory and apply it to practice? How do APN educators and preceptors read nursing theory and apply it to practice? What is the best way to teach and incorporate nursing theory into practice? These are theoretical questions that need to receive priority and be examined.

Acton, Irvin, and Hopkins (1996) believe that the limited research that specifically tests nursing models is a deterrent to the advancement of nursing science. In order to identify and validate a body of knowledge that is uniquely related to nursing, support for nursing in the form of testing must be established. Moody (1988) found that between 1977 and 1986, only 3% of 720 studies tested theory, concepts, or hypotheses from a conceptual or theoretical framework. Silva (1986) also reported a limited number of research articles classified as theory-testing. More work has been done on the development of theory

than on its testing. Fawcett (2000) stresses that nursing must continue to work on testing theory; this means that conceptual-theoretical-empirical structures need to be devised so that it is possible to test constructs and propositions. Since theories are dynamic, testing will evolve and change over time. Theory-testing research evaluates how well the explanations and predictions that evolve from a theory hold up and thus refines the theory into a clearer and more useful depiction of reality (Acton et al, 1996). Silva (1986) determined that the purpose of theory research is to examine the underlying validity of the assumptions or propositions of the select nursing model. In addition, the research must use a nursing-related theoretical framework. The authors of the research should present the details of the research and explicitly discuss how the data explains, supports, or refutes the model or theory. Chinn and Kramer (1995) call this research *theory-linked*. By virtue of developing or testing theory, it sets the stage to contribute to the knowledge of the discipline. Isolated research, on the other hand, does not develop or test theory. The idea for research may come from many different sources, but it does not directly test theory. It may provide direction for future theory development and testing. Figure 26-1 shows the classic graphic depiction of how research and theory are linked. The spiral represents the interaction between theory and research. Chinn and Kramer (1995) explain that, "If you begin with theory, research derived from the theory is used to clarify

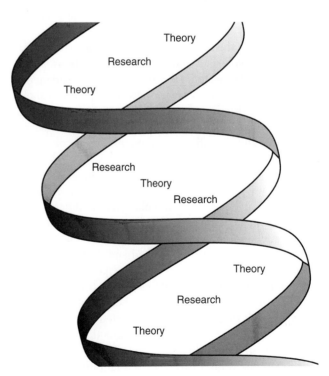

Figure 26-1 Theory-research spiral of knowledge. (From Chin, P., & Kramer, M. [1995]. *Theory and nursing: a systematic approach* (4th ed.). St. Louis: Mosby.)

and extend the theory. If you begin with research, theory that is formed from the findings can be subsequently used to direct research. In order for this spiral process to continue, research must be conducted with the specific aim of contributing to theory development."

There are two types of research that contribute to theory testing. One is theory-generating research. This type of research is usually considered an inductive approach. The researcher intends to approach the world with no preconceived notions of what the events in the world mean. Observations are made with as open a mind as possible, and most often this type of research is qualitative in nature. Grounded theory is an example of this type. (Box 26-1 shows other research methods that are used for theory generation.) A study of this type of research was conducted by Price (1993). In this research, a grounded theory approach and ethnographical interviewing were used to generate a hypothesis about parents' perceptions of quality nursing care for their hospitalized children.

Theory-testing research examines how well a theory depicts phenomena and their relationships. In most instances, a single study is based on one or two relational statements; no one study can test all the propositions that can be derived from a theory. A deductive approach is usually used in theory-testing research. The research starts with an abstract relational statement and then proceeds to specific hypotheses or research questions for the situation. This type of research is usually conducted using descriptive or correlational designs when research questions are used. When hypotheses are developed, experimental designs are more likely used, particularly when an intervention is tested. If the theory is complex, multiple studies are needed to provide data to support the propositions. Schorr (1993) used a repeated measures analysis of variance to analyze the effect of music on perceived pain thresholds of women with chronic pain. (Table 26-1 shows a comparison of clinical problems, research purposes, research problems, and hypothesis statements in theory-linked research.)

In most cases, once a study is completed, more questions are generated about the involved theory. These questions can be used to stimulate more research. The theory may need to be revised, or a new concept may need to be added based on the research findings. Theory-generating research can be applied and useful in practice because the question is of an inductive nature and derived from practice. It is less likely that theory-testing research can be immediately applied to practice, although new approaches in practice may be suggested by the data.

Acton et al (1996) propose 15 criteria that can be used to evaluate theory-testing research. These criteria were developed based on a review of the literature specific to theory testing. (Box 26-2 identifies the 15 criteria.)

As APNs conduct either theory-generating or theory-testing research, it is important for them to identify their

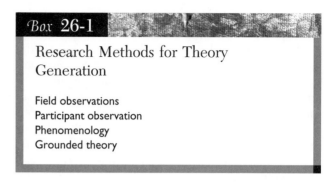

Box 26-1

Research Methods for Theory Generation

Field observations
Participant observation
Phenomenology
Grounded theory

study as theory-linked. This recognition facilitates the identification of theory-linked research, and APNs need to continue to contribute to the nursing knowledge base by participating in such research.

IMPLICATIONS FOR MSN EDUCATION AND ADVANCED PRACTICE

A major responsibility exists for nursing educators to examine the place of nursing theory in advanced practice programs. How can nursing educators convey to APN students the need for nursing theory and nursing identity? Should APN programs include separate courses on nursing theory in the curriculum? Whall (1996) argues that Master's-level courses that present nursing theories should serve as the foundation for APN knowledge. If a separate course is not provided, can careful integration of this theory throughout an APN program be achieved?

Historically, members of oppressed groups tend to identify with the oppressor (Roberts, 1983). Given that medicine has long held a dominant position in the health care setting, how can nurse educators help APN students recognize the inherent tendency for the oppressed group (nurses) to take on the values and identity of the dominant group (physicians)? Preferring medical theory to nursing theory can be interpreted as one example of oppressed-group behavior. Nursing educators need to help point out these behaviors and their attendant risk to APNs and the nursing profession as a whole.

An implication for practice is derived from the question: Is it important to differentiate APN practice from the practice of others such as physicians or PAs? If little difference can be found in the theoretical preparation between APNs and PAs, how can APNs achieve differentiation in their practices from those of PAs? Already health care systems such as the Planned Parenthood Association classify PAs and nurse practitioners (NPs) together as midlevel practitioners. The perception that APNs and PAs provide the same service in the same fashion is held by health care systems and some health care providers, and

Table 26-1

Comparison of Clinical Problems, Research Purposes, Research Problems, and Hypothesis Statements in Theory-Linked Research

TYPE OF STATEMENT	WHAT THE STATEMENT CONVEYS	THEORY GENERATING	THEORY TESTING
Clinical problem	Specifies the experiential observations that generated or influenced the study.	How do parents of hospitalized children perceive their care?	What can be done to alleviate chronic pain?
Research purpose	Specifies whether the study is theory-generating or theory-testing.	Generates substantive theory that explains parental perceptions when their child is hospitalized.	To test music as a unitary tranformative means of altering the perception of chronic pain within the context of Newman's theory (1986) of health as an expander of consciousness (Schorr, 1993).
Research problem	Leads to a question to be answered. Is less general than the purpose and makes clear how the purpose is to be achieved. Expresses the nature of the variable or events to be studied. Implies the empiric possibilities for the abstract concepts given in the purpose. Expresses the relationships between concepts if the relationship is the focus for the study.	What does quality nursing care mean to parents of hospitalized children (Price, 1993)?	Does music change the pain perception threshold?
Hypothesis	Indicates the specific choices made in relation to the variable for the study. Implies the design of the study. Implies the type of analysis used.	Quality nursing care involves a process of parent and child interaction with the nurse that leads to the establishment of a positive relationship and ultimately results in the satisfaction of the biophysical needs of the parents and child (Price, 1993).	The pain perception threshold will increase with the use of music as a unitary transformative nursing intervention (Schorr, 1993)

From Chinn P.L., & Kramer M.K. (1995). *Theory and nursing.* St. Louis: Mosby.

this perception has serious implications. Currently, APNs are licensed by state boards of nursing and certified by nursing organizations. If the theory to guide practice that is provided in APN programs is the same as that in the PA programs, what is there to eventually stop a movement from including both groups under the supervision of state medical boards? To prevent the negative consequences of being labeled midlevel practitioners or physician extenders, APNs must be able to do what all other practice disciplines are required to do—demonstrate the viability of their unique theoretical knowledge.

Denial of nursing theory's relevance to the APN role may have serious consequences for the profession. As more aspects of medicine are integrated into the APN's role, and

Box 26-2

Criteria for Evaluating Theory-Testing Research

1. The purpose of the study is to examine the empirical validity of the constructs, concepts, assumptions, or relationships from the identified theoretical frame of reference.
2. The theoretical frame of reference must be explicitly described and summarized.
3. The constructs and concepts to be examined must be theoretically defined.
4. An overview of previous studies that are based on the theoretical framework or clearly show the derivation of the concepts being tested must be included in the review of the literature.
5. The research questions or hypotheses must be logically derived from the definitions, assumptions, or propositions of the theoretical frame of reference.
6. The research questions or hypotheses must be specific enough to place the theoretical frame of reference at risk for falsification.
7. The operational definitions must be clearly derived from the theoretical frame of reference.
8. The design must be congruent with the level of theory described in the theoretical frame of reference.
9. The instruments must be theoretically valid and reliable.
10. The theoretical frame of reference must guide the sample selection.
11. The statistics used must be the most robust possible.
12. The analysis of data must provide evidence for supporting, refuting or modifying the theoretical framework.
13. The research report must include an interpretive analysis of the findings in relation to the theory being tested.
14. The significance of the theory for nursing must be discussed.
15. Ideally the researcher must make recommendations for further research on the basis of the theoretical findings.

Data from Acton, Irvin, Hopkins (1996). Theory testing research: building the science. In J. Kenney (Ed.), *Philosophical and theoretical perspectives for advanced nursing practice* (pp. 338-347). Sudbury, MA: Jones and Bartlett.

as the role of nursing and nursing theory is diminished or devalued, the nursing practice will be more derivative of medicine than nursing. Loss of a theoretical grounding in nursing will result in loss of the APN's identity as a nurse. Without careful and deliberative efforts to theoretically ground the APN role in nursing knowledge, the work of APNs may become labeled as "medicine" and be placed under the regulatory control of state medical boards and the educational auspices of medical organizations. This change would pave the way for a further loss of identity as hospitals and other health care systems continue to conceal the work of nursing under the broad rubric of patient care services departments or titles such as midlevel practitioner.

If theory is going to be used in practice, it must be developed cooperatively with those who practice nursing. Having the perspective of the reality of practice is crucial when developing a theory that will be useful in practice. Timpson (1996) says many APNs believe that most nursing theorists are removed from the realities of the practice setting. In addition, the semantic ambiguity of their writings contributes to the notion that theories are not useful in practice. Timpson suggests that a practice-led perspective by which nursing theory can be better articulated and assimilated might help the adoption and use of theory within the discipline.

King's Theory of Goal Attainment (1981) presents concepts that address transactions and goal attainment. King believes that systematic and planned transactions between nurse and patient enhance health. This theory is very useful for APNs because many of their interactions and transactions with patients are systematic. In many situations, APNs are communicating information to patients. Goal attainment is a means for prescribing or intervening to facilitate a change in patient behavior. For example, Hanna (1993) used King's theory to test the effect of a nurse-patient transactional intervention on 51 adolescent females. This intervention was based on action, reaction, an identified problem, mutual goal-setting, and exploration of and agreement on the means to achieve the goal—the basics of a nurse-patient transaction according to King (1981). Once the experimental group was prescribed contraceptives, the intervention was completed. All subjects had their contraceptive perceptions assessed immediately after usual care or the intervention, and their compliance was measured at the 3-month follow-up. Hanna found a significant difference in contraceptive adherence in those adolescents who participated in the transactional intervention and those who did not. This theory fits nicely with the goal of involving patients in the decision-making of primary care.

Another example that is an exemplar of nursing theory involves Jackie. Jackie is a MSN-prepared nurse who is a certified massage therapist and has opened her own business. She uses Parse's Man-Living-Health Theory (1981) as the basis of her practice. Her business is even named using the tenets of the theory . Her interaction with patients is based on the notion that Man chooses meaning in situations and bears the responsibility for the decision-making. According to Parse, health is reflective of Man's chosen way of living. By offering baby massage classes to mothers, Jackie is contributing to health as the mothers learn how to comfort and massage their babies.

Suggestions for Further Learning

- Review a number of websites for PA programs and for NP, certified registered nurse anesthetist (CRNA), and certified nurse midwife (CNM) programs to compare the curricula. What are the similarities and differences?
- Start a dialogue on a NP site about the role of nursing theory in advanced practice. Review the responses.
- Survey APNs in your community and ask whether they are able to identify elements of nursing theory in their practice.
- Review NP, CRNA, and CNM websites. How many references to nursing theory are found? What are contributing factors for the results obtained?
- Get the classic article: Silva, M. (1986). Research testing nursing theory: state of the art. *Advances in Nursing Science* 9(10): 1-11. In this article Silva reports on three exemplary cases of empirical research that tested theoretical constructs or propositions from a nursing theory.
- Get one of the following articles: Braden, C. (1990). A test of the self-help model: learned response to

chronic illness experience. *Nursing Research, 39*(1): 42-47; Smith, M. (1988). Testing propositions from Rogers' conceptual system. *Nursing Science Quarterly, 1*(2): 60-67; and Frey, M (1989). Social support and health: a theoretical formulation derived from King's conceptual framework. *Nursing Science Quarterly, 2*(3): 138-148. These studies meet 14 of 15 or 15 of 15 of the criteria identified for theory-testing research (see Box 26-2).

- Review the following websites for references to APNs. How many references are found? What are contributing factors for the results obtained?
  - Nursing Theory Link Page at Clayton College and State University (healthsci.clayton.edu/eichelberger/nursing.htm)
  - Nursing Theory Page at Valdosta State University College of Nursing (www.valdosta.edu/nursing/history_theory/theory.html)
  - Nursing Theory Page by Judy Norris (www.ualberta.ca/~jrnorris/nt/theory.html)

Theory allows for a clearer, more unified understanding of phenomena of unique interest to the discipline. It contributes to the description, explanation, and prediction of phenomena and ultimately allows the discipline to prescribe a course of action that will bring about a desired result. Nursing theories represent a broad range of purposes. Grand theories attempt to explain the mission and goals of nursing care. Microtheories provide nurses with precise practice directives and specified patient goals. A discipline's efforts in the realm of theory culminate in the development of an integrated, larger body of knowledge that underpins and directs the activities of the discipline. Lack of conceptual clarity regarding roles and theoretical directives are significant professional concerns for the future of advanced nursing.

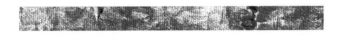

DISCUSSION QUESTIONS

These questions can be used to promote critical thinking and encourage discussion.

1. Select one of the critical issues discussed in the chapter. Do you agree or disagree with the position of the authors? Explain your position.
2. Identify a theory that you are currently using in clinical practice. What are the origins of this theory? What is

the level (i.e., descriptive, explanatory, predictive, prescriptive) of the theory? Explain. What elements of the theory correspond with the characteristics described by Torres (1990)?
3. Describe your perception of nursing theory in an APN program. How can students best merge medical and nursing theories for the best of both worlds? Some people believe that nurses have a sense of what nursing is about, so that in an APN program, most of the time needs to be spent learning the new role (i.e., the medical perspective) so that APN graduates can merge the two components when finished. Do you agree or disagree with this notion?

REFERENCES/BIBLIOGRAPHY

Acton, G., Irvin, B., & Hopkins, B. (1996). Theory testing research: building the science. In J. Kenney (Ed.), *Philosophical and theoretical perspectives for advanced nursing practice* (pp. 338-347). Sudbury, MA: Jones and Bartlett.

American Association of Colleges of Nursing (1996). *The essentials of Master's education for advanced practice nursing.* Washington, DC: American Association of Colleges of Nursing.

American Association of Colleges of Nursing (1998). *Certification and regulation of advanced practice nurses (online).* Available online at www.aacn.nche.edu/Publications/positions/cerreg.htm.

American Nurses Association (1995). *Social policy statement.* Kansas City, MO: American Nurses Association.

Bellack, J.P., Graber, D.R., O'Neil, E.H., Musham, C., & Lancaster, C. (1999). Curriculum trends in nurse practitioner programs: current and ideal. *Journal of Professional Nursing, 15*(1), 15-27.

Brown, S.J. (1998). A framework for advanced practice nursing. *Journal of Professional Nursing, 14*(3), 157-164.

Chinn, P.L., & Kramer, M.K. (1991). *Theory and nursing: a systematic approach.* St. Louis: Mosby.

Chinn, P.L., & Kramer, M. (1995). *Theory and nursing: a systematic approach* (4th ed.). St. Louis: Mosby.

Christman, L. (1998). Advanced practice nursing: is the physician's assistant an accident of history or a failure to act? *Nursing Outlook, 46*(2), 56-59.

Dickoff, J., James, P., & Wiedenbach, E. (1968). Theory in a practice discipline: part I. Practice oriented theory. *Nursing Research, 17*(5), 415-435.

Ehrenreich, B., & English, D. (1973). *Witches, midwives and nurses: a history of women healers.* Old Westbury, NY: The Feminist Press.

Fawcett, J. (2000). Contemporary nursing knowledge: nursing models and theories (3rd ed.). Philadelphia: FA Davis.

Fawcett, J., & Downs, F. (1992). *The relationship of theory and research* (2nd ed.). Philadelphia: FA Davis.

Fitzpatrick, J.J., & Whall, A.L. (1996). Conceptual models of nursing: analysis and application. Stamford, CT: Appleton & Lange.

Hanna, K. (1993). Effect of nurse-client transaction on female adolescents' oral contraceptive adherence. *Image: Journal of Nursing Scholarship 25*(4): 285-290.

Holder, P.J., & Chitty, K.K. (1997). Theory as a basis for professional nursing. In K.K. Chitty (Ed.), *Professional nursing: concepts and challenges* (pp. 211-231). Philadelphia: WB Saunders.

Jacox, A. (1974). Theory construction in nursing: an overview. *Nursing Research, 23*(1), 4-13.

Johnson, D. (1964). Nursing and health education. *International Journal of Nursing Studies, 1,* 219.

Keck, J.F. (1998). Terminology of theory development. In A. Marriner-Tomey & M.R. Alligood (Eds.), *Nursing theorists and their work* (4th ed.). St. Louis: Mosby.

King, I. (1981). *A theory of nursing: system, concepts, process.* New York: John Wiley & Sons.

Komnenich, P. (1998). The evolution of advanced practice in nursing. In C.M. Sheehy & M.C. McCarthy (Eds.), *Advanced practice nursing: emphasizing common roles.* Philadelphia: FA Davis.

Lazarus, R., & Folkman, S. (1984). *Stress, appraisal, and coping.* New York: Springer.

Marriner-Tomey, A., & Alligood, M.R. (1998). *Nursing theorists and their work* (4th Ed). St. Louis: Mosby.

Meleis, A.I. (1997). *Theoretical nursing: development and progress* (3rd ed.). Philadelphia: JB Lippincott.

Mishel, M. (1988). Uncertainty in illness. *Image: Journal of Nursing Scholarship, 20*(4), 225-232.

Moody, L., Wilson, M., Smyth, K., Schwartz, R., Tittle, M., & Van Cott, M. (1988). Analysis of a decade of nursing practice research: 1977-1986. *Nursing Research. 37*(6): 374-379.

Nelson-Marten, P., Hecomovich, K., & Pangle, M. (1998). Caring theory: a framework for advanced practice nursing. *Advanced Practice Nursing Quarterly, 4*(1), 70-77.

Newman M. (1986). *Health as expanding consciousness.* St. Louis, Mosby.

Nichols, E.F. (1997). Educational patterns in nursing. In K.K. Chitty (Ed.), *Professional nursing: concepts and challenges* (pp. 33-58). Philadelphia: WB Saunders.

Parse, R. (1981). *Man-living-health: a theory of nursing.* New York: John Wiley & Sons.

Pfettscher, S.A., deGraff, K.R., Marriner-Tomey, A., Mossman, C.L., & Slebodnik, M. (1998). Florence Nightingale: modern nursing. In A. Marriner-Tomey & M.R. Alligood (Eds.), *Nursing theorists and their work* (4th ed.) (pp. 67-85). St. Louis: Mosby.

Powers, B.A., & Knapp, T.R. (1990). *A dictionary of nursing theory and research.* Thousand Oaks, CA: Sage Publications.

Price, P. (1993). Parents' perceptions of the meaning of quality nursing care. *Advances in Nursing Science, 16*(1): 33-41.

Reverby, S. (1987). *Ordered to care: the dilemma of American nursing, 1850-1945.* New York: Cambridge University Press.

Roberts, S. (1983). Oppressed group behavior: implications for nursing. *Advances in Nursing Science, 5*(4): 21-30.

Rosenstock, I.M. (1966). Why people use health services. *Milbank Memorial Fund Quarterly, 11*(4): 246-252.

Salussolia, M. (1997). Is advanced nursing practice a post or a person? *British Journal of Nursing, 6*(16), 928-933.

Schorr, J. (1993). Music and pattern change in chronic pain. *Advances in Nursing Science, 15*(4): 27-36.

Silva, M. (1986). Research testing nursing theory: state of the art. *Advances in Nursing Science. 9*(10): 1-11.

Timpson, J. (1996). Nursing theory: everything the artist spits is art? *Journal of Advanced Nursing, 23*(5): 1030-1036.

Torres, G. (1990). The place of concepts and theories within nursing. In J.B. George (Ed.), *Nursing theories: the base for professional nursing practice* (3rd ed.). East Norwalk, CT: Appleton & Lange.

Walker, L.O., & Avant, K.C. (1995). *Strategies for theory construction in nursing.* Norwalk, CT: Appleton & Lange.

Whall, A.L. (1996). Current debates and issues critical to the discipline of nursing. In J.J. Fitzpatrick & A.L. Whall (Eds.), *Conceptual models of nursing: analysis and application* (3rd ed.) (pp. 2-12). Stamford, CT: Appleton & Lange.

Chapter 27

Evaluation of Theory

Anne M. Dollins, Louise M. Niemer, & Denise Robinson

Theory description, analysis, and testing are important activities in the support of a discipline's work. However, a discipline must also evaluate theory. Advanced practice nurses (APNs) must evaluate theory from their frame of reference. This chapter discusses the importance of theory evaluation and provides different approaches for the evaluation of theoretical works for their applicability to advanced practice.

CRITICAL ISSUES: EVALUATION OF THEORY IN ADVANCED PRACTICE

Informal theory evaluation is often conducted by nurses during the course of basic and advanced nursing studies and through continuing education efforts. Informal theory evaluation is simplistic and entails an almost intuitive acceptance of a theory based on its "match" with the nurse's own practice or particular view of nursing. Formal theory evaluation, however, is a rigorous process and does not occur as often. Formal theory evaluation is a necessary element of an individual's professional nursing practice. Meleis (1991) says that this form of evaluation is also a critical element in the discipline's knowledge development in that it:

1. Serves as an appropriate framework for research, teaching, administration, or consultation.
2. Identifies effective theories in exploring some aspect of practice or guiding a research project.
3. Compares and contrasts different explanations of the same phenomenon.
4. Enhances the potential of constructive changes and further theory development.
5. Identifies epistemological approaches of a discipline through attention to the sociocultural context of the theorist and the theory.
6. Assesses the ontological beliefs in a discipline.
7. Identifies schools of thought in a discipline.
8. Affects changes in clinical practice, defines research priorities, and identifies content for teaching and guidelines for nursing administration.
9. Uses nursing frameworks to explain nursing to the public.
10. Defines a discipline's domain.
11. Allows the nurse to be a critical consumer of theories.

Models for Evaluation of Nursing Theory

Different models exist for the evaluation of nursing theory. Meleis (1991), Barnum (1990), Chin and Kramer (1995), Fawcett (1989), Parse (1987), and others have described differing frameworks for the evaluation of theory. Similarities and differences exist within each framework. Meleis (1991) provides an evaluative framework that she identifies as the critique of a theory. Meleis' critique requires examination of a theory for three major criteria: relationship between structure and function, a diagram of the theory, and its circle of contagiousness. Elements that are considered within the area of the relationship between structure and function include clarity, consistency, simplicity or complexity, and tautology. The theory's diagram criterion evaluates its visual and graphic presentations, logical representation, and clarity. The circle of contagiousness refers to the theory's spread of geographical acceptance. This criterion also is used to differentiate between the influence of the theorist and the influence of the theory.

Barnum (1990) recommends an evaluative framework that classifies criteria into two major characteristics. The first characteristic focuses on internal criticism, the second on external criticism. Internal criticism attends to aspects of the theory that relate to the internal construction of the theoretical work. Internal criticism judges a theory for its clarity, consistency, adequacy, logical development, and level of theory development. External criticism judges a theoretical work for reality convergence, utility, significance, discrimination, scope of theory, and complexity.

Chin and Kramer (1995) propose an evaluative framework that examines five major criteria: clarity, simplicity, generality, accessibility, and significance. Clarity is determined by considering semantic and structural clearness and consistency. Simplicity addresses the number of conceptual elements and their relationships. Generality is determined by the scope of situations explained by the theory. Accessibility asks: To what extent are the theory's elements grounded in empirically verifiable phenomena? Significance is determined by the degree to which the theoretical work results in the attainment of accepted goals for nursing practice, research, and education.

Fawcett (1989) differentiates between the analysis and evaluation of theory and conceptual models. Analysis entails an intensive examination to determine exactly and concretely what the author is saying. It is conducted in an objective manner without inferences regarding what statements might mean or referring to others' interpretations of the theory or conceptual model. In contrast, evaluation of a theory or model "involves judgments about the value and logical structure [and] draws conclusions about its credibility" for the discipline (Fawcett, 1989). Evaluation entails appraisal of the extent to which the theory or model meets certain external criteria and standards.

Parse's (1987) evaluation criteria are derived from Kaplan (1964). Kaplan believes that a valid theory is one worth publishing, teaching, researching and using. The two major areas of evaluation criteria include structure and process criteria. (Box 27-1 delineates the evaluation criteria.)

Structure criteria refer to those elements of the basic structure of the theory. These elements help one to discover the historical grounding of the theory and identify the essential elements. Process criteria include correspondence, coherence, and pragmatics. *Correspondence* refers to the semantic integrity of the theory (Parse, 1987). It implies that the meanings of the terms are consistent, clear, and congruent with the philosophical assumptions. Assumptions are ideas that are given currency and considered to be true. Philosophical assumptions reflect the particular worldview of a theorist. Assumptions may be derived from commonly accepted knowledge or an individual's personal beliefs and values (Powers & Knapp, 1990). The source of commonly accepted knowledge may be previous research. Fundamental assumptions serve as the initial points of a theorist's conceptualization. One measure of correspondence is how well the theory fits within the paradigm of nursing. *Coherence* refers to the theory's syntax, logic, and consistency in the flow of ideas (Kaplan, 1964). *Pragmatics* refers to the practical nature of the theory. A practical nature is evidenced by a theory's use in research and practice and its contribution to nursing science. The work of APNs blends the work of nurses and physicians. In evaluating theory for APNs, one can acknowledge this blending by examining a theory for assumptions that support both disciplines. One must determine whether the assumptions support both the traditional work of nurses and the newly integrated work previously done only by physicians. Given this necessarily broader range of knowledge, familiarity with a wide range of literature on the part

---

Box 27-1

Criteria for Evaluation of Nursing Theories

Structure Criteria Questions

- How is the historical evolution of the theory described?
- Are the philosophical assumptions underpinning the theory explicitly stated?
- Are the principles, concepts, and propositions of the theory explicitly stated?
- How is "person" or "human" defined in the theory?
- How is health defined in the theory?
- Does the theory explicate the relationship between person or human and health?

Process Criteria Questions

Correspondence

- Does the theory fit with the established general knowledge about person and health?
- Does the theory interrelate concepts at the same level of discourse to describe, explain, or predict regarding person and health?
- With what paradigmatic perspective does the theory correspond?
- Does the theory correspond with the philosophical assumptions?

- Are the principles, concepts, and propositions described parsimoniously in abstract terms?
- Are the meanings of the principles, concepts, and propositions clear?
- Is the meaning of each concept of the theory at a consistent level of discourse?

Coherence

- How do the principles of the theory relate to other theories?
- Is there a logical flow from philosophical assumptions to propositions?
- Is the theory structured in a symmetrically aesthetic way?

Pragmatics

- Can the theory be moved down the ladder of abstraction for use in theory and practice?
- Does the theory generate research questions for investigation?
- Does the theory offer guidelines for practice?
- Is there evidence of support for the theory in research and practice?
- How can the contribution of the theory to nursing science be described?

From Parse, R. (1987). *Nursing science*. Philadelphia: WB Saunders.

of an APN is required so as to more adequately recognize and consider assumptions, be they implied or explicit.

One must also consider another element of assumptions when evaluating theory for use by APNs. Common use of the word *advanced* implies a quality or state of being at a higher level of difficulty or complexity (Morris, 1981). Given that the work of APNs is viewed as having a complex nature, one must consider whether the assumptions support this common belief. In addition, one must determine whether the assumptions are consistent with nursing philosophy. Assumptions about humans, health, the environment, and nursing must be consistent with the basic beliefs and values of the discipline. Theoretical works that are derived from assumptions incompatible with nursing philosophy need to be recognized as such. Any of the models just discussed can be used to evaluate nursing theory. For the purpose of illustration, this chapter uses Parse's framework for theory evaluation. Other models are discussed in more depth in Chapters 30 and 31.

Theory Evaluation: Martha Rogers' Science of Unitary Human Beings Structure

The first step in evaluating theory describes the historical evolution of the theory and the model's assumptions. Assumptions that underpin a theoretical work should be made explicit by the theorist. Identifying theoretical assumptions allows one to consider the values held by the theorist. It also enables one to recognize ideas that are of specific relevance to the phenomenon and the theory or model.

Historical evolution

Martha Rogers is as integral to the development of the Science of Unitary Human Beings as the environment is integral to human beings in her theory. One can not write of the historical development of this theory or nursing theory in general without writing of Martha Rogers. Through her lifetime commitment to the development of a theoretical basis for nursing, she earned the deserved recognition as an icon of nursing theory. Through her theoretical work, the development and testing of nursing theory was recognized as a major concern and priority for the profession of nursing in the 1970s.

Rogers' formal educational credentials were obtained from 1936 until 1954. She earned a diploma in nursing from the Knoxville General Hospital School of Nursing in Knoxville, Tennessee in 1936. In the next year, she earned a Bachelors of Science from George Peabody College in Nashville. She went on to earn a Master's in nursing from Teachers' College and a Master's in public health from Johns Hopkins University. Rogers completed her doctoral degree of science at Johns Hopkins University in 1954.

Rogers' early nursing work was in the area of public health. She worked as a staff nurse and as a visiting nurse

supervisor; later, Rogers brought her experience to education as a visiting lecturer. She eventually came to hold the positions of Professor and Head of the Division of Nurse Education at New York University.

As a scholar, Rogers was able to draw upon an extensive knowledge of the humanities, arts, and sciences. Her life experiences and education helped her conceive a vision that called for a scientific basis for nursing practice. In the early 1960s, Rogers argued that the science of nursing was unique and pioneered the profession's development of a theoretical framework. In 1970, Rogers provided the first view of this unique theoretical framework through the book *An Introduction to the Theoretical Basis of Nursing*. Through the years elements of the theory underwent reexamination and refinement. In 1983, these changes were described in her second major publication, *Science of Unitary Human Beings,* and in 1986, Rogers further expanded the theory.

Other nurses have contributed to the development, refinement, and dissemination of this theory. The following theories were derived from Rogers' work: Barrett's (1989) Theory of Power, Carboni's (1995) Enfolding Health-as-Wholeness-and-Harmony theory, and Newman's (1986) Health as Expanded Consciousness Theory. Parse (1998) believes the Human Becoming Theory to be consistent with elements of Rogers' theory. Other nurses who have contributed to work related to this theory include Malinski, Phillips, and Meehan.

To understand the development of a theory it is important to know the major influences of those that developed and proposed the theory. First, when proposing or refining theory a theorist should identify significant theoretical influences. Identification of these influences enhances understanding and appropriate application of a theory, allowing one to better recognize and understand the underlying assumptions of the theory. This increased understanding can facilitate comprehension of its major concepts and theoretical propositions. Thus, as the major developer of the Science of Unitary Human Beings, it is important to know the major influences on Martha Rogers. Rogers viewed the theory as coming from a number of sources. Sarter (1988) identifies the works of von Bertalanffy, de Chardin, Russels, Polyani, Lewin, Dobzhandsky, and Einstien as major influences on Rogers' theorizing. Exposure to this knowledge was partially gained during her university education before her nursing studies. During this time Rogers studied the sciences and liberal arts. Her keen interest and extensive knowledge of the sciences, humanities, and arts provided a rich and fertile theoretical ground from which the theory developed. She attributed its development to a "creative synthesis" (Rogers, 1992) of ideas and contemporary knowledge.

Philosophical assumptions underlying theory

In 1970, Rogers proposed five major assumptions. The essential meaning of the assumptions has undergone little change over the intervening years, and the assumptions are as follows:

1. Each human being is a unified whole. A human being possesses a distinctive integrity and evidences attributes that are greater than and different from the sum of his or her parts.
2. Matter and energy are constantly exchanged between human beings and the environment.
3. The life process of human beings progresses along a space-time continuum in a manner that is not reversible and is unidirectional.
4. The identity of individuals and their innovative wholeness is recognized through life patterns.
5. Human being is distinguished from the being of other entities through the following potentials: abstraction and imagery; language; and thought, sensation, and emotion (Rogers, 1970; Falco & Lobo, 1995).

Principles, concepts, and propositions

Nursing theories and models traditionally identify (and should always identify) four domains that constitute nursing's metaparadigm: person, health, environment and nursing. Explicit definitions and descriptions regarding the theorized nature of these four domains facilitate description completeness. In addition the theory should identify theoretical propositions that link the four domains of nursing's metaparadigm. These theoretical propositions should identify the relationships and interrelationships between and among person, health, environment, and nursing. For example, it is not sufficient for a nursing theory to just define health and environment. The theory must propose a link between the two domains. Finally, when considering whether a theory sufficiently describes and explains the phenomenon of interest, one must determine whether the proposed concepts are adequate to describe and explain the phenomenon given the scope of the theory and the phenomenon chosen. Would the addition of other elements make the theory seem plausible and the explanation understandable? Would the addition of other elements make the theory seem complete? For APNs this question is especially relevant. Recognizing the integration of previously physician-claimed responsibilities into the work of APNs, does a theory used for advanced practice need to identify other domains to be included in the metaparadigm for advanced practice? If other domains should be considered for inclusion into this metaparadigm, what should they be? This question needs to be confronted and studied within the discipline.

In the Science of Unitary Human Beings, five major concepts are introduced into the body of nursing theory. These concepts are energy field, openness, pattern, pandimensionality, and unitary human being. These concepts represent a new way to conceptualize the focus of nursing.

The major fundamental concept of this theory is energy field (Rogers, 1992). The energy field is the fundamental unit of living and nonliving entities. Both human beings and the environment are identified as energy fields. The word *field* is meant to reflect the unifying aspect of this concept. An energy field can not be reduced to the simple sum of its parts. The word *energy* identifies the field as dynamic. An energy field is considered to be in continuous motion, always changing, and infinite (Rogers, 1992). It is understood to have no boundaries.

Because the energy field is recognized as being without boundaries and infinite, it is characterized as being open (Rogers, 1992). Openness is viewed as a continuous way of existing that allows for the integrality of human and environmental energy fields. This openness describes all energy fields. The concept of openness allows for a different understanding of humans and their environment, enabling one to see that humans and their environment are constantly changing and evolving in relation to one another. The concept of openness precludes the acceptance of the concepts of adaptation, causality, and equilibrium (Rogers, 1992).

Pattern is the unique attribute of an energy field that is recognized as a single wave (Rogers, 1992). Thus pattern provides the energy field with a recognizable identity. It is not something that can be directly observed. Instead, patterns are recognized through observable occurrences that are the manifestations of field patterns. The patterns of energy fields are constantly changing.

Pandimensionality, another significant concept, is "a non-linear domain without spatial or temporal attributes" (Rogers, 1992). Pandimensionality reflects the synthesis of energy field aspects such as infinity; flowing wholeness; innovative, ongoing patterns without boundaries; nonlinearity; and unpredictability (Phillips, 1994). Pandimensionality lends credence to the belief in multiple realities and multiple methods of awareness (Butcher, 1994).

The unitary human being is defined as an irreducible, indivisible, pandimensional energy field (Rogers, 1992). A unitary human being is recognized through patterns and manifestations unique to the whole being. These manifestations cannot be predicted from an understanding of the parts.

Environment is defined as an irreducible, pandimensional energy field (Rogers, 1992). This energy field is recognized through patterns; it is integral to the human energy field.

Principles of homeodynamics are Rogers' proposed scientific principles related to the life process (Rogers, 1970). These theoretical formulations provide a framework to describe and explain unitary human being life events that are relevant to life processes. Rogers identifies three principles of homeodynamics: integrality, resonancy, and helicy. Integrality is the "continuous mutual human field and environmental field process" (Rogers, 1992). Resonancy is the "continuous change from lower to higher frequency wave patterns in human and environmental fields" (Rogers, 1992). Helicy is the "continuous, innovative, unpredictable, increasing diversity of human and environmental field patterns" (Rogers, 1992).

Definitions

The recipient of nursing care is seen as person within this theory. A person is understood to be a unitary human being that exists as an energy field (Rogers, 1992). As an energy field, person is defined as an irreducible, indivisible, and pandimensional entity (Rogers, 1992). A person is recognized by the patterns and attributes evidenced as specific to the whole being. Understanding of the parts does not allow for predictions relative to the individual. Person is theorized to possess the potential for abstraction and imagery, language and thought, and sensation and emotion (Rogers, 1992).

Environment is theorized as the energy field that is integral to the unitary human being (Rogers, 1992). This energy field, like all energy fields, is theorized to be irreducible, indivisible, and pandimensional. Environment can be identified by patterns evidenced through manifestations of the environment's characteristics.

Nursing is a unique learned profession that is recognized as science and art (Rogers, 1990). Rogers purposefully differentiates nursing as science from the use of the word *nursing* to imply its practice (Rogers, 1990; Rogers, 1994). Nursing's uniqueness resides in its phenomenon of concern—unitary human beings existing in a pandimensional world that expands to wherever unitary humans exist. Nursing as a humanistic science is directed toward describing and explaining the unitary human being environmental field process and in developing the hypothetical generalizations and predictive principles basic to knowledgeable practice. The art of nursing resides in the innovative application of nursing science to promote human betterment.

Within this theory, health is not explicitly defined. For Rogers the word *health* is ambiguous; she prefers the word *well-being* (Rogers, 1994). However, implicit within the theory, health may be recognized as an interpretation of the interaction evidenced between unitary human beings and the environment (Rogers, 1970). This interpretation reflects a valuing that may be culturally or individually determined (Rogers, 1980). In addition, propositions are not explicitly stated in any of Rogers' work.

Process Criteria

Correspondence: relationship between person and health

The relationship between person and health is implied, not explicitly described. Rogers says, "Health and sickness, however defined, are expressions of the process of life" (1970). Whall (1987) believes that Rogers' declined to be more explicit with the definition of *health* because it is value laden and varies from culture to culture. The definition of *person* is congruent with the assumptions and principles.

From the five assumptions, Rogers developed the aforementioned major concepts of the theory: energy field, openness, pattern, pandimensionality, and unitary human being. The principles of homeodynamics also are derived from the five assumptions. The three principles are integrality, resonancy, and helicy. The assumptions all have internal congruence and demonstrate Rogers' holistic, nonmechanistic view (Whall, 1987). The concepts and principles are explicitly stated. They are also broad and abstract but at a consistent level of discourse. This model has great explanatory power; however, because the concepts are abstract it may be more difficult to measure predicted outcomes (Whall, 1987).

Theory is developed within a perspective or worldview. This perspective limits what assumptions may effectively function as a foundation for a theory. In turn these assumptions limit the theoretical concepts and the nature of the theoretical propositions. These elements assist in the classification of the theory.

The criterion of logical congruency evaluates the logical consistency of the theory. Logical consistency is evaluated in two ways. First, the explicit and implicit elements of the theory are examined to determine whether the theory is representative of the worldview from which it is derived. Second, congruency of the theory's explicit and implicit elements with features of the theory classification must also be determined. Answers to the following questions assist in determining the logical congruency of a theory:

1. Is the internal structure of the theory or conceptual model logically congruent?
2. Does the theory or model reflect more than one contrasting worldview?
3. Does the theory or model reflect characteristics of more than one category of model?
4. Do the components of the theory or model reflect a logical translation of diverse perspectives? (Fawcett, 1989)

Theories or models that posses internal structures that are not logically consistent, that are derived from more than one perspective or worldview, or that possess characteristics from multiple theory or model categories are not usually considered logically congruent. Theoretical works that possess logically inconsistent structures need further refinement. Also, theoretical works that represent more than one worldview or possess characteristics representative of multiple theory or model classifications need to undergo refinement. During the theorizing process, diverse concepts and propositions must be examined for elements that need to be adapted or translated to one perspective. This translation requires a redefinition process that results in the theoretical elements being representative of one theoretical perspective and classification (Fawcett, 1989).

Rogers' approach uses a simultaneity worldview. This means that person is seen as "mutually living and evolving with the environment" (Whall, 1987). Rogers' focus is on the whole. Whall believes that there is a close integration between the principles and assumptions, and thus they are logically consistent. Butcher (1999) describes Rogers' worldview "which entails a recognition that there is a deep interconnectedness and oneness of everything, the living and nonliving. Humans are coextensive with the universe and are coparticipating in its continuous creative evolution."

One of the major purposes of theories and models for practice disciplines is to develop knowledge to improve the nature and outcomes of practice. For this type of knowledge to be developed, a theoretical work must generate concepts and proposed relationships between and among the concepts. These concepts and relationships must be carefully and clearly articulated so they can undergo rigorous testing. This testing either supports or refutes aspects of the theory. Theoretical works that are refuted through research necessarily lose currency and are not considered credible. Because the concepts in Rogers' theory are so abstract, they are able to encompass the nature of person and life process. This abstractness does limit the theory's utility by APNs in practice because much work must be done to define the concepts and relationships to make them useable for testing. In addition, Rogers' theory is somewhat difficult to understand due to its abstractness and new terminology; some APNs may feel that this also limits its utility.

Coherence

Although Rogers' theory does not appear to be related to most other nursing models, it does have certain similarities to them, and the theories of Newman (1986) and Parse (1987) are closely related and based upon Rogers' model. However, some concepts defined by Rogers (such as helicy) are not used in any other models. Because Rogers' theory uses five concepts, three principles, and five assumptions, her framework is very simplistic. It has clarity, and its beauty, according to Whall (1987), lies in its simplicity and balance.

Pragmatics: use in practice and research

Theoretical works that are considered relevant for advanced practice need to be challenged appropriately. Theoretical concepts or propositions relative to the nature of advanced practice that have been tested for non–advanced practice nursing may need to be retested in settings where an APN provides care. The discipline needs to consider whether retesting of a theory regarding its applicability to APNs must be conducted before findings can be generalized to the practice. Because Rogers' theory is so broadly defined, numerous research phenomena can be examined, such as patterns, energy, power of knowledge, temporal experience, and healing touch.

In regard to theories, there are three social considerations. Social congruence exists when a theory recommends nursing activities that meet society's expectations (Fawcett, 1989). Evaluating theory that is relevant for APNs is an issue here; patients used to receiving certain types of care from physicians may be initially reluctant to receive this care from APNs. When evaluating theory in this area, one must consider whether the theory-generated practice recommendations are acceptable to society. In some cases the discipline may need to help patients and society create new expectations. Also, future theoretical works relevant to APNs need to take social congruence into consideration.

Social significance is the second social consideration. Social significance exists when application of a theory results in an outcome desired by a patient (Fawcett, 1989). Butcher (1999) stresses that this is the core value of human uniqueness that has emerged from Rogers' theory. This value is certainly important and has significance to APNs and patients. Determination of a theory's social significance is usually provided through research. Thus, when evaluating theory for social significance, research literature needs to be studied.

The third social consideration is social utility. Social utility exists when a theory provides comprehensive guidelines for education, practice, research, and administration. These guidelines need to be sufficiently explicit so as to facilitate adherence (Fawcett, 1989). To meet this criterion a theorist must necessarily consider a broad range of nursing situations and activities when developing the theory. To evaluate this criterion, one must examine the theory in light of APN activities and situations and determine whether sufficient direction is given for the different arenas where APNs provide care. Rogers' theory has served as the cornerstone for several research methodologies, including Cowling's (1997) Pattern Profiling and Case Study method, Butcher's (1994) Unitary Field Pattern Portrait, and Barrett's (1998) Pattern Manifestation Knowing and Voluntary Mutual Patterning.

The final consideration when evaluating theory relates to the theory's capacity to contribute to and increase APN knowledge. To make this determination requires a review of the literature relating to the theory. After a review of the literature, one can determine the level to which APN knowledge is increased. Kaplan (1964) proposes that value of a theory "lies not only in the answers it gives, but in the new questions it raises." In this regard, Rogers' Science of Unitary Human Beings has contributed to nursing science. It has raised many questions and is currently being used to seek answers to those questions.

In nursing literature the significance of the Science of Unitary Human Beings for nursing research, theory, and practice has been recognized, and a number of indicators of this acceptance have been identified (Phillips, 1997). In the last decade there has been an increase in work to develop and test Rogerian theory (Phillips, 1997). Rogers' theory offers a uniquely new way of looking at nursing and continues to stimulate many research questions to test the theory. Rogerian conferences provide scholars with opportunities to communicate their insights and findings related to Rogers' theory. The Society of Rogerian Scholars publishes a journal, *Visions: The Journal of Rogerian*

Nursing Science, to promote the dissemination of the theory. Other journals have also published numerous studies and articles about the Science of Unitary Human Beings (Phillips, 1997). The Science of Unitary Human Beings served as the theoretical grounding for the development of other nursing theories such as Health as Expanding Consciousness (Newman, 1986) and the Human Becoming Theory (Parse, 1998)

Rogers' theory offers new ways for APNs to conceptualize the science that serves as a foundation for practice. The theory also offers a practice methodology called a *health patterning practice method.* This practice methodology was designed to help one come to know and distinguish human health patterns and assist patients to participate in their well-being (Barrett, 1998). New noninvasive treatments are also available to APNs and are consistent with this theory. Examples include therapeutic touch, meditation, imagery, and visualization (Phillips, 1990).

PRIORITIES FOR RESEARCH

Development of nursing theory through research warrants particular attention at all levels of nursing. Clearer theoretical direction for practice, research, and education that is uniquely related to nursing serves to better define the discipline. Theoretical development through research has particular importance for APNs. APN curricula that emphasize a medically based practice may fail the discipline in its need for definition and autonomy. Theoretical research relative to advanced practice should appropriately examine and systematically evaluate theoretical models of nursing in practice and education arenas. For example, how do APNs practice nursing? If an APN uses Rogers' theory as a worldview on how to approach patients and provide care, how would it affect outcomes?

Meehan (1991) used Rogers' theory as the basis for her research on therapeutic touch and postoperative pain. A single-trial, three-group design with 108 patients was conducted comparing therapeutic touch, a placebo control intervention that mimicked therapeutic touch, and the standard intervention of a narcotic. The degree of pain was measured using a visual analogue scale. No decrease in postoperative pain was found in the therapeutic touch group, although the group waited a significantly longer time to request further analgesic medication. Further research is needed to explore the relationship between therapeutic touch and Rogers' theory.

McEvoy (1990) evaluated the process of dying within the conceptual model of unitary human beings. Twenty-eight adults with a diagnosis of cancer and a life expectancy of 1 month participated in the dying group. The nondying group consisted of 28 adults who were free of life-threatening disease. McEvoy predicted that the dying group would experience more paranormal experiences than the nondying group. This hypothesis was supported in the final week of life, but not before. Based on Rogers' theory, it would be expected that as the human field and the environmental field were engaged in simultaneous, mutual process, additional perceptional modalities might become present. More paranormal events were experienced in the last week before death, but additional research is needed to clearly understand the human experience of dying (McEvoy, 1990). Other research has used Rogers' theory as a theoretical framework to evaluate the notion of temporal experiences (Paletta, 1990), guided imagery (Butcher & Parker, 1990), and patterning of time experience and human field motion (Rapacz, 1990). Future studies need to be conducted to demonstrate the ability to operationalize Rogers' theory.

IMPLICATIONS FOR MSN EDUCATION AND ADVANCED PRACTICE

For nursing theory to be used effectively in advanced practice, graduates must be exposed to and acknowledge the significance of nursing theory. One way to approach the curricular process is to analyze all concepts and knowledge within that framework. Mathwig, Young, and Pepper (1990) stress the notion that it is not a case of having nursing's science content integrated into other knowledge or concepts; rather, it is using the nursing theory as a mechanism within which to analyze the concepts and knowledge. Use of a Rogers' nursing science–based education places the nursing process within an expanded frame of reference and focuses on the individual as a unitary being and the individual-environment field process. When nursing theory serves as the worldview for a curriculum it is comprehensively reflected in the philosophy, mission, course objectives, and student learning experiences. This same perspective gives APN students the opportunity to look at their patients from a different perspective.

It is difficult to conceive of any one existing theory that meets all of the criteria for applicability for advanced practice. This dilemma resides in the work of the APN. The responsibilities of this position blend the work of two disciplines, nursing and medicine. Because of this, the evaluation of theory for APNs becomes more difficult and political than that of evaluation of theory for non-APNs. While acknowledging this concern and examining the different elements of theory evaluation for advanced practice, significant questions arise. One question is whether there is a need to reevaluate nursing theory for generalizability to advanced practice. This question and the others posed in the search for theory open up a new area of concern for nursing. Dialogue that seeks to find the answers to these questions may help to generate new ideas about the nature of the discipline.

Paradoxically, the work of evaluating theories developed

Suggestions for Further Learning

- Get the article: Frik, S., & Pollock, S. (1993). Preparation for advanced nursing practice. *Nursing and Healthcare, 14*(4), 190-195. This article discusses the preparation of APNs. What role do they identify for nursing theory in that preparation?

- Go to the Rogers website (www.uwcm.ac.uk/uwcm/ns/martha/homepage.html) or obtain a copy of the journal *Visions: The Journal of Rogerian Nursing Science* to further explore Rogers' theory.

- Marcia Anderson uses Rogers' theory as the basis for her practice with substance abuse. See her website at www.pnc-wbi.com/. Here are some publications related to her work:

  - Andersen, M.D., & Braunstein, M.S. (1992). Conceptions of therapy: personalized nursing LIGHT model with chemically-dependent female offenders. In T. Mieczkowski (Ed.), *Drugs, crime, and social policy: research, issues, and concerns* (pp. 250-262). Needham Heights, MA: Allyn & Bacon.

  - Andersen, M.D., & Hockperson, E.M. (1997). Well-being and high-risk drug use among active drug users. In M. Madrid (Ed.), *Patterns of Rogerian knowing.* New York: National League for Nursing Press.

  - Andersen, M.D., Hockperson, E.M., & Smereck, G.A.D. (1996). Effect of a nursing outreach intervention to drug users in Detroit, Michigan. *Journal of Drug Issues, 26*(3), 619-634.

  - Andersen, M.D., & Smereck, G.A.D. (1989, Fall). Personalized nursing LIGHT model. *Nursing Science Quarterly, 2*(3), 120-130.

  - Andersen, M.D., & Smereck, G.A.D. (1992, Summer). The consciousness rainbow: An explication of Rogerian field pattern personifestations. *Nursing Science Quarterly, 5*(2), 72-79.

  - Andersen, M.D., & Smereck, G.A.D. (1994). Personalized nursing: a science-based model of the art of nursing. In M. Madrid & E.A.M. Barrett (Eds.), *Rogers' scientific art of nursing practice* (pp. 261-283). New York: National League for Nursing.

  - Andersen, M.D., & Smereck, G.A.D. (1994). *The art of nursing: the personalized nursing practice model* (Videotape). Plymouth, MI: Personalized Nursing Corporation.

  - Andersen, M.D., & Smereck, G.A.D. (1994). *The art of nursing: the personalized nursing practice model workbook.* Plymouth, MI: Personalized Nursing Corporation.

  - Andersen, M.D., Smereck, G.A.D., & Braunstein, M.S. (1993). LIGHT model: an effective intervention model to change high-risk behaviors among hard-to-reach urban drug users. *The American Journal of Drug and Alcohol Abuse, 19*(3), 309-325.

- Another nurse scholar that uses Rogers' theory is Elizabeth Barrett. She is interested in health patterning. Information from her website indicates her interest in this topic (www.uwcm.ac.uk/uwcm/ns/martha/Barrett.htm). According to Barrett, "Health patterning is a process of facilitating unitary well-being by assisting clients with their knowing participation in change. The focus includes lifestyle changes, struggles with illness, and resolution of difficulties in living and dying. In the health patterning process, people are helped to become aware of feelings, thoughts, and attitudes within a gentle, life-affirming environmental context that involves meaningful use of theory and associated health patterning modalities. These modalities include therapeutic touch, imagery, and meditation as well as use of sound, light, color, and motion. Meaningful dialogue and centering are integral to persony of these approaches as well as knowledgeable caring, authenticity and love.

- W. Richard Cowling has used Rogers' Unitary Person Theory as the basis of his investigations into despair. Check out his website at views.vcu.edu/son/faculty/wcowling/cowling.html, or some of the following publications:

  - Cowling, W.R. (1990). Chronological age as an anomalie of evolution. In E.A. Barrett (Ed.), *Visions of Rogers' science-based nursing* (pp. 143-149). New York: National League for Nursing.

  - Cowling, W.R. (1990). A template for unitary pattern-based nursing practice. In E.A. Barrett (Ed.), *Visions of Rogers' science-based nursing* (pp. 45-65). New York: National League for Nursing.

  - Cowling, W.R. (1993). Unitary knowing in nursing practice. *Nursing Science Quarterly, 6,* 201-207.

  - Cowling, W.R. (1993). Unitary practice: Revisionary assumptions. In M.S. Parker (Ed.), *Nursing theories in practice* (Vol. 2). New York: National League for Nursing.

  - Cowling, W.R. (1997). A unitary conceptual and theoretical legacy. *Visions: The Journal of Rogerian Nursing Science, 6*(1), 19-21.

  - Cowling, W.R. (1997). Unitary pattern appreciation: the unitary science/practice of reaching for essence. In M. Madrid (Ed.), *Patterns of Rogerian knowing.* New York: National League for Nursing.

  - Cowling, W.R. (1998). Unitary case method. *Nursing Science Quarterly, 11*(4), 139-141.

  - Cowling, W.R. (1999). A unitary-transformative nursing science: potentials for transcending dichotomies. *Nursing Science Quarterly, 12*(2), 132-135.

  - Cowling, W.R. (in press). Healing as appreciating wholeness. *Advances in Nursing Science.*

  - Cowling, W.R., Barrett, E.A.M., Carboni, J.T., & Butcher, H.K. (1997). Unitary perspectives on methodological practices. In M. Madrid (Ed.), *Patterns of Rogerian knowing.* New York: National League for Nursing.

  - Langston, N., Cowling, W.R., & McCain, N.L. (1998). Transforming academic nursing: from balance through integration to coherence. *Journal of Professional Nursing, 15*(1), 28-32.

- Vidette Todaro-Franceschi's work has looked at the concept of energy, and she has written a publication on the subject: Todaro-Franceschi, V. (1999). *The enigma of energy: where science & religion converge.* New York: Crossroad Publishing. You can also find out more at her website (www.uwcm.ac.uk/uwcm/ns/martha/vidette.htm).

in the past and present is driven by a need to look to the future. The act of evaluating theory requires recognition of what exists currently and what will be experienced by the discipline in the future. Henchley (1978) identifies four ways of conceptualizing the future: possible future, plausible future, probable future, and preferable future. The preferable future is the vision of the future that is most desirable. When evaluating nursing theory for advanced practice, one must consider to which future a given theory will take the discipline. Does the theory make nursing's preferable future more likely?

DISCUSSION QUESTIONS

These questions can be used to promote critical thinking and encourage discussion.

1. Select one of the nursing theories or models from Chapter 30. Identify how you would evaluate it. How would this evaluation assist you to look at it from an APN framework?
2. Given that professional nursing requires currency in the literature, discuss the different types of literature with which APNs need to be familiar to be able to evaluate new theoretical assumptions.
3. For APNs, should new concepts be added to the four traditional theoretical domains of nursing? Provide a rationale for your position.

REFERENCES/BIBLIOGRAPHY

Barnum, B.J.S. (1990). *Nursing theory: analysis, application, evaluation* (3rd ed.). Glenview, IL: Scott, Foresman and Company.

Barrett, E.A.M. (1989). A nursing theory of power for nursing practice: derivation from Rogers' paradigm. In J. Riehl-Sisca (Ed.), *Conceptual modes for nursing practice* (3rd ed.) (pp. 207-217). Norwalk, CT: Appleton & Lange.

Barrett, E. (1998). A Rogerian practice methodology for health patterning. *Nursing Science Quarterly, 11,* 136-138.

Butcher, H., & Parker, N. (1990). Guided imagery within Rogers' Science of Unitary Human Beings: an experimental study. In E.A.M. Barrett (Ed.), *Visions of Rogers' science-based nursing* (pp. 269-286). New York: National League for Nursing.

Butcher, H.K. (1994). The unitary field portrait method: development of a research method for Rogers' Science of Unitary Human Beings. In M. Madrid & E.A.M. Barrett (Eds.), *Rogers' scientific art of nursing practice* (pp. 397-429). New York: National League for Nursing.

Butcher, H. (1996). A unitary field pattern portrait of dispiritedness in later life. *Visions: The Journal of Rogerian Nursing Science, 4,* 41-58.

Butcher, H. (1998). Crystallizing the processes of the unitary field pattern portrait research method. *Visions: The Journal of Rogerian Nursing Science, 6,* 130-136.

Butcher, H. (1999). Rogerian ethics: an ethical inquiry into Rogers' life and science. *Nursing Science Quarterly, 12*(2),111-118.

Carboni, J (1995). A Rogerian process of inquiry. *Nursing Science Quarterly, 8,* 22-27.

Chin, P.L., & Kramer, M.K. (1995). *Theory and nursing: a systematic approach* (4th ed.). St. Louis: Mosby.

Cowling, W. (1997). Pattern appreciation: the unity science/practice of reaching essence. In M. Madrid (Ed.), *Patterns of Rogerian knowing* (pp. 129-142), New York: National League for Nursing.

Falco, S.M., & Lobo, M.L. (1995). Martha Rogers. In J.B. George (Ed.), *Nursing theories: the base for professional nursing practice* (pp. 229-248). Norwalk, CT: Appleton & Lange.

Fawcett, J. (1989). *Analysis and evaluation of conceptual models of nursing* (2nd ed.). Philadelphia: FA Davis.

Henchley, N. (1978). Making sense of the future. *Alternatives, 7*(24).

Kaplan, A. (1964). *The conduct of inquiry.* Scranton, PA: Chandler Publishing.

Mathwig, G., Young, A., & Pepper, J. (1990). Using rogerian science in undergraduate and graduate nursing education. In E.A.M. Barrett (Ed.), *Visions of Rogers' science-based nursing* (pp. 319-334). New York: National League for Nursing.

McEvoy, M. (1990). The relationships among the experience of dying, the experience of paranormal events, and creativity in adults. In E.A.M. Barrett (Ed.), *Visions of Rogers' science-based nursing* (pp. 209-228). New York: National League for Nursing.

Meehan, T. (1991). Therapeutic touch and postoperative pain: a Rogerian research study. *Nursing Science Quarterly, 6,* 69-78

Meleis, A.I. (1991). *Theoretical nursing: development & progress* (2nd ed.). Philadelphia: JB Lippincott.

Morris, W. (Ed.). (1981). *The American heritage dictionary of the English language* (1st ed.). Boston: Houghton Mifflin.

Newman, M.A. (1986). *Health as expanding consciousness.* St. Louis: Mosby.

Paletta, J. (1990). The relationship of temporal experience to human time. In E.A.M. Barrett (Ed.), *Visions of Rogers' science-based nursing* (pp. 229-254). New York: National League for Nursing.

Parse, R. (1987). *Nursing science.* Philadelphia: WB Saunders.

Parse, R.R. (1998). *The Human Becoming School of Thought.* Thousand Oaks, CA: Sage.

Phillips, J.R. (1990). Changing human potential and future visions for nursing: a human field image perspective. In E.A.M. Barrett (Ed.), *Visions of Rogers' science-based nursing* (pp. 13-25). New York: National League for Nursing.

Phillips, J.R. (1994). The open-ended nature of the Science of Unitary Human Beings. In M. Madrid & E.A.M. Barrett (Eds.), *Rogers' scientific art of nursing practice* (pp. 11-25). New York: National League for Nursing.

Phillips, J.R. (1997). Martha E. Rogers: an icon of nursing. *Nursing Science Quarterly, 10*(1) 39-41.

Powers, B.A., & Knapp, T.R. (1990). *A dictionary of nursing theory and research* (1st ed.). Thousand Oaks, CA: Sage Publications.

Rapacz, K. (1990). The patterning of time experience and human field motion during the experience of pleasant guided imagery: a discussion. In E.A.M. Barrett (Ed.), *Visions of Rogers' science-based nursing* (pp. 287-294). New York: National League for Nursing.

Rogers, M.E. (1970). *An introduction to the theoretical basis of nursing*. Philadelphia: FA Davis.

Rogers, M.E. (1980). *The Science of Unitary Person* (Videotape). New York: Media for Nursing.

Rogers, M.E. (1983). Science of Unitary Human Beings. In L.W. Clements and F.B. Roberts (Eds.), *Family health: a theoretical approach to nursing care*. New York: Wiley.

Rogers, M.E. (1986). Science of Unitary Human Beings. In V. Malinki (Ed.), *Explorations on Martha Rogers' Science of Unitary Human Beings* (pp. 3-8). Norwalk, CT: Appleton-Century Crofts.

Rogers, M.E. (1990). Nursing: science of unitary, irreducible, human beings: update 1990. In E.A.M. Barrett (Ed.), *Visions of Rogers' science-based nursing* (pp. 5-10). New York: National League for Nursing.

Rogers, M.E. (1992). Nursing science and the space age. *Nursing Science Quarterly, 5*(1), 27-34.

Rogers, M.E. (1994). The Science of Unitary Human Beings: current perspectives. *Nursing Science Quarterly, 7*(1), 33-35.

Sarter, B. (1988). Philosophical sources of nursing theory. *Nursing Science Quarterly, 1*(2), 52-59.

Whall, A. (1987). A critique of Rogers' framework. In R. Parse (Ed.), *Nursing science* (pp. 147-158). Philadelphia: WB Saunders.

Chapter 28

Nursing's Utilization of Theory

Ann W. Keller

S cience is a body of knowledge organized with particular attitudes and methods and concerned with human beings and their worlds (Phillips, 1996). The goal of science is the discovery of truths (Jacox, 1974). To understand nursing and its development, science's place in relation to human knowledge must be understood. A nursing pattern of knowing has been identified by nursing scholars as necessary to differentiate nursing science from other disciplines, and this chapter addresses nursing's utilization of theory.

DEFINITIONS

Gortner (1980) has defined **nursing science** as reflecting nursing's understanding of human biology, behavior, health, and illness. In her definition, she includes the process necessary to bring about changes in health status and the behavior patterns associated with normal and critical life events, as well as the principles governing life states and processes. The goal of nursing science is to understand, explain, and represent human nature (Gortner & Schultz, 1988). Nursing science consists of defined concepts describing human responses to health, illness, and therapeutic nursing actions (Hinshaw, 1989). Nursing science in relationship to practice, then, is the body of knowledge with a nursing prospective that produces and tests knowledge gained in nursing work.

The discussion of the relationship of human knowledge to nursing knowledge can occur within the discussion of what constitutes a discipline. The *Oxford English Dictionary* defines **discipline** as "a branch of instruction or education; a department of learning or knowledge; a science or art in its educational aspect." This is important because this framework is used to organize what the discipline's perspective will be; what is questioned and answered; how the discipline will be studied; and to what criteria the discipline will be held (Donaldson & Crowley, 1978). Within these particulars is what differentiates this discipline from others.

Academic disciplines are traditionally mathematics, history, philosophy, physics, physiology, and sociology. The **professional disciplines** include nursing, law, and medicine. Meleis (1997) identifies the discipline of nursing as based in practice, research, philosophy, and theory. She proposes that the development of nursing in the last 30 years has occurred due to the effect nursing theory development has had on the discipline of nursing. Theory is now imbedded in all arenas of nursing: practice, administration, and education (Meleis, 1997).

CRITICAL ISSUES: UTILIZATION OF THEORY

The formal education of nursing practice evolved while working within procedural formats first advocated by Florence Nightingale. This evolution later included nursing education and administration as practice arenas. Nursing educators and administrators began to explore ways to teach and administer care, searching for answers to questions to improve the quality of teaching for students and caring for patients. In the decades that followed, schools of nursing opened in the United States and Europe, some which were based on Nightingale's plan. Nursing education became recognized as a profession and form of higher education.

At the turn of the century, the number of nursing schools was approximately 400 (Doheny, Cook, & Stopper, 1997). At that time, teaching issues of major concern were of a technical nature, predominantly driven by medical discoveries. Nursing's technical skill was additionally influenced by physician-authored texts on management of the sick. Physicians replaced superintendents of nursing as instructors, and they became governing board members. Despite these influences, nursing education was still slow in finding a place in the university setting, though number of diploma programs continued to increase.

At the outset of World War I, a limited body of educated nurses was prepared. With the ravages of war, the demand for nurses increased. To meet this demand for nurses, as many as 100 schools of nursing opened during the war (Doheny et al, 1997). With such a rapid proliferation, the programs lacked a strong academic foundation and did not use the developed body of nursing knowledge. These deficits were documented in Goldmark's report, published in 1923. This report was instrumental in initiating changes that resulted in the closure of weaker nursing schools. Consequently, nursing education began to move slowly back to the university.

World War II also increased the need for nurses. Federal money was made available to increase enrollment in established programs. Although nurses graduated in large numbers at this time, a shortage continued until the war ended. Throughout the war years, the inability to prepare the necessary number of nurses showcased nurses' importance to society.

Nursing for the Future, published by Brown in 1948, called for nursing education to include a two-tiered system of preparation. The first level of nursing education provided graduates with a higher level of communication skill that facilitated interactions with others and data collection skills that would lead to complex problem analysis and resolution. Included in Brown's report were recommendations for increased research for nursing practice and the development of clinical specialists. The second level of nursing education provided graduates with a more technically oriented preparation. Brown envisioned both levels of nursing education occurring in institutions of higher learning (Brown, 1948).

Advanced practice went through similar growing pains. The American Nurses Association (ANA) has identified four groups of clinical advanced practice nurses (APNs): certified registered nurse anesthetists (CRNAs), clinical nurse specialists (CNSs), certified nurse midwives (CNMs), and nurse practitioners (NPs). Nurse anesthetists have been a professional group since the 1800s. Their initial training was primarily by physicians in certificate programs, and it was not until the 1980s that most were prepared in a graduate nursing program. Because most of their training was by physicians, many nurse anesthetists were not fully accepted by the nursing profession. APNs experienced this same lack of acceptance because their training occurred the same way. In the 1970s, schools of nursing began to offer Master's programs for APNs.

Initially, CNS programs focused primarily on psychosocial needs, but today programs address all specialty areas. CNSs were always educated in Master's degree programs. These differences in the way APNs were educated created a dichotomy among persons within the profession, hindered progress, and introduced divisiveness within the discipline of nursing.

Today, according to the ANA's Council of Nurses in Advanced Practice, APNs are experts in assessment, diagnosis, and treatment of complex responses of individuals, families, and communities to actual or potential problems in wellness and/or acute or chronic health issues. They function as multidisciplinary colleagues and health team members, integrating leadership, education, and research into their role as clinicians and/or consultants (Pokorny & Barnard, 1992). The National Council of State Boards of Nursing (1992) identified credentials for APNs as: (1) basic education and licensure, (2) graduate degree in nursing, and (3) experience in the area of specialization. Since most of the initial educational programs for APNs were not within schools of nursing, many programs did not include information on nursing theory. However, as more of the APN programs have become part of nursing schools, theory has been integrated into the curricula or added as a separate course.

As the discipline of nursing matured, nurses engaged in identifying what they knew and what they needed to know. The number of nurses with advanced preparation increased, and scholarly inquiry was generated amongst these scientist/theorists. Questions were raised, some of which asked how to enrich nursing education. Nurses turned to research to find the answers. This inquiry led to an expanded body of knowledge of nursing about nursing work and nursing interventions. The examination of this and other ongoing theoretical work produced a formalized structured body of nursing knowledge. This knowledge was amplified into a meaningful, whole nursing theory (Chinn & Kramer, 1995; Benoliel, 1997; Meleis, 1997). Rogers (1985) asserts that this organized body of theoretical knowledge is what identified nursing as a profession. APNs need to understand the historical background of how advanced practice and nursing theory were integrated. This provides a perspective of where and how nursing theory might best fit in today's advanced practice.

Chinn and Kramer (1995) describe theory as a creative and rigorous structuring of ideas that projects a shorthand way to identify concepts and the characteristics that give phenomena their identity. Barnum (1994) states that a theory is similar to a territorial map that differs from an aerial view of the same territory in that it points out and describes the parts important for travelers.

Nursing theory is part of nursing knowledge. Nursing theory, as defined by Meleis (1997), is a "conceptualization of some aspect of nursing reality communicated for the purpose of describing phenomena, explaining relationships between phenomena, predicting consequences, or prescribing nursing care." Nursing theory seeks to describe or explain nursing and is a tentative, purposeful, and systematic view of phenomena. Rutty (1998) suggests that the ultimate direction of theory development is to positively influence nursing practice.

Patterns of Knowing

To understand how nursing uses theory, one must become familiar with the relationship between the structure and patterns of nursing phenomena. One must recognize how these elements together constitute the body of knowledge that is nursing. In one vision, Carper (1978) identifies four fundamental patterns of knowing: empirics, the science of nursing; aesthetics, the art of nursing; personal knowledge in nursing; and ethics, the moral knowledge of nursing. (Figure 28-1 demonstrates these concepts graphically.)

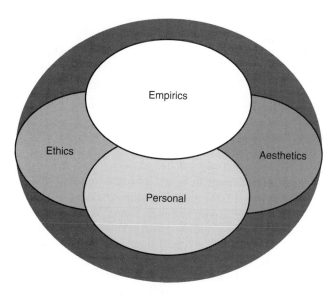

Figure 28-1 The whole of knowing. (From Chinn, P., & Kramer, M. [1995]. *Theory and nursing: a systematic approach* [4th ed.]. St. Louis: Mosby).

Empirical knowledge (empirics) in nursing is used to describe, explain, and predict phenomena (Carper, 1978; Jacobs-Kramer & Chinn, 1988). Those nurses who use empirical knowledge, which is highly valued in Western cultures, claim to *know* because of their belief in traditional science. Traditional science advocates the use of systematic problem-solving methods employed by many academic disciplines (Chinn & Kramer, 1995). Empirical knowing is constructed from this traditional pattern of science, where reality is constructed as verifiable phenomena. Phenomena are verified through the use of the senses.

The second pattern of knowing is aesthetic knowing (aesthetics). For nursing, aesthetic knowing is the art of providing a patient with whatever is required to restore or extend coping capabilities. The skilled nurse can choose from past experiences to connect and collaborate with patients in their care. The increased experience of the nurse broadens the field of experiential choices and the complexities of the applications of other experiences to the current one (Carper, 1978; Benner, 1984). Aesthetic knowing involves the creative processes of engaging, intuiting, and envisioning (Chinn & Kramer, 1995). The nurse-patient interaction is the engaging of self directly in a situation. Within this situation, intuition, based on the collection of experiences, is drawn upon. Benner identifies this manner of practice as the art form of nursing (1984).

The third pattern of knowing is personal knowledge. Personal knowledge is a type of knowing that scholars in many fields have used as they struggle to describe the interpersonal interaction that occurs between self and other. In nursing, personal knowledge is an area of great importance because it embodies the concept of health through the interaction of nurse and patient. Experienced, mature, caring nurses use "therapeutic use of self" to engage with patients, whom they acknowledge as complex, whole beings. This type of engagement brings about positive interactions, characterized by integrity, that produce change in their lives (Carper, 1978).

The fourth pattern of knowing is moral knowledge or ethics. The moral knowledge of nursing identifies the obligation of service. *Moral knowing* refers to all judgments involved with and created in response to choices and goals conceived within the framework of service to patients. As a nurse becomes experienced, choices broaden. The nurse learns to identify the philosophical and moral positions available for application to each individual served.

Chinn and Kramer (1995) believe the four patterns of knowing provide ways to share wisdom and understanding that can be used in practice. The critical component is the integration of the four patterns of knowing into practice. For example, if an APN has a problem that he or she wants to solve related to how effective a nursing intervention is, it would be logical to develop a research strategy to describe the intervention. If the intervention was based on comfort or caring, the APN would explain how comfort is achieved and what steps need to take place for it to occur. It might even be possible to predict when it would occur. As the research process develops and is refined, theories of comfort are investigated and evaluated to see how they fit with the APN's own theory of comfort. Finally, as the research process is carried out, the meaning of comfort, the personal insight of how comfort is experienced, and the ethical obligation related to comfort are addressed.

Nursing Theory–Guided Practice: What It Is and Is Not

The issue of exactly what constitutes nursing theory is still being debated. Cody (1994) argues that much of what is considered nursing theory is really not. He believes that some use the term *nursing theory* but in reality mean any theory that nurses use. His premise is that any knowledge that is useful in general health care or the care of a specific population is not necessarily nursing theory. Cody posits that general knowledge, just by virtue of being written by a nurse or used by nurses, does not constitute nursing theory. He postulates that the definition of nursing theory that should be used is "a distinct and well-articulated system of concepts and propositions rooted explicitly in a philosophy of nursing and intended solely to guide nursing practice and research. Nurses, by virtue of being nurses, have an obligation to concentrate and focus on theory that is specific to their discipline, participate in its development and refinement, and guide its use. This may be a particular issue for APNs because the line between nursing and medical care is very blurred. Medicine still has a strong influence on nursing actions, and many APNs believe that mastery of the medical framework is essential to advanced practice. However, as more APNs recognize the distinction between medicine and nursing and contribute to nursing's knowledge base, nursing will progress more consistently toward recognition as a full profession.

It is interesting that most APNs believe that research findings should guide practice. In reality, it should be theory supported through empirical testing (Cody, 1994). Because nursing theories identify the value of the human, values guide practice. Cody also argues that much of the research that has constituted nursing is concerned more with practical problem-solving (e.g., dressings, positioning) and does not contribute to the advancement of knowledge in the discipline. Cody gives the example of two different interventions to heal a decubitus ulcer. The intervention that heals the ulcer faster could be recommended for future use, but this procedure does not really guide practice. What guides practice is putting value on promoting health and desiring to do so without harming the patient. Nursing theory–guided practice is based on theory specific to nursing, rooted in the philosophy of nursing, and intended solely to guide nursing research and practice. Cody (1994) continues, "True theory guided practice is far more comprehensive and more complex than mere applications of the results of problem solving investigations. Only when nurses are guided in their practice by a theory base specific to nursing will nursing have achieved parity with other scholarly disciplines."

Theory and Practice

Chinn and Kramer (1995) define *nursing practice* as the experiences a practicing nurse encounters during the process of caring for people. In nursing, theory is used to enlighten nurses about nursing practice situations and to guide research. The interaction of practice and theory shapes practice and helps in establishing guidelines for practice (Meleis, 1997). These practice experiences are oriented from the views of both nurse and patient. The experiences are interactive, individual, and framed by the environment.

APNs do not obtain from theory the same structure and guidance they previously obtained from the principles and procedures that exist to standardize practice. Theory challenges existing practice by creating new ways to think and practice (Chinn & Kramer, 1995). From nursing experience and nurses' perceptions of their world, nursing theorists and APNs develop conceptual meanings. These conceptual meanings are arrived at through reflection, discussion, and attempts to make sense of the meanings. APNs and theorists communicating between and among themselves develop language and tools to communicate about the meaning of the experiences.

Much has been written about the difficulty of putting theory into practice (Kim, 1993; Kim 1994; Phillips, Mousseau-Gershman, & Powell, 1998). The individual nurse must come, with knowledge, to the individual patient in each nurse-patient interaction. Or, simply stated,

the nurse must choose a nursing intervention that is appropriate for that particular situation. It is at this point that the nurse brings all past experience and knowledge to bear; he or she makes a choice of action and then applies the theory chosen (Kim, 1993). It is in this dynamic interaction that theory and practice are integrated for patient care.

An idea's meaning is constructed of the sum of the thing, its name or label, the feelings and values associated with it and its label, and perceptions of the thing. Words may possess multiple meanings. Extracting the exact meaning is important in creating conceptual meaning. A *concept* is a mental abstraction of experience. Nurses in practice observe, name, and make sense of what happens in their experiences, and they use their senses to verify and share their experiences. Communication of these meanings and empiric testing of the evidence of their experience has contributed, and continues to contribute, to theory development by providing a foundation for discourse about meanings.

Theories provide a view of a patient situation that can be accessed by an APN to map the organization of data. Theory helps an APN establish an information and relationship hierarchy for the collected data. From this mapping, care and outcomes can be planned. This systematic collecting and organizing of data leads to working efficiently and purposefully (Raudonis & Acton, 1997).

Utilization of Theory in Advanced Practice

Nurse executives and APNs can use and supervise the use of theoretical models. An effective way to employ theoretical models would be to coordinate the choice of nursing theoretical models with the process of measuring outcomes derived from the unit's mission, nursing standards of practice, and use of resources (Smith, 1993; Simms, Price, & Ervin, 1994). While outcomes research is a critical piece of advanced practice, Gioiella (1996) cautions that it is meaningless without being linked to a theoretical model. She believes that if data are only gathered, it is just reporting and not doing science. Only if data are used to measure or describe relationships and linked to a theoretical framework can an activity be considered research and good science.

When working within a practice that requires theoretical applications, an understanding of the discipline's major concepts and definitions is important. This understanding should help guide an APN to evaluate the theoretical fit to the patient situation. Is the theory clear and simple? Do the assumptions make sense in this situation? How does the theorist see the concepts relating to each other and to situations? Has the theory been tested in situations that are of a similar nature to the one to which the theory will be applied? Are the patients and environment similar to that reflected in the theory? What follows is an example of how an APN might evaluate the usefulness of Orem's Self-Care Deficit Theory of Nursing.

Orem's (1995) Self-Care Deficit Theory is known to be useful in many settings, but it has most frequently been applied to the care of ill adults and well and ill children (Mariner-Tomey & Alligood, 1998). This theory offers a view of practice that is well suited to the phenomena for advanced practice. The match between the theory and practice is enhanced because the theory directs nursing action. Orem proposed the existence of three types of nursing systems: wholly compensatory (doing self-care for the individual), partially compensatory (assisting the individual with self-care), and supportive and educative (supporting and educating the individual in self-care performance) (Mariner-Tomey & Alligood, 1998).

Because the theory is patient centered and explains the systems within which the patient and nurse interact, the theory would seem appropriate for direct care or as a philosophical foundation for models of care. One must ask: Are the goals of this theory and the goals of the APN consistent? Examine the standards of practice to clarify what the unit's practice goals are. As nursing executives, APNs could develop their institutional or departmental mission and philosophy using Orem's Self-Care Deficit Theory. Nursing consultants can use Orem's framework in their practice or in their educational work with colleagues (Mezinskis, 1998). Would these situations be similar to the theory's described situations?

A review of the literature reveals that Orem's Self-Care Deficit Theory has been the subject of nursing research for many years. It has been used in studies of nursing care and delivery (Harris, 1980), nursing administration (Walker, 1993), postoperative recovery (Hanucharurnkui & Vinya-Nguag, 1991), and clinical practice (Taylor, 1988; Taylor & McLaughlin 1991). Does the research evidence support the use of the theory (Chinn & Kramer, 1995)? A review of these studies would further inform a potential user.

It is after this level of familiarity with a theorist and the theorist's work has been reached that scholarly discussions with other APNs and colleagues should occur. Would APNs feel comfortable using this theory? Collecting this data and reflecting on its previous use with colleagues should include how the use of this theory will affect practice in terms of resource and time usage, recordkeeping, and evaluative activities. For example, Linda is a CNS who is working with Larry, a patient with diabetes. He has type 1 diabetes and takes insulin three times a day. He is currently in the hospital because of an infection and hyperglycemia. Using Orem's theory as a theoretical framework with which to approach his care, Linda evaluates his therapeutic self-care demand. Larry needs to adjust his self-care to obtain better control of his diabetes and engage in preventive care. However, Linda realizes that until Larry's blood sugar is under better control, it will not be meaningful for him to discuss all available strategies. Larry's self-care capabilities are good when his blood sugar is in control. When it is uncontrolled, he is unable to think

clearly and make good decisions. Larry does have the psychomotor skills to administer the insulin. He currently uses urine testing and wants to switch to blood monitoring. It will be important for Linda to go over "what if" questions to help prepare him to make decisions related to meeting self-care demands. At this point, the type of nursing required by Larry is partially compensatory because he needs assistance in meeting his health care needs. After meeting with Linda, Larry is interested in working out a self-care regimen that will work for him and prevent him from only reacting to crisis situations. A written plan is developed, and an evaluation will take place once he returns for a follow-up visit in a couple of weeks. Depending on how well Larry is able to meet his self-care needs, this plan may necessitate involving his wife more in his day-to-day management. This is just a simple example of how a theoretical framework can be used to approach patient care.

Another example of how to choose a theory could involve an evaluation of King's Theory of Goal Attainment. Imogene King's (1981) Theory of Goal Attainment has an open systems approach directed toward goal attainment. This theory views the patient and nurse as a personal system that coexists with other personal and group systems within the whole of the system of society. King's theoretical framework includes three systems: personal, interpersonal, and social. The nurse-patient system collaborates and communicates to set and attain goals for patient satisfaction through the use of effective nursing care. Concepts are explicated in relation to specific systems. The concepts are included in the social system and include organization, boundary identification of roles, power, authority, decision-making, status, and mechanisms to regulate rules. One should examine the concepts and the theory's view of their relationships. Would these help to obtain the desired results in this specific practice? Are the goals of the practice and the goals of King's theory aligned? These answers clarify issues of the theory's appropriateness as a theoretical framework.

After reviewing the theory, an APN should conduct a literature search to determine previous use and evaluation of the theory. In this case, the APN would learn that King's conceptual framework has been used at Ohio State University for curriculum design of the nursing program, and that Loyola-University of Chicago's Department of Medical-Surgical Nursing is using portions of the theory's nursing process steps (Marriner-Tomey & Alligood, 1998). Other areas for application of King's Theory include nursing research (King, 1987; Laben, Dodd, & Sneed, 1991; Rosendahl & Ross, 1982), administration (King, 1989), education (Daubenmire, & King, 1989; King, 1984; Rooke, 1995), and multiple practice settings (Martin, 1990; Temple & Fawdry, 1992; Norgan, Ettipio, & Lasome, 1995; Meiner, 1998). How was the theory applied? Was it clear, or were practice and theory variables incongruous? Can nursing actions be based on what is known? Will this result in nursing care that will meet patients' needs and expectations? Hanna (1993) used King's Theory of Goal Attainment to direct her research with female adolescents and contraceptive adherence. King's nurse-patient transactional communication directed the intervention. The researcher found that female adolescents who had the transactional intervention had greater levels of contraceptive adherence than those who did not. King's Theory of Goal Attainment seems to fit very well in an advanced practice environment where the plan of care is mutually agreed upon by the APN and the patient. The patient is the one ultimately responsible for carrying out the plan of care. Using Goal Attainment has the potential to affect a patient's adherence to or involvement with the care regimen.

Kim (1996) believes that there are two issues related to the use of theory in practice. First, she notes putting theory into practice involves transforming the symbolic knowledge into actions. This is based on the notion that theory is the knowledge that explains things and practice is where things get done. The second issue is the ability to sort and choose between the multitudes of theories, which are sometimes both contradictory and complementary. It is deemed helpful if the work of science (theory) is placed within the realm of nursing practice. Phillips (1996) suggests bringing APNs and researchers closer together to work collaboratively on identifying problems and generating knowledge. APNs need to recall that nursing theory is a matter that applies to all nurses in practice. As an APN approaches a specific patient situation, multiple factors come into play: knowledge in the public and private domain, the APN's perception of the situation, the APN's framing of the situation, and the choice of interventions or strategies appropriate to the situation (Kim, 1996). These factors make each situation different for each patient, because each APN brings specific frameworks and meanings to the encounter. It is at this point that nursing theories provide a framework with which to classify phenomena. This framework helps an APN ask the appropriate questions. An example might be a patient who comes to the office very frequently. One APN, based on her theoretical perspective, considers this person someone who does not want to work and who tends to be hypochondriacal. Another APN looks at the frequent visits as those of someone who needs help because he is anxious or depressed. This situation would have drastically different solutions for each APN. While there are differences in the interventions and strategies, there are similarities because they are directed toward the same outcomes. In this scenario, the ultimate outcome would be to address the problem and decrease clinic visits, regardless of the cause. The step at which an APN chooses an intervention has been most often identified as the time for application of nursing theory in practice. At this time, the APN would need to review all the appropriate theories that might guide care.

Kim (1996) identifies four modes of theory application in practice (Table 28-1). These four modes describe the different ways APNs may seek out and use theory in their practice. APNs should consider the following criteria when applying theory to practice. First, the best-tested theory should be used for application to practice whenever possible. This adds to the knowledge base of the particular theory. Second, when using theory in practice, APNs must use ethical decision-making to guide its use. Third, APNs must remember that once the theory is applied, there is not a way to reverse actions. Finally, APNs must reflect on the effectiveness of the theory.

IMPLICATIONS FOR MSN EDUCATION AND ADVANCED PRACTICE

The demand for nurses has been altered by increased demand for health and wellness care linked to technological advances, a demographical trend toward an older population, and an identified need for gender-specific and culturally sensitive care. The balance between measures used by managed care to control costs and the need for quality care and continued patient access is the current challenge to the health care delivery system. To date, facilities have merged and aligned to produce a mix of services projected to keep them economically healthy. Within facilities, in addition to establishing an economically sound mix of services, staff mix is seen as a way to control the cost of quality care. The actual provision of care has become more complex. Awareness of the APN's role and skills has increased; this has enabled the health care system to find another way to meet the demand for cost-effective care delivery. It is within this context that advanced practice has found a niche, a place to develop practices and function to its broadest capacity. It falls to nursing educators in advanced practice to continuously collaborate with other APNs and continue developing models of practice in which practical skills evolve, enabling growth of the discipline (Autar, 1996). Educators must address competency, efficiency, and evidence-based practice for APNs. This has direct ramifications for curriculum development and educational programming. Educators must be able to address rapid changes in both the content and the delivery methods for nursing education. New ideas must be considered to keep APN programs flexible and innovative. Lifelong learning must be stressed, and research must be emphasized differently. Sackett, Richardson, Rosenberg, and Haynes (1998) note that most clinicians do not keep up to date with clinical information. This means that evidence-based practice needs to be stressed in APN curricula.

Research is a vital skill; if it is not developed during the educational process, it is unlikely to develop after graduation (Downs, 1998). Walker and Redman (1999) recommend the use of reflective practice along with

Table 28-1	
Four Modes of Theory Application	
MODEL	**EXAMPLE**
Coherence	This mode requires the APN's commitment to a particular theory or framework (i.e., using a specific theory to direct his or her worldview). This means the APN approaches the whole situation from the perspective of the given theory. This theory directs the assessment of the situation and the choice of interventions. For example, if an APN used Rogers' Science of Unitary Human Beings for his or her orientation to practice, then only strategies that fit within that theory could be considered as choices. The use of the coherence mode may create dogmatism in practice.
Integrative	In this situation the APN incorporates new theories and techniques into his or her practice, beliefs, and patterns. This mode tends to be more evolutionary because the APN incorporates an ever-expanding practice paradigm. For example, one APN integrated Orem's Self-Care Deficit and the Theory of Nursing transtheoretical model of exercise behavior with the facts concerning populations at risk to help reduce the risk of heart disease and promote health. The critical issue with this mode is the need to continually test and research the theories that are integrated.
Pragmatic or eclectic	In this mode the use of theory is not based on the APN but on the patient and his or her problems. In this situation the APN chooses the theory that is most applicable to the patient's problems. Thus the name *eclectic* is appropriate because APNs can choose from a variety of theories. In fact, Kristjanson, Tamblyn, and Kuypers (1987) propose that multiple theories be used in practice; they reject the notion of a single model approach for nursing practice.
Reflective	In this approach the theory choice is embedded in reflections by the APN. New theories are chosen based on their appropriateness for the situation, the APN's reflection of the situation, his or her capabilities, and reflections with the patient.

Data from Kim, H. (1996). Putting theory into practice: problems and prospects. In J. Kenney (Ed.), *Philosophical and theoretical perspectives for advanced practice* (pp. 353-363), Sudbury, MA: Jones and Bartlett.

evidence-based practice to encourage appropriate and effective research utilization. Reflective practice includes nursing process skills such as assessment; therapeutic intervention; evaluation; utilization of philosophy, theory, and research as the basis for practice; critical thinking; use of multiple patterns of knowing; and self-corrective reasoning. It is this reflection that brings together the essence of nursing with the evidence that supports it. The University of Colorado has developed a new curriculum designed to meet the needs of the next 100 years and the changing roles and responsibilities of nurses to provide evidence-based, theory-guided nursing care. A theoretical framework was developed for all nursing programs within the school of nursing. This competency-based curriculum promotes movement from one program to another and decreases barriers that force students to drop out. The outcomes identified for programs include the ability to reflect; competent, effective practice; generation of nursing knowledge and leadership skills; and social changes to improve health for individuals and communities. Each program may have a different emphasis, but the outcomes apply to all programs. The central foundation is a theory-guided, evidenced-based reflective practice with an emphasis on respect for diversity, culture, relationship-centered caring, and social justice and responsibility. The definition of reflective practice is "a nursing practice competency characterized by professional nursing that uses deliberate action integrating theoretical, research and philosophical bases for practice" (Walker and Redman, 1999). The associated outcome of competency is practiced reflectively, guided by theory, based on the best evidence, and integrated with creative and critical thinking.

It is at this time that the strengths of the past must be emphasized in APN education. Nurse educators must build on nursing's uniqueness as described by the many nursing theories. These theories can serve as the basis for theory-guided, evidence-based practice and form the core of nursing education. This is particularly important as patients are demanding more than the fragmented depersonalized care provided by many in medicine and other disciplines. While it is tempting to mimic medicine's position in health care, Baumann (1998) asserts it would be a mistake for nursing. He writes that the missing ingredient in nursing education is frequently nursing theory, yet that theory gives center stage to holism, caring, comfort, families, and communities, to name just a few core concepts. Nursing can not become just one more competitor in the health care market; rather, it should offer an alternative that "integrates relevant outcomes driven practice and education with the art and science of relationship centered caring and healing" (Walker and Redman, 1999).

The development of midrange theories may prove to be more useful in practice and is an alternative to the development of grand theories. Another possibility might be the development of integrative theories based on the grand theories. Ray (1998) suggests that these integrative theories might better reflect the interdependent and collaborative nature of nursing without losing the unique contribution of nursing.

As APN numbers increase and more care is provided by APNs, it is likely that more research and application of theory will occur. Barriers to the use of theory in practice include lack of knowledge of nursing theories and their complex and confusing language. It will be vital in the upcoming years to merge the nursing theory and nursing practice paths. As these paths merge and nursing theory becomes a regular and expected part of practice, a distinct and strong scientific base will be created.

PRIORITIES FOR RESEARCH

As the twentieth century closes, a literature review for the last three decades evidences enormous strides in the development of nursing theory. Brilliant nurse theorists are currently reflecting on, testing, and evaluating what nurses know now. These theorists have taught APNs where they have been, taught APNs how to evaluate what is known and how it has come to be known. As the twenty-first century dawns, the discipline of nursing is engaged in theoretical thinking and scholarly discourse about the nature of theory and practice. Nursing should continue to test theories that are currently being used. Fawcett (1999) expresses her view that much of the research conducted by nurse scientists in recent years has employed non-nursing methodologies to generate new theories guided by non-nursing conceptual frameworks. She notes that only 6 of the 73 studies (8%) reported in *Nursing Research* and *Research in Nursing and Health* in 1998 involved the generation or testing of nursing theories using nursing methodologies. However, of those 6, 4 studies tested ad hoc theories that integrated nursing and other non-nursing theories, leaving just 2 of 73 (3%) involving solely nursing theories. Those two studies were guided by Leininger's Theory of Culture Care Diversity and Pender's Theory of Health Promotion. It should be noted that the two journals mentioned do not require that research utilize a conceptual model of nursing or nursing theory when describing advances in nursing science. *Nursing Science Quarterly* and *Visions: The Journal of Rogerian Nursing* both require the use of theoretical frameworks in all research that is published. Fawcett (1999) recommends that APNs end their fascination with non-nursing theories. She predicts that nursing will survive and flourish if all nurses become nurse scholars. There no longer is a big division between nursing researchers and practicing nurses; rather, all nurses will come to perform a single role—that of a scholar. The research-practice gap can be eliminated if all nurses (especially APNs) engage in integrated practice-research activities.

While agreeing to some extent with Fawcett's evaluation of theory-guided nursing research, Rawnsley (1999) introduces some other salient points. She suggests the rethinking of the issue of integration of nursing theories and relevant findings from other fields. Her premise is that these relevant findings could enrich the original theoretical frameworks that are derived from the core of nursing science. However, she too recognizes the need to begin and end with nursing theories. In this way, knowledge is generated and refined but always centered on nursing science.

Theory links research and practice and connects nursing experiences with frameworks that help interpret nurses' interactions with patients (Silva, 1986). These nursing-specific frameworks define practice values and help develop further knowledge (Meleis, 1997). APNs and theorists can collaborate to develop situation-specific explanatory models to increase nursing's understanding of care in context. Outcome measurement research will become a priority to demonstrating cost-effective care delivery.

The most powerful factor in health care and advanced practice is the demand for cost-effective delivery of health care and its economic responses. Nursing must continue to rethink the traditional ways of doing and viewing nursing care. Interdisciplinary practice will increase boundary issues and concerns for nursing in all practice settings. Tanner, Benner, Chesla, and Gordon (1993) conducted a research study evaluating the phenomenology of knowing patients. This study was conducted to look at the development of expertise in critical care nursing. The purpose was to review analyses related to knowing the patient and its role in nursing practice. Nurses from adult, pediatric and neonatal intensive care units (130 nurses in all) gave exemplars from their practice. Based on analyses, this data reveals that knowing a patient means both knowing the patient's normal responses and knowing the patient as a person. This knowing of patients is essential for skilled clinical nursing judgment. This type of research can be considered theory generating and is a way of knowing. Knowing a patient can make quite a difference in the nursing care the patient receives. It is related to specific nursing skills, clinical judgment, advocacy, and the need to learn about specific patient populations.

It has become cliché to speak of future technology as exploding. However, nursing practice continues to be shaped by theses rapid-fire technological advances. The discipline of nursing will be called upon to handle instant information that is constructed in ways different from those of the past. Understanding how scholarly reflection has influenced knowledge and theory development over the last three decades, nursing must thoughtfully monitor how to incorporate new information into the existing body of knowledge. New theories must be developed and researched to help APNs deliver care to patients in ways that are innovative, culturally sensitive, and patient centered. With increased numbers of APNs and doctorally prepared nurse scientists graduating with working knowledge of theory and research, nursing's move into the twenty-first century will bring an unparalleled period of knowledge development.

DISCUSSION QUESTIONS

These questions can be used to promote critical thinking and encourage discussion.

1. If nursing theory is part of nursing knowledge, and part of its purpose is to describe or explain nursing, what changes in nursing knowledge would you recommend to reflect the work of APNs?
2. When applying theory to practice, an understanding of its major concepts and definitions is intended to help guide APNs to evaluate the fit of the theory to patient situations. Consider the four core concepts of nursing theory (person, health, environment, and nursing) derived from a specific nursing theory, and recall a patient situation from your APN experience. How could the four concepts, as explicated in the theory, have directed your practice activities?
3. Do you agree or disagree with the premise of Fawcett and others that only nursing theory should be used as the basis for nursing?
4. Keller identifies the most powerful factors in health care and advanced practice as the demand for cost-effective delivery of health care and its resulting economic responses. What aspects of advanced practice should be reconsidered, given these pressures? What role do interdisciplinary boundary issues play in this debate? How can nursing theory help in the consideration of these questions?

Suggestions for Further Learning

- For additional information on the philosophy of science and theory in nursing, read Rutty, J. (1998). The nature of philosophy of science, theory, and knowledge relating to nursing and professionalism. *Journal of Advanced Nursing, 28*(2), 243-250.
- For additional information on theory-based advanced nursing practice, read Kenney, J.W. (1999). *Philosophical and theoretical perspectives for advanced nursing practice.* Sudbury, MA: Jones and Bartlett.
- For additional information on nursing theorists and their work, read Marriner-Tomey, A., & Alligood, M.R. (1998). *Nursing theorists and their work* (4th ed.). St. Louis: Mosby.

REFERENCES/BIBLIOGRAPHY

Autar, R. (1996). Role of the nurse teacher in advanced nursing practice. *British Journal of Nursing , 5*(5), 298-301.

Barnum, B. (1994). *Nursing theory: analysis, application, evaluation.* Philadelphia: JB Lippincott.

Baumann, S. (1998). Nursing: the missing ingredient in nurse practitioner education. *Nursing Science Quarterly, 11,* 89-90.

Benner, P. (1984). *From novice to expert: excellence and power in clinical nursing practice.* Menlo Park, CA: Addison-Wesley.

Benoliel, J. (1997). The interaction between theory and research. *Nursing Outlook, 25*(2), 108-113.

Botoroff, J.L. (1991). Nursing: a practical science of caring. *Advances in Nursing Science, 14*(1), 26-39.

Brown, E.L. (1948). *Nursing for the future.* New York: Russell Sage Foundation.

Carper, B. (1978). Fundamental patterns of knowing in nursing. *Advances in Nursing Science, 1*(1), 13-23.

Chinn P., & Kramer, M. (1995). *Theory and nursing: a systematic approach.* St. Louis: Mosby.

Cody, W. (1994). Nursing theory-guided practice: what it is and what it is not. *Nursing Science Quarterly, 7*(4), 144-145.

Daubenmire, M., & King, I. M. (1989). A baccalaureate nursing curriculum based on King's conceptual framework. In J. P. Riehl-Sisca (Ed.), *Conceptual models for nursing practice* (3rd ed.). Norwalk, CT: Appleton & Lange.

Doheny, M. O., Cook, C. B., & Stopper, M.C. (1997). *The discipline of nursing: an introduction* (4th ed.). Stamford, CT: Appleton & Lange.

Donaldson, S., & Crowley, D. (1978). The discipline of nursing. *Nursing Outlook, 26*(2), 113-120.

Downs, F. (1998). The rightful place of research in academia. *Nursing Outlook, 46*(5), 246-247.

Fawcett, J. (1999). The state of nursing science: hallmarks of the 20th and 21st centuries. *Nursing Science Quarterly, 12*(4), 311-318.

Gioiella, E. (1996). The importance of theory-guided research and practice in the changing health care scene. *Nursing Science Quarterly, 9*(2), 47.

Goldmark, J. (1923). *Nursing and nursing education in the United States* (Report of the Committee for the Study of Nursing Education and report of a survey by Josephine Goldmark). New York: MacMillan.

Gortner, S.R. (1980). Nursing science in transition. *Nursing research, 29*(3), 180-183.

Gortner, S.R., & Schultz, P. (1988). Approaches to nursing science methods. *Image: Journal of Nursing Scholarship, 20*(1), 22-24.

Hanna, K. (1993). Effect of nurse-client transaction on female adolescents' oral contraceptive adherence. *Image: Journal of Nursing Scholarship, 25*(4), 285-290.

Hanucharurnkui, S., & Vinya-Nguag, P. (1991). Effects of promoting patients' participation in self-care on postoperative recovery and satisfaction with care. *Nursing Science Quarterly, 4*(1), 14-20.

Harris, J. (1980). Self-care is possible after delivery. *Nursing Clinics of North America, 15*(1), 191-194.

Hinshaw, A. (1989). Nursing science: the challenge to develop knowledge. *Nursing Science Quarterly, 2*(4), 162-171.

Ingram, R. (1991). Why does nursing need theory? *Journal of Advanced Nursing, 16,* 350-353.

Jacobs-Kramer, M., & Chinn, P. (1988). Perspectives on knowing: a model of nursing knowledge. *Scholarly Inquiry in Nursing Practice, 2*(2), 129-139.

Jacox, A. (1974). Theory construction in nursing: an overview. *Nursing Research, 23*(1), 4-13.

Kenney, J.W. (1999). Theory-based advanced nursing practice. In J. W. Kenny (Ed.), *Philosophical and theoretical perspectives for advanced nursing practice* (pp. 327-343). Sudbury, MA: Jones and Bartlett.

Kenny, J.W. (Ed.). (1999). *Philosophical and theoretical perspectives for advanced nursing practice*. Sudbury, MA: Jones and Bartlett.

Kim, H.S. (1993). Putting theory into practice: problems and prospects. *Journal of Advanced Nursing, 18*(10), 1632-1639.

Kim, H.S. (1994). Practice theories in nursing and a science of nursing practice. *Scholarly Inquiry for Nursing Practice, 8*(2), 145-166.

Kim, H.S. (1996). Putting theory into practice: problems and prospects. In J.W. Kenney (Ed.), *Philosophical and theoretical perspectives for advanced nursing practice* (pp. 353-363). Sudbury, MA: Jones and Bartlett.

Kimnenich P. (1998). The evolution of advanced practice in nursing. In C. Sheehy and M. McCarthy (Eds.), *Advanced nursing practice*. Philadelphia: FA Davis.

King, I. M. (1981). *A theory for nursing*. New York: John Wiley & Sons.

King, I. M. (1984). Philosophy of nursing education: a national survey. *Western Journal of Nursing Research, 6*(4), 387-406.

King, I. M. (1987). Translating research into practice. *Journal of Neuroscience Nursing, 19*(1), 44-48.

King, I. M. (1989). King's system framework for nursing administration. In B. Henry, C. Arndt, M. DiVincenti, & A. Marriner-Tomey (Eds.), *Dimensions of nursing administration: theory, research, education, practice* (pp. 35-45). Boston: Blackwell Scientific Publications.

Kristjanson, L, Tamblyn, R., & Kuypers, J. (1987). A model to guide the development and application of multiple nursing theories. *Journal of Advanced Nursing, 12*, 523-529.

Laben, J., Dodd, D., & Sneed, L. (1991). King's theory of goal attainment applied in group therapy for inpatient juvenile sexual offenders, maximum security state offenders, and community parolees, using visual aids. *Issues in Mental Health Nursing, 12*(1), 51-64.

Leininger, M. (1978). *Transcultural nursing: concepts, theories, and practices*. New York: John Wiley & Sons.

Marriner-Tomey, A., & Alligood, M.R. (1998). *Nursing theorists and their work* (4th ed). St. Louis, MO: Mosby.

Martin, J. (1990). Male cancer awareness: impact of an employee education program. *Oncology Nursing Forum, 17*, 59-64.

Meiner, S. (1998). Interactionist theory. In A.S. Luggen, S.S. Travis, & S. Meiner (Eds.), *NGNA core curriculum for gerontological advanced practice nurses* (pp. 13-15). Thousand Oaks, CA: Sage.

Meleis, A.I. (1986). Theory development and domain concepts. In P. Moccia (Ed.), *New approaches to theory development*. New York: National League for Nursing.

Meleis, A.I. (1997). *Theoretical nursing: development and progress*. Philadelphia: JB Lippincott.

Merton, R. (1957). *Social theory and social structure*. Glencoe, IL: The Free Press.

Mezinskis, P.M. (1998). Orem's self-care deficit theory. In A.S. Luggen, S.S. Travis, & S. Meiner (Eds.), *NGNA core curriculum for gerontological advanced practice nurses* (pp. 13-15). Thousand Oaks, CA: Sage.

National Council of State Boards of Nursing (1992). *Position paper on the licensure of advanced practice nursing*. Chicago: National Council of State Boards of Nursing.

Newman, M.A. (1993). Theory for nursing practice. *Nursing Science Quarterly, 7*(4), 153-157.

Nightingale, F. (1859). *Notes on nursing: what it is, and what it is not*. London: Harrison and Sons.

Nolan, M., & Grant, G. (1992). Mid-range theory building and the nursing theory practice gap: a respite care case study. *Journal of Advanced Nursing, 17*, 217-223.

Nolan, M., Lundh, U., & Tishelman, C. (1998). Nursing's knowledge base: does it have to be unique? *British Journal of Nursing, 7*(5), 270-276.

Norgan, G., Ettipio, A., & Lasome, C. (1995). A program plan addressing carpal tunnel syndrome: the utility of King's goal attainment theory. *AAOHN Journal, 43*(8), 407-411.

Orem, D.E. (1995). *Concepts of practice* (5th ed.). St. Louis: Mosby.

Parse, R.R. (1981). *Man-Living-Health: a theory of nursing*. New York: John Wiley & Sons.

Peplau, H.E. (1952). *Interpersonal relations in nursing*. New York: GP Putnam & Sons.

Phillips, J.R. (1996). What constitutes nursing science? In J.W. Kenney (Ed.), *Philosophical and theoretical perspectives for advanced nursing practice* (pp. 95-97). Sudbury, MA: Jones and Bartlett.

Phillips, R., Donald, A., Mousseau-Gershman, Y., & Powell, T. (1998). Applying theory to practice—the use of 'ripple effect' plans in continuing education. *Nurse Education Today, 18*, 12-19.

Pokorny, B., & Barnard, K. (1992). ANA to revise nursing statement. *American Nurse, 6*.

Raudonis, B.M., & Acton, G.J. (1997). Theory-based nursing practice. *Journal of Advanced Nursing, 26*, 138-145.

Rawnsley, M. (1999). Response to Fawcett's "The state of nursing science." *Nursing Science Quarterly, 12*(4): 315-318.

Ray, M., (1998). Complexity and nursing science. *Nursing Science Quarterly, 11*, 91-93.

Rogers, M. (1985). The nature and characteristics of professional education for nursing. *Journal of Professional Nursing, 1*, 382-383.

Rooke, L. (1995). Focusing on King's theory and systems framework in education by using an experiential learning model: a challenge to improve the quality of nursing care. In M.A. Frey & C. Sieloff (Eds.), *Advancing King's framework and theory for nursing* (pp. 278-293). Newbury Park, CA: Sage.

Rosendahl, P., & Ross, V. (1982). Does your behavior affect your patient's response? *Journal of Gerontological Nursing, 8*, 575-75.

Rutty J. (1998). The nature of philosophy of science, theory and knowledge relating to nursing and professionalism. *Journal of Advanced Nursing, 28*(2), 243-250.

Sackett, D., Richardson, W., Rosenberg, W., & Haynes, R. (1998). *Evidence based medicine: how to practice and teach EBM*. London: Churchill Livingstone.

Sheehy, C., & McCarthy, M. (1998). *Advanced nursing practice*. Philadelphia: FA Davis.

Silva, M.C. (1986). Research testing nursing theory: state of the art. *Advances in Nursing Science, 9*(1), 1-11.

Simms, L.M., Price, S.A., & Ervin, N.E. (1994). *The professional practice of nursing administration.* Albany, NY: Delmar.

Smith, M. (1993). The contribution of nursing theory to nursing administration practice. *Image: Journal of Nursing Scholarship, 25*(1), 63-67.

Tanner, C., Benner, P., Chesla, C., & Gordon, D. (1993). The phenomenology of knowing the patient. *Image: Journal of Nursing Scholarship, 24*(4): 273-280.

Taylor, S. (1988). Nursing theory and nursing process: Orem's theory in practice. *Nursing Science Quarterly, 1*(3), 111-119.

Taylor, S., & McLaughlin, K. (1991). Orem's general theory of nursing and community nursing. *Nursing Science Quarterly, 4*(4), 153-160.

Temple, A., & Fawdry, K. (1992). King's theory of goal attainment: resolving filial caregiver role strain. *Journal of Gerontological Nursing, 18*(3), 11-15.

Titler, M., Kleiber, C., Steelman, V., Goode, C., Rakel, B., Barry-Walker, J., Small, S., & Buckwalter, K. (1994). Infusing research into practice to promote quality of care. *Nursing Research, 43*(5): 307-313.

Ulbrich, S. (1999). Nursing practice theory of exercise as self-care. *Image: Journal of Nursing Scholarship, 31*(1): 65-70.

Upton, D.J. (1999). How can we achieve evidence-based practice if we have a theory-practice gap in nursing today? *Journal of Advanced Nursing, 29*(3), 542-548.

Walker, D. (1993). A nursing administration perspective on use of Orem's Self-Care Deficit nursing theory. In M.E. Parker (Ed.), *Patterns of nursing theories in practice* (pp. 252-263). New York: National League for Nursing.

Walker, L.O., & Avant, K.C. (1995). *Strategies for theory construction in nursing.* Norwalk, CT: Appleton & Lange.

Walker, P., & Redman, R. (1999). Theory guided, evidence based reflective practice. *Nursing Science Quarterly, 12*(4): 298-303.

Chapter 29

Integrating Conceptual Models, Theories, Research, and Practice

Jacqueline Fawcett

The professional discipline of nursing is mandated by society to develop and disseminate nursing knowledge and use that knowledge to improve the well-being of human beings. Nursing knowledge is formalized in conceptual models of nursing and nursing theories. The credibility of conceptual models and the empirical adequacy of theories is determined by means of nursing research. Credible conceptual models and empirically adequate theories are linked and applied in nursing practice as conceptual-theoretical-empirical systems (C-T-E systems) of nursing knowledge.

In a classic article, Donaldson and Crowley (1978) proclaim that nursing is a professional discipline. As such, nursing has a social mandate to develop, disseminate, utilize, and evaluate knowledge. In contrast, academic disciplines (e.g., physics, physiology, sociology, psychology, philosophy) are mandated only to develop and disseminate knowledge.

The professional discipline of nursing has two major dimensions: nursing science and the nursing profession. Nursing science is accomplished by means of nursing research, and the product of nursing research is C-T-E system development and dissemination. The nursing profession is actualized through nursing practice, and the major activity of nursing practice is C-T-E system utilization and clinical evaluation. The development, dissemination, utilization, and clinical evaluation of nursing knowledge in the form of explicit nursing discipline–specific C-T-E systems can best be fostered through the integration of nursing research and nursing practice. This integration can best be fostered through the combination of nursing science and the nursing profession. Figure 29-1 presents an integrated view of the dimensions of the professional discipline of nursing and the activities associated with these dimensions. The dimensions of nursing science and the nursing profession are regarded as integrated, as are the research and practice activities that flow from those integrated dimensions and the C-T-E system activities that flow from the integration of research and practice. Note that the integra-

tion of nursing research and practice means that research is practice and practice is research.

DEFINITIONS

Each C-T-E system is made up of a conceptual model, one or more theories, and empirical indicators. A **conceptual model** is defined as "a set of relatively abstract and general concepts that address the phenomena of central interest to a discipline, the propositions that broadly describe those concepts, and the propositions that state relatively abstract and general relations between two or more of the concepts" (Fawcett, 2000).

A conceptual model provides a distinctive frame of reference—"a horizon of expectations" (Popper, 1965)—and "a coherent, internally unified way of thinking about . . . events and processes" (Frank, 1968) that tells its adherents how to observe and interpret the phenomena of interest to the discipline. Each conceptual model, then, presents a unique focus that has a profound influence on individuals' perceptions. The unique focus of each conceptual model is an approximation or simplification of reality that includes only those concepts that the model author considers relevant and useful as aids to understanding (Lippitt, 1973; Reilly, 1975). Thus certain aspects of the phenomena of interest to a discipline are regarded as particularly relevant, and other aspects are ignored. Each conceptual model also provides a structure and rationale for the scholarly and practical activities of its adherents. The works of several nurse scholars currently are recognized as conceptual models; among the best known are Johnson's Behavioral System Model, King's General Systems Framework, Levine's Conservation Model, Neuman's Systems Model, Orem's Self-Care Framework, Rogers' Science of Unitary Human Beings, and Roy's Adaptation Model (Johnson, 1990; King, 1990; Rogers, 1990; Levine, 1991; Neuman, 1995; Orem, 1995; Roy & Andrews, 1999).

A **theory** is defined as "one or more relatively concrete

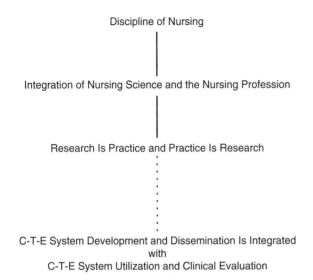

Discipline of Nursing

Integration of Nursing Science and the Nursing Profession

Research Is Practice and Practice Is Research

C-T-E System Development and Dissemination Is Integrated
with
C-T-E System Utilization and Clinical Evaluation

Figure 29-1 The professional discipline of nursing: integration of nursing science and the nursing profession, nursing research and nursing practice, and C-T-E system development/dissemination and C-T-E system utilization/evaluation. (From Fawcett, J. [2000]. *Analysis and evaluation of contemporary nursing knowledge: nursing models and theories.* Philadelphia: FA Davis.)

and specific concepts that are derived from a conceptual model, the propositions that narrowly describe those concepts, and the propositions that state relatively concrete and specific relations between two or more of the concepts"(Fawcett, 2000). This definition of a theory indicates that a conceptual model always is the precursor to a theory. Indeed, the belief that theory development proceeds outside the context of a conceptual frame of reference is "absurd" (Popper, 1965). Moreover, in as much as each theory deals only with a limited aspect of reality, many theories are needed to deal with all of the phenomena encompassed by a conceptual model. Each conceptual model, then, is more fully specified by several theories.

Theories vary in their level of abstraction and scope. A more abstract and broader theory is referred to as a **grand theory**. A more concrete and narrower theory is referred to as a **midrange theory**. Grand theories are rather broad in scope. They are made up of concepts and propositions that are less abstract and general than the concepts and propositions of a conceptual model, but they are not as concrete and specific as the concepts and propositions of a midrange theory. Midrange theories are narrower in scope than grand theories. They are made up of a limited number of concepts and propositions written at a relatively concrete and specific level. Each midrange theory addresses a more or less relatively concrete and specific phenomenon by describing what the phenomenon is, explaining why it occurs, or predicting how it occurs.

A few nurses have presented their ideas about nursing in the form of explicit grand theories. The most widely known are Leininger's (1991) Theory of Culture Care Diversity and Universality, Newman's (1994) Theory of

Health as Expanding Consciousness, and Parse's (1998) Theory of Human Becoming. A few other nurses have presented their ideas about nursing in the form of explicit midrange theories. The most widely known are Orlando's (1961) Theory of the Deliberative Nursing Process, Peplau's (1952) Theory of Interpersonal Relations, and Watson's (1985) Theory of Human Caring.

An **empirical indicator** is defined as "a very concrete and specific real world proxy for a middle-range theory concept; an actual instrument, experimental condition, or clinical procedure that is used to observe or measure a middle-range theory concept" (Fawcett, 2000). Empirical indicators provide the means by which middle-range theories are generated or tested. Empirical indicators that are instruments yield data that can be sorted into qualitative categories or calculated as quantitative scores. Empirical indicators that exist as experimental conditions or clinical procedures tell a researcher or clinician exactly what to do. They are, in effect, protocols or scripts that direct actions in a very precise manner.

Empirical indicators are most frequently associated with nursing research. **Nursing research** is "a formal, systematic, and rigorous process of inquiry used to generate and test the concepts and propositions that comprise [nursing] middle-range theories, which are derived from or linked with a conceptual model [of nursing]" (Fawcett, 1999). Nurses have developed a plethora of empirical indicators in the form of research instruments directly derived from various conceptual models of nursing and nursing theories (Fawcett, 2000). Most such research instruments are paper and pencil questionnaires; others are interview guides.

Empirical indicators also take the form of clinical tools used in nursing practice. **Nursing practice** is "the use, by a [nurse], of knowledge and skill to provide a service" (Thomas, 1997). Nurses have developed many clinical tools that are directly derived from various conceptual models of nursing and nursing theories (Fawcett, 2000). These clinical tools encompass standards for nursing practice, assessment formats, diagnostic taxonomies, patient classification systems, intervention protocols, and clinical information systems.

CRITICAL ISSUES: CONCEPTUAL MODELS, THEORIES, RESEARCH, AND PRACTICE

Research and practice always start with a conceptual model. The influence of a conceptual model on research is explained by Batey (1997), who points out that although two investigators may observe the same situation or event, "their notions of why it occurs, their conceptual organization about the problem, [and] the knowledge base they select for studying that problem may differ." In other words, each investigator views situations and events through a particular lens or frame of reference, which is encapsulated in a conceptual model. The same may be said for the influence of a conceptual model on practice.

Research and practice frequently are viewed as systematic processes employed to answer questions and solve problems. The process often is regarded as sterile, a linear series of steps to be surmounted in the search for solutions to problems. Research and practice, however, are much more than methods of problem-solving. Indeed, the function of research is to generate or test midrange theories; more specifically, research is the vehicle for the development of midrange theories and the refinement of conceptual models. In particular, research is one part of a cycle—the part that supplies the data. The other parts of the cycle—the conceptual model and the theory—give meaning to the data. The function of practice is to utilize and evaluate conceptual models and midrange theories in real-world clinical situations. In such situations, the observations and documentation of the activities of the clinical practice supply the data, and the conceptual model and the theory give meaning to those data. The cycle is completed when the meanings ascribed to the research data and/or the clinical practice data are used to draw conclusions regarding the empirical adequacy of the theory and the credibility of the conceptual model.

Integrating C-T-E Systems, Nursing Research, and Nursing Practice

Recognition of nursing as a distinct professional discipline confers a certain status that is especially attractive to advanced practice nurses (APNs). The status conferred by being a member of the professional discipline of nursing, rather than of an occupation or a trade, carries with it the responsibility to develop, disseminate, utilize, and evaluate explicit nursing discipline–specific C-T-E systems. More specifically, the responsibility of members of the professional discipline of nursing is to conduct discipline-specific research (Mitchell, 1994) using discipline-specific research methodologies (Thorne, Kirkham, & MacDonald-Emes, 1997) and engage in discipline-specific practice (Smith, 1995) using discipline-specific nursing practice processes.

Integrating C-T-E systems, research, and practice is a seemingly complex activity that has, to date, eluded most nurses, as it has most members of other professional disciplines. Integration, however, can be quite straightforward. To integrate C-T-E systems, research, and practice, one must use an explicit nursing discipline–specific C-T-E system to guide nursing practice and use clinical information gained from the implementation of that C-T-E system as research data for single-case studies. In other words, every nursing situation for the purpose of the delivery of nursing services is also for the purpose of research. Every nursing situation, then, is a single-case study of an experiment in which the intervention is hypothesized to have a certain outcome (Wood, 1978). Thus the clinical

---

Box 29-1

Single-Case Study Approach to Integrating Nursing Research and Practice within the Context of a C-T-E System of Nursing Knowledge

- Develop a prototype C-T-E system of nursing knowledge for a clinical population.
- Develop an individualized C-T-E system for a particular patient.
- Provide nursing in accordance with the nursing practice process of the C-T-E system.
- Use the documented information about C-T-E system–based nursing actions and the outcomes for a patient as single-case–study research data.

Adapted from Fawcett, J. (2000). *Analysis and evaluation of contemporary nursing knowledge: nursing models and theories.* Philadelphia: FA Davis.

---

data available in every nursing practice situation are used to refine or reject existing C-T-E systems and develop new C-T-E systems (Box 29-1).

Drawing from Wood's (1978) discussion of social work research and casework processes, the steps of the nursing practice process can be viewed as the steps of the nursing research process. APNs, then, are researchers (Rolfe, 1993), and patients are their own controls in quasi-experimental single-case studies guided by explicit nursing discipline–specific C-T-E systems. Within the context of a particular C-T-E system, the nursing practice process is the same as the nursing research process (Table 29-1). Thus the results of assessment make up the baseline data. The labeling used to summarize a patient's health status represents the statement of the problem to be studied. Goal-setting represents the hypothesis that specifies the desired nurse-sensitive outcome and the means to achieve that outcome. The desired outcome is the dependent variable, and the means to achieve that outcome is the independent variable. Implementation is of the intervention or the experimental treatment, which is the independent variable. The experimental treatment (i.e., the intervention) should be written in the form of a clinical script that specifies exactly how the goal will be achieved for a particular patient. The clinical script is then viewed as a research protocol. Any necessary deviations from the *a priori* script for the intervention should be recorded so that it is possible to link what was to be done with what actually was done and with what outcome actually occurred. Evaluation is analysis of the nurse-sensitive outcome (i.e., the dependent variable). Written or computerized documentation of each step of the nursing practice process provides the actual data from which a conclusion regarding the hypothesis may be drawn.

Table 29-1

Parallels between the Nursing Practice Process and the Nursing Research Process

NURSING PRACTICE PROCESS	NURSING RESEARCH PROCESS
Assessment	Baseline data
Labeling	Statement of the problem
Goal-setting	Hypothesis
• Desired nurse-sensitive outcome	• Dependent variable
• Means to achieve outcome	• Independent variable
Implementation of intervention	Experimental treatment
	• Independent variable
Evaluation	Nurse-sensitive outcome
• Outcome actually achieved	• Dependent variable
Documentation of clinical information	Record of data to be analyzed
	Conclusion regarding hypothesis

From Fawcett, J. (2000). *Analysis and evaluation of contemporary nursing knowledge: nursing models and theories.* Philadelphia: FA Davis.

Using the Roy Adaptation Model in Practice

The generic nursing practice process listed in Table 29-1 can be replaced by the components of the particular practice process associated with the nursing conceptual model of the C-T-E system. The nursing practice process associated with the Roy Adaptation Model (Roy & Andrews, 1999) serves as an example. Baseline data in Roy's model encompass the assessment of behaviors in the physiological, self-concept, role function, and interdependence modes, as well as the assessment of environmental stimuli. The statement of the problem is the nursing diagnosis, which in Roy's model is a statement of behaviors within each adaptive mode and their relevant stimuli, or a label that summarizes a behavioral pattern across adaptive modes that is affected by the same stimuli. The hypothesis is the Roy Adaptation Model nursing process step of goal-setting. The experimental treatment is nursing intervention, which in Roy's model is the management of stimuli. The nurse-sensitive outcome is the nursing process step of evaluation of behaviors following intervention. The clinical tools and research instruments derived from Roy's model are used to collect and record the data for the assessment, nursing diagnosis, goal-setting, intervention, and evaluation steps of the nursing practice process that then will be used for the single-case study (Table 29-2). Thus clinical tools are useful for research purposes, and

research instruments can be examined for their utility in clinical situations.

Consider the following example of a single-case study. Joan is an APN at Redbud Community Health Center. She uses the Roy Adaptation Model to guide her nursing practice and has developed a prototype C-T-E system of nursing knowledge for patients who have ineffective responses in the oxygenation dimension of the physiological mode of adaptation. Joan develops an individualized C-T-E system for Mr. Bradley, who complains of "gasping for breath" when he climbs a flight of stairs. Using the Roy Adaptation Model nursing process (assessment of behaviors, assessment of stimuli, nursing diagnosis, goal-setting, intervention, evaluation), Joan finds out that Mr. Bradley is a "healthy 80-year-old guy" who "races up stairs to get to the top quickly, just like [he] always [has] done." Mr. Bradley agrees that he should try to walk, rather than run up stairs, and calls Joan a week later to tell her that he no longer "gasps for breath" and feels much better walking up stairs; he adds that "even my feet feel better now that I'm not pounding down on them." Joan documents the successful implementation of the C-T-E protocol with Mr. Bradley and prepares a written single-case study research report that is accepted for publication in *Nurse Practitioner*.

The key to the integration of nursing research and nursing practice is recognition and acceptance of the similarity between the process of research and the process of practice, as well as recognition and acceptance that both research and practice are guided by the same C-T-E system. The previous example illustrates Joan's ability to integrate practice and research within the context of an explicit C-T-E system.

Single-case studies can be aggregated for the purposes of quality assurance programs. The use of an explicit nursing discipline–specific C-T-E system to guide each case study ensures that the outcome is a nurse-sensitive outcome (i.e., that the outcome is directly associated with a nursing assessment, a nursing label, and a nursing intervention). Thus nursing quality assurance programs will yield data that are relevant to nursing. Long-sought-after and much desired evidence-based best practices (Anderson, 1998; Fagin, 1998) are the collective result of both single-case studies and quality assurance programs.

IMPLICATIONS FOR MSN EDUCATION AND ADVANCED PRACTICE

The rapid growth of APN education programs (especially nurse practitioner [NP] programs) in recent years has diverted attention away from nursing discipline–specific C-T-E systems and toward the medical model as the basis for research and practice. As a result, the human experience of health and nursing itself have been medicalized

Table 29-2

Research Instruments and Clinical Tools Derived from the Roy Adaptation Model

INSTRUMENT	DESCRIPTION
Research Instruments	
Health-Illness (Powerlessness) Questionnaire (Roy, 1979)	Measures hospitalized patients' perceptions of powerlessness in illness.
Hospitalized Patient Decision-Making (Roy, 1979)	Measures hospitalized patients' perceptions of decisions they actually make while in a hospital, as well as the decisions they would prefer to make.
Cognitive Adaptation Processing Scale (Roy & Andrews, 1999)	Measures cognitive adaptation strategies for patients with spinal cord injury, patients with sensory and motor deficits from neurosurgery, and older adults with hearing loss.
Inventory of Functional Status—Antepartum Period (IFSAP) (Tulman, Higgins, Fawcett, Nunno, Vansickel, Haas, & Speca, 1991)	Measures the extent to which women continue to perform their usual household, social, community, personal care, child care, occupational, and educational activities during pregnancy.
Inventory of Functional Status—Fathers (Tulman, Fawcett, & Weiss, 1993)	Measures the extent to which expectant and new fathers continue to perform their usual household, social, community, personal care, child care, occupational, and educational activities.
Parental Roles Questionnaire (Varnell, 1990)	Measures parentization, which is operationalized as an expectant parent's and his or her spouse's perceptions of parental role behaviors, including mothering behaviors, fathering behaviors, incorporation of norms, and childhood background.
Interdependence Questionnaire (Short, 1994)	Measures the giving and receiving behaviors of Roy's interdependence adaptive mode in the categories of significant other, support systems (friendships and extended family), and the experience of feeling alone in new mothers.
Inventory of Functional Status—After Childbirth (Fawcett, Tulman, & Myers, 1988)	Measures the extent to which women resume performance of their usual household, social, community, personal care, and occupational activities and assume infant care responsibilities following childbirth.
Inventory of Functional Status—Caregiver of a Child in a Body Cast (Newman, 1997)	Measures the extent to which parental caregivers or their surrogates continue their usual household, social, community, child care, personal care, and occupational activities while caring for a child in a body cast.
Self-Perceived Adaptation Level (Ide, 1978)	Measures the perceived ability of well older adults to manage or cope with changes in their internal or external environment within the context of Roy's role function and interdependence adaptive modes.
Inventory of Functional Status in the Elderly (Paier, 1994)	Measures the extent to which independent, community-dwelling older adults perform personal care, household, social, community, volunteer, work, care of another, and leisure activities.
Sleep/Activity Behavior Log (O'Leary, 1991)	Records sleep and activity patterns of persons with Alzheimer's disease.
Inventory of Functional Status—Cancer (Tulman, Fawcett, & McEvoy, 1991; Fawcett & Tulman, 1996)	Measures the extent to which women continue their usual household, social, community, personal care, and occupational activities following a diagnosis of cancer.
Adaptation After Surviving Cancer Profile (Dow, 1993)	Measures transcendence after cancer, uncertainty over the future, mastery of cancer, family relationships, work disclosure, and risk-taking in women who are survivors of breast cancer.
Health Outcomes Questionnaire (Lewis, Firsich, & Parsell, 1978, 1979)	Measures the health outcomes of nursing care in the areas of nausea and vomiting, self-image, anxiety, and functional effectiveness for adult cancer patients receiving chemotherapy.
Varricchio-Wright Impact of Cancer Questionnaire—Parents (Wright, 1993)	Measures perceptions of quality of life for parents of children with cancer in Roy's physiological, self-concept, role function, and interdependence adaptive modes.
Inventory of Functional Status—Dialysis (Thomas-Hawkins, Fawcett, & Tulman, 1998)	Measures the extent to which men and women receiving hemodialysis continue their usual household, social, community, and personal care activities.
Structured Interview Guide (LeMone, 1995)	Collects data regarding the psychosexual concerns of individuals with diabetes mellitus within the context of Roy's physiological, self-concept, role function, and interdependence adaptive modes.
Prosthetic Problem Inventory Scale (Huber, Medhat, & Carter, 1988)	Identifies problem areas in the use of prostheses by lower-extremity amputees in the areas of activities of daily living, social participation, sexual activity, and athletic participation.

From Fawcett, J. (2000). *Analysis and evaluation of contemporary nursing knowledge: nursing models and theories.* Philadelphia: FA Davis.

Table 29-2

Research Instruments and Clinical Tools Derived from the Roy Adaptation Model—cont'd

INSTRUMENT	DESCRIPTION
Clinical Tools	
Nursing Manual: Assessment Tool According to the Roy Adaptation Model (Cho, 1998)	Guides assessment of behaviors and stimuli for the physiological, self-concept, role function, and interdependence adaptive modes.
Questions for Nursing Assessment of Sensory Impairment (Roy & Andrews, 1999)	Provides a list of questions to ask when assessing the senses aspect of the physiological/physical adaptive mode.
Adaptation Assessment Form (Rambo, 1984)	Guides assessment within the context of Roy's physiological adaptive mode and the growth and developmental tasks associated with the person's primary role within the context of the role function adaptive mode.
Admission History and Assessment Form (Jakocko & Sowden, 1986)	Guides assessment of hospitalized children within the context of Roy's physiological, self-concept, role function, and interdependence adaptive modes.
Family Development/Nursing Intervention Identifier (Hinman, 1983)	Guides Roy Adaptation Model–based assessment of school age children and their families.
Admission Assessment Form (Hamner, 1989)	Guides assessment of adults hospitalized in a coronary care unit within the context of Roy's physiological, self-concept, role function, and interdependence adaptive modes.
Nursing History Tool (Robitaille-Tremblay, 1984)	Guides assessment of hospitalized psychiatric patients within the context of Roy's physiological, self-concept, role function, and interdependence adaptive modes.
Postanesthesia Care Unit Preoperative Assessment Tool (Jackson, 1990)	Guides assessment of preoperative assessment of surgical patients within the context of Roy's physiological, self-concept, role function, and interdependence adaptive modes.
Comprehensive Sexual Assault Assessment Tool (Burgess & Fawcett, 1996)	Guides documentation of the assessment of sexual assault victims by sexual assault nurse examiners; taps the Roy Adaptation Model stimuli, coping processes, and adaptive modes, and its data can be used for clinical agency statistical analyses.
Joseph Continence Assessment Tool (Joseph & Lantz, 1996)	Permits assessment of factors that may affect the success or failure of incontinence treatment within the context of Roy's physiological, self-concept, role function, and interdependence adaptive modes; particularly useful for providers in ambulatory care or community settings.
Osteoporosis Assessment (Doyle & Rajacich, 1991)	Guides assessment of individuals with osteoporosis within the context of Roy's self-concept, role function, interdependence, and physiological adaptive modes.
Questions for Assessing Emotional and Social Adaptation to Dialysis (Frank, 1988)	Guides assessment of renal dialysis patients within the context of Roy's self-concept, role function, interdependence, and physiological adaptive modes.
Community Health Assessment (Hanchett, 1988)	Guides assessment of a community in the areas of survival, continuity, growth, transactional patterns, and member control.
Typology of Indicators of Positive Adaptation (Roy & Andrews, 1999)	Provides a list of the indicators of positive adaptation for individuals and groups in the physiological/physical, self-concept/group identity, role function, and interdependent adaptive modes.
Typology of Commonly Recurring Adaptation Problems (Roy & Andrews, 1999)	Provides a list of the common adaptation problems for individuals and groups in the physiological/physical, self-concept/group identity, role function, and interdependence adaptive modes.
Nursing Diagnostic Categories (Roy & Andrews, 1999)	Provides a list of generic nursing diagnoses within the context of indicators of positive adaptation, common adaptation problems, and NANDA nursing diagnoses for all aspects of the physiological/physical adaptive mode, self-concept/group identity, role function, and interdependence adaptive modes.
Potential Nursing Diagnoses (Frank, 1988)	Provides a list of potential nursing diagnoses, relevant for patients receiving renal dialysis, within Roy's self-concept, role function, interdependence, and physiological adaptive modes.
Nursing Diagnoses for MI Patients (Hamner, 1989)	Provides a list of nursing diagnoses and associated focal and contextual stimuli that are relevant for patients who have had a MI.

MI, Myocardial infarction; *NANDA*, North American Nursing Diagnosis Association.

Continued

Table 29-2

Research Instruments and Clinical Tools Derived from the Roy Adaptation Model—cont'd

INSTRUMENT	DESCRIPTION
Clinical Tools—cont'd	
A Parent's Guide to Cesarean Birth (Fawcett & Burritt, 1985; Fawcett & Henklein, 1987)	Prepares expectant parents for unplanned or planned cesarean birth; provides procedural, sensory, and coping strategy information about the labor (in the case of unplanned cesarean birth), delivery, and postpartum periods, organized according to the four Roy Adaptation Model adaptive modes.
The Patient's Guide to Preterm Labor (Taylor, 1993)	Helps women deal with preterm labor; provides procedural, sensory, and coping strategies information about home- and hospital-based treatment of preterm labor, organized according to the four Roy Adaptation Model adaptive modes.
Standards of Nursing Practice (Rogers, Paul, Clarke, Mackay, Potter, & Ward, 1991)	Provides descriptions of performance expectations for provision of high-quality nursing that reflects the Roy Adaptation Model in the areas of nursing assessment, nursing care planning, implementation of nursing care, evaluation of nursing, and professional development and accountability.
Perinatal Standards of Care (Weiss & Teplick, 1993, 1995)	Provides separate guidelines and expectations for nursing practice and desired patient outcomes for antepartal patients, intrapartum laboring patients, postpartum patients, neonates, and NICU patients. Standards are made up of adaptation goals, outcome criteria, and relevant nursing interventions.
Nursing Judgment Method (Roy & Andrews, 1999)	Provides a format for use of the McDonald and Harms (1966) method of judging the probability of attaining goals and value of alternative nursing interventions.
COPD Outcome Criteria (Laros, 1977)	Provides outcome criteria for patients with COPD, listed for each adaptive mode in a progressive sequence of days following hospital admission.
MCN Developmental/Diagnostic Model Nursing Care Plan Format (Starn & Niederhauser, 1990)	Provides a nursing care plan format for childbearing and childrearing families.
Nursing Process Format for Families (Whall, 1986)	Guides the use of a Roy Adaptation Model–oriented nursing process for families.
Documentation System (Weiss & Teplick, 1993, 1995)	Facilitates recording of nursing assessments, interventions, and progress toward patient outcomes; provides consistency (through use of flow sheets) between desired patients outcomes and nursing interventions included in the relevant patient standard of care.
Nursing Care Plan (Rambo, 1984)	Provides a general form for documentation of Roy Adaptation Model–based nursing practice, including medical problems, medical treatment, associated nursing actions, nursing problems, associated focal and contextual stimuli, goals, nursing interventions, and evaluation.
Nursing Care Plan Form (Fawcett, 1992)	Provides a general form for documentation of Roy Adaptation Model–based nursing assessment, intervention, and evaluation of outcomes.
Kardex Form Flow Sheet Care Plan Charting Form (Peters, 1993)	Provide organized worksheets and documentation forms for Roy Adaptation Model-based assessment, goal-setting, interventions, and evaluation for use on a general medical unit.
Nursing Care Plan Form(Hamner, 1989)	Permits documentation of Roy Adaptation Model–based assessment of behaviors and stimuli, nursing diagnoses and goals, intervention, and evaluation for use on a coronary care unit.
STRESS Tool (Modrcin-McCarthy, McCue, & Walker, 1997)	Permits documentation of signs of stress, touch interventions, reduction of pain, environmental considerations, state, and stability in medically fragile preterm infants.
Nursing Job Descriptions (Rogers et al, 1991)	Provides Roy Adaptation Model–based job descriptions for nurse administrators (e.g., directors of nursing departments, unit managers), RNs, registered nursing assistants, and technicians.
Quality Assessment Tools (Weiss & Teplick, 1993, 1995)	Provides a Roy Adaptation Model–based method for quality assessment and monitoring, with separate tools available for particular patient populations.
Performance Appraisal System (Rogers et al, 1991)	Provides a Roy Adaptation Model–based system for appraisal of nurses' performance of their responsibilities.
Intershift Report Format (Riegel, 1985)	Provides guidelines for presenting intershift reports organized according to the Roy Adaptation Model's nursing diagnosis, stimuli, and adaptive mode responses.

From Fawcett, J. (2000). *Analysis and evaluation of contemporary nursing knowledge: nursing models and theories.* Philadelphia: FA Davis. *COPD,* Chronic obstructive pulmonary disease; *MCN,* maternal child nursing; *NICU,* neonatal intensive care unit; *RN,* registered nurse.

(Chinn, 1999), and independent functioning has been equated with physician skills (McBride, 1999). In turn, some NPs, clinical nurse specialists (CNSs), certified nurse midwives (CNMs), and certified registered nurse anesthetists (CRNAs) strive to become physician assistants (PAs), junior doctors, pseudo doctors, or physician substitutes (Meleis, 1993; Huch, 1995; Watson, 1996; Kendrick, 1997; McBride, 1999).

Those nurses who emulate physicians most likely do so because "the lure of following the medical model is sanctioned and well rewarded in some settings" (Hawkins & Thibodeau, 1996). Consequently, the value of using nursing discipline–specific C-T-E systems to guide nursing research and nursing practice needs to be underscored so that all APNs can become senior nurses with freedom and autonomy (Meleis, 1993; Hawkins & Thibodeau, 1996; Watson, 1997). Chalmers (Chalmers, Kershaw, Melia, & Kendrich, 1990) points out, "Nursing models [and theories] have provided what many would argue is a much needed alternative knowledge base from which nurses can practice in an informed way. An alternative, that is, to the medical model which for so many years has dominated many aspects of health care." Nursing discipline–specific C-T-E systems also provide an alternative to the institutional model of practice in which "the most salient values [are] efficiency, standardized care, rules, and regulations" (Rogers, 1989). The institutional model, moreover, typically upholds, reinforces, and supports the medical model (Grossman & Hooton, 1993).

Nursing discipline–specific C-T-E systems collectively identify the distinctive nursing territory within the vast arena of health care (Feeg, 1989). Each conceptual model of nursing and nursing theory provides a holistic orientation that reminds APNs of the focus of nursing on people, their environments, and their health (Fawcett, 2000) and reinforces the view that nursing research and nursing practice ultimately are for patients' sakes (Dabbs, 1994). Moreover, although some APNs hold the "unfortunate view [that nursing conceptual models and theories] are the inventions and predictions only of scholars and academics [that have] little significance for their own practice environments," at least some other APNs recognize the beneficial effects of nursing models and theories (Hayne, 1992; Neil, 1995). Indeed, C-T-E system–based nursing practice helps APNs better communicate what they do and why they do it (Neff, 1991).

In particular, nursing discipline–specific C-T-E systems provide a nursing knowledge base that has a positive effect on practice "by enabling well-coordinated [nursing] to take place, by providing a basis for the justification of [nursing] actions and by enabling [advanced practice] nurses to *talk nursing*" (Chalmers et al, 1990), *think nursing* (Perry, 1985; Nightingale, 1993), and engage in *thinking nursing* (Allison & Renpenning, 1999), rather than just doing tasks and carrying out physicians' orders (Le Storti, Cullen, Hanzlik, Michiels, Piano, Ryan, & Johnson, 1999).

However, APNs are able to talk nursing and think nursing only if they use nursing conceptual models, theories, and empirical indicators, which provide a distinctive nursing language. The lack of a nursing language when nursing conceptual models and theories are not used "has been a handicap in nurses' communications about nursing to the public as well as to persons with whom they work in the health field" (Orem, 1997). APNs must learn about nursing models and theories before they can use them to guide practice. Most graduate programs include a required course on contemporary nursing knowledge, including conceptual models of nursing and nursing theories. The responsibility to provide such courses and integrate the content into the rest of the APN curriculum falls to nurse educators. If a course addressing nursing models and theories is not included in the curriculum, or if the content is not integrated into APN clinical courses, APN students, as consumers of education, should request it. APNs who have not had the opportunity to take a course on nursing models and theories or have not had the opportunity to learn how to implement C-T-E systems in practice have the professional responsibility to undertake independent study by reading relevant textbooks and journal articles. (Fawcett [2000] provides comprehensive bibliographies.) All APNs have the responsibility to seek continuing education programs that present strategies to implement C-T-E systems.

Thinking nursing within the context of nursing discipline–specific C-T-E systems helps APNs "clarify their thinking on their role, especially at a time when the roles of many health professionals are becoming blurred" (Nightingale, 1993). Moreover, thinking nursing within the context of nursing discipline–specific C-T-E systems can shape the way in which advanced practice is viewed. For example, APNs may elect to specialize in the use of a particular nursing conceptual model or theory as the starting point for construction of C-T-E systems, or they may elect to specialize in a particular concept of a nursing model or theory. An APN could, for example, specialize in one behavioral subsystem of Johnson's Behavioral System Model (Rogers, 1973).

Clearly, the use of nursing discipline–specific C-T-E systems distinguishes nursing as an autonomous health profession and represents "nursing's unique contribution to the health care system" (Parse, 1995). The use of explicit C-T-E systems as guides for nursing practice already is a hallmark of professional nursing practice (Fawcett & Carino, 1989). However, it is important for APNs to continue to utilize and evaluate explicit nursing discipline–specific C-T-E systems if the professional discipline of nursing is to retain a place in the multidisciplinary health care arena.

PRIORITIES FOR RESEARCH

Research findings indicate that nurses feel vulnerable and experience a great deal of stress as they attempt to achieve their professional aspirations within a rapidly changing, medically dominated, bureaucratic health care delivery system (Graham, 1994). As structures for critical thinking within a distinctively nursing context, nursing discipline–specific C-T-E systems provide the intellectual skills that APNs need to survive at a time when cost-containment through reduction of professional nursing staff is the modus operandi of managed care and administrators of health care delivery systems, including hospitals, home health care agencies, and health maintenance organizations (HMOs).

Johnson (1990) notes that although individual APNs and nursing departments take risks when the decision is made to use an explicit nursing discipline–specific C-T-E system to guide nursing practice, the rewards far outweigh the risks. Johnson states that "to openly use a nursing model is risk-taking behavior for the individual nurse. For a nursing department to adopt one of these models for unit or institution use is risk-taking behavior of an even higher order. The reward for such risk-taking for the individual practitioner lies in the great satisfaction gained from being able to specify explicit concrete *nursing* goals [with] patients and from documenting the actual achievement of the desired outcomes. The reward for the nursing department is having a rational, cohesive, and comprehensive basis for the development of standards of nursing practice, for the evaluation of practitioners, and for the documentation of the contribution of nursing to patient welfare."

Anecdotal and empirical evidence indicates that some additional rewards of using explicit nursing discipline–specific C-T-E systems to guide practice include reduced staff nurse turnover, more rapid movement from novice to expert nurse, increased patient and family satisfaction with nursing, increased nurse job satisfaction, and considerable cost savings (Fawcett, 2000). Furthermore, as the use of C-T-E systems moves nursing practice from a base of implicit knowledge to one of explicit nursing knowledge, both APNs and patients are empowered. Indeed, "[nursing] knowledge is power" (Orr, 1991) that can be used to empower individuals, families, and communities to fully participate in decisions about their health care (Lister, 1991; Malin & Teasdale, 1991).

The development, dissemination, utilization, and clinical evaluation of explicit nursing discipline–specific C-T-E systems will end the journey (along the "dependent path") that has led to APNs functioning primarily as "assistants to physicians or as quasi practitioners of medicine" (Orlando, 1987). It will facilitate the beginning of a journey along the independent path of professional nursing (Orlando, 1987). Furthermore, development, dissemination, utilization, and clinical evaluation of explicit nursing discipline–specific C-T-E systems is the only way that advanced practice can move from being a "silent service" recognized primarily by its absence (Allison & Renpenning, 1999) to a very public service, the need for which is widely recognized. The challenge to each APN is to adopt an explicit nursing discipline–specific C-T-E system and use that C-T-E system to integrate nursing research and nursing practice.

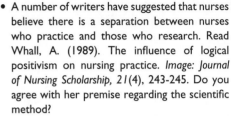

Suggestions for Further Learning

- A number of writers have suggested that nurses believe there is a separation between nurses who practice and those who research. Read Whall, A. (1989). The influence of logical positivism on nursing practice. *Image: Journal of Nursing Scholarship, 21*(4), 243-245. Do you agree with her premise regarding the scientific method?
- Get the article: Brown, S. (1998). A framework for advanced practice nursing. *Journal of Professional Nursing, 14*(3), 157-164. How does Brown address the issue of nursing theory in advanced practice? Brown proposes a framework for advanced practice—do you agree with concepts she proposes?
- Get the article: Mitchell, G. (1997). Questioning evidence-based practice for nursing. *Nursing Science Quarterly, 10*(4), 154-155. How does this view correspond to all you have read regarding the need for evidence-based practice?

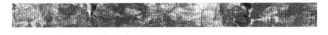

DISCUSSION QUESTIONS

These questions can be used to promote critical thinking and encourage discussion.

1. How do C-T-E systems of nursing knowledge influence your conceptualization of your work as an APN?
2. Fawcett (2000) cautions APNs on the risk of medicalizing human experiences of health and nursing and equating advanced practice with the skills of physicians. Reflect on your perceptions of advanced practice. What is your response to this concern?
3. Select a nursing discipline–specific C-T-E system and review one of your clinical experiences from this framework. Identify ways this C-T-E system could guide your nursing practice.

REFERENCES/BIBLIOGRAPHY

Allison, S.E., & Renpenning, K. (1999). *Nursing administration in the 21st century*. Thousand Oaks, CA: Sage.

Anderson, C.A. (1998). Does evidence-based practice equal quality nursing care? *Nursing Outlook, 46*, 257-258.

Andrews, H.A., & Roy, C. (1986). *Essentials of the Roy Adaptation Model*. Norwalk, CT: Appleton-Century-Crofts.

Batey, M.V. (1997). Conceptualizing the research process. In L.H. Nicoll (Ed.), *Perspectives on nursing theory* (pp. 684-692). Philadelphia: JB Lippincott.

Burgess, A.W., & Fawcett, J. (1996). The Comprehensive Sexual Assault Assessment Tool. *Nurse Practitioner, 21*(4), 66, 71-72, 74-76, 78, 83, 86.

Chalmers, H., Kershaw, B., Melia, K., & Kendrich, M. (1990). Nursing models: enhancing or inhibiting practice? *Nursing Standard, 5*(11), 34-40.

Chinn, P.L. (1999). From the editor. *Advances in Nursing Science, 21*(4), v.

Cho, J. (1998). *Nursing manual: assessment tool according to the Roy Adaptation Model.* Glendale, CA: Polaris Publishing.

Dabbs, A.D.V. (1994). Theory-based nursing practice: for our patients' sake. *Clinical Nurse Specialist, 8*, 214, 220.

Donaldson, S.K., & Crowley, D.M. (1978). The discipline of nursing. *Nursing Outlook, 26*, 113-120.

Dow, K.H.M. (1993). An analysis of the experience of surviving and having children after breast cancer. *Dissertation Abstracts International, 53*, 5641B.

Doyle, R., & Rajacich, D. (1991). The Roy Adaptation Model: health teaching about osteoporosis. *American Association of Occupational Health Nursing Journal, 39*, 508-512.

Fagin, C.M. (1998). Nursing research and the erosion of care. *Nursing Outlook, 46*, 259-260.

Fawcett, J. (1992). Documentation using a conceptual model of nursing. *Nephrology Nursing Today, 2*(5), 1-8.

Fawcett, J. (1999). *The relationship of theory and research* (3rd ed.). Philadelphia: FA Davis.

Fawcett, J. (2000). *Contemporary nursing knowledge: nursing models and theories.* Philadelphia: FA Davis.

Fawcett, J., & Burritt, J. (1985). An exploratory study of antenatal preparation for cesarean birth. *Journal of Obstetric, Gynecologic, and Neonatal Nursing, 14*, 224-230.

Fawcett, J., & Carino, C. (1989). Hallmarks of success in nursing practice. *Advances in Nursing Science, 11*(4), 1-8.

Fawcett, J., & Henklein, J. (1987). Antenatal education for cesarean birth: extension of a field test. *Journal of Obstetric, Gynecologic, and Neonatal Nursing, 16*, 61-65.

Fawcett, J., & Tulman, L. (1996). Assessment of function. In R. McCorkle, M. Grant, M. Frank-Stromborg, & S.B. Baird (Eds.), *Cancer nursing: a comprehensive textbook* (2nd ed.) (pp. 66-73). Philadelphia: WB Saunders.

Fawcett, J., Tulman, L., & Myers, S. (1988). Development of the Inventory of Functional Status after Childbirth. *Journal of Nurse-Midwifery, 33*, 252-260.

Feeg, V. (1989). From the editor: is theory application merely an intellectual exercise? *Pediatric Nursing, 15*, 450.

Frank, D.I. (1988). Psychosocial assessment of renal dialysis patients. *American Nephrology Nurses Association Journal, 15*, 207-232.

Frank, L.K. (1968). Science as a communication process. *Main Currents in Modern Thought, 25*, 45-50.

Graham, I. (1994). How do registered nurses think and experience nursing: a phenomenological investigation. *Journal of Clinical Nursing, 3*, 235-242.

Grossman, M., & Hooton, M. (1993). The significance of the relationship between a discipline and its practice. *Journal of Advanced Nursing, 18*, 866-872.

Hamner, J.B. (1989). Applying the Roy adaptation model to the CCU. *Critical Care Nurse, 9*(3), 51-61.

Hanchett, E.S. (1988). *Nursing frameworks and community as client: bridging the gap.* Norwalk, CT: Appleton and Lange.

Hawkins, J.W., & Thibodeau, J.A. (1996). *The advanced practice nurse: current issues* (4th ed.). New York: Tiresias Press.

Hayne, Y. (1992). The current status and future significance of nursing as a discipline. *Journal of Advanced Nursing, 17*, 104-107.

Hinman, L.M. (1983). Focus on the school-aged child in family intervention. *Journal of School Health, 53*, 499-502.

Huber, P.M., Medhat, A., & Carter, M.C. (1988). Prosthetic problem inventory scale. *Rehabilitation Nursing, 13*, 326-329.

Huch, M.H. (1995). Nursing and the next millennium. *Nursing Science Quarterly, 8*, 38-44.

Ide, B.A. (1978). SPAL: a tool for measuring self-perceived adaptation level appropriate for an elderly population. In E.E. Bauwens (Ed.), *Clinical nursing research: its strategies and findings* (Monograph series 1978: Two) (pp. 56-63). Indianapolis, IN: Sigma Theta Tau.

Jackson, D.A. (1990). Roy in the postanesthesia care unit. *Journal of Post Anesthesia Nursing, 5*, 143-148.

Jakocko, M.T., & Sowden, L.A. (1986). The Roy Adaptation Model in nursing practice. In H.A. Andrews & C. Roy (Eds.), *Essentials of the Roy adaptation model* (pp. 165-177). Norwalk, CT: Appleton and Lange.

Johnson, D.E. (1990). The behavioral system model for nursing. In M.E. Parker (Ed.), *Nursing theories in practice* (pp. 23-32). New York: National League for Nursing.

Joseph, A., & Lantz, J. (1996). A systematic tool to assess urinary incontinence parameters: a closer look at unfamiliar parameters. *Urologic Nursing, 16*, 93-98.

Kendrick, K. (1997). What is advanced nursing? *Professional Nurse, 12*(10), 689.

King, I.M. (1990). King's conceptual framework and theory of goal attainment. In M.E. Parker (Ed.), *Nursing theories in practice* (pp. 73-84). New York: National League for Nursing.

Laros, J. (1977). Deriving outcome criteria from a conceptual model. *Nursing Outlook, 25*, 333-336.

Leininger, M.M. (1991). The theory of culture care diversity and universality. In M.M. Leininger (Ed.), *Culture care diversity and universality: a theory of nursing* (pp. 5-65). New York: National League for Nursing.

LeMone, P. (1995). Assessing psychosexual concerns in adults with diabetes: pilot project using Roy's modes of adaptation. *Issues in Mental Health Nursing, 16*, 67-78.

Le Storti, L.J., Cullen, P.A., Hanzlik, E.M., Michiels, J.M., Piano, L.A., Ryan, P.L., & Johnson, W. (1999). Creative thinking in nursing education: preparing for tomorrow's challenges. *Nursing Outlook, 47*, 62-66.

Levine, M.E. (1991). The conservation principles: a model for health. In K.M. Schaefer & J.B. Pond (Eds.), *Levine's conservation model: a framework for nursing practice* (pp. 1-11). Philadelphia: FA Davis.

Lewis, F.M., Firsich, S.C., & Parsell, S. (1978). Development of reliable measures of patient health outcomes related to quality nursing care for chemotherapy patients. In J.C. Krueger, A.H. Nelson, & M.O. Wolanin (Eds.), *Nursing research: development, collaboration, and utilization* (pp. 225-228). Germantown, MD: Aspen Publishers.

Lewis, F.M., Firsich, S.C., & Parsell, S. (1979). Clinical tool development for adult chemotherapy patients: process and content. *Cancer Nursing, 2*, 99-108.

Lippitt, G.L. (1973). *Visualizing change: model building and the change process*. Fairfax, VA: NTL Learning Resources.

Lister, P. (1991). Approaching models of nursing from a postmodernist perspective. *Journal of Advanced Nursing, 16,* 206-212.

Logan, M. (1990). The Roy adaptation model: are nursing diagnoses amenable to independent nurse functions? *Journal of Advanced Nursing, 15,* 468-470.

Malin, N., & Teasdale, K. (1991). Caring versus empowerment: considerations for nursing practice. *Journal of Advanced Nursing, 16,* 657-662.

McBride, A.B. (1999). Breakthroughs in nursing education: looking back, looking forward. *Nursing Outlook, 47,* 114-119.

McDonald, F.J., & Harms, M. (1966). Theoretical model for an experimental curriculum. *Nursing Outlook, 14*(8), 48-51.

Meleis, A.I. (1993, April). Nursing research and the Neuman model: directions for the future (Panel discussion at the Fourth Biennial International Neuman Systems Model Symposium [B. Neuman, A.I. Meleis, J. Fawcett, L. Lowry, M.C. Smith, A. Edgil, participants]). Rochester, NY.

Mitchell, G. (1994). Discipline-specific inquiry: the hermeneutics of theory-guided nursing research. *Nursing Outlook, 42,* 224-228.

Modrcin-McCarthy, M.A., McCue, S., & Walker, J. (1997). Preterm infants and STRESS: a tool for the neonatal nurse. *Journal of Perinatal and Neonatal Nursing, 10*(4), 62-71.

Neff, M. (1991). President's message: the future of our profession from the eyes of today. *American Nephrology Nurses Association Journal, 18,* 534.

Neil, R.M. (1995). Evidence in support of basing a nursing center on nursing theory: the Denver Nursing Project in Human Caring. In B. Murphy (Ed.), *Nursing centers: the time is now* (pp. 233-246). New York: National League for Nursing.

Neuman, B. (1995). *The Neuman Systems Model* (3rd ed.). Norwalk, CT: Appleton and Lange.

Newman, D.M.L. (1997). The Inventory of Functional Status—Caregiver of a Child in a Body Cast. *Journal of Pediatric Nursing, 12,* 142-147.

Newman, M.A. (1994). *Health as expanding consciousness* (2nd ed.). New York: National League for Nursing Press.

Nightingale, K. (1993). Editorial. *British Journal of Theatre Nursing, 3*(5), 2.

O'Leary, P.A. (1991). Family caregivers' log reports of sleep and activity behaviors of persons with Alzheimer's disease. *Dissertation Abstracts International, 51,* 4780B.

Orem, D.E. (1995). *Nursing: concepts of practice* (5th ed.). St. Louis: Mosby.

Orem, D.E. (1997). Views of human beings specific to nursing. *Nursing Science Quarterly, 10,* 26-31.

Orlando, I.J. (1961). *The dynamic nurse-patient relationship*. New York: GP Putnam's Sons.

Orlando, I.J. (1987). Nursing in the 21st century: alternate paths. *Journal of Advanced Nursing, 12,* 405-412.

Orr, J. (1991). Knowledge is power. *Health Visitor, 64,* 218.

Paier, G.S. (1994). Development and testing of an instrument to assess functional status in the elderly. *Dissertation Abstracts International, 55,* 1806B.

Parse, R.R. (1995). Commentary: Parse's theory of human becoming: an alternative guide to nursing practice for pediatric oncology nurses. *Journal of Pediatric Oncology Nursing, 12,* 128.

Parse, R.R. (1998). *The human becoming school of thought: a perspective for nurses and other health professionals*. Thousand Oaks, CA: Sage.

Peplau, H.E. (1952). *Interpersonal relations in nursing*. New York: G.P Putnam's Sons.

Perry, J. (1985). Has the discipline of nursing developed to the stage where nurses do "think nursing"? *Journal of Advanced Nursing, 10,* 31-37.

Peters, V.J. (1993). Documentation using the Roy Adaptation Model. *American Nephrology Nurses Association Journal, 20,* 522.

Popper, K.R. (1965). *Conjectures and refutations: the growth of scientific knowledge*. New York: Harper and Row.

Rambo, B. (1984). Adaptation nursing: assessment and intervention (pp. 385-395). Philadelphia: WB Saunders.

Reilly, D.E. (1975). Why a conceptual framework? *Nursing Outlook, 23,* 566-569.

Riegel, B. (1985). A method of giving intershift report based on a conceptual model. *Focus on Critical Care, 12*(4), 12-18.

Robitaille-Tremblay, M. (1984). A data collection tool for the psychiatric nurse. *The Canadian Nurse, 80*(7), 26-28.

Rogers, C.G. (1973). Conceptual models as guides to clinical nursing specialization. *Journal of Nursing Education, 12*(4), 2-6.

Rogers, M. E. (1989). Creating a climate for the implementation of a nursing conceptual framework. *Journal of Continuing Education in Nursing, 20,* 112-116.

Rogers, M.E. (1990). Nursing: science of unitary, irreducible, human beings: update 1990. In E.A.M. Barrett (Ed.), *Visions of Rogers' science-based nursing* (pp. 5-11). New York: National League for Nursing.

Rogers, M.E., Paul, L.J., Clarke, J., Mackay, C., Potter, M., & Ward, W. (1991). The use of the Roy Adaptation Model in nursing administration. *Canadian Journal of Nursing Administration, 4*(2), 21-26.

Rolfe, G. (1993). Closing the theory-practice gap: a model of nursing praxis. *Journal of Clinical Nursing, 2,* 173-177.

Roy, C. (1979). Health-illness (powerlessness) questionnaire and hospitalized patient decision making. In M.J. Ward & C.A. Lindeman (Eds.), *Instruments for measuring nursing practice and other health care variables* (Vol. 1) (pp. 147-153). Hyattsville, MD: US Department of Health, Education, and Welfare.

Roy, C. (1984). *Introduction to nursing: an adaptation model* (2nd ed.). Englewood Cliffs, NJ: Prentice-Hall.

Roy, C. (1989). The Roy Adaptation Model. In J.P. Riehl-Sisca (Ed.), *Conceptual models for nursing practice* (3rd ed.) (pp. 105-114). Norwalk, CT: Appleton and Lange.

Roy, C., & Andrews, H. A. (1999). *The Roy Adaptation Model* (2nd ed.). Stamford, CT: Appleton and Lange.

Short, J.D. (1994). Interdependence needs and nursing care of the new family. *Issues in Comprehensive Pediatric Nursing, 17,* 1-14.

Smith, M.C. (1995). The core of advanced practice nursing. *Nursing Science Quarterly, 8,* 2-3.

Starn, J., & Niederhauser, V. (1990). An MCN model for nursing diagnosis to focus intervention. *American Journal of Maternal Child Nursing, 15,* 180-183.

Taylor, C. (1993). *The patient's guide to preterm labor*. Woodbury, NJ: Underwood-Memorial Hospital.

Thomas, C.L. (1997). *Taber's cyclopedic medical dictionary* (18th ed.). Philadelphia: FA Davis.

Thomas-Hawkins, C., Fawcett, J., & Tulman, L. (1998). The Inventory of Functional Status—Dialysis: development and testing. *American Association of Nephrology Nurses Journal, 25,* 483-490.

Thorne, S., Kirkham, S.R., & MacDonald-Emes, J. (1997). Interpretive description: a noncategorical qualitative alternative for developing nursing knowledge. *Research in Nursing and Health, 20,* 169-177.

Tulman, L., Fawcett, J., & McEvoy, M.D. (1991). Development of the Inventory of Functional Status—Cancer. *Cancer Nursing, 14,* 254-260.

Tulman, L., Fawcett, J., & Weiss, M. (1993). The Inventory of Functional Status—Fathers: development and psychometric testing. *Journal of Nurse-Midwifery, 38,* 117-123.

Tulman, L., Higgins, K., Fawcett, J., Nunno, C., Vansickel, C., Haas, M.B., & Speca, M.M. (1991). The Inventory of Functional Status—Antepartum Period: development and testing. *Journal of Nurse-Midwifery, 36,* 117-123.

Varnell, G.M.P. (1990). Parental role perceptions: instrument development. *Dissertation Abstracts International, 51,* 1197B.

Watson, J. (1985). *Nursing: human science and human care: a theory of nursing.* Norwalk, CT: Appleton-Century-Crofts.

Watson, J. (1997). The theory of human caring: retrospective and prospective. *Nursing Science Quarterly, 10,* 49-52.

Watson, M.J. (1996). Watson's theory of transpersonal caring. In P. Hinton Walker & B. Neuman (Eds.), *Blueprint for use of nursing models: education, research, practice, and administration* (pp. 141-184). New York: National League for Nursing.

Weiss, M.E., & Teplick, F. (1993). Linking perinatal standards, documentation, and quality monitoring. *Journal of Perinatal and Neonatal Nursing, 7*(2), 18-27.

Weiss, M.E., & Teplick, F. (1995). Linking perinatal standards, documentation, and quality monitoring. *Neonatal Intensive Care, 8*(1), 38-43, 58.

Whall, A.L. (1986). Strategic family therapy: nursing reformulations and applications. In A.L. Whall (Ed.), *Family therapy theory for nursing: four approaches* (pp. 51-67). Norwalk, CT: Appleton-Century-Crofts.

Wood, K.W. (1978). Casework effectiveness: a new look at the research evidence. *Social Work, 23,* 437-458.

Wright, P.S. (1993). Parents' perception of their quality of life. *Journal of Pediatric Oncology Nursing, 10,* 139-145.

Portions of this chapter were adapted, with permission, from Fawcett, J. (2000). *Analysis and evaluation of contemporary nursing knowledge: nursing models and theories.* Philadelphia: FA Davis.

Chapter 30

Grand Nursing Theories and Conceptual Models

Theresa Beery, Anne M. Dollins, Mary Gers, Linda LaCharity, Denise Robinson, & Lisa Spangler Torok

A significant number of advanced practice nurses (APNs) view themselves as different than physicians (Baumann, 1998). The main difference is viewed as the ability of nurses to offer care that is unique and specific to a patient. Many APNs attribute this difference to the belief that nursing knowledge is constitutive to the care they provide. As part of this nursing knowledge, nursing theories and conceptual models enable APNs to conceptualize and understand information in a fashion different than that offered by the traditional biomedical model (Baumann, 1998). Thus it is important for APNs to be knowledgeable in the area of nursing theory and conceptual models. Smith (1994) states that, in the future, nursing will no longer only be directed toward cure, symptom relief, prevention, or rehabilitation. In addition, APNs will strive to achieve or promote quality of life, health, and healing as defined and directed by their patients. This requires a nursing practice that is grounded in nursing knowledge, which means the use of nursing theory must be acknowledged as the base in nursing. All APNs need to articulate the beliefs and values that serve as the foundation of their practice. Nursing schools need to include nursing theory not just as a single academic course, but as the substance of nursing. Doing so prepares nursing for the twenty-first century.

The focus of this chapter is to briefly describe a select group of grand, or broad, nursing theories and identify how they have been or could be used in advanced practice. Theory can be categorized in many ways. Grand nursing theories tend to define general parameters on which nursing function is based, while midrange theories give more specific guidance related to nursing practice. The grand theories presented here represent a variety of theories that are applicable across a broad spectrum of practice settings and are not intended to represent the full range of current nursing theories. Readers are encouraged to seek out and study nursing theories other than those presented here.

CRITICAL ISSUES: EVALUATING THE MERITS OF GRAND THEORIES AND CONCEPTUAL MODELS

Orem's Self-Care Deficit Theory of Nursing

Dorothea E. Orem, who has a background in nursing and nursing education, is considered a trailblazer in the development of distinct nursing knowledge. The initial impetus for her model was the need to develop a curriculum for a practical nursing program in 1959, which required identification of the domain and boundaries of nursing. For this, she drew on her years of experience as a nursing consultant in the Division of Hospital and Institutional Services of the Indiana State Board of Health. Orem searched for an answer to the question, "What is nursing?" For this search, Orem credits her ability to reflect and search for meaning to her experiences in nursing, her study of formal logic and metaphysics, and the use of resources from the fields of human organization and action theory. Her search for the meaning of nursing and the boundaries of nursing was structured by three more specific questions: What do nurses do and what should nurses do as practitioners of nursing? Why do nurses do what they do? What results from what nurses do as practitioners of nursing? (Orem, 1991)

Using her three questions to guide her, Orem introduced the Self-Care Framework. She identified two phases in the development of her theory. The first ended in 1972, when the essential ideas were identified, relationships were defined, and the first book was published. The second phase began in late 1972, when the focus was on diffusion and refinement of the theory. Orem maintained that human limitations for self-care associated with health situations give rise to a requirement for nursing (Orem, 1991). This general theory of nursing is an account of relationships that serve to organize the outlook of nurses.

Assumptions

Five general assumptions or generalizations about human beings relate to all three questions and have been implicit in Orem's thinking from the beginning. Orem now refers to these five assumptions as the guiding premises for her conceptualization of nursing. They are referred to as *premises* because they are advanced as true, not merely assumed. The five premises are:

1. Human beings require continuous deliberate inputs to themselves and their environments to remain alive and function in accord with natural human endowments.
2. Human agency, the power to act deliberately, is exercised in the form of care of self and others in identifying needs and making needed inputs.
3. Mature human beings experience privations in the form of limitations of action in the care of self and others involving the making of life-sustaining and function-regulating inputs.
4. Human agency is exercised in discovering, developing, and transmitting to others ways and means to identify needs and make inputs to self and others.
5. Groups of human beings within structured relationships cluster tasks and allocate responsibilities for providing care to group members who experience privations for making required deliberate inputs to self and others (Orem, 1995).

Major concepts

Orem describes her theory as a general theory comprised of three articulating theories: theory of self-care, theory of self-care deficit, and theory of nursing systems. Orem called her general theory the Self-Care Deficit Theory of Nursing (SCDTN). To Orem, the word *deficit* does not indicate a limitation but rather an imbalance between the capabilities of the individual and the needs for action. Orem explains her use of three theories by contending that the theory of nursing systems is not meaningful in the absence of subsumed theories of self-care and self-care deficit (Orem, 1991). Each of the interrelated theories has a central idea, a set of propositions, and a set of presuppositions.

To understand Orem's theory, one must examine several key concepts. Orem defines **self-care** as the practice of activities that individuals initiate and perform on their own behalf in maintaining life, health, and well-being. Persons who engage in self-care have the requisite action capabilities, agency, or power to act deliberately to regulate factors that affect their own functioning and development (Orem, 1991). Input of required materials and the provision of needed conditions when deliberately made or sought by persons for themselves is referred to as *self-care*. When these provisions are made by others for persons dependent on them, it is referred to as *dependent-care*. When these provisions are made by nurses for individuals with health-derived or health-associated incapacities for self-care, it is an aspect of nursing (Orem, 1996).

Self-care agency is described as the power of individuals to engage in self-care, reflecting their capability for self-care. Self-care agency is an acquired ability that is affected by conditions and factors in the environment (Orem, 1991). Self-care agency is the name assigned to the internal enabling conditions of human beings that make it possible for them to perform the estimative, transitional, and productive operations through which self-care is effected. In the SCDTN, these internal enabling conditions were identified during a search for understanding of the underlying structure of the theoretical concept of self-care agency (Orem, 1996). Three types of enabling conditions are identified. *Foundational capabilities and dispositions* refers to the ability to engage in all types of deliberate action, not only self-care. *Power components* are the capabilities that allow for the initiation and performance of self-care operations. Without the development and operational readiness of the power components, no self-care operation could be performed (Orem, 1995). *Capabilities for estimative, transitional and productive operations* are necessary to meet existent and projected self-care requisites (Orem, 1995).

Therapeutic self-care demand is defined as the summation of measures of self-care required at moments in time and for some duration (Orem, 1991). This totality of care actions is performed to meet what Orem calls *self-care requisites*, or generalized purposes for which an individual performs self-care. Orem identifies three types of self-care requisites. **Universal self-care requisites** are associated with life processes and are common to all human beings. **Developmental self-care requisites** include actions to maintain conditions to support life and development. **Health deviation requisites** are required when injury or illness is present. An example of a universal self-care requisite would be to maintain a sufficient intake of water. What is sufficient must be determined for individuals in relation to prevailing internal and external conditions in some time, place, and frame of reference (Orem, 1995). An example of a developmental requisite is to supply and maintain conditions that permit and foster sensory-motor development in infancy. A health deviation requisite would be the monitoring of individuals for signs and symptoms of bleeding and for changes in vital processes following a surgical procedure performed under general anesthesia (Orem, 1996).

Orem defines **self-care deficit** as the relationship between self-care agency and therapeutic self-care demands of individuals in which capabilities for self-care, because of existent limitations, are not equal to meeting some or all of the components of their therapeutic self-care demands (Orem, 1991). Orem is clear that the deficit itself is not a disorder or problem but an expression of the relationship between the two concepts. This self-care deficit or potential deficit must exist for nursing to be legitimate. **Nursing agency,** or **collective nursing capabilities,** is defined as the complex property or attribute of persons educated and trained as nurses that is enabling when exercised for knowing and helping others meet their therapeutic self-care demands (Orem, 1991). Nursing agency is a complex, acquired ability that is learned and performed with a goal in mind. When nursing agency is activated, a nursing system is produced. **Nursing system** is defined as all the actions and interactions of nurses and patients in nursing practice situations (Orem, 1991). Orem describes three types of nursing systems, and the type of nursing system used is dependent upon the self-care needs and abilities of a patient. The first system is a wholly compensatory nursing system, used when a patient cannot participate in any self-care (i.e., the nurse performs all necessary actions). This might be used for a patient in intensive care and on a ventilator. The second system is a partly compensatory nursing system, used when a patient and nurse both make contributions toward self-care. This might refer to a patient who is hypertensive and diabetic, with the diabetes being out of control. The patient is able to care for himself but needs assistance from the APN to do so. The third system is a supportive-educative nursing system in which a patient performs all self-care actions requiring ambulation and movement, while the nurse provides support and information (Orem, 1995). A good example might be a patient who wishes to quit smoking. The APN provides information about the ways in which a patient can stop, strategies for stopping, and support once the patient does stop smoking.

Theory of self-care. *Self-care* is described as behavior that is learned from interaction and communication in larger social groups. The theory of self-care is both descriptive and explanatory. It describes actions and events that are recognized as self-care and identifies the relation of performed self-care actions to human functioning and development (Orem, 1996). Orem identifies presuppositions (assumptions) on which the theory of self-care rests. Self-care actions vary by cultural and social experiences. It is also assumed that all individuals have the potential ability and motivation necessary to provide care for themselves and dependents. However, having the ability or potential does not guarantee that all will seek knowledge or take action. In situations where all or some abilities are underdeveloped or inoperable, someone must perform the self-care. When a family member or responsible adult performs such care, it is termed *dependent care*. When care is performed by a nurse, it is referred to as *specialized care*.

The structure of the process of self-care is viewed as those enduring elements that characterize the meeting of each and every self-care requisite. This structure is hypothesized to consist of three types of operations—estimative operations, transitional operations, and production operations. An operation is a process or action that is part of some work to be done. In this situation, the work is knowing and meeting each existent self-care

requisite (Orem, 1996). The three operations are defined as follows:

1. Estimative self-care operations investigate existent relevant human and environmental conditions in a time and place of reference. They investigate the meaning of conditions for the lives, health, and well-being of individuals.
2. Transitional operations include selecting and appraising results achieved through performance of estimative operations, making judgments about what can and should be done, and making decisions about what will be done in meeting specific self-care requisites.
3. Production operations are actions to secure needed resources, bring about necessary conditions in self and environment, and perform the measures of care associated with using specific methods in meeting each self-care requisite (Orem, 1996).

Theory of self-care deficit. The central idea of self-care deficit theory is that individuals are affected from time to time by limitations that do not allow them to meet their self-care needs. These limitations may occur because of a health condition or because of factors that are internal or external to the individual. These limitations may incapacitate a person and hinder the ability to meet general or specific human needs. Orem is clear that nursing must be legitimate (i.e., the relationship between the individual and nurse is based on the condition that establishes a need for nursing) (Orem, 1991). Self-care deficits are understood in terms of the relationship between the amount and kind of required self-care (therapeutic self-care demand) and the action capabilities and limitations of individuals for knowing what care is needed and producing this care. When individuals' action capabilities are not adequate to know and meet their therapeutic self-care demands, a deficit relationship exists. Nurses not only must be knowledgeable about self-care, self-care requisites, and therapeutic self-care demands, they must also understand the human power called self-care agency (Orem, 1996).

Theory of nursing system. Understanding Orem's theory of nursing system is the key to understanding her general theory of nursing. The major components of the theory of self-care and the theory of self-care deficit are incorporated within the theory of nursing system (Orem, 1991). The central idea is that nurses have skills that they use to determine if nursing help is necessary or legitimate. When limitations for performing self-care have their origins in the health states of individuals or in the nature of individuals' health care requirements, nursing is the required health service. The proper object of focus of nursing is not health, disease, or care; it is human beings with health-derived or health-associated self-care deficits (Orem, 1996). If a deficit relationship exists, the nurse should design a plan of care that clearly identifies what is to be done and by whom—nurse, patient, or family member. These actions of the nurse and of the patient and/or dependent caregiver are collectively called the *nursing system*. The goal of the nursing system is to increase a patient's capabilities to meet a need or requisite or to decrease the demands on the patient (Orem, 1991).

Core nursing concepts

Recipient of nursing care. Orem (1991) refers to *person* as a unity that can be viewed as functioning biologically, symbolically, and socially. Orem is concerned with a person's ability to perform self-care; if he or she is unable to perform self-care, nursing is needed. Persons under the care of nurses, as well as persons under hospital care, have been identified by the term *patient*. Orem describes a patient as a receiver of care—someone who is under the care of a health care professional at this time in some place or places.

Health. Orem (1991) differentiates health and well-being in her SCDTN. Health is used in the sense of a person's state that is characterized by soundness or wholeness of developed human structures and of bodily and mental functioning. Well-being is used in the sense of an individual's perceived condition of existence (Orem, 1991). She defines *disease* as an abnormal biological process with characteristic symptoms. Orem's discussion of the various health-related terms and her categories of health-related nursing situations suggest that she views health both as a continuum from excellent to poor and a dichotomy of presence or absence (Fawcett, 1995a). Orem believes that nurses should view the health state of a patient as a basic conditioning factor influencing a patient's potential for self-care.

Environment. Orem (1991) believes that human beings are never isolated from their environments; they exist in them. Human environments are analyzed and understood in terms of physical, chemical, biological, and social features. Examples of features Orem included in the human environment are: (1) atmosphere of the earth, (2) animals in the world, (3) family and family dynamics, (4) availability of resources, and (5) cultural practices. She states that environmental conditions can positively or negatively affect the health and well-being of individuals, families, and communities.

Nursing. Orem (1991) sees nursing as a human service that has its foundations in persons with needs for self-care. Nursing is legitimate only when individuals can not meet their own self-care requisites. Nursing, a specialized health service, is distinguished from other human services by its focus on persons unable to provide the amount and quality of time-specific care necessary to regulate their own functioning and development. Practitioners of nursing perform

---

Box 30-1

Six Components of a Nursing Focus

1. The nurse's perspective of the health situation
2. The patient's perspective of the health situation
3. The patient's state of health
4. The health results sought for the patient
5. The therapeutic self-care demand of the patient's self-care requisites
6. Whether or not the patient can engage in self-care

---

estimative, transitional, and productive operations in order to: (1) know what exists in concrete nursing practice situations, (2) know what can be changed, and (3) make decisions about what can and should be done (Orem, 1991). Nurses are concerned with the continuing therapeutic care a patient requires. There are six components of a nursing focus (shown in Box 30-1). A patient's health state not only gives rise to requirements for health care, it also affects that patient's ability to engage in self-care activities (Orem, 1991).

Self-Care Deficit Theory of Nursing and the advanced practice nurse

A number of schools of nursing have adopted Orem's theory as the framework on which their curriculum is based. The framework also has been used as a conceptual framework for nursing in various institutions (Crews, 1972; Allison, 1973; Backscheider, 1974). Orem's Self-Care Model has been used in many nursing practice areas, including ambulatory clinics (Crew, 1972; Allison, 1973; Backscheider, 1974), nursing homes (Anna, Christensen, Hohon, Ord, & Wells, 1978), and acute care units (Mullin, 1980), as well as with various populations of patients, including children (Gaffney & Moore, 1996), adolescents (Dashiff, 1992; Anderson & Olnhausen, 1999), families (Mapanga & Andrews, 1995; Fawdry, Berry, & Rajacich, 1996; Baker, 1998; Geden & Taylor, 1999), older adults (Ward-Griffin & Bramwell, 1990; Lile & Hoffman, 1991), various ethnic groups (Meleis & Lipson, 1992; Villarruel, 1995), and people with various diseases (Allison, 1973; Robinson, 1991; Aish & Isenberg, 1996; Conner-Warren, 1996). APNs need to be knowledgeable and skilled at identifying self-care demands and deficits and in determining the potential for regulation of self-care abilities and powers for the development of self-care agency.

While frequently APNs do not couch assessment in these terms, determining the level of self-care for patients is a large part of what they do. For example, Kendra brings her 4-month child in for an examination because the boy does not feel well. He is not eating well and seems to have trouble sleeping due to his coughing. Kendra is not able to clearly tell the APN what she has done for him. She knows something is not right but is not clear exactly what it is. The baby has scattered rhonchi and wheezing throughout; retracting; and nasal flaring. A nebulizer treatment improves his condition, but based on the mother's apparent inability to care for him and his condition, he is sent to the hospital and admitted.

Over the years, the three theories discussed previously have been developed to answer two questions that must have answers for APNs to understand what nurses encounter and what they do. The first question is: Why do people need nursing, or what human condition brings about a need for nursing? The theories of self-care and self-care deficit provide hypothesized answers. The second question is: What is the structure of the entity referred to as *nursing*? The theory of nursing system provides a hypothesized answer (Orem, 1996). Because Orem believes that self-care is a learned ability and a deliberate action, an APN must be able to assess for self-care deficits and identify if one exists. Knowing that a patient has a self-care deficit has a direct effect on what interventions are then used. Emphasizing a person's ability to care for self could lead to less indiscriminate use of the health care system and more efficient use of resources. This is an important issue in this era of cost-containment. The ability of a nurse or patient to identify when a patient is unable to care for self makes the theory behind the ability a utilitarian theory. When in an ambulatory setting, an APN's role may be that of providing support and education because the thrust is toward teaching.

Neuman Systems Model

Betty Neuman is recognized as the major theorist of the Neuman Systems Model (NSM). Neuman received her nursing education from a diploma program from Peoples Hospital in Akron, Ohio in 1947. Ten years later she earned a Bachelor's of Science in public health nursing from the University of California at Los Angeles (UCLA). During the 1960s, she made significant contributions to the community mental health movement. It was during that time that Neuman obtained a Master in Science degree as a public health/mental health nurse consultant, also from UCLA. In 1985, Pacific Western University granted her a doctorate in clinical psychology. Neuman's clinical expertise encompassed many areas, including school, industrial, office, and community nursing.

Neuman identified a number of influences from which her model was derived. One source was her wide range of clinical experiences. Neuman's personal philosophy was also fundamental to the model's development. She believed that it was important for people to help others so they may live (Neuman, 1995). The writings of de Chardin and other philosophers helped inform her personal philosophy. Neuman also drew from Gestalt theory, Selye's theory of stress and stress responses, and general systems theory.

Neuman developed the NSM in the 1970s. It initially served as a framework to organize course content at the request of graduate students in community health at UCLA (Fawcett, 1989; Fitzpatrick & Whall, 1989; Wesley, 1994; George, 1995; Neuman, 1996). In 1988, in order to protect and promote the integrity of the model, Neuman incorporated the Neuman Systems Model Trustees Group. According to George (1995), any changes to the model must have unanimous approval by the trustees unless Neuman herself promulgates the changes.

Assumptions

In the early development of this model, Neuman identified a set of assumptions from which the theory was derived. In 1995, she considered the assumptions to be propositions of the model and renamed them as such. The propositions that Neuman identified as fundamental to the theory are identified in Box 30-2.

Major concepts

"The Neuman Systems Model provides a comprehensive, flexible, holistic, and systems-based perspective for nursing" (Neuman, 1996). The major focus of the NSM is the recognition of stress or stressors and the stressor-induced reaction occurring in the patient system. Major concepts of the theory are derived from this focus. The major concepts of the theory are basic structure, patient variables, lines of resistance, flexible line of defense, normal line of defense, stressors, reconstitution, environment, and prevention.

The *basic structure* is the central core of the patient system (Neuman, 1995). This structure is composed of the system's variables, genetic features, and all the strengths and weaknesses of the particular organism. The central core contains all elements required for survival. A steady state is sought as the system seeks to regulate itself. If too much energy is expended in system regulation, disequilibrium occurs.

While Neuman views patients holistically, there is a recognition of different aspects of a patient. These patient aspects, or *patient variables*, include the physiological, psychological, sociocultural, developmental, and spiritual (Neuman, 1996). The physiological variable represents the functional component of the human body (George, 1995). The psychological variable addresses cognitive process and relationships. The sociocultural variable speaks to social and cultural expectations, while lifespan development constitutes the developmental variable. Spiritual beliefs and their effect on the individual are recognized through the spiritual variable.

Lines of resistance encircle the basic structure's energy resources. This buffer functions as the last line of defense for the organism. The lines of resistance become activated only if the normal line of defense is invaded. Reconstitution can occur only if the lines of resistance are successful

Box 30-2

Neuman's Fundamental Propositions

1. Each patient or patient system is recognized as unique. Given this uniqueness, however, there are commonalties that constitute all patients. These commonalties usually find expression within a usual, identified range of responses possessed by the basic structure.

2. The existence of environmental stressors is recognized. Not all stressors are identified and understood. Stressors may exert their influence singly or in combination. These stressors possess varying capacities to disturb a patient's normal line of defense. The degree to which a patient is guarded by this line of defense depends upon the specific interrelationships of the following patient variables: physiological, psychological, sociocultural, developmental, and spiritual.

3. The normal line of defense is interpreted to be the usual wellness/stability state. This line of defense is constituted by a range of usual responses to the environment. Due to the need to attend to varying stress situations, the line of defense may change over time. Changes in health status can be identified by comparing patient responses to a baseline normal line of defense.

4. The integrity of the usually responsive normal line of defense may be disrupted by an environmental stressor. The nature and extent of the system's response to the stressor is dependent upon the interrelationships among the physiological, psychological, sociocultural, developmental, and spiritual variables.

5. Wellness exists within a range of available energy that sustains the patient system in a peak state of system balance. A patient, regardless of wellness/illness status, is constituted by the interrelationship of physiological, psychological, sociocultural, developmental, and spiritual variables.

6. Each patient or patient system possesses internal resistance factors recognized as lines of resistance. The purpose of the lines of resistance is to return the patient or patient system to an improved level of stability after exposure to an environmental stressor.

7. Primary prevention pertains to the prevention of negative reactions subsequent to patient exposure to environmental stressors through the identification and amelioration of potential or actual risk factors by using accepted knowledge for patient assessment and intervention.

8. Secondary prevention pertains to symptoms subsequent to stressor-induced reactions, prioritization of interventions, and care intended to lessen the negative effects of stressors.

9. Tertiary prevention pertains to the adaptive processes of early reconstitution and the maintenance influences that return a patient to primary prevention efforts.

10. A patient is characterized as a system that is engaged in a fluid, constant exchange of energy with the environment.

Data from Neuman, B. (1995). *The Neuman Systems Model* (3rd ed.). Norwalk, CT: Appleton & Lange.

in fighting off the stressor. The *flexible line of defense* serves as a buffer to protect a patient from illness or environmental stressors (Neuman, 1995). It is conceptualized as the outer boundary of the patient system. The purpose of the flexible line of defense is to expand or contract. The expanded flexible line provides good defense and protection to the normal line of defense. When the flexible line of defense contracts, disequilibrium may occur. Gigliotti (1996) equates the response of the flexible line of defense to Selye's alarm reaction.

The *normal line of defense* is the patient's level of wellness, developed over time. The normal line of defense develops as a result of the patient coping with stressors in the environment (Neuman, 1995). If the flexible line of defense fails, the normal line of defense will be compromised. If the normal line of defense is invaded, illness occurs and the body may not be able to deal with additional stressors (George, 1995).

A *stressor* is described as an environmental force that may cause system instability. Stressors may occur at any time, as a single one-time stressor or as multiple stressors that may be present at any given time. Neuman classifies stressors as intrapersonal, interpersonal, and extrapersonal.

Intrapersonal stressors are experienced within the individual as anger, fear, or anxiety. Interpersonal stressors occur between individuals. Extrapersonal stressors are those stressors that occur outside of the person; an example would be financial pressures. Adaptation to a stressor is called *reconstitution* (Neuman, 1995).

Environment is recognized as forces, internal and external, that surround and influence the patient system, while the realm of activities that promote system balance constitutes *prevention*. Primary prevention is used before the patient system responds to a stressor, and the goals of primary prevention are health promotion and illness prevention. Primary prevention seeks to make the flexible line of defense as strong as possible by prevention of stress and promotion of risk reduction. Intervention occurs as soon as the risk factor is identified, thereby preventing a reaction to the stressor. Wesley (1994) uses the example of a special diet for a breastfeeding mother as a primary prevention intervention. Secondary prevention is used if primary prevention is not possible or is ineffective and symptoms occur. The goal is alleviation of symptoms so that reconstitution may occur. Secondary prevention focuses on strengthening of the internal lines of resistance.

If reconstitution is not possible, death may occur. Tertiary prevention takes place once stabilization of the system occurs during secondary prevention. The goal of the tertiary prevention is to maintain reconstitution, which will eventually return the patient to the primary prevention stage.

Core nursing concepts

Recipient of nursing care. The recipient of nursing care is the patient system, and the patient system can be interpreted to include "individuals, families, groups, communities, and organizations, or collaborative relationships between two or more individuals" (Neuman, 1996). As previously stated, the recipient of nursing care or patient system is composed of core structures consisting of physiological, psychological, sociocultural, developmental, and spiritual variables. The system is dynamic, intent on maintaining health or moving away from illness in varying degrees.

Health. Health is defined by Neuman (1995) as system stability that exists on a continuum from illness to optimal wellness. She describes health as a condition in which the level of wellness is related to the balance that exists within the system. Illness occurs when imbalance within the system occurs. Equilibrium can be returned to the system through the process of reconstitution. If reconstitution does not occur, system resources may become depleted, which could result in death.

Environment. Environment is constituted by all factors that influence the patient system and are influenced by the patient system. The environment exists at different levels: internal, external, and created. These environments surround the patient at any given time (Neuman, 1995). The internal environment is made up of those influences that exist totally within the boundaries of the patient system; it is by nature intrapersonal. Conversely, the external environment is made up of those influences that exist outside the patient system; it is extrapersonal. As exchange occurs between the internal and external environments, a created environment is developed unconsciously by the patient system. The created environment is necessary for the integrity and stability of the system. The objective of the created environment is to promote the health of the patient. If the maintenance of the created environment by the patient system requires too much energy, stressors invade the lines of resistance and illness may occur.

Nursing. Neuman recognizes nursing as a unique profession (1972). The goal of nursing is to assist patients in the attainment of optimal wellness through promotion of patient-system stability. The role of nursing is to prescribe specific actions for patients experiencing or potentially experiencing either situations that are influenced by stressors or stressor-induced reactions.

Systems Model and the advanced practice nurse

The NSM was conceptualized to assist graduate students in their understanding of integrated nursing care; its first use was at UCLA (Neuman & Young, 1972). The NSM was later used to guide an entire baccalaureate program in Pennsylvania (Mirenda, 1995). The model is flexible and broad so that educators can be creative in how they use it to guide curricula (Lowry, Hinton-Walker, & Mirenda, 1995). The model is also organized so that courses can be logically placed. Beynon, Chadwich, Chang, Craig, Fawcett, Frese, Henton-Walker, and Neuman (1997) predict the model will be useful for nursing education into the twenty-first century. They state that, "Nurses who are taught to use NSM will have the requisite competencies to provide holistic, patient centered care that emphasizes wellness for individuals, families and communities in a variety of settings."

Given this history, the NSM offers a sound theoretical framework for those nurses who practice at an advanced level. The model provides APNs with "an opportunity to increase the scope of nursing practice because of its breadth and flexibility, and its focus which is congruent with emerging health care trends" (Neuman, 1996). The model directs attention to holistic patient perspectives, patient perceptions, involvement in health care decisions, and primary prevention.

The NSM is a highly developed nursing model. Like the Roy Adaptation Model, this model offers nursing a framework to view nursing from a systems theory orientation. The model provides a very organized framework to guide nursing practice. For this reason, it contributes significantly to nursing education and nursing practice. To successfully implement it in practice, an APN needs to have a congruent philosophical stance on nursing and a holistic approach to nursing care.

Reed (1993) used Neuman's model as a framework for her research of families. Her first step was to identify how the model was being used with families in the practice settings. She found that the NSM had served as a framework for a public health unit in Canada for over 5 years. At this practice site, Reed was able to identify the issues surrounding the gap between theory and practice. Identified problems included the difficulty in translating abstract concepts from the model into concrete terms. After meeting with Neuman and others, more flexible and expanded definitions of the family were developed. Each of the five Neuman variables (physiological, spiritual, developmental, psychological, and sociocultural) were conceptualized so that each area could be clearly identified for patients, and each variable served as an organizational structure for gathering data. Nurses with the clinic felt that the new assessment data were much more thorough, based on the clarified definitions. The nurses could clearly see how the model could be used to assist in identifying lines of defense for families.

Newman's Health as Expanding Consciousness Theory

Before Margaret Newman entered nursing, she witnessed a powerful and profound experience of health. Her mother was coping with the challenge of physical debilitation due to amyotrophic lateral sclerosis. During the time she cared for her mother, Newman came to realize that health was not something that was separate from her mother; in fact, the experience of illness was a part of health for her mother, creating a unique patterning in her life (Newman, 1986). Newman perceived that health was more than and different from its accepted definition, which at that time was "the absence of disease." The idea of health puzzled Newman, and she chose to enter nursing to find some meaning in the concepts and reality of health and disease (Newman, 1997a).

Newman came to believe that health can be found even within illness. She proposed that there is no dichotomy in which health is separated from illness and no continuum that places health (a disease-free state) on one end and illness on the other (Newman, 1986). Disease, for Newman, is simply a manifestation of health. Health and disease are not separate, so one must not be valued over the other. The potential for growth and consciousness evolution is present throughout and may coexist with pathology. Health can be seen as a process and pattern in the holistic view of health.

Newman (1997a) wrote that her theory evolved out of the awareness that every person, no matter how debilitated or diseased, is engaged in a process of uncovering meaning and interconnectedness with others. She pointed to evidence that people in life-threatening crises often describe characteristics of higher consciousness. It is her belief that the concept of pattern recognition has profound implications for both practice and research. This theory offers nurses a perspective for practicing both within the context of expansion and growth of others and within the context of personal growth.

Early work

Newman began preliminary work on her theory while in graduate school at New York University, where she was initially a student and later a colleague of Martha Rogers. Newman reported that the Theory of Health as Expanding Consciousness grew out of the Rogerian view of nursing science (Newman, 1997a). She cited the broad range of both philosophical and scientific literature upon which Rogers based her theory. Newman's own work evolved from the thoughts of a similar group of scientists and philosophers. Newman described the evolution of her theory: "My long-time compelling interest in the meaning of illness and my nursing practice with partially immobilized persons brought about the study of movement, time and space, and eventually consciousness, as parameters of health" (Newman, 1997a).

Newman first presented her theory of health in 1978 and first published work on the theory in 1979. Since then, she has continued to prolifically describe and expand her work over a 20-year period, demonstrating how expanding consciousness can be found in theory evolution itself. In her more recent work, she underscores the relevance of her theory for clinical practice by noting that nursing's commitment is to the care of the whole person and not merely the treatment of pathology (Newman, 1997b).

Newman's work was heavily influenced by Martha Rogers, but she was also inspired by philosophers such as Theilhard de Chardin and scientists such as physicist David Bohm and mathematician Arthur Young. She built on Young's theory of human evolution and his mechanism for movement from potential to real freedom. Newman was able to apply this process to her ideas about expanding consciousness, writing that the beginning of potential consciousness moves through time and space, to infinite space and timelessness, and on to absolute consciousness (Newman, 1986).

Assumptions

In her 1979 work, Newman described the assumptions underlying her theory.

1. Health encompasses conditions heretofore described as *illness* or (in medical terms) *pathology*.
2. These pathological conditions can be considered a manifestation of the total pattern of the individual.
3. The pattern of the individual that eventually manifests itself as pathology is primary and exists before structural or functional changes.
4. Removal of the pathology in itself will not change the pattern of the individual.
5. If becoming "ill" is the only way an individual's pattern can manifest itself, then that is health for that person.
6. Health is the expansion of consciousness.

Over time, additional assumptions have been identified. These assumptions follow directly from work by Rogers. First, human beings are open energy systems interconnected with and inseparable from the environment. Second, humans are continuously evolving, and this evolution presents a pattern that is unique for every individual person. The last assumption is that humans are not merely thinking and feeling beings; they possess an intuitive capacity as well. Newman wrote that there is no real difference between mind and matter; they are both manifestations of energy. The difference between the two manifestations (that humans can recognize) is related to the speed and intensity of the energy's movement, with mind energy making rapidly moving waves and matter energy reflecting waves that are lower and slower (Newman, 1994a, 1994b).

Newman has stated that these assumptions reflect works by Martha Rogers on ideas of wholeness and patterns, as well as work by Itzhak Bentov. Bentov depicts life as an ongoing process of consciousness expansion (Newman, 1997a). Additional credit is given to Bohm's (1980) theory of implicate order, Prigogine's (1976) theory of dissipative structures, and Young's (1976) theory of consciousness evolution. Newman makes it clear that her theory has been enriched by the work of these individuals but was not based on it. Rather, it emerged from the science of unitary beings (Newman, 1997a).

Major concepts

The major concepts of the theory evidence its derivation from the work of Martha Rogers, though Newman offers a unique definition of consciousness. Newman defines *consciousness* as "information of the system . . . the capacity of the system to interact with the environment" (Newman, 1994a, 1994b). Consciousness is the essence of all matter; it is not something possessed or not possessed by a specific person—all people are consciousness. Understanding this definition is a necessary step in understanding Newman's theory of nursing.

When one typically thinks of consciousness, sensations, thoughts, and feelings come to mind, but Newman's definition casts a much wider net than this. For Newman, consciousness subsumes the entire informational capacity of the human—all information processed by a person. This includes the information capacity of all bodily systems—the endocrine and neurological systems, the immune system and the entire human genome (Newman, 1994a, 1994b).

The concepts presented by Newman in her 1979 work describe the interrelationship of consciousness, movement, space, and time. Reemergence of these concepts in later writings (Newman, 1999) demonstrates the power of the evolving pattern of the theory itself. Major assumptions of the theory have been expanded to include the following:

1. Time and space have a complementary relationship.
2. Movement is a means by which space and time become a reality.
3. Movement is a reflection of consciousness.
4. Time is a function of movement.
5. Time is a measure of consciousness.

The concept of pattern is also pivotal. Newman views the total pattern of person in interaction with environment as a network of consciousness. Pattern recognition provides the APN with important information that can depict what is going on with the whole (Newman, 1994a, 1994b). For Newman, consciousness is much more that the ability

to maintain alertness and orientation. Seeing consciousness as information capacity makes these concepts somewhat more tangible (Newman, 1986).

Newman (1986) writes about the potential of absolute consciousness and notes that it has an ability to organize itself and possesses an order that is implicit. She sees the human potential to evolve to a higher consciousness as consistent with Rogers' work on the movement of living systems to increasing complexity. Newman proposes the evolution of consciousness as the process of health. She states, "The human being comes from a state of potential consciousness into the world of determinate matter and has the capacity for understanding that will enable him or her to gain insight regarding his/her pattern."

Illness, then, is a reflection of the person-environment interaction. The ultimate step in the evolutionary progression is attainment of absolute consciousness, which Newman says has been equated with love. This is a state where all is accepted and there is no dichotomy of good and bad, pain and pleasure, disease and nondisease.

Core nursing concepts

Recipient of nursing care. Newman uses the terms *person* or *patient* to identify the recipient of care. She sees people as dynamic patterns of energy—open systems in constant connection with the environment. There is no separation of person and consciousness; they are one. In addition, Newman asserts that humans are not separate individuals with isolated diseases. Humans are in constant interaction with each other. Though a pattern that evidences disease affects one individual, those effects are not limited to that person; the pattern affects that person's family and the community (Newman, 1994a, 1994b).

People are seen as centers of consciousness with patterns of energy and an overriding pattern of expanding consciousness. One can not isolate a single person because each life is a part of a continually widening whole. An individual's pattern interacts in mutuality with the pattern of the family and the immediate environment. This pattern then widens to include the community, work, and school. The interactions of each of these growing patterns ultimately merge into a world pattern, or pattern of the whole, which Newman sees as the phenomenon of nursing's practice (Newman, 1994a, 1994b).

Health. Health is the expansion of consciousness and is expressed as an evolving pattern. It includes both disease and nondisease in a movement toward synthesis. Newman presents a problem associated with this way of articulating what health is: if health includes disease, it is problematic when one says that nurses engage in health promotion. Newman recognizes that her view of health, which includes disease, is fairly radical because it negates the idea that health and disease are on opposite ends of a continuum or that dichotomy exists between them. To increase understanding of this concept, Newman describes this view of health as a fusion of opposites and relates it to work by Hegel on the dialectical fusion of opposites. "One point of view fuses with the opposite point of view and brings forth a new, synthesized view. In this case, DISEASE fuses with its opposite, the absence of disease, NON-DISEASE, and brings forth a new concept of HEALTH" (Newman, 1994a). This is a way of envisioning a health that includes disease. Newman asserts that people have difficulty with this concept in part because people are conditioned through language and culture to see fragments rather than the whole. Viewing reality as fragmented makes it more difficult for people to abandon the dichotomous view of health as something separate from disease (Newman, 1997). APNs can use this information when working with patients who have chronic illness; a good example is hypertension. While the patient certainly has a chronic illness, many times the patient does not know he or she has a problem until sequelae of the disease process occur. Even when the patient is aware of the disease, most patients would not describe themselves as having a chronic illness, especially if the hypertension is well controlled. To approach the patient with controlled hypertension as an "ill" person would not be using Newman's model as it is described.

Environment. Environment is linked to the person in a person-environment dyad. Newman included both near and far environment in her conceptualization of health. Additionally, health is recognized as a pattern of person-environment interaction that acknowledges the importance of family and society. Newman wrote:

> When we begin to think of ourselves as centers of energy within an overall pattern of expanding consciousness, we can begin to see that what we sense of our lives is part of a much larger whole. First the pattern of consciousness that is the person interacts within the pattern of the consciousness that is the family and physical surroundings and within the pattern that is the person's larger environmental affiliation, such as work or school, and then within the pattern of the local community, and continuing on within the pattern of the universe. (Newman, 1986)

The environment is made up of open systems extending throughout the universe. Disability that results in physical restriction can lead to expanding consciousness because it reframes a person's assumptions about movement, space, and time. Newman (1986) reports research discussing the way circadian rhythms affect the sleep-wake cycle, temperature regulation, and productivity. One study she describes found a lessening of depression when intensive care unit (ICU) patients were allowed to control their environments by requesting procedures or visitors at certain times and arranging the cards in their rooms.

Nursing. Nursing's task is to assist people in their movement toward expansion of consciousness. The ability to see the pattern within a frame of movement, space, and time is essential. The nurse enters a person's pattern in a way of rhythmic connection that may allow clarity of the pattern to develop. There is a partnership between the nurse and the patient, which Newman describes as *nonintervention.*

The professional enters into a partnership with the patient with a mutual goal of participating in an authentic relationship, trusting that in the process of its evolution, both will grow and become healthier in the sense of higher levels of consciousness (Newman, 1986). The nurse must not control the situation, but he or she must function in a true spirit of mutuality with the patient, sharing in the discovery and expansion of patterning. Health is a process, and the nurse can facilitate that process but must not try to control it. Newman described a holographic model of intervention to support the understanding of mutual and simultaneous interaction that is described in Martha Rogers' work. This model depicts interpersonal interactions as the merging of patterns of energy into the pattern of the whole. This is helpful because it eliminates the separation of the person performing the intervention and the person receiving it. Newman writes, "It precludes an instrumental approach of action-reaction or observer-observed and emphasizes the sensing into the whole of one's own (interactive) pattern in order to 'see' the pattern of the other. It recognizes the unity of the pattern" (Newman, 1997a).

In describing the dominant paradigms of nursing science, Newman refers to her earlier writings that depict the focus of nursing as "caring in the human health experience." Newman believed at the time that this purpose was beyond the constriction of individual worldviews (Newman, 1997b). However, she later clarified that it is essential that nursing move away from any paradigm that includes a power differential between the nurse and the recipient of care. She urges a movement toward a view of "reflective, compassionate consciousness" (Newman, 1997b) with no elements of control involved.

In a description of the integrative model of nursing practice, Newman (1994a) outlines the responsibilities of the nurse. These responsibilities begin with the development of a primary relationship with a patient. The purpose of this relationship is to ascertain the person's health care needs and support the patient's decisions and actions. Newman sees the professional nurse's role as that of nursing clinician/case manager (1994a) and has supported the professional doctorate as the appropriate preparation for this role. Two other roles for nurses are included in her new paradigm—a staff role that comes mainly from a medical paradigm and a team leader/liaison role that integrates the other roles and coordinates a program of care for each patient (Newman, 1994). Her writings on these two additional roles evolved from a discussion of the effect of cost-containment on the ability to provide nursing care. The APN role can subsume the other roles identified by Newman. In many ways, an APN does serve as a case manager to facilitate patient movement through the health care system. The leadership role is also evident as the APN coordinates the plan of care for each patient.

Health as Expanding Consciousness Theory and the advanced practice nurse

The creative conceptualization of the theory of Health as Expanded Consciousness offers nursing a broader view of phenomena related to nursing theory, practice, and research, and this expanded view allows for more creativity. Health is conceptualized in a manner that allows for the recognition and further development of concepts not previously attended to by nursing. These new concepts may lead to new research questions to be tested. Nursing practice is informed uniquely by this theory in that it offers nurses another way to view their relationships with patients and to enter into such relationships. This theory's attention to the phenomena of movement, time, space, freedom, and consciousness also allows a nurse to see a patient's experience in a different light. This different way of seeing may lead to different ways of interacting with patients and their families. Practice within this theory is driven by mutuality of interaction (with no power differential), discovery of the unique pattern of each person, and movement of that person through life processes toward the development of higher consciousness. Newman's work demonstrates commitment to practice. She has written that nursing is both dynamic and relational but cannot be understood without being experienced. When one looks at nursing, one must look at the process from the inside. This theory applies not only to a person who comes into the health care system with a particular pathology, it also includes the patterning of all who are engaged in that person's care and environment. APNs should approach patients as open and responsible beings; this means working with a patient (for example) who chooses to diet, exercise, and use stress reduction as a way to approach an elevated blood pressure.

Yamashita, Jensen, and Tall (1998) describe how a nurse may incorporate principles from Newman's theoretical approach into practice. In their scenario, a 29-year-old patient has had an automobile accident and is suffering from severe pain in her neck, shoulder, and arm, as well as having migraines for the first time in her life. The patient describes herself as being unfocused since the injury. The nurse scans the patient's energy field and finds thick congestion over her right neck, shoulder, and arm. The nurse then uses therapeutic touch to address the areas of congestion and the patient's lack of balance. The patient indicates that the therapeutic touch is helpful and after 18 sessions, feels much more like she did before the accident. As part of the process the nurse teaches the patient how to address areas of pain by herself. In this example, by using

Newman's perspective the nurse recognized the changed energy pattern and helped move it to one of a higher level of consciousness.

Another important aspect of Newman's theory for APNs is the patient-APN relationship. An APN must be fully "present" with a patient; this means focusing fully on the patient in an act of unconditional love and compassion. This perspective certainly adds a different facet to how a patient might normally be approached by a primary care provider (PCP).

Newman (1994a, 1994b) suggests that the prevailing scientific paradigm in nursing today is one that combines the holistic view with the objectivity and predictability of a post-positivist philosophy. This is probably an accurate description of the need to objectively address patient outcomes but also include the nature of the human experience and the interactions that take place along the way. It behooves APNs to acknowledge the subjectivity, multidimensionality, and context-dependent nature of patients within each encounter. Newman believes that her theory is not external to APNs but is lived by them and manifested in practice. APNs must be transformed by the theory and become transforming partners in interactions with patients (Newman, 1994a, 1994b). Implications for Master of Science in Nursing (MSN) education include the opportunity to learn about the theory and its application to APN practice; this means presenting a variety of theories and allowing students to pick theories that "call" to them—the ones that might fit with their philosophical perspectives and approaches.

Paterson and Zderad's Humanistic Nursing Theory

When the Humanistic Nursing Theory was first formally presented, its uniqueness resided in its existential phenomenological orientation. This orientation was derived from the phenomenological orientation of Josephine Paterson and Loretta Zderad. By looking at nursing through this philosophical orientation, they provided subsequent theorists a new way to conceptualize nursing.

Influenced by their respective nursing backgrounds and their study of the existential works of Husserl, Marcel, and Buber, Paterson and Zderad began to formulate their Humanistic Nursing Theory in the early 1950s. Their original purpose in examining the phenomenon of nursing was not so much an attempt to develop formal nursing theory as it was a collaborative effort to answer questions related to nursing as it was experienced by themselves and other practicing nurses. Paterson described this work as a "long-sought haven" (1978).

Paterson's professional experience included work as a public health nurse and mental health consultant for New York, Massachusetts, and Maryland. Zderad worked as a psychiatric staff nurse and clinical instructor in Illinois. Both were interested in the experiences and feelings of nurses and patients as they interacted with each other. Independently, they began to utilize a phenomenological orientation to explore and research nursing as they perceived it. In the 1970s, both held faculty positions at Catholic University and at Ohio State University. It was during this time that they met and began to share their beliefs and research interests related to the phenomenon of nursing. As a result of this sharing of ideas and beliefs, their Humanistic Nursing Theory was conceptualized. In 1976, the theory was published in their book *Humanistic Nursing*, which was rereleased in 1988. Their legacy—phenomenological nursology—provides a mechanism for concept and theory development within nursing (Paterson & Zderad, 1988).

Assumptions

The assumptions that underpin this theory are primarily of a philosophical nature. They are derived from the nursing experiences of Paterson and Zderad and their study of phenomenology, existential philosophy, and humanistic psychology. Scholars such as Marcel, Buber, Bergson, de Chardin, Frankl, Jung, and Hesse are referenced throughout *Humanistic Nursing*. Box 30-3 outlines the assumptions found in their work.

Major concepts

The phenomenon of interest for Paterson and Zderad was the lived experience of human interaction in nursing situations. Nursing situations are human encounters shared by nurses and patients as human beings. The major concepts of the theory are derived from this particular focus, and a significant number of concepts have been identified within the work.

A *nurse* is a human being that hears and responds to the call of patients in need of assistance relative to the health-illness aspect of their existence. The nurse frames a response from the belief that patients possess the possibility for well-being and more-being. A *patient* is a human being incarnate who presents as a person in need of help related to the health-illness aspect of life.

A mode of being with other human beings in which humans are open, available, and knowable to each other is called *intersubjective relating*. Another human being is recognized as a human being and a subject, not an object. *Well-being* is a potential way of existing related to the patient's health-illness quality of life that draws from that which is both probable and sought by the patient and nurse. *More-being* is a potential way of existing related to the patient's health-illness quality of life that draws from that which is possible and viewed by the patient and the nurse as highly desirable. Other concepts identified by Meleis (1991) are listed in Box 30-4.

Core nursing concepts

Recipient of nursing care. While the recipient of nursing care is never explicitly defined, the recipient is identified as a patient and human being, a human in need of help. Within Paterson and Zderad's work, it is recognized that humans are unique beings marked by the singularity of their own situated existence and their capacity to make choices. Humans possess an awareness of self and others. This awareness sends out a call for humans to strive for a sense of authenticity with others. Humans, along their fellow humans, struggle to live, confirm their existence, and come to an understanding of the meaning of their existence.

Health. Paterson and Zderad do not provide an explicit definition of health; however, one can make inferences about their concept of health from their writings. Paterson and Zderad (1988) describe the contemporary view of

---

Box 30-3

Assumptions Underlying Paterson and Zderad's Humanistic Nursing Theory

1. Each human being is unique.
2. Human beings are total biopsychosocial beings and possess the capacity for more being through intersubjectivity and exercising choices.
3. Human beings possess an inherent drive to know their angular worldviews and the angular worldviews of others.
4. Lived experiences of the moment are influenced by the past, present, and future and are constituted by more than these temporal elements.
5. Encounters between human beings have the potential to be open and significant and characterized by great intimacy. Participants of these encounters may be profoundly influenced by these human situations.
6. Humans beings exist as free beings and make decisions and participate in matters relating to their own care.
7. Nurses and patients are human beings who coexist independently and interdependently.
8. Nursing requires two human beings willing to establish and participate in an existential relationship with each other.
9. The nature or quality of life and/or the experience of death are influenced by nursing acts.
10. Nurses must recognize and acknowledge the intrinsic confusion of human existence and the inherent human need to respond as if poised, controlled, and joyful.

Data from Meleis, A. (1991). *Theoretical nursing: development and progress* (2nd ed.). Philadelphia: JB Lippincott.

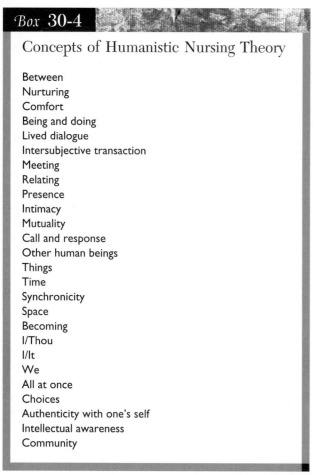

From Meleis, A. (1991). *Theoretical nursing: development and progress* (2nd ed.). Philadelphia: JB Lippincott.

health as "the absence of disease" as narrow. They view health as that which is necessary for human survival. Consistent with the theory's existential orientation, health is proposed to be a process of well-being and striving for more well-being. Paterson and Zderad recognize health as the major focus of nursing.

Environment. The environment is constituted by two spheres or worlds: the inner world of the patient and/or nurse and the objective world. The outer world is identified as the *real world*. The real world consists of humans and things existing in time and space (Paterson & Zderad, 1988); time and space are aspects of a world. Time is viewed not only as measured time but also as time lived or experienced by humans. Space is conceptualized as both a physical setting or space that can be measured and a space that is lived or experienced by humans. Humans are able to affect this world and are conversely affected by it. Through experiencing this real world, humans are able to create their own inner world. This inner world is named the *angular world*. The angular world is a reality unique to each person and is described as biased and shaded.

Nursing. Nursing exists as a discipline whose practitioners hear the purposeful call of humans in need of help and respond to this call to assist patients to a state of well-being and more-being. This help is delimited to health-illness situations and is provided through lived dialogue. Lived dialogue requires a meeting of patient and nurse; relating; and presence. The nurse contributes his or her whole self to the nursing situation. According to Paterson and Zderad (1998), "This involves a living out of the nurturing, intersubjective transaction with all of one's human capacities."

Paterson and Zderad (1988) set humanistic nursing as a goal to be achieved by nurses. Humanistic nursing can help a nurse come to know self, family, and community and achieve self-actualization. Humanistic nursing is "a major value shaping one's nursing practice."

Humanistic Nursing Theory and the advanced practice nurse

Many APNs provide care in a setting that calls for repeated encounters with patients over time. This type of contact requires the establishment of an ongoing relationship between the APN and patient, and this theory offers a framework in which to view that relationship. The theory identifies the elements of the relationship and ways to relate to the patient so as to establish, develop, and maintain the relationship. As such, this theory is significant for the practice of APNs.

Humanistic nursing calls for APNs to be aware of each person's uniqueness, as well as their commonality with others. For example, Lisa, an APN who has hypertension, has found it helpful to share with her patients how it has been for her since she was diagnosed with hypertension and the steps she has taken to address the disease process. Sharing this story with her patients is not to say "do as I did," but to say "I also have a problem, so we have that in common." Humanistic nursing also means that APNs present all choices to patients and discuss the pros and cons of each. The ability of a patient to make choices based on awareness and knowledge of such choices is a concern of humanistic nursing according to Chin and Kramer (1995). An APN who is able to offer these types of choices and interactions to his or her patients offers genuine presence to patients. It is an acknowledgment by the APN that the patient is in need. Minicucci (1998) extends the notion of the nurse's presence not only to individuals but to families as well. Many times when a patient is depressed, it involves not only the patient, but also interaction between the patient and his or her family system.

Humanistic theory could be very useful when APNs are working with patients who are suffering depression or other mental health issues. In many practices, these patients make up a third or more of the patient base, and the notion of an APN's use of self may play an important role in working with them. Paterson and Zderad (1976) discourage nurses from viewing patients as diagnoses or cases.

Roy's Adaptation Model

In 1964, as a graduate student, Sister Callista Roy was challenged by her mentor, Dorothy E. Johnson, to develop a conceptual model for nursing (Andrews & Roy, 1986). Adaptation theorists who influenced the development of Roy's model include Helson, Dohrenwend, Lazarus, Mechanic, and Selye. Additional influences include Bertalanffy's general systems theory, Rapoport's theory of systems, and Maslow's theory of human needs (Lutjens, 1991). Roy has described her model as primarily a systems model that contains interactionist levels of analysis (Riehl & Roy, 1980) and a focus on outcomes (Lutjens, 1991). Since its initial conception, the Roy Adaptation Model has continued to undergo dynamic evolution.

Assumptions

The Roy Adaptation Model was derived from scientific and philosophical assumptions, with the eight scientific assumptions based on systems and adaptation theory (Roy, 1980). (These original assumptions are listed in Box 30-5.) The eight assumptions were updated in 1999 to ensure applicability in the twenty-first century and are as follows:

1. Systems of matter and energy progress to higher levels of complex self-organization.
2. Consciousness and meaning are constitutive of the integration of person and environment.
3. Awareness of self and environment is rooted in thinking and feeling.
4. Human decisions are accountable for the integration of creative processes.
5. Thinking and feeling mediate human action.
6. System relationships include acceptance, protection, and fostering of interdependence.
7. Persons and the earth have common patterns and integral relationships.
8. Person and environment transformations are created in human consciousness. Integration of human and environment meanings result in adaptation. (Roy, 1999)

Eight philosophical assumptions also underpin the Roy Adaptation Model (Roy, 1988). Four of these assumptions are based on the principle of humanism and four are based on a principle developed by Roy called *veritivity*.

Roy (1988) states that humanism recognizes the person and subjective dimensions of human experience as central to knowing and valuing. Maslow's ideas influenced Roy's view of humanism. The four assumptions based on the principle of humanism are:

1. The individual shares in creative power.
2. The individual behaves purposefully, not in a sequence of cause and effect.
3. The individual possesses intrinsic holism.
4. The individual strives to maintain integrity and to realize the need for relationships.

Box 30-5

Underlying Assumptions of Roy's Adaptation Model

1. A person is a biopsychosocial being.
2. A person is in constant interaction with a changing environment.
3. To cope with a changing world, a person uses both innate and acquired mechanisms that are biological, psychological, and social in nature.
4. Health and illness are one inevitable dimension of life.
5. To respond positively to environmental changes, a person must adapt.
6. A person's adaptation is a function of the stimulus one is exposed to and one's adaptation level.
7. A person's adaptation level is such that it comprises a zone that indicates the range of stimulation that will lead to a positive response.
8. A person is conceptualized as having four modes of adaptation: physiological, self-concept, role function, and interdependence.

Roy developed the principle of veritivity. This term is derived from the Latin word *veritas*, which means *truth*. Veritivity has been defined as a principle of human nature that affirms a common purposefulness of human existence (Roy, 1988). In the adaptive person, veritivity reflects activity, creativity, unity, purpose, and value (Roy, 1987). Roy (1988) expressed a belief that there is an absolute truth. The philosophical assumptions underlying this principle include:

1. The individual is viewed in the context of purposefulness of human existence.
2. There exists unity of purpose of humankind.
3. There exist activity and creativity for the common good.
4. There is value and meaning to life.

Roy has also adapted the philosophical assumptions for the model to be more congruent with the twenty-first century. Her revised philosophical assumptions are:

1. Persons have mutual relationships with the world and with a god figure.
2. Human meaning is rooted in an omega point convergence with the universe.
3. God is intimately revealed in the diversity of creation and is the common destiny of creation.
4. Persons use human creative abilities of awareness, enlightenment, and faith.
5. Persons are accountable for the processes of deriving, sustaining, and transforming the universe. (Roy, 1997)

Major concepts

Adaptation is the core concept of Roy's model. Adaptation can be viewed as a process or as a product or outcome. The process aspect of adaptation involves positive responses by individuals to changes in the environment. Individuals, as adaptive systems, are viewed as possessing the ability to adjust effectively to changes in the environment and, conversely, to affect the environment itself (Andrews & Roy, 1991). The individual's coping mechanisms or adaptive modes can facilitate or hinder the process of adaptation. Adaptation, as an outcome, is the end-state of the adaptation process and has been defined by Roy as the condition of the person with respect to the environment (Roy, 1990). A person's *adaptation level* is the extent to which the individual is able to react, in a positive manner, to changes in the environment. This level, described as fluid and constantly changing, is influenced by an individual's internal resources. An individual's adaptation level is made up of focal, contextual, and residual stimuli (Andrews & Roy, 1991; Lutjens, 1991). An individual can change his or her adaptation level by learning effective coping strategies. A newer definition of adaptation is proposed by Roy (1999) for accountability for the future; in this new definition, *adaptation* is defined as "the process and outcome whereby the thinking and feeling person uses conscious awareness and choice to create human and environmental integration."

Coping refers to routine or accustomed patterns of behavior employed to deal with daily situations, as well as the development of new behaviors when drastic changes challenge familiar responses (Roy & McLeod, 1981). A coping mechanism is defined as an innate or acquired way of responding to the changing environment (Andrews & Roy, 1991). Roy proposed the existence of two forms of coping—the regulator and cognator subsystems of coping mechanisms. *Regulator coping mechanisms* are useful primarily when coping with physiological stimuli. The regulator subsystem works primarily through the autonomic nervous system to organize a reflex action that prepares an individual to respond and adapt to the environment (Meleis, 1991). Through neural, chemical, and endocrine processes, regulator mechanisms respond automatically to stimuli from the internal and external environment. The regulator coping mechanisms also play a role in the formation of perception (Andrews & Roy, 1986).

Cognator coping mechanisms are brought into action to cope with psychosocial stimuli (Roy, 1984). The cognator subsystem identifies, stores, and relates stimuli so that a symbolic meaning can be attached to the behavior (Meleis, 1991). Cognator coping responses occur through four cognitive-emotive channels: perceptual/information processing, learning, judgment, and emotion. The perceptual/information processing channel includes selective attention, coding, and memory. The learning channel involves imitation, reinforcement, and insight. The judgment channel includes problem-solving and decision-making, while the emotion channel includes seeking relief from anxiety and making affective appraisals and attachments (Andrews & Roy, 1986). Failure of either the regulator or cognator subsystems can result in maladaptation (Roy, 1984).

The four *adaptive modes* of the model were developed in response to the need for a method to organize assessment data. Roy defines the adaptive modes as ways of coping that show the activity of the regulator and cognator systems (Andrews & Roy, 1986). The four adaptive modes identified by Roy are physiological, self-concept, role function, and interdependence.

The *physiological adaptive mode* is associated with the way a person's physical body responds to environmental stimuli. Andrews and Roy (1991) identify five primary needs for physiological integrity: oxygen, nutrition, elimination, activity/rest, and protection. Regulator coping mechanisms are primarily accountable for the maintenance of physiological integrity. Examples of regulator mechanisms include fluid and electrolyte balance and neurological and endocrine system functions. An example of the physiological adaptive mode is when a patient who has chronic pulmonary obstructive disease plans a day's activities based on how well he or she is breathing. Activities occur, but they are spaced so that breathing is not compromised.

Self-concept, role function, and interdependence are psychosocial adaptive modes. The self-concept mode is concerned with psychological and spiritual aspects of a person. Underlying this mode is the basic human need for psychic integrity, defined as the need to know who one is so that one may exist with a sense of unity (Andrews & Roy, 1986; Roy & Andrews, 1991). Self-concept has been defined as the composite of beliefs and feelings one has about oneself at a given time (Andrews & Roy, 1986). Two areas form the self-concept: the physical self, including body sensation and body image, and the personal self, made up of self-consistency, self ideal, and moral-ethical-spiritual self (Andrews & Roy, 1991). For example, Malia is an 18-year-old girl who has had self-concept problems for a number of years. She does not think she is worthy of the love or affection her family gives her. This low self-concept affects her when she makes decisions and choices about activities. Because she does not care much for herself, the choices she makes are not in her best interest, such as being sexually promiscuous, lying, and stealing. Treatment for Malia can not be effective until the issue of her poor self-concept is resolved. This means that antidepressants, while helping with the symptoms of depression, will not address the underlying problem. A treatment that can affect Malia's inner core will need to be undertaken.

Role function and interdependence modes focus on the roles of an individual in society. The role function mode focuses on the basic human need for social integrity. *Social integrity* is defined as knowing who one is in relation to others. Roles are sets of expectations about how a person in a particular position behaves toward others in different positions (Andrews & Roy, 1986). Instrumental and expressive behaviors are associated with each role. Instrumental behaviors are generally physical and long term in nature, while expressive behaviors are usually emotional (Lutjens, 1991).

The interdependence mode centers on the need of affectional adequacy or the feeling of security in nurturing relationships (Andrews & Roy, 1986). Relationships consistent with this mode include significant others, or persons of the highest importance to an individual, and support systems, or continuing social collectives such a groups, organizations, or networks (Lutjens, 1991). Andrews and Roy (1986) describe two major areas of behavior associated with the interdependence mode. *Receptive behaviors* include receiving, taking-in, and assimilating nurturing behaviors offered by others. *Contributive behaviors* are the behaviors of an individual that give or supply nurturing to significant others or one's support systems (Lutjens, 1991). In the case of Malia, the self-concept mode also affects her interdependence mode; she is not able to have effective and giving relationships with her family or other teenage peers.

Adaptive responses are those behaviors that promote the integrity of a person and contribute to the person's general goals (e.g., survival, growth, reproduction, mastery). Adaptive responses result in the end-state of adaptation. Behaviors that do not contribute to personal integrity or the goals of adaptation are called *ineffective responses* (Andrews & Roy, 1986).

Core nursing concepts

Recipient of nursing care. The recipient of nursing care may be an individual, a family, a group, a community, or society as a whole. The basis for any family, group, community, or society is the individual (Andrews & Roy, 1986). For this reason, discussions of the Roy Adaptation Model primarily focus on the person and concepts related to one-on-one relationships with nursing. Roy views the person as a holistic adaptive system. Systems are described as sets of parts connected to function as a whole for some purpose; each system functions by virtue of the interdependence of its parts (Andrews & Roy, 1986).

In this model a person is an active participant who interacts with the environment and formulates adaptive responses, which contribute to the goals of survival, growth, reproduction, and mastery (Lutjens, 1991). Growth involves the physiological, cognitive, psychological, emotional, and spiritual aspects of the individual. Reproduction is not limited to child-bearing, but encompasses *generativity*, or "bringing forth" by a variety of human activities, such as creating works of art (Lutjens, 1991).

Health. Health is a state, as well as a process of becoming an integrated and whole person (Andrews & Roy, 1991). Health has further been described as a reflection of the interaction of the person with the environment, also called the adaptation process. Health is evidenced by adaptation within each of the four adaptive modes. The integration of these modes is viewed as a reflection of an individual's wholeness. Lack of integration results in lack of health (Roy, 1984). Within the process of health, individuals strive to achieve their maximum potential (Lutjens, 1991). The process of health is applicable to both healthy people and people who are ill. Individuals who are healthy may eat well-balanced diets, exercise, lose weight, and not smoke. Individuals who are ill may seek to control their symptoms and integrate their relationships with significant others (Lutjens, 1991).

Environment. Environment encompasses all conditions, circumstances, and influences that surround and affect the development and behavior of a person (Andrews & Roy, 1991). Environmental changes stimulate individuals to make adaptive changes. All internal and external stimuli are instrumental in forming a person's environment. Stimuli are classified into three types: focal, contextual, and residual. Focal stimuli are immediate, provoking situations or events confronting a person, demanding attention, and prompting one to seek relief (Lutjens, 1991). Focal stimuli, mediated by contextual and residual factors, are also called *stressors*. A stressor has also been defined as a demand for an adaptive response (Roy & McLeod, 1981).

Contextual stimuli include all other stimuli present and identified as influencing the current situation (Andrews & Roy, 1986). Residual stimuli may influence the adaptation level, but their effect has not been confirmed (Andrews & Roy, 1986). Residual stimuli are general, vague, ambiguous factors. A residual stimulus whose influence is confirmed becomes either a focal or contextual stimulus (Lutjens, 1991). Focal, contextual, and residual stimuli may all be external or internal factors. Roy's model allows for a change in the stimulus's classification depending on the setting. Factors considered to be focal stimuli in one situation may be considered contextual stimuli in another setting (Andrews & Roy, 1986). Of importance to nursing is understanding which factors are influencing any given situation and determining how a person perceives and responds to the influencing stimuli (Lutjens, 1991).

Nursing. Nursing is seen as a science and as the application of knowledge from nursing science to nursing practice (Andrews & Roy, 1986). One goal of nursing is to promote adaptation in each of the four modes, thereby contributing to a person's health, quality of life, and dying with dignity (Andrews & Roy, 1991). When a person is in an adaptive state, he or she is free to respond to other stimuli (Lutjens, 1991). Another goal of nursing is to decrease ineffective responses. Nursing is needed when the adaptive system of a person confronts unusual stresses or when weakened coping mechanisms cause the person's usual attempts at coping to become ineffective (Chinn & Kramer, 1991; Meleis, 1991).

The nursing process describes nursing activities within

the Roy Adaptation Model. The six steps in the nursing process include: assessment of behavior, assessment of stimuli, nursing diagnosis, goal setting, intervention, and evaluation (Mastal & Hammond, 1980; Lutjens, 1991). There are two levels of assessment within the nursing process. The first level is assessment of behavior within the four adaptive modes. The second level centers on identification of focal, contextual, and residual stimuli influencing behaviors. Based on the nurse's interpretation of assessment information, nursing diagnoses are chosen. Nursing diagnoses reflect the nurse's clinical judgment about a person's adaptation status. The formulation of goals must be mutually agreed on by the person and the nurse (Lutjens, 1991). Nursing interventions involve the management of stimuli by altering, increasing, decreasing, removing, or maintaining focal, contextual, or residual stimuli (Andrews & Roy, 1991). During the evaluation phase of the nursing process, the nurse determines whether or not planned interventions have been successful in meeting established goals (Andrews & Roy, 1986). An example of patient assessment with urinary incontinence is described in Jirovec, Jenkins, Isenberg, and Baiardi (1999), and Figure 30-1 shows the model of urine control that is substructed from Roy's Adaptation Model. It indicates the concepts of focal, contextual, and residual stimuli and identifies coping mechanisms and adaptive modes, and it

can serve as a way to evaluate a patient with urinary continence difficulties.

Adaptation Model and the advanced practice nurse
The Roy Adaptation Model is one of the most highly developed nursing models. It offers a framework to view nursing from a systems theory orientation. This model also offers nurses a very organized framework to guide nursing practice and has been widely used both in practice and in education. For example, Brower and Baker (1976) describe the model as used in a geriatric nurse practitioner (GNP) program. The four adaptive modes serve as the organizing focus for the program, and the authors note that the framework is helpful for students to make the conceptual differentiation of advanced (nursing) practice from medical practice. Camooso, Greene, and Reilly (1981) also describe how Roy's model was used to guide their journey as graduate students in an adaptive mode.

Weiss, Hastings, Holly, and Craig (1994) used a qualitative research methodology to determine the utility of Roy's model in practice. The researchers found that the model was useful in focusing, organizing, and directing nurses' thoughts and actions regarding patient care. There appeared to be four levels of integration of theory into practice. Conscious integration included those nurses who incorporated identifiable components into their care. One

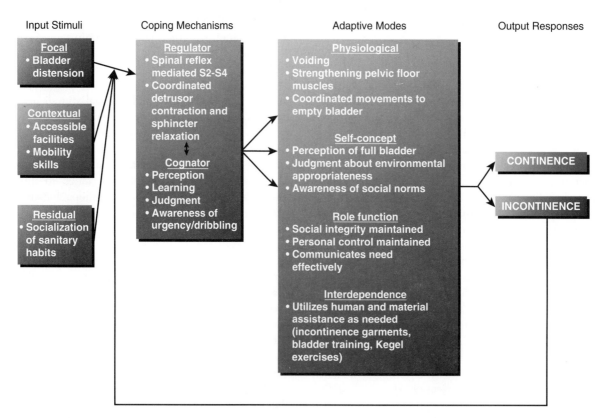

Figure 30-1 Conceptual model of urine control substructed from Roy's Adaptation Model. (From Jerovec, M., Jenkins, J., Isenberg, M, & Barardi, J. [1999]. Urine control theory derived from Roy's conceptual framework. *Nursing Science Quarterly, 12*[3]: 251-255. Reprinted by permission of Sage Publications, Inc.)

nurse described her patient assessment: "I look at their interdependence. Where are they at? Who's going to be there for them? Are they looking to go back to work? What is their role function?" A second level of integration was unconscious integration. These nurses used the model concepts but did not specifically relate them to the framework. Directed integration was the third level of integration and seemed to revolve mainly around documentation and care planning. This was directed because the documentation forms provided structure in performing assessment and creating plans of care. The last level of integration was the lack of integration. These subjects felt the model was not a way of thinking—it was only related to the paperwork they filled out. In general, the integration into practice was more the integration of theory concepts than use of the language of the model. Those who learned about the model in their nursing program were more likely to integrate the framework into care. Most nurses felt the framework was of benefit to nurses and patients. It helped them provide comprehensive, holistic care. Disadvantages to using the model included the possibility of limiting critical thinking (i.e., just doing rote thinking) and the theoretical nature of the language; some nurses felt it was confusing and not relevant to the actual care of patients. Of the subjects, 17 out of 20 felt that continued use of the model was in the best interest of nurses and patients.

When using the updated definition of adaptation, Roy (1999) identifies the role of nursing as accepting, protecting, and fostering integral relationships of persons and environment. This newer definition has introduced the notion of social accountability into play; Roy feels this increases the utility of the theory for nursing application.

PRIORITIES FOR RESEARCH

Once one has become familiar with several nursing theorists or chosen one on which to base a practice, it is important to use the theory in practice and begin collecting data on how effective the framework is to guide the practice. This leads to the ultimate goal for APNs: optimizing the health status of patients. This section presents research implications for the five theories discussed in this chapter.

Orem's Self-Care Deficit Theory of Nursing

Orem's SCDTN has been used as the framework for practice and research at the Aging Health Care Institute in Washington (Evans, 1983). Numerous studies have also been conducted using the theory as the framework for study (see References/Bibliography at the end of the chapter for some of these). This extensive use verifies that the theory has premises that are useable in the clinical area and testable through research. Concepts that are embedded in Orem's theory include motivation, decision-making, energy, and the knowledge necessary to carry out self-care

actions to maintain health and well-being. These concepts seem very applicable to advanced practice. Another area ripe for research includes the notion of self-concept and its relationship with self-care agency. Smits and Kee (1992) found a correlation between self-concept and self-care agency, but no significant differences in self-care agency when compared to age, income, gender, or employment status. Dodd and Dibble (1993) found that the basic conditioning factors of support, education, and anxiety were significantly correlated with self-care agency scores. Studies by Hart (1995) revealed that multiparous women had lower self-care agency scores than primiparous women, perhaps indicating that women who already have children have less ability to provide self-care during pregnancy. All of the basic conditioning factors have been researched, but with mixed results. Orem (1995) points out that "different basic conditioning factors influence self-care agency at different times."

Neuman Systems Model

Because of its organized framework, the NSM serves as an excellent model for nursing research. Research based on this model would involve inquiry into the influence of stressors on the various patient systems' lines of defense and how nursing may use various levels of preventative interventions. A survey done by Louis and Koertvelyessy (1989) revealed that the NSM is one of the three most frequently used conceptual models of nursing for research, and it continues to be used often today. According to Neuman, as of 1997, 150 Neuman-based studies had been published. International use is increasing, as is the utility of NSM interdisciplinary research.

One purpose of the NSM is to predict the effects of primary, secondary, and tertiary interventions on patient stability. Another purpose is to determine the cost, benefit, and utility of prevention interventions. These areas are critical for APNs to research because in effect they support the notion of the APN role. Neuman has identified rules related to research with this model (Box 30-6).

Research based on Neuman's model has generally followed the rules for research. The research includes qualitative to quantitative studies and has addressed such patient issues as substance use by men and women with traumatic spinal cord injuries; the incidence of seat belts; and the health needs of the homeless. Studies have been descriptive, correlational, and experimental. Neuman believes that the research is sensitive to social political trends such as health care reform, primary prevention, and rural health care (Neuman, 1996). Research instruments have been identified to assist with assessment based on the Neuman model (Quayhagen & Roth, 1989).

APNs can use the NSM to approach patient care by focusing on lines of prevention. Research related to primary prevention is particularly timely and important. Gigliotti (1999) evaluated role stress in women. She found

Box 30-6

Research Rules for the Neuman Systems Model

- Phenomena to be studied include the following: physiological, psychological, sociocultural, developmental, and spiritual variables; properties of the central core of the patient system; properties of flexible and normal lines of defense; characteristics of the environment; and elements of primary, secondary, and tertiary prevention interventions.
- Problems to be studied are those that deal with patient system stability. Research will advance understanding of the influence of prevention on stressors and patient system stability.
- Subjects can be individuals, groups, communities, and organizations. Data can be collected in inpatient, ambulatory care, home, and community settings.
- One needs an appropriate research base for both inductive and deductive research using either qualitative or quantitative designs. Data-analysis techniques associated with both qualitative and quantitative research designs are appropriate.

Data from Neuman, B. (1996). The Neuman systems model in research and practice. *Nursing Science Quarterly, 9*(2), 67-70.

women who were both mothers and students to be at higher risk for experiencing multiple role stress, because these role behaviors are opposed. A sample of 191 women who were mothers and students participated, and the data revealed that interaction between two of the variables—psychological and sociocultural—invaded the normal line of defense only in the presence of increasing age (the developmental variable). Gigliotti notes that the research was complex due to the complexity of the variables, but significant differences were found based on the interaction of these variables. Practice implications from this study include the notion of stressors for women with multiple roles, especially if they are older than 37 years. This might mean that APNs need to talk with patients about ways to decrease stress (e.g., time management, relaxation techniques, exercise). Knowing the potential for increased stress and the invasion of the normal lines of defense for women with multiple roles probably has implications even for the majority of APNs themselves.

Newman's Health as Expanding Consciousness Theory

Newman offers three tenets based on her theory that can guide research into the phenomena of real concern to nursing. These tenets can also guide theory-based practice.

The tenets are mutuality of interaction between nurse and patient, uniqueness and wholeness of pattern in each patient situation, and movement of the life process toward higher consciousness (Newman, 1997b). These tenets may serve as areas for future investigation. Yamashita, Jensen, and Tall (1998) believe that therapeutic touch could be a means to facilitate the establishment of authentic relationships, linking APNs' and patients' energy fields.

Published research applying the theory has addressed diverse populations including women with ovarian and breast cancer (Moch, 1990; Endo, 1998), homosexual men with human immunodeficiency virus (HIV) (Kendall, 1996), adults with chronic lung disease (Jonsdottir, 1998) or coronary artery disease (Newman & Moch, 1991), adolescents with insulin-dependent diabetes mellitus (Schlotzhauer & Farnham, 1997), and people with terminal illness (Fryback, 1993).

All experiences are considered meaningful by Newman. This means the data a patient has to share is rich with meaning from the patient's perspective. Given this approach, Newman's hermeneutic dialectic method and hermeneutic phenomenology are methodologies that might be used more often with Newman's theory. These approaches focus on understanding from a patient's perspective and examine how events take on historical, social, and cultural meaning within a patient's life; they are also more true to the theory. The researcher using these methods must be open to new perspectives and can not impose a predetermined view on a patient's experience. In-depth interviewing invites patients to share their experiences.

Jonsdottir (1998) used these methods to describe the experiences of 10 people with chronic obstructive pulmonary disease. When the patients described their experiences, a number of themes emerged—a sense of resignation to the situation as a way to survive, difficulties in expressing oneself and relating to others, and difficulties with breathing and activity restrictions. Life patterns were described as isolated and closed in. Jonsdottir explains the meaning of these patterns as the patients working hard to maintain as stable and unchanging a life situation as possible given the health limitations. Even sharing the information in the interviews was difficult for the patients. In such situations, APNs need to be nonjudgmental and respecting of people's experiences. This also may mean accepting the unpredictability of patients' lives. Each situation can serve as a stimulus to realize a fuller sense of self.

Moch (1990) evaluated the patterns experienced by women after they had been diagnosed with breast cancer. The women identified that, after diagnosis, they were more attuned to their own needs and more aware of the caring actions of the people around them. In general, the women felt more appreciative and connected to life than before the diagnosis. In Newman's terms, these interactions can be taken as evidence of expanding consciousness.

Paterson and Zderad's Humanistic Nursing Theory

Humanistic nursing has been researched in a more limited way than most of the broad or grand nursing theories. Research specifically looking at the nursing presence has been very limited, yet those studies that have been done have supported the presence of the nurse as a powerful force for effecting change with patients, families, and communities (Wilson, 1986; Pettigrew, 1988; Fuller, 1991; Mohnkem, 1992). More recently, Lubchuk, (1996) used humanistic care as a basis of her research with two patients suffering from cancer. The role of the nurse as a "carer", entering into a relationship with the person for whom he or she cares, was examined. This experience helped the author become aware of existential experiences of herself and the patient.

Stubblefield and Murray (1999) looked at parents' perceptions and expectations of health care providers who were involved with their children's lung transplant experiences. A phenomenological approach was used to interview 15 parents. The parents identified two types of care: concerned care and collaborative care. Components of concerned care included being treated as an individual, seeing familiar faces, feeling that their children really mattered, and/or (conversely) feeling abandoned. Collaborative care reflected the parents' views of being part of the team and at the same time feeling caught in the middle. The authors identified the needs that parents have for continuity of care. Humanistic nursing was used as the link between the study results and nursing practice. Stubblefield and Murray (1998) also used humanistic nursing as a means to explore what it was like to live with children who had undergone a lung transplant. Parents identified the lung transplant as a way to create hope for their child, a way to create normalcy, and a way to develop a new perspective on life.

Several instruments have been developed to assist in research related to humanistic nursing. O'Connor, (1989) used the Humanistic Nursing Behaviors (HNB) Scale to look at service in nursing and patient satisfaction. The HNB Scale evaluates group norms about interactions with patients. O'Connor also used the LaMonica-Oberst Patient Satisfaction Scale (LOPSS), Rathus Assertiveness Schedule (RAS) and the Barrett-Lennard Relationship Inventory (BLRI) to look at patients' satisfaction and relationship with nursing. The nurse-patient relationship was shown to be important. A number of design issues related to the HNB Scale and RAS questionnaires emerged and need further investigation.

Another research instrument developed based on the conceptualization of humanistic nursing is the Measurement of Presence Scale (MOPS) (Hines, 1991). The scale was developed based on attributes that related to the essential structure of presence. These attributes were then further defined through systematic theory analysis and

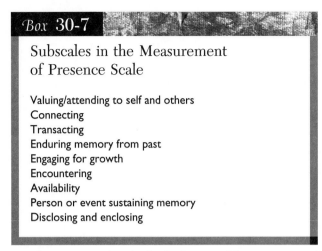

Box 30-7

Subscales in the Measurement of Presence Scale

Valuing/attending to self and others
Connecting
Transacting
Enduring memory from past
Engaging for growth
Encountering
Availability
Person or event sustaining memory
Disclosing and enclosing

Data from Hines, D. (1991). *The development of the measurement of presence scale* (Unpublished doctoral disseration UMI PUZ9203067). Dallas, TX: Texas Women's University.

construction. The instrument was tested to determine psychometrical properties, including content validity, internal consistency (cronbach alpha .932), and subscales with correlation coefficients all greater than .6. Factor analysis indicated that there were nine subscales (identified in Box 30-7). Hines recommends that further testing occur on the MOPS. APNs might find that using MOPS is helpful in practice because it may give a sense of how patients perceive an APN to be present within the APN-patient encounter.

Future research related to humanistic nursing needs to be conducted, especially in relation to advanced practice. APNs' use of presence in stimulating healing of patients may reveal important concepts about the role of APNs in providing care.

Roy's Adaptation Model

Because of its organized framework, Roy's model serves as an excellent framework for nursing research. Research focuses on persons or groups adapting and on the adaptive processes that affect health status (Roy, 1987). Research based on this model should involve inquiry into basic life processes and how nursing enhances these processes (Roy, 1987). Basic research should focus on investigation of human life processes, with emphasis on adaptation, which occurs when a person interacts with the environment (Fawcett & Tulman, 1990). This model is appropriate for use with both qualitative and quantitative research designs. Examples of nursing research with Roy's Adaptation Model as a theoretical background have included studies of changes in functional status after childbirth (Tulman & Fawcett, 1990), human-pet interactions and loneliness (Morrison, 1989), women with coronary heart disease

(Varvaro, 1990), urine incontinence (Jirovec et al, 1999), Mexican American family processes (Niska, 1999), pain research (Calvillo & Flaskerud, 1993), coping processes of widows (Robinson, 1995), chronic illness (Pollock, 1993), and the nursing perspective (Weiss, Hastings, Holly, & Craig, 1994), to name but a few. By 1995, Roy had well over 187 research studies recorded (Roy, 1999). (Table 29-2 provides a more thorough listing of research instruments and clinical tools using Roy's Adaptation Model.)

Krouse and Krouse (1999) used Roy's adaptation framework to guide their study of complementary therapeutic practices in patients with chronic sinusitis. Many of the patients (81%) used physical exercise to relieve symptoms, while herbal therapy was used 32% of the time. Other modalities included acupuncture, chiropractic therapy, biofeedback, and chelation therapy. Nurse practitioners (NPs) may want to incorporate effective complementary therapies into their care of patients with chronic sinusitis, and pediatric nurse practitioners (PNPs) have used Roy's adaptation framework to help adolescents adapt to asthma.

Levesque, Ricard, Ducharme, Duquette, and Bonin (1998) have developed a program of research evaluating the tenets of Roy's model. They are specifically trying to understand a person's adaptation to various environmental stimuli and the nursing interventions that promote adaptation. Pollock (1993) found in her research with patients with diabetes, multiple sclerosis, rheumatoid arthritis, and hypertension that hardiness, an ability to tolerate stress, and health promotion activities were positively correlated with physiological and psychosocial adaptation. There also did not appear to be any differences among the groups; this may mean that while each chronic illness has specific issues, the process of psychosocial adaptation is similar. An important variable in determining a person's ability to adapt is his or her perception of the disability caused by the illness. For APNs, it is unrealistic in most chronic illnesses to alter the disease process, so emphasis is on altering the contextual stimuli. Pollock (1993) notes that for a person with low hardiness, it may be important to address educational and health resources to promote adaptation. If hardiness can be learned, then patients with chronic illnesses are prime candidates to learn how to adapt and maximize quality of life. Continued research can focus on the effectiveness of nursing interventions in promoting adaptive responses.

IMPLICATIONS FOR MSN EDUCATION AND ADVANCED PRACTICE

As the twenty-first century begins, Silva (1999) challenges nurses to answer two questions: What is the present state of nursing science? What does one envision as the future of nursing science? To consider these questions it is

necessary to look at several things. Many APNs look at the grand nursing theories developed in the 1950s and find them meaningless and irrelevant. However, it was these theories that served to move nursing away from the medical model and into ways of knowing nursing that are more congruent with nursing values and phenomena. Other APNs would be just as happy if all nursing theory was deleted or eliminated because it does not "speak to them." Silva (1999) posits that it is more critical than ever to be able to understand and articulate the theoretical basis of nursing. Rutty (1998) agrees and recommends that for nurses to successfully work in the interdisciplinary teams of the twenty-first century, the convoluted and difficult language in existing nursing theories needs to be simplified.

What is nursing and nursing science? These questions have been raised numerous times, and most nurses would be hard pressed to give a cogent response. Silva (1999) believes a more appropriate and telling question to ask is, "How should nursing science be defined?" Silva proposes that APNs (and all nurses) "let go." "Letting go" refers to giving up some aspect of nursing science and moving on to another aspect when the timing seems right. Letting go means looking at the degree of investment and commitment to a nursing science goal, determining what is timely and cutting edge, and looking at the related disciplines in a similar manner. Nursing can not be isolated. Silva's discussion challenges APNs to raise questions about nursing science and the APN's role within that science. Professional practice is "logic in use; moving between the patient data base and the abstracted information of research and theory to hypothesize ways in which problems are solved and goals are achieved" (Rawnsley, 1999).

DISCUSSION QUESTIONS

These questions can be used to promote critical thinking and encourage discussion.

1. Determine which one of the theories described in this chapter best matches your current practice. Identify which elements or aspects of this theory are most consistent with your practice and explain.
2. Select one nursing theory or model that you believe has the most to offer the future of the discipline in the areas of practice, research, and theory. Identify and share arguments that support your position.
3. Do you think broad or grand theories are useful in advanced practice? Why or why not? How do they compare with the midrange theories (see Ch. 31) in application and research?
4. What other nursing theories are appropriate for use in advanced practice? How would you envision incorporating them into your practice?

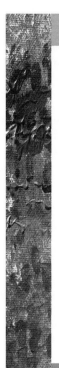

Suggestions for Further Learning

- Get the article: Baumann, S.L. (1998). Nursing: the missing ingredient in nurse practitioner education. *Nursing Science Quarterly 11*(3), 89-90. Identify the major premise of the article. Do you agree with Baumann's position? Do you believe his position is shared by the majority of APNs? What significance does this position hold for APNs and the discipline of nursing?
- Visit these websites for various nursing theorists and examine the information presented:
  - Dorthea Orem (www.muhealth.org/~nursing/scdnt/scdnt.html)
  - Margaret Newman (www.tc.umn.edu/~hoym0003/index.html)
  - Betty Neuman (www.neumann.edu/nursing/NSM Home.htm)
  - Callista Roy (www.bc.edu/bc_org/avp/son/theorist/nurse-theorist.html)
- To further research the NSM, read Gigliotti, E. (1997). Use of Neuman's lines of defense and resistance in nursing research: conceptual and empirical considerations. *Nursing Science Quarterly, 10*(3), 136-142.
- Get the article: McQuiston, C., & Campbell, J. (1997). Theoretical substruction: a guide for theory testing research. *Nursing Science Quarterly, 10*(3), 117-123.
- Go to this generic nursing theory website for information on a number of nursing theories: www.wholenurse.com/Student_Nurse/Nsg-theory.shtml.
- Get the article: McKinnon, N. (1991). Humanistic nursing: it can't stand up to scrutiny. *Nursing and Health Care, 12*(8), 414-416. What is your response to this article? Do you agree or disagree?
- Get the following article: Glazer, S. (2000, Summer). *Post modern nursing.* Available online at www.thepublicinterest.com/. Glazer presents rather scathing comments about therapeutic touch and nursing theorists. She also argues that nursing needs the objective view of scientific research. What are your views after reading this article? How would you support or refuse to support the use of therapeutic touch and other less scientific treatments?

REFERENCES/BIBLIOGRAPHY

Aish AE, & Isenberg M. (1996). Effects of Orem-based nursing intervention on nutritional self-care of myocardial infarction patients. *International Journal of Nursing Studies, 33,* 259-270.

Allison, S. (1973). A framework for nursing action in a nurse conducted diabetic management clinic. *Journal of Nursing Administration, 3*(4), 53-60.

Allison, S.E., & Renpenning K. (1999). *Nursing administration in the 21st century: a self-care theory approach.* Thousand Oaks, CA: Sage.

Anderson, J.A., & Olnhausen, K.S. (1999). Adolescent self-esteem: a foundational disposition. *Nursing Science Quarterly, 12,* 62-67.

Andrews, H., & Roy, C. (1986). *Essentials of the Roy Adaptation Model.* Norwalk, CT: Appleton-Century-Crofts.

Andrews, H., & Roy, C. (1991). Essentials of the Roy Adaptation Model. In C. Roy & H. Andrews (Eds.), *The Roy Adaptation Model: the definitive statement.* Norwalk CT: Appleton-Century-Crofts.

Anna, D., Christensen, D., Hohon, S., Ord, L., & Wells, S. (1978). Implementing Orem's conceptual framework. *Journal of Nursing Adminstration, 8*(11), 8-11.

Backsheider, J. (1974). Self care requirements, self care capabilities and nursing systems in the diabetic nurse management clinic. *American Journal of Public Health, 64,* 1138-1146.

Baker, S. (1998). The relationships of self-care agency and self-care to caregiver strain as perceived by female family caregivers of elderly parents. *Journal of the New York State Nurses Association, 28,* 7-11.

Banfield, B.E. (1997). *A philosophical inquiry of Orem's self-care deficit nursing theory* (Unpublished doctoral dissertation). Ann Arbor, MI: Wayne State University.

Baumann, S.L. (1998). Nursing: The missing ingredient in nurse practitioner education. *Nursing Science Quarterly, 11*(3), 89-90.

Beach E.K., Smith A., Luthringer L., Utz S.K., Ahrens S., & Whitmire V. (1996). Self-care limitations of persons after myocardial infarction. *Applied Nursing Research, 9,* 24-28.

Beynon, C., Chadwich, P., Chang, N., Craig, D., Fawcett, J., Frese, B., Henton-Walker, B, & Neuman, B. (1997). The Neuman Systems Model: reflections and projections. *Nursing Science Quarterly 10*(1), 18-21.

Bohm, D. (1980). *Wholeness and the implicate order.* London: Routledge & Kegan Paul.

Brouse, S.H., & Laffrey, S.C. (1989). Paterson and Zderad's humanistic nursing framework. In J. Fitzpatrick & A. Whall (Eds.), *Conceptual models of nursing: analysis and application* (2nd ed.) (pp. 205-225). Norwalk, CT: Appleton and Lange.

Brower, H., & Baker, B. (1976). Using the adaptation model in a practitioner curriculum. *Nursing Outlook, 24,* 686-689.

Calvillo, E., & Flaskerud, J. (1993). The adequacy and scope of Roy's Adaptation Model to guide cross cultural pain research. *Nursing Science Quarterly, 6*(3), 118-129.

Camooso, C., Greene, M., & Reilly, P. (1981). Students' adaptation according to Roy. *Nursing Outlook, 29,* 108-109.

Chinn, P., & Kramer, M. (1991). *Theory and nursing: a systematic approach* (3rd ed.). St. Louis: Mosby.

Chin, P., & Kramer, M. (1995). *Theory and nursing: a systematic approach* (4th ed.). St. Louis: Mosby.

Conner-Warren, R. (1996). Pain intensity and home pain management of children with sickle cell disease. *Issues in Comprehensive Pediatric Nursing, 19,* 183-195.

Crews, J. (1972). Nurse managed cardiac clinics. *Cardiovascular Nursing, 8,* 15-18.

Crockett, M. (1982). Self reported coping histories of adult psychiatric and non-psychiatric subjects and controls. *Nursing Research, 31,* 122.

Dashiff, C. (1992). Self care capabilities in black girls in anticipation of menarche. *Health Care for Women International, 13,* 67-76.

Denyes, M. (1982). Measurement of self care agency in adolescents. *Nursing Research, 31,* 63.

Dodd, M., & Dibble, S. (1993). Predictors of self care: a test of Orem's model. *Oncology Nursing Forum, 20*(6), 895-901.

Drew, F., Craig, D., & Beynon, C. (1989). The Neuman Systems Model for community health administration and practice: provinces of Manitoba and Ontario, Canada. In B. Neuman (Ed.), *The Neuman Systems Model* (2nd ed.) (pp. 315-341). Norwalk, CT: Appleton and Lange.

Ducharme, F., Ricard, N., Dugquette, A., Levesque, L., & Lanchance, L. (1998). Empirical testing of a longitudinal model derived from the Roy Adaptation Model. *Nursing Science Quarterly, 11*(4), 149-159.

Endo, E. (1998). Pattern recognition as a nursing intervention with Japanese women with ovarian cancer. *Advances in Nursing Science, 20*(4), 49-61.

Fawcett, J. (1989). *Analysis and evaluation of conceptual models of nursing* (2nd ed.). Philadelphia: FA Davis.

Fawcett, J. (1995a). *Analysis and evaluation of conceptual models of nursing* (3rd ed.). Philadelphia: FA Davis.

Fawcett, J. (1995b). Constructing conceptual-theoretical-empirical structures for research: future implications for use of the Neuman systems model. In B. Neuman (Ed.), *The Neuman Systems Model* (3rd ed.) (pp. 459-471). Norwalk, CT: Appleton and Lange.

Fawcett, J., & Tulman, L. (1990). Building a program of research from the Roy Adaptation Model of nursing. *Journal of Advanced Nursing, 15,* 720-725.

Fawdry M.K., Berry M.L., & Rajacich D. (1996). The articulation of nursing systems with dependent care systems of intergenerational caregivers. *Nursing Science Quarterly, 9,* 22-26.

Fitzpatrick, J., & Whall, A. (1989). *Conceptual models of nursing: analysis and application* (2nd ed.). Norwalk, CT: Appleton and Lange.

Fryback, P.B. (1993). Health for people with terminal diagnosis. *Nursing Science Quarterly, 6*(3), 147-159.

Fuller, J. (1991). *A conceptualization of presence as a nursing phenomenon* (Unpublished doctoral dissertation). Salt Lake City, UT: University of Utah.

Gaffney, K., & Moore, J. (1996). Testing Orem's theory of self-care deficit: dependent care agent performance for children. *Nursing Science Quarterly, 9*(4), 160-164.

Geden E., & Taylor S.G. (1991). Construct and empirical validity of the self-as-carer inventory. *Nursing Research, 40,* 47-50.

Geden E.A., & Taylor S.G. (1999). Theoretical and empirical description of adult couples' collaborative self-care systems. *Nursing Science Quarterly, 12,* 329-334.

George, J. (1995). *Nursing theories: the base for professional nursing practice.* Norwalk, CT: Appleton & Lange.

Gigliotti, E. (1997). Use of Neuman's lines of defense and resistance in nursing research: conceptual and empirical considerations. *Nursing Science Quarterly, 10*(3), 136-142.

Gigliotti, E. (1999). Women's multiple role stress: testing Neuman's flexible line of defense. *Nursing Science Quarterly, 12*(1), 36-44.

Hagopian, G.A. (1996). The effects of informational audiotapes on knowledge and self-care behaviors of patients undergoing radiation therapy. *Oncology Nursing Forum, 23,* 697-700.

Harper, B. (1984). Application of Orem's theoretical construct to self care medication behaviors in the elderly. *Advances in Nursing. 2,* 29-46.

Hart, M. (1995). Orem's self care deficit theory: research with pregnant women. *Nursing Science Quarterly, 8*(3), 120-126.

Hart M.A., & Foster, H.N. (1998). Self-care agency in two groups of pregnant women. *Nursing Science Quarterly, 11,* 167-171.

Helson, H. (1964). *Adaptation level theory.* New York: Harper & Row.

Hinds, P., & Young, K. (1987). A triangulation of methods and paradigms to study nurse given wellness care. *Nursing Research, 36,* 195-198.

Hines, D. (1991). *The development of the measurement of presence scale* (Unpublished doctoral dissertation UMI PUZ9203067). Dallas, TX: Texas Women's University.

Hiromoto B.M., & Dungan J. (1991). Contract learning for self-care activities: a protocol study among chemotherapy outpatients. *Cancer Nursing, 14,* 148-154.

Horn, B., & Swain, M. (1977). *Development of criterion measures of nursing care.* Springfield, VA: National Center for Health Services Research, National Technical Information Service.

Jaarsma T., Halfens R., Senten M., Abu Saad H.H., & Dracup K. (1998). Developing a supportive-educative program for patients with advanced heart failure within Orem's general theory of nursing. *Nursing Science Quarterly, 11,* 79-85.

Jasper, M. (1994). Issues in phenomenology for researchers of nursing. *Journal of Advanced Nursing, 19,* 309-314.

Jirovec, M., Jenkins, J., Isenberg, M., & Baiardi, J. (1999). Urine control theory derived from Roy's conceptual framework. *Nursing Science Quarterly, 12*(3), 251-255.

Jonsdottir, H. (1998). Life patterns of people with chronic obstructive pulmonary disease: Isolation and being closed in. *Nursing Science Quarterly, 11*(4), 160-166.

Kearney, B., & Fleischer, B. (1979). Development of an instrument to measure exercise of self care agency. *Research in Nursing and Health, 2,* 25-34.

Kendall, J. (1996). Human association as a factor influencing wellness in homosexual men with immunodeficency virus disease. *Applied Nursing Research, 9*(4), 195-203.

Krouse, H., & Krouse, J. (1999). Complementary therapeutic practices in patients with sinusitis. *Clinical Excellence for Nurse Practitioners, 3*(6), 346-352.

Lancaster, D., & Whall, A. (1989). The Neuman Systems Model. In J.J. Fitzpatrick & A. Whall (Eds.), *Conceptual models Of nursing: analysis and application* (2nd ed.) (pp.255-269). Norwalk, CT: Appleton and Lange.

Levesque, L., Ricard, N., Ducharme, F., Duquette, A., & Bonin, J. (1998). Empirical verification of a theoretical model derived from the Roy Adaptation Model: findings from five studies. *Nursing Science Quarterly, 11*(1), 31-39.

Lile, J., & Hoffman, R. (1991). Medication taking by the frail elderly in two ethnic groups. *Nursing Forum, 26*(4), 9-24.

Lobchuk, M. (1996). Humanistic nursing: discussing nursing with myself. *Pflege, 9*(2), 120-126.

Louis, M. (1995). The Neuman model in nursing research: an update. In B. Neuman (Ed.), *The Neuman Systems Model* (3rd ed. pp. 473-495). Norwalk, CT: Appleton and Lange.

Louis, M., & Koertvelyessy, A. (1989). The Neuman Model in research. In B. Neuman (Ed.), *The Neuman Systems Model* (2nd ed.) (pp. 93-114). Norwalk, CT: Appleton and Lange.

Lowry, L., & Anderson, B. (1993). Neuman's framework and ventilator dependency: a pilot study. *Nursing Science Quarterly, 6*(4), 195-200.

Lowry, L., Hinton-Walker, P., & Mirenda, R. (1995). Through the looking glass back to the future. In B. Neuman (Ed.), *The Neuman Systems Model* (3rd ed.) (pp. 64-65). Norwalk, CT: Appleton and Lange.

Lutjens, L. (1991). *Callista Roy: An adaptation model*. Thousand Oaks, CA: Sage.

Mapanga, K., & Andrews, C. (1995). The influence of family and friends' basic conditioning factors and self care agency on unmarried teenage primiparas' engagement in contraceptive practice. *Journal of Community Health Nursing, 12*(2), 89-100.

Marchione, J.M. (1993). *Margaret Newman: health as expanding consciousness*. Thousand Oaks, CA: Sage.

Mastal, M., & Hammond, H. (1980). Analysis and expansion of the Roy Adaptation Model: A contribution to holistic nursing. *Advances in Nursing Science, 2*(4), 71-81.

McCaleb, A., & Edgil, A. (1994). Self concept and self care practices of health adolescents. *Journal of Pediatric Nursing, 9*(4), 233-238.

McDermott, M. (1993). Learned helplessness as an interacting variable with self care agency: testing as a theoretical model. *Nursing Science Quarterly, 6*(1), 28-38.

McKinnon, N. (1991). Humanistic nursing: it can't stand up to scrutiny. *Nursing and Health Care, 12*(8), 414-416.

Meleis, A. (1991). *Theoretical nursing: development and progress* (2nd ed.). Philadelphia: JB Lippincott.

Meleis, A., Lipson, J., & Paul, S. (1992). Ethnicity and health among five middle eastern immigrant groups. *Nursing Research, 41*(2), 98-103.

Minicucci, D (1998). A review and synthesis of the literature: the use of presence in the nursing care of families. *Journal of the New York State Nurses Association, 29*(3/4), 9-15.

Mirenda, R. (1995). *A conceptual theoretical strategy for curriculum development in baccalaureate nursing programs* (Unpublished doctoral dissertation). Chester, PA: Widener University.

Moch, S. (1990). Health within the experiences of breast cancer. *Journal of Advanced Nursing, 15*, 1426-1435.

Mohnkem, S. (1992). *Presence in nursing: its antecedents, defining attributes, and consequences* (Unpublished doctoral dissertation). Austin, TX: University of Texas at Austin.

Moore, J., & Pichler, V. (2000). Measurement of Orem's basic conditioning factors: a review of published research. *Nursing Science Quarterly, 13*(2), 137-142.

Morrison, M. (1989). Human-pet interaction and loneliness: a test of concepts from Roy's adaptation model. *Nursing Science Quarterly, 2*, 194-202.

Mosher R.B., & Moore J.B. (1998). The relationship of self-concept and self-care in children with cancer. *Nursing Science Quarterly, 11*, 116-122.

Mullin, V. (1980). Implementing the self care concept in the acute care setting. *Nursing Clinics of North America, 15*, 177-190.

Neuman, B. (1995). *The Neuman Systems Model* (3rd ed.). Norwalk, CT: Appleton & Lange.

Neuman, B. (1996). The Neuman systems model in research and practice. *Nursing Science Quarterly, 9*(2), 67-70.

Neuman, B. (1997). The Neuman Systems Model: reflections and projections. *Nursing Science Quarterly, 10*(1), 18-21.

Neuman, B., & Young, R. (1972). A model for teaching total person approach to patient problems. *Nursing Research, 21*, 264-269.

Newman, M.A. (1979). *Theory development in nursing*. Philadelphia: FA Davis.

Newman, M.A. (1986). *Health as expanding consciousness*. St. Louis: Mosby.

Newman, M.A. (1994a). *Health as expanding consciousness* (2nd ed.). New York: National League for Nursing Press.

Newman, M.A. (1994b). Theory for nursing practice. *Nursing Science Quarterly, 7*(4): 153-157.

Newman, M.A. (1997a). Evolution of the theory of health as expanding consciousness. *Nursing Science Quarterly, 10*(1), 22-25.

Newman, M.A. (1997b). Experiencing the whole. *Advances in Nursing Science, 20*(1), 34-39.

Newman, M.A., & Moch, S.D. (1991). Life patterns of persons with coronary heart disease. *Nursing Science Quarterly, 4*(4), 161-167.

Nicoll, L. (1986). *Perspectives on nursing theory*. Boston: Little, Brown, and Company.

Niska, K. (1999). Mexican American family processes: nurturing, support and socialization. *Nursing Science Quarterly, 12*(2), 138-142.

O'Connor, P. (1989). *Service in nursing: correlates of patient satisfaction* (Unpublished doctoral disseratation UMI PUZ9002681). Cleveland, OH: Case Western Reserve.

Orem, D.E. (1991). *Nursing: concepts of practice* (4th ed.). St. Louis: Mosby.

Orem, D.E. (1995). *Nursing: concepts of practice* (5th ed.). St. Louis: Mosby.

Orem, D.E. (1996). The world of the nurse. *The International Orem Society Newsletter, 3*(1), 1-6.

Orem, D.E. (1997). Views of human beings specific to nursing. *Nursing Science Quarterly, 10*(1), 26-31.

Orem, D.E., & Vardiman, E. (1995). Orem's nursing theory and positive mental health: practical considerations. *Nursing Science Quarterly, 8*(4), 165-174.

Paterson J.G. (1978). The tortuous way toward nursing theory. In National League for Nursing, *Publication theory development: what, why, how?* New York: National League for Nursing.

Paterson J., & Zderad, L. (1988). *Humanistic nursing*. New York: National League for Nursing.

Pettigrew, J. (1988). *A phenomenological study of the nurse-presence with person experiencing suffering* (Unpublished doctoral dissertation). Dallas, TX: Texas Women's University.

Pollock, S. (1993). Adaptation to chronic illness: a program of research for testing nursing theory. *Nursing Science Quarterly, 6*(2), 86-92.

Pollock, S., Frederickson, K., Carson, M., Massey, V., & Roy, C. (1994). Contribution to nursing science: synthesis of findings from adaptation model research. *Scholarly Inquiry for Nursing Practice, 8*, 361-372.

Praeger, S.G. (1995). Josephine E. Paterson & Loretta T. Zderad. In J.B. George (Ed.), *Nursing theories for professional nursing practice* (pp.301-315). Norwalk, CT: Appleton and Lange.

Prigogine, I. (1976). Order through fluctuation: self-organization and social system. In E. Jantsch & C.H. Waddington (Eds.), *Evolution and consciousness* (pp. 93-133). Reading, MA: Addition-Wesley.

Quayhagen, M., & Roth, P. (1989). From models to measures in assessment of mature families. *Journal of Professional Nursing, 5*, 144-151.

Rawnsley, M. (1999). Commentary. *Nursing Science Quarterly, 12*(3): 224-226.

Raymond, D.P. (1995). Esthetic and personal knowing through humanistic nursing. *Nursing and Health Care: Perspectives on Community, 16*(6), 332-336.

Reed, K. (1993). Adapting the Neuman systems model for family nursing. *Nursing Science Quarterly, 6* (2), 93-97.

Riehl, J., & Roy, C. (1980). *Conceptual models for nursing practice* (2nd ed.). New York: Appleton-Century-Crofts.

Robinson, C. (1994). Nursing interventions with families: a demand or an invitation to change. *Journal of Advanced Nursing, 19*, 897-504.

Robinson, D. (1991). *The effect of nursing follow-up on self care abilities of post myocardial infarction patients* (Dissertation). Austin, TX: University of Texas at Austin.

Robinson, J. (1995). Grief responses, coping processes, and social support of widows: research with Roy's model. *Nursing Science Quarterly, 8*(4), 158-164.

Roy, C. (1980). The Roy adaptation model. In J. Riehl & C. Roy (Eds.), *Conceptual models for nursing practice* (2nd ed.). New York: Appleton-Century-Crofts.

Roy, C. (1984). *Introduction to nursing: an adaptation model* (2nd ed.). Englewood Cliffs, NJ: Prentice-Hall.

Roy, C. (1987). Roy's Adaptation Model. In R. Parse (Ed.), *Nursing science: major paradigms, theories and critiques*. Philadelphia: WB Saunders.

Roy, C. (1988). An explication of the philosophical assumptions of the Roy Adaptation Model. *Nursing Science Quarterly, 1*(1), 26-34.

Roy, C. (1990). Strengthening the Roy Adaptation Model through conceptual clarification: response. *Nursing Science Quarterly, 3*(2), 64-66.

Roy, C. (1997). Future of the Roy model: challenge to redefine adaptation. *Nursing Science Quarterly, 10*(1), 42-48.

Roy, C., & Andrews, H. (1991). *The Roy Adaptation Model: the definitive statement*. Norwalk, CT: Appleton-Century-Crofts.

Roy, C., & McLeod, D. (1981). Theory of person as an adaptive system. In C. Roy & S. Roberts (Eds.), *Theory construction in nursing: an adaptation model*. Englewood Cliffs, NJ: Prentice-Hall.

Rutty, J. (1998). The nature of philosophy of science, theory and knowledge relating to nursing and professionalism. *Journal of Advanced Nursing, 28*, 243-250.

Schlotzhauer, M., & Farnham, R. (1997). Newman's theory and insulin dependent diabetes mellitus in adolescence. *Journal of School Nursing, 13*(3), 20-23.

Silva, M. (1999). The state of nursing science: reconceptualizing for the 21st century. *Nursing Science Quarterly, 12*(3), 221-226.

Smith, M. (1994). Beyond the threshold: nursing practice in the next millennium. *Nursing Science Quarterly, 7*(1), 6-7

Smits, M., & Kee, C. (1992). Correlates of self care among the independent elderly: self concept affects well being. *Journal of Gerontological Nursing, 18*, 13-18.

Stubblefield, C., & Murray, R. (1998). Parent's perceptions of their children's lung transplant experiences. *Journal of Family Nursing, 4*(4), 367-386.

Stubblefield, C., & Murray, R. (1999). Parents call for concerned and collaborative care. *Western Journal of Nursing Research, 21*(3), 356-371.

Taylor S.G. (1988). Nursing theory and nursing process: Orem's theory in practice. *Nursing Science Quarterly, 1*, 111-119.

Taylor S.G. (1989). An interpretation of family within Orem's general theory of nursing. *Nursing Science Quarterly, 2*, 131-137.

Taylor, S.G., Geden, E., Isaramalai, S., & Wongvatunyu, S. (2000). Orem's Self Care Deficit nursing theory: its philosophic foundation and the state of the science. *Nursing Science Quarterly, 13*(2), 104-110.

Taylor S.G., & Godfrey N.S. (1999). The ethics of Orem's theory. *Nursing Science Quarterly 12*, 202-207.

Taylor S.G., & McLaughlin K. (1991). Orem's general theory of nursing and community nursing. *Nursing Science Quarterly, 4*, 153-160.

Taylor S.G., Renpenning K., Geden E., Neuman B., & Hart M.A. (in press). A theory of dependent-care: A corollary theory to the theory of self-care. *Nursing Science Quarterly*.

Tulman, L., & Fawcett, J. (1990). Changes in functional status after childbirth. *Nursing Research, 39*(2), 70-75.

Varvaro, F. (1991). Women with coronary heart disease: an application of Roy's adaptation model. *Cardiovascular Nursing, 27*(6), 31-35.

Villarruel, A. (1995). Mexican American cultural meanings, expression, self care and dependent care actions associated with experiences of pain. *Research in Nursing and Health, 18*, 427-436.

Walker, L., & Grobe, S. (1999). The construct of thriving in pregnancy and postpartum. *Nursing Science Quarterly, 12*(2), 151-157.

Ward-Griffin, C., & Bramwell, L. (1990). The congruence of elderly client and nurse perceptions of the clients' self care agency. *Journal of Advanced Nursing, 15*, 1070-1077.

Weiss, M., Hastings, W., Holly, D., Craig, D. (1994). Using Roy's adaptation model in practice: nurses' perspective. *Nursing Science Quarterly, 7*(2): 80-86.

Wesley, R. (1994). *Nursing theories and models* (pp. 94-101). Springhouse, PA: Springhouse.

Wilson, H. (1986). Presencing social control of schizophrenia in an anti-psychiatric community: doing grounded theory. In P. Munhall & C. Oiler (Eds.), *Nursing research* (pp. 131-144). Norwalk, CT: Appleton-Century-Crofts.

Yamashita, M., Jensen, E., & Tall, F. (1998). Therapeutic touch: applying Newman's theoretic approach. *Nursing Science Quarterly, 11*(2): 49-50.

Young, A.M. (1976). *The reflexive universe: evolution of consciousness*. San Francisco: Robert Briggs.

Zderad, L.T. (1978). From here-and-now to theory: reflections on "how." In *Theory development: what, why, how?* New York: National League for Nursing.

Chapter 31

Midrange Nursing Theories and Related Non-Nursing Theories

Linda Baas, Lisa Bradshaw, Kathy Kolcaba, Louise M. Niemer, & Denise Robinson

This chapter explores the significance of some midrange nursing theories and selected non-nursing theories relevant to the discipline of nursing. It provides brief descriptions of three midrange nursing theories regarding comfort, uncertainty, and modeling and role modeling. The non-nursing theories include diffusion of innovation and stress/adaptation theories. Readers are encouraged to read the original primary sources for a broader understanding of these theories.

Initial theory development may be derived from practice, research, or another theory (Meleis, 1997). This other theory may be a nursing theory; two examples of this type of theory development are Newman's Theory of Health as Expanded Consciousness and Barrett's Theory of Power—both were derived from Rogers' Science of Unitary Human Beings. It is also possible for the other theory to be a non-nursing theory, as a number of nursing theories have been partially derived from non-nursing knowledge. Neuman's System Theory was based on general systems theory, and Roy's Adaptation Model was based on adaptation theory. Other examples include Peplau's use of psychoanalytic theory for her theory of interpersonal relations in nursing and Benner's use of the Dreyfus model of skill acquisition as a theoretical source (Benner, 1984).

DEFINITIONS

Nursing theory is identified as knowledge that contributes to the total collection of the unique body of nursing knowledge (Meleis, 1997). Theory can be categorized in many ways. One way relates to whether is it grand (broad) or midrange theory. **Grand (broad) nursing theories** define general parameters on which nursing function is based, while **midrange theories** give more specific guidance related to nursing practice. Broad theories provide direction for practice by identifying the ideal of practice, which then serves as a guide for research and education. The concepts in midrange theories are grounded in a practice context. Midrange theory coincides with research questions directly linked to practice problems. Chin and Kramer (1995) state that midrange theory avoids a focus on methodology and shifts the focus to understanding phenomena. Midrange theory tends to cluster around a concept of interest, such as comfort, caring, fatigue, pain, or social support. In general, the midrange theories were developed later than most of the broad nursing theories.

Many nurse leaders believe that the future of nursing theory development lies in the area of midrange theory. These theories are constructed to describe, explain, and predict a single common phenomenon or a limited number of phenomena. Blegan and Tripp-Reimer (1997) assert, "Middle range theory, when developed from research and thoughtful consideration of practice and tested by research projects, represents the most valid and useful type of knowledge available." There is disagreement by nurse scholars as to what exactly a midrange theory is and which of the current theories is to be considered a midrange theory. Other scholars discuss whether the burgeoning of midrange theories contributes to nursing science. Cody (1999) attempts to classify midrange theories into three types. One type is developed from the grand theories. These theories and the resulting research help provide support and clarity for the grand theories. Another type of midrange theory is original frameworks developed by thoughtful working-through of a health phenomenon or clinical problem. In general, the author of such a theory has some connection to one extant school of thought (grand theory). It is imperative that the author identify the philosophical underpinnings and conduct research that is methodologically congruent with the theory itself. The last type of midrange theory is borrowed from another discipline with little or no alteration. Most scholars acknowledge the need and desire to use knowledge from many different sources in one's day-to-day activities (Cody, 1999). However, Cody cautions that these non-nursing midrange theories do not contribute to the distinct core knowledge of nursing science, nor can practice guided by these theories be considered uniquely nursing practice. Cody believes that midrange theory tied or linked to the grand theories makes the most sense in terms of making a substantive contribution to nursing science. Midrange theories that are engulfed in nursing philosophy and open to scholarly inquiry also foster the development of nursing science.

A *non-nursing theory* is a theory that does not focus primarily on the domain of nursing knowledge. It may include some elements of nursing's domain, but it does not include others and may not place the same importance on such nursing elements as nursing does. A theory, or elements of a theory, determined to be non-nursing theory but serving as a basis for the development for a nursing theory is known as *borrowed theory* (Powers & Knapp, 1990). It is given this name because the theory is in a sense borrowed by nursing from another discipline or a basic science. A borrowed theory does not share the worldview of and practice of the borrowing discipline. Some theories or theory elements that are borrowed are also given the name *related theories*. Related theories have a focus on phenomena that have the potential to be very fruitful for explanations for similar phenomena of interest to nursing. The more aligned a theory is with the domains of interest and the perspective of nursing, the more a theory is considered to be related to nursing theory.

CRITICAL ISSUES: EVALUATING THE MERITS OF MIDRANGE AND RELATED THEORIES

The classification of theory as either discipline-specific, related, or unrelated is based upon the assumption that a discipline can lay claim to a specific and unique body of knowledge. It has been traditionally perceived that a discipline does maintain ownership of a unique body of knowledge that guides its practice and research. Given this perception, some propose that the use of borrowed theory in the development of nursing theory is a less-than-desirable strategy. This view comes from the recognition of the problems that may result from the use of borrowed theory. These problems include misinterpretation of the original theory, resulting in its misapplication; continued use of the theory after the original theory is discredited; and inappropriate matching of the theory with a nursing context or nursing intent (Barnum, 1990). On the other hand, the assumption that a discipline does maintain ownership of a unique body of knowledge can be seen as an outdated way of viewing knowledge in an information age. Given more contemporary methods of information dissemination (such as the Internet), access and use of information has changed significantly. This broad dissemination has implications for classification of knowledge. The use of borrowed theory can be a legitimate approach for the development of nursing theory (Walker & Avant,

1995). Concept, statement, and theory derivation can be successful strategies in the borrowing of non-nursing theory, and the problems cited by Barnum (1990) can be prevented. Purposeful consideration in the early development of the nursing theory as to its appropriateness of fit to nursing can help (Barnum, 1990). The use of borrowed theory can lead to the development of nursing theory that enhances advanced practice nurse (APN) practice and research.

The more nurses recognize that they use theory, the better they can become at examining assumptions for nursing validity. These assumptions provide the basis on which nurses practice. Some of the basic beliefs that underscore nursing practice include:

- Nursing practice is interdisciplinary.
- Nurses deal with many disciplines in practice and in the educational setting.
- Nursing courses are frequently taught in an integrated format. This allows nurses to get outside of their practice to see how others might see them. This also allows nurses to watch for licensure dangers so that nursing can continue to exist.
- Nurses realize that patients' faith in health care providers and scientists is derived from the belief that the "depth of knowledge these experts possess gives them legitimate power and authority" (Martin, Oaks, Taussig, & Vanderstraten, 1997).

Nursing theory–based practice affirms the value that nursing brings to health care. The following sections present information related to midrange nursing and non-nursing theories and describe how APNs might incorporate this information into their practices.

Kolcaba's Theory of Comfort

Entailed in the Theory of Comfort is the hope that nurses will, in part, reembrace their historic mission of providing comfort to those who need it. This is a theory for a type of practice that is skillful yet holistic, technical yet nurturing. Perhaps it is best suited to APNs who have the experience, abilities, and intuition to combine all of these elements in the art of comfort care.

As early as 1869, nursing was called an art and a science, although the latter definition was yet to be defined or developed. Various semantics of comfort were used to describe the art of nursing. For example, Nightingale (1859) exhorted, "It must never be lost sight of what observation is for. It is not for the sake of piling up miscellaneous information or curious facts; [it is] for the sake of saving life and increasing health and comfort." From 1900 to 1929, comfort played a pivotal role in nursing care (McIlveen & Morse, 1995). The nurse was considered to have time to attend to the details influencing patient comfort. Aikens (1908) stated that there was nothing concerning the comfort of the patient that was small enough to ignore. Comfort of the patient was the nurses' first and last consideration. A good nurse was one who made patients comfortable, and the provision of comfort tested the nurses' desirability and character as nurses (Aikens, 1908).

In 1926, Harmer stated that nursing care was concerned with providing a "general atmosphere of comfort" and that personal care of patients included attention to "happiness, comfort, and ease, physical and mental" in addition to "rest and sleep, nutrition, cleanliness, and eliminations." Goodnow (1935) devoted a chapter in her book *The Technique of Nursing* to "The Patient's Comfort." She wrote, "A nurse is judged always by her ability to make her patient comfortable. Comfort is both physical and mental, and a nurse's responsibility does not end with physical care." In textbooks dated 1904, 1914, and 1919, emotional comfort was called "mental comfort" and was achieved mostly by providing physical comfort and modifying the environment for patients (McIlnveen & Morse, 1995).

In these examples, the reader may gain a vague understanding that comfort is positive; achieved with the help of nurses; and, in some cases, indicates an improvement from a previous state or condition. The reader may associate comfort intuitively with a nurturing activity. However, comfort's meaning is actually implicit, hidden in context, and often ambiguous.

Comfort in early nursing theories

Orlando (1961) focuses on the needs of patients and the ability of nurses to assess and meet those needs. Nurses accomplish care through effective nurse-patient relationships. This process consists of careful observation and utilization of the principles of nursing that Orlando developed in her theory. Nurses were to assess their patients' physical and mental comfort before and after a comfort measure was delivered. In *Humanistic Nursing* (Paterson & Zderad, 1988), Paterson calls comfort a construct that communicates "the nature or experience of nursing." She believes that comfort is an "umbrella under which all the other terms—growth, health, freedom, and openness— could be sheltered." Because Paterson was a psychiatric nurse, she defines comfort from a mental perspective rather than a physical one. She believes, however, that mental discomforts can lead to physical discomforts. Thus her definition of comfort is "a state valued by a nurse as an aim in which a person is free to be and become, controlling and planning his own destiny, in accordance with his potential at a particular time in a particular situation." Paterson uses comfort as a stable and positive state but with existential properties of transcendence into freedom. This type of comfort frees patients to be "all that they [can] be" at that time.

In her theory of caring, Watson (1979) claims that patients' environments are critical for their mental and physical well-being. Therefore, when possible, nurses provide comfort through environmental interventions. Watson also lists specific comfort measures that nurses utilize in this regard. She uses the term *comfort measures* synonymously with *interventions*.

Comfort was an important construct in at least one grand nursing theory. For example, Roy built her theory of adaptation around nursing actions that help patients adapt to four categories of needs: physiological, self-concept, role-function, and interdependence (Roy & Roberts, 1981). Nurses are to employ traditional comfort measures to achieve comfort in the physiological mode. Like Watson (1979), Roy's comfort measures are synonymous with interventions. If one of a patient's basic physiological needs is compromised, nurses assess the problem and provide comfort, thereby relieving the discomforts of physiological compromise. In the aforementioned references to comfort in nursing, three meanings of the concept emerge that are congruent with modern and archaic dictionary definitions and with the concept analysis that follows.

While early nurse theorists and authors viewed comfort as a positive and holistic concept, nursing textbooks described comfort unidimensionally as the absence of certain discomforts. This was congruent with the North American Nursing Diagnosis Association's (NANDA's) nursing diagnoses of that era, in which altered comfort was noted to be the state in which an individual experiences an uncomfortable sensation in response to a noxious stimulus. This is a circular definition, but Carpenito (1987) further describes the discomforts as acute pain, chronic pain, pain in children, pruritus (intense itching), and nausea/vomiting. Here, there is no indication that comfort is a positive state. However, in her book about nursing diagnoses for wellness, Campbell (1984) states, "Comfort evolves from an awareness that comfort needs will be met and that previously experienced comfort will be repeated." Thus the dimension of the patient's anticipation that physical comfort needs will be met provides psychological comfort, a positive state.

Comfort and modern inquiry

The seeds of modern inquiry about comfort were sown in the 1980s, marking a period of collective but separate awareness about the concept of holistic comfort. Morse (1983) began observing the comforting actions of nurses and described comfort as "the most important nursing action in the provision of nursing care for the sick." Hamilton (1989) made a leap forward by exploring the meaning of comfort from patients' perspectives. She used interviews to ascertain how each patient in a long-term care (LTC) facility defined comfort. The theme that most frequently emerged was "relief from pain," but patients also identified good positioning in well-fitting furniture and a feeling of being independent, encouraged, worthwhile, and useful. At the end of the article, Hamilton stated, "The clear message is that comfort is multi-dimensional, meaning different things to different people."

In a formal concept analysis of comfort, Kolcaba and Kolcaba (1991) explicated meanings of the term as it had been used in psychology, psychiatry, medicine, ergonomics, and nursing. They found that one meaning of comfort was a *relief* from discomfort. A second meaning was comfort as a state of *ease* and peaceful contentment. A third meaning was comfort as a renewing and strengthening mechanism, which Paterson (Paterson & Zderad, 1988) called *transcendence*. These three meanings were later incorporated into Kolcaba's (1991) taxonomic structure of comfort. A fourth meaning of comfort was a cause of relief from discomfort and/or of the state of comfort. This meaning was entailed in the term *comfort measure*, or a nursing intervention intended to enhance patient comfort. The third and fourth meanings were later used in Kolcaba's Theory of Comfort (1994) that describes how nurses respond to the needs of patients.

While the concept analysis was being conducted (a process that took about 4 years), Morse continued to focus on comforting as a nursing action and believed that this action was central to nursing and had to be described. She used a qualitative, observational approach to study nurses at work. The comforting actions that Morse described consisted of touching, talking and, to a lesser extent, listening (1994). Although she did not specify semantic senses or definitions, and often used the terms *comfort*, *comforting*, *comfortable*, and *comforted* interchangeably, she was describing the process of comfort by nurses. Kolcaba concentrated on comfort as an outcome of nursing care. She incorporated the literature about holism in nursing into her description of comfort and explicated four contexts of human experience in which comfort was experienced (1991). When the three types of comfort—relief, ease, and transcendence—were juxtaposed with the four contexts—physical, psychospiritual, social, and environmental—the taxonomic structure was created, a map of the content domain of the outcome of comfort.

Definitions for the context of the experience of comfort are as follows. Physical comfort pertained to bodily sensations and physiological mechanisms inherent to health (e.g., oxygenation, elimination, electrolyte and fluid balance, metabolism). Psychospiritual comfort pertained to internal awareness of self, including esteem, concept, sexuality, and meaning in one's life; it also pertained to one's relationship to a higher order or being. Environmental comfort pertained to external surroundings, condition, and influences. Social comfort pertained to interpersonal, family, and societal relationships (Kolcaba, 1992; Kolcaba & Fisher, 1996). The content domain of comfort thus consisted of 12 cells, each of which represented a unique aspect of human experience.

From this map, the General Comfort Questionnaire (GCQ) was developed, to which 253 patients responded in an instrumentation study (Kolcaba, 1992). This marked the first time comfort had been quantified for nursing research. The working definition of comfort that has evolved is "the immediate state of being strengthened by having needs for relief, ease, and transcendence met in the physical, psychospiritual, social, and environmental contexts of experience" (Kolcaba & Fisher, 1996). The idea of patient comfort being a strengthening factor was entailed in the third meaning of comfort. From the *Oxford English Dictionary*, one may learn that the term *comfort* was derived from the Latin word *confortare*, meaning "to strengthen greatly." McIlveen and Morse (1995) point out that early dictionary definitions included "to strengthen" and "to make strong." The idea of comfort being a strengthening force has been noted in current nursing literature as well (Cameron, 1993; Schuiling & Sampselle, 1999).

Theory of Comfort

Because a nursing outcome has little meaning when it stands alone, Kolcaba embedded comfort in a midrange theory for nursing (1994). The theory was developed for nursing from Murray's (1981) holistic and abstract theory of human behavior, as shown in Figure 31-1. Lines 1 through 3 represent Murray's constructs, and line 4 represents the constructs and their relationships entailed in Kolcaba's Theory of Comfort. Line 5 can be further delineated by nurses for their own research or practice setting. Line 5 represents a practice-level theory, and, in this example, was the theoretical basis for Kolcaba's intervention study with women going through radiation therapy for early-stage breast cancer (Kolcaba & Fox, 1999). In that study, comfort was operationalized as the Radiation Therapy Comfort Questionnaire (RTCQ), an adaptation of the GCQ. The theory is that interventions are designed and implemented to meet comfort needs of specified populations of patients. Patients, families, and/or communities judge the effectiveness of interventions in light of existing intervening variables. Intervening variables are positive and negative factors that recipients bring to the situation and over which nurses have little influence, such as poverty, strong social networks, or chronic illness. The recipients of nursing care judge the effectiveness of interventions. The distinction between comfort as process and product is discussed in depth in Kolcaba's 1995 work. Comfort is the immediate desired outcome of nursing interventions.

Enhanced comfort strengthens recipients to engage in healthy behaviors that are operationalized as health-seeking behaviors (HSBs). Schlotfeldt defines *health-seeking behaviors* as a range of acquired physiological, psychological, social, cultural, institutional, philosophical, and spiritual activities of patients that are necessary for achieving optimal health (Glazer & Pressler, 1989). The range includes internal and external behaviors and/or a peaceful death (Schlotfeldt, 1981) and are the subsequent desired outcomes of nursing care. They have a positive, reciprocal correlation with comfort because, as HSBs are engaged, comfort is further enhanced. The assumptions

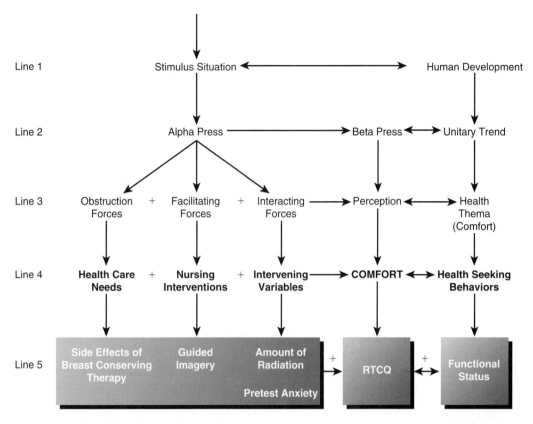

Figure 31-1 Kolcaba's midrange Theory of Comfort. (From Kolcaba, K. [1991]. A taxonomic structure for the concept comfort. *Image: Journal of Nursing Scholarship, 23*[4], 237-240.)

underpinning the Theory of Comfort come from a humanistic perspective and are presented in Box 31-1.

Analysis of basic considerations

A nursing theory can be considered a perspective for examining and practicing nursing; it is predictive and descriptive. Relationships that are predicted in theory must be testable, and the relationships between the first two boxes of Line 5, Figure 31-1, were tested in an experimental design (Kolcaba & Fox, 1999). In this study, women with early-stage breast cancer who received guided imagery (GI) had higher comfort during radiation therapy (RT) than those who did not receive GI. The relationship between comfort and functional status was inconclusive due to problems utilizing the functional status questionnaire. Common to nursing theories are definitions and considerations of recipients of nursing care (formally called *persons*), health, environment, and nursing (Pieper, 1983). Those concepts are defined below, consistent with the Theory of Comfort.

Recipient of nursing care. Comfort theory views recipients of care in the broadest sense and the most individual sense. As Donahue (1989) states, "It is through comfort and comfort measures that nurses provide strength, hope, solace, support, encouragement, and assistance to indi-

> ### Box 31-1
>
> ## Humanistic Assumptions for the Theory of Comfort
>
> - Human beings each perceive stimuli simultaneously (holistically).
> - Human beings strive to meet or have met their basic comfort needs, which are interrelated.
> - Striving for comfort consists of continued active involvement of recipients facilitated, when necessary, by coaching from nurses and health care teams.
> - In acute health care situations, enhanced comfort (compared to a preintervention baseline) usually is more realistic than total comfort.
> - Enhancing the comfort of patients is an altruistic goal of nursing care and a worthy end in and of itself. However, it is also a means to the end of engaging in HSBs (which may be more visible).

viduals, groups, and communities as they experience a multitude of life circumstances." She describes the work of nurses for the Red Cross in national and international relief societies where disasters such as floods, fires, tornadoes, mine cave-ins, and epidemics occur. Thriving

422 Section VI *Theoretical Foundations of Nursing Practice*

today are countless parish nurse organizations that minister to congregations. Nurses also comfort families and patients when they face difficult life circumstances. Persons together and persons individually have their own energy and energy fields. Energy fields are part of the persons and sometimes need to be manipulated by nurses (who have their own energy fields) to achieve enhanced comfort and desired HSBs. However, whole persons do not disappear into ever-larger wholes; they are distinguished from their settings (Kolcaba, 1997). In Line 5, Figure 31-1, recipients of care were the women with early-stage breast cancer.

Health. Health is conceptualized as an individual's or group's state of being, representing the totality or essence of people at any moment in time. This state is constantly changing and can be inferred from the individual or group's level of physical and psychosocial functioning. According to Schlotfeldt (1981), health may include the presence of disease, and health and illness are not on a single continuum. A realistic health goal for one person is quite different from a realistic health goal for another. People use HSBs in their quest for optimal health. Criteria for optimal health include physical and emotional comfort; physiological, emotional, and social function; and achievement and self-fulfillment (Glazer & Pressler, 1989). In Line 5, Figure 31-1, health is operationalized as functional status.

Environment. The environment surrounds recipients of care (Kolcaba, 1997). It includes historical, social, and physical factors. Health care occurs in the context of an often stressful environment. When possible, the environment should be altered or repaired to enhance comfort and improve subsequent HSBs. Modifications in the environment that achieve HSBs (or attempt to do so) are comfort measures. This view of the environment is consistent with Nightingale's view (1859) of the environment. The environment provides context for understanding the needs of recipients. It is rich with "intervening variables" that affect the success of nursing interventions. In Line 5, Figure 31-1, the environment consists of the women's homes, perceived support, and the related milieu.

Nursing. Nursing is the attention paid to recipients' needs for enhanced holistic comfort. Nurses design interventions to address such needs, and this includes special attention to physical comfort needs related to medical problems. There are times when comfort needs can be met by recipients' existing support systems, and there are times when comfort is not the most urgent need. However, nurses sense when comfort needs exist in their recipients; addressing those needs will bring better subsequent outcomes. In Line 5, Figure 31-1, the nursing intervention is a GI audiotape designed to meet the holistic comfort needs of women with early-stage breast cancer.

Theory of Comfort and the advanced practice nurse

Kolcaba's Theory of Comfort has much to offer nursing theory, practice, and research. The merit of this theory is due to two significant strengths: relevance and purposeful development. Kolcaba's historical analysis documents the relevance of this theory to nursing theory and practice. This midrange theory can be used to develop practice level theory that can be readily applied, and this applicability demonstrates the theory's high level of relevance and thus increases its significance for nursing practice. The theory's conceptualization was purposefully derived from a nursing theory of a broader scope, and it lends itself to practice applications due to its clarity and explicitness, which allow for the easy development of research questions and testing.

Knowing that specific patient populations have different comfort needs makes it easier for APNs to address the comfort needs of patients. For example, Kolcaba describes an oncology patient who is not in physical pain but needs comfort in the transcendental and psychospiritual sense. Once these specific needs are identified, comfort measures can be designed. Schuiling and Sampselle (1999) describe the specific comfort needs of women in labor. Enhancement of comfort is a valued outcome of nurse midwifery care. Research questions that would provide valuable data for midwifery practice include: Does comfort exist as a phenomenon in labor? Does the use of comfort measures provide for better physical outcomes, especially as related to perineal tissues? What are the biological and physiological markers of comfort, which could quantify the physiological effect of providing comfort? (Schuiling & Sampselle, 1999). Having data to address these questions would likely improve the care and comfort midwives could provide.

Uncertainty-in-Illness Theory

Uncertainty-in-illness is a midrange theory of nursing. It was developed by Mishel (1984) to explain how individuals cognitively process and find meaning in the events associated with illness and disease. It is based on theories of cognitive appraisal and predominantly reflects the theory of Lazarus and Folkman (1984). Further development of the model has included situations of chronic illness, as well as parents of critically ill children. The Uncertainty-in-Illness Theory is nursing based and has applicability in nursing situations involving patients and families in the diagnostic and treatment phases of debilitating or life-threatening diseases. It provides a framework for assessing and intervening when patients or their family members experience uncertainty.

Major concepts

Uncertainty is defined as "the inability to determine the meaning of illness-related events" (Mishel, 1990). It occurs when there are insufficient or meaningless stimuli such that an individual is unable to determine the meaning of illness-related events and/or unable to predict illness outcomes. Illness-related uncertainty is postulated to have four forms: (1) ambiguity regarding the disease condition, (2) degree of complexity regarding treatment and system of care, (3) lack of information regarding the disease and its severity, and (4) unpredictability regarding how the disease will unfold (Mishel, Hostetter, King, & Graham, 1984; Mishel, 1988).

The Uncertainty-in-Illness Model depicts a theoretical process by which individuals establish the meaning of illness-related events. The process consists of four stages: antecedents, appraisal, coping, and adaptation (Figure 31-2). When illness-related stimuli (antecedents) are confusing, unexpected, or preclude prediction of outcomes, uncertainty arises. Appraisal of the significance of the uncertainty influences the coping strategies that are mobilized and the adaptation that results.

Antecedents. Stimuli frame, the first antecedent, relates to the symptoms of the event itself. For patterns to be established, symptoms must be clarified and assigned to a category composed of like attributes. This facilitates *pattern recognition.* The first element of the stimuli frame is symptom patterns, which are needed for a person to identify their perception of an event as uncertain, not recognized, or misperceived.

Event familiarity, the second element of the stimuli frame, refers to the repetitiveness of events that occur in the health care environment. The novelty of the experience, especially related to the perceived complexity of treatment and system of care, is particularly evocative of uncertainty (Mishel, 1988; Mishel & Braden, 1988). As novelty diminishes, event familiarity develops and uncertainty declines. However, when the treatment experience remains variable and precludes establishment of event familiarity, uncertainty about treatment and system of care complexity remains high (Mishel, 1988).

For example, Joyce was a 49-year-old woman who was recently diagnosed with lung cancer. She had been very healthy for the last 20 years and was very proactive in her healthy lifestyle. She never smoked, ate a low-fat diet, and exercised vigorously 5 to 6 days a week. She noticed that while exercising her breathing tolerance was not normal, and she started the diagnostic process. A tumor was found next to the mediastinum and deemed inoperable. She had two courses of chemotherapy, and the tumor appeared to have shrunk by about 15%. The next stage was where uncertainty appeared. When trying to decide what the next phase of treatment would entail, another physician was consulted and more tests were run. At this point, surgery was still not an option. However, the surgeon wanted to know exactly where the tumor was and if it had encroached into the mediastinum. He felt no further treatment should be attempted until the exact location of the tumor was determined. This could not be determined by a computed tomography (CT) scan, so Joyce was to have an exploratory surgery. During this time of waiting, Joyce was very nervous and scared. She knew that the outcome of the surgery would have a great effect on her overall prognosis.

Event congruence, the final aspect of the stimuli frame, is the degree of consistency between what a person expects from the illness experience and what in fact occurs. Event congruence occurs when the disease and treatment experiences correspond with the individual's expectations. When event congruence is high, uncertainty is low. Conversely, incongruency between anticipated and actual experiences creates uncertainty regarding the predictability and stability of the situation. Disease relapse or reoccurrence, failure to achieve control of a disease process within a predetermined period, and failure of treatment to decrease symptoms contribute to incongruency resulting in uncertainty (Mishel, 1988).

Physiological malfunction associated with illness is postulated to reduce an individual's cognitive capacity. Cognitive processes requiring attention are the most susceptible to disruption. As a progenitor to uncertainty, the inability to

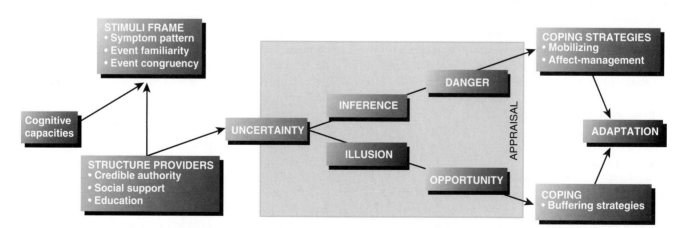

Figure 31-2 Uncertainty-in-Illness Model. (From Mishel, M. [1988]. Uncertainty in illness. *Image: Journal of Nursing Scholarship, 20*[4], 225-232.)

fully attend to stimuli interferes with an individual's ability to sufficiently process illness-related events. The resultant schema is confusing, lacks meaning, and creates uncertainty (Mishel, 1988). Physical illness demands its own attention and can reduce cognitive efficiency. The effects of experiences such as pain and discomfort, drugs, and sleep deprivation can further weaken cognitive abilities and heighten uncertainty (Mishel, 1988).

Structure providers constitute the second antecedent variable to uncertainty. Later research demonstrates that structure providers contribute more significantly to uncertainty than does the stimuli frame (Mishel & Braden, 1988). Structure providers indirectly assist an individual to determine the meaning of illness symptoms and events. They provide direct influence when the individual relies on them to interpret uncertain illness-related events. Structure providers are comprised of credible authority, social support, and education. In Joyce's situation the structure provider was the physician. He had a direct influence on the level of uncertainty in her case.

Credible authority refers to the confidence and trust that an individual has in the health care provider (Mishel, 1988). Nurses or physicians as sources of credible authority indirectly influence the stimuli frame by providing information regarding symptoms that can be anticipated and the expected course of the illness. Structure providers directly influence uncertainty through the assumption of power and prestige bestowed upon them by society; this is particularly true of physicians (Mishel, 1988). An individual will not attempt to comprehend technical explanations of the disease process but will adopt the perspectives of a credible authority figure at face value. Mishel and Braden (1988) later found that credible authority, in the form of physician credibility, was a direct antecedent of uncertainty.

Social support is proposed to indirectly influence uncertainty through its effect on the stimuli frame. Through discussion and interactions with one's social network, symptoms and events are interpreted to create a meaningful illness schema. The effect of the direct influence of social support "is the modification of three types of uncertainty: (a) the ambiguity concerning the state of the illness, (b) the complexity perceived in treatment, and (c) the unpredictability of the future" (Mishel, 1988). Later research demonstrates that social support has a significant influence on symptom appraisal but does not exert a significant direct effect on uncertainty (Mishel & Braden, 1988). Social support through assistance with everyday tasks may also assist an individual to better process illness-related events (Mishel & Braden, 1987).

Education, the third structure variable, is theorized to "enlarge a patient's knowledge base" (Mishel, 1988) by providing the individual with a broader frame of reference for interpretation of illness-related events. Education affects the stimuli frame to indirectly influence uncertainty. It is theorized that individuals with a limited educational background might have more difficulty interpreting the stimuli frame symptoms and events. Similarly, education is theorized to directly influence uncertainty in an inverse manner; individuals with more education require less time to construct meaning from the illness situation and thus experience uncertainty for shorter periods of time than do individuals with less education (Mishel, 1988).

Appraisal. Although uncertainty bears a negative connotation depending upon the implications, uncertainty can also provide hope for a positive illness outcome. Determination of uncertainty as either threat or opportunity is theorized to be the product of two appraisal processes: inference and illusion (Mishel, 1990). Inference involves factors such as a person's personal disposition (e.g., locus of control, resourcefulness), knowledge, beliefs, and life experiences. These attributes play into the value attributed to the uncertainty. Hypothetically, an individual with a strong external locus of control would depend on environmental stability and predictability and perceive uncertainty as a threat (Mishel, 1988).

Negative certainty denotes a known undesirable outcome. However, when an illness is characterized by a downward trajectory, uncertainty regarding the illness is often deemed desirable. Illusion is the construction of positive beliefs regarding outcomes of the illness and is proposed to occur in illness situations associated with deterioration (Mishel, 1988). Through the generation of an illusion, appraisal of a positive potential for a hopeful outcome is recognized. Physiological changes associated with a given disease may bear the potential threat of serious disability. Uncertainty that this will actually occur enables the individual to construct an illusion for the optimistic possibility that it may not happen.

Coping. Appraisal determines whether uncertainty is perceived as danger or opportunity. "A danger appraisal occurs when the predictive accuracy of the inference is unknown" (Mishel, 1988). When uncertainty is a threat, coping strategies are directed at decreasing the uncertainty and controlling the stress response. Mobilizing strategies of direct action, vigilance, and information-seeking are directed at reducing uncertainty. Affect-management tactics of faith, disengagement, and cognitive restructuring are implemented when mobilization is ineffective at reducing uncertainty. These tactics play a major role in managing anxiety resulting from the perceived inability to moderate uncertainty (Mishel, 1988).

When uncertainty is appraised as opportunity (as was discussed previously), the possibility for a positive outcome is anticipated. The nebulous nature of uncertainty allows an individual to create illusions of optimistic outcome possibilities rather than dwell on the negative ones. To maintain hope, buffering strategies that enable a person to sustain uncertainty are employed. The individual may avoid or ignore information or selectively attend to reinforcing stimuli. The individual may also see himself or herself as being different from others with the same illness, thus potentially exempting himself or herself from similar outcomes. In a study conducted by Deane and Degner (1998) with women who experienced a benign breast biopsy, the most important information need for the women was to find out when they would learn the diagnosis. In this situation, there was a possibility for a positive outcome (i.e., a benign lesion), so the women could focus on the potential for a positive diagnosis.

Adaptation. The notion of uncertainty being a tolerable or preferable situation is generally discounted in the literature. Coping strategies emanating from illusion are usually labeled *denial* and considered maladaptive responses (Mishel, 1988). However, according to the Uncertainty-in-Illness Theory, adaptation can and does occur in situations of uncertainty when there is a sense of relative stability that enables goal-directed behavior to continue. Adaptation is regarded to be a biopsychosocial function within the person's "individually defined range of usual behavior" (Mishel, 1988).

Assumptions

The Uncertainty-in-Illness Theory implicitly supports the notion that certainty regarding illness situations and outcomes is preferred over uncertainty. Furthermore, the theory assumes that people can control uncertainty and actively seek to do so. There is a clear influence of Western culture with its emphasis on control and logical and linear thinking on the derivation of the theory (Mishel, 1990). Positive uncertainty—that which contributes to adaptation through the use of buffering strategies—is even presented as a controlling mechanism in this regard. There is an assumption of the existence of a causal relationship among the variables comprising the Uncertainty-in-Illness Model. The model explicitly assumes that an individual's actions to control uncertainty are the result of a cognitive thought process and emphasizes the influence of immediate situational variables that impel the individual to find meaning in uncertainty. However, the model does not clearly integrate the possible influence of emotions, beliefs, and experience on the individual's interpretation of the uncertainty situation.

An important assumption of the theory is that individuals seek to imbue experiences with meaning and will actively seek to find meaning in an illness situation. Many health-related and nursing theories support the notion of the individual as a responsive and reactive being. However, few theories have advanced the idea that finding meaning is a significant component of the health and illness experience. In this regard, this theory serves to further nursing's humanistic focus.

Nursing concepts

The Uncertainty-in-Illness Theory was developed to explain how individuals cognitively process illness-related events that contribute to uncertainty in order to ascertain meaning from the event. Although the Uncertainty-in-Illness Model is a nursing theory, the concepts of recipient of care, health, environment, and nursing are not explicated. However, the attributes of these concepts as they relate specifically to the Uncertainty-in-Illness Theory can be deduced.

Individuals are future-oriented, goal-directed beings who actively seek to find meaning in their daily experiences. Meaning is cognitively derived from previous experience and influenced by interactions with others significant to the individual. Certainty means that one is able to anticipate events and related outcomes and engage in activities accordingly. Uncertainty is engendered when an individual is unable to deduce meaning from current events. It precludes the individual's ability to anticipate outcomes and engenders a sense of instability and inability to engage in goal-directed activities. However, when future expectations are discouraging, uncertainty can mean the possibility for a more desirable future.

Health is a felt state of relative stability that enables the individual to engage in goal-directed activities. Uncertainty regarding future events impedes goal-directed actions. Illness and disease are not opposites of health. However, uncertainty regarding illness- or disease-related events can contribute to a diminished sense of health if an individual is unable to find meaning in the events associated with an illness or disease. Uncertainty regarding the outcomes of a potentially devastating illness or disease may serve to sustain hope for a positive future. The potential for growth following an experience of uncertainty is not explicated in the model.

The environment is composed of present and previous experience (the stimuli frame) and others who are significant to an individual in particular circumstances (the structure variables). The individual draws on environmental cues to cognitively process events and determine their meaning. In the context of illness or disease situations, an individual relies on what he or she knows and has experienced, as well as on discourse with family, friends, and health care providers to determine the meaning of related events.

Nursing strives to assist individuals in illness or disease situations toward health, toward achieving a felt sense of stability and direction. Assessment of environmental factors that affect an individual's appraisal of illness-related events is necessary. Evaluation of the stimuli frame (e.g., individual perceptions of symptoms and events relative to the illness or disease experience), the structure variables (e.g., social support, knowledge), and the individual's ability to cognitively process events provides a basis for intervention that will assist the individual to construct meaning from the experience. The nurse, as a credible authority, employs interventions that facilitate the individual's appraisal of the events. Controlling pain, providing information regarding symptom progression or the pattern of events, and promoting the family's participation in the experience exemplify appropriate nursing interventions.

Uncertainty-in-Illness Theory and the advanced practice nurse

This theory was developed from a nursing perspective. It posits a view of adaptation to the illness experience that is mediated by an individual's ability to place illness-related events into a meaningful schema. As such, it is congruent with humanistic nursing because it emphasizes individual meaning as the focus of nursing. APN students need to be introduced to the concepts of uncertainty theory as part of their exposure to a variety of nursing theories.

APNs often encounter situations in which patients and families seek to know what to expect. However, many individuals experience long-term and chronic illness conditions. Uncertainty theory does not specifically address situations in which individuals experience continual uncertainty. Furthermore, the theory may reflect class and cultural biases that preclude its applicability to minority populations and other cultural groups.

An example of how to incorporate the basic findings from uncertainty research into practice is that of Steve. Steve, an APN working in the critical care unit, knows that when he cares for patients on ventilators beginning the weaning process, there is much uncertainty in how the weaning will progress. Using uncertainty theory as a framework with which to approach patients, he tries to reduce patient stress during the process and seeks input from patients to help decrease the amount of uncertainty experienced.

Modeling and Role-Modeling

Modeling and Role Modeling (MRM) was developed by Erickson, Tomlin, and Swain (1983), a team of three clinicians, educators, and researchers. The theory was derived from their lived experiences, clinical practice, education in nursing and the social sciences, and research. Two of the original authors conducted theory-testing research, and two applied the theory to practice. In addition, they served as mentors for many who have studied and applied the theory in diverse settings with people across the lifespan (Frisch & Bowman, 1995).

The theorists wrote *Modeling and Role-Modeling: A Theory and Paradigm for Nurses* (1983) at a time when they were colleagues at the University of Michigan. In this first publication of the theory as a whole, MRM is described as a holistic framework that integrates assumptions about persons, nursing, health, and environment with extant theories of psychosocial and cognitive development (Erikson, 1968; Piaget, 1969), basic and growth needs (Maslow, 1968), loss and attachment (Bowlby, 1980), and stress and adaptation (Engel, 1962; Selye 1974). Although decades have passed since many of these psychosocial theories were first proposed, the core concepts continue to

be used today. In some cases the original psychosocial theories have been updated or refined for current relevance; however, they are still widely discussed and taught in nursing and the social sciences as the basis for understanding similarities and differences among people. Although MRM openly recognizes the contributions of non-nursing theories, Erickson, Tomlin, and Swain (1983) provide a unique conceptual perspective of patient self-care, nursing, and the nurse-patient interaction. Because the work of many familiar psychosocial scientists and theorists is woven into MRM, it is a familiar and comfortable theory for many nurses to adopt for their practice (Frisch & Bowman, 1995; Sappington & Kelly, 1996).

Other major influences on the development of this theory were growth in the holistic nursing movement and the science of psychoneuroimmunology (PNI). The holistic approach advocated in MRM leads nurses to understand how each person is unique, while the science of PNI provides the integration of the mind and body. Erickson described her interest in body-mind connections as first occurring early in her nursing career and resulting from clinical observations and personal experiences (Erickson, 1998).

Perhaps the most important influence on the development of this theory was Milton Erickson, a noted psychiatrist and the father-in-law of Helen Erickson. Milton Erickson was a master teacher and clinician. He frequently spoke on the use of hypnosis, analogy, and storytelling, and many of these lectures were published. The senior Erickson stressed the need to focus on the whole patient, make a thorough assessment of the patient's world, and provide brief targeted intervention (Erickson, 1988).

Helen Erickson was honored with the position of Professor Emeritus at the University of Texas at Austin. She articulated the theory and has conducted research that tested aspects of MRM in healthy persons, people with hypertension, and families with Alzheimer's disease (Erickson & Swain, 1990; Acton, Irvin, Jensen, Hopkins, & Miller, 1997). Her research was funded by a variety of external sources including the National Institute of Health. Along with Jean Watson, Dr. Erikson was honored by the American Holistic Nurses Association as the first certified holistic nurse. Her expertise as a holistic nurse was also recognized by inclusion in the book *Nurse Healers* (Keegan & Dossey, 1998). Dr. Erickson has guided many graduate students conducting research on aspects of the theory. She has consulted internationally on the application of MRM to practice and the curriculum. Serving as the first President of the Society for the Advancement of Modeling and Role-Modeling, she has remained active in the organization. In 1996, Dr. Erickson was inducted as a Fellow in the American Academy of Nursing.

Evelyn Tomlin has a varied background in nursing practice settings. She was one of the early certified nurses in critical care. International nursing practice in Afghanistan and European countries provided a unique perspective to development of her personal view of nursing. Tomlin has taught at the University of Michigan and provided continuing education offerings for nurses in other settings. With several colleagues, she established one of the first independent nursing practices in Michigan. She has pursued an interest in developing the interface between MRM, Judeo-Christian principles (Tomlin, 1990), and healing prayer (Erickson, Caldwell-Gwin, Carr, Harmon, Hartman, Jarlsberg, McCornnick, & Noone, 1998).

Mary Ann Swain, an educational psychologist, has had a close relationship to nursing throughout her career. For many years she served on the faculty at the University of Michigan College of Nursing and held the positions of Director of the Doctoral Nursing Program and Chairperson for Nursing Research. She eventually assumed the position of Associate Vice President for Academic Affairs at the University of Michigan. Dr. Swain served as the Provost for the New York University System (Erickson et al., 1998). Over the past 15 years she has been a coinvestigator on many MRM studies. In addition, she has guided numerous students in the conduct of theses or dissertations that tested theoretical relationships of MRM.

MRM is one of the eight nursing theories recognized as a basis for practice by the American Holistic Nurses Association (Dossey, 1998). MRM has been classified as a conceptual model by George (1995) and as a midrange theory by Marriner-Tomey and Allingood (1998). In a review of the literature, Liehr and Smith (1999) identified twenty-two midrange theories. Two of the constructs from MRM, affiliated-individuation (Irvin & Acton, 1996; Acton, 1997; Acton et al, 1997) and developmental residual (Kinney, 1990; Kinney & Erickson, 1990), were included among the recognized midrange theories contributing to the growth of nursing science. The Society for the Advancement of Modeling and Role-Modeling has hosted biennial conferences and supported a website and listserve. MRM has been adopted by several institutions, agencies, and schools as a guide for practice and curriculum.

Major concepts/constructs

Before discussing the major concepts/constructs of the theory, it is important to explain the name of the theory. Following that, four major constructs of the theory are presented. Relationships among these constructs are described to illustrate how the theory can be applied by APNs in varied clinical settings.

The title Modeling and Role-Modeling provides a succinct description of two major roles of the nurse. *Modeling* refers to the complete and holistic assessment that encompasses building a "model of the patient's world." This model starts with the acquisition of primary data from an individual's perspective (e.g., what the person believes is enhancing, maintaining, or threatening health). Secondary information is obtained from nursing observations and the patient's family members and friends.

Tertiary data comes from the health care team. All three levels of data obtained during the assessment are important, but the emphasis is placed on what the patient tells the nurse. This does not discount the need for a thorough description of the patient's present symptoms or health complaint and a review of systems and physical examination performed by the APN. However, this approach to data collection emphasizes the importance of understanding the patient's world. Information related to the patient's world is the foundation for a trusting relationship. Using this approach to assessment, similarities and differences among people are recognized and valued. Additionally, the nurse builds a model of the patient's environment to better understand the stressors that threaten health and identify perceived external supportive resources (Erickson & Swain, 1982; Erickson et al, 1983; Erickson, 1990a). It is important to note that the patient can be an individual, family, or group.

For example, Darla is an APN who is seeing Laura (42 years old) for her annual checkup. Laura is discussing her fear and concern about breast cancer. Laura has noticed a small lump in her breast. Darla reviews how to do a breast self-examination with Laura and conducts a very thorough examination of Laura's breasts. She notes that the lump is small, approximately 1 centimeter, movable, and nontender. It is soft and compressible. Laura does not have family history of breast cancer. Darla sends Laura for a mammogram. The mammogram is within normal limits, with a recommendation for follow-up in 6 months. Laura is still quite concerned. She feels that she knows her body and having the lump frightens her; it is constantly on her mind. Darla makes a referral to a surgeon to do a biopsy. They are unable to do a fine needle aspiration, and the surgeon wants to just watch the lump. Darla calls and talks with the surgeon about Laura's all-consuming fear about breast cancer. The surgeon agrees to do an incision biopsy; unfortunately, the outcome is not positive; Laura does have a cancerous lesion. However, the lesion is small and the prognosis is much better because Darla listened to what her patient had to say and served as her advocate in getting more definitive treatment. According to MRM theory, Darla took into account the patient's view of her own health, the patient's primary perspective of what was happening to her body. This is a key point with MRM theory.

Role-modeling refers to the actions of the nurse as he or she works with a patient to promote growth, health, and quality of life. The role of the nurse is to assist the patient in the pursuit of health through a role-modeling process that facilitates growth. Role-modeling may be viewed as more of a remodeling process that comes about through enhancing the patient's internal and external resources in an effort to restore adaptive equilibrium and promote self-care actions. Five aims for all interventions can be used to achieve the overall outcomes of maintaining or achieving health goals (Erickson et al, 1983; Erickson,

1990a). These guidelines for developing an individualized plan of care are described later in this section.

Self-care is a major element within MRM, and it is viewed quite differently from Orem's theory. In MRM, *self-care* is defined as the capacity of the individual to mobilize sufficient resources to cope with the stress of a health-related problem. Self-care has three concepts: self-care knowledge, self-care resources, and self-care action. Self-care knowledge is what a person perceives has threatened his or her health as well as what is needed to recover. It is not the knowledge of the disease process and treatment modalities prescribed. Instead, it is a personal understanding of the stressors and threats to one's holistic health status. Self-care resources buffer the effect of stress and help restore or maintain health; they can be derived either from internal or external sources. For instance, resources can include the external support obtained from friends and family and the internal resource of hope. Based on the perception of what is needed (self-care knowledge) and available (self-care resources), the patient and nurse work together to formulate a plan of self-care actions designed to restore, maintain, or gain health (Erickson, 1990b; Erickson et al, 1983). Erickson and Swain (1990) found a profound improvement in blood pressure in persons with hypertension treated with an individualized self-care intervention. In studies of persons after a myocardial infarction and those with heart failure or transplant, self-care knowledge of what was needed and the resources that were available predicted quality of life (Baas, 1992; Baas, Fontana, & Bhat, 1997).

A second element within MRM is affiliated-individuation. This construct describes the dual needs of being connected (affiliated) with others and being autonomous (individuation). While these needs appear to be conflicting, for most people they actually coexist in a dynamic equilibrium that is situationally based. MRM proposes that affiliated-individuation provides resources that aid in coping. Loss of a person or object to which a person has been attached can be viewed as a loss of coping resources. People grieve for the loss and, unless grief is resolved and a new attachment made, the person may experience the morbid grief of chronic depression (Engel, 1962; Bowlby, 1980). In a study of family members of persons with Alzheimer's disease, affiliated-individuation was a significant buffer of stress that helped caregivers cope with the burden of providing for a loved one with many needs (Irvin & Acton, 1996; Acton, 1997; Acton et al, 1997).

The third element in MRM, the Adaptive Potential Assessment Model (APAM), is based on Selye's (1974) physiological response to stress and Engel's (1962) psychosocial response to stress. Stressors may be real or perceived, but either leads to a state of arousal. When coping resources are mobilized, a person adapts and returns to a state of equilibrium. If unable to muster the resources needed to cope with the stressor, the person becomes impoverished. Long-term impoverishment results in de-

pression and morbid grief. Adaptive resources can be external (e.g., social support, physical or financial assistance) or internal (e.g., hope, self-efficacy, autonomy). Affiliated-individuation is an adaptive resource, and mobilization of adaptive (self-care) resources is the basis of self-care actions. Through a series of studies, characteristics of arousal, equilibrium, and impoverishment have been identified (Erickson & Swain, 1982; Barnfather, Swain, & Erickson, 1989; Barnfather, 1990).

The fourth element within MRM is developmental residual. According to Erikson (1968), a person goes through a series of stages of psychosocial development. At each stage the person meets a challenge, and if he or she overcomes the challenge, the person gains new coping skills. For instance the person develops trust or autonomy from the early developmental stages. However, throughout life, one continuously faces stressors or challenges that require dealing with the conflicts of earlier developmental stages. If one has successfully met the previous challenges, there is positive developmental residual that can be an adaptive resource in this new situation. For instance, a person is suddenly hospitalized and forced to be dependent on the health care team. This person can more readily develop trust if he or she has done so in the past. However, if the person has unresolved issues, lacks a secure attachment, has little developmental residual, or is in a state of arousal, he or she might have a high degree of mistrust of health care providers. If the nurse initially focuses on building trust, other interventions may be more successful (Erickson et al, 1983). Developmental residual has been studied in older adults (Curl, 1992; Baas, Curl, Hertz, Robinson, 1994; Hertz, 1996), adults (Darling-Fischer & Leidy, 1988; Kinney, 1990; MacLean, 1992; Baas, Beery, Fontana, & Wagoner, 1999), and adolescents (Miller, 1986).

Assumptions

Erickson (1990a) delineated the major assumption of MRM. Many of the assumptions describe the nature of people and the role of nursing. People have self-care knowledge, and nurses can identify this by modeling the person's world. All behaviors are motivated by needs, which can be either basic or growth-promoting. Another inherent need is for affiliated-individuation. An object or person that provides a secure attachment can fulfill needs. Transitional entities that are concrete or abstract can be used by the nurse to secure attachments or transfer attachments to fulfill needs (Beery & Baas, 1996). Other resources come from the successful completion of developmental challenges. Growth entails meeting the developmental challenges of a particular stage, but a positive developmental residual, such as trust or autonomy, can be a valuable coping resource when faced with a stressor later in life. Based on the original work, Erickson (1990a) further delineated 13 propositions derived from the theoretical assumptions and providing linkages among the major concepts (Box 31-2).

Basic Propositions of Modeling and Role Modeling Theory

1. An individual's ability to contend with new stressors is directly related to the ability to mobilize the necessary resources.
2. An individual's ability to mobilize resources is directly related to his or her need deficits and assets.
3. Distressors are related to unmet basic needs; stressors are related to unmet growth needs.
4. Objects that repeatedly facilitate the individual in need satisfaction take on significance for the individual. When this occurs, attachment to the object results.
5. Secure attachment produces feelings of worthiness.
6. Feelings of worthiness result in a sense of futurity.
7. Real, threatened, or perceived loss of the attachment object results in the grief process.
8. Basic need deficits coexist with the grief process.
9. An adequate alternative object must be perceived as available for the individual to resolve the grief process.
10. Prolonged grief due to an unavailable or inadequate object results in morbid grief.
11. Unmet basic and growth needs interfere with growth processes.
12. Repeated satisfaction of basic needs is a prerequisite to working through developmental tasks and resolving related development crises.
13. Morbid grief is always related to need deficits.

Major divisions according to core nursing concepts

Recipient of care. In MRM, people are viewed as holistic beings with biophysical, psychological, social, and cognitive systems in constant interaction. These components are described as overlapping and intertwining spheres with a spiritual drive and genetic base that serves as the central core of the system. A clear distinction is made between wholism (the sum of the parts) and holism (more than the sum of the parts). Within this theory, similarities and differences among people are identified. All people are unique individuals, but there are common and shared needs, experiences, processes, and challenges. The similarities that all humans encounter include fulfilling basic needs, facilitating growth and development, and meeting affiliation and individuation needs. Differences include the manner in which people adapt to stress and self-care (Erickson et al, 1983; Erickson, 1990a; Erickson et al, 1998).

Health. Several definitions of health are offered. The first definition of health comes from the World Health Organization (WHO). The WHO defines health as a state of physical, mental, and social well-being, not merely the absence of disease or infirmity. An additional definition of

health relies on the APAM and describes health as a state of dynamic equilibrium among the various subsystems. This implies that a less-than-ideal state of health exists when a person is in the state of arousal or impoverishment (Erickson et al, 1983). Furthermore, health is viewed as a personally derived model based on a person's self-care knowledge.

Environment. The environment is not specifically addressed in this theory. However, it is implied that a person is in constant interaction with others and the environment as he or she uses available external and internal resources to cope with stressors and perform self-care actions.

Nursing. Nursing is an interactive relationship with patients. The nurse performs a holistic assessment by building a model of a patient's world. This includes assessing what the patient expresses as the problem and his or her goals, resources, and strengths. Also, the nurse identifies basic needs, affiliated-individuation, the APAM, developmental residual, and self-care knowledge and resources. After constructing a model of the patient's world, the nurse intervenes through role-modeling.

There are five identified strategies for all interventions within MRM. First and foremost, the nurse builds trust with the patient. A trusting relationship allows the patient to meet affiliation needs. Second, the nurse provides patient-control, which facilitates meeting individuation needs. Third, the nurse and patient develop mutual goals. Fourth, the nurse promotes the patient's strengths and uses them as the basis for remodeling interventions designed to achieve health goals. Last, the nurse provides a positive orientation by reframing. Reframing allows the patient to see the "half-full glass" instead of the "half-empty one." The nurse promotes these five strategies by providing nurturance, facilitation, and unconditional acceptance of the patient (Erickson et al, 1983).

Modeling and Role-Modeling and the advanced practice nurse

MRM has appeal to many in advanced practice because it provides a framework in which nurses and patients can meet individualized health goals. The holistic health assessment goes beyond a health history and physical examination by obtaining a model of the patient's world. This theory provides a framework for practice that fosters holistic care that complements APNs' knowledge of disease prevention and treatment. Patients are particularly responsive to the personalized approach to care (Erickson, 1990a). For example, Nancy is a 61-year-old patient who is concerned that she has a blood clot in her leg. Her past medical history is unremarkable except for well-controlled hypertension and hypothyroidism. She is complaining of having soreness in her right calf. She denies any trauma to the area and says it feels as if the muscle is sore. She admits to usually taking several aspirin a day, but she has decided that she needs to stop taking so much aspirin; she believes this might have led to a blood clot in her leg (patient perspective and cause of illness). Nancy has two sisters who have blood clot problems, and her father did as well. Her husband recently died suddenly of complications from lung cancer (stressor). She has two daughters that she is very close to and gets support from; they are both nurses. Nancy's physical examination is unremarkable except for mild tenderness with palpation. There is no heat, erythema, increased size, or positive Homan's sign. While the signs and symptoms are not clearly pointing to a deep vein thrombosis (DVT), Nancy feels sure this is what is going on. The APN orders Doppler studies, and the test is positive for DVT. Based on MRM, the APN has incorporated the major points of the theory: patient perception and support system and the notion that the patient has the best knowledge of her body and knows when something is wrong. This experience shows how the APN essentially built a model of the patient's world and used this data to promote a positive outcome.

Stress/Adaptation Theories

The term *stress* has infiltrated much of the current scientific and popular literature. The concept of stress has been extensively researched and written about in relation to illness as well as daily life. Theorists have tried to define stress and describe how people deal or "cope" with stress. The most notable of these theorists are Hans Selye, who developed the General Adaptation Syndrome (GAS), and Richard Lazarus and Susan Folkman, who developed the theory of stress, adaptation, and coping. Their research and the resulting theories have influenced studies in nursing, psychology, and medical science.

Selye's General Adaptation Syndrome

Selye has been described as the father of modern stress work (Pearson & Vaughan, 1986). In 1926, as a second-year medical student, Selye observed that patients suffering from diverse diseases seemed to have many signs and symptoms in common (Selye, 1974, 1976). He described this phenomenon as a "syndrome of just being sick" (Selye, 1974) and asserted that in the early stages of disease it is difficult to differentiate between specific diseases because the symptoms are very much alike. This observation stayed with Selye. In 1935, as a young research assistant at McGill University, he observed a pattern of stereotyped reactions that occurred in response to stress while studying the effect of injected hormones on rats (Selye, 1956, 1974). He used the term *stress* to define an orchestrated set of bodily reactions against a noxious stimuli; the reactions were considerable enlargement of the adrenal cortex, atrophy of the lymphatic structures, and development of peptic ulcers (Selye, 1956). He called his conceptualization of this set of bodily reactions the General Adaptation Syndrome, and he published his findings on stress research in his landmark book *The Stress of Life* in 1956.

Major concepts. Stress, as Selye defines it, is not an imposed environmental demand; rather, it is the body's response to imposed demands. Stress is the wear and tear of the body caused by demands upon it (Selye, 1956, 1974). Selye's theory, with its emphasis on the hypothalamic-pituitary-adrenocortical axis, postulates that a person's body responds to stress through a series of nonspecific processes that continue until adaptation occurs or death ensues (Henneman, 1989; Polit & Hungler, 1995).

Stress activates the GAS. Selye (1956) explains that this name was chosen because the syndrome is general, produced only by agents that have a general effect on large portions of the body; adaptive, stimulating defense reactions to aid in the restoration of homeostasis; and a syndrome consisting of individual manifestations that are coordinated and partly dependent on each other. The GAS has three phases: the alarm phase, the phase of adaptation or resistance, and the phase of exhaustion.

The alarm phase occurs when the body shows initial signs of exposure to a stressor (Selye, 1976). The individual's defense forces are mobilized as the person prepares for "fight or flight." The adrenal cortex discharges hormones into the bloodstream to increase metabolism, access energy reserves, and decrease inflammation (Selye, 1956). During this phase, resistance is low, and if the stressor is sufficiently strong, death may result (Selye, 1974, 1976).

The phase of adaptation or resistance occurs when the body starts to show signs of adaptation to the stressor. The bodily signs of the alarm phase disappear, and resistance increases as the individual fights back (Selye, 1976, 1974; Sutterly & Donnelly, 1981). During this phase, the adrenal cortex accumulates an abundant reserve of hormones (Selye, 1956).

If the body is exposed to prolonged stress, the phase of exhaustion may occur. The symptoms are strikingly similar to those of the alarm reaction (Selye, 1956). Adaptation energy is depleted, the body is overwhelmed, the signs of alarm are irreversible, and death may ensue (Selye 1974, 1976; Sutterly & Donnelly, 1981). It is not necessary for all three of the phases of the GAS to develop, only the most severe stress that leads to the phase of exhaustion. Most stressors only produce changes manifesting in the alarm and resistance phases.

Assumptions. According to Selye (1956), it is through the GAS that an individual's body enables one to adjust to the constant changes and stressors occurring around him or her. Selye (1974) asserts that stress is not something to be avoided. It occurs even while an individual is sleeping. In fact, complete freedom from stress is only achieved through death. From Selye's point of view, the stressor itself is immaterial; although stress is a specific syndrome, it is nonspecifically induced (Selye, 1956, 1974). It is the intensity of the demand for adaptation that influences the body's reaction. Individuals differ in their reaction to stress, and the same stimulus or degree of stress may produce diverse reactions in different people. This is attributed to "conditioning factors" that can selectively enhance or inhibit the stress effect (Selye, 1974). These conditioning factors explain why individuals react somewhat differently to stress depending on their acquired characteristics. Conditioning factors may be internal (e.g., genetic predisposition, age, sex) or external (e.g., drug treatment, dietary factors).

Selye's General Adaptation Model and the advanced practice nurse.
Selye's theory may aid in the assessment and treatment of patients. Application of this theory contributes to a holistic view of the individual receiving care. For example, a patient hospitalized in the intensive care unit (ICU) for respiratory distress may develop peptic ulcers during a traumatic and extensive hospital stay as a result of the body's stress response. Many Master of Science in Nursing (MSN) programs utilize stress theory when discussing diseases and their sequelae.

Selye (1974) believes that stress plays a role in the development of every disease. Thus any stressor can lead to the development of disease and poor health, ranging from hypertension to peptic ulcer disease. Theoretically, management of stress may lead to a decreased incidence of some diseases. Many have recognized the importance of stress in the development of ill health when the stress is excessive (Pearson & Vaughan, 1986). This perspective may be helpful to an APN as he or she addresses the management of some illnesses, such as coronary artery disease and anxiety. Selye asserts that it is the individual's reaction to his or her environment that determines the stressor's effect. Thus control of the environment may lead to decreased stress reactions. The nurse often controls the hospital environment of patients. Controlling physiological or psychological stress can impede or exacerbate the body's response.

Lazarus and Folkman's Stress, Appraisal, and Coping
World War I and the Korean War renewed interest in stress research due to the recognition of stress's significance to military combat. In the 1960s, Richard Lazarus, a professor of psychology at the University of California at Berkley, and his colleagues began an effort to study how people react and adapt to stress (Lazarus & Folkman, 1984). Whereas Selye concentrated on the body's reaction to stress, Lazarus focused on the psychological components of stress, mainly appraisal and coping. Susan Folkman, a fellow research psychologist, joined him in this research, and together they published many studies, including the classic book *Stress, Appraisal, and Coping* (Lazarus & Folkman, 1984).

Lazarus and Folkman's theory asserts that there are important differences in how individuals respond to stress based on how stressful the situation is appraised to be or its personal significance. What may be stressful for one person may not be stressful for another. Stressors can range from cataclysmic episodes to daily hassles. The way a person appraises a stressful encounter influences how one copes and emotionally reacts. Although daily hassles may be far less dramatic than major life events, it is the everyday stressors that may be more important in adaptation and health (Lazarus & Folkman, 1984).

Major concepts. Lazarus and Folkman (1984) define psychological stress as "a particular relationship between the person and the environment that is appraised by the person as taxing or exceeding his/her resources and endangering his/her well-being." Their definition of stress takes into account the relationship between the individual and the environment, including the characteristics of the individual and the nature of the environmental event. Their theory emphasizes two major processes as mediators in the person-environment relationship: cognitive appraisal and coping (Lazarus & Folkman, 1984).

Cognitive appraisal is the evaluative process that determines the magnitude of stress an event causes an individual, considering what is at stake for the individual (primary appraisal) and what coping resources and options are available (secondary appraisal) (Folkman & Lazarus, 1980, 1984). Primary and secondary appraisal together influence the degree of stress and the emotional reaction the individual experiences. Appraisal is a potent predictor of coping response. Coping is the effort of the individual to manage the specific internal and external demands of the person-environment relationship and the appraised stress and emotional reactions they illicit (Lazarus & Folkman, 1980, 1984). Coping is a dynamic process involving ongoing appraisal and reappraisal of the person-environment relationship (White, Richter, & Fry, 1992). Coping efforts serve two main functions: the management or alteration of the environment that is the source of stress (problem-focused coping) and the regulation of stressful emotions in an attempt to change the meaning of the event (emotion-focused coping). Problem-focused coping strategies are more appropriate in situations appraised as within one's personal control and amenable to change, whereas emotion-focused coping strategies are more likely utilized when the situation is appraised as overwhelming and beyond one's control (Lazarus & Folkman, 1980, 1984; White et al, 1992). For example, one may use problem-focused coping by dropping a class during a stressful semester. Emotion-focused coping is often used to make life more bearable by avoiding confrontation with reality (e.g., denying a disease by being noncompliant or delaying treatment). Thus inherent to Lazarus and Folkman's stress theory is appraisal of the event and the coping methods utilized.

Assumptions. Intrinsic to Lazarus and Folkman's theory are the following assumptions: (1) coping is bounded by meanings, and (2) coping is a dynamic process. The theory is described as phenomenological; that is, individuals are understood to constitute and be constituted by meanings. When these meanings are disrupted, stress results. Coping is what an individual does to manage the disruption (Marriner-Tomey, 1989). The extent to which a person experiences stress is dependent on the appraised threat to one's meanings. When the threat is perceived to be great, the event may be appraised as extremely stressful, regardless of the availability and effectiveness of resources (Lazarus & Folkman, 1980, 1984; White et al, 1992). Lazarus and Folkman (1980, 1984) also emphasize that coping is a dynamic process. Coping involves the continuous appraisal and reappraisal of the shifting person-environment relationship, with the individual at times relying on one form of coping and at other times relying on another as the significance of the situation is assessed and reassessed.

Stress, appraisal, and coping and the advanced practice nurse. Knowing that an individual's appraisal of stress can affect coping forces nurses to particularize care toward the coping styles and needs assessed. This is also true for the individual and his or her perception of health. How a person perceives or appraises the quality of his or her mental and physical health affects how he or she copes with the stresses of daily living (Polit & Hungler, 1995). Those who feel more in control of their health are more likely to gather information about disease and health maintenance when alerted to possible hazards than those who feel that their health and well-being are beyond their control (Lazarus & Folkman, 1984). Lazarus and Folkman (1984) suggest that there are three ways that coping can influence health: (1) by influencing the frequency, intensity, duration, and patterning of neurochemical stress reactions; (2) by influencing the presence of injurious substances in the body (released in the stress reaction) and their risk to health; and (3) by impeding or promoting health- or illness-related behaviors. Lazarus and Folkman (1984) maintain that some studies of coping suggest that different coping styles influence specific health outcomes (e.g., control of anger and hypertension).

Stress is the consequence of the relationship between the person and the environment. Thus manipulation or alteration of the environment may have a major effect on appraised stress as well as the quality of coping. On the other hand, environmental factors that cannot be modified must be internally dealt with or adapted to. The environment is one of the key elements in evaluating stress.

Rogers' Diffusion of Innovations Theory

The Diffusion of Innovations Theory was developed in the 1970s when it became evident that much of the research supported by government funds was not being used. A think tank of experts in the area of research utilization was convened by the government to evaluate this issue. This group began to develop strategies and ways to examine the process of utilization. In education, a National Diffusion Network was established through the U.S. Department of Education, and a journal called *Knowledge: Creation, Diffusion, Utilization* was founded to publish the works of this think tank.

Major concepts

The Diffusion of Innovations Theory was developed by Rogers as a modification of Lewin's change theory to describe behaviors commonly seen by people when they are engaged in change. There are differences between change and innovation. Change deals with any modification in operations, structure, or ends. Innovation is narrower. Rogers (1983) defines *innovation* as "an idea, practice or object that is perceived as new by an individual or other unit of adoption." The idea or item might not be new but must be considered new by those considering adoption. Thus all innovation is change, but not all change is innovation. Change for an individual occurs over five phases (discussed shortly). Diffusion is the "process by which an innovation is communicated through certain channels over time among the members of a social system. The main elements in diffusion include an innovation, communication channels, time and a social system.

Communication channels include a variety of methods, such as one-to-one communication, communication within a group, or mass media such as books or television. Although mass media is effective in diffusion, interpersonal channels tend to be most effective in adopting an innovation. Such communication is most efficacious when the two people are similar in values, beliefs, and social status.

According to Burns and Grove (1997), time is another important element in understanding the innovation adoption process. There are three factors that influence this process: (1) the timespan from the point at which the person hears about the innovation to the point a decision is made concerning the innovation, (2) the innovativeness of the person or agency that determines the time to achieve adoption, and (3) the number of people within the social system who adopt an innovation within a given period.

Rogers (1983) defines *social system* as "a set of interrelated units that is engaged in joint problem solving to accomplish a common goal." Diffusion occurs within the social system, and the process of diffusion is affected by the structure of the system. The system is affected both by formal leaders (those in positions related to authority and power) and informal leaders. Informal leaders share their opinion with others in the organization through interactions. Change agents are professionals outside the social system who enter it for the purpose of influencing the adoption of innovation within a system. Change agents link the social system (change agency) to the patient system (innovation or change recipient) (Figure 31-3). The change agents assist the innovation flow from the change agency to

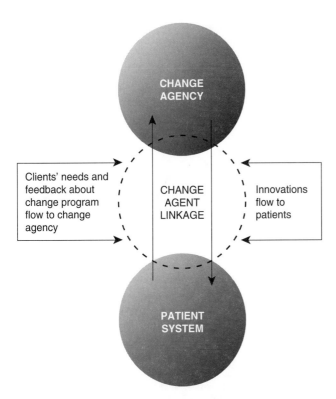

Figure 31-3 Change agents provide linkages between a change agency and a patient system. (Reprinted with permission of the Free Press, a division of Simon and Schuster. From Rogers, E.M. [1983]. *Diffusion of innovations* [3rd ed.]. New York: Free Press.)

the patient system. The patient system provides feedback on the innovation process to the agency. Change agents typically use informal leaders to assist in diffusion campaigns. For example, an APN might make sure that the informal leader of an organization is supportive of a new documentation form being proposed. The APN knows that this person's view is valued by other employees and can help in the diffusion process.

While most people believe that innovation is positive, this is not always the case. Many times, those without power, the poor, and minorities are not considered in the consequences of adopting the innovation. An innovation at one office (e.g., reengineering) may not work at another office.

Stages of the innovation process

Rogers (1983) conceptualizes five stages of the innovation process (depicted in Figure 31-4). These stages are knowledge, persuasion, decision, implementation, and confirmation. The knowledge stage is the first awareness of the existence of an innovation. Knowledge of the innovation can occur in a variety of ways, such as formal communication (e.g., through mass media or publications). Informal communication within an agency also can provide awareness of the innovation. Factors such as previous practice, needs and problems, and norms of the social system can affect the knowledge stage.

Rogers defines *innovativeness* as the "degree to which an individual or unit of adoption is relatively earlier in adopting new ideas than are the other members of a system." As people are exposed to change, they typically adopt one of six behaviors as a response to change based on their degree of innovativeness (shown in Table 31-1). The adopter distribution resembles a normal curve (Figure 31-5). The innovators, early adopters, and laggards are deviated from the mean as would be expected in a normal curve. Knowing this distribution can help if an APN is involved in change within the organization. The early adopters and early majority form a powerful group and can serve to promote change in the late majority. When the behavior of the system is oriented to change, the early adopters tend to be opinion leaders and supportive of change. When the normal behavior of the system is opposed to change, then early adopters tend to be opinion leaders against change, creating barriers against the innovation. During the knowledge phase, the characteristics of a unit need to be examined. Factors such as the socioeconomic variables, personalities, and communication behaviors can influence the innovation process.

The persuasion stage occurs when an individual forms an opinion of the innovation, developing a favorable or unfavorable outlook. There are characteristics of the innovation that determine the likelihood that it will be adopted, as well as the speed of the adoption. First, the *relative advantages* of the innovation need to be determined. In other words, is the innovation better than current practice? *Compatibility* is the degree to which the innovation is compatible with values, processes, past experiences, and priority of needs. *Complexity* is the notion of how complicated or difficult the innovation is to use or understand. *Trialability* is the availability of the innovation to be tried out before full acceptance is needed. *Observability* is the degree to which the results of adoption of the innovation are visible to others; innovations that are more visible are more readily adopted. Communication is less effective via mass media at this stage of the process. People involved in the adopting process want to know the details and ask: Have you used it? How did it work? Did you have problems with it? What are the advantages and disadvantages of using it? Interactions with peers are more likely to influence individuals during this phase and later phases.

A decision occurs when an individual decides to adopt or reject the innovation. Adoption means full acceptance of the innovation and implementation of the ideas in practice. Adoption continues indefinitely or until the evaluation process reveals that there are problems. Rejection is the decision not to adopt the innovation. Rejection can be active, as when after examining the innovation a decision is made to reject it. Rejection can also be passive, as when the innovation is never seriously considered but no one makes a specific decision about it. There might be enough opposition so that a decision is never made. The rate of

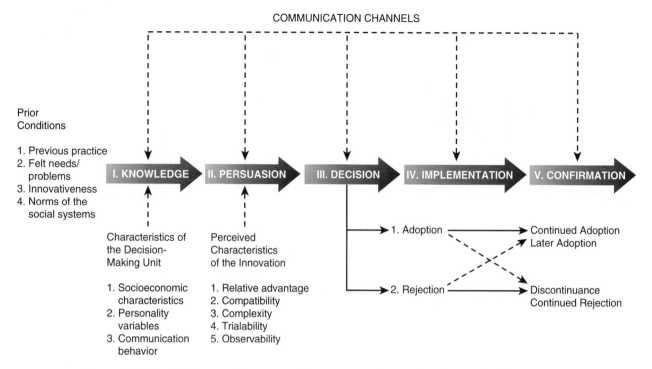

Figure 31-4 A model of states of the innovation-decision process. (Reprinted with permission of the Free Press, a division of Simon and Schuster. From Rogers, E.M. [1995]. *Diffusion of innovations* [4th ed.]. New York: Free Press.)

Table **31-1**	
Categories of Adopters	
BEHAVIOR	**DESCRIPTION**
Innovators	These are enthusiastic individuals who embrace and thrive on change. They are the first ones to adopt the change, usually amid much controversy within the organization. Innovators might even be the change agents that an agency hires to implement an innovation. Innovators can cope with high levels of uncertainty. They tend to be less linked with others in the system and to have less influence on adoption of an innovation within their own system. *Mavericks* might be an appropriate term for them.
Early adopters	These people are open and receptive to ideas, though they are less obsessed with adventure and change. These people tend to be opinion leaders. They rapidly learn about new things, use them, and then serve as role models in their use. In a hospital, early adopters might be the CNSs or educators.
Early majority	These are the largest number of people, those who prefer the status quo but will make a change when they see it is inevitable. They are a little ahead of the "average Joe" in adopting changes. These people are rarely leaders, but they are active followers and will readily follow in the use of a new idea.
Late majority	These people are followers, skeptical of innovation and change. They generally have negative views about change and will only accept it after the majority of people have already accepted it or because of group pressure.
Laggards	These people are the last to adopt changes. They are dedicated to tradition and generally opposed to any form of change. They are very security conscious and often isolated without a strong support system. By the time they adopt an idea, it is no longer considered new.
Rejecters	These people openly resist change and encourage others to oppose it as well. These people are generally covert in their activities and can cause major disruptions within a system, even to the point of sabotaging an innovation.

Data from Rogers, E. (1995). *Diffusion of innovation*. New York: The Free Press; Bushy, A., & Kamphuis, J. (1989). Rogers' adoption model in the implementation of change. *Clinical Nurse Specialist*, 3(4), 188-191; Marquis, B., & Huston, C. (1996). *Leadership and management functions in nursing*. Philadelphia: JB Lippincott; and Burns, N., & Groves, S. (1993). *The practice of nursing research* (2nd ed.). Philadelphia: WB Saunders.

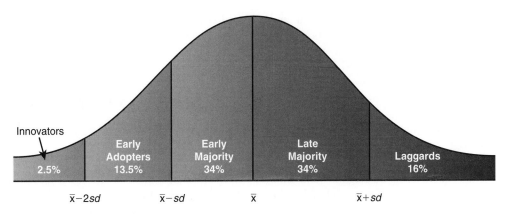

Figure 31-5 Adopter categorization on the basis of innovativeness. (Reprinted with permission of the Free Press, a division of Simon and Schuster. From Rogers, E.M. [1995]. *Diffusion of innovations* [4th ed.]. New York: Free Press.)

adoption is measured by the length of time it takes for the system to adopt the innovation. At the beginning, diffusion is slow, with only innovators accepting the innovation. As more and more people accept the innovation, the length of time decreases and the diffusion rate increases. When most people have adopted the innovation, the rate of diffusion once again decreases as the number of people remaining who have not accepted the innovation become fewer and fewer.

Implementation occurs when a person uses the innovation. Depending on the complexity of the innovation, an implementation plan may need to be developed, especially if it is critical that all people adopt the innovation for use exactly as it was developed. In other situations, it is less critical that all people use the innovation in exactly the same manner, so some people reinvent and modify the innovation to meet their own needs. Uncertainty is one of the repercussions of innovation; there is not a specific way to predict exactly what the outcomes will be when the innovation is adopted. However, information and education reduce uncertainty.

During the confirmation phase, the effectiveness of the innovation is evaluated. Confirmation follows when a person seeks the opinions of others regarding the innovation. It is possible that the person may change his or her decision based on the feedback. The innovation can be discontinued because a better innovation came along, or disenchantment may occur when the user is dissatisfied with its outcome.

Rogers' theory can be used in multiple situations. Haller, Reynolds, and Horsley (1979) suggest the use of this framework to facilitate implementation of procedures. Coyle and Sokop (1990) looked at innovation behavior among nurses. Furthermore, several projects were undertaken using Rogers' theory as a way to improve the adoption of innovations in nursing practice. These were the Western Interstate Commission for Higher Education (WICHE) nursing research development project, the Conduct and Utilization of Research in Nursing (CURN)

project, and the Nursing Child Assessment Satellite Training (NCAST) project. In these projects, nurse researchers used Rogers' theory as a framework to design and implement strategies for utilization.

The WICHE project addressed research utilization in nursing and developed the first model for utilization of nursing research. However, they were limited by the number of clinical studies that could be implemented in practice (Krueger, 1978, Krueger, Nelson, & Wolanin, 1978). The CURN project was a 5-year project to increase the utilization of nursing research findings by disseminating findings and encouraging research that could be directly implemented in practice. Research utilization was visualized as an organizational process rather than one that just applied to individuals, and 10 areas were identified that had been sufficiently researched to warrant implementation in the clinical areas. A year after implementing the process, significant differences were found in terms of research utilization in the experimental groups.

The NCAST project was developed and implemented for individual nurses. Nurses were taught about child assessment techniques, and of these nurses, 85% adopted the assessment technique; this high adoption rate continued for at least 4 years after the program was initiated. Furthermore, the assessment procedures are still taught today.

Diffusion of Innovations Theory and the advanced practice nurse

There are a number of implications for education when considering Rogers' Diffusion of Innovations Theory. First, the theory can be used as a part of teaching nursing research and looking at the utilization of research in practice. According to Burns (1993), students need a background in utilization theory and guidance in developing and implementing research utilization projects.

Second, the theory can be taught as part of the larger topic of change. Students should become familiar with one of the theories of change, such as that of Lewin, Lippitt,

Havelock, or Rogers, because they are so useful and applicable in advanced practice. For example, Lori is an APN at Redbud Community Health Center. She is the chairman of the medical records committee. The committee wants to implement several flowsheet-type documentation forms. Input is sought from all APNs and physicians and incorporated into the new forms, and using Rogers' theory helps the committee plan its strategies to get the forms adopted. First they conduct a literature review to find any research that supports the use of flowsheet documentation in terms of accuracy and time saving. They also obtain the statistics collected by the quality assurance committee that indicate how well the practices in the Center are doing in terms of documenting the care provided. Lori and her colleagues on the committee all test the flow sheets ahead of time and record cycle times to indicate how much time the form takes to complete. The committee also evaluates the personality variables of each office. Several people are identified as innovators and early adopters; these people are targeted as opinion leaders and will be approached as key people in the process. Probable laggards or rejecters are also identified, and their influence on the process is considered. The committee discusses the best way to communicate with all the APNs and physicians. They decide to announce the development of the forms in the monthly provider meeting. They know that in the knowledge phase, mass media is an effective means of communication. This choice also means that the minutes of the monthly meeting will contain information about the forms.

During the persuasion phase, each of the committee members targets other providers and makes contact with them. The committee members stress the advantages of the proposed system, including how compatible the forms are with the others used within the system, how the forms are simple, and how they can be tested before implementation. Communication during this phase is one on one, with the committee members sharing their experiences with the forms.

During the decision phase the providers decide whether they accept or reject the forms. The flow sheets are formally voted and approved at the monthly meeting. Several APNs and physicians comment that after being able to test the forms, they are much more likely to adopt them. During the implementation phase, all committee members are available for assistance or comments. The committee conducts spot checks to see how well the forms are being utilized. One office put the new forms in all charts and has a 100% adoption rate. Another office has one physician who loves the forms and uses them consistently, while her colleague does not use the forms at all; this is not surprising as he does not use any of the forms developed previously.

The evaluation phase reveals that most of the APNs and physicians like the forms. The committee begins collecting data to determine how well the flowsheets are being utilized. After a 6-month trial, the committee plans to have data concerning its use and present the information in the monthly provider meeting.

IMPLICATIONS FOR MSN EDUCATION AND ADVANCED PRACTICE

The utility of a theory is reflected in its congruence with the philosophical perspectives of the discipline, as well as how well it can guide practice and research. For a theory to be used in practice, APNs must have a working knowledge about the basics of the theory, the underlying assumptions of the theory, and how the theory can be used in practice and research. This means that schools of nursing should include theoretical content in the curricula of APNs. Ideally, it also means that APNs will see the use of theory in practice by their preceptors and faculty. For APN students to see how a theoretical model can be translated into practice is very helpful and increases the chances that the particular theory (or another theory) will be used. In programs where theory is not emphasized, it is less likely that the use of theory in practice will be an important component of practice.

The ultimate outcome or objective of including theory in APN curricula is the development of theory-guided, evidence-based reflective practice. This type of practice helps address the historical gap between research and practice. Meleis (1997) states, "A discipline's progress is measured by its theoretical developments and the ability of its members to raise significant questions, to solve central problems, and to answer questions that have social significance." According to Walker and Redman (1999), grand theories allow nursing to define itself, and development needs to continue in this regard. Walker and Redman go on to say that theory-guided practice is the future of nursing. Ray (1998) suggests that midrange theory and its application may be a new avenue to investigate. The use of midrange and related theories in APN practice would help contribute to reflective practice. Reflective practice incorporates nursing process skills and critical thinking; multiple ways of knowing; philosophy, research and theory as the basis for practice; and self-corrective reasoning (Walker & Redman, 1999).

Barnum's (1990) concerns for borrowed theory can guide the determination of inquiry priorities. Nursing theory should be examined for: (1) misinterpretations of the original theory, resulting in its misapplication, (2) continued use of discredited non-nursing theory, and (3) inappropriate matches with nursing context and nursing intent. Findings from this examination can guide nursing theory development. A metaanalysis of nursing theory to identify the most frequently used sources of borrowed theory should also be conducted. Given the identification of these sources, a philosophical inquiry can then be conducted to identify what these sources say about nursing and advanced practice. Research should also be conducted to identify which other disciplines are informed by these same related theories. How do other disciplines integrate these related theories into their discipline?

PRIORITIES FOR RESEARCH

Kitson (1997) believes that true reflective practice is when nursing learns that "discriminating between knowledge based on opinion and practice, as opposed to scientific evidence, is an important stage in the development of a professional group." While some nurse scholars believe that evidence-based research is the biggest sell-out for nursing and focuses only on the medical model, others disagree. When considering the definition of reflective practice, the components of self-corrective reasoning and critical thinking are included. Self-corrective reasoning includes the ability to take a theoretically based look at practice, evaluate the values and needs of patients based on that theory, and be realistic enough to look at the specific outcomes of one's practice. This means being able to define the outcomes of APN practice, both in terms of its disease focus and its economic focus. To ignore this vital piece of research is like a person ignoring a leg; both legs are needed for best functioning. The same is true with theoretically focused, evidence-based reflective practice. This section presents research that provides information for APNs to see utilization of theory in practice. Information is presented by which APNs can make self-corrections as needed based on the research findings.

Kolcaba's Theory of Comfort

The construction of Kolcaba's theory was the result of inductive and deductive methods applied during different stages of theory development. This midrange theory is evaluated from the perspective of recipients of care. That is, do recipients experience enhanced comfort as a result of nursing interventions? As a result of nursing care, are they strengthened to engage in subsequent HSBs? The theory is congruent with outcome-based practice and is an example of a new orientation for theories—from an emphasis on what nurses do to an emphasis on patient outcomes (Nolan & Grant, 1992). The Theory of Comfort is focused on what patients want and need from nursing. If nurses deliver what patients want and need, recipients of care will more readily identify and value nursing as a key to their health.

The taxonomy structure of comfort has been developed. The next step in the advancement of this theory is the development of objective and subjective indicators for comfort in various nursing specialties. For example, for a patient who has a closed head injury, the patient can not

say he or she is uncomfortable, but the APN knows that he or she is because restlessness, hostility, or withdrawal is visible. Subjective indicators are helpful for the patient to complete on a pretest/posttest basis to see if nursing interventions have met the patient's comfort needs. There are times when patients can not tell anyone that they are uncomfortable. In such cases, an APN must be able to use objective and subjective clues to identify the patient's discomfort. As the midrange theory of comfort is further developed and researched, APNs will have another tool in their arsenal to address patient concerns.

Uncertainty-in-Illness Theory

The concepts and constructs of this theory are well developed and have enabled viable research questions that have helped refine the theory. Since its inception, instrumentation has been developed and refined (Mishel, 1981, 1983), various aspects of the model have undergone testing (Mishel & Braden, 1987), and related theoretical associations have been tested (Mishel, Padilla, Grant, & Sorenson, 1991). Uncertainty has been examined in men with prostate cancer (Germino, Mishe, Belyea, Harris, Ware, & Mohler, 1998); adolescents with cancer (Neville, 1998); people with human immunodeficiency virus (HIV) infection (Santacroce, 2000), life-threatening arrhythmias (Carroll, Hamilton, & McGovern, 1999), heart failure (Winters, 1999), asthma (Sexton, Calcasola, Bottomley, & Funk, 1999), and breast cancer (Deane & Degner, 1998; Mast, 1998); and ventilator patients (Wunderlich, Perry, Lavin, & Katz, 1999). Ongoing research among diverse populations and across varied settings will refine the theory and more definitively delineate its scope and credibility for nursing practice. Some preliminary implications from the research indicates that there may be ethnic differences in how African-American and Caucasian males respond psychologically to prostate cancer. Germino et al (1998) point out that much of the education related to prostate cancer is based on Caucasian individuals. However, the differing cultural perspectives of patients and their families influence the uncertainty that is experienced during illness.

Santacroce (2000) looked at the uncertainty mothers felt when taking their children in for HIV testing. The results suggested that when a mother has HIV, health care providers can address her needs and HIV status during the baby's screening visits. Carroll et al (1999) conducted a study looking at uncertainty among men and women with life-threatening arrhythmias. The subjects were tested before treatment and 6 months after treatment with an implantable defibrillator. While the patients' perception of health status improved, the improvements did not appear to translate into improvements in quality of life and the psychological state, as these were lower 6 months after the arrhythmias. This study has implications for APNs in caring for not only patients with arrhythmias, but people with other diseases as well. Most APNs would guess that after an illness has been successfully treated, patients would perceive their health as better, and their spirits would rise accordingly. The Carroll et al (1999) study indicates that this may not be the case. The notion of uncertainty is still present and affecting patients, and APNs need to consider this. Continued research with the uncertainty model will help identify the role of uncertainty in both acute and chronic illnesses.

Modeling and Role-Modeling

The application of components of MRM have been studied in patients ranging from newborns to older adults and in settings ranging from critical care to the home. The theory has been applied when patients could not communicate, as in intensive care settings, cases of prespeech development, and cases of dementia; in these instances, the modeling of a patient's world must be done through others' descriptions and keen observations. In this time of self-care demand and consumer-focused health care delivery, MRM provides a useful and satisfying basis for holistic advanced practice. Finally, MRM theory has a scientific foundation, with a developing body of knowledge consistent with midrange theory. It is this level of theory that provides a focus that may actually guide practice (Baas et al, 1994; Sappington & Kelley, 1996; Acton et al, 1997; Liehr & Smith, 1999).

Stress/Adaptation Theories

Selye's influence can be seen in nursing models. For example, his theory was very instrumental in forming Roy's Adaptation Model (Randell, Tedrow, & Van Landinghan, 1982), and some nurse researchers have used Selye's GAS as their contextual framework. Henneman (1989) used the GAS to explore the effect of direct nursing contact on the stress response of patients being weaned from mechanical ventilation. Cahill (1998) did the same while examining the differences in cortisol levels of women with low symptom patterns of premenstrual symptoms versus those with magnified patterns of premenstrual symptoms. Selye's influence is apparent in both research and practice. Selye's GAS theory is one of the most widely accepted stress theories. Its influence can be seen throughout the medical and nursing sciences and constitutes an essential element of a holistic view of patient care.

Like their colleague Selye, Lazarus and Folkman's stress theory has had an immense effect on nursing theory, practice, and research. Their studies and works are cited throughout nursing literature. Their theory's practical application aids in the assessment and implementation phases of the nursing process. Clearly, appraisal and coping influence how a person manages and reacts to disease. Consideration of these principles emphasizes the importance of individualized nursing care and implicates the

application of holistic principles. Some researchers have used Lazarus and Folkman's theory as their conceptual framework. White et al (1992) used their theory when examining coping and social support in relation to adaptation to chronic illness. Farran (1997) considered Lazarus and Folkman's theory when exploring theoretical perspectives concerning the positive aspects of caring for older adults with dementia, and Hansell, Hughes, Caliandro, Russo, Budin, Hartman, & Hernandez (1998) also drew on their work when investigating stress, coping, and social support among caregivers of children with acquired immune deficiency syndrome (AIDS). For APNs who work in an acute care setting, research using MRM and Lazarus and Folkman's theory with ventilator-dependent patients might be relevant (Lowry & Anderson, 1993). Four subjects who were patients in an ICU participated in Lowry and Anderson's pilot study. Factors that were identified as being important to the patients included social support, fear of being ventilated, and hope. The notion that the ventilator was a cause of stress confirms findings of other research, as does the realization that as a patient grows accustomed to the machine, fear decreases. The ventilator was perceived as an extrapersonal stressor. Knowing the results of stress on the body assists APNs to anticipate problems or prevent problems from occurring. Thus Lazarus and Folkman's work has influenced nursing theory and research and can be integrated into advanced practice.

Rogers' Diffusion of Innovations Theory

Rogers' Diffusion of Innovations Theory has great applicability for use in research. Coyle and Sokop (1990) used the framework in their study of nursing adoption behaviors, while Stetler and DiMaggio used it to evaluate research utilization among clinical nurse specialists (CNSs). Landrum (1998a, 1998b) looked at marketing innovations for nurses, while Brett (1989) and Maher (1992) evaluated the adoption of information systems.

A number of researchers used Rogers' theory as a basis for evaluating nursing practice; these researchers include Barker (1990); Carter (1995); Gingiss, Gottlieb, and Brink (1994); Joyce, Keck, and Gerkensmeyer (1999); Pearcey and Draper (1996); Smith, Zhang, and Colwell (1996); Taylor-Piliae (1998); and Winter (1988). A frequent use for Rogers' theory was to look at research utilization by nurses (Dabbs, 1992; Berggren, 1996; Stiefel, 1996; Youngstrom, 1996; Beaumont, 1997). Cline (1996) used the theory as the framework for her research concerning nurse practitioner (NP) acceptance by the consumer. She conducted her study at a Midwestern university to determine how the employees of the university perceived NPs. The subjects completed a questionnaire identifying their perceptions about NPs and also rated themselves in terms of adoption of innovation behaviors. Schulte (1996) conducted a similar study with baccalaureate graduates.

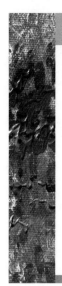

Suggestions for Further Learning

- Review Bothamley, J. (1993) *Dictionary of theories.* Detroit, MI: Gale Research International Limited. Select two theories that are not familiar and examine them for applicability to advanced practice. Are any specific nursing theories included in this text? Why or why not?
- Get the article: Brown, S. (1998). A framework for advanced practice nursing. *Journal of Professional Nursing,* 14(3), 157-164. What types of theories does Brown assert should be used in advanced practice?
- Go to Comfort Line at uakron.edu/~kolcaba.
- Get the article: Kolcaba, K. (1991). A taxonomic structure for the concept comfort. *Image: Journal of Nursing Scholarship, 23*(4), 237-240. What guidelines does this article provide in terms of research using this theory?
- Get the article: Whall, A. (1993). Let's get rid of all nursing theory. *Nursing Science Quarterly,* 6(4), 164-165. What is your reaction to this article? Do you agree or disagree with the author's premise?
- Cody (1999) disagrees that midrange theory such as that described in Good, M., & Moore, S. (1996). Clinical practice guidelines as a new source of middle-range theory: focus on acute pain. *Nursing Outlook, 44,* 74-79 contributes to nursing science. Do you agree or disagree?
- Go to the discussion board on the MRM website at mrm.globalmax.com. It addresses how to implement MRM theory into curriculum.

Rogers' theory appears to have great relevance and applicability for nursing research. APNs have the opportunity to use this theory in practice and to evaluate its effectiveness.

DISCUSSION QUESTIONS

These questions can be used to promote critical thinking and encourage discussion.

1. Review the nursing theory descriptions in Chapter 30. Identify non-nursing theories that influenced the development of the nursing theories or models. Identify non-nursing theories that have largely influenced nursing education and practice. How might this affect your future practice?
2. Consider the perception that the work of advanced practice is not uniquely nursing but rather reflects an overlap between medicine and nursing. What non-nursing theories hold increased relevance for APNs? Do any nursing theories lose currency in light of this overlap of practice with medicine?
3. Describe how you might use Rogers' Diffusion of Innovation Theory in your practice.
4. Can nursing theory serve as a source for borrowed theory for other practice disciplines? Which disciplines do you believe would benefit from integrating nursing theory into their body of knowledge? Why?
5. Should nursing use non-nursing theories as a basis for practice? Why or why not?

REFERENCES/BIBLIOGRAPHY

Acton, G.A., Irvin, B.L., Jensen, B.A., Hopkins, B.A., & Miller, E.W. (1997). Explicating middle-range theory through methodological diversity. *Advances in Nursing Science, 19*(3), 78-85.

Acton, G.J. (1997). Affiliated-individuation as a mediator of stress and burden in care givers of adults with dementia. *Journal of Holistic Nursing, 15*(4), 336-357.

Aikens, C. (1908). Making the patient comfortable. *Canadian Nurse and Hospital Review, 4*(9), 422-424.

Baas, L.S. (1992). The relationship among self care knowledge, self care resources, activity level and life satisfaction in persons three to six months after a myocardial infarction (Dissertation University Microfilms No. 9225512). *Dissertation Abstracts International, 53.*

Baas, L.S., Beery, T.A., Fontana, J.A., & Wagoner, L. (1999). An exploratory study of developmental growth in adults with heart failure. *Journal of Holistic Nursing, 17*(2), 117-138.

Baas, L.S., Curl, E., Hertz, J., & Robinson, K. (1994). Innovative approaches to theory based measurement: modeling and role-modeling research. *Advances in Nursing Science Series: Advances in Methods of Inquiry for Nursing, 5,* 147-159.

Baas, L.S., Fontana, J.A., & Bhat, G. (1997). Relationship between self care resources and the quality of life of persons with heart failure. *Progress in Cardiovascular Nursing, 12*(10), 25-38.

Barker, E. (1990). Use of diffusion of innovation model for agency consultation. *Clinical Nurse Specialist, 4*(3), 163-166.

Barnfather, J.S. (1990). An overview of the ability to mobilize coping resources related to basic needs. In H.C. Erickson & C. Kinney (Eds.), *Modeling and role-modeling: theory, practice and research* (pp. 156-169). Austin: Society for the Advancement of Modeling and Role-Modeling.

Barnfather, J.S., Swain, M.A., & Erickson, H. (1989). Construct validity of an aspect of the coping process: potential adaptation to stress. *Issues in Mental Health Nursing, 10,* 23-40.

Barnum, B.J.S. (1990). Nursing theory: analysis, application, evaluation. Glenview, IL: Scott, Foresman and Company.

Beaumont, E. (1997). *Dissemination of research-based knowledge among home care nurses: a Q methodology study* (Dissertation UMI PUZ9728471). Chicago, IL: University of Illinois at Chicago.

Beery, T.A., & Baas, L.S. (1996). Medical devices and attachment: holistic healing in an age of invasive technology. *Issues in Mental Health Nursing, 17*(3), 233-243.

Benner, P. (1984). *From novice to expert.* Menlo Park, CA: Addison-Wesley.

Berggren, A. (1996). Swedish midwives' awareness of attitudes to and use of selected research findings. *Journal of Advanced Nursing, 23*(3), 462-470.

Blegen, M., & Tripp-Reimer, T. (1997). Implications of nursing taxonomies for middle range theory development. *Advances in Nursing Science, 19*(3), 37-49.

Bouve, L., Rozmus, C., & Giordano, P. (1999). Preparing parents for their child's transfer from the PICU to the pediatric floor. *Applied Nursing Research, 12*(3), 114-120.

Bowlby, J. (1980). *Attachment and loss: Vol. 3. Loss, sadness, and depression.* New York: Basic Books.

Brett, J. (1989). Organizational integrative mechanisms and adoption of innovations by nurses. *Nursing Research, 38*(2), 105-110.

Burns, N., & Grove, S. (1993). *The practice of nursing research* (2nd ed.). Philadelphia: WB Saunders.

Burns, N., & Grove, S. (1997). *The practice of nursing research* (3rd ed). Philadelphia: WB Saunders.

Bushey, A., & Kamphuis, J. (1989). Rogers' adoption model in the implementation of change. *Clinical Nurse Specialist, 3*(4), 188-191.

Bushey, A., & Kamphuis, J. (1993). Response to innovation: behavioral patterns. *Nursing Management, 24*(3), 62-64.

Cahill, C. (1998). Differences in cortisol, as stress hormone, in women with turmoil-type premenstrual symptoms. *Nursing Research, 47*(5), 278-284.

Cameron, B. (1993). The nature of comfort to hospitalized medical surgical patients. *Journal of Advanced Nursing, 18,* 424-387.

Campbell, C. (1984). *Nursing diagnoses and interventions in nursing practice* (2nd ed). New York: Wiley & Sons.

Carpenito, L. (1987). *Nursing diagnosis: application to clinical practice* (3rd ed.). Philadelphia: JB Lippincott.

Carroll, D., Hamilton, G., & McGovern, B. (1999). Changes in health status and quality of life and the impact of uncertainty in patients who survive life threatening arrhythmias. *Heart and Lung, 28*(4), 251-260.

Carter, J. (1995). *Implementation of the Nursing Interventions Classifications in five clinical sites* (Dissertation UMI PUZ9536177). Iowa City, IA: University of Iowa.

Chin, P., & Kramer, M. (1995). *Theory and nursing* (4th ed.). St. Louis: Mosby.

Cline, J. (1996). *Public perception of nurse practitioners* (Unpublished Master's thesis). Highland Heights, KY: Northern Kentucky University.

Cody, W. (1999). Middle range theories: do they foster the development of nursing science? *Nursing Science Quarterly, 12*(1), 9-13.

Coyle, L., & Sokop, A. (1990). Innovation adoption behavior among nurses. *Nursing Research, 39*(3), 176-180.

Curl, E.D. (1992). Hope in the elderly: exploring the relationship between psychosocial developmental residual and hope (Dissertation University Microfilms No. 92-25, 559). *Dissertation Abstracts International, 53,* 1782B.

Dabbs, C. (1992). *Baccalaureate nursing faculty utilization of nursing research in curricula* (Dissertation UMI PUZ9314460). St. Louis: St. Louis University.

Darling-Fischer, C., & Leidy, N. (1988). Measuring Eriksonian development of the adult: the modified Erikson Psychosocial Stage Inventory. *Psychological Reports, 62,* 747-754.

Deane, K., & Degner, L. (1998). Information needs, uncertainty and anxiety in women who had a breast biopsy with benign outcome. *Cancer Nursing, 21*(2), 117-126.

Donahue, P. (1989). *Nursing: the finest art* (Master prints). St. Louis: Mosby.

Dossey, B.M. (1998). *Core curriculum for holistic nursing.* Rockville, MD: Aspen Publishers.

Engel, G.S. (1962). *Psychological development in health and disease.* Philadelphia: WB Saunders.

Erickson, H.C. (1988). Modeling and role-modeling: Ericksonian techniques applied to physiological problems. In J. Zeig & S. Lankton (Eds.), *Developing Ericksonian therapy: state of the art.* New York: Brunner/Mazel.

Erickson, H.C. (1990a). Theory based practice. In H.C. Erickson & C. Kinney (Eds.), *Modeling and role-modeling: theory, practice and research* (pp. 1-27). Austin, TX: Society for the Advancement of Modeling and Role-Modeling.

Erickson, H.C. (1990b). Self-care knowledge: an exploratory study. In H.C. Erickson & C. Kinney (Eds.), *Modeling and role-modeling: theory, practice and research* (pp. 178-202). Austin, TX: Society for the Advancement of Modeling and Role-Modeling.

Erickson, H. C. (1998). Nurse healers in education: Helen Erickson. In L. Keegan & B.M. Dossey (Eds.), *Profiles of nurse healers* (pp. 117-122). Albany NY: Delmar.

Erickson, H.C., & Swain, M.A.P. (1982). A model for assessing potential adaptation to stress. *Research in Nursing and Health, 5,* 93-101.

Erickson, H.C., & Swain, M.A.P. (1990). Mobilizing self-care resources: a nursing intervention for hypertension. *Issues in Mental Health Nursing, 11,* 217-235.

Erickson, H.C., Tomlin, E., & Swain, M.A. (1983). *Modeling and role-modeling: theory and paradigm for nursing.* Lexington, SC: Pine Press of Lexington.

Erickson, M.E, Caldwell-Gwin, J.A., Carr, L.A., Harmon, B.K., Hartman, K., Jarlsberg, C.A., McCormick, J., & Noone, S. (1998). Helen C. Erickson, Evelyn M. Tomlin, Mary Ann P. Swain: modeling and role-modeling. In A. Marriner-Tomey & M.A. Allingood, (1998). *Nursing theorists and their works* (4th ed). St. Louis: Mosby.

Erikson E. (1968). *Identity, youth, and crisis.* New York: WW Norton.

Farran, C. (1997). Theoretical perspectives concerning positive aspects of caring for elderly persons with dementia: stress/adaptation and existentialism. *The Gerontologist, 37*(2), 250-256.

Frisch, N.C., & Bowman, S.S. (1995). Helen C. Erickson, Evelyn M. Tomlin, and Mary Ann P. Swain. In J. George (Ed.), *Nursing theories: the base for professional nursing practice.* (4th ed.). Norwalk, CT: Appleton & Lange.

Funk, S., Tornquist, E., & Champagne, M. (1989a). Application and evaluation of the dissemination model. *Western Journal of Nursing Research, 11*(4), 486-491.

Funk, S., Tornquist, E., & Champagne, M. (1989b). A model for improving the dissemination of nursing research. *Western Journal of Nursing Research, 11*(3), 361-367.

George, J.B. (1995). *Nursing theories: the base for professional nursing practice* (4th ed.). Norwalk, CT: Appleton & Lange.

Germino, B., Mishel, M., Belyea, M., Harris, L., Ware, A., & Mohler, J. (1998). Uncertainty in prostate cancer: ethnic and family patterns. *Cancer Practice, 6*(2), 107-113.

Gingiss, Gottlieb, & Brink, S. (1994). Measuring cognitive characteristics associated with adoption and implementation of health innovation in schools. *American Journal of Health Promotion, 8*(4), 294-301.

Glazer, G., & Pressler, J. (1989). Schlotfeldt's Health Seeking Nursing Model. In J. Fitzpatrick & A. Whall (Eds.), *Conceptual models of nursing: analysis and application* (pp. 241-253). Norwalk, CT: Appleton & Lange.

Goodnow, M. (1935). *The technique of nursing.* Philadelphia: WB Saunders.

Haller, K., Reynolds, M., & Horsley, J. (1979). Developing research based innovation protocols: process, criteria and issues. *Research in Nursing and Health, 2*(1), 45-51.

Hamilton, J. (1989). Comfort and the hospitalized chronically ill. *Journal of Gerontological Nursing, 15*(4), 28-33.

Hansell, P., Hughes, C., Caliandro, G., Russo, P., Budin, W., Hartman, B., & Hernandez, O. (1998). The effect of a social support boosting intervention on stress, coping, and social support in caregivers of children with HIV/AIDS. *Nursing Research, 47*(2), 79-86.

Harmer, B. (1926). *Methods and principles of teaching the principles and practice of nursing.* New York: MacMillan.

Havelock, R., (1973). *The change agent's guide to innovation in education.* Englewood Cliffs, NJ: Educational Technology Publications.

Henneman, E. (1989). Effect of nursing contact on the stress response of patients being weaned from mechanical ventilation. *Heart & Lung, 18*(5), 483-489.

Hertz, J. (1996). Conceptualization of perceived enactment of autonomy in elderly. *Issues in Mental Health Nursing, 17*(3), 261-273.

Hickey, M. (1990). The role of the clinical nurse specialist in the research utilization process. *Clinical Nurse Specialist, 4*(2), 93-96.

Horsley, J., Crane, J., & Bingle, J. (1978). Research utilization as an organizational process. *Journal of Nursing Administration, 8*(7), 4-6.

Horsley, J., Crane, J., Crabtree, K., & Wood, D. (1983). *Using research to improve nursing practice* (CURN Project). New York: Grune & Stratton.

Hunt, M. (1987). The process of translating research into nursing practice. *Journal of Advanced Nursing, 12*(1), 101-110.

Irvin, B.L., & Acton, G. (1996). Stress mediation in care givers of cognitively impaired adults: theoretical model testing. *Nursing Research, 45*(3), 160-166.

Joyce, B., Keck, J., & Gerkensmeyer, J. (1999). Evaluating the implementation of a pain management flow sheet. *Journal of Pediatric Nursing, 14*(5), 304-312.

Keegan, L., & Dossey, B.M. (1998). *Profiles of nurse healers.* Albany, NY: Delmar.

King, D., Barnard, K., & Hoehn, R. (1981). Disseminating the results of nursing research. *Nursing Outlook, 29*(3), 164-169.

Kinney, C. K. (1990). Facilitating growth and development: a paradigm case for modeling and role-modeling. *Issues in Mental Health Nursing, 11,* 375-395.

Kinney, C.K., & Erickson, H.C. (1990). Modeling the client's world: a way to holistic care. *Issues in Mental Health Nursing, 11,* 93-108.

Kitson, A. (1997). Using evidence to demonstrate the value of nursing. *Nursing Standard, 11*(28), 34-39.

Kolcaba, K. (1991). A taxonomic structure for the concept comfort. *Image: Journal of Nursing Scholarship, 23*(4), 237-240.

Kolcaba, K. (1992). Holistic comfort: Operationalizing the construct as a nurse-sensitive outcome. *Advances in Nursing Science, 15*(1), 1-10.

Kolcaba, K. (1994). A theory of holistic comfort for nursing. *Journal of Advanced Nursing, 19,* 1178-1184.

Kolcaba, K. (1995). Comfort as process and product, merged in holistic nursing art. *Journal of Holistic Nursing, 13*(2), 117-131.

Kolcaba, K., & Fisher, E. (1996). A holistic perspective on comfort care as an advance directive. *Critical Care Nursing Quarterly, 18*(4), 66-76.

Kolcaba, K., & Fox, C. (1999). The effects of guided imagery on comfort of women with early stage breast cancer undergoing radiation therapy. *Oncology Nursing Forum, 26*(1), 67-72.

Kolcaba, K., and Kolcaba, R. (1991). An analysis of the concept of comfort. *Journal of Advanced Nursing, 16*(1), 1301-1310.

Kolcaba, R. (1997). The primary holisms in nursing. *Journal of Advanced Nursing, 25,* 290-296.

Krueger, J. (1978). Utilization of nursing research. *Journal of Nursing Administration, 8*(1), 6-9.

Krueger, J., Nelson, A., & Wolanin, M. (1978). *Nursing research: development, collaboration and utlization.* Germantown, MD: Aspen Publishers.

Landrum, B. (1998a). Marketing innovations to nurses, part 1: how people adopt innovations. *Journal of Wound, Ostomy, and Continence Nursing, 25*(4), 194-199.

Landrum, B. (1998b). Marketing innovations to nurses, part 2: marketing's role in the adoption of innovations. *Journal of Wound, Ostomy, and Continence Nursing, 25*(5), 227-232.

Lazarus, R., & Folkman, S. (1980). An analysis of coping in a middle aged community sample. *Journal of Health and Social Behavior, 21*(9), 219-239.

Lazarus, R., & Folkman, S. (1984). *Stress, appraisal, and coping.* New York: Springer.

Lenz, E., Pugh, L., Milligan, R., Gift, A., & Suppe, F. (1997). The middle range of unpleasant symptoms: an update. *Advances in Nursing Science, 19*(3), 14-27.

Lewin, K. (1951). *Field theory in social science.* New York: Harper and Row.

Liehr, P., & Smith, M.J. (1999). Middle range theory: spinning research and practice to create knowledge for the new millennium. *Advances in Nursing Science, 21*(4), 81-91.

Lippitt, R., Watson, J., & Westley, B. (1958). *The dynamics of planned change.* New York: Harcourt, Brace, and World.

Lowry, L., & Anderson, B. (1993). Neuman's framework and ventilator dependency: a pilot study. *Nursing Science Quarterly, 6*(4), 195-200.

Lutjens, L., & Tiffany, C. (1994). Evaluating planned change theories. *Nursing Management, 94*, 38-42.

MacLean, T. (1992). Influence of psychosocial development and life events on the health practices of adults. *Issues in Mental Health Nursing, 13*, 403-414.

Maher, M. (1992). *Selected factors influencing the implementation of a computerized nursing care plan system* (Dissertation UMI PUZ9222134). Buffalo, NY: State University of New York at Buffalo.

Marquis, B., & Huston, C. (1996). *Leadership and management functions in nursing* (2nd ed.). Philadelphia: JB Lippincott.

Marriner-Tomey, A. (1989). *Nursing theorists and their work* (2nd ed.). St. Louis: Mosby.

Marriner-Tomey, A., & Alligood, M.A. (1998). *Nursing theorists and their works* (4th ed.). St. Louis: Mosby.

Martin, E., Oaks. L., Taussig, K., & Vanderstraten, A. (1997). AIDS: knowledge and discrimination in inner city. In G. Downey and J. Dummit (Eds.), *Cybers and Citadel: antropological interventions in emergency sciences and technology* (pp. 50-65). Sante Fe, NM: Society of American Research.

Maslow, A.H. (1968). *Toward a psychology of being.* New York: VanNostrand Reinhold.

Mast M. (1995). Adult uncertainty in illness: a critical review of research. *Scholarly Inquiry for Nursing Practice, 9*(1), 3-24.

Mast, M. (1998). Survivors of breast cancer: illness trajectory, positive reappraisal, and emotional distress. *Oncology Nursing Forum, 25*(3), 555-562.

McIlveen, K., & Morse, J. (1995). The role of comfort in nursing care: 1900-1980. *Clinical Nursing Research, 4*(2), 127-148.

Meleis, A.I. (1997). *Theoretical nursing: development & progress* (3rd ed.). Philadelphia: Lippincott, Wilkins, and Williams.

Miller, S.H. (1986). The relationship between psychosocial development and coping ability among disabled teenagers ((University Microfilms No. 87-02, 793). *Dissertation Abstracts International, 47*, 4113B.

Mishel, M. (1981). The measurement of uncertainty in illness. *Nursing Research, 30*(5), 258-263.

Mishel, M. (1983). Parents' perception of uncertainty concerning their hospitalized child. *Nursing Research, 32*(6), 324-330.

Mishel, M. (1988). Uncertainty in illness. *Image: Journal of Nursing Scholarship, 20*(4), 225-232.

Mishel, M. (1990). Reconceptualization of the uncertainty in illness theory. *Image: Journal of Nursing Scholarship, 22*(4), 256-262.

Mishel, M. (1995). Response to adult uncertainty in illness: a critical review of research. *Scholarly Inquiry for Nursing Practice, 9*(1), 25-29.

Mishel, M. (1999). *Mishel Uncertainty in Illness Scale.* Glendale, CA: CINAHL

Mishel, M., & Braden, C. (1987). Uncertainty: a mediator between support and adjustment. *Western Journal of Nursing Research, 9*(1), 43-57.

Mishel, M., & Braden, C. (1988). Finding meaning: antecedents of uncertainty in illness. *Nursing Research, 37*(2), 98-127.

Mishel, M., Hostetter, T, King, C., & Graham, V. (1984). Predictors of psychosocial adjustment in patients newly diagnosed with gynecological cancer. *Cancer Nursing, 7*, 291-299.

Mishel, M., Padilla, G., Grant, M., & Sorenson, D. (1991). Uncertainty in illness theory: a replication of the mediating effects of mastery and coping. *Nursing Research, 40*(4), 236-240.

Morse, J. (1983). An ethnoscientific analysis of comfort: a preliminary investigation. *Nursing Papers, 15*, 6-19.

Morse, J., Botdorff, J., & Hutchinson, S. (1994). The phenomenology of comfort. *Journal of Advanced Nursing Science, 20*, 189-195.

Murray, H. (1981). *Explorations in personality.* New York: Oxford Press.

Neville, K. (1998). The relationship among uncertainty, social support and psychological distress in adolescents recently diagnosed with cancer. *Journal of Pediatric Oncology Nursing, 15*(1), 37-46.

Nightingale, F. (1859). *Notes on nursing.* London: Harrison.

Nolan, M., & Grant, G. (1992). Mid-range theory building and the nursing theory practice gap: a respite care case study. *Journal of Advanced Nursing, 17*(2), 217-223.

Olsen, J., & Hancett, E. (1997). Nurse-expressed empathy, patient outcomes, and development of a middle range theory. *Image: Journal of Nursing Scholarship, 29*, 71-76.

Orlando, I. (1961). *The dynamic nurse-patient relationship: function, process, and principles.* New York: GP Putnam's Sons.

Paterson, J., & Zderad, L. (1988). *Humanistic nursing.* New York: National League for Nursing.

Pearcey, P., & Draper, P. (1996). Using the diffusion of innovation model to influence practice: a case study. *Journal of Advanced Nursing, 23*(4), 714-721.

Pearson, A., & Vaughan, B. (1986). *Nursing models for practice.* Rockville, MD: Aspen Publishers.

Pelz, D., & Horsley, J., (1981). Measuring utilization of nursing research. In J. Ciarlo (Ed.), *Utilizing evaluation.* Beverly Hills, CA: Sage.

Piaget, J. (1969). *The psychology of the child.* New York: Basic Books.

Pieper, B. (1983). Levine's nursing model. In J. Fitzpatrick & A. Whall (Eds.), *Conceptual models of nursing: analysis and application* (pp. 101-115). Norwalk, CT: Appleton & Lange.

Polit, D., & Hungler, B. (1995). *Nursing research* (5th ed.). Philadelphia: JB Lippincott.

Powers, B.A., & Knapp, T.R. (1990). *A dictionary of nursing theory and research.* Thousand Oaks, CA: Sage.

Randell, B., Tedrow, M., & Van Landinghan, J. (1982). *Adaptation nursing: the Roy conceptual model applied.* St. Louis: Mosby.

Ray, M. (1998). Complexity and nursing science. *Nursing Science Quarterly, 11*, 91-93.

Rogers, E. (1995). *Diffusion of innovation* (4th ed.). New York: The Free Press.

Roy, C., & Roberts, S. (1981). *Theory construction in nursing: an adaptation model.* Englewood Cliffs, NJ: Prentice Hall.

Santacroce, S. (2000). Support from health care providers and parental uncertainty during the diagnosis phase of perinatally acquired HIV infection. *Journal of Association of Nurses in AIDS Care, 11*(2), 63-75.

Sappington, J., & Kelley, J.H. (1996). Modeling and role-modeling theory: a case study of holistic care. *Journal of Holistic Nursing, 14*(2), 130-141.

Schlotfeldt, R. (1981). Nursing in the future. *Nursing Outlook, 29*, 295-301.

Schuiling, K., & Sampselle, C. (1999). Comfort in labor and midwifery art. *Image: Journal of Nursing Scholarship, 31*(1), 77-81.

Schulte, B. (1996). *Nurse perception of nurse practitioners* (Unpublished Master's thesis). Highland Heights, KY: Northern Kentucky University.

Sexton, D., Calcasola, S., Bottomley, S., & Funk, M. (1999). Adults' strategies with asthma and their reported uncertainty and coping strategies. *Clinical Nurse Specialist, 13*(1): 8-17.

Selye, H. (1956). *The stress of life*. New York: McGraw-Hill.

Selye, H. (1974). *Stress without distress*. Philadelphia: JB Lippincott.

Selye, H. (1976). *Stress in health and disease*. New York: McGraw-Hill.

Smith, D., Zhang, J., & Colwell, B. (1996). Pro-innovation bias: the case of the giant Texas smoke screen. *Journal of School Health, 66*(6), 210-213.

Stetler, C., & Dimaggio, G. (1991). Research utilization among clinical nurse specialists. *Clinical Nurse Specialist, 5*(3), 151-155.

Stiefel, K. (1996). *Career commitment, nursing unit culture and nursing research utilization* (Dissertation UMI PUZ9623126). Columbia, SC: University of South Carolina.

Suppe, F. (1993). *Middle range theories: what they are and why nursing science needs them* (Proceedings of the American Nurses Association's Council of Nurse Researchers Scientific Session). Washington, DC: American Nurses Association.

Sutterley, D., & Donnelly, G. (1981). *Coping with stress*. Rockville, MD: Aspen Publishers.

Tahan, T. (1998). Patients waiting for heart transplantation: an analysis of vulnerability. *Critical Care Nurse, 18*(4), 40-48

Taylor-Piliae, R. (1998). Establishing evidence based practice: issues and implications in critical care nursing. *Intensive & Critical Care Nursing, 14*(1), 30-37.

Tomlin, E.M. (1990). Spiritual concerns in nursing: The interface of Modeling and Role- modeling with professional nursing's Christian roots and values. In H. Erickson & C. Kinney (Eds.), *Modeling and Role-Modeling: theory, practice and research* (pp. 40-66). Austin, TX: Society for the Advancement of Modeling and Role-Modeling.

Walker, L.O., & Avant, K.C. (1995). *Strategies for theory construction in nursing*. Norwalk, CT: Appleton & Lange.

Walker, P., & Redman, R. (1999). Theory guided evidenced based reflective practice. *Nursing Science Quarterly, 12*(4), 298-303.

Watson, J. (1979). *Nursing: the philosophy and science of caring*. Boulder: Colorado Associated University Press.

Weiss, C. (1980). Knowledge creep and decision accretion. *Knowledge: Creation, Diffusion, Utilization, 1*(3), 381-404.

White, N., Richter, J., & Fry, C. (1992). Coping, social support, and adaptation to chronic illness. *Western Journal of Nursing Research, 14*(2), 211-224.

Winter, J. (1988). *Relationship between research and practice: nurses' attitudes about relaxation therapy* (Dissertation UMI PUZ8824432). New York: Columbia University Teachers College.

Winters, C. (1999). Heart failure: living with uncertainty. *Progress in Cardiovascular Nursing, 14*(3), 85-91.

Wunderlich, R., Perry, A., Lavin, M., & Katz, B. (1999). Patient's perceptions of uncertainty and stress during weaning from mechanical ventilation. *Dimensions of Critical Care Nursing, 18*(1), 2-10.

Youngstrom, L. (1996). *Nursing staff development educators and research utilization* (Dissertation UMI PUZ9709112). Chester, PA: Widener University.

Section VII

Human Diversity and Social Issues

Ann Schmidt Luggen & Sue E. Meiner

The face and accent of America is changing, and each person looks out at these changes from his or her own cultural lens. The central message of this unit for advanced practice nurse (APN) practice and education is the inestimable value of making culture a more visible phenomenon of concern in health care and reshaping the cultural lens of APNs to that end.

Chapter 32, the first chapter of the unit, examines the need for inclusion of social and cultural issues in educating APNs so that their view of the health care arena comes from a multicultural lens. This chapter provides justification for including multiculturalism in APN education and reviews the guidelines that have been proposed by various groups for doing so.

In Chapter 33, the basic concepts that frame the dimensions of culture are reviewed. The concepts of cultural stereotyping and ethnocentrism are considered with their potential effect on patient experiences of health and illness and APN assumptions about practice. This chapter provides a background for appreciating and celebrating diversity.

The theoretical basis that informs the practice of transcultural nursing is the focus of Chapter 34. Leininger's Culture Care Diversity and Universality Theory, Purnell's Cultural Competence Theory, and examples of applicability in the real world of advanced practice are prominent features of the chapter. Other models that guide intervention and evaluation of APN practice in direct care and administration are also included.

As the demography of the United States changes to a more multicultural mix, APNs and educators need to understand the educational needs of diverse students as learners and prospective practicing APNs. Chapter 35 explores cultural diversity and what it means to Master of Science in Nursing (MSN) education, both in terms of curriculum and instruction. There are guidelines for what should be included in a curriculum to prepare APNs for the reality of practice in the twenty-first century as it is anticipated to be. Also included are strategies for admission and progression that contribute to success of culturally diverse students in universities.

According to Harris and Myers (1996), "Workplace diversity can either cause ruptures in the fabric of an organization; or, if handled correctly, it can be woven into strong fibers to support that same organization." The central issue of Chapter 36 is the multicultural perspective of the organization and how it affects and is affected by the changing multicultural workforce.

One's normative assumptions about health and illness are framed on one's experiences. Accordingly, as anyone in clinical practice knows firsthand, racial and ethnic issues remain significant in health and illness patterns, epidemiology and disease risk, and the experiences of illness and suffering. These are the issues of concern in Chapter 37.

The crosscultural view of varied ethnic populations continues in Chapter 38, which examines the health and illness experiences of women in a gender-dichotomized society. More than half of the American population is made up of women; they spend more health care dollars and make more health care visits than men. However, their care has been both fragmented and without research initiatives until recent decades. This chapter explores gender issues in health care and how care and marketing of care can be implemented to the advantage of women patients.

In Chapter 39, one finds a perspective on the aging population and how the experience of aging differs across cultural groups. Aging individuals form a new, flourishing group with a strong voice across America. The demographics of this group and the implications of aging on health care are a focus of this chapter.

Chapter 40 provides a comprehensive view of the social problem and tragedy Americans call domestic violence. The chapter explores spouse/partner abuse, child abuse, and older adult abuse from a theoretical understanding of abuse and the human dynamics involved. It also addresses remedies used by APNs to help the abused heal and take back their lives.

Throughout this unit, the message is congruent with the words of Kelley and Fitzsimons (2000) that community is the ultimate laboratory for appreciating "the reality of culture as a human experience." Before one finds the rightful place in the community to make that possible, one must first understand how human diversity and sociocultural problems affect the way individuals live their lives. Mishler (1984) acknowledges that two voices are prominent in health care; some providers listen only to the voice of medicine, the technological/bioscientific perspective, even as patients and families speak from their "lifeworld." Unit VII is written to enhance understanding of human diversity and to promote APNs' special capacity to engage other discourse—the patient's "lifeworld" story, which provides the rich, sociocultural perspective for care that is so meaningful.

REFERENCES/BIBLIOGRAPHY

Harris, A.W., & Myers, S. (1996). *Tools for valuing diversity*. Irvine, CA: Richard Chang Associates.

Kelley, M.L., & Fitzsimons, V.M. (2000). *Understanding cultural diversity: culture, curriculum, and community in nursing*. Boston: Jones & Bartlett & National League for Nursing Press.

Mishler, E.G. (1984). *The dynamics of medicine: dialects of medical interviews*. Norwood, NJ: Ablex.

Chapter 32

Cultural Diversity: An Issue for MSN Education

Ann Schmidt Luggen & Cheryl Pope Kish

$\mathbf{C}$ ulture represents a person's way of viewing the world and serves to guide that person's beliefs, actions, and practices, including those related to health and illness. At the point of contact between advanced practice nurse (APN) and patient, the way in which they perceive each other and relate is affected by their respective cultural worldviews. APNs need to be able to work sensitively with patients and families, understanding their uniqueness and diversity as humans as is demanded by holistic practice.

Every 10 years, the U.S. Bureau of the Census counts the population of the United States, with the most recent census conducted in the year 2000. Every day, the face of America changes; the population becomes more multicultural. Currently, one of four persons living in the United States is a member of a minority population, and this trend is expected to continue. The growing diversity in the U.S. population makes education for working with culturally diverse populations part of the practice reality of today's APN.

Why should higher education in nursing be concerned with diversity? If the goal of higher education is indeed to teach critical thinking, social responsiveness, effectiveness in communication, and appreciation of differences, then diversity becomes a necessity (Santovec, 1994; Kelley & Fitzsimons, 2000). This chapter examines factors that justify issues of cultural diversity in graduate education as a necessity to accomplishing the goals of higher education in nursing. In addition, it provides guidance for introducing diversity into APN nursing education that has been provided by varied non-nursing and nursing groups.

DEFINITIONS

Culture refers to "a way of perceiving, behaving, and evaluating the world. It provides a blueprint or guide for determining people's values, beliefs, and practices, including those pertaining to health and illness" (Andrews, 1999). Culture, then, reflects one's preferred way of relating with the world, provides life with order and meaning, and guides actions and interactions. The ways of one's culture are passed from generation to generation. While it is flexible, culture tends toward stability over time. The term *cultural diversity* is simply a reference to the differences or variations noted within the population. Habayeb (1995) explores eight themes relevant to cultural diversity—immigrant status, noncompliant behavior, diversity in susceptibility to disease, differences in population groups, demographical changes, urban and rural contexts, workforce diversity, and methodological issues related to studying those from diverse backgrounds—noting finally that there is no reliable definition as yet because of the complexity of the concept. Talabrere (1996) takes issue with the term *cultural diversity*, seeing it as ethnocentric. For example, as the Caucasian panethnic group is so often used as an example, it sets a norm against which others are measured, focusing on how different other people are from Caucasians than on how different Caucasians are from them.

An *ethnic group* is a collection of individuals within a "larger social system whose members have common ancestral, racial, physical or national characteristics and who share cultural symbols such as language, lifestyle, religion, and other characteristics that are not fully understood or shared by outsiders" (Andrews, 1999). At times, such groups are referred to as *ethnic minorities*, implying that they receive different, sometimes unequal treatment by virtue of their physical or cultural characteristics. Members of ethnic minorities often perceive this difference in treatment as a kind of collective discrimination; indeed, they may find the term *minority* an offensive one because of its connotation of something inferior or marginal (Andrews, 1999).

Five panethnic population groups have been officially recognized by the United States government: Caucasian (considered the majority), African American, Hispanic, Asian/Pacific Islander, and American Indian/Alaska Native. These population groups were defined to enable systematic data collection to serve decision-makers in equitable allocation of resources and public policy. Over time, there has been a tendency to view the groups homogenously, failing to appreciate their many subgroups and their differences; this stance increases the potential for stereotyping. Andrews (1999) asserts that instead of embracing the prevailing panethnic population classification system, professionals should ask patients to identify the specific cultural group or groups with which they identify. For example, with which of the 550 American Indian/Alaska Native groups does the patient identify? Does the Latino patient identify with a specific group from Central America or from Spain? Does the European Caucasian immigrant see herself as Polish or German? Italian or Irish?

Stereotyping is a process of applying exaggerated, fixed, inflexible notions about groups, notions based on incomplete or distorted information from limited personal experience with the particular group or from outside sources (Harris & Myers, 1996). Stereotypes are central to prejudice because they block one's ability to see an individual as such. Instead, all characteristics about a particular group, however mistaken, are associated with everyone in that group. Early life experiences begin to shape stereotypes, which can be sustained by selective perception and selective forgetting if one is not careful or if one's education or experience does not reshape the stereotypical beliefs. For example, Patti, whose mother has never worked outside the home, believes that this is true for all women. Tom, who consistently hears his father utter racial epithets in the home, begins to believe the comments being made. However, as people are exposed to a wider circle of people, attend school, and participate in other life events, stereotypes can be shattered and replaced by a more accurate view; however, open-mindedness is a necessary requisite to shattering stereotypes.

Race refers to biological variations presumed to be significant. Race has been defined as "an inbreeding group of individuals with a specific geographic locus. Superficial physical similarity can coexist with drastic differences in cultural-behavioral patterns" (Zuckerman, 1990). Although three races have been identified (negroid, mongoloid, and caucasian), there is now ample genetic evidence of more differences within the races than between races (Ramer, 1992).

Clearly, everyone has a cultural heritage. Having a degree of pride in membership in a particular cultural group can have positive aspects. Conversely, **ethnocentrism** refers to a belief that one's own culture or ethnic group is superior to all others. With ethnocentrism comes a subconscious expectation that others should act as we do, believe what we do, and value what we do because our superior standard is the one against which all should be measured. Clearly, this misdirected notion has no place in the professional worldview of APNs. Instead, APNs should seek **cultural competence**. Roberts (1990) defines cultural competence as "a program's (and person's)

ability to honor and respect [the] beliefs, interpersonal styles, attitudes, and behaviors" of patients. Purnell and Paulanka (1998) view cultural competence as a conscious process along a continuum. At the stage of unconscious incompetence, one is unaware of a knowledge deficit about another culture, a kind of cultural blindness. At the level of conscious incompetence, there is awareness of a knowledge deficit. Conscious competence involves learning about another person's culture, verifying generalizations about the culture, and providing culturally sensitive interventions in behalf of the other person. Finally, unconscious competence refers to an automatic provision of culturally competent care to those who are culturally different.

Cultural competence is an expectation of **transcultural nursing**. As that name implies, transcultural nursing transcends cultural boundaries in professional practice. Nurse anthropologist, Madeline M. Leininger coined the term *transcultural nursing*. Dr. Leininger (1970), who was the first to note the significance of culture on patients' health and illness, envisioned a blending of both theory and practice from nursing and anthropology; "sharing their special knowledge and experiences, both would undoubtedly see new pathways in thinking and research." In the decades since transcultural nursing was conceived, it has become a highly specialized arena of clinical practice supported by its own organization and journal. Not all APNs become transcultural nurses; however, all need an ability to provide culturally sensitive care free of bias. To this end, APNs need to be able to collect cultural assessment data to enable understanding of the cultural context of patients and families and to problem-solve on behalf of culturally diverse patients, families, aggregates, and communities (Andrews & Boyle, 1999).

Ethnocentrism can also involve perceptions that a particular age or gender is superior to another, contributing to the potential for discriminatory interactions and actions. At the least, this kind of ethnocentrism is associated with insensitivity to the unique needs of those individuals, which is certainly problematic when one is a nursing professional. Any assumption that contributes to judging others "according to similarity with or dissimilarity from a standard considered ideal or normal are called 'isms.'" For example, **ageism** refers to the assumption that members of one age group are superior to those of other age groups. Robert Butler (1990), who coined the term *ageism* in the mid-1960s as he noted a culturally rooted discomfort with aging and a negative perception of older adults, believes that ageism persists today despite increased numbers of older adults. A belief or assumption that one gender is superior to the other is known as **sexism.** For example, there are stereotypes that women are less rational and more emotional than men. Too often in health care, this translates to women's symptoms being trivialized by male physicians.

CRITICAL ISSUES: JUSTIFYING A NEED FOR GRADUATE CULTURAL DIVERSITY EDUCATION

Advanced practice, with its intimate relationships with patients in all levels of care and in all care settings, is bound to feel the effect of the evolving diversity of the U.S. population. Presently, racial and ethnic minorities make up 28% of the population (American Association of Colleges of Nursing [AACN], 1998). Older adults account for 12%. For each of these populations, their values and beliefs intertwine with health behaviors and experiences of illness. APNs must have cultural competence when dealing with such diverse cultural groups.

Population Trends

The majority population of the United States continues, at present, to be Caucasian. This group, then, continues to predominate in the APN practice population. However, this is subject to change within the first half of the new millennium. Louie (1998) acknowledges a number of societal factors that have affected the patient population for nursing. First, minority groups are traditionally among the poorest of population groups. One's economic reality affects both access to and payment for health care. As never before, APNs are challenged to recognize the economic aspects of health care and be fiscally responsible providers. Second, there has been a major population shift secondary to immigration. Between 1980 and 1990, the Caucasian population decreased 6%; it now represents 69% of the U.S. population. The African-American population increased 13.2% and is now 14.5% of the population. The Hispanic population increased 53% and now represents 6.5%. Asian Americans are projected to account for 9.9% of the U.S. population by 2025. The changes in the minority population projected by the U.S. Department of Health and Human Services (DHHS) (1996) are shown in Table 32-1.

Aging Trends

The proportion of older adults is increasing in North America and other developing countries. Life expectancies are increasing, and in some areas of the world, including the United States, fertility rates are declining. At the beginning of the twentieth century, life expectancy was about 47 years; however, a Caucasian baby born at the millennium in the United States has a life expectancy of 75.8 years. Projections indicate that by 2025, 19% of the population of the United States will be 65 years of age or older (U.S. Bureau of the Census, 1993). Additionally, the percentage of the "old-old" (those who are ages 85 to 94)

Table 32-1

Minority Population Projections: 1995 to 2050

POPULATION GROUP	1995	2050
Caucasians	74%	53%
African Americans	12%	14%
Hispanics	10%	24%
Asians	3%	8%
Native Americans	1%	1%

Data from U.S. Department of Health and Human Services (1996). *Health United States: 1995* (Publication No. PHS96-1242). Hyattsville, MD: U.S. Department of Health and Human Services.

is a rapidly growing component of the population, and the numbers of centenarians (those over the age of 100) are increasing (National Institute on Aging, 1993).

Aging adults are a remarkably heterogeneous group; although many have chronic illnesses that complicate their aging and require considerable health care, many others are surprisingly robust (Manton, Stallard, & Len, 1993). A priority for APNs who work with older adults is the ability to recognize individuality in the aging process. Primary care with emphasis on assessment of aging and functional status; health promotion; functional maintenance; and illness and injury prevention or risk reduction is important when caring for aging adults, irrespective of the setting in which they live.

Gender Trends

According to the U.S. Bureau of the Census (1996), women account for 52% of the population of the United States. They make 60% of all visits to physicians (Braus, 1997) and 75% of all health care decisions in American households; they also spend almost two of every three health care dollars (Smith Barney Research, 1998). So not only are women an important patient population for APNs, they also represent a crucial market niche. Understanding gender-specific care, therefore, is an essential component of APN education.

Aging women represent a large percentage of the population, with the peak projected in 2030, when there will be more than 37.7 million women ages 65 and older. Projections indicate that in that same year, there will be more than five million women ages 85 and older in the United States (Braus, 1997). The number of women approaching midlife is expected to peak at 22.2 million; this has implications for program development related to the transition to menopause and the inherent risk reduction.

Workforce Trends

With the change in population, one would expect that the nursing profession would begin to reflect those percentages; however, such is not the case. In fact, approximately 92% of the nursing workforce is Caucasian, and the majority of nurses are women. According to statistics from the AACN (2000), approximately 10% of the 2.5 million registered nurses (RNs) in the United States represent minority groups. In 1992, the DHHS specified 9% (206,400 individuals) of 2.24 million RNs with a racial/ethnic distribution as follows: African American, 90,000; Hispanic, 30,400; Asian/Pacific Islander, 76,000; and Native American, 10,000. Clearly, the workforce percentages have not kept pace with the population percentages.

Educational Enrollment Trends

Enrollment trends in basic nursing programs reveal that individuals from panethnic population groups other than Caucasian are underrepresented (Table 32-2). Also of particular concern is the attrition rate for certain minority groups in basic nursing programs; for example, in 1990, African American students made up 10.4% of the nursing student population, and in 1995, 9.4%. Asians made up 3% of the basic nursing student population in 1990 and 4% in 1995. For those years, retention for Hispanic nursing students was favorable, although the overall percentage of Hispanic enrollment was low.

To create a population of nursing professionals that matches the patient population anticipated in the next decades, basic nursing programs must recruit and retain students from currently underrepresented groups. Although there was a slight increase in graduations for minority students between 1991 and 1994, minority groups clearly continue to have limited enrollments in Master's programs. Fortunately, attrition in Master's programs is not the critical issue; the critical issue is in undergraduate nursing education. Those statistics, shown in Table 32-3, clearly indicate that graduate educators must quickly attend to the lack of representation of minority students in advanced practice to enable cultural congruence of APNs and their patient populations.

The percentage of Hispanics has increased by 40% in the United States since 1990, now accounting for 11.7% of the total population; however, less than 2% of RNs are Hispanic. In the fall semester of 1999, only 4.5% of baccalaureate students in the country were Hispanic; slightly more than 5% of Master's degree and doctoral students in that same semester were Hispanic in origin. Concerned about these disparities between prospective nurses and the patient populations they serve, the AACN announced (on June 15, 2000) their collaboration with the two major Hispanic nursing organizations to provide Hispanic students with "expanded access to nursing education" (AACN, 2000).

Transcultural nursing has emerged as a formal area of study over the past 25 years (Louie, 1998). In 1970, the University of Washington started a Master's program in transcultural nursing; Penn State opened theirs in 1974 (Louie, 1998). The University of Utah started Master's and doctoral programs in transcultural nursing in 1977, and the University of Miami has incorporated transcultural nursing in their undergraduate and graduate nursing curricula and has a Distinguished Chair of Transcultural Nursing and a Transcultural Nursing Research Institute (Louie, 1998).

Approximately one fourth of nursing programs have a crosscultural program at the undergraduate level (Meleis, 1995). Only 8% of Master's programs have such coursework, and less than 2% of doctoral students in nursing have access to a seminar on crosscultural nursing or diversity. Programs need to shift from "unicultural" to multicultural approaches to nursing (Meleis, 1995).

According to Abraham (1998), by the year 2000, one third of college students and more than one third of the nation's workforce will be people of color (i.e., not Caucasian). However, projections indicate that minorities will represent only 10% of full-time faculty in higher

---

Table 32-2

Minority Graduation from Basic Nursing Programs: 1990 and 1995

MINORITY GROUP	1990	1995
African Americans	6.8%	7.0%
Hispanics	3.1%	3.1%
Asians	2.4%	3.0%

Data from Center for Research in Nursing Education and Community Health (1996b). *Nursing datasource. Volume I: trends in contemporary nursing education* (Publication No. 19-6932). New York: National League for Nursing Press.

Table 32-3

Minority Graduation from MSN Programs: 1991 and 1994

MINORITY GROUP	1991	1994
African Americans	4.9%	6.0%
Hispanics	2.1%	3.3%
Asians	2.2%	3.2%

Data from Center for Research in Nursing Education and Community Health (1996). *Nursing data review* (Publication No. 19-6851). New York: National League for Nursing Press.

education in 2000. If there are to be culturally diverse faculty to educate students for professional nursing roles as either generalists or APN specialists, attention must be given to preparing more of such individuals for roles in higher education.

National Support for Cultural Diversity Education

In 1998, the Association of American Colleges and Universities (AACU) conducted its first national poll related to diversity in higher education. The results of this survey are supportive of content and process education related to cultural diversity. (Box 32-1 provides an overview of the survey findings.)

The DHHS established a Task Force on Black and Minority Health to examine disparities in health care in 1984 (Andrews, 1997). Since then, although great strides have been made in the improvement of health and longevity, a persistent disparity in health indicators in subgroups of the population continues. Today, the Office of Minority Health (OMH) coordinates all federal efforts to improve health care of racial and ethnic minority populations (Andrews, 1997).

On an international scope, the World Health Organization (WHO) (1978) proclaimed health for all by the year 2000. While this is far from realized, progress continues; however, inequities and barriers still exist (Meleis, 1995). Having their own plans for 2000, the OMH contributes to a public-private effort of the states to improve minority health.

With the publication of *Healthy People 2000: National Health Promotion and Disease Prevention* (US DHHS, 1991), there was national evidence of the value placed on meeting the health care needs of diverse and socially "needy" populations. There are 49 specific objectives for improvements in minority health status (Andrews, 1997), and five goals are delineated: (1) increase life expectancy to at least 78 years, (2) increase the number of healthy years of life to at least 65, (3) decrease infant mortality to no more than 7 per 1000 live births, (4) decrease the disparity in life expectancy between Caucasian and minority populations to no more than 4 years, and (5) decrease disability caused by chronic conditions to no more than 7% of all people. Clearly, vulnerable groups are a predominant concern of this national initiative.

The Pew Health Professions Commission (1998), in its report *Recreating Health Professional Practice for a New Century*, delineated 21 competencies necessary to clinical practice in the twenty-first century. (Box 32-2 lists the competencies.) Although only one competency specifically addresses cultural competence, many others imply the need for culturally sensitive care and respect for the worth, dignity, and uniqueness of individuals.

Nursing sources

The American Nurses Association (ANA) supports education related to cultural diversity, implied with the following statement from president Beverly Malone, "Nurses who are prepared to deal with differences in people are prepared to deal with diversity. Non-majority populations seek respect, not tolerance; [they] do not wish to 'melt' into a cultural 'pot' of minorities and become indistinguishable from majority Americans" (ANA, 1998). In addition, the ANA's *Scope and Standards of Advanced Practice Registered Nursing* (1996) speaks minimally to culture and diversity. Standard health promotion, health maintenance, and health teaching are to be appropriate to a patient's developmental level, learning needs, readiness and ability to learn, and culture. The Southern Council on College Education (1991), along with the Southern Regional Education Board, developed a position paper resulting from a 3-year federally sponsored–effort—*Faculty Preparation to Teach Gerontological Nursing Project*. The consensus of this work is a pressing need to develop a new worldview of aging. Other aspects identified for caring for the aging population include: (1) a new wellness model, (2) reduced reliance on pharmaceuticals, (3) increased nutrition interventions, natural treatments, and activity, (4) increased attention to those at risk, and (5) recognition and value for wisdom as a legacy of the aged. The American Academy of Nursing (AAN) has an Expert Panel on Culturally Competent Care. This group contributed to a monograph geared toward leaders in nursing to provide a framework of culturally competent care. The AAN focuses not only on ethnic minorities, but on "marginalized" groups—those different from the mainstream (Meleis, 1995). The AACN (1998) is a partner in a coalition of health profession organizations called Health Professionals for Diversity.

Box 32-1

Results of a National Poll Related to Cultural Diversity

- Two of three Americans believe colleges should prepare people to function in a diverse society.
- One of three people believe diversity programs raise, rather than lower, academic standards.
- 71% of people believe that diversity education helps bring society together.
- 94% of people believe the nation's growing diversity makes it more important for us to understand people different from ourselves.
- 22% of Americans believe the United States is doing a good job in meeting diversity challenges.
- 75% of people believe that a diverse student body has a positive effect on student education.

From Association of American Colleges and Universities (1998). *Results of first ever national poll on diversity in higher education.* Washington, DC: Association of American Colleges and Universities.

Box 32-2

Twenty-One Competencies for the Twenty-First Century

1. Embrace a personal ethic of social responsibility and service.
2. Exhibit ethical behavior in all professional activities.
3. Provide evidence-based, clinically competent care.
4. Incorporate the multiple determinants of health in clinical care.
5. Apply knowledge of the new sciences.
6. Demonstrate critical thinking, reflection, and problem-solving skills.
7. Understand the role of primary care.
8. Rigorously practice preventive health care.
9. Integrate population-based care and services into practice.
10. Improve access to health care for those with unmet needs.
11. Practice relationship-centered care with individuals and families.
12. Provide culturally sensitive care to a diverse society.
13. Partner with communities in health care decisions.
14. Use communication and information technology effectively and appropriately.
15. Work in interdisciplinary teams.
16. Ensure care that balances individual, professional, system, and societal needs.
17. Practice leadership.
18. Take responsibility for quality of care and health outcomes at all levels.
19. Contribute to continuous improvement of the health care system.
20. Advocate for public policy that promotes and protects the health of the public.
21. Continue to learn and help others learn.

Data from Pew Health Professions Commission (1998, December). *Recreating health professional practice for a new century* (Fourth report of the Pew Health Professions Commission). San Francisco: The Center for the Health Professions. Available online at www.futurehealth.uscf.edu/pewcomm/competen.html.

The AACN has as a long-term goal the assurance of culturally relevant curricula to reflect the 2050 projection that minorities will make up nearly 50% of the U.S. population.

Nursing education sources

The AACN's 1997 vision paper *Statement on Diversity and Equality of Opportunity* incorporates the need for culturally competent care with the need for cultural knowledge and care of patients across the age spectrum. There is also an AACN task force on diversity and opportunity that proposes that schools of nursing recruit and retain students who reflect the diversity of the population they serve. The AACN's *Nursing Education Agenda for the 21st Century*, a product of the task force, expresses concern about the nursing profession being mainly Caucasian, middle-class females and the need for a message to potential students that the profession embraces diversity (AACN, 1993). This source also identifies national issues, many of which are related to human diversity; these issues include:

- Uninsured or underinsured Americans (numbering 60 million in 1991)
- Aging of Americans and of the world population
- High costs of health care
- Increasing incidence of avoidable conditions (e.g., chronic diseases)
- Increasing incidence of newborns with low birth weights and the high infant mortality (10 per 1000 live births)
- Lack of access to preventative health care by culturally diverse populations

- Shorter life expectancy for African Americans (12%) than for the overall population (69.4 versus 75 years)
- Higher risk for African Americans and Hispanics than for Caucasians for five leading causes of death: heart disease, cancer, stroke, injury, and homicide

The AACN (1996) proposed a framework for educators who design, implement, and evaluate Master's education for APNs, defining those elements considered essential. The resulting product was *The Essentials of Master's Education for Advanced Practice Nursing*, which suggests the necessity of a global awareness as an underpinning for culturally sensitive care and an appreciation of the kinds of problems associated with social issues and lifestyle choices, many of which are preventable. In ensuring appropriate and sensitive health care that appreciates human diversity, objectives are delineated that specify that APN graduates should be able to:

- Differentiate and compare the wide range of cultural norms and health care practices of groups of varied racial and ethnic backgrounds
- Define, design, and implement culturally competent health care
- Ensure that systems meet the needs of the populations served and are culturally relevant
- Recognize the variants in health, including physiological variations, in a wide range of cultural, racial, ethnic, age, and gender groups, which may influence assessment and plans of care
- Practice in collaboration with a multicultural task force

The *Curriculum Guidelines and Program Standards for Nurse Practitioner Education* developed by the National Organization of Nurse Practitioner Faculties (NONPF) (1995) to define and guide APN education suggest that "cultural competence in the provision of health care is a basic value in nurse practitioner practice. The growing diversity of our nation's population necessitates that professionals develop the attitudes, behaviors, and policies that enable professionals to work effectively in cross-cultural situations."

Neither the National League for Nursing Accrediting Commission (NLNAC) nor the Commission on Collegiate Nursing Education (CCNE), which accredit Master of Science in Nursing (MSN) programs, prescribe the way in which cultural diversity should be addressed in a curriculum. However, the self-study documents, prepared for program review by these agencies, are expected to delineate the way in which prospective MSN graduates are educated to acquire the wisdom, technical abilities, and ethical qualities for their selected advanced practice roles. The programs evaluated by the NLNAC (1999) are expected to articulate their "commitment to [the] culturally, racially, and ethically diverse community in which the institution and nursing unit exist." Both of the accrediting agencies support the curriculum guidelines and program standards established by the NONPF (1995), which suggest that cultural aspects of advanced practice be integrated throughout the curriculum.

IMPLICATIONS FOR MSN EDUCATION AND ADVANCED PRACTICE

Those who educate APNs and those who practice as APNs need to be futurists, able to determine how projections about the cultural mix of society and the professional workforce will shape their respective work settings and plan accordingly. Otherwise, nursing educates and practices to maintain the status quo rather than gain a preferred future.

Both clinicians and educators will do well to be informed about the cultural groups that predominate their practice communities as appropriate underpinning for cultural competence. While not all APNs will practice transcultural nursing to the fullest extent of the growing specialty, they should all practice culturally sensitive and culturally competent care. Although the basics for understanding cultural diversity and gaining cultural competence are ideally provided during the MSN program, the richness and uniqueness of a particular culture can only be experienced as people work together to understand each other and value each other's similarities and differences. APN students need clinical experience with patients from different cultures to incorporate culturally sensitive care into their management plans. (Chapter 35 offers specific

suggestions for incorporating cultural diversity education into the curriculum and instruction of APN programs.)

Nursing education, both undergraduate and graduate, must continue to recruit qualified students from diverse cultures and provide the academic, financial, and other support services to affect retention. A 4-year project called the Transcultural Leadership Continuum (TLC) for the Robert Wood Johnson Foundation, initiated at a group of nursing programs in New Jersey, determined that the following elements were associated with retention of minority students on all levels (Kelly & Fitzsimons, 2000): (1) inclusion of incentive learning strategies early in the program, (2) promotion of relationships and a sense of connectedness, (3) provision of mentorship options, (4) accommodation of work and family loads by flexible schedules and academic loads, and (5) early introduction of educational mobility. Faculty members need to be educated about educational biculturalism in order to better understand students' life needs and academic needs.

PRIORITIES FOR RESEARCH

Anyone who designs research related to advanced practice, whether in clinical practice or education, should be careful to ensure that the research sample is inclusive of an appropriate cultural mix. It is important to determine if the "truths" uncovered by nursing and health care research are transportable across cultures. Research could be designed to discover the best practices for teaching cultural diversity in graduate programs. What are the similarities and differences in educating an APN anticipating primary care practice versus those like the certified registered nurse anesthetist (CRNA) and clinical nurse specialist (CNS) who might practice in hospital settings? How does an APN who encounters a patient from an unfamiliar culture learn to meet that individual's cultural needs? What folk treatments do various cultures embrace, and how are these incorporated into a APN's management plan?

Qualitative studies might examine the experience of APN students learning to work with diverse individuals and how they progress through the phases of cultural competence development. Evaluation studies might examine the extent to which members of various cultural groups are satisfied with APN care delivered by a member of a different culture. For example, is a patient's perception of care more positive if he or she and the APN are of the same racial, ethnic, and cultural group? Is there a perception that "something is missing" in care delivered by someone from a different culture? Does patient compliance change as a result of having a more culturally competent APN? Will having access to such evaluation data contribute to a change in APN behavior toward a more culturally sensitive practice?

Research is needed to help those in education, design, marketing and support services enhance minority recruit-

Suggestions for Further Learning

- Consult the following websites for additional information about cultural sensitivity:
  - Cross Cultural Health Care Program (www. xculture.org/)
  - EthnoMed (healthlinks.washington.edu/clinical/ethno med)
  - Alternative Medicine Home Page (www.pitt.edu/ ~cbw/altm.html)
  - Diversity RX (www.diversityrx.org/HTML/DIVRX. htm)
  - Transcultural Nursing (www.megalink.net~vic/)
- Locate a patient assessment and employ it to assess yourself as a member of a familiar culture. Employ the assessment instrument again to assess someone from a different culture. The following resources have excellent examples of patient cultural assessment instruments: Andrews, M.M., & Boyle, J.S. (1999). *Transcultural concepts in nursing care* (3rd ed.). Philadelphia: JB Lippincott; Giger, J.N., & Davidhizar, R.E. (1995). *Transcultural nursing: assessment and intervention* (2nd ed.). St. Louis: Mosby; and Purnell, L., & Paulanka, B. (1998). *Transcultural health care*. Philadelphia: FA Davis.
- Have APNs representing different specialty practices locate admission assessment instruments. Bring these into a group setting where they can be subjected to critique and revision to better reflect cultural sensitivity. For example, the certified nurse midwife (CNM) may access a prenatal and labor assessment; the nurse practitioner (NP) may access a primary care assessment; the CRNA may access a preoperative assessment; and

the CNS may access a hospital admission instrument. In the revision process, be sure to appreciate the practical realities of the environment in which the "new instruments" would be used. For example, do not make them overly cumbersome or time consuming, such that they would not be used appropriately.
- Using the same guidelines as in the previous point, access different types of discharge summaries for critique and modification.
- For APN or other nursing educators, read the following sources specific to cultural diversity and higher education: Fitzsimons, V., & Kelley, M. (1996). *The culture of learning*. New York: National League for Nursing Press; Kelley, M.L., & Fitzsimons, V.M. (Eds.) (2000). *Understanding cultural diversity: culture, curriculum, and community in nursing*. New York: National League for Nursing Press; Santovec, M. (1994). *Recruitment and retention in higher education*. Madison, WI: Magna Publications; and Task Force on Cultural Diversity (1998). *Preparing graduates to meet the needs of diverse populations*. Atlanta, GA: Southern Regional Education Board.
- Read Alvord, L.A., & Van Pelt, E.C. (1999). *The scalpel and the silver bear—the first Navajo woman surgeon combines western medicine and traditional healing*. New York: Bantam. This remarkable book tells the story of Dr. Alvord's struggles to balance the Navajo healing philosophy of balance and "walking in beauty" with traditional western medicine and surgery. It is a wonderful review of the interconnectedness that best heals people, as well as an appreciation of gender and ethnic diversity in the clinical world of medicine.

---

ment and retention. Tremendous insights for program evaluation and curriculum design would be gained from qualitative research that seeks to understand the experience of a student from a minority group on a majority campus. For example, what is it like to be the only Asian student in a graduate class? What is the experience of an African-American student in a primary care clinical site where there are no other African Americans? What is it like to be the only man in a women's health course or a nurse midwifery program? Does a student who returns to graduate school at age 45 face particular challenges related to being a diverse student in a population of 30-year-old students?

DISCUSSION QUESTIONS

These questions can be used to promote critical thinking and encourage discussion.

1. Obtain data from your local community about the population. Determine what cultural groups you are most likely to see in your clinical practice or classroom. Search the literature for information about those groups that can guide practice decisions. One excellent source of such information is Giger, J.N., & Davidhizar, R.E. (1999). *Transcultural nursing: assessment and intervention* (3rd ed.). St. Louis: Mosby.

2. Identify individuals from each of the major cultural groups in your practice community. Invite them to a class or continuing education seminar to share information with APNs about the essential aspects of working with someone of that culture.

3. In a small group setting of APNs, discuss the level of cultural education you had in your basic nursing education program and those cultural practice experiences you have had thus far in your nursing career. Consider what graduate education for APNs should add to your cultural sensitivity and cultural competence. In the discussion, be sure to address the seminal question: What should the experience of classroom and clinical

education bring to the cultural competence of graduate nursing students?

4. Read the following reference as an impetus for discussion: Quinless, F. (2000). Primary care, education, and research integration: a vehicle for a culture of health. In M.L. Kelley & V.M. Fitzsimons (Eds.), *Understanding cultural diversity: culture, curriculum, and community in nursing* (pp. 133-148). New York: National League for Nursing Press. How might the experiences of this faculty be used to guide similar health care services for culturally diverse populations in your setting? What would you do differently? The same?

5. On June 10, 1963, President John F. Kennedy made the following statement: "Let us not be blind to our differences—but let us also direct attention to our common interests and the means by which those differences can be resolved. And if we cannot end now our differences, at least we can help make the world safe for diversity." How can that notion be applied to the development of cultural competence for APNs?

REFERENCES/BIBLIOGRAPHY

Abraham, A.A. (1998). *Diversity in college faculty: SREB states address a need*. Atlanta, GA.: Southern Regional Education Board.

Alvord, L.A., & Van Pelt, E.C. (1999). *The scalpel and the silver bear—the first Navajo woman surgeon combines western medicine and traditional healing*. New York: Bantam.

American Association of Colleges of Nursing (1993). *AACN's nursing education agenda for the 21st century*. Washington, DC: American Association of Colleges of Nursing.

American Association of Colleges of Nursing (1996). *The essentials of Master's education for advanced practice nursing*. Washington, DC: American Association of Colleges of Nursing.

American Association of Colleges of Nursing (1997a). *Statement on diversity and equality of opportunity*. Washington, DC: American Association of Colleges of Nursing.

American Association of Colleges of Nursing (1997b). *Vision of baccalaureate and graduate nursing education*. Washington, DC: American Association of Colleges of Nursing. Available online at www.aacn.nche.edu.

American Association of Colleges of Nursing (1998). Improving health care through diversity. *Syllabus, 24*(5), 3-4, 8.

American Association of Colleges of Nursing. (2000). *News bulletin*. Available online at www.aacn.nche.edu.

American Nurses Association (1996). *Scope and standards of advanced practice registered nursing*. Washington, DC: American Nurses Association.

American Nurses Association (1998, January-February). The dynamics of difference. *The American Nurse*.

Andrews, M.M. (1997). Cultural diversity and community health nursing. In J.M. Swanson, & M.N. Nies (Eds.), *Community health nursing* (2nd ed.) (pp. 435-476). Philadelphia: WB Saunders.

Andrews, M.M. (1999). Theoretical foundations of transcultural nursing. In M.M. Andrews, & J.S. Boyle (Eds.), *Transcultural concepts in nursing care* (3rd ed.) (pp. 3-22). Philadelphia: JB Lippincott.

Andrews, M.M., & Boyle, J.S. (1999). *Transcultural concepts in nursing care* (3rd ed.). Philadelphia: JB Lippincott.

Association of American Colleges and Universities (1998). *Results of first ever national poll on diversity in higher education*. Washington, DC: Association of American Colleges and Universities.

Banks, J.A., & Banks, C.M. (1997). *Multicultural education: issues and perspectives*. London: Allyn & Bacon.

Braus, P. (1997). *Marketing health care to women*. Ithaca, NY: American Demographic Books.

Brislin, R. & Yoshida, T. (1994). *Improving intercultural interactions: modules for cross-cultural training*. Thousand Oaks, CA.: Sage.

Burns, J. (1992, July 6). Health programs targets needs of mature adults. *Modern Healthcare,* 31.

Bushy, A. (1992). Cultural considerations for primary health care: where do self-care and folk medicine fit? *Holistic Nursing Practice, 6*(3), 10-18.

Butler, R. (1990). Editorial: a disease called ageism. *Journal of the American Geriatric Society, 38*(2), 178-180.

Campion, E. (1994). The oldest old. *New England Journal of Medicine, 330*(23), 1819-1820.

Center for Research in Nursing Education and Community Health (1996a). *Nursing data review* (Publication No. 19-6851). New York: National League for Nursing Press.

Center for Research in Nursing Education and Community Health (1996b). *Nursing datasource. Volume I: trends in contemporary nursing education* (Publication No. 19-6932). New York: National League for Nursing Press.

Council on Collegiate Education for Nursing (1999). *Preparing the work force for the 21st century: the nurse educator's challenge*. Atlanta, GA.: Southern Regional Education Board.

Dienemann, J. (Ed.) (1998). *Cultural diversity in nursing: issues, strategies, and outcomes*. New York: American Academy of Nursing.

Falkenhagen, K. (1998). *Cultural competence in nursing*. Sacramento, CA: CME Resource.

Faulkner & Gray (1998). *Women's health chartbook. Wellness & prevention sourcebook*. New York: Faulkner & Gray.

Fitzsimons, V., & Kelley, M. (1996). *The culture of learning*. New York: National League for Nursing Press.

Galanti, G. (1997). *Caring for patients from different cultures: case studies from American hospitals* (2nd ed.). Philadelphia: University of Pennsylvania Press.

Gary, F.A. (1998). Preparing for the 21st century diversity in nursing education, research, and practice. *Journal of Professional Nursing, 14*(5), 272-279.

Giger, J.N., & Davidhizar. R.E. (1995). *Transcultural nursing: assessment and intervention* (2nd ed.). St. Louis: Mosby.

Habayeb, G.L. (1995). Cultural diversity: a nursing concept not yet reliably defined. *Nursing Outlook, 43*(5), 224-227.

Hahn, M.S. (1995, November). Providing health care in a culturally complex world. *ADVANCE for Nurse Practitioners,* 43-45.

Harris, A.W., & Myers, S.G. (1996). *Tools for valuing diversity*. Irvine, CA: Richard Chang Associates.

Kelley, M.L., & Fitzsimons, V.M. (2000). *Understanding cultural diversity: culture, curriculum, and community in nursing.* Boston: Jones & Bartlett & National League for Nursing Press.

Leininger, M. (1970). *Nursing and anthropology: two worlds to blend.* New York: John Wiley and Sons.

Leininger, M. (1997). Transcultural nursing research to transform nursing education and practice: 40 years. *Image: Journal of Nursing Scholarship, 29*(14), 341-347.

Louie, K. B. (1998). Cultural influences on nursing. In G. Deloughery (Ed.), *Issues and trends in nursing* (3rd ed.) (pp. 171-194). St. Louis: Mosby.

Manton, K., Stallard, E., & Len, K. 91993). Forecasts of active life expectancy: policy and fiscal implications. *Journal of Gerontology, 48,* 11-28.

Mattson, S. (2000). Providing care for the changing face of the U.S. *AWHONN Lifelines, 4*(3), 49-52.

Meleis, A.I. (Ed.) (1995). *Diversity, marginalization, and culturally competent health care issues in knowledge development.* Washington, DC: American Academy of Nursing.

Nance, T. (1995). Intercultural communication: finding common ground. *Journal of Obstetric, Gynecologic, and Neonatal Nursing, 24*(3), 249-255.

National Institute on Aging (1993). *In search of the secrets of aging.* Washington, DC: U.S. Department of Health & Human Services.

National League for Nursing Accrediting Commission (1999). *Interpretive guidelines for standards and criteria—baccalaureate and higher degree programs.* New York: National League for Nursing Accrediting Commission.

National Organization of Nurse Practitioner Faculties (1995). *Curriculum guidelines and program standards for nurse practitioner education.* Washington, DC: National Organization of Nurse Practitioner Faculties.

Pew Health Professions Commission (1998, December). *Recreating health professional practice for a new century* (Fourth report of the Pew Health Professions Commission). San Francisco: The Center for the Health Professions. Available online at www.futurehealth.uscf.edu/pewcomm/competen.html.

Purnell, L., & Paulanka, B. (1998). *Transcultural health care.* Philadelphia: JB Lippincott.

Ramer, L. (1992). *Culturally sensitive caregiving and childbearing families: series 4. Nursing issues for the 21st century.* White Plains, NY: March of Dimes Birth Defects Foundation.

Roberts, R. (1990). *Developing culturally competent programs for families and children with special needs.* Washington, DC: Georgetown University Child Development Center, Maternal and Child Health Bureau.

Santovec, M. (1994). *Recruitment and retention in higher education.* Madison, WI: Magna.

Smith Barney Research (1998). *The new women's movement: women's health care.* Available online at www.smithbarney.com/index_.html.

Southern Council on College Education (1991). *Faculty preparation to teach gerontological nursing project paper.* Atlanta, GA: Southern Council on College Education.

Talabere, L.R. (1996). Meeting the challenge of culture care in nursing: diversity, sensitivity, and congruence. *Journal of Cultural Diversity, 3*(2), 53-61,

Task Force on Cultural Diversity (1998). *Preparing graduates to meet the needs of diverse populations.* Atlanta, GA: Southern Regional Education Board.

Torres, S. (1993, July). Cultural sensitivity: a must for today's primary care provider. *ADVANCE for Nurse Practitioners,* 16-18.

Tripp-Reimer, T., Brink, P., & Saunders, J. (1984). Cultural assessment: content and process. *Nursing Outlook, 32,* 78-82.

U.S. Bureau of the Census (1993). *General population characteristics.* Washington, DC: U.S. Government Printing Office.

U.S. Bureau of the Census (1996). *General population characteristics.* Washington, DC: U.S. Government Printing Office.

U.S. Department of Health and Human Services (1991). *Healthy people 2000: national health promotion and disease prevention.* Washington, DC: U.S. Government Printing Office.

U.S. Department of Health and Human Services (1992). *National sample survey.* Hyattsville, MD: U.S. Department of Health and Human Services.

U.S. Department of Health and Human Services (1996). *Health United States: 1995* (Publication No. PHS96-1242). Hyattsville, MD: U.S. Department of Health and Human Services.

Washington, L.J. (1999). Expanding opportunities in graduate education for minority nurses. *Journal of National Black Nurses, 10*(1), 68-80.

World Health Organization (1978). *Primary health care: report of the International Conference on Primary Health Care.* Geneva, Switzerland: World Health Organization.

Zuckerman, M. (1990). Some dubious premises in research and theory on racial differences. *American Psychologist, 45*(12), 1297-1303.

Chapter 33

Basic Concepts in Cultural Diversity

Diane Eigsti Gerber, Ann Schmidt Luggen, & Gracie S. Wishnia

By the year 2010, many readers of this text will be reporting to a Hispanic, Asian, or African-American woman at their workplace, and some of their neighbors will likely be Hispanic or Asian families. Readers will be utilizing their skills with employees in multinational corporations or in companies with international branches (Johnson, 1994). Women, people of color, immigrants, and those with physical limitations are rapidly becoming the norm, rather than the exception, in the workplace. Communication, industrial, and transportation technologies are shaping the view of the world as a global village. The devastation from nighttime earthquakes in Turkey is seen live on American television the next morning at breakfast, jets can convey the Ebola virus from Africa to New York in 24 hours, and pollution from factories in China and lawn mowers in the United States contributes to global warming, a situation affecting all humankind. It is imperative that students, neighbors, and citizens of a city, state, nation, and the world know more than the customs, facts, foods, and languages of other cultures. People must have the skills to work in and adapt to a rapidly changing national and international society and appreciate the resources and contributions of a diverse population.

For health care providers, working with diversity means that advanced practice nurses (APNs) need to respect their patients as complete human beings living within their own unique cultural heritage; this not only helps patients to get well or stay well, it also provides them with a sense of well-being. Cultural competence is not about tolerance—tolerance is neutral. To view cultural diversity as a vehicle to wholeness, a shift in personal perspectives and values must occur; such changes occur with increased knowledge, first of oneself and then of others (Erickson, 1997). The ultimate goal is the realization that diversity provides richness and promotes power and creativity in our professional and personal lives and contributes to the building of a global village that is positive for everyone.

DEFINITIONS

The study of culture is associated with many definitions. A common dictionary definition of **culture** is the integrated pattern of human knowledge, belief, and behavior that depends upon man's capacity and learning to transmit knowledge; the customary beliefs, social forms, and material traits of a racial, religious, or social group. Thus culture can be viewed at many levels (e.g., the culture of a reader's classroom, specific university, city, or country). A fish may discover its need for water only when it is no longer in it, and a mammal may only realize its need for air when it is under water. One's own culture is like water to a fish or air to a mammal; it nurtures and sustains. One lives and breathes through one's own culture almost without realizing it. Therefore what one culture regards as essential may not be essential to another culture. In fact, what is vital to one culture may be regarded by another culture as antagonistic, threatening, or contemptible (Trompenaars, 1994).

Diversity is the term used to explain differences between cultures (Catalano, 1996). Diversity has two associated levels of characteristics: primary and secondary. Primary characteristics include those obvious traits, such as nationality, race, gender, age, and color; religious preference, though not physically obvious, is also considered a primary characteristic of cultural diversity. Secondary characteristics include socioeconomic status; duration of time away from one's country of origin; residential status, gender, age, and sexual orientation issues; and education (Catalano, 1996).

The social group whose members dominate by controlling the most important positions or places in society is known as the **dominant culture.** In the United States, at the present time, the dominant culture is the Caucasian panethnic group. There is some indication that by 2080, Caucasians will be in the minority, accounting for 48.9% of the total population (Catalano, 1996). The **minority culture**, then, is a social group that potentially faces discriminatory treatment from the dominant group. Disproportionate numbers of individuals in the minority group are often within the lower socioeconomic classes; many live in abject poverty.

When individuals adapt the beliefs, values, attitudes, and practices of the dominant culture, they are said to have experienced **acculturation.** That process is associated with an individual "fitting in" more in the mainstream. Some individuals publicly assume those cultural behaviors and attitudes that allow them to fit in but behave differently in private. This may lend security to the individual but may also increase stress. Mr. Chang, the owner of several Chinese restaurants, is an interesting example of partial blending. When he works as cashier, Mr. Chang totals customers' bills on an IBM cash register, then pulls an abacus from underneath the desk and checks the total before rendering the exact bill.

Culture shock is a normal phenomenon and happens to all individuals in new situations where values are different and the usual symbols and signs are markedly different. International travel and hospitalization are two common experiences that contribute to culture shock. An APN reared and educated in the farmlands of Kansas who comes to an inner city ghetto of South Philadelphia to practice will likely experience culture shock. There may be an initial honeymoon phase where the new setting feels positive and impressive, but over time the individual will become disenchanted with the changes. Then there is a slow process of adaptation and resolution of the conflicts associated with the change in setting or situation (Padilla, 1980). "Although knowing about culture shock can help to control one's negative social or therapeutic behavior, it doesn't make the culture shock any less s-h-o-c-k-i-n-g, just as knowing the stages of grief doesn't make loss less painful" (Ramer, 1992).

The belief that one's own way, one's own culture, is superior or better than others (a phenomenon known as *ethnocentrism*) contributes to *stereotypes,* generalizations made about the data one processes every day. This is a prejudiced, often preconceived, and often false view about groups of people.

There are notable variations within and between cultures with respect to time orientation and sense of space. *Polemics* is the study of how persons of different cultures relate to their physical space and territory (Hall, 1963). *Monochromatic time* refers to the tendency to place high value on keeping to a timed appointment, while *polychromic time* refers to a tendency to place less value on timed appointments and more value on completion of business and involvement with people (Hall, 1983).

CRITICAL ISSUES: CULTURAL DIVERSITY FOR ADVANCED PRACTICE NURSES

The framework used to examine culture is one that examines systems and characteristics. There are eight systems, or societal structures, and nine characteristics, or dimensions, of living that are expressed in every dominant culture in one form or another. People learn how to live in these systems and express these characteristics from the first sights and sounds they experience as babies, thus making

parents the first teachers, the first programmers. From smiles and frowns, people learn acceptable and unacceptable ways of doing things. When people leave their families, they continue this learning—this programming process—in kindergarten, school, and college, through television and other forms of media, and from day-to-day life experiences. (The *characteristics* that are inherent in a culture are depicted in Table 33-1. *Systems* that are part of a culture are depicted in Table 33-2. Both provide examples from the mainstream of various cultures.)

To discuss culture, it is necessary to make some generalizations about the way things are done; however, it is important to remember that there are variations and exceptions to generalizations. These systems and characteristics can be used to examine the differences in cultures both within the United States and around the world. They guide behavior ranging from when to make eye contact and when to smile to how children are reared and when and how to deal with conflict. No society exists without these systems and characteristics, and no individual is free of culture.

Time and Space

Time may be perceived quite differently by people in different cultures. Some cultures are more oriented to the present, while others look to the future and plan and save accordingly. For example, time in Latin America and the Middle East is *polychromatic* and stresses the involvement of people and the completion of business rather than keeping to strict schedules. The result is that a physician's appointment time may not be taken seriously and the physician or patient may be late or the appointment may be broken. A dinner party set for 8:00 PM may well find a Brazilian guest more than fashionably late because of time perception. In the United States, time is *monochromatic*; keeping the exact time for the appointment is seen as important for both physician and patient (Hall, 1983). Waiting in lines or for appointments has a negative perception. Over time, if health care providers are consistently late, many individuals will find a new provider, believing that their time is too valuable to wait (sometimes interpreted as "too valuable to waste").

Making sense of differences such as the way appointments are kept, the amount of distance between two people who are conversing, or whether or not eye contact is made during conversation can be confusing and uncomfortable without knowledge and appreciation of differences in peoples. It is comfortable to be with individuals who "do things the way we do." In a classroom or meeting, people tend to sit in the same spot time after time. At a party, acquaintances tend to gather together.

Individuals of different cultures have a different perception of space or territoriality. In America, distance between individuals is considered intimate at 0 to 18

Table 33-1		

Concepts of Culture: Characteristics (with Examples from Mainstream Culture)

CONCEPT	DEFINITION	EXAMPLES
Communication and language	The communication system, verbal and nonverbal, that distinguishes one group from another	Dialects and specific languages Facial expressions and eye contact
Dress and appearance	Hair, outward garments, and adornments (or a lack thereof), as well as body decorations that tend to be distinctive by culture	"Dressing for success" The dress code at "J. Crew University" Saris in India Jeans and cowboy boots in Texas
Food and eating habits	The manner in which food is selected, prepared, presented, and eaten	Kosher food laws Belching to the cook in Asia Use of chopsticks in China
Time and time consciousness	Sense of time differs by culture, so that times in some cultures are exact and others are relative	"Time is money" The Arab word *In shallah*, which means *whenever it comes to pass*
Rewards and recognition	The manner and method of offering praise for good deeds, length of service, and various accomplishments	Merit raises or tips for good service in the United States Emphasis on the good of the group in Japan
Relationships	Cultures set human and organizational relationships by age, sex, status, wealth, power, and wisdom	The democratic nature of families in the Unites States The head of an extended gypsy family makes all family decisions in Hungary
Values and standards	The priorities attached to certain behaviors; the acceptable norms for the group	The individual freedom expected in the Unites States The dominance of the group ensures harmony in Asia
Sense of self and space	Some cultures are very closed to others, determining the physical aspect of how closely people relate to each other and the amount of formality expected in relationships	"Too close for comfort" "Get out of my space"
Beliefs and attitudes	The major ethics of a group of people and how it influences their feeling toward themselves and others	The Judeo-Christian foundation of the Unites States The position of women in society Views on abortion

From Gardenswartz, L., & Rowe, A. (1993). *Managing diversity: a complete desk reference and planning guide.* Burr Ridge, IL: Irwin Professional Publishing; and International Negotiations Management (1993). *Global awareness.* Loudon, TN: International Negotiations Management.

inches; at this distance, visual details, smell, body heat, and touch are possible. Friends and acquaintances respect personal distance, usually giving 1.5 to 4 feet. Social distance is considered to be 4 to 12 feet, while anything over 12 feet is considered public space (Andrews & Boyle, 1999). For individuals accustomed to these distances, invasion of space can be distressing.

Bennett (1986), a crosscultural specialist, asserts that intercultural sensitivity is not normal; however, failure to develop this sensitivity is not an option. Failure to exercise intercultural sensitivity is not simply bad morality—it is self-destructive. Box 33-1 displays three fundamental facts about cultural understanding.

Conflict

Conflict may result when people interpret the behavior of others as different from their own. Explaining another person's behavior based on one's own assumptions results in errors. According to Adler and Kiggunder (1983), people find it necessary to make sense of others' behaviors, and the following three steps take place: (1) people de-

Table 33-2

Concepts of Culture: Systems (with Examples from Mainstream Culture)

CONCEPT	DEFINITION	EXAMPLES
Kinship	Family relationships and the way people reproduce and train and socialize their children	Emphasis on the nuclear family in the United States Care of aging parents within households in India
Education	How young or new members of a society are provided with information, knowledge, skills, and values	Schools readying children for kindergarten in Japan Open admission to universities in the United States
Economics	How society produces and distributes its goods and services	Use of the dollar for currency in the United States Use of cigarettes as currency in some developing countries
Politics	The dominant means of governance for maintaining order and exercising power or authority	Democracy in the United States Theocracy in Iran
Religion	The means for providing meaning and motivation beyond the material aspects of life (i.e., the spiritual side of a culture or its approach to the supernatural)	Hinduism in India Catholicism in Brazil
Association	The network of social groupings that people form	Athletic clubs and church potlucks in the United States
Health	The way a culture prevents and cures disease or illness or cares for victims of disasters or accidents	Emphasis on the scientific basis for disease in the West Holism in Eastern cultures "Walking in beauty" among the Navajos
Recreation	The ways in which people socialize or use their leisure time	Watching television in the United States Taking walks in Germany

From Gardenswartz, L., & Rowe, A. (1993). *Managing diversity: a complete desk reference and planning guide*. Burr Ridge, IL: Irwin Professional Publishing; and International Negotiations Management (1993). *Global awareness*. Loudon, TN: International Negotiations Management.

Box 33-1

Cultural Understanding

- Culture is the unique lifestyle of a particular group of people. Unlike good manners, it is not something possessed by some and not by others—it is possessed by all human beings.
- Humans create culture not only as an adaptive mechanism to their biological or geographical environment, but as a means of contributing to their social evolution. Our heredity combines both genes and culture traits, which influence one another.
- The effects of our cultural conditioning are so great that people whose experience has been limited to the rules of one culture have difficulty understanding communication based on another set of rules.

From International Negotiations Management (1993). *Global awareness*. Loudon, TN: International Negotiations Management.

scribe the behavior (e.g., the patient was late to an appointment); (2) people interpret the behavior (e.g., the patient is too lazy to get there on time); and (3) people evaluate the behavior (e.g., the patient really does not care about getting needed health care). Steps two and three are the troublesome ones when people are trying to get along with others who do things differently.

Understanding the cultural programming of Middle Eastern or Asian patients would help nurses know that keeping appointments at an exact time is simply not the way they do things. Family and friends who help a patient get to the clinic are much more important than the time of the appointment. Furthermore, many cultures see men as responsible for the well-being of women and may not know how to interpret the actions of a female caregiver who is trying to teach men about health care. It is natural for nurses to come to the professional setting with the assumption that they and their patients view time and their professional contributions in the same way. However, this is not the situation, and conflict can result.

Ethnocentrism

When people look at other cultures and ways of functioning that are different from their own, they tend to make judgments. It is usual for a nurse to believe that being on time for an appointment is the "right" way to do things. However, believing that one's own way or culture is superior to other ways is ethnocentric. The problem with making ethnocentric judgments is that often the tendency is to see others in a less-than-favorable light. To view

Middle Eastern patients as lazy or inattentive is a barrier to them receiving *culturally competent care*, care that not only helps them get well but also helps them feel well.

Each culture's way of doing things has advantages and disadvantages; culturally competent caregivers are able to state and understand these. For example, placing a priority on relationships with one's family is a behavior that can facilitate high-level wellness; constant concern with numerous appointments that crowd the schedules of many people can lead to high levels of stress. Culturally competent caregivers are also aware of their own stereotypes and prejudices.

Stereotypes and Prejudices

Stereotypes are generalizations people make about the huge amount of data processed every day. Stereotypes can be helpful. For example, the generalization that streets full of cars are potentially dangerous keeps us from getting hit crossing the street. However, generalizations about individuals or groups of people (e.g, the physically disadvantaged, athletes, homeless women, those living in poverty, immigrants) are damaging and limiting because they ignore the variety of people that make up any group of people. Prejudice, or having preconceived and often false views about groups of people, is a common feeling; however, prejudice is the foundation for stereotypes that are often damaging.

Stereotypes come from one's experiences and information and often capture some characteristics that can be seen in a group. However, stereotypes are frequently charged with negative assumptions. They do not change, even when information exists that proves them wrong; usually when stereotyping occurs, people are not interested in the facts (Gardenswartz & Rowe, 1993).

All people hold stereotypes. Try finishing the following sentences: _____ are very fine athletes. _____ are lazy and unreliable. _____ are excellent in mathematics. _____ are dangerous. Stereotypes become self-fulfilling prophecies. People look for data to prove them. Every time a nurse in a clinic cares for patients from a certain country or ethnic group, the nurse expects them to be late (for example), and every time they are, they prove that the nurse's experience is correct. Because the nurse places a high value on keeping to the appointment schedule, he or she subtly communicates displeasure to both the patients and his or her coworkers. Gradually, receiving nonverbal and perhaps verbal communication that their way of doing things is not acceptable, the patients come to the clinic only when it is absolutely essential, when they are acutely ill.

Because generalizing is a human reaction, ridding one-

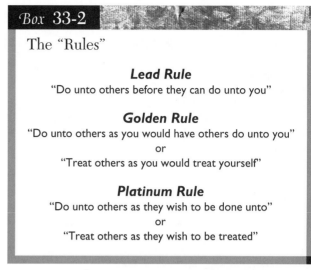

From International Negotiations Management (1993). *Global awareness.* Loudon, TN: International Negotiations Management.

self of damaging stereotypes can be difficult. However, it can be done. The first step, often painful, is to recognize one's own stereotypes. Then, one should try to find data to disprove the stereotypes. If, for example, one thinks that athletes are not scholars, one should find athletes who are. Getting rid of stereotypes means being aware, on a daily basis, of one's own thoughts about others and the negative influence they can have. Learn the "Platinum Rule" in Box 33-2. Truly culturally competent caregivers utilize it with all of their family, patients, friends, and neighbors on a regular basis.

Communication and Cultural Understanding

All people are versatile communicators, having a wide range of communication skills that go beyond words and include facial and hand gestures as well as sounds and smells. Needs, values, standards, explanations, and ideals are communicated. Perceptions of people, things, and situations communicated via body language, bearing, appearance, tone of voice, choice of words, and content of the language are also common. If clinic staff disapprove of the conduct of a group of people who come for care, their disapproval cannot help but be communicated to that group. (Principles about the communication process are depicted in Box 33-3.)

Crosscultural communication is a "people process." Communication is the most important tool people have for getting things done and is the basis for understanding and cooperation. It can transfer information, get things done, and meet people's needs. It can also distort messages, cause frustrations, and make people, organizations, and families hurtful and ineffective.

The Communication Process

- Communication involves a sender, receiver, and message. The message conveys meaning through the medium used to send it (the how) and its content (the what). Individuals selectively comprehend all new data. They determine what is relevant to and consistent with their own needs. This is why two people can receive the same message and derive two entirely different meanings from it.

- No matter how hard one tries, one cannot avoid communicating. When we are silent, our body language is communicating something. We communicate by our activity or our inactivity—by what we do or do not do. All behavior is communication because it contains a message, whether intended or not.

- Communication does not necessarily mean understanding. Understanding takes place only when individuals have the same interpretation of the symbols used in the communication process, whether the symbols are words or gestures. When we communicate, only three things can happen (two of which are bad!):
  - What we are communicating is completely understood
  - What we are communicating is misunderstood
  - What we are communicating is not understood

- Communication is irreversible. One cannot take back a communication. It can be explained, clarified, or restated, but it cannot be wiped out. It becomes part of our experience and influences present and future meanings.

- Communication always occurs in a context. One cannot ignore the circumstances surrounding the communication process. The location, timing, and surroundings form the environment.

- Communication is a dynamic process. It is a continuous and active process without a beginning or an end. One is both a sender and receiver at the same time.

Adapted from International Negotiations Management (1993). *Global awareness*. Loudon, TN: International Negotiations Management.

Cultural Concept of Health

The way in which individuals view health and illness, learned through the processes of growth and maturation, has its base in their culture. What is defined as a health problem or illness, when and where to seek health care and preventive services, what is expected from treatment, and the way in which the sick role is enacted are a part of one's culture. Many cultural groups view illness as a distortion of balance in some aspect of their lives; a large number of the world's people view illness as a result of *mal occhio*—the evil eye—or as a result of an evil spirit. In fact, in some cultures, surgery is feared because it may allow an evil spirit to enter the body. Clearly, without an understanding of these diverse beliefs, health care providers, who practice from a traditional western medicine framework, will be confused about the meaning of these beliefs and practices for their patients. It is important that these views and their associated health care practices are not trivialized or discounted and that the rules of western medicine are not imposed on patients. When providers are not knowledgeable about the health beliefs and practices of other cultures, misdiagnosis or ineffective treatment may occur, with dangerous, even life-threatening consequences and a waste of health care dollars. Patients have been institutionalized with misdiagnosed schizophrenia and parents submitted to police because of suspected child abuse because of cultural practices unfamiliar to providers. It is important to explore a patient's explanatory model for the illness and what kind of treatment is expected.

Most cultures have traditional healers that engage with patients through what is known as *folk medicine*. A patient may use these individuals for the majority of care, or they may blend folk medicine approaches with more traditional western medicine. Traditional healing, often called *alternative* or *holistic*, focuses on the body's ability to heal itself and the interrelatedness of mind, body, and spirit. Traditional healing is less costly than the biomedical/scientific approach to health care; in fact, many members of the current cultural majority in the United States engage in alternative medicine of some type, either as a substitute for or supplement to scientific medicine. Herbal therapy, for example, has become a mega-business, and alternative medicine as a whole in the United States is a billion-dollar business (Wallis, 1991). Patient assessment should include a respectful discussion of any home and folk remedies being used as preventive and treatment measures. However, one should remember that some patients are reluctant to discuss alternative healing methods; this is especially true if they have had previous negative experiences with providers who have "disapproved" of such remedies. Culturally competent APNs will not be "disappointed by" or disapproving of patients' use of folk healing. Traditional healing should be included in the management plan to the extent possible.

Developing Strength through Diversity

Diversity means simply the state of being different. Evolution produces diversity because lack of diversity in biology means (for example) fewer types of plants and, as a result, weakness. Diversity is the natural order of life. No human being is exactly like another, just as no snowflake is like another. Differences in biology through evolution give strength to life.

The United States is a diverse country. The landscape across the United States varies from mountains to plains, from deserts to rainforest. The people's ethnic origins mirror the world, and their educational institutions, technology, and socioeconomic structures, are varied. Still, living and being comfortable with diversity can be difficult.

Culture is so powerful that it often takes effort to learn to be comfortable with people who do things differently. How often do people shut themselves off from learning new ways of carrying out the activities of daily life? How often do health care providers subtly communicate their disregard for patients who are different?

Given contemporary demographical changes in the workforce in this country, including increases in the number of women, minorities, immigrants, and older adults, nurses do not have choices about interacting with or giving care to people who are different. Nurses do have choices about how they interact. Viewing differences as negative, or being so immersed in one's own culture that there is little sense of other valid ways of thinking and acting, results in hostility and alienation.

It is the premise of this chapter that seeing differences as positive is a route to growth. Persons who appreciate diversity are not fenced in by the norms of one culture but are continually being molded by new cultural contacts and relationships. Working together with many different viewpoints, people may begin to find solutions to the health, environmental, social, and economic problems that face this nation and the world. Ultimately, people do not have a choice to get along with others who are different. If people wish to have a sense of security about the future, they must build a democratic, multicultural society where accepted difference is the norm. The alternative is a world that is increasingly divided and violent.

There are four attitudes that assist in learning about other cultures (Hess, 1994). These include a high regard for the diversity of people on the earth; an eagerness to learn and be challenged by new experiences; a desire to make connections with other people; and a readiness to give of oneself and receive in return in the process of making new connections. These kinds of attitudes will help everyone bridge differences and make this a world of differences that are positive as well as enjoyable.

IMPLICATIONS FOR MSN EDUCATION AND ADVANCED PRACTICE

The practice of APNs must be informed by an understanding of cultural diversity and its implication for managing health care. Self-awareness, with recognition of one's own stereotypes and biases, is an important prerequisite. An APN should determine which cultural groups predominate his or her practice area and learn as much as possible about those cultures. The importance of a willingness to learn from dialogues with patients and families cannot be overemphasized; it is impossible to learn everything about a culture from a book. Sensitive communication is important to the process of becoming culturally aware, especially the skill of careful and respectful listening.

While in graduate school, students should learn how to work with interpreters to optimize both assessment and intervention. Ideally, a trained medical interpreter or bilingual health care provider will be available to help bridge the cultural gap between a foreign (or non–English-speaking) patient and provider. Not only do medical interpreters have familiarity with the other culture that can be invaluable, they understand medical terminology, agency policy, and ethics (Andrews & Boyle, 1999). With a trained interpreter, confidentiality is also not an issue, as it would be if a family member or friend were serving as interpreter. Although the provider remains in control of the content and process flow of the interview, the interpreter is an invaluable member of the team. It is usually surprising to novices that communication through an interpreter takes considerably longer than providing the same information directly to an English-speaking patient. The interpreter must be given time about every sentence or two to provide a response. Use of simple language, with as little medical jargon as possible, facilitates the process of making the message as close to verbatim as possible. Since gender is such an important issue in many cultures, an interpreter of the same gender as the patient is preferred.

On occasion, no interpreter will be available. At such times, a polite, formal, and unhurried approach is important. Also, even if the APN can only use a few words of the patient's language, using them shows sensitivity and respect. Simple language and pantomimed words might suffice, and a calm, unhurried, and moderate voice is important. Under stress, there is a tendency to speak faster; with a listener who does not understand, there is also a tendency to speak louder, which sometimes connotes anger. Drawings of spoons or pills may help in discussing medication doses; simple actions given in their appropriate sequences may help in teaching about care (e.g., wash hands, open package, rub medicine onto skin, wash hands). Sticking to one idea at a time is important. For example, one should not ask both "Are you hurting and nauseated?" "Do you hurt?" (with pantomime) followed by "Are you sick at your stomach?" (also with pantomime) would be more easily understood. Phrasebooks or flash cards for common phrases can be helpful additions in these circumstances (Andrews & Boyle, 1999). Knowing about a culture's nonverbal communication (e.g., use of eye contact and touch) and spatial orientation is also helpful for accurate interpretation of patient behavior, as well as guidance for appropriate behavior in the patient's presence. These are important aspects of what Andrews and Boyle (1999) call *cultural courtesy*. Knowledge of the cultural time orientation of a patient can be important to making and keeping scheduled appointments. For some patients, walk-in appointment options can be helpful. Tolerance for differences in a patient's sense of time is important to the nurse-patient relationship.

Clearly, APNs need an understanding about how patients of diverse cultures prevent or care for illness. They need to understand lifeways, folk remedies, and the involvement of a healer. The ability to ask about these aspects of care can be roleplayed before an actual encounter if there is concern about how to conduct sensitive assessments. Because health promotion and management of illness often necessitate dietary changes, it is important for APNs to understand the dietary preferences and practices of a particular culture and be able to incorporate the patient's cultural practices and preferences into the dietary management plan.

The way in which different cultures view medications can also be a crucial component of management. For example, for some people, certain foods or drinks must be taken with medications to ensure "balance"; this is fine unless the food or beverage affects the medication in some way. Tea or milk, for example, taken with oral iron therapy would minimize the effectiveness of the drug. When medication is necessary to control chronic problems like diabetes mellitus or hypertension, regardless of continuing symptoms, careful explanation is necessary. For some patients, such as certain Chinese Americans, the cultural tradition is that medication is necessary only as long as symptoms persist (Andrews & Boyle, 1999).

In many cultures, it is not the patient who makes the ultimate decisions about treatment; other family members may make such decisions. In some cases, the family will consult an outside authority in an effort to reach a decision about medical intervention or treatment. This is important information for APNs, who may be expecting all patients to be autonomous in health care decisions.

Andrews and Boyle (1999) warn about the negative connotations of the terms *compliant* and *noncompliant* with respect to culturally diverse patients. With a patient of a different culture, the extent of compliance with treatment might be an issue of cultural preference, failure to understand the provider's instructions, or uncertainty in the nurse-patient relationship.

Information about the biological variations and differences in disease risks among and between patients of different cultures is critical to APN practice. Additional details about this component of cultural diversity are included in Chapter 37.

PRIORITES FOR RESEARCH

Although cultural aspects of care continue to be widely studied, research directed at the management of culturally diverse patients by APNs is sorely lacking. Since APNs are known for providing holistic care, they may come to be preferred providers for patients from diverse cultures, and this could serve as a legitimate question for study: Do patients from different cultures prefer APNs over physicians for health care? What characteristics of the APN are perceived as positive by diverse patients?

Ethnographical studies directed at discovering cultural themes and determining "cultural programming" of patients of particular cultures are needed (Streubert & Carpenter, 1995). Case studies can also continue to contribute to the knowledge base about varied cultural groups and their health.

Research is also needed about how best to assess patients for evidence of cultural beliefs, attitudes, and practices on busy units. The transcultural assessment instruments, albeit compelling for getting answers about cultural phenomena, are not practical for consistent use in all settings for all patients. What questions are essential to gain data for safe and effective practice by APNs? How are these questions best phrased?

Methods for provision of informed consent and teaching materials also need methodological and empirical testing to ensure cultural, age, and educational level appropriateness. Because pharmacological management is so critical to effective care and so easily misunderstood, particular emphasis should be placed on testing materials about drug treatment. Attention should be given to potential diet/drug interactions and drug/folk remedy interactions.

APNs are in a unique position to share the practical wisdom gained when working with patients of diverse cultures. Best practices and evidence-based practices need dissemination so that the cultural competence of all APNs can be enhanced. What works in the day-to-day practice setting to lend comfort to patients and families and strengthen the nurse-patient relationship can be invaluable. Too often, APNs believe that the simple measures that work for them are universally known, so exemplary practices are not shared. When this is the case, everyone loses.

DISCUSSION QUESTIONS

These questions can be used to promote critical thinking and encourage discussion.

1. Discuss cultural groups in your area whose health promotion needs are not adequately met and identify specific outcomes to improve their health care.
2. Compare methods of teaching various cultural groups. Consult a text on transcultural nursing to facilitate this activity.
3. Read Galanti, G. (1997). *Caring for patients from different cultures: case studies from American hospitals* (2nd ed.). Philadelphia: University of Pennsylvania

Suggestions for Further Learning

- Consult the following resources for learning about strength in diversity:
  - Highsmith Multicultural Bookstore, W5527 Highway 106, PO Box 800, Fort Atkinson, WI 53538; phone (800) 558-2110
  - HR Press, PO Box 28, Fredonia, NY 14063; phone (716) 672-4254
  - Intercultural Press, PO Box 700, Yarmouth, ME 04096
  - International Women's Tribute Centre, 777 United Nations Plaza, New York, NY 10017; phone (212) 687-8633
  - Summerfield, E (1993). *Crossing cultures through film.* Yarmouth, ME: Intercultural Press
  - Women Make Movies, Inc., 426 Broadway, Suite 500C, New York, NY 10013; phone (212) 925-0606
  - Complete Cultural Diversity Library, ODT Inc., PO Box 134, Amherst, MA 01004
- Examine one of the following resources: Eliades, D.C., & Suitor, C.W. (1994). *Celebrating diversity: approaching families through their food.* Arlington, VA: National Center for Education in Maternal Child Health (available at 2000 15th Street North, Suite 701, Arlington, VA. 22201-2617; phone [703] 524-7802); May, L., & Sharratt, S.C. (1994). *Applied ethics: a multicultural approach.* Englewood Cliffs, NJ: Prentice-Hall; Real, M.R. (1996). *Exploring media culture: a guide.* Thousand Oaks, CA, Sage; and Simons G.F., & Abramms, B. (1992). *The question of diversity assessment tools for organizations and individuals.* Amherst, MA: ODT, Inc.
- Seek out information from the following organizations:
  - A World of Difference Institute, Anti-Defamation League, 823 United Nations Plaza, New York, NY 10017; website www.adl.org
  - Institute for Social and Cultural Change (SPEAK OUT), PO Box 99096, Emeryville, CA 94662
  - International Society for Intercultural Education Training and Research, SIEDTAR USA, 573 Bayview, Yarmouth, ME 04096; phone (207) 846-9598
  - Southwest Center for Human Relations Studies (sponsor of the Annual National Conference on Race and Ethnicity in American Higher Education), University of Oklahoma, 555 E. Constitution, Suite 209, Norman, OK 73072

Press. Discuss some of the cases you find compelling. Suggest how a culturally competent APN might prevent such cases or provide an appropriate remedy.

4. In a small group setting, discuss a time in which a patient encounter was complicated by an issue of culture. What happened? What would you do differently if it happened again? Why?

REFERENCES/BIBLIOGRAPHY

Adler N., & Kiggunder M.K. (1983). Awareness at the crossroad: designing translator-based training programs. In D. Landes & R. Breslin (Eds.), *Handbook of intercultural training* (Vol. 2). New York: Pergamon.

Andrews, M.M., & Boyle, J.S. (1999). *Transcultural concepts in nursing care* (3rd ed.). Philadelphia: JB Lippincott.

Bennett, M (1986). Toward ethnorelativism: a developmental model of intercultural sensitivity. In M. Paige (Ed.), *Cross cultural orientation: new conceptualizations and applications.* New York: University Press of America.

Catalano, J.T. (1996). *Nursing now! Today's issues, tomorrow's trends* (2nd ed.). Philadelphia: FA Davis.

Eliades, D.C., & Suitor, C.W. (1994). *Celebrating diversity: approaching families through their food.* Arlington, VA: National Center for Education in Maternal Child Health.

Erickson, J.I. (1997). Culturally competent care: viewing diversity as a vehicle to wholeness. Caring headlines. *MGH Patient Care Services,* 3(21), 1.

Galanti, G. (1997). *Caring for patients from different cultures: case studies from American hospitals* (2nd ed.). Philadelphia: University of Pennsylvania Press.

Gardenswartz, L., & Rowe, A. (1993). *Managing diversity: a complete desk reference and planning guide.* Burr Ridge, IL: Irwin Professional Publishing.

Giger, J.N., & Davidhizar, R.E. (1995). *Transcultural nursing—assessment and intervention* (2nd ed). St. Louis: Mosby.

Hall, E. (1963). Proxemics: the study of man's spacial relationships. In I. Gladstone (Ed.), *Man's image in medicine and anthropology* (pp. 109-120). New York: International University Press.

Hall, E. (1983). *The dance of life: the other dimension of time.* New York: Doubleday.

Hess, D. (1994). *The whole world guide to culture learning.* Yarmouth, ME: Intercultural Press.

International Negotiations Management (1993). *Global awareness.* Loudon, TN: International Negotiations Management.

Johnson, W.B. (1994). Workforce 2000: executive summary. In G.R. Weaver (Ed.), *Culture, communication and conflict: readings in intercultural relations.* Needham, MA: Simon & Schuster

Madrid, A. (1990, November-December). Diversity and its discontents. *Academe,* 15.

Padilla, A. (1980). Acculturation: theory, models, and some new findings. *Colorado Westview Press,* 47-84.

Potter, P.A., & Perry, A.G. (1993). *Fundamentals of nursing: concepts, process, and practice* (3rd ed.). St. Louis: Mosby.

Ramer, L. (1992). *Culturally sensitive caregiving and childbearing families. Module 1—nursing issues for the 21st century.* White Plains, NY: March of Dimes Birth Defects Foundation.

Streubert, H. J., & Carpenter D. R. (1995). *Qualitative research in nursing.* Philadelphia: JB Lippincott.

Torres, S. (1993, July). Cultural sensitivity: a must for today's primary care provider. *ADVANCE for Nurse Practitioners,* 16-18.

Trompenaars, F. (1994). *Riding the wave of culture—understanding diversity in global business ethics.* Burr Ridge, IL: Professional Publications.

Wallis, C. (1991, November 4). Why alternative health care medicine is catching on. *Time,* 68-74.

Zagorsky, E.S. (1993). Caring for families who follow alternative health care practices. *Pediatric Nursing, 19*(1), 71-75.

Chapter 34

Theories and Models of Transcultural Nursing

Ann Schmidt Luggen & Cheryl Pope Kish

Nursing is a transcultural care profession. It involves caring for unique individuals across many cultures. As the population of this country becomes more diverse, advanced practice nurses (APNs) will have a greater need than ever to understand cultural diversity and provide care that is sensitive and culturally congruent. To that end, APNs need a framework in transcultural theory to inform their clinical practice. This chapter presents Leininger's Theory of Culture Care Diversity and Universality and Purnell's Model for Cultural Competence in some detail and then summarizes other conceptual models related to transcultural nursing.

DEFINITIONS

Although Section VI of this book provided a comprehensive view of nursing theories and defined the relevant terms, it is appropriate here to offer several definitions again to set a context for examining conceptualizations about transcultural care. Definitions specific to each theory or model are provided in that theory's section.

A *theory* is a "construct that accounts for or organizes some phenomenon" (Barnum, 1998). Therefore a nursing theory provides a way of organizing the phenomenon called nursing, describing and explaining it through a set of salient points that are critical to understanding nursing as a discipline. Leininger (1991) continues to define theory, as in her early works, as "patterns or sets of interrelated concepts, expressions, meanings and experiences that describe, explain, predict, and can account for some phenomena or domain of inquiry procured through an open creative and naturalistic discovery process." In an overview of her theory, Leininger (1991) writes, "Theories are creative ways to discover new 'truths,' refute inadequate explanations, and gain in-depth insights about a phenomenon in order to advance discipline knowledge and improve human conditions."

A *conceptual framework* or *model* is defined as a set of concepts and related principles that are integrated into a configuration that is meaningful (Marriner-Tomey & Alligood, 1998). Conceptual frameworks tend to be less formal in providing an identity for the phenomenon of interest—in this case the discipline of nursing. Like theories, conceptual frameworks are useful for guiding clinical practice, education, and research.

Transcultural nursing is a term coined by Leininger in the mid-1950s as she envisioned blending the disciplines of anthropology and nursing in both theory and practice to enable a cultural perspective to patient care. Transcultural nursing is defined by Andrews (1999) as "a specialty within nursing focused on the comparative study and analysis of different cultures and subcultures . . . with respect to caring behavior, nursing care, health-illness values, beliefs, and patterns of behavior." As the name suggests, "Transcultural nursing goes across cultural boundaries, seeking to find the essence of nursing."

Giger and Davidhizar (1995) define transcultural nursing as "a culturally competent practice field that is client centered and research focused." Clearly, not all APNs will engage in the full spectrum of transcultural nursing. However, all are encouraged to provide culturally sensitive care that appreciates patients' uniqueness and is free of inherent biases based on race or ethnic group, religion, gender, age, or philosophy.

CRITICAL ISSUES: UNDERSTANDING TRANSCULTURAL THEORIES AND MODELS

A theory or conceptual model to guide one's clinical practice is advantageous because it provides a systematic view or map that organizes the many pieces of information for practice into an orderly, meaningful pattern that enables competent, individualized, quality care. A theoretical or conceptual base for practice and research also increases an APN's credibility and practice by enabling new perspec-

tives. Transcultural theories and models, whether embraced in their entirety or used in part, are valuable to any professional whose clinical practice involves culturally diverse clients. Knowledge about specific cultures—their value systems and lifeways—is an excellent starting point for providing culturally appropriate care as a certified registered nurse anesthetist (CRNA), clinical nurse specialist (CNS), certified nurse midwife (CNM), or nurse practitioner (NP).

Leininger's Theory of Culture Care Diversity and Universality

In the 1950s, during work in a child guidance setting with emotionally disturbed children of diverse cultural backgrounds, professional nurse Dr. Madeline Leininger became convinced that their behavior was culturally determined. Her clinical experience and her questions about cultural aspects of care served as an impetus for her graduate study in anthropology at the University of Washington at Seattle. Her education and subsequent 2-year experience with the indigenous people of Gadsup in the Eastern Highlands of New Guinea served as a beginning point for the Theory of Culture Care Diversity and Universality. Leininger also developed an appreciation, shared in her classic 1970 work *Nursing and Anthropology: Two Worlds to Blend*, that "the fields of anthropology and nursing must be interdigitated so that each field will profit from the contribution of the other. It is apparent that if these two fields were sharing their special knowledge and experiences, both would undoubtedly see new pathways in thinking and research." This first book served as the foundation for not only her theory but also for the specialty practice of transcultural nursing. Leininger's second book, *Transcultural Nursing: Concepts, Theories, Research and Practice*, published in 1979, was the first definitive manuscript published on the topic.

Over the past 47 years, Dr. Leininger has explicated her theory, which is derived from holistic nursing and anthropological perspective of persons living in different places in the world and in different contexts, and seen it studied in cultures in Western and non-Western areas. The theory was constructed within a qualitative discovery paradigm with largely person-centered (*emic*) views rather than other-centered (*etic*) views. In her words, "It was natural to theorize about the diversities of human care to explain the differences that might prevail within and among cultures" and to discover about nursing "what was universal or that which commonly existed and could be identifiable about human care in all or most cultures worldwide [which would be] critical if nursing was to be a global or universal profession and discipline"(Leininger, 1991).

Over her long and distinguished career as a nursing educator, Dr. Leininger established transcultural nursing programs at four universities, the last being Wayne State University in Detroit, until her semiretirement in 1995.

She initiated the Transcultural Nursing Society in 1974 and the *Journal of Transcultural Nursing* in 1989 (Welch, Alexander, Beagle, Butler, Dougherty, Andrews-Robards, Solotkin, and Velotta, 1998).

The major concepts and definitions associated with the Theory of Culture Care Diversity and Universality are shown in Box 34-1. Leininger (1991) proposes three major modes as guides to nursing judgments, decisions, and actions: (1) cultural care preservation and/or maintenance; (2) cultural care accommodation and/or negotiation; and (3) cultural care repatterning or restructuring. These modes were experientially derived and "were care-centered and based on the use of generic (emic) care knowledge along with professional (etic) care knowledge obtained from research using the theory." All care modes require that nurse and patient become "co-participants" for the kind of culturally congruent care that is "beneficial, satisfying, and meaningful to people nurses serve."

Major assumptions

The premises of the theory are as follows and were taken directly from Leininger's definitive work, *Culture Care Diversity and Universality: A Theory of Nursing* (1991):

1. Care is the essence of nursing and a distinct, dominant, central, and unifying focus.
2. Care (caring) is essential for well-being, health, healing, growth, survival, and to face handicaps or death.
3. Culture care is the broadest holistic means to know, explain, interpret, and predict nursing care phenomena to guide nursing care practices.
4. Nursing is a transcultural humanistic and scientific care discipline and profession with the central purpose of serving human beings worldwide.
5. Care (caring) is essential to curing and healing, for there can be no curing without caring.
6. Culture care concepts, meanings, expressions, patterns, processes, and structural forms are both different (displaying diversity) and similar (leaning toward commonalties or universalities) among all cultures of the world.
7. Every human culture has generic (lay, folk, or indigenous) care knowledge and practices and usually professional care knowledge and practices; these vary transculturally.
8. Cultural care values, beliefs, and practices are influenced by and tend to be embedded in the language, religious (spiritual), kinship (social), political (legal), educational, economic, technological, ethnohistorical, and environmental context of a particular culture.
9. Beneficial, healthy, and satisfying culturally based nursing care contributes to the well-being of individuals, families, groups, and communities within their environmental context.
10. Culturally congruent or beneficial nursing care can only occur when an individual's, group's, family's,

Box 34-1

Major Concepts & Definitions of Leininger's Theory

Leininger has developed many terms relevant to the theory; the major ones are defined here. The reader can study her full theory from her definitive book on the theory.

1. *Care* refers to abstract and concrete phenomena related to assisting, supporting, or enabling experiences or behaviors toward or for others with evident or anticipated needs to ameliorate or improve a human condition or lifeway.

2. *Caring* refers to actions and activities directed toward assisting, supporting, or enabling another individual or group with evident or anticipated needs to ameliorate or improve a human condition or lifeway, or to face death.

3. *Culture* refers to the learned, shared, and transmitted values, beliefs, norms, and lifeways of a particular group that guides their thinking, decisions, and actions in patterned ways.

4. *Cultural care* refers to the subjectively and objectively learned and transmitted values, beliefs, and patterned lifeways that assist, support, facilitate, or enable another individual or group to maintain their well-being and health, improve their human condition and lifeway, or deal with illness, handicaps, or death.

5. *Cultural care diversity* refers to the variabilities and/or differences in meanings, patterns, values, lifeways, or symbols of care within or between collectivities that are related to assistive, supportive, or enabling human care expressions.

6. *Cultural care universality* refers to the common, similar, or dominant uniform care meanings, patterns, values, lifeways, or symbols that are manifest among many cultures and reflect assistive, supportive, facilitative, or enabling ways to help people. (The term *universality* is not used in an absolute way or as a significant statistical finding.)

7. *Nursing* refers to a learned humanistic and scientific profession and discipline that is focused on human care phenomena and activities in order to assist, support, facilitate, or enable individuals or groups to maintain or regain their well-being (or health) in culturally meaningful and beneficial ways, or to help people face handicaps or death.

8. *Worldview* refers to the way people tend to look out on the world or their universe to form a picture or a value stance about their life or the world around them.

9. *Cultural and social structure dimensions* refers to the dynamic patterns and features of interrelated structural and organizational factors of a particular culture (subculture or society), which includes religious, kinship (social), political (and legal), economic, educational, technological, and cultural values and ethnohistorical factors, and how these factors may be interrelated and function to influence human behavior in different environmental contexts.

10. *Environmental context* refers to the totality of an event, situation, or particular experience that gives meaning to human expressions, interpretations, and social interactions in particular physical, ecological, sociopolitical, and/or cultural settings.

11. *Ethnohistory* refers to those past facts, events, instances, and experiences of individuals, groups, cultures, and institutions that are primarily people-centered (*ethno*) and that describe, explain, and interpret human lifeways within particular cultural contexts and over short or long periods.

12. *Generic (folk or lay) care system* refers to culturally learned and transmitted, indigenous (or traditional), folk (home-based) knowledge and skills used to provide assistive, supportive, enabling, or facilitative acts toward or for another individual, group, or institution with evident or anticipated needs to ameliorate or improve a human lifeway or health condition (or well-being) or deal with handicaps and death situations.

13. *Professional care system* refers to formally taught, learned, and transmitted professional care, health, illness, wellness, and related knowledge and practice skills that prevail in professional institutions, usually with multidisciplinary personnel to serve consumers.

14. *Health* refers to a state of well-being that is culturally defined, valued, and practiced and that reflects the ability of individuals (or groups) to perform their daily role activities in culturally expressed, beneficial, and patterned lifeways.

15. *Cultural care preservation or maintenance* refers to those assistive, supporting, facilitative, or enabling professional actions and decisions that help people of a particular culture retain and/or preserve relevant care values so that they can maintain their well-being, recover from illness, or face handicaps and/or death.

16. *Cultural care accommodation or negotiation* refers to those assistive, supporting, facilitative, or enabling creative professional actions and decisions that help people of a designated culture adapt to or negotiate with others for a beneficial or satisfying health outcome with professional care providers.

17. *Cultural care repatterning or restructuring* refers to those assistive, supporting, facilitative, or enabling professional actions and decisions that help patients reorder, change, or greatly modify their lifeways for new, different, and beneficial health care patterns while respecting the patients' cultural values and beliefs and still providing a beneficial or healthier lifeway than before the changes were coestablished with the patients.

18. *Cultural congruent (nursing) care* refers to those cognitively based assistive, supportive, facilitative, or enabling acts or decisions that are tailored to fit with individual, group, or institutional cultural values, beliefs, and lifeways in order to provide or support meaningful, beneficial, and satisfying health care or well-being services.

From Marriner-Tomey, A., & Alligood, M.R. (1998). *Nursing theorists and their work* (4th ed.). St. Louis: Mosby.

community's, or culture's care values, expressions, and patterns are known and used appropriately and in meaningful ways by the nurse.

11. Culture care differences and similarities between professional caregivers and patients, or care-receivers, exist in any human culture worldwide.

12. Patients who experience nursing care that fails to be reasonably congruent with their beliefs, values, and caring lifeways will show signs of cultural conflicts, noncompliance, stress, and ethical or moral concerns.

13. The qualitative paradigm provides new ways of knowing and different ways to discover epistemic and ontological dimensions of human care transculturally.

The Sunrise Model

The Sunrise Model depicting Leininger's theory is shown in Figure 34-1. The rising sun symbolizes care (Leininger, 1991). One might begin at the top of this model with the worldview and social structure features to consider the revealing ways in which these affect health and care or at

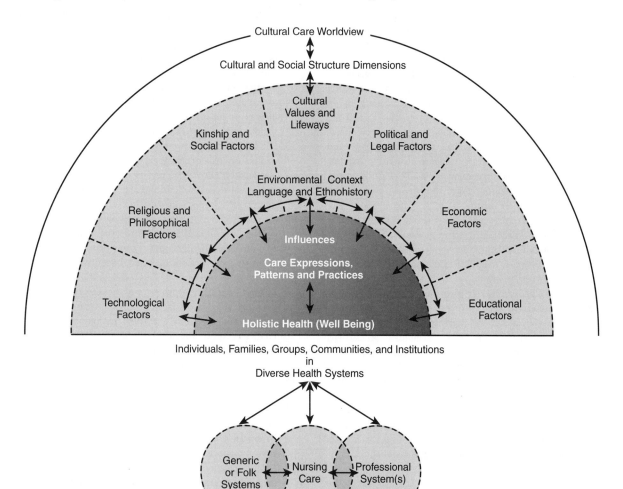

Figure 34-1 Leininger's Sunrise Model to depict the Theory of Culture Care Diversity and Universality. (From Leininger, M. [1991]. *Culture care diversity and universality: a theory.* New York: Jones & Bartlett [www.jbpub.com] and National League for Nursing.)

the bottom to explore the focus on professional nursing care and generic health care systems. At the midpoint of the model is nursing, which incorporates the folk/generic care system with the professional care system. The arrows denote influencers but not causal or linear relationships. Dotted lines in the model indicate an open system. The model depicts human beings as inseparable from their culture.

One will note that the terms *nursing interventions* and *nursing problems* are absent from both the theory and the model. This was a purposeful exclusion on Leininger's part because those terms are associated with Western professional nursing ideologies. Nursing interventions selected without value for a patient's lifeways or values would be perceived as interfering; likewise, nursing problems are not always congruent with what patients view as problems. This model is a productive one for guiding assessment, culturally congruent care, and scientific inquiry.

Welch et al (1998) critique Leininger's theory. They judge the theory as holistic and comprehensive. A basic knowledge of anthropology and a significant basis in transcultural nursing are needed for one to use the theory and accompanying model in an accurate and scholarly manner. The theory is well organized and highly useful to clinical practice in a variety of settings, in education, and in research with the qualitative paradigm. "Grounded data derived with the use of ethnomethods or from an emic or people's viewpoint is leading to high credibility, confirmability, and a wealth of empirical data" (Welch et al, 1998).

Use of the theory in practice, education, and research

Leininger's theory has been used more widely in the last couple of decades than previously. When the theory was first introduced in the 1950s, few nurses were prepared in anthropology or nursing theory to the extent needed to understand or apply the theory. Publications related to the theory were limited because of a lack of appreciation for its relevance or value to practicing professionals. Furthermore, the qualitative research paradigm was undervalued. However, with the realization of transcultural nursing as a specialty area at the graduate level in the late 1970s and a push toward autonomous nursing practice from a nursing model (instead of a medical model), the theory gained prominence (Leininger, 1995; Welch et al, 1998). With increased globalization of the United States, there is an expectation that the theory will be perceived as urgently needed and applicable to practice in a variety of clinical settings.

For example, Kay is a CNM. The patient population in her nurse-midwifery–run clinic is predominantly Caucasian and African American; there are also a few Asian-American and Hispanic patients. Kay, who is Caucasian herself, finds Leininger's theory of cultural care valuable to guide her care for diverse patients. In one case, Kay uses the theory to care for Ashanda, a 16-year-old African-American patient presenting to the prenatal clinic. Using the Sunrise Model as an assessment guide, Kay determines a culture care view of the patient. Ashanda lives in a small apartment within public housing with her mother Florence and two sisters, ages 13 and 10. Her father is not in the picture. There is a large extended family in the area; in fact, Ashanda is worried about how news of her pregnancy will be received during the family reunion this weekend; she tells Kay that they are expecting "40-something family" at the reunion. She goes on, "I've really disappointed a lot of people, most especially my Grandma, who has always been my champion." Ashanda's mother is still very angry with Ashanda for getting pregnant and worries about how she will manage the additional expenses for the baby. She expresses concern as well about how she will provide care. Florence says Ashanda knows nothing about baby care and will not be able to attend school and be a full-time mother too. The baby's father is a teen and cannot provide for the baby, and he and Ashanda are no longer together. There is Medicaid coverage for health care, but financial concerns are persistent. Florence is candid about her disappointment in her daughter. "This girl makes all As and is an award-winning track star; all her teachers say she will get scholarships to colleges and may be good enough for the Olympics one day. I don't know now, though . . . seems as though she's ruined her future with this foolishness." Florence consulted her preacher and several deacons when she learned about the pregnancy, seeking their advice about what to do. She continues to "pray to sweet Jesus every day to help us get through this pregnancy." Ashanda's mother works the evening shift in a large manufacturing company. Ashanda, as the oldest, oversees her sisters while their mother works, and a neighbor "listens out" for the girls while their mother is working.

A diet assessment reveals that Ashanda regularly eats grits and bacon or sausage and juice for breakfast. Her school lunch program provides nutritious food, but she does not drink the milk and discloses that she rarely eats more than a quarter of the lunch. At night, she usually eats vegetables and corn bread. There is occasional pork or chicken, usually fried. The green leafy vegetables are plentiful but cooked with fat back. Florence complains that Ashanda "eats like a bird, plus she runs that off on the track. When she gets truly hungry, she runs to the hamburger joint near our house and gets herself French fried potatoes and coca cola." Mrs. Price acknowledges that the family does use home remedies; the grandmother can be counted on to suggest "old standards." For example, they consistently use sassafras tea and wrap the chest with "liniment" and flannel cloth for colds and use vanilla flavoring on an aching tooth. Prayer is also considered a way to treat illness; "good living" is considered a preventive strategy.

Kay's management plan, guided by the three modes for

nursing decisions and actions, follows. (Note that this is not the total plan of care; it represents only a few examples that are related to cultural competence).

Culture care preservation and maintenance. According to Leininger's theory, this mode is appropriate to retain cultural beliefs and values when possible. Kay realizes that Ashanda's cultural food pattern and poor eating habits place her at some risk for anemia. The lack of protein and calories is of concern as well during pregnancy. Kay does diet counseling, provides written materials appropriate for teenagers, and refers Ashanda to WIC . She also prescribes prenatal vitamins. While she preserves Ashanda's cultural pattern for "soul food," she suggests limiting the amount of fried foods (including fat back in the vegetables) and suggests ways to obtain protein in the diet. Ashanda agrees to try yogurt, cheese, and peanut butter as well as some chocolate milk. Since the home remedies mentioned by Florence are not harmful in pregnancy, these may be preserved if desired. Kay points out that no medications should be taken without consulting the caregiver first. As both Ashanda and the baby's father are African Americans, an ethnic group at risk for having sickle cell trait, screening for sickle cell anemia will be a part of the management under this category.

Accommodation and negotiation. The theory suggests that some cultural practices may need to be negotiated for an optimal outcome. One example of this mode occurs at the initial prenatal visit when Kay and Ashanda discuss her level of exercise and the nurse's concern about safety for her and the fetus (related to extreme fatigue, increased body temperature, and possible falls related to a changing center of gravity later in pregnancy). Kay refers Ashanda to the athletic trainer for the track team to plan an exercise program safe for pregnancy and provides written information from the American College of Obstetricians and Gynecologists (ACOG) data bank on exercise in pregnancy. A second example occurs later in pregnancy when it becomes evident that Ashanda expects to have her mother, her new boyfriend, some church members, and several aunts in the labor ward with her. Kay and Ashanda discuss the hospital regulations about labor coaches and other visitors, and Kay suggests that she will need to select one or two significant persons to remain with her throughout labor, knowing that the staff may wish for others to remain in a waiting area until after the birth. She promises Ashanda that she can speak with these people by a telephone at her bedside in the labor room.

Restructuring and patterning. This mode suggests reordering or modifying some lifeways for a more healthful outcome. Kay uses this mode from the theory later in Ashanda's pregnancy. Despite prenatal vitamins, Ashanda becomes severely anemic. Kay determines that Ashanda is eating starch because several aunts have informed her that

it will make her baby healthier and more beautiful. Kay provides detailed information to Ashanda and her mother about pica and its hazards. Ashanda agrees to stop eating starch, agrees to take her iron supplements consistently, and chooses from a list of iron-rich foods those that she likes and is willing to eat more of in her daily diet. Kay also orders ferrous sulfate and provides appropriate education about taking the drug. She follows up on the anemia throughout the pregnancy.

Studies utilizing the theory

Dr. Leininger herself (1995) cites eight factors as influential in establishing transcultural nursing (and hence the theory) in practice, education, and research (Box 34-2).

In 1981, Leininger conducted a survey of schools of nursing incorporating transcultural nursing into nursing curricula in the United States; results showed that only 34% of National League for Nursing (NLN)–accredited baccalaureate programs, 15% of Master of Science in Nursing (MSN) programs, and 2% of doctoral programs had substantive coursework in transcultural nursing. She cited the following reasons for such limited numbers: (1) lack of sufficient numbers of qualified faculty, (2) failure to value and promote such programs by academicians and nurse leaders, (3) dominance of traditional "unicultural" curriculum models, (4) meager funding for such programs, (5) dominance of biomedical and psychological content, (6) fear, and (7) ignorance, prejudice, and biases among administrators and educators (Leininger, 1995).

Currently there are several universities that offer

Box 34-2

Factors Influencing the Use of Transcultural Nursing in Practice, Education, and Research

1. Marked increase in worldwide migration, necessitating differential health care services
2. Increase in multicultural identities, with people expecting respect and understanding for their unique health values, beliefs, and lifeways
3. Increase in technology with diverse effects
4. Increase in cultural conflicts, clashes, and violence, which affects health care as more cultures interact
5. Increase in world travel and employment
6. Increase in litigation related to cultural conflict, negligence, ignorance, and imposition practices in health care
7. Increase in feminism and gender issues, which place inherent demands on the health care system
8. Increase in demand for community- and culture-based health care services in diverse environmental contexts

Data from Leininger, M. (1995). *Transcultural nursing: concepts, theories, research, and practices* (2nd ed.). New York: McGraw-Hill.

transcultural specialization at the Master's or doctoral level: the University of Utah (the first such program), the University of Washington at Seattle, the University of California at Los Angeles (UCLA), the University of Miami in Florida, and Wayne State University in Detroit (the largest such program). Several other colleges and universities offer courses in transcultural nursing. Leininger (1995) estimates that over her lifetime as a nurse educator, she has personally taught transcultural concepts to at least 10,000 undergraduate and graduate students through formal coursework or conferences around the world. Clearly, the theory is applicable to education. The Transcultural Nursing Society initiated certification in transcultural nursing (CTN) in 1988, further indicating the extent to which this theory educates specialists.

During the past 3 decades, the theory has been used worldwide to guide scholarly inquiry; it has been tested in 100 cultures and subcultures, where 172 constituent patterns have been identified by transcultural researchers in 75 Western and non-Western countries (Leininger, 1995). Although many nursing journals invite theoretical and empirical manuscripts related to transcultural aspects of nursing, the *Journal of Transcultural Nursing* is the main publisher of manuscripts related to transcultural research

In her book *Culture Care Diversity and Universality: A Theory* (1991), Leininger includes seven complete ethnonursing studies within the following contexts: Philippine- and Anglo-Americans in hospitals; Old Order Amish; urban Mexican Americans; pregnancy and childbearing in Ukrainians; the Gadsup Akuna from New Guinea; dying patients in hospitals and hospices; and Greek-Canadian widows. In an appendix, she also provides the bibliographical references for 36 known research studies using her theory. As additional evidence of the wide range of studies using Leininger's theory, there have been several doctoral dissertations using the theory and/or the associated ethnonursing approach in the last few years. A variety of them are summarized here to indicate the scope of inquiry within the context of the theory.

Gibson (1995) conducted an exploratory descriptive study related to the quality of life for adult patients experiencing hemodialysis (n = 20), looking at *a priori* categories that included life satisfaction, socioeconomic status, general health, and functional status. Three categories emerged inductively: spirituality, caring and health care professionals, and coping. The findings suggested a need for inclusion of content related to these themes, as well as a need for cultural and legislative accessibility in curriculum. Drury (1995) spent 2 years on a field study with homeless, chronically mentally ill individuals attempting to leave the streets, noting interactions between their needs and community resources. This group made direct requests for care infrequently and were noted to have unmet needs related to disrupted community life, household moves, legal disputes, and bureaucratic problems. Culturally based

lifeways and patterns of mutual avoidance between them and caregivers limited delivery of services.

Miller (1997) examined professional and generic care patterns, expressions, and meanings within a political context for Czech immigrants. The capitalist market and economic structure in the United States influenced lifeways in all dimensions. Care patterns were based on "choice," "responsibility," and "helping each other." In an ethnonursing study relating to the humor, care, and well-being of Lithuanian Americans, Gelazis (1994) discovered that cultural humor helps this group bear life's burdens, meet survival functions, and diffuse confrontational situations. Humor was found to support well-being.

Schweiger (1992) used case study methodology with a professional nurse with 20 years of clinical experience to explore commitment to clinical practice. Using a life history research method that included interviews with the nurse, her family, and friends and examination of memorabilia, the researcher found the recurring and dominant theme to be caring. Recurring patterns found to be related to commitment to clinical practice included humor, determination, loyalty, efficiency, responsibility, dependability, and devotion. Subthemes included nostalgia, work ethic, and bonding.

Spangler (1991) conducted a study of nursing care values and practices of Anglo-American and Philippine-American nurses in a 200-bed general hospital. She found that the Anglo-American nurses' care was characterized by promotion of autonomy based on informed decision-making, assertiveness, and control of situations. For Philippine-Americans, nursing care was characterized by an "obligation to care" based on core values of physical comfort, respect, and patience. Cultural differences between the two groups of nurses were found to generate nurse-to-nurse conflict. Two universal themes were discovered that indicated the significant influence of environment, social structure, and the cultural values of the hospital on the nurses' practices. These themes were: (1) a nursing shortage leading to heavy workloads, frustration for the nurses, and an inability to provide the professional nursing ideal, and (2) institutional norms, standards, and regulations strongly influencing nursing practice. This study was included in Leininger's 1991 book.

Miers (1993) conducted a phenomenological study addressing professional nurse caring as experienced by family members of critically ill patients. Parents or spouses (n = 9) described meaningful caring and noncaring behaviors and how they felt with each experience. Four themes emerged: the way the nurse is, meeting patients' needs first, meeting family members' needs, and feelings evoked by caring and noncaring. The "way the nurse is" theme included personal characteristics of the nurse, expressions, behaviors, and professional attitudes. "Meeting patients' needs first" was evidenced by the nurse's providing continuous and vigilant monitoring, communicating emotional care and encouragement, giving physical comfort, assisting with healing, maintaining dignity, and providing privacy. "Meeting family members' needs" was shown with nursing behaviors such as offering honest and consistent information, facilitating access to the physician and to the patient, allowing the family to participate in care, providing physical and spiritual support and comfort, and recognizing and acknowledging the family. "Feelings evoked by caring and noncaring" related to caring behaviors that relieved stress, provided security and safety for the patient, and made the family feel connected and cared for; it also related to noncaring behaviors that caused uneasiness and fear of sanctions.

Leininger's theory has received support in study after study, and the ethnonursing approach to data collection has shown a remarkable ability to enable rich and meaningful data that enhance understanding of other cultures and lend direction to nursing care.

Welch et al (1998) assert that limited research dollars for transcultural studies seriously affects ongoing research. Two factors are identified as causes: biomedical and technical research proposals receiving priority funding, and research needing federal money requiring quantitative objective measurement to be competitive. In the 1990s, national and international organizations began to fund ethnonursing research; national conferences, such as the recent National Organization of Nurse Practitioner Faculties (NONPF) Conference in California, also promote persistence in research related to transcultural nursing and application of transcultural research findings to practice and education.

Purnell's Model for Cultural Competence

Purnell's evolving interactional model provides a concise, systematic framework for learning inherent dimensions of culture. The empirical framework enables culturally competent health and illness care across educational and practice settings. The model (depicted in Figure 34-2) reveals four circles. The first (outer) circle represents the global society, the second represents community, the third represents family, and the fourth (inner) represents the person. Inside the circles are 12 pie-shaped wedges indicating cultural domains and their associated phenomena (discussed in the next section). The metaparadigm concepts of the model are global society, community, family, person, and conscious competence. The dark center represents unknown phenomena. The jagged (erose) line along the bottom of the circular structure represents cultural consciousness as a nonlinear concept. The model incorporates the following fields of inquiry: biology, anthropology, sociology, economics, geography, history, ecology, psychology, physiology, political science, pharmacology, and nutrition, as well as selected theories from communication, family development, and social support (Purnell & Paulanka, 1998). Box 34-3 summarizes the operational definitions for the model's metaparadigm concepts.

Microaspects

At a microlevel, Purnell's model has an organizational framework consisting of 12 domains common to all cultures and with interconnections that affect health; these are: (1) overview, inhabited localities, and topography; (2) communication; (3) family roles and organization; (4) workforce issues; (5) biocultural ecology; (6) high-risk health behaviors; (7) nutrition; (8) pregnancy and childbearing practices; (9) death rituals; (10) spirituality; (11) health care practices; and (12) health care practitioners. Phenomena of interest are listed with each domain (see Figure 34-2). This concise structure is useful and applicable to a range of empirical experiences that use either inductive or deductive inquiry in assessing cultural domains. Once APNs have collected and analyzed assessment data along these domains, they can delineate a culturally appropriate management plan in concert with a patient's needs. The concept of health in this model is viewed as "a state of wellness defined by people within their ethnocultural group" and includes physical, mental, and spiritual components. Health can be defined individually, locally, regionally, nationally, or globally in this model (Purnell & Paulanka, 1998).

Concept of cultural competence

A broader understanding of culture with an attendant increase in awareness of cultural diversity improves the probability that an APN will provide culturally competent care. In Purnell's model, acquisition of **cultural competence** involves the following: "(1) developing an awareness of one's own existence, sensations, thoughts and environment without letting it have an undue influence on those from other backgrounds; (2) demonstrating knowledge and understanding of the client's culture; (3) accepting and respecting cultural differences; and (4) adapting care to be congruent with the client's culture. Cultural competence is a conscious process and not necessarily linear" (Purnell & Paulanka, 1998).

Acquisition of cultural competence is a progressive process beginning with a state of unconscious incompetence; in this state, a caregiver has a knowledge deficit about other cultures. At the next level, the conscious incompetence level, there is awareness about other cultures. The consciously competent person is learning about culture, verifying with patients what would best meet their needs, and employing culturally specific interventions. Most APNs are at this level of cultural competence. At the final level, the unconsciously competent level, an APN automatically provides culturally competent care to culturally diverse patients (Purnell & Paulanka, 1998).

For example, Carol is a family nurse practitioner (FNP) who works in a Migrant Health Project Clinic in the peach belt of Georgia, where there is a large population of Mexican-American migrant workers. She subscribes to Purnell's cultural competence model of transcultural

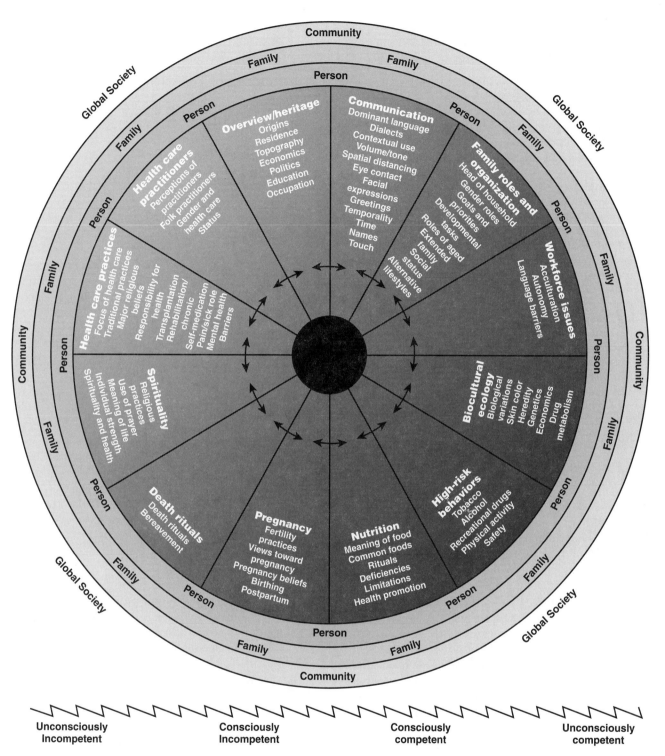

Figure 34-2 Purnell's Model for Cultural Competence. (From Purnell, L.D., & Paulanka, B.J. [1998]. *Transcultural health care: a culturally competent approach.* Philadelphia: FA Davis.)

nursing and uses it extensively in her practice. The patient assessment on which she bases her management plan is structured around the 12 domains for assessing ethnocultural attributes. One of her assigned patients today is Susa, a 20-year-old woman with a fever and sore throat. (Chart 34-1 indicates portions of the ethnocultural patient history on Susa, collected using Purnell's assessment domains.)

Planning care for patients like Susa is difficult because of their long working hours; for optimal care of the migrant population, clinics need to be accessible in the evenings,

Data from: Purnell, L.D., & Paulanka, B.J. (1998). *Transcultural health care*. Philadelphia: FA Davis.

Box 34-3

Definitions for the Selected Metaparadigm Concepts in Purnell's Cultural Competence Model

Global society—One large community of multicultural individuals who consciously or unconsciously alter their worldviews and lifeways in response to global events and chaos.

Community—A group of people who have a common interest or identity and live in a specified locality. Community includes physical, social, and symbolic characteristics that cause people to connect.

Family—Two or more people who are emotionally involved with each other. They may or may not live in close proximity. This includes blood-related and non–blood-related significant others who are either physically or emotionally close or distant.

Person—A biopsychosociocultural human being who is constantly adapting to the environment in biological, physiological, psychological, social, and ethnocultural ways.

Cultural competence—Having the knowledge, understanding, and skills regarding a diverse culture that allows one to provide acceptable, congruent care.

after dusk, when the fieldwork ends. Susa can be (and is) treated for her tonsillitis at this visit. Her visual problem necessitates referral to an optometrist or ophthalmologist, depending on what Carol discovers on examination. Without funds or insurance, referral can be difficult. Carol refers Susa to the local Lion's club, an organization well known for supporting visual care in the community. She also attends to Susa's request for information on contraception; another visit is planned for after Susa reads the pamphlets and talks with her husband. At that visit, Carol will discuss more health screening and promotion. Carol will also discuss Susa's concerns about using her sister's pain medicine from Mexico, where drugs are sold over the counter without prescriptions and the content of the drugs and quality of their manufacture are not controlled. Carol tells Susa to report further backaches, with treatment to be provided at the clinic; Susa will not need her sister's medication. Carol plans to continue collecting ethnocultural data at subsequent visits when Susa is feeling better. Since there is not an exact translation for the words *nurse practitioner* in Spanish, it will be important for Carol to help Susa understand as much as possible about the NP's role in her care.

Purnell's model has been used extensively in the United States, Canada and Europe. It has been tested in long-term care (LTC), acute care, and home care settings (Purnell, 2000).

Other Models of Transcultural Nursing

Other models also direct practice, education, and research; most are less well developed than those discussed thus far.

APNs might use one of these models in its entirety or merge the most relevant features of each to form a model that fits with their own practice sites or provides guidelines for research.

The Giger and Davidhizar Transcultural Assessment Model

The Giger and Davidhizar Transcultural Assessment Model (1995), developed by two educators, provides an approach to assessment that minimizes time for comprehensive assessments that would enable culturally competent care (Figure 34-3). The metaparadigm identified for the model includes several components. Transcultural nursing is conceptualized as a culturally competent practice field where patients are central and research is a focus. Culturally diverse nursing care considers six variable cultural phenomena that are evident in all cultural groups: communication, space, social organization, time, environmental control, and biological variation. All people are culturally unique individuals who are products of their experiences, cultural beliefs, and cultural norms. Culturally sensitive environments define places where primary, secondary, or tertiary care is provided. The Giger and Davidhizar Transcultural Assessment Model has been widely used in a variety of clinical settings since its inception in 1991.

CONFHER Model

The CONFHER model, proposed by Fong (1985), identifies key aspects of a cultural profile with the potential to affect a patient's health status. It provides a systematic assessment framework for gathering cultural background data of value to developing a culturally specific plan of care. An APN familiar with a patient's cultural group will know some of the general information for the model; other data will be very specific to the patient.

The CONFHER assessment guide covers several cultural components: **C**ommunication style, **O**rientation, **N**utrition, **F**amily relationships, **H**ealth beliefs, **E**ducation, and **R**eligion (Fong, 1985). Communication style includes language and dialect preferences, nonverbal behaviors, and social customs. Orientation includes ethnic identity, acculturation, and value orientation. Nutrition covers both the symbolism of food and food preferences and taboos. Family relationships are defined by family structure and role, dynamics and decision-making styles, and lifestyle and living arrangements. Cultural components of health beliefs include thoughts on alternative health care; health,

Chart 34-1

Example of a Partial Patient Assessment of Ethnocultural Attributes Based on Purnell's Cultural Competence Model

Patient
Susa, age 20

Overview, Inhabited Localities, and Topography
Married to Hector, a 26-year-old Mexican American; has a 3-month old son named Tomas.

Migrated 5 months ago from Juarez, Mexico, the place of birth for both spouses (baby born in the United States).

Lives in a two-room apartment furnished by the farmer for whom they work harvesting peach and pecan crops; in-laws live nearby, while patient's parents remain in Mexico; came to the area to be near Hector's family.

Patient has ninth-grade education; husband has seventh-grade education.

Communication
Speaks little English; sister-in-law, who is bilingual (in English and Spanish), serves as the patient's interpreter. (Additional cultural communication patterns and temporal relationships will be assessed at later visits).

Prefers to be called Susa.

Family Roles and Organization
Husband is head of household and primary decision-maker; he seeks frequent advice from his father.

Earning an adequate living is the goal of the family, as is the safety and wellbeing of the child: "Our baby is the world to us."

Discloses homesickness; she especially misses her mother and sisters; there is limited money for mailing letters or making telephone calls.

Now that patient is past childbirth and "back in the fields," there is 12-year-old girl taking care of the baby (potential older babysitters are required to work in the fields); patient worries about the level of knowledge of this child care provider, but her husband says they can not survive on his wages alone. (Additional data about family issues will be added at subsequent visits).

Workforce Issues
Family works 7 days a week from approximately 7 AM to 7 PM; most work associates are also Mexican-American migrant workers; patient works near her mother- and sisters-in law; otherwise, she does not communicate much with other workers, having only two or three female friends among them; there is no time for leisure activities.

Employer is very kind and generous with his workers, but the work is grueling and causes backaches; very hot in the fields; patient sometimes works in a shed sorting peaches on conveyor belts; she worries about accidents because hand injuries are common.

Biocultural Ecology
Skin and hair are consistent with Mexican-American culture.

Patient is at particular risk for pesticide-related illness, sun-related cancers, and farm injuries

Caution: Review drug metabolism variations (if applicable) with the patient before prescribing anything.

Patient's ethnic group risks include infections, communicable disease, parasites, sexually transmitted diseases, tuberculosis, and pesticide-related problems.

High-Risk Behaviors
Denies use of tobacco, alcohol, or other drugs; has had a mutually monogamous sexual relationship for 18 months.

Infrequent visits to health care; did not have a postpartum follow-up visit.

Nutrition
24-hour diet recall:
Breakfast: scrambled egg on tortilla, coffee with cream
Mid-morning: glazed donut and apple juice
Lunch: burrito and soda
Midafternoon: banana
Supper: fried chicken (one leg, one thigh; from take-out), refried beans, rice, tortilla, tomato and lettuce, iced tea. (Will collect additional data on diet later.)

Pregnancy and Childbearing
G I P I A 0; normal spontaneous delivery of 6-pound, 2-ounce boy 3 months ago, with local anesthesia, "drug in vein" for pain control, and midline episiotomy; wants birth control but her husband is opposed; has used vaginal film since delivery without her husband's knowledge but is concerned about its efficacy; husband refuses to use condoms.

Restrictions and taboos related to childbearing: not applicable.

Death Rituals
Not applicable at present.

Note: This is only a portion of an ethnocultural assessment. It is meant to supplement a traditional history and physical examination, not be substituted for it.

Continued

Chart 34-1

Example of a Partial Patient Assessment of Ethnocultural Attributes Based on Purnell's Cultural Competence Model—cont'd

Spirituality

Patient and spouse are Catholic, but their job precludes attending mass; patient occasionally goes to confession; patient has a small statue of the Virgin Mary on a small, homemade altar used for daily prayers; sometimes her in-laws and others join in prayer time.

Patient proudly showed a wooden rosary given to her by her family on her wedding day.

Health Care Practices

Does not get routine health care; sees a provider only when too sick to work; did get some prenatal care; last Pap test was at a prenatal visit; last dental visit was 2 years ago (with a toothache); no vision screen; not certain about immunization status. (Will access records of obstetric care, where she thinks immunizations are recorded.)

Uninsured and not eligible for Medicaid.

Long hours and 7-days-a-week schedule are a barrier to care.

Has no routine medications; takes generic ibuprofen for headache and backaches; mentions that her sister recently sent her some pain medicine for her bad backaches; it was bought in a pharmacy in Juarez. (Will continue to collect data related to culture and health/illness.)

Has noted a recent change in vision.

Health Care Practitioners

Prefers female provider. Husband refuses to let her see male provider.

Note: This is only a portion of an ethnocultural assessment. It is meant to supplement a traditional history and physical examination, not be substituted for it.

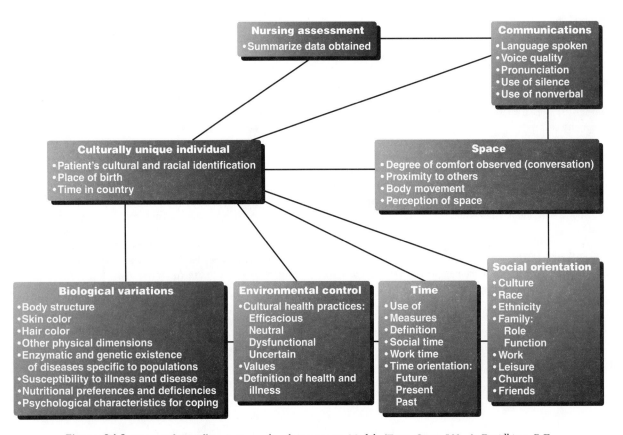

Figure 34-3 Giger and Davidhizar's Transcultural Assessment Model. (From Giger, J.N., & Davidhizar, R.E. [1995]. *Transcultural nursing: assessment and intervention.* St. Louis: Mosby.)

crisis, and illness beliefs; response to pain and hospitalization; and disease predisposition and resistance. When examining cultural components of education, one must consider learning style, informal and formal education, and occupation and socioeconomic level. Lastly, religion includes preferences, beliefs, rituals, and taboos.

Spector's Health and Illness Model

The phenomenon of concern in Spector's model is the differing perceptions of health and illness held by providers and patients. These differences may contribute to misunderstandings on the part of providers; APNs may believe that patients are misusing the system in some way or not taking advantage of certain services for which they are eligible, while patients may not understand the meaning of the service, may not understand that it is affordable, or may not envision that particular service as helpful. For example, the Sherwoods, an African-American family who recently experienced a stillbirth, do not follow up on their referral to a perinatal support group. The APN group leaders know from the literature that African Americans tend to be underrepresented in support group membership. If they allow that stereotype to interfere with their follow up with the Sherwoods, this family may miss out on a strategy for positive grief resolution.

Educating oneself to change personal and professional stereotypes so that culturally appropriate care may be provided is not always an easy or direct process, and it takes time. Spector (1996) describes a multistep process in which one must explore one's own cultural identity and heritage and confront biases and stereotypes; develop an awareness and understanding of the complexities of the modern health care delivery system—its philosophy, problems, biases, and stereotypes; develop keen awareness of the socialization process that brings providers into this complex system; and develop the ability to "hear" things that transcend language and foster an understanding of patients, their cultural heritage, and the resilience found within each culture that supports family and community structures.

Spector (1996) advises assessment of each patient's health beliefs and health traditions. Health in the traditional context includes physical, mental, and spiritual facets in constant flux within the context of family, culture, work, community, history, and environment. The traditional ways of maintaining health, protecting health (preventing illness), and restoring health often differ from the prevailing Western scientific philosophy of care. Health maintenance includes the "active everyday ways people go about living and attempting to stay well"; health protection includes avoiding harm, illness, and misfortune; and health restoration involves traditional remedies and special foods.

In her view of health and illness, Spector (1996) also introduces an expanded, empirically based perspective of heritage consistency. The concept of heritage consistency was developed by Estes and Zitzow (1980) as "the degree to which one's lifestyle reflects his or her respective tribal culture." Spector's expansion refers to the degree that a person's lifestyle reflects his or her traditional culture, be it European, African, Hispanic, Native American, or Asian. The values indicating heritage consistency exist along a continuum from consistent (traditional) to inconsistent (acculturated). Assessment of heritage consistency includes data related to socialization, religion, and ethnicity. Factors indicative of heritage consistency that help to determine ethnic group differences in health beliefs and practices include:

1. Childhood development that occurred in the person's country of origin or in a U.S. immigrant neighborhood of the same ethnic group
2. Extended family members who encouraged participation in traditional religion or cultural activities
3. Individuals who engage in frequent visits to their country of origin or to the "old neighborhood" in the United States
4. Family homes that are within the ethnic community
5. Individual participation in ethnic cultural events, such as religious festivals and national holidays
6. Individuals who were raised in an extended family setting
7. Individuals who maintain regular contact with their extended family
8. Individuals whose names have not been Americanized
9. Individuals who were educated in a parochial (nonpublic) school with a religious or ethnic philosophy similar to that of the family
10. Individuals who engage in social activities primarily with others of the same ethnic background
11. Individuals who have knowledge of the culture and language of origin
12. Individuals who possess elements of personal pride about their heritage (Spector, 1996)

Campinha-Bacote's Culturally Competent Model

The model designed by Campinha-Bacote (1994a) utilizes the following concepts, each of which is represented in the model by a circle that intersects all of the others: (1) cultural awareness, or respect for patients from diverse backgrounds; (2) cultural knowledge, or a caregiver's ability to gather cultural information from a patient; (3) cultural skills, or the ability to make a cultural assessment and collect relevant data; (4) cultural encounter, or nursing skills utilized in interactions with patients from diverse cultures; and (5) cultural desire, or the motivation of health care providers to want to engage in the process of cultural competence.

This model and the Cultural Sophistication Framework that follows represent an APN's progression along a continuum from minimal sensitivity to an understanding of the uniqueness of patients from diverse cultures and then to the optimal state of cultural competence. These two models are more useful in an evaluation context than as models to guide nursing decisions and actions; APNs may place themselves along the continuum, seeing a need for change in their approach to diverse patients. At other times, someone in a supervisory position may point out a need for change. For example, Jane, a CNS new to working with the Amish, finds that she initially feels awkward with these patients. She treats them with warmth and positive regard and appreciates that their lifestyle, beliefs, and values are different than her own, but she is concerned that her lack of knowledge will cause her to say or do something wrong—something that would be insensitive or even offensive. Because Jane does not yet know all the health beliefs and practices of the Amish, she cannot incorporate their cultural beliefs into their plans of care. Over time, Jane learns more about this patient population; she reads about health care for the Amish, talks with knowledgeable staff members, and begins to feel more comfortable asking the patients themselves about their culture and how she can work with them to improve health care. She says to one woman, "I am trying to learn more about your way of life. Please bear with me and help me learn so I can be a better caregiver for you and others. If I say something wrong, please tell me."

Jane finds that her assessments begin to include more cultural data; for example, she consistently asks about home remedies. She remembers that a particular farmer with diabetes, who rises at 4:30 in the morning, will need his medication schedule adapted to different meal times than most other patients. She also begins to feel more comfortable inviting coparticipation by patients in managing their care. The nurse-patient relationships thrive and Jane desires to become even more culturally aware so she can become a more informed advocate for this population. A self-review using the Campinha-Bacote model would enable Jane to acknowledge the differences in her performance over time and give her some direction for how to further move toward cultural competence.

Orlandi's Cultural Sophistication Framework

Orlandi's model is a continuum of cultural competence with three components or dimensions: (1) cultural incompetence (e.g., cognitively oblivious, affectively apathetic, unskilled), (2) cultural sensitivity (e.g., cognitively aware, affectively sympathetic, skills lacking), and (3) cultural competence (e.g., cognitively knowledgeable, affectively committed to change, highly skilled) (Louie, 1998).

A comparison of the practices of three APNs shows how providers find themselves at different points along the continuum of cultural sophistication. Vivien is technically capable as an APN; she has an expansive knowledge base and is an excellent diagnostician. However, her patient management is less than optimal because her plan is the same for all patients and dependent on their diagnosis alone, without regard for their culture, views, health beliefs, values, or lifeways. She is not aware that this is the case; in fact, Vivien sees herself as a holistic APN; she does

not realize that her lack of cultural awareness is destructive to what might be accomplished on behalf of her patients, nor does she realize that she is missing something very special in her nurse-patient relationships that comes with culturally congruent care. However, Vivien may ultimately "get it" and change the way she practices; a supervisor's evaluation that points out the deficit might help Vivien understand where and how she could improve.

Teresa is culturally sensitive and is beginning to incorporate the more obvious cultural factors into her care plans. However, she is still unable to ask questions in a way that enables collection of the meaningful, less obvious data about patients' cultures as a basis for care.

Jack is at the third level in this model; in fact, his inclusion of culture in patient care is such that Teresa asks him for advice about improving her skill at cultural assessment. She has noticed that when Jack does not know about how a treatment option will fit into the beliefs and health patterns of a particular patient, he knows how to sensitively ask the patient. When the health practice of the patient is at odds with the treatment goal, Jack knows how to communicate this effectively without appearing insensitive. Early in his practice, Jack used a translator to communicate with the numerous Hispanic patients he was seeing. When he did use the few Spanish words he knew and saw how much patients appreciated his effort to communicate with them, Jack enrolled in a Spanish course for health care professionals. Now he communicates with minimal help from an interpreter.

Knowledge of a cultural competence continuum can help strengthen one's practice base on behalf of those from diverse cultures. The ultimate goal is to increase one's responsibility for knowledge of cultural diversity and one's behavior toward those who are culturally different. Many APNs note that as they become more culturally competent, they experience a different sense of "connection" with patients. This change enhances clinical decision-making and enriches practice.

Organizational Culture—a Model of Conflict

In the 1970s, management theorists began to study organizational culture to determine how people interact in an organization. The interest in organizational cultural research was fueled by economic successes in industry in Japan. The realization that other cultures operated differently and successfully prompted research and changes in management. Organizational culture theory is written from three perspectives (Coehling, 1994): the anthropologist perspective, which is descriptive; the organization/management theorist perspective, which provides a better conceptualization of organizational life to facilitate worker and manager responses; and the organizational manager perspective, the purpose of which is guiding or controlling organizational operations and seeking formulas for success to function more effectively.

The Lowenstein-Glanville Model is useful for managers who work with employees of different backgrounds. This may include different age groups, ethnic or racial groups, or socioeconomic groups (Lowenstein, 1998). The model identifies how minor disputes can grow into major ones through varied perceptions of an incident. The model has a continuum from unperceived injurious experience (UNPIE) to naming-blaming-claiming to legal dispute.

The effect of social position, perception of prejudice, attributions to others, risk of punishment, degree of reward, and the perception of an institution's caring or rejection all contribute to continuum evolution. Nurse managers are in a position to identify, label, and deal with cultural differences and assist in conflict resolution. Communication patterns may be established through cultural conditioning; employees from different cultures and age groups may use different means to communicate the same message. People from different cultural backgrounds and socioeconomic groups may not view organizational goals the same way. However, if differences are recognized, diverse groups can work together to ensure similar goals and develop unit norms.

IMPLICATIONS FOR MSN EDUCATION AND ADVANCED PRACTICE

"It is believed that demography is destiny, demographic change is reality, and demographic sensitivity is imperative" (Giger & Davidhizar 1995). If this statement is true, there is no time like the present, as the country's demography changes, for APNs to expand their worldview of culture. Culture is more than a backdrop in patients' lives; culture critically and intimately affects every aspect of their lives, including their health. Therefore helping patients achieve and maintain optimal health demands attention to culture. Transcultural nursing theories and conceptual models lend direction to nursing for that purpose.

Many of the theories and models related to transcultural nursing provide assessment instruments or direction for inclusion of cultural queries into practice. Depending on an APN's practice setting, the comprehensiveness of the instruments can be prohibitive for use with all patients, given the time constraints in most clinics today and the push to see more patients each day. APNs may prefer to critique the different instruments and the lists of cultural assessment questions and devise shorter, more practical, and time-efficient tools for daily practice.

Transcultural theories and models provide new insights about the differences in perception of health and illness among caregivers and patients. APNs must guard against a paternalistic view that they know best regarding what patients and families need and want from health care and from them as providers of that care. Instead, APNs are advised to listen to patients, even when it necessitates listening "between the lines" to understand a patient's perceptions.

APNs are advised to frame the question raised by Spector (1996) in terms of their own practice settings: How can APNs "change the method of operations and provide care for the emerging majority and at the same time for the population at large?" With today's emphasis on managed care, case management, and health care teams and a continued impetus for APNs to distinguish their practice, the question becomes even more provocative.

In education settings, transcultural models can be utilized in curriculum development, whether schools favor integrated curricula or a separate course. Transcultural models can also enhance faculty understanding of students from differing cultures and guide instructional strategies that enhance student achievement. Chapters 32 and 35 in this book relate specifically to cultural diversity in curricula and education.

In administration/management situations, models can be used to assess organizational culture and workforce issues among staff (Purnell, 2000). Ethics committees can use transcultural models to assess appropriateness of care. All facilities can use the models to guide care plan development for groups of patients (e.g., orthodox Jewish patients).

Quinless (2000) describes the problematic beginnings for a primary care clinic associated with a nursing program that was designed to meet both the health needs of the community, mostly a Hispanic population, and the clinical and service needs of the university. The program was imposed by outsiders—the university—without an emic perspective and almost failed. When the insiders—the patients and families—were consulted and their feedback was incorporated, patients indicated satisfaction, and health care for the community was positively affected by the clinic. APNs and educators, envisioning a service learning or community health initiative, would do well to heed the practical wisdom of those, like Quinless (2000), who have led successful ventures.

PRIORITIES FOR RESEARCH

Leininger developed a research approach in the 1960s to facilitate study—her Theory of Culture Care Diversity and Universality. In her words (1991), *ethnonursing* is a "qualitative research method using naturalistic, open discovery, and largely inductively derived emic modes and processes with diverse strategies, techniques, and enabling tools to document, describe, understand, and interpret the people's meanings, experiences, symbols, and other related aspects bearing on actual or potential nursing phenomena."

The major features of Leininger's ethnonursing research approach are described here from the perspective of her own descriptions of the methodology (Leininger, 1991, 1995). Over time, she has developed several *enablers*, or guides or models that facilitate the method. These are the Stranger-Friend, Observation-Participation-Reflection, Acculuration, Life-History Health Care, Phases of Ethnonursing Data Analysis, Cultural Care Values and Meanings, Culturalogical Care Assessment, Audio-Visual, and Professional Care Enabler guides.

In addition, she has collaborated in developing a qualitative software program, the Leininger-Templin-Thompson (LTT) Ethnoscript Qualitative Software, to process large amounts of data; this software is also considered an enabler. The program is useful for other qualitative approaches where large amounts of naturalistic data need to be processed systematically.

Leininger suggests a sequence for conducting ethnonursing research (Box 34-4). The researcher is encouraged to modify this sequence to fit the setting or context of the study. Furthermore, Leininger (1991) delineates the following five summative principles to guide use of the method:

1. Maintain open discovery, active listening, and a genuine learning attitude in working with informants in the total context in which the study is conducted.
2. Maintain an active and curious posture about the "why" of whatever is seen, heard, or experienced, with appreciation of whatever informants share.

3. Record whatever is shared by informants in a careful and conscientious way for full meanings, explanations, or interpretations to preserve informant ideas.
4. Seek a mentor who has experience with the ethnonursing research method to act as a guide.
5. Clarify the purposes of additional qualitative research methods if they are combined with the ethnonursing method (e.g., when combining life histories, ethnography, phenomenology, or ethnoscience).

Most qualitative researchers would likely concur with these principles and appropriate guides for all such research. All would also agree that ethnonursing and other qualitative approaches should employ substance and rigor and be subjected to critique using appropriate standards for evaluating qualitative inquiry.

As nursing attempts to build the science of transcultural care, studies of any cultural or subcultural group that explain an informant's world would be advantageous. An emic view of marginalized and disenfranchised groups will continue to develop transcultural nursing science. Having an accurate view of a cultural group and an understanding of what practices work best at protecting, maintaining, and

---

Box 34-4

Leininger's Phases of Ethnonursing Research

1. Identify the general intent or purpose(s) of your study with focus on the domain(s) of inquiry phenomenon under study, area of inquiry, or research questions being addressed.
2. Identify the potential significance of the study to advance nursing knowledge and practices.
3. Review available literature on the domain or phenomena being studied.
4. Conceptualize a research plan from beginning to the end with the following general phases or sequence factors in mind.
   - Consider the research site, community, and people to study the phenomena.
   - Deal with the informed consent expectations.
   - Explore and gradually gain entry (with essential permissions) to the community, hospital, or country where the study is being done.
   - Anticipate potential barriers and facilitators related to gatekeepers' expectations, language, political leaders, location, and other factors.
   - Select and appropriately use the ethnonursing enabling tools with the research process (e.g., Leininger's *Stranger-Friend Guide* and *Observation-Participation-Reflection Guide*. The researcher may also develop enabling tools or guides for study).
   - Chose key and general informants.

   - Maintain trusting and favorable relationships with the people conferring with ethnonurse research expert(s) to prevent unfavorable developments.
   - Collect and confirm data with observations, interviews, participant experiences, and other data. (This is a continuous process from the beginning to the end and requires the use of qualitative research criteria to confirm findings and credibility factors).
   - Maintain continuous data processing on computers, with field journals reflecting active analysis and reflections, and with discussions with research mentor(s). Computer processing with Leininger, Templin, and Thompsons's software is a helpful means to handle large amounts of qualitative data.
   - Frequently present and reconfirm findings with the people studied to check credibility and confirmability of findings.
   - Make plans to leave the field site, community, and informants in advance.
5. Do final analysis and writing of the research findings soon after completing the study.
6. Prepare published findings in appropriate journals.
7. Help implement the findings with nurses interested in findings.
8. Plan future studies related to this domain or other new ones.

From Leininger, M. (1991). *Culture care diversity and universality: a theory.* Sudbury, MA: Jones & Bartlett [www.jbpub.com] and National League for Nursing.

restoring health decreases the likelihood that care for the culturally diverse will continue to be intuitive. An example of descriptive research reinforces this point. Austin, Gallop, McCay, Peterneli-Taylor, and Bayer (1999) surveyed a stratified sample of 3423 mental health nurses from across Canada about their attitudes, knowledge, and cultural competence in caring for psychiatric patients with a history of sexual abuse. Their final sample consisted of 1701 nurses (a 49.8% response rate). Of these, 96% reported frequent care of patients with a history of sexual abuse and 19% reported a personal history. Data were collected using a sexual abuse comfort scale, the sexual attitude scale, and an instrument designed to address education. Although most nurses had experiences with those from different cultures, only 4.6% perceived themselves as very culturally competent in this arena of practice. The majority believed that the central issue was the sexual abuse history, not the culture, and predicted that the difficulty they would face in caring for a particular patient would be related not to the patient's culture, but to the sexual abuse. Although culture was not perceived as the central issue, many respondents focused on the extent of sexual abuse and incest in First Nations (Native Canadians) and its relationship to substance abuse, self-harm, poverty, and isolation; spirituality was also seen as important to the First Nation population, and therefore, to the patients of interest in the study. Interestingly, despite a resounding stated desire to learn more about the First Nations culture, few, if any, respondents suggested asking members of the culture to be informants.

Purnell suggests (2000) that cultural competence be viewed as an outcome of care. There has been minimal research conducted on the effects of cultural competence training (Chrisman & Schultz, 1997) and how best to accomplish the progression from unconscious incompetence along the continuum to competence. Purnell and Paulanka (1998) suggest that most professionals never get to the final or unconscious stage of cultural competence; a study might be designed to explore the reason for this and how to enable further progression.

Ethnonursing research might be conducted with culturally diverse nursing students at the graduate and undergraduate levels to determine the way in which culture relates to their learning process as well as how programs might plan recruitment and retention strategies to better meet the needs of diverse students. Few studies have been done with minority faculty to determine best practices for recruitment and retention measures for their preferred future and job satisfaction.

Phillips, Palmer, Wetting, and Fenwick (2000) conducted survey research that examined the relationships between gender, age, ethnicity, education, and income level and the attitude toward using a NP for care. While there was no significance found for the gender and race variables, increased income, increased education, and age significantly increased the positive inclination for NP care,

as did previous experience with a NP provider. This study deserves replication with a different, more ethnically diverse population (of the total respondents [n = 238], 163 were Caucasian) and with a more representative geographical sample. Would similar findings hold for an inclination toward seeing other APN providers, like a CNM? Does the specialty of the NP matter? Studies of this type have implications for education and for marketing the APN role.

As the workforce diversifies, additional study is warranted in organizational culture and how different aspects of leadership and management affect recruitment, retention, satisfaction, and job performance of various groups. Has management attempted to go beyond stereotyping and a persistent etic view to determine what is best for staff? Would an emic perspective change the nature of the workplace?

DISCUSSION QUESTIONS

These questions can be used to promote critical thinking and encourage discussion.

1. Spector (1996) invites the question, "Is there a difference between curing and healing?" How would you answer that question? Support your answer.
2. Have you ever had a personal experience where you and your health care provider had a different perception as to health or illness? What was that experience like for you? How was it resolved?
3. When you hear the words *marginalized* and *disenfranchised* in regard to groups, what individuals come to mind? What about such individuals places them in their particular category? Where are the gaps in health services for those individuals? How might these be remedied? What researchable problems do you see for this population? How might an ethnonursing study address these problems?
4. Collect copies of several cultural assessment instruments. Critique them for use in your clinical practice. Pay particular attention to the similarities and differences in the instruments. How might you blend their best parts for a time-efficient and practical assessment that can be used with culturally diverse patients? In what situations might you wish to use a particular instrument in its entirety? What makes this situation different?
5. Some would argue that chapters in texts about transcultural nursing that deal with the particulars of a cultural group lead to a "cookbook" nursing approach based on stereotypes (e.g., "The Amish patient is . . . ," "Filipino women are . . . "). Respond to this criticism.

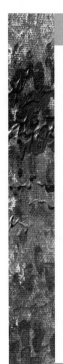

Suggestions for Further Learning

- Learn more about Dr. Madeline Leininger and her Cultural Care Diversity and Universality Theory in Marriner-Tomey, A., & Alligood, M.R. (1998). *Nursing theorists and their work.* St. Louis: Mosby.
- Choose a qualitative study mentioned in this chapter and critique it using the criteria for evaluating qualitative studies. These may be found in most research texts, or you may consult Meleis, A.. (1996). Culturally competent scholarship: substance and rigor. *Advances in Nursing Science, 19*(2), 17-26.
- Obtain the videotape *The Nurse Theorists: Portraits of Excellence. Madeline Leininger* to get a personal glimpse of Dr. Leininger and hear about her work in her own words. This 44-minute color videotape is available from FITNE, 5 Depot Street, Athens, OH 45701; phone (740) 592-2511.
- Read Fadiman, A. (1997). *The spirit catches you and you fall down: a Hmong child, her American doctors, and collision of two cultures.* New York: Farrar, Straus, & Giroux. (The paperback version was printed in 1998.) You can read an excerpt and review of this book at most Internet booksellers' websites.
- Read Gropper, R.C. (1996). *Culture in the clinical encounter: an intercultural sensitizer for the health professional.* Thousand Oaks, CA: Intercultural Press.
- Conduct a web search on cultural competence. Note that this topic spans many disciplines. Read some references from disciplines outside nursing for insights that might be useful to your nursing practice.
- Select a cultural assessment from one of the models mentioned in this chapter. Obtain a copy and use with a minority patient in your clinical population. What was the experience like? How long did the assessment take? What do you perceive as the advantages of the assessment instrument? Are there any disadvantages?
- Investigate the programs and services of the Transcultural Nursing Society, Madonna University College of Nursing & Health, 36600 Schoolcraft Road, Livonia, MI 48150-1173; website: www.transculturalcare.org/.

---

6. Leininger (1995) frames two questions relevant to worldwide transcultural nursing. How would you answer them? First, what factors are keeping nurses from getting to know the cultural health needs of people in different communities and the ways to change health services for them? Second, why are patients from different cultures relying so much on their generic or folk health practices, especially when professional services are accessible to them?

REFERENCES/BIBLIOGRAPHY

Andrews, M.M. (1999). Theoretical foundations of transcultural nursing. In M.M. Andrews & J.S. Boyle (Eds.), *Transcultural concepts in nursing care* (3rd ed.) (pp. 3-22). Philadelphia: JB Lippincott.

Austin, W., Gallop, R., McCoy, E., Peterneli-Taylor, C., & Bayer, M. (1999). Culturally competent care for psychiatric clients who have a history of sexual abuse. *Clinical Nursing Research, 8*(1), 5-24.

Barnum, B.S. (1998). *Nursing theory: analysis, application, evaluation* (5th ed.). Philadelphia: JB Lippincott.

Bushy, A. (1999). Social and cultural factors affecting health care and nursing practice. In J. Lancaster (Ed.), *Nursing issues in leading and managing change.* St. Louis: Mosby.

Campinha-Bacote, J. (1994a). *The process of cultural competence: a culturally competent model of care* (2nd ed.). Cincinnati, OH: Transcultural CARE Associates Press.

Campinha-Bacote, J. (1994b). Transcultural psychiatric nursing: diagnostic and treatment issues. *Journal of Psychosocial Nursing, 32*(8), 41-46.

Campinha-Bacote, J. (1999). A model and instrument for addressing cultural competence in health care. *Journal of Nursing Education, 38*(5), 203-207.

Chrisman, N., & Schultz, P. (1997). Transforming health care through cultural competence training. In J. Dieneman (Ed.), *Cultural diversity in nursing* (pp. 70-79). Washington, DC: American Academy of Nursing.

Coehling, H.V.E. (1994). Organizational culture. In L. Simms, S. Price, & N. Ervin (Eds.), *The professional practice of nursing administration* (2nd ed.). Albany, NY: Delmar.

Davidhizar, R., & Giger, J.N. (1997). Canadian transcultural nursing: applying the Giger & Davidhizar model. *Journal of Cultural Diversity, 4*(1), 26-31.

DeSantis, L. (1994). Making anthropology clinically relevant to nursing care. *Journal of Advanced Nursing, 20,* 707-715.

Drury, L.J. (1995). *Lifeways of homeless chronically mentally ill individuals in a community housing program* (Doctoral dissertation UMI # PUZ9525250). Chicago: Rush University College of Nursing.

Eliason, M.J. (1993). Ethics and transcultural care. *Nursing Outlook, 41*(5), 225-228.

Emblen, J.D., & Halstead, L. (1993). Spiritual needs and interventions: comparing the views of patients, nurses, and chaplains. *Clinical Nurse Specialist, 7*(4), 175-182.

Estes, G., & Zitzow, D. (1980, November). *Heritage consistency as a consideration in counseling Native Americans.* Dallas, TX: National Indian Education Association Convention.

Fong, C.M. (1985). Ethnicity and nursing practice. *Topics in Clinical Nursing, 7*(3), 1-10.

Gelazis, R. (1994). *Humor, care, and well-being of Lithuanians-Americans: an ethnonursing study using Leininger's Theory of Culture Care Diversity and Universality* (Doctoral dissertation UMI # PUZ 9234710). Detroit, MI: Wayne State University.

Gibson, M.H. (1995). *The quality of life of adult hemodialysis patients* (Doctoral dissertation UMI # PUZ 9603848). Austin, TX: University of Texas at Austin.

Giger, J.N., & Davidhizar, R.E. (1995). *Transcultural nursing: assessment and intervention*. St. Louis: Mosby.

Hahn, J.A. (1997). Transcultural nursing in home health care: learning to be culturally sensitive. *Home Health Care Management and Practice, 10*(1), 66-71.

Harsburgh M., & Foley, D. (1990). The phenomenon of care in Sicilian-Canadian culture: an ethnographic nursing case study. *Nursing Forum, 25*(3), 14-20.

Kreps, C., & Kunimoto, Y. (1994). *Effective communication in multicultural health care settings*. Thousand Oaks, CA: Sage.

Leininger, M. (1970). *Nursing and anthropology: two worlds to blend*. New York: John Wiley & Sons.

Leininger, M. (1981). *Survey of schools of nursing incorporating transcultural nursing in undergraduate and graduate programs in the USA* (Unpublished manuscript). Detroit, MI: Wayne State University.

Leininger, M. (1984). *Care: the essence of nursing and health*. Thorofare, NJ: Slack.

Leininger, M. (1990). The significance of cultural concepts in nursing. *Journal of Transcultural Nursing, 2*(1), 22-26.

Leininger, M. (1991). *Culture care diversity and universality: a theory* (Publication #15-2402). New York: National League for Nursing Press.

Leininger, M. (1995). *Transcultural nursing: concepts, theories, research and practices* (2nd ed.). New York: McGraw-Hill.

Lester, R. (1998). Cultural competence: a nursing dialogue. *American Journal of Nursing, 98*(2), 26-33.

Lowenstein, A.J. (1998). Cultural diversity in the workplace. In J.A. Dienemann (Ed.), *Nursing administration: managing patient care* (pp. 101-124). Stamford, CT: Appleton & Lange.

Louie, K.B. (1998). Cultural influences on nursing. In G. Deloughery (Ed.), *Issues and trends in nursing* (3rd ed.) (pp. 171-194). St. Louis: Mosby.

Mahon, P.Y. (1997). Transcultural nursing: a source guide. *Journal of Nursing Staff Development, 13*(4), 218-222.

Marriner-Tomey, A., & Alligood, M.R. (1998). *Nursing theorists and their work* (4th ed.). St. Louis: Mosby.

Masi, R. (1995) Multicultural health: principles and policies. In R. Masi, L. Mensah, & K. McLeod (Eds.), *Health and cultures: Vol. I. Policies, professional practice and education* (pp. 11-22). New York: Mosaic.

McCance, T.V., McKenna, H.P., & Boore, J.R.P. (1999). Caring : theoretical perspectives of relevance to nursing. *Journal of Advanced Nursing, 30*(6), 1388-1395.

McDonald, M.R., & Miller-Grolla, L. (1995). Developing a collective future: creating a culture specific nurse caring practice model for hospitals. *Canadian Journal of Nursing Administration, 3*(3), 78-95.

Meleis, A. (1996). Culturally competent scholarship: substance and rigor. *Advances in Nursing Science, 19*(2), 17-26.

Meleis, A.I. (Ed.). (1995). *Diversity, marginalization, and culturally competent health care issues in knowledge development*. Washington, DC: American Academy of Nursing.

Miers, L.J. (1993). *The meaning of professional nurse caring: the experience of family members of critically ill patients* (Doctoral dissertation UMI # PUZ 9419296). Birmingham, AL: University of Alabama at Birmingham.

Miller, J.E. (1997). *Politics and care: a study of Czech American within Leininger's theory of culture care diversity and universality* (Doctoral dissertation UMI # PUZ 9725851). Detroit, MI: Wayne State University.

Motwani, J., Hodge, J., & Crampton, S. (1995). Managing diversity in the health care industry: a conceptual model and an empirical investigation. *Holistic Care Supervisor, 13*(3), 16-23.

Nkongho, N. (1992). Teaching health professionals transcultural concepts. *Holistic Nursing Practice, 6*(3), 29-33.

Peters, T., & Waterman, R. (1987). *In search of excellence*. New York: Harper & Row

Phillips, C.Y., Palmer, C.V., Wetting, V.S., & Fenwick, J. (2000). Attitudes toward nurse practitioners: influence of gender, age, ethnicity, education, and income. *Journal of the American Academy of Nurse Practitioners, 12*(7), 255-259.

Price, J., & Cordell, B. (1994). Cultural diversity and patient teaching. *Journal of Continuing Education in Nursing, 25*(4), 163-166.

Purnell, L. (2000). A description of the Purnell model for cultural competence. *Journal Transcultural Nursing, 11*(1), 40-46.

Purnell, L.D., & Paulanka, B. J. (1998). Purnell's model for cultural competence. In L.D. Purnell & B.J. Paulanka (Eds.), *Transcultural health care* (pp.7-51). Philadelphia: FA Davis.

Quniless, F. (2000). Primary care, education, and research integration: a vehicle for a culture of health. In M.L. Kelley & V.M. Fitzsimons (Eds.), *Understanding cultural diversity: culture, curriculum, and community in nursing*. Boston: Jones & Bartlett & National League for Nursing Press.

Randall, T. (1991). Key to organ donation may be cultural awareness. *Journal of the American Medical Association, 285*(2), 176-178.

Santiago-Irizarry, N. (1996). Culture as cure. *Cultural Anthropology, 11*(1), 3-24.

Schweiger, J.L. (1992). *Commitment to clinical nursing practice* (Doctoral dissertation UMI # PUZ 9306310). Columbia, NY: Columbia University Teacher's College.

Spangler, Z.D.L. (1991). *Nursing care values and caregiving practices of Anglo-American and Philippine-American nurses in a hospital context* (Doctoral dissertation UMI # PUZ 9127270). Detroit, MI: Wayne State University.

Spector, R. (1996). *Cultural diversity in health and illness* (4th ed.). Stamford, CT: Appleton & Lange.

Spector, R. (2000). *Cultural diversity in health and illness* (5th ed.). Upper Saddle River, NJ: Prentice Hall.

Welch, A.Z., Alexander, J.E., Beagle, C.J., Butler, P., Dougherty, D.A., Andrews-Robards, K.D., Solotkin, K.C., & Velotta, C. (1998). Madeline Leininger—culture care: diversity and universality theory. In A. Marriner-Tomey & M.R. Alligood (Eds.), *Nursing theorists and their work* (4th ed.) (pp. 439-462). St. Louis: Mosby.

Wenger, A.F.Z. (1996), Cultural context, health, and health care decision-making. *Journal of Transcultural Nursing, 7*(1), 3-14.

Zoucha, R., & Husted, G.L. (2000). The ethical dimensions of delivering culturally congruent nursing and health care. *Issues in Mental Health Nursing, 21*(3), 325-340.

Chapter 35

Education, the Nursing Profession, and Cultural Diversity

Ann Schmidt Luggen & Cheryl Pope Kish

At U.S. universities today, student bodies are becoming an increasingly vibrant mix of ethnic and racial minority students. This is not surprising given that while the U.S. population has grown 10% between 1980 and 1990, specific ethnic groups have increased their numbers many times (Poss, 1999). Hispanics have increased by more than 50%, and Asian/Pacific Islanders have grown more than 100%. In the face of these data, education of nurses in culturally competent care does not appear to be the norm that it should be. According to the American Academy of Nursing (AAN), only about one fourth of nursing schools in the United States offer a meaningful curriculum emphasizing cultural competency (Meleis, 1995). Fewer than 10% of Master's programs have cultural diversity courses.

At the same time that the adequacy of educating the prospective workforce for culturally competent care is being questioned, there is growing concern that culturally diverse students are not proportionally represented in graduate and professional education. This chapter examines both of these dimensions of culture and education and what it all means to curriculum and instruction.

DEFINITIONS

Culture refers to the "totality of socially transmitted behavioral patterns, arts, beliefs, values, customs, lifeways, and all other products of human work and thought characteristics of a population of people that guide their worldview and decision making" (Purnell & Paulanka, 1998). Culture is learned within the context of one's family and, though it influences the way an individual views the world and relates to it and other people, it is largely unconscious.

Cultural diversity refers to the "variations and differences among and between cultural groups due to differences in lifeways, language, values, norms, and other cultural aspects" (Leininger, 1995). As this country becomes more culturally diverse, encountering others from a culture different than one's own is inevitable. "When individuals of dissimilar cultural orientations meet in a work or therapeutic environment, the likelihood for developing a mutually satisfying relationship is improved if both parties in the relationship attempt to learn about each other's culture" (Purnell & Paulanka, 1998). This would also be the case if individuals met within the context of higher education. The greater the cultural mix on campuses, the richer the educational experience in providing cultural sensitivity and awareness.

Culture is particularly important to the educational enterprise because culture influences how one learns how to learn. Culture is the "medium of our individuality . . . the way we express our self. It is the medium of our human relationships" (Spector, 1996). For minority graduate students who are enrolled in courses with faculty who represent a different cultural group, there exists a potential for ***biculturalism***, which refers to a dual sense of identity and often divided loyalty (LaFromboise, Coleman, & Gerton, 1993). After all, faculty members teach from the context of their culture; students learn from the context of theirs.

Educators must guard against ***cultural bias***, which is a "firm position or stance that one's own values or beliefs must govern the situation and decision" (Leininger, 1995). They must also guard against what Leininger (1995) refers to as ***cultural blindness,*** or "the inability of an individual to recognize one's own lifestyle, values, and modes of behavior and those of another individual because of strong attitude to make them invisible due to ethnocentric tendencies."

To appreciate the way in which issues of cultural diversity affect the educational process, two definitions pertinent to education are appropriate. ***Curriculum*** is defined by Bevis (1989) as "the totality of learning activities that are designed to achieve specific educational goals." For advanced practice nurse (APN) programs, curriculum would include both the content and the processes involved to prepare prospective graduates with the knowledge, values, and skills necessary to inform specialization in nursing practice and allow ethical clinical decision-making to meet the holistic needs of their respective patient populations. Working with Jean Watson in proposing a more caring curriculum that captured the rich interactions between faculty and students, Bevis suggested that curriculum be redefined to account for the many interactions and transactions between teachers and learners (Bevis & Watson, 1989). In that direction, Nelms (1991) defined curriculum as an "educational journey, in an educational environment in which the biography of the person (the student) interacts with the history of the culture of nursing through the biography of another person (the faculty) to create meaning and release potential in the lives of the participants."

Instruction refers to the processes for implementation of the curriculum. What faculty members do before, after, and at the time of the teaching occasion to increase the probability that students will learn is all part of the process of instruction. Dr. Bretland, for example, is teaching a course in women's health in a nurse practitioner (NP) program. For the unit on childbearing, she plans specific reading assignments, places materials on reserve, identifies related websites and notes them on the course syllabus, and locates women from several cultural groups to form a panel in class to discuss childbearing in their cultures. During the class period, if the panel has not been asked about a particular aspect of childbearing she considers important to student learning, the professor raises the question for the panel. She gauges student participation, notes where there might be confusion, and attempts clarification. After the class session, the professor reads class-related assignments and responds to student reactions in their course journal. When Dr. Bretland learns that there has been an influx of more Vietnamese patients into the community, she makes a note to add a Vietnamese woman to the group next semester. All of these behaviors are part of instruction.

CRITICAL ISSUES: SUPPORTING CULTURAL DIVERSITY IN CURRICULUM AND INSTRUCTION

Over time, APNs have gained a positive reputation for their holistic approach to patient care. The population trends that are making the United States a more global nation necessitate an APN community capable of providing culturally sensitive and knowledgeable care that continues to appreciate individualization. For example, by 2050, nearly one half of the United States population will represent groups that are considered ethnic and racial minorities today. The implications for curriculum seem obvious. In fact, Ketefian and Scisney-Matlock (1999) state that nursing has a social mandate to provide care for

Table 35-1		
Minority Population Projections: 1995 to 2050		
POPULATION GROUP	**1995**	**2050**
Caucasians	74%	53%
African Americans	12%	14%
Hispanics	10%	24%
Asians	3%	8%
Native Americans	1%	1%

Data from U.S. Department of Health and Human Services (1996). *Health United States: 1995* (Publication No. PHS96-1242). Hyattsville, MD: U.S. Department of Health and Human Services.

patients who are culturally and racially different. (Table 35-1 indicates the projected population change from 1995 to 2050, which serves to justify the social mandate for nursing.)

Between 1960 and 1990, the percentage of women earning baccalaureate degrees increased from 35% to 54%, while the percentages of women earning doctoral degrees increased from 10% to 37% (Naughton, 2000). While these figures are not specific to nursing, they give nursing educators some notion about the gender diversity in academe today.

There is a noticeable presence of first-generation college students on campuses today, many from cultural backgrounds largely underrepresented in higher education until now. These students will need additional help not only in adapting to biculturalism in education but also in understanding the educational system and how it works. One student from Latin America explained that he missed an academic advisement session because he did not understand what that meant. He explained to the faculty advisor: "I asked my girlfriend. She wasn't sure either but her mother, who is a college graduate, knew what to tell us. Nobody in my family ever went to college. I couldn't ask my mother or father for help with this."

Attending to human diversity in curriculum, however, extends beyond racial and ethnic differences to the inclusion of age and gender diversity. By 2025, 19% of the United States' population is expected to be persons 65 years of age and older, with increasing numbers of those 85 years of age and older (National Institute on Aging, 1993). Women continue to account for nearly 52% of the population. Within the other categories of human diversity, students will have opportunities to meet the needs of those whose religious philosophy differs from their own, to care for those with varied disabilities, and to work with patients with diverse sexual preferences. Curriculum, therefore, must prepare students for such experiences.

The National League for Nursing (NLN) (1996), through its accrediting commission, proposes that cultural content be evident in undergraduate nursing curricula and that the mission and goals of all nursing programs reflect a commitment to a culturally, racially, and ethnically diverse community. The American Association of Colleges of Nursing (AACN), which also has an arm that accredits nursing programs, concurs that curricula need to be culturally relevant to minority populations (AACN, 1996).

The nursing program must be able to show congruence between the nursing unit's mission or philosophy statement and that of the parent institution's mission. It is common in these days for a university's mission to reflect the value for cultural diversity and internationalization in its community of scholars. The first issue of *Change* in 1992 reported on the extent of multiculturalism on American college and university campuses with a survey representative of higher education (n = 196 institutions). That report generated the following findings indicative of multiculturalism in curriculum (Naughton, 2000):

- Of colleges and universities, 34% offer a multicultural general education requirement.
- Coursework in gender and ethnic studies is offered by at least 33% of these institutions; programs and departments related to these specializations were rare.
- Inclusion of diversity in course offerings occurs in 54% of these institutions.
- Public colleges and universities are ahead of private institutions in introducing multiculturalism to the curriculum.
- Multiculturalism has been introduced in colleges and universities in every region of the country.
- Provision of multiculturalism in the curriculum is cited by 72% of administrators as a topic of concern for their respective institutions.

Based on their collective philosophy, nursing faculty select an organizing framework to structure their curriculum. The faculty's collective philosophies about teaching, learning, and evaluating, as well as how the discipline of nursing should be envisioned, explained, and evaluated, guide the construction of a curriculum framework. Faculty may envision the phenomenon of nursing from a single theory framework or from an eclectic view that renders a more conceptual framework. Classically, when faculty develop an organizing framework, they consider not only the content to be included in the curriculum but also the setting in which the program will operate and the characteristics of students. An examination of setting necessarily includes recognition of those illnesses and disorders commonly seen in the school's patient population; this would include disorders more common in certain ethnic and racial groups. The student aspect of an organizing framework might consider such cultural aspects as preferred learning styles, time orientation, English as a second language, mean grade point average, employment status, other role demands, and length of time in the country.

The AAN, in its work *Diversity and Marginalization and Cultural Competent Care* (1995), developed the following priorities, all of which relate to the content aspect of a program's organizing framework or curriculum:

- Synthesis of theory and research related to marginalized populations and the nursing mission
- Utilization and testing of models of culturally sensitive, competent care
- Creation of environments for dialogue about marginalization, values, cultural sensitivity, and competency to bridge practice, research, and theory gaps
- Analysis and development of methodologies congruent with diversity, marginalization, and culturally competent care
- Development of a common language to enhance comparative research and theory related to culturally competent care
- Development, refinement, and testing of effective models for recruitment and retention of marginalized and vulnerable populations in research, education programs, and service agencies

In the same document, the AAN makes recommendations that have clear implications for nursing curriculum and instruction. They insist on: (1) commitment to quality culturally competent care that is equitable and accessible; (2) development, support, and maintenance of a knowledge base and expertise in cultural competence; (3) development of mechanisms to synthesize theory and research knowledge of nursing care of different ethnic, stigmatized, and disenfranchised populations; (4) creation of a knowledge base reflecting heterogeneous health care practices of cultural groups; (5) development of common strategies to provide a foundation for education and research; (6) identification, description, and examination of methods, theories, and frameworks for knowledge development in the health care of minorities and stigmatized and disenfranchised populations; (7) description and identification of principles of organizations that provide an environment that enhances effective working relationships and knowledge; (8) development related to marginalization and disenfranchised students, faculty, and clinicians; (9) identification of models effective in health care delivery to minorities and stigmatized and disenfranchised populations; (10) development of mechanisms that lead to improved systems of health care delivery; (11) support for regulation of content reflecting diversity in the nursing curriculum, with specific attention given to state boards of nursing examinations and continuing education, as well as graduate and undergraduate curricula; (12) establishment of ways to teach and guide faculty and nursing students to provide culturally specific and culturally competent nursing care to patients in clinical areas in local, regional, national, and international arenas; and (13) collaboration with ethnic and minority nursing organizations to develop models for recruitment, education, and retention of nurses from their constituency.

In the process of curriculum development, once the philosophy is articulated and the organizational framework is specified, the faculty identifies program outcomes and objectives. Traditionally, this process is carefully guided by a determination of what a graduate of the program should be able to do as a result of the program—what cognitive, affective, and technical abilities will result from this particular educational experience. APN faculty who practice have a realistic sense of what the real world of clinical practice requires from an APN in a particular specialty. Some programs use advisory committees or councils consisting of those knowledgeable about clinical practice, and having racial and ethnic minorities as members of advisory committees can be helpful for providing a fuller understanding of the contemporary workforce.

Guidelines from specialty organizations and literature can also be helpful to designing culturally inclusive curriculum and designating program competencies or outcomes. *The Essentials of Master's Education for Advanced Practice Nursing* (AACN, 1996) has been of inestimable value to curriculum planning for APN education; it clearly states the expectation that while Master's-prepared nurses are capable of functioning in a nursing faculty or nursing administration role, "the primary focus of the Master's education program should be the clinical role." This document suggests core content in theory; research; policy, organization, and financing of health care; ethics; professional role development; human diversity and social issues; and health promotion and disease prevention. For those preparing for direct care roles in advanced practice, knowledge of health assessment, physiology/pathophysiology, and advanced pharmacology is an expectation. These three courses would serve students' understanding of biological variations among cultural groups and how these affect management of illness.

Demonstrating value for diversity requires that faculty attend not only to curriculum content but also to instructional methods and strategies used in the program. "Traditional, didactic lecture and evaluation of individual performance is not a culturally neutral approach to teaching. These methods favor students from the dominant culture who have been socialized in an 'individualistic, competitive, man-can-control-nature' world-view" (Salmond, 2000). Students who have not been socialized to this instructional approach often experience anxiety, self-doubt, and confusion—aspects of biculturalism—as they attempt to balance traditional college approaches with their own norms (Adams, 1992; Pacquiao, 1996). Strategies that enable active participation and interactive learning, with faculty adding content not covered by student discussion and providing handouts that facilitate organization, are a more appropriate choice for minority students. Case study, storytelling, and simulations benefit all cultural groups and help in linking theory and reality if the faculty

design such aids with fidelity to the clinical setting (Salmond, 2000). Smith (2000) suggests journaling, family history, and cultural autobiography as valuable strategies for facilitating a cultural identity. Kirkpatrick, Brown, & Atkins (1998) and Bradshaw (1996) promote use of the Internet to integrate cultural diversity and global awareness in the curriculum; they link students with international partners.

Male students at all levels of nursing education continue to constitute a minority, and faculty are advised to be aware of the unique needs of this group to minimize their sense of biculturalism. Attending to what an educational experience is like for male students in a predominantly female discipline is always appropriate. Moreover, faculty should ask themselves to what extent they minimize the role of men in the profession. For example, are the APNs in all the case studies women? On exams, do the scenarios in the questions always relate to female APNs? Are there male faculty or male APNs as clinical preceptors or mentors?

One might question how even the most comprehensive curriculum could enable a student to learn about all cultures well enough to care for any patient. The answer is that this is not possible and also unnecessary. Cultural competence is an educational process of developing working relationships across lines of difference; this includes "self-awareness, cultural knowledge about illness and healing practices, intercultural communication skills, and behavioral flexibility" (Lester, 1998).

Some poignant examples demonstrate the need for cultural content in nursing education programs (Lester, 1998):

- An emergency department nurse was caring for a Vietnamese baby. The baby had a tight string on its wrist, which the nurse cut off. The family became distressed because the string was to protect the baby from evil and harm.
- Russian patients at one U.S. hospital were seen as very aggressive and demanding. However, these people had come from Russian concentration camps, where they had to fight for every basic requirement. Nurses found that it took a long time for the Russian immigrants to learn that the nurses would help them without such behaviors.
- A certified nurse midwife (CNM) learned that the way to teach nutrition and good eating habits to pregnant adolescents was to teach that they "will look good when they have the baby." This is part of the adolescent self-image and important in the United States. However, this did not work for Chinese mothers; their focus was entirely on the baby's health.
- A nurse who was teaching Japanese families in Hawaii was never able to establish eye contact and did not feel he was establishing a relationship with his patients. After much time, he learned that eye contact was confrontational for this culture. At that point, he began

looking at the wall behind the families, or at their shoulders, with success.

- A young woman from Haiti was in the emergency department, suffering from abdominal pain. She had very recently lost her mother and was also suffering from this loss. As she waited, she performed traditional mourning; she talked aloud to the spirits and planned a barefoot walking pilgrimage in Haiti. No one in the emergency department spoke Haitian Creole, but one staff member knew French, understood her words, and assumed her to be psychologically disturbed. She was admitted to a locked ward and given an antipsychotic treatment for 3 days until a Haitian physician was able to see her.

- A Russian child treated for pneumonia had numerous black-and-blue bruises on his back, and the mother was charged with abuse. In fact, she had been using suction cups to treat the pneumonia, a standard practice in Russia. It was a lengthy process to deal with this cultural error, and the family was left with a fear of U.S. hospitals.

These are excellent examples of inappropriate care from a discussion panel on cultural competence (Lester, 1998). With more knowledge, flexibility, time, and resources, these kinds of serious problems can be avoided.

Preparing Advanced Practice Nurses for the Multicultural Workplace

In 1977, the American Nurses Association (ANA) and the United States Department of Health and Human Services (DHHS) surveyed nurses to determine their racial and ethnic backgrounds. The survey found that 6.2% of active registered nurses (RNs) were of ethnic minority backgrounds. The ANA adopted Resolution 52 in 1980, which addressed recruitment, retention, and graduation of minorities in baccalaureate and higher degree programs (Louie, 1998). Table 35-2 shows a comparison of the RN population in 1992 and 1996, as reported by Deloughery (1998).

The ANA (1998) reported data from their 1996 survey related to other aspects of the RN workforce: 4.9% were males, up from 4% in 1992; 60% worked in hospitals, down from 66.5% in 1992; and 8.1% worked in long-term care (LTC), up from 7% in 1992. The average age of RNs, 44.3 years in 1996, was an increase (from 42.3) from the 1992 survey. Moreover, new RNs were older—33.5 years of age at graduation; in 1980, the average age at graduation was 27 years.

As the country becomes more multicultural, the workforce will become more diverse; however, it is not likely to mirror the population proportionately. As students are educated for APN roles and the different perspective specialization brings to practice, they need to understand the dynamics of cultural diversity in the workplace. One example of variations by culture is related to collectivism versus individualism and the potential conflict this difference engenders. It has been noted that nurse managers in the United States tend to give more difficult assignments to international nurses because they are perceived to be more cooperative. The international nurses often resent the harder assignment, but they do not demand fairness because of a collectivistic orientation. Over time, the response to such unfair work assignments may result in a higher turnover of international nurses. An orientation of collectivism tends to promote interpersonal harmony, while an individualistic orientation places greater emphasis on individual rights, autonomy, self-sufficiency, and achievement. The United States and most European countries tend to be individualistic, while the countries of Asia and South America tend towards collectivism (Mack, 1996).

According to Mack (1996), gender can also affect assignments in the workplace. Men and women are socialized differently and often bring communication and negotiation styles borne of those differences into the practice setting. For example, socialization may make women more intuitive listeners and men more competitive. Since nursing requires negotiation in many situations, understanding this kind of gender perspective may be helpful. However, it is critical not to be swayed by such stereotypes when making clinical assignments.

Table **35-2**					
Comparison of Ethnicity of the Registered Nurse Population: 1992 and 1996					
YEAR	**CAUCASIAN NON-HISPANIC**	**AFRICAN AMERICAN**	**ASIAN/PACIFIC ISLANDER**	**HISPANIC**	**NATIVE AMERICAN/ ALASKA NATIVE**
1992	90.3%	4.2%	3.4%	1.6%	0.5%
1996	90.1%	4.0%	3.4%	1.4%	0.4%

Data from Deloughery G., (1998). *Issues and trends in nursing* (3rd ed.). St. Louis: Mosby.

Supporting Multiculturalism in Academia

At this time, about 32 million people in the United States speak languages other than English at home; half of these speak Spanish (Poss, 1999). Faculty members in nursing programs, as they aspire to cultural competence, need to appreciate the challenges faced by students who have a language barrier that affects their learning. In graduate education, where so much of outcome evaluation and grading is derived from writing scholarly papers and presenting a well-organized, well-articulated position verbally, this can be especially problematic. Students for whom English is a second language often need tutorials or additional faculty support in developing an organized idea and writing a scholarly paper.

Today, college students are older than they used to be; 15% are older than 35 years of age (Roberts, 1994). Many more are female; 55% of undergraduate students are women. Racially and ethnically, college students are also increasingly becoming more diverse; one in five college students in the United States is from a racial or ethnic minority (Roberts, 1994). (Box 35-1 indicates the enrollment of diverse students in American higher education.)

Research and survey data indicate that today's nursing students are less representative of the population in terms of diversity (McCloskey, 1994). According to the first national poll on diversity in higher education, two out of three Americans say it is very important that universities prepare students to function in a diverse society (Association of American Colleges and Universities [AACU], 1998). Furthermore, nearly 58% say our nation is growing apart, and 71% say that diversity education on college campuses helps bring society together.

Borchert (1994) suggests that the "typical Master's degree student in the 1990s attends school part-time, is older, probably has worked after obtaining the baccalaureate, and is more likely to be female." This description certainly presents a striking resemblance to many Master of Science in Nursing (MSN) students. Further information about adults returning to school for a Master's degree reveals that women account for 50% of students and that the mean age is 33, with about one fifth of students over the age of 40. More than half of students are married, and many have dependents. Almost 90% work more than 30 hours a week (National Center for Education Statistics, 1993). Another common role demand for older graduate students is dealing with aging and chronically ill parents who may be geographically distant; this necessitates time away from studies. These competing role demands, so common for graduate students in nursing, are inherently difficult for all, but they may compound the challenges faced by minority students.

Cultural and racial diversity can be a deterrent to a college education. For the many people who do enter college, failure is not uncommon. The Center for Research in Nursing Education and Community Health (1996) indicates a significant attrition rate for minority students. Minority representation in graduate education in nursing is also limited; in 1994, for example, only 6% of those graduating from MSN programs were African American; 3.3% were Hispanic, and 3.2% were Asian. Even smaller numbers of Native Americans graduated (Center for Research in Nursing Education and Community Health, 1996). Clearly, these percentages of graduates do not reflect the global community that is the United States today; that is a concern for nursing education. It is also a concern for nursing practice because the numbers of MSN graduates fail to add significantly to the diversity of the existing health care workforce, wherein minorities are underrepresented (only 9%).

Reentry programs such as the federally funded Trio programs of Upward Bound, Student Support Services, and Talent Search (Higher Education Act of 1963 [Title IV, Subpart 4]) can advocate for undergraduate students, secure admissions, and provide support during the university experience. Graduate students have less national support during their education; most efforts to remedy their academic or lifeway concerns are university-based and require administrators and faculty committed to supporting culturally diverse students.

Culturally diverse faculty in higher education

Of 15,000 full-time nursing faculty in academia, only 890 are African American (McNeal, 1998). Other racial and ethnic groups are also underrepresented among the ranks of nursing faculty. These low numbers exist despite affirmative action hiring practices. Small colleges and universities lack the financial incentives to be competitive with major universities and health science centers in hiring minority faculty. Very little has been published about the minority faculty group and what factors are associated with successful recruitment and retention. McNeal (1998) did find increased satisfaction among African-American faculty in historically African-American nursing schools and less satisfaction in predominantly Caucasian schools. This finding exists despite the fact that the faculty had heavier teaching loads, fewer publications and grants, and less access to research information and communication technology in the African-American schools.

Box 35-1

Enrollment of Racial/Ethnic Minorities in U.S. Colleges: 1980-1990

All Enrollments	Up 18%
Hispanics	Up 66%
African Americans	Up 13%
Native Americans	Up 23%
Asian/Pacific Islanders	Up 100%

From National Center for Education Statistics (1991). Washington, DC: Department of Education.

Fewer minority faculty translates to a lack of role models for minority students, a lack of individuals who truly understand their bicultural experience. Also, a multicultural understanding is best achieved when students and faculty are from varied cultures. Hence, without multicultural faculty, a rich cultural experience is lacking for all students and faculty. Having part-time faculty and clinical preceptors engaged with student learners enhances their cultural exposure to some extent. Another option is mentoring assignments between diverse students and community partners, who can be helpful as role models. For example, MSN student Hesa Xiu, an Asian student who immigrated to attend graduate school, was introduced to John Chen, an Asian-American clinical nurse specialist (CNS), as a mentor. Not only did John mentor Hesa about academic and clinical concerns, he and his family included Hesa in special occasions that provided a well-rounded education for her and minimized homesickness.

Admission and retention strategies that support multiculturalism

Admission and retention in a university can be problematic for culturally diverse students. Traditionally, universities have used admission criteria that are believed to predict academic achievement, such as grade point average and standardized tests. However, women and minorities, especially those from lower socioeconomic groups, do not perform as well on standardized admission tests (Vaseleck, 1994); this appears to be true even if their undergraduate grade point averages are equivalent to those of non-minority students. Admission formulae that use multiple weighted factors, portfolio assessment, and onsite interviews are measures that may be helpful to many minority students (Hagedorn & Nora, 1996).

Persistence or retention rates for minority students continue to concern educators. Constructive faculty-student relationships, mentoring programs, tutoring and other academic support, economic support, and academic development activities (e.g., orientations, handbooks, writing seminars) appear to be helpful to persistence in graduate school. Nerad and Miller (1996) offer these additions to the list of how to enhance retention in graduate and professional schools: (1) monitor progress rates carefully and have dialogues with students any time problems arise and always at the end of the initial year; (2) devise an advising and mentoring effort that includes written guides, newsletters, and websites to keep students informed; (3) work with students in orientation-to-school sessions, grant proposal workshops, and interdisciplinary research retreats; and (4) provide academic job search assistance.

Instructional strategies that support multiculturalism

Many faculty teach ethnically diverse students in a generic way, described by students as "the English way" or "the general way," but the faculty is unaware of their biases (Yoder, 1996). Students in one study stated that nursing faculty assume the perspective of the dominant group and teach it as the truth, or the general way. Many faculty have no formal preparation relative to cultural issues other than a basic course in sociology (Yoder, 1997). Multicultural understanding is relatively new as a concern to higher education, and programs preparing prospective faculty may not have included cultural aspects of education in coursework. Faculty may have little experience interacting with those from other countries or other cultures. It is well established that faculty tend to teach as they were taught. Faculty may need continuing education in understanding multicultural issues and promoting success for minority students. Faculty must be committed to a multicultural student population and willing to examine policies and procedures for any inflexibility that impedes multiculturalism. They must check with stakeholders regarding their perceptions of the cultural environment of the university. Like the manager of an organization, it is the faculty who are leaders in creating a culture supportive of diversity (Salmond, 2000) and an appreciation that "diversity is not egalitarianism. Treating everyone the same and following the 'golden rule' works in homogeneous groups"; this paradigm permits cultural blindness when a given group is culturally inclusive.

Even if students have difficulty with the way in which they are taught, they may be reluctant to come forward with their grievances (Bowser, Auletta, & Jones, 1993). The conflict will, however, be expressed, sometimes as students "adopt an attitude"; they may perform poorly on exams, come late to class, fall asleep in class, or fail to turn in required work on time. Such students may be sending signals that there is conflict. The faculty needs to resist labeling and judging students and instead be open to indirect messages from students and reach out privately to students who appear to be in conflict. For students who are not culturally prepared for class, faculty may wish to consider adapting the syllabus early in the semester and attending to how evaluation strategies might affect the culturally diverse students. The usual midterm evaluations can be punishments rather than opportunities to learn for these students (Bowser et al, 1993).

Just as there is concern in U.S. grade schools about content written from a Euro-American viewpoint and omitting African-American, Hispanic, Asian, and Native-American experiences, college texts are only beginning to exhibit a crosscultural context. Nursing research, which provides the basis for nursing knowledge, has rarely incorporated cultural contexts. This is probably due to the fact that nurses have rarely been educated with a crosscultural curriculum. Researchers cannot assume that measures used in research are equivalent across cultures (Amick, Levine, Tarlov, & Walsh, 1995). "Even seemingly robust, well-established variables such as stressful events and social support, whose impact on health is well documented, may have varying meanings and may manifest their influence in diverse ways depending on the context." For example, the acceptance of help may be perceived as stressful by some, not as the buffer and support that others believe it to be.

Salmond (2000) describes the process of unlearning and challenging commonly held ideas and beliefs as a measure for cultural education. To risk this kind of confrontational, albeit gentle, process, students need to feel secure. One way to build a sense of trust for students is to structure courses with consistent cohorts of students. As the students come to know each other and the faculty, they will feel more comfortable challenging ethnocentric or judgmental statements. It is possible for both faculty and students alike to have cultural blindness and to experience anxiety when confronted with evidence that this is indeed the case. According to Salmond (2000), "It is a trusting climate and a nonjudgmental confrontation that leads to the unlearning and learning which is needed for multicultural competence." Salmond suggests that faculty and students contract to inform each other when comments or insights with ethnocentric connotations are shared.

Pacquaio (1996) discovered that students from ethnically diverse backgrounds tend to equate hard work and persistence with success and could not understand why time spent on an assignment and working hard did not produce an acceptable grade. Salmond (2000), who acknowledges similar experiences with students from nondominant cultures, suggests that faculty acknowledge the effort made by such a student in preparing the assignment, letting that provide the lead-in to specific feedback about the merits and limitations of the work.

Support services for multiculturalism

A more diverse population of students requires support systems to enable academic success and an otherwise meaningful educational experience. As universities admit international students or those from nondominant cultures in this country, there should be assurance of a variety of support services with qualified staff in place. Ideally, staff would either reflect culturally diverse groups or be specially trained to work with students of varied cultures. Support might include counseling and crisis management; academic services; advisement; language, writing, and mathematics tutorials; health and wellness care; and employment assistance services. Innovative scheduling; distance learning; assistantships that provide tuition funding and stipends; and mobility options can also be supportive. Careful profiling of students is important to designing innovative and relevant support systems. Frequent evaluations of support services for evidence of perceived accessibility and adequacy is also important; current students as well as alumni should be surveyed for this purpose.

The presence of culturally diverse students on many campuses has led to establishment of support groups and formal organizations to meet their unique needs. For example, one university has an international student organization that includes not only students whose permanent home is in another country but also persons from nondominant cultures in this country. Students from around the world engage in dialogue and activities, both academic and otherwise, with African-American, Hispanic-American, Asian-American, and Native-American students whose permanent home is the United States. Some nursing schools also have special associations for minority students; interestingly, these commonly invite male students for membership, because men are considered a minority in the nursing population.

Nursing students can also be referred to the professional organizations specific to their cultural groups. For example, there is a group for Hispanic nurses (accessible at www.nahn.org), a Philippine Nursing Association (www.pna-american.org), and a Black Nurses Association (www.nbna.org). The former is primarily a forum group, but the latter two have more formal programs that influence legislation and promote policy, meet educational needs, unify nurses, and advocate for quality health care for members of their cultural group.

IMPLICATIONS FOR MSN EDUCATION AND ADVANCED PRACTICE

The cultural aspects of advanced practice may be addressed in a separate course in an MSN curriculum or as an integrated component throughout the educational program. The shared vision of the faculty will determine which of these options is most appropriate within the context of a program's mission. An isolated seminar, however, is no longer adequate. Placing crosscultural perspectives within a theoretical context, which is then applied in the clinical setting, is optimal for enabling students to appreciate the different ideas and ideals that affect health and illness in diverse populations.

Because APNs need to learn more about diseases that are more prevalent in racial and ethnic populations, this content is often integrated in settings where there is already a separate course on cultural competency. Sickle cell anemia, seen in African Americans, is an example of a disease that is present mainly in a single racial group. Content on culturally based assessment is also of concern; for example, assessing cyanosis and jaundice in dark-skinned patients may be difficult for a nurse experienced only with light-skinned patients (Louie, 1998). Cultural expression of illness is different from group to group. Stoicism may be seen in young Amish men suffering pain, while a low tolerance to pain may be exhibited by Philippine women. Faculty development activities need to be instituted in colleges to promote sensitivity to cultural differences and assist faculty in incorporation of this content into course curricula.

At some point in their APN education, students should also be given information and clinical experience with

Guidelines for Using an Interpreter to Communicate with Patients

1. Determine the interpreter's time constraints.
2. Determine if the patient needs a same-sex interpreter because of cultural beliefs.
3. Plan a preconference and a postconference with the interpreter.
   a. Clarify any concerns through the interview.
   b. Determine if dialects or accents are a problem.
   c. Determine if the patient is coherent or if there are signs of mental aberrance.
   d. Discuss interpretation style and interpretation:
      • Phrased interpretation (easiest; use short phrases)
      • Simultaneous interpretation
      • Summary interpretation (patient and/or nurse make long statements; interpreter summarizes; usually laden with errors)
   e. Ask interpreter to provide feedback:
      • Ask if he or she understands the terms.
      • Ask him or her to tell you and explain when culturally related ideas are expressed.
4. Arrange seating so that the patient can see the interpreter and the nurse. Having the interpreter stand behind or next to nurse works well.
5. Introduce yourself to the family and the interpreter.
6. Establish the context of the patient visit. For example, explain to a new patient whose complaint is recent onset of abdominal pain, "I will ask you for some information by asking questions, and then I will do a physical examination."
7. In the progress notes, write down the interpreter's name and language.

Courtesy of Harborview Medical Center, University of Washington.

using an interpreter to interview patients or provide teaching. Guidelines for working with an interpreter, developed by the Massachusetts General Hospital, are shown in Box 35-2.

A new role being used in many clinic settings is that of the health promoter. APNs need to be familiar with this role and what it provides to the health care team working with culturally diverse patients and families. Although it is invaluable when nurses can learn a patient's language and fully understand the culture, this is not always feasible. The health promoter is a supplement to nurses acquiring cultural competence. (Poss, 1999). Health promoters are persons of the same race or ethnic group as the patients served. The health promoter forms a needed link between the health care system and the community, filling a vital communication gap that currently exists in many settings. In many major centers, children of family members are used to interpret their parents' descriptions of health problems (Lester, 1998). An example would be an 8-year-old child describing his grandmother's vaginal discharge. However, this situation can affect the family's power structure and responsibility. The presence of an informed health promoter would eliminate or minimize such problems.

There is already considerable information available on utilizing the health promoter role. The National Cancer Institute, Indian Health Service, W.K. Kellogg Foundation, March of Dimes, Office of Minority Health, Health Resources and Service Administration, DHHS, Robert Wood Johnson Foundation, and Centers for Disease Control and Prevention (CDC) have all funded health promoters for clinical practice.

This chapter has provided specific strategies related to enhancing multiculturalism in MSN programs through curriculum design, instructional methods, and support systems. The bottom line, however, is the assessment of outcomes and to what extent these outcomes are affected by student characteristics, program objectives, instructional setting, economic resources devoted to the program, a supportive milieu on campus, and the educational process. Master's-prepared APNs are being educated for direct care of patients through roles as NPs, CNSs, CNMs, and certified registered nurse anesthetists (CRNAs). Furthermore, they are being educated for the nonclinical roles of educator, collaborator, researcher, leader, consultant, and change agent. Cultural sensitivity pervades all these roles, and institutional data, student interviews, and longitudinal surveys with alumni and employers can provide invaluable data to determine if a program has prepared students in a way appropriate to actualizing them.

Haworth and Conrad (1996) believe that for too long, assessment of educational quality has focused on the "prestige" model. In this model, educational quality has been associated with factors such as: (1) numbers and "scholarliness" of doctorally-prepared faculty and their level of external research funding, actual research, and publication; (2) selectivity of a critical mass of outstanding students; (3) a solid financial foundation; and (4) impressive physical facilities and resources, including library holdings. The Association of Governing Boards (1992) asserts that this view of quality "stoke[s] academic egos instead of students' dreams." Terenzini and Pascarella (1994) would concur. In their words,

> After taking into account the characteristics, abilities, and backgrounds students bring with them to college, we found that how much students grow or change has only inconsistent and, perhaps in a practical sense, trivial relationships with such traditional measures of institutional "quality" as educational expenditures per student, student/faculty ratios, faculty salaries, percentage of faculty with the highest degree in their field, faculty research productivity, size of the library, admissions selectivity, or prestige rankings.

Haworth and Conrad (1997) provide a contrasting framework for a learning-centered view of quality assessment that focuses on student learning. Their perspective is based on interviews with stakeholders of Master's-degree education that included students, alumni, and employers; moreover, their data include not only prestigious research universities but also smaller universities. The model proposed by Haworth and Conrad (1997) suggests that high-quality programs are those that, from the perspective of diverse stakeholders, provide education that positively affects student learning and preparation for practice roles. The faculty in such programs would need to ensure that activities, actions, and resources are directed toward optimal student learning and role preparation (Bergquist, 1995). Building on the perspective of their nearly 800 interviews in 47 Master's-degree programs in 31 institutions across the nation, Haworth and Conrad (1997) identified characteristics of programs with the potential to enrich learning and bring meaning to the educational experience. Using a constant comparative methodology, they constructed the Engagement Theory, which describes a high-quality Master's-degree program. (The authors provide the caveat that no program has all of the ideal qualities.) The theory is organized around the central concept of student, faculty, and administrative engagement in teaching and learning. (A capsule summary of the "diverse and engaged students" aspect of the theory is provided in Table 35-3.) Faculty that care about students as unique and holistic individuals and are culturally sensitive are ideal examples of the theory in practice. Other attributes of the ideal program include (Haworth & Conrad, 1996):

- *Participatory program cultures*—There must be an environment where there is collegiality and support for creation of a shared program and direction, an involved community of learners, and safety for questioning orthodoxies and exploring alternative viewpoints and possibilities
- *Interactive teaching and learning*—There must be considerable emphasis by faculty and administrators for critical dialogue, experiential learning, cooperative peer learning, mentoring, and out-of-class learning.
- *Connected program requirements*—There must be curricula requirements that bridge theory and practice wherein there is planned breadth and depth of course work, a residency (e.g. internship, practicum), and a tangible final product that shows synthesis. This product, whether thesis, project, or some other option, needs to show that a student has developed analytical and written communication skills; is capable of "big picture" thinking and strategizing; and has developed an independent, self-assured professional self.
- *Adequate resources*—There must be evidence of monetary and nonmonetary support for students, faculty, and the institution's infrastructure.

Table 35-3	

Criteria and Indicators for the Attribute "Diverse and Engaged Students"

Criterion	Indicators
Student diversity	Students with a variety of educational, life, and professional workplace experiences are represented in the program.
	Male and female students from a variety of racial, ethnic, and socioeconomic backgrounds are represented.
Engagement in teaching and learning	Students actively contribute diverse perspectives on knowledge and practice to class discussions.
	Students demonstrate a visible commitment to their own and others' learning (via their participation in classroom discussions, cooperative learning activities, individual and group projects, independent studies, and research).
Departmental policies and practices	Departmental student admission policies emphasize a variety of criteria, including educational background, life experience, professional nonuniversity workplace experience, cultural diversity, academic achievement, and motivation for learning.
	Admission decisions are based heavily on the "goodness of fit" between student goals and those of the faculty and program.

From Haworth, J.G., & Conrad, C.F. (1997). *Emblems of quality in higher education: developing and sustaining high quality programs.* Needham Heights, MA: Allyn & Bacon.

One can easily envision this model as an appropriate framework for assessing multiculturalism in a nursing program and its parent institution. Two questions would predominate that assessment: (1) What are the distinguishing features in this program or university that promote multiculturalism? (2) How do these features affect student learning and the overall quality of the educational experience for students? The perceptions of multiple stakeholders, using both quantitative and qualitative approaches, would be necessary to find answers to these important queries.

PRIORITIES FOR RESEARCH

Transcultural nursing is a fairly recent specialty area in higher education, and few programs prepare educators and clinicians for roles as transcultural nurses; however, all Master's programs are obligated to prepare students for the global workplace that is the present reality for advanced practice. Many questions are as yet unanswered and would be appropriate for empirical study. For example, what are the unique needs of culturally diverse students as learners? What are their preferred learning styles? What instructional methods are correlated with academic success and clinical competence in these learners? What are the needs of first-generation college students in both the majority and minority populations? What are the best practices for meeting those needs? What are the unique experiences of male APN students in a predominantly female specialty?

Attention should be given to curricula that offer a crosscultural perspective of advanced practice in an attempt to answer questions such as: What is the best way to teach cultural diversity? Is a single course better as a foundation, or is an overall integration of cultural concepts more effective? To what extent do existing program philosophies and objectives address cultural competence? Does this differ when faculty members have had courses in transcultural nursing? In what ways are diverse student populations considered in program planning?

There is a dearth of studies of culturally diverse faculty, and this needs to be remedied. For example, what are the experiences of minority faculty in majority institutions? In schools where the minority faculty represent the dominant culture? What factors are correlated with recruitment, job satisfaction, and retention of minority faculty? What professional development strategies are most effective for preparing faculty to assume a more multicultural perspective? Questions should address the enrollment and retention of diverse students. What admission requirements are being used across the nation? Which are predictive for minority students? What are the best practices for retaining minority students?

Learning assessment studies might well focus on ways to ensure quality evaluation data from multiple stakeholders. A common problem is low returns on alumni and employer surveys; research could focus on what measures would work most effectively. For example, does a particular incentive increase the probability that an alumni respondent will return a survey related to program quality? Is a telephone- or web-based survey more productive than a written one? The Engagement Theory could be tested through research.

Suggestions for Further Learning

- In a group of your peers, designate what should be included in a curriculum to prepare culturally competent APNs. Does the group support a separate culturally related course or integration of crosscultural perspectives throughout the program? Support your answer. Be specific about what concepts should be included.
- Consult Haworth, J.G., & Conrad, C.F. (1997). *Emblems of quality on higher education: developing and sustaining high-quality programs.* Needham Heights, MA: Allyn & Bacon. Critique the qualitative methodology used by these researchers to construct their theory. Critique the theory.
- Read more about educating individuals to understand diversity in Fitzsimons, V.M., & Kelley, M.L. (1996). *The culture of learning.* Boston: Jones & Bartlett & National League for Nursing Press; and Kelley, M.L., & Fitzsimons, V.M. (2000). *Understanding cultural diversity: culture, curriculum, and community in nursing.* Boston: Jones & Bartlett & National League for Nursing Press.
- Compare and contrast why and how customs practiced by one student are different from those practiced by another student and discuss.

- Read a current book or article and identify the cultural biases.
- Describe a nurse or faculty member who "fits in" in the unit (or setting). Describe a nurse or faculty member who does not fit in. Discuss.
- The Agency for Health Care Policy and Research (AHCPR) has two pocket-sized health guides available in Spanish-language versions. These are evidence-based information guides, dating from 1999, on the prevention of avoidable health problems. They are also available in English. They may be obtained from the AHCPR Clearinghouse, PO Box 8547, Silver Springs, MD 20907; website: www.ahcpr.gov, and are titled:
  - *Guia de salud infantil* (a child health guide) (APPIP-99-0013)
  - *Guia de salud personal* (a personal health guide) (APPIP-99-0012)
- Consult the following reference for educators and researchers: da Gloria Miotto Wright, M., & Korniewicz, D.M. (1998). *New perspectives in international health and nursing education.* Washington, DC: Pan American Health Organization, World Health Organization, and Georgetown University.

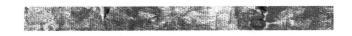

DISCUSSION QUESTIONS

These questions can be used to promote critical thinking and encourage discussion.

1. Invite a group of graduate students from different cultures to discuss what education has been like in their respective experiences. Share your commonalities and differences. Speculate on how the experiences of each individual shape their current way of learning.

2. Survey a university for a list of student services and organizations that have meeting a particular need of culturally diverse students as an objective. What are the gaps in services? What available community resources might fill the gaps? What services might be added?

3. Interview a graduate student from a different culture. What has been his or her experience in the APN program? What does the student perceive as the positive crosscultural aspects of the program? The negative ones?

4. Interview a male student about his experiences in the predominantly female world of nursing education. What has helped him? What have been barriers that needed to be overcome?

5. Break down sample stereotypes and share your descriptions with the class. Discuss possible stereotypes of the following:

   - A person named Jose, Anh, or Chandelier
   - A person who cleans houses
   - An engineer
   - A nurse

REFERENCES/BIBLIOGRAPHY

Adams, M. (1992). *Promoting diversity in college classrooms: innovative responses for the curricula, faculty, and institutions.* San Francisco: Jossey Bass.

American Academy of Nursing (1995). *Diversity, marginalization, and culturally competent health care* (Publication # 189). Washington, DC: American Academy of Nursing.

American Association of Colleges of Nursing (1996). *The essentials of Master's education for advanced practice nursing.* Washington, DC: American Association of Colleges of Nursing.

American Association of Colleges of Nursing (1998). Improving health care access through diversity. *Syllabus, 24*(5), 3-4, 8.

American Nurses Association (1995). ANA addressing cultural diversity in the profession. *The American Nurse, 30*(1), 25.

Amick, B., Levine, S., Tarlov, A., & Walsh, D. (1995). *Society and health.* New York: Oxford University Press.

Association of American Colleges & Universities (1998, October 24). Memo from Carol Geauy Schneider, President, to AAC&U member presidents. Washington, DC: Association of American Colleges & Universities.

Association of Governing Boards of Universities & Colleges (1992). *Trustees and troubled times in higher education.* Washington, DC: Association of Governing Boards of Universities & Colleges.

Banks, J.A., & Banks, C.M. (1997). *Multicultural education: issues and perspectives.* London: Allyn & Bacon.

Bergquist, W. (1995). *Quality through access, access with quality: the new imperative for higher education.* San Francisco: Jossey Bass.

Bevis, E.O. (1989). *Curriculum building in nursing: a process* (3rd ed.). New York: National League for Nursing.

Bevis, E.O., & Watson, J. (1989). *Toward a caring curriculum: a new pedagogy for nursing.* New York: National League for Nursing.

Boston, P. (1992). Understanding cultural differences through family assessment. *Journal of Cancer Education, 7*(3), 261-266.

Borchert, M.A.E. (1994). *Master's education: a guide for faculty and administrators. A policy statement.* Washington, DC: Council of Graduate Schools.

Bowser, B., Auletta, G., & Jones, T. (1993). *Confronting diversity issues on campus.* Thousand Oaks, CA: Sage.

Bradshaw, L.L (1996). Using the Internet to create international experiences for students. *International Review, 6*(1), 77-87.

Buchanan, B. (2000, third quarter). Bridging the retention gap. *Reflections on Nursing Leadership,* 28-30.

Campbell, A.P., & Davis, S.M. (1996). Faculty commitment: retaining minority nursing students in majority institutions. *Journal of Nursing Education, 35*(7), 298-303.

Campinha-Bacote, J. (1990). *Readings in transcultural care.* Wyoming, OH: Campinha-Bacote

Campinha-Bacote, J., Yahle, T., & Langenkamp, M. (1996). The challenge of cultural diversity for nurse educators. *Journal of Continuing Education for Nurses, 27*(2), 59-64.

Capers, C.F. (1992). Teaching cultural competence: a nursing education imperative. *Holistic Nursing Practice, 6*(3), 19-28.

Center for Research in Nursing Education and Community Health. (1996). *Nursing data review* (Publication # 19-6851). New York: National League for Nursing Press.

Center for Research in Nursing Education and Community Health (1996). *Nursing datasource: volume I. Trends in contemporary nursing education* (Publication # 19-6932). New York: National League for Nursing Press.

Cohen, C. (1998, April 29). *Race preferences in college admissions* (Heritage Lectures #611). Washington, DC: The Heritage Foundation.

Conrad, C.F., Haworth, J.G., & Millar, S.B. (1993). *A silent success—Master's education in the United States.* Baltimore & London: Johns Hopkins University Press.

Cook, P.R., & Cullen, J.A. (2000). Diversity as a value in undergraduate nursing education. *Nursing and Health Care Perspectives, 21*(4), 178-183.

Courage, M., &Godbey, K. (1992). Student retention: policies and services to enhance persistence to graduation. *Nurse Educator, 17*(2), 29-32.

Culley, L.A. (1995). A critique of multiculturalism in health care: the challenge for nurse education. *Journal of Advanced Nursing, 23*(2), 564-570.

Davidhizar, R., Dowd, S.B., & Giger, J.N. (1998). Educating the culturally diverse healthcare student. *Nurse Educator, 23*(2), 38-42.

Deloughery, G. (1998). *Issues and trends in nursing* (3rd ed.). St. Louis: Mosby.

Dienemann, J. (Ed.) (1998). *Cultural diversity in nursing: issues, strategies, and outcomes*. New York: American Academy of Nursing.

Doll, R.C. (1996). *Curriculum improvement: decision making and process* (9th ed.). Boston: Allyn & Bacon.

Eliason, M.J., & Macy, N.J. (1992). A classroom activity to introduce cultural diversity. *Nurse Educator, 17*(3), 32-36.

Falkenhagen, K. (1998). *Cultural competence in nursing*. Sacramento, CA: CME Resource.

Giger, J. N., & Davidhizar, R. E. (1995). *Transcultural nursing*. St. Louis: Mosby.

Hadwiger, S.C. (1999). Cultural competence case scenarios for critical nursing care. *Nurse Educator, 24*(5), 47-51.

Hagedorn, L.S., & Nora, A. (1996). Rethinking admission criteria in graduate and professional programs. *New Directions for Institutional Research, 62,* 31-44.

Haworth, J.G., & Conrad, C.F. (1996). Refocusing quality assessment on student learning. *New Directions for Institutional Research, 62,* 45-60.

Haworth, J.G., & Conrad, C.F. (1997). *Emblems of quality in higher education: developing and sustaining high quality programs*. Needham Heights, MA: Allyn & Bacon.

Kelefian, S., & Scisney-Matlock, M. (1999, September-October). Diversity in nursing education: part I. *Journal of Professional Nursing, 301.*

Kirkpatrick, M.K., Brown, S., & Atkins, T. (1998). Using the Internet to integrate cultural diversity and global awareness. *Nurse Educator, 23*(2), 15-17.

LaFromboise, T., Coleman, L.K., & Gerton, J. (1993). Psychological impact of biculturalism: evidence and theory. *Psychological Bulletin, 14*(3), 395-413

Leininger, M. (1995). *Transcultural nursing: concepts, theories, research, and practices*. New York: McGraw-Hill.

Leininger, M. (1997). Transcultural nursing research to transform nursing education with practice: 40 years. *Image: Journal of Nursing Scholarship, 29*(4), 341-347.

Lester, N. (1998). Cultural competence: a nursing dialogue. *American Journal of Nursing, 98*(8), 26-34.

Long, P. (2000, May). Multicultural care—meeting the challenge. *ADVANCE for Nurse Practitioners,* 79-80.

Louie, K.B. (1998). Cultural influences on nursing. In G. Deloughery (Ed.), *Issues and trends in nursing* (3rd ed.) (pp. 171-188). St. Louis: Mosby.

Mack, E. (1996). The effects of cultural factors. In R. Jones & S. Beck (Eds.), *Decision making in nursing* (pp. 87-96). Cincinnati, OH: Delmar.

Massachusetts General Hospital (1997). Working with interpreters: guidelines. *Caring Headlines, 3*(21), 13.

Mattson, S. (2000). Striving for cultural competence—providing care for the changing face of the U.S. *AWHONN Lifelines, 4*(3), 48-52.

McCloskey, J. (1994). *Current issues in nursing*. St. Louis: Mosby.

McNeal, G. (1998, third quarter). Study shows technology is key to African American faculty success. *Reflections on Nursing Leadership,* 28.

Meleis, A. (Ed.). (1995). *Diversity, marginalization, and cultural competent health care: issues in knowledge development*. Washington, DC: American Academy of Nursing.

Minnick, A., Roberts, M., Young, W., Marcontonio, R., & Kleinpell, R. (1997). Ethnic diversity staff nurse employment in hospitals. *Nursing Outlook, 45*(1), 35-40.

National Center for Education Statistics (1993). *U.S. Department of Education 1992-1993. National postsecondary student aid study (NPSA 93). Graduate data analysis system*. Washington, DC: Government Printing Office.

National League for Nursing Accrediting Commission (1996). *Criteria and guidelines for the evaluation of baccalaureate and higher degree programs*. New York: National League for Nursing.

Naughton, F. (2000). Bringing diversity into curriculum: successes and problems. In M.L. Kelley & V.M. Fitzsimons (Eds.), *Understanding cultural diversity: culture, curriculum, and community in nursing* (pp. 125-131). Boston: Jones & Bartlett & National League for Nursing Press.

Nelms, T. (1991). Has the curriculum revolution revolutionized the definition of curriculum? *Journal of Nursing Education, 30*(1), 5-8.

Nerad, M., & Miller, D.S. (1996). Increasing student retention in graduate and professional programs. *New Directions for Institutional Research, 62,* 61-76.

Pacquiao, D. (1996). Educating faculty in educational biculturalism. In V. Fitzsimons & M. Kelley (Eds.), *The culture of learning* (pp. 129-162). New York: National League for Nursing.

Poss, J.E. (1999). Providing culturally competent care: is there a role for nurse promoters? *Nursing Outlook, 47*(1), 30-36.

Purnell, L., & Paulanka, B (1998). *Transcultural health care*. Philadelphia: FA Davis.

Roberts, H. (1994). Diversity and change on campus. In H. Roberts (Ed.), *Teaching from a multicultural perspective*. Thousand Oaks, CA: Sage.

Salmond, S.W. (2000). Culture learning and unlearning: creating a culture supporting the development of transcultural nurse managers. In M.L. Kelley & V.M. Fitzsimons (Eds.), *Understanding cultural diversity: culture, curriculum, and community* (pp. 149-160). Boston: Jones & Bartlett & National League for Nursing Press.

Sims, G., & Baldwin, D. (1995). Race, class, and gender considerations in nursing education. *Nursing and Health Care: Perspectives on Community, 16*(6), 316-320.

Smith, L.S. (2000). Teaching to a diverse student group: transcultural concepts. In L.J. Scheetz (Ed.), *Nursing faculty secrets* (pp. 123-129). Philadelphia: Hanley & Belfus.

Spector, R.E. (1996). *Cultural diversity in health and illness* (4th ed). Stamford, CT: Appleton & Lange.

Sue, D.W., & Sue, D. (1990). *Counseling the culturally diverse*. New York: Wiley Interscience Publications.

Terenzini, P.T., & Pascarella, E.T. (1994). Living with myths: undergraduate education in America. *Change, 26,* 28-32.

Vance, C., & Olson, R.K. (Eds.). (1998). *The mentor connection in nursing*. New York: Springer.

Vaseleck, J. (1994). Stop working and put down your pencils: the use and misuse of standardized admission tests. *Journal of College & University Law, 20*(4), 405-415.

Washington, L.J. (1999). Expanding opportunities in graduate education for minority nurses. *Journal of National Black Nurses, 10*(1), 68-80.

Witterchein, G. (1998, July). Ready or not, here comes multicultural care. *Physicians Management,* 34-39.

Yoder, M.K. (1996). Instructional responses to ethnically diverse nursing students. *Journal of Nursing Education, 35*(7), 35-321.

Chapter 36

Organizations: Culture and Diversity

Ann Schmidt Luggen & Gracie S. Wishnia

In today's rapidly evolving health care system, where patients are "in sicker and out quicker," nursing staff often feel frustrated and unable to give quality care. In this same workplace, diversity of the workforce has become an issue; the workforce is aging, and the ethnic diversity of the workforce pool is changing—from "yesterday's" 87% non-Hispanic Caucasian base to the 75% of today (Koch, 1998). Add to this the cultural environment of an organization, and one sees, at times, a chaotic, disorganized system that responds to stimuli dysfunctionally. It is the goal of this chapter to present the essence of organizational culture, some of the problems encountered therein, and some research ideas for problem resolution.

DEFINITIONS

Organizational culture refers to values and attitudes about health care, work, and relationships between the corporate office and the staff in various divisions. Consistency of values and attitude of staff throughout an organization equates to corporate well-being. Inconsistency leads to confusion and discord (Byers, 1997). Organizations may also have subcultures. ***Organizational subcultures*** are similar to corporate cultures, but they may differ in emphasis (Coeling, 1997). For example, an organization may value innovation and teamwork; a particular unit may value these but emphasize teamwork more and place less value on innovation. Curran and Miller (1990) found that there was little "connectedness" between corporate culture and nursing units. Nurses seemed almost unaware of issues until there was an administrative change.

Corporate or organizational culture is different from organizational climate. ***Organizational climate*** refers to ways in which an organization is perceived and the feelings evoked by the organization's atmosphere (Flarey, 1993). The perception may be accurate or inaccurate, and different employees in the organization may perceive their employing organization very differently. For example, Donald, an adult nurse practitioner (ANP), perceives team spirit and great cooperation in his community clinic, but Lydia, a clinical nurse specialist (CNS), perceives a sense of competition and believes that the providers and staff "don't always pull in the same direction in this clinic."

CRITICAL ISSUES: UNDERSTANDING ORGANIZATIONAL CULTURE

The Joint Commission on Accreditation of Health Care Organizations (JCAHO) has 12 essential principles that characterize a health care organization's commitment to quality of care (Rowland & Rowland, 1997). These indicators serve as a basis for measuring effectiveness. The second of these essential principles is *organizational culture*, which specifies:

> The organization fosters a culture that promotes a high degree of commitment to quality patient care. In promoting this culture, the organization seeks the involvement of all those who use or provide its services. The organization encourages self-assessment, open communication, appropriate participatory decision-making, and fair conflict resolution among all levels of clinical and managerial personnel.

Sovie (1993) further describes organizational culture to be the shared values and beliefs that affect leaders; perceptions of work; approaches to work; the way in which people go about their work; and organizational interrelatedness. According to Hagberg and Heifetz (1998), organizational culture is the human dimension of an organization. It is not the values list developed by the top administration and framed in the lobby of the institution. What the organization strives for and values may actually be different from the values, beliefs, and norms expressed in its behavior and practice. Organizational culture comprises broadly shared, deeply held values of the organization (Rowland & Rowland, 1997). This includes values that persist over time even when group members change (Sorrel-Jones, 1999).

The organizational or corporate culture drives the organization and its actions (Hagberg & Heifetz, 1998). It is the "operating system" that guides how employees think, feel, talk, and act. It is the special competencies that group members display and that are passed on from generation to generation (e.g., emotional and aesthetic responses, behavior patterns).

Subcultures in the Organization

Most organizations have a dominant culture that is pervasive throughout—across units, departments, and even regions in the case of multiorganization alliances (Hagberg & Heifetz, 1998). This is known as *cultural integration*. Many successful companies have strived for this (e.g., IBM, Procter & Gamble). However, organizations can and do vary widely in their degree of cultural integration. Subcultures coexist; they may share characteristics and norms of the dominant culture or may be quite different (Hagberg & Heifetz, 1998). They can be cooperative or in conflict. They may differ by department (laboratory versus marketing), occupation (physician versus nurse), level of hierarchy (management versus staff), or regional site (e.g., multicampus hospitals) (Hagberg & Heifetz, 1998).

One characteristic of cultures is that they encourage *ethnocentrism*, or dominance of one culture. This can be problematic—people who endorse one set of values or ideas may distrust, dislike, and fear those with ideas different from their own (Trice & Beyer, 1993). The stronger the ideas and values, the more intolerant toward those with other ideas and values. This interferes with coordination and cooperation in teams, units, and entire organizations. To understand the dynamics of a culture's growth and change, one must first examine what happens in any group or organization as it grows and develops. As groups mature they develop subgroups that share their own cultures; from the point of view of a larger organization, these are subcultures (Schein, 1992).

Assessment of Organizational Culture

Cultural assessment can provide measurable data about real organizational values and norms (Hagberg & Heifetz, 1998). It can demonstrate the disparity between the lists of ideal values in the lobby and the real organizational culture.

Fisher (1996) identifies core dimensions of an organization's culture as: (1) clarity of direction (formality of planning systems), (2) decision-making (where decision-making occurs and the extent of information available to facilitate decisions), (3) integration (coordination, cooperation, and communication among the organization's units),

(4) management style (ethics and patterns of support), (5) ambience (distinct atmosphere), (6) performance orientation (level of accountability), (7) vitality (responsiveness to change), (8) management compensation (internally equitable, externally competitive, and tied to performance), (9) management and staff development (opportunities), (10) identity (internal and external image), (11) quality of care (focus on quality and resources), and (12) rituals (weekly management meetings and who sits in which chair).

There are many instruments for assessment of organizational culture. (One example is provided in Box 36-1.) The culture of educational institutions can be assessed by examining the values, attitudes, and behaviors of the institution evident in the following categories: structure, mission/governance, cultural representativeness, faculty and students, curriculum/instruction, resources, and ethical practices. Box 36-2 shows questions that are useful to assessing the organizational culture of a nursing program. An organization can be identified as functional or dysfunctional. Table 36-1 includes some organizational aspects for functional and dysfunctional cultures (Fisher, 1996).

Two important areas of culture in an organization are its sacred cows and its taboos. Sacred cows are revered rules in an organization and represent the minimum standard of conduct (Fisher, 1996). The rules are usually unwritten, yet everyone knows and respects them. A sacred cow at a major medical center might be requiring senior management to belong to a professional organization. An expectation of promptness or a certain dress code might be an organizational sacred cow. In some organizations, devotion to an attitude that "the needy are our priority" is a kind of sacred cow.

Taboos, expectations of how employees must not behave, are revered also. Fisher (1996) identifies these common organizational taboos: (1) physicians are the most important employees, and as such, should never be antagonized; (2) the chain of command must always be followed; (3) unions are not welcome; (4) inconsistencies of values and actions are not discussed; and (5) conflict should be avoided.

In actuality, what management values, rewards, and gives time and attention to is often the strongest indicator of an organization's culture (Hagberg & Heifetz, 1998). For example, does management encourage risk-taking? Does it challenge old ways of doing things? Does it punish those who challenge established norms? Do mavericks fit into the organization? Is rapid change the norm? Does the organization value excellence? Does management value employees as individuals, or is the focus entirely on profit or task performance? Do managers make most decisions, or is there participatory governance in the organization? Interestingly, outsiders or new employees can "see" an organization's culture better than people who "grew up in it" and can more easily answer these questions (Hagberg & Heifetz, 1998).

Box 36-1

Assessing the Organizational Culture

How does the organization view the physical environment?
1. Is the environment attractive?
2. Does it appear that there is adequate maintenance?
3. Are nursing stations crowded or noisy?
4. Is there an appropriate-sized lobby? Are there quiet areas?
5. Is there sufficient seating for families in the dining room?
6. Are there enough conference rooms?

What is the organization's social environment?
1. Are many friendships maintained beyond the workplace?
2. Is there an annual picnic or holiday party that is well attended by the employees?
3. Do employees seem to generally like each other?
4. Do all shifts and all departments get along fairly well?
5. Are certain departments disliked or resented?
6. Are employees on a first-name basis with coworkers, doctors, charge nurses, and supervisors?

How supportive is the organization?
1. Is educational reimbursement available?
2. Are good low-cost meals available to employees?
3. Are there adequate employee lounges?
4. Are funds available to send employees to workshops?
5. Are employees recognized for extra effort?
6. Does the organization help pay for the holiday party or other social functions?

What is the organizational power structure?
1. Who holds the most power in the organization?
2. Which departments are viewed as powerful? Which are viewed as powerless?
3. Who gets free meals? Who gets special parking places?
4. Who carries beepers? Who wears lab coats? Who has overhead pages?
5. Who has the biggest office?
6. Who is never called by his or her first name?

How does the organization view safety?
1. Is there a well-lighted parking place for employees arriving or departing after dark?
2. Is there an active and involved safety committee?
3. Are security guards needed?

What is the communications environment?
1. Is upward communication usually written or verbal?
2. Is there much informal communication?
3. Is there an active grapevine? Is it reliable?
4. Where is important information exchanged (e.g., the parking lot, the doctors' surgical dressing room, the nurses' station, the coffee shop, in surgery, the delivery room?)

What are the organizational taboos and sacred cows?
1. Are there special rules and policies that can never be broken?
2. Are certain subjects or ideas forbidden?
3. Are there relationships that cannot be threatened?

The *culture audit*, conducted by a task force of employees and managers (possibly with the assistance of an outside firm or consultant), is a critical tool for cultural transformation in health care organizations (Wilkoff & Ziegenfuss, 1995). Box 36-3 shows the five phases of a culture audit.

Creating Organizational Culture

New alliances, departments, and units are opportunities for creating new cultures. The nurse executive is a primary force in creating a new culture that reflects the changing health care environment (Rowland & Rowland, 1997). The nurse executive role-models a positive attitude, openly communicates, and has a clear view of the organization's or department's mission. The executive communicates expectations, values, and direction for the nursing department in accord with the overall institutional goals and vision.

The leader does not micromanage; this conveys the message that a decision has been imposed "from the top" (Bruhn, 1996). Some of the mechanisms that leaders use to communicate their beliefs, values, and assumptions are conscious, deliberate actions. Other mechanisms may be unintended (e.g., in those cases where culture may become a defense mechanism against anxieties unleashed by inconsistent leader behavior).

Mentoring the manager at the next lower level promotes a positive culture (Rowland & Rowland, 1997). This behavior cascades down to the staff level and helps staff feel valued and empowered. Empowered staff members are vital in creating a team. One means of changing the culture and promoting diversity is the empowerment of staff who have good interpersonal skills (Bruhn, 1996).

Leader characteristics and eccentricities will also be reflected in others. A chief nursing officer who avoids conflict will see that this behavior shapes the behaviors of others (Hagberg & Heifetz, 1998). What the leader espouses, values, rewards, and punishes will serve as the model for others. When an organization faces a crisis, the manner in which leaders and others deal with it creates new norms, values, and working procedures. So much of an organization's culture is tied up with hierarchy, authority, power, and influence that the mechanisms of conflict resolution have to be constantly worked out and consensually validated. No better opportunity exists for leaders to send signals about their own assumptions about human

Box 36-2

Assessing Organizational Culture in Nursing Programs

Institutional Structure

1. What type of institution is the university? Public or private? Secular or nonsecular?
2. What is the organizational structure of the university? Of the nursing program?

Mission and Governance

1. What values are evident in the university's mission/philosophy?
2. Does the mission/philosophy of the university support multiculturalism?
3. Is the mission/philosophy of the nursing unit consistent with that of the university?
4. What evidence exists that the mission/philosophy of the nursing unit guides policies, procedures, and practices?
5. What evidence exists that the administration supports the nursing unit?
6. In what way do faculty and students participate in institutional governance? Is there a student nursing organization? A chapter of Sigma Theta Tau, International? A faculty senate? A chapter of the American Association of University Professors?

Cultural Representativness

1. What is the cultural mix of students in the university? In the nursing unit? By program (e.g., baccalaureate, MSN)?
2. What percentage of the full-time faculty represents culturally diverse backgrounds?
3. What percentage of those in administrative positions represents culturally diverse backgrounds?
4. Does the cultural mix at the university (e.g., students, faculty, staff, administrators) represent the cultural mix of the surrounding community?

Faculty

1. Are the numbers of qualified faculty adequate for reasonable classroom enrollments, safe and state-mandated faculty-student clinical ratios, and a reasonable faculty workload?
2. Are faculty qualified by educational or experiential backgrounds?
3. Is there a system for faculty development?
4. Are nursing faculty treated equitably in comparison to faculty in other disciplines?
5. What evidence is there that the following faculty performance factors are valued?
   - Scholarship
   - Research
   - Publication
   - Service
   - Student advisement
   - Clinical practice
6. Is affirmative action and/or nondiscrimination evident with respect to recruitment, employment, salary, and performance evaluation?

Students

1. What support services are evident for students?
   - Health/wellness
   - Counseling
   - English as second language
   - Academic tutoring and mentoring
   - Special needs
   - Financial aid
   - Orientation programs
   - International and cultural needs
2. Are student-specific policies fair, nondiscriminatory, and equitable on campus in terms of selection, admission, grading, progression, and graduation?
3. What programs are in place to maximize nursing student retention?

Curriculum/Instruction

1. What evidence exists that the baccalaureate program properly prepares a nursing generalist? That the MSN program properly prepares nursing specialists in the majors or program options?
2. Do the programs meet national standards and state board requirements? Are they accredited?
3. What evidence exists that the programs prepare graduates for appropriate roles in contemporary health care settings?
4. To what extent are cultural diversity content and clinical learning opportunities integrated in the curriculum?
5. What instructional methods predominate in the programs?
6. What evidence exists that the programs are appropriate in length, scope, and depth to prepare the specified professional? What evidence exists that there is a clear difference in levels (e.g., baccalaureate degree, MSN degree)?
7. How are the following factors included in the program?
   - Technology
   - Service learning
   - International exchanges
   - Flexible scheduling options
   - Distance learning

Resources

1. Are fiscal resources equitably distributed so that the nursing unit receives its fair share?
2. Is there financial support of cultural diversity programs?
3. Are instructional resources, including library holdings, appropriate to meet the program goals?
4. Is the environment safe and conducive to academic achievement and a positive educational experience?

Ethical Practices

1. Are individuals treated fairly and with regard for their inherent worth and dignity?
2. Is human diversity merely managed, or is it celebrated?

Courtesy of Cheryl Pope Kish.

Table 36-1

Comparison of Functional and Dysfunctional Organizational Cultures

ISSUE	FUNCTIONAL CULTURE	DYSFUNCTIONAL CULTURE
Service	Patient focused	Provider focused
Standards	Clear	Not clear
Decision-making	Participative	Top down
Outcomes	Frequently measured	Not measured
Education	Ongoing	Not valued
Teamwork	Team culture	Turf wars
	Cooperative departments	Competitive
Conflict	Open and dealt with	Hidden

From Fisher, M.L. (1996). *Quick reference to redesigning the nursing organization.* Cincinnati, OH: Delmar (a division of Thomson Learning; fax [800] 730-2215).

Box 36-3

Five Phases of the Organizational Culture Audit

1. Needs awareness
   - Recognize need (e.g., organization facing major change, managed care).
   - Develop audit objectives.
2. Diagnosis
   - Select data-gathering methods.
   - Carry out data collection and analysis.
   - Develop a model of culture and get feedback on the model.
3. Planning
   - Determine if the culture enhances or impedes needed changes for health care reform and the competitive environment.
4. Action
   - Note if the culture moves toward the future.
   - Note if the culture affects all systems (e.g., technology, structure, reward, decision-making, budget, management).
5. Evaluation
   - Assess the effect of the culture on performance.
   - Use the original diagnosis as a baseline.

Data from Wilkoff, M., & Ziegenfuss Jr., J.T. (1995, May). Culture audits: a tool for change. *Health Progress,* 34-38.

nature and relationships than when they themselves are challenged. For example, a leader may criticize a subordinate during a presentation. Then, after realizing a mistake was made about a culturally sensitive issue, the leader apologizes, but the damage is done. Leaders do well to role-model their communication skills and their control of what they say, because words have implied and explicit consequences regarding assumptions based on culture and subcultures.

Personal cultures can arise in an organization. They come from ethnicity, race, religion, socioeconomic status, position, or occupation (Fisher, 1996). When these cultural contexts conflict with organizational norms, problems appear. One way to protect an organization from these conflicts is promotion of a caring environment (Fisher, 1996). This caring is individualized rather than generalized; patients are treated as individuals rather than "cases," and employees are valued and perceive that they are valued.

Changing Organizational Culture

Many management theorists believe that one cannot create or change a culture (Trice & Beyer, 1993). Others believe one can deliberately change it, but only a little and only with great difficulty. Still others believe that corporate cultures can be readily manipulated like any other management task. However, the culture of an organization is steeped in its history (Hughes, 1990). Strong organizational cultures are formed when there is a long, definable history. For example, one Jewish hospital, whose roots began in the late nineteenth century, developed when Jewish physicians were not given practice privileges at other local hospitals. Over time, the situation changed, but this history continues to dictate certain attitudes and expectations. Complex social understandings develop over time into cultural norms and values. One may note, for example, that promotions in a strong culture go only to "insiders," which perpetuates the organizational culture (Hughes, 1990).

Rowland and Rowland (1997) describe the following plan for change of organizational culture. To plan change requires that one first identify both positive and negative perceptions operating within the culture of the institution. Second, organizational structure is assessed and the organizational chart examined to determine the way in which the structure facilitates or hinders goal achievement. One should assess the flow of information and determine how to make it better. A third issue is consideration of the climate of the organization. An assessment of the way in which management rewards and reinforces behavior can be helpful. For example, what symbolic behaviors are punished? What behaviors get attention? Which behaviors do not get attention? It can be helpful to look for evidence of "mixed messages," resulting in confusion for employees, and determine which strategies need clarification. Finally, any barriers that create a sense of "us versus them" and interfere with smooth relationships should be identified.

Fisher (1996) emphasizes other aspects of successful change in organizational culture, starting with an examination of the clarity of its purposes, goals, and tasks. Is cultural diversity in the mission statement? Is there unity among leaders of the organization? Are those affected by change involved in the plans for change? Is there participatory governance? Is a win-win approach in place? Are both short-term and long-term goals set for the organization, and is their emphasis on sustainable cultural changes? Clearly, once these data are available, strategies begin to remedy any problems so that cultural changes in the organization may go forward.

A strong commitment from the leadership needs to be present for organizational change or redesign to occur. Communication of new values needs to reach every unit, and everyone needs to be committed to the values and to the changes (Sovie, 1993). Whenever organizations make a major change, some employees see the change as chaotic. However, this chaos can free a person from past constraints; chaos opens the organization to the possibility of a new culture.

The authors of *Reengineering the Corporation*, Michael Hammer and James Champy, estimate that over half of the radical changes they advocate "fade into oblivion" (Stewart, 1994). One reengineering consultant states that "people and culture—the human systems of a company—are what makes or breaks any change initiative" (Stewart, 1994). The most often cited barriers to change are employee resistance and dysfunctional corporate culture. For example, shared values and behaviors can be at odds (e.g., celebrating star performers when teamwork is the expressed value).

As an organization matures, it becomes more bureaucratic. The more the structure, procedures, rituals, and espoused values work in making the organization successful, the more they become the criteria for selection of new leaders. As a result, "The likelihood of new leaders becoming cultural change agents declines as the organization matures" (Schein, 1992).

Communication networks are imperative for planning change and redesign (Fisher, 1996). Knowledge of the timing of change and inclusion of those involved supports change. Other factors that are helpful to ensure success in change and redesign include the following (Fisher, 1996):

- Make new assumptions explicit (e.g., perform bedside rounds that include the family).
- Change the physical environment (e.g., eliminate registered nurse [RN] stations for bedside charting).
- Challenge sacred cows (e.g., eliminate routine vital signs every 4 hours).
- Change the structure to facilitate new goals (e.g., give the nursing council the same authority as the medical council).
- Target rewards to the new goals (e.g., pay staff bonuses for performance using the new standards of quality).
- Eliminate barriers that block goals (e.g., institute crossdiscipline committees).
- Coach for success (e.g., identify necessary skills and attitudes, target education with an outcome focus, and value education).

Reorganization or redesign can mean hiring many new employees. Regardless of why new employees are needed, it is critical that new hires fit the new culture (Hagberg & Heifetz, 1998). They need to be receptive to diversification. It is possible to make hiring decisions based on compatibility of a candidate's personality, values, and behaviors and the current and desired culture. A goal of the hiring practices should be to support an increasing workforce diversity that resembles the community (Veninga, 1994).

Creating an Organizational Climate for Multiculturalism

The goal of modern society is to keep abreast of change, anticipate and plan for change, and keep inequities of all kinds minimized so that citizens may fully participate in the society in which they live and work (Bruhn, 1996). The workplace should be a model for achieving goals of representativeness, parity, and multiculturalism (Bruhn, 1996), and diversity is the first step in the process of achieving multiculturalism in organizations. Organizations are changing and becoming more heterogeneous, and they are currently engaged in first-generation efforts to manage diversity—they have mandates to diversify and rely on numbers to justify attempts to do so (Bruhn, 1996).

Second-generation efforts are beyond numerical goals. Their goal is retention of high-performance employees with diverse characteristics. A third-generation multicultural organization capitalizes on the advantages of diversity. "An organization cannot be considered multicultural if it only tolerates diversity" (Bruhn, 1996). Organizations must value diversity, promote it, and proactively manage differences to minimize conflict and maximize advantages.

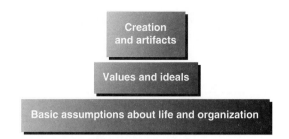

Figure 36-1 The 3-Tiered Model of organizational culture. (Data from Rowland, H.S., & Rowland, B.L. [1997]. *Nursing administration handbook.* [4th ed]. Gaithersburg, MD: Aspen Publishers.)

Organizational Culture Models

All organizations are unique, just as each individual within them is unique. However, there are various ways to assess or analyze organizations. Several models are presented here.

3-Tiered Model

In the 3-Tiered Model, basic assumptions about life (in general) and the organization (in particular) serve as the bottom or foundational tier and include assumptions about human nature, human relationships, the environment, reality, and time (Figure 36-1). The second level, values and ideals, includes nonobservable, reportable attitudes about helping others and the importance of employee growth and development. The upper tier, creations and artifacts, includes what Hagberg & Heifetz (1998) address as the visible expressions of the culture—the policies, rituals, and practices, like work schedules and work conditions, symbols and ceremonies, jargon, work attire, technologies, work processes, architecture and décor, and slogans.

Typology Model

Management researchers Trice and Beyer (1993) have advanced various typologies of organizational cultures. There is, however, little consensus about how to categorize them. (The Trice and Beyer Typology Model is shown in Table 36-2.)

Vestal, Fralicx, and Spreier (1997) describe four models: (1) functional culture, or steady, dependable individual accomplishment that helps employees work up the corporate ladder; (2) process culture, or team culture with a focus on customer satisfaction; (3) time-based culture, or culture evolved from the need for speed in marketing changes, which requires employees who are confident self-starters and flexible; and (4) network culture, or the creation of strategic alliances to achieve goals; employees in this culture need to be highly skilled facilitators with strength in negotiation.

Model for Guiding Organizational Change for Multiculturalism

Bruhn (1996) has synthesized Cox's ideas (1993) and created a stepwise process toward the goal of a multicultural organization (Figure 36-2). The chief executive officer (CEO) or president establishes the climate for diversity (Bruhn, 1996), and management's top ranks need to be committed. The CEO attends the diversity training courses. Goals are developed with measurable outcomes (e.g., zero age-discrimination grievances). Employees should be rewarded for practicing diversity principles and "not punished for failing to follow them" (Bruhn, 1996).

The underlying premise for managing diversity is understanding, not denying, differences among employees. Differences are valued and dealt with openly and constructively. Sameness fosters resistance to change. Training sessions should involve those from successful diversity programs. Employees need to learn what constitutes prejudice, sexism, and racism. According to Bruhn (1996), employees need to learn group dynamics, conflict resolution, and prevention of grievances.

There are many more models identified in the management literature. These include Process, Tough-Guy-Macho, Work Hard–Play Hard, Sensation-Thinking, Intuition-Thinking, Intuition-Feeling, Sensation-Feeling, Apathetic, Caring, Exacting, Integrative, Paranoid, Avoidant, Charismatic, Bureaucratic, and Schizoid. Cultural models that focus on individuals, not organizations, may also be utilized.

Organizational Culture Research

A history of organizational culture research begins in the 1930s with the Hawthorne studies at the Western Electric Company in Chicago (Trice & Beyer, 1993). A Harvard Business School faculty member and an Anthropology Department faculty member collaborated on research examining social structure, friendships, cliques, and formal prescribed relationships among employees. They examined ideological relations, the workers' culture, and shared beliefs and understandings of the organization.

For the next 40 years, similar studies were conducted, although no consistent theory emerged. Much of the work involved quantitative surveys, a technique developed to measure employee morale. Organizational sociologists became less interested in groups and more interested in formal structure. The computer revolution that enabled handling large volumes of data diminished the qualitative work that was being done—descriptions and interpretations of cultural forms, such as myths and rites in the workplace (Trice & Beyer, 1993).

In the 1980s, organizational culture became a management fad (Trice & Beyer, 1993). Peters and Waterman's *In Search of Excellence* (1982) and Ouchi's *Theory Z* (1981) garnered much attention. Major conferences began to

Table 36-2

Trice and Beyer Typology Model

TYPE A	TYPE J	TYPE Z
Hierarchical control	Clan control	Clan control
High specialization	Low specialization	Moderate specialization
Short-term employment	Lifetime employment	Long-term employment
Individual responsibility	Collective responsibility	Individual responsibility
Individual decision-making	Collective decision-making	Consensus decision-making

From Trice, H.M.T., & Beyer, J.M.B. (1993). *The culture of work organizations.* Englewood Cliffs, NJ: Prentice-Hall.

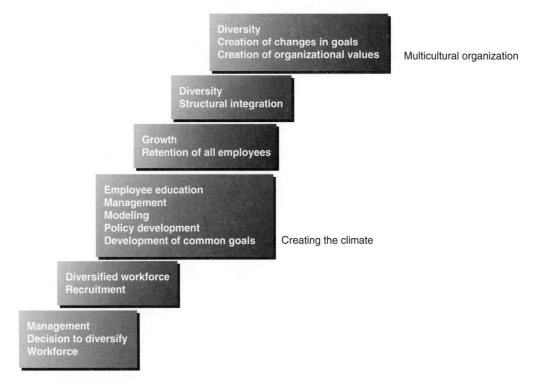

Figure 36-2 Stepwise process towards a multicultural organization. (Data from Bruhn, J.G. [1996]. Creating an organizational climate for multiculturalism. *Health Care Supervisor, 4*[4], 11-18.)

focus on corporate culture, and organizational folklore and symbolism brought managers and scholars together. To understand group culture, Kotter and Heskett (1992) studied strong and weak corporate cultures and found that those strong cultures that were able to adapt to their changing environments had a set of care beliefs about the importance of people.

Future Organizational Cultures

The time from the 1960s to the early 1990s had a number of underlying assumptions that defined organizational culture (Wilkoff & Ziegenfuss, 1995). Hospitals competed independently. New technology was automatically acquired. Physicians' practices were autonomous, and spe-

cialists were king. Nurses were in chronic short supply, and patients would come to health care settings for their care.

Now the picture of organizational culture includes Internet meetings, office furniture on wheels, and smiling employees. According to some literature (Caudron, 1998), the vocabulary is new: *cool* is *ku, clutch,* or *tasty* (meaning the same as *far out* and *groovy* used to). Companies are interested in being cool places to work, and cool is no longer just appropriate for the entertainment or high-tech industries. Cool is a culture and a subject of research (Caudron, 1998). It refers to out-of-the-box, nontraditional thinking and to corporate America. In an effort to be cool, progressive companies have implemented flexible schedules, onsite day care, and processes that enable employees to express opinions.

Cultivating cool is an art more than a science (Caudron, 1998). The dimensions needed to become *kew-el* include respect for balance between one's work and one's life; a sense of purpose; diversity, which is increasingly important; integrity; participatory management; and a learning environment. Young employees want to have a life outside the office. Blurring the lines between work and life can be accomplished through flexible work schedules, including part-time and job-sharing options; telecommuting and sabbaticals; and onsite day care. For example, Brian, 31 years old and involved in a special project over many months, learned that the administrators were planning to send the project team to a professional ballgame and dinner as a reward for their overtime and hard work. Brian went privately and asked the supervisor to consider a half-day off instead. "Look around, most of these guys are married with young children. They've seen little of their families lately because of the overtime. Even though they like each other and enjoy social activities together, they would probably rather go home and do something with their kids than go to a game." The next day, at noon, the supervisor came to the group, thanked them for a job well done thus far, and sent them home with this expectation, "Go spend some time with your families." This, reported Brian and his colleagues, was the "ultimate example of cool."

A coauthor of the *Fortune 100* list of best companies to work for states, "Cool companies are those in which employees feel connected to the product, to the corporate mission, or to the overall vision of the industry" (Caudron, 1998). Employees are energized by making a contribution. Merck, the pharmaceutical company, has created a devoted workforce by "putting patients before profits." Employees are proud of their low-cost medication for acquired immune deficiency syndrome (AIDS) and their company's donation of medication to developing countries.

Being part of the real world and not just a politically correct world is important to employees (Caudron, 1998). Employees feel safe expressing differences, whether those are related to gender, sexual orientation, or opinion. Allstate Insurance Company has received national recognition for its provision of opportunities for women, Hispanics, and disabled people. According to Caudron, (1998), integrity is a new "turn on" for employees who are tired of checking their value systems at the front door. Companies are working more toward high ethical standards.

Participatory management approaches recognize that employees on the front lines (e.g., staff nurses) may have the best ideas. It is not productive to tell front-line employees how to do their jobs. One research company searched for the "coolest" company (Caudron, 1998) and found it to have no established hierarchy and no secretaries. Also, cool companies promote lifelong learning. Human resource departments provide opportunities for growth for all employees.

Community Links

More and more, health care organizations are forming partnerships with local and regional communities (Hunt, 1994). The community provides patients and is a labor resource. Educational partnerships can be formed with local universities and health care organizations. This helps in development of educational programs for aides, orderlies, and other lower-wage semiprofessionals to earn degrees.

Executives who know their community can alter services to better meet community needs (Hunt, 1994). For example, new immigrants have a difficult time negotiating the health care system bureaucracy, but creative problem-solving can construct services that provide a solution to such community needs. The local culture inevitably shapes the geographical subculture as well. One finds a different blend of assumptions in each geographical area, reflecting not only the local national culture but also the business conditions and customer requirements of the local bureaucracy. Building an effective organization is ultimately a matter of meshing the different subcultures through a common language and common procedures for solving problems (Schein, 1992).

Workplace Violence

Regrettably, violence in the workplace has become a part of the organizational culture for health care settings; more than a million U.S. workers are assaulted in the workplace every year—40,000 assaults per week. In the 1990s, this problem has increased by 300%, and the epidemic nature of the problem has been attributable to declining relationships between labor and management, lack of timely and effective support in stressful situations, inadequacy of pre-employment screening to identify violence potential, shortages of staff, and the ease of obtaining guns (Speer, 1997). Some speculate that depersonalization of the current health care environment exacerbates the problem. Workplace violence costs the industry billions of dollars annually.

Workplace violence has become so common, especially in emergency departments and psychiatric settings, that many nurses tolerate or even ignore it, leaving it unreported and considering it a part of a patient's symptomatology or a family member's reactions to stress and therefore part of the job of nursing. Examples include the man who pushes the advanced practice nurse (APN) to the floor when he learns she thinks he has been abusing his wife and children, the woman with delirium tremens (DTs) who injures a staff member while trying to rid her clothing of "bugs," and the gun-toting gang members who descend on the emergency department after a knife fight sends other members there by ambulance. These are all people encountered in the daily practice of APNs.

Workplace violence, though, is not limited to those clinical settings; it can occur anywhere there are troubled patients and families under stress. For example, at Redbud

Primary Care Center, Mr. Warren, worried that he has cancer, became upset when a patient who he thinks arrived after him is seen first. He lashes out at the other man, and when the APN attempts to calm him down, he pushes her to the floor, causing her to break her glasses and cut her face. Across town, Mr. Edwards grabs the shirt of an insurance clerk and threatens her because he is upset about a clinic bill. Mrs. Johannson, who has dementia, scratches the CNS who is caring for her; and Mrs. Cowen, a laboring patient with a history of crack cocaine use, kicks the certified nurse midwife (CNM). While these incidences of assault are serious and of concern, the Occupational Safety and Health Administration (OSHA, 2000) notes that as many as 1000 workers across this country are murdered in the workplace every year.

There should be a zero tolerance policy for workplace violence. All staff members need to be educated to recognize volatile situations and know how to respond to de-escalate the volatile situation in order to safeguard patients and others, as well as themselves. An escalating situation can often be defused with therapeutic listening and open-ended communication that invites the patient or family to express their frustrations, fears, anger, or other emotions to a provider who remains calm and does not respond with anger, argumentative remarks, or defensiveness. Acknowledging the genuine emotions being expressed can be valuable (Rakoczy, 2000b). For example, in the Redbud clinic example, the APN or another staff member might say to Mr. Warren, "You seem upset that the other gentleman got called back before you. I know you have been waiting a long time. That's hard when you're sick or feeling worried. Let me see how long it will be until we can get you back to see the nurse practitioner."

In situations where the patient or family has a known history of violent behavior, an increased, highly visible security presence can be helpful. Many clinics have a code word that means "call for help!" Generally, a staff member should not attempt to restrain a combative individual without help. Most training for medical settings recommends an entire team for hands-on management of this kind of patient or family member. The least restrictive method to ensure the safety of all concerned should be the objective of the health care team (Katz, 2000).

All threats of violence, even those that appear to be made in jest, should be taken seriously. There are red flags and cues that a person is becoming volatile: intoxication, swearing, a demanding tone, profanity, hand wringing, fist clenching, striking objects, and especially pacing. In addition to trying to defuse the situation, a caregiver should send for help and then manage the situation calmly in accord with the agency's policy and procedures. Careful documentation of the incident is important for tracking outcomes and justifying costs for treating injuries sustained, as well as for meeting OSHA requirements (Rakczoy, 2000b; Speer, 1997).

Katz (2000), a psychotherapist turned expert on prevention of workplace violence, reminds nurses that denial and minimization of the risk of workplace violence is irrational and dangerous. Nurses should be proactive, taking advantage of training and becoming familiar with policy and preventive procedures. They can also have important role in an assessment of site security (Box 36-4).

"Every organization has its own unique history and culture, its own successes and internal challenges, and its own ways of dealing (or not dealing) with stress" (Katz, 2000). The ideal response by the organization to the threat of workplace violence is a proactive program that includes: (1) site analysis for hazards in the environment that can be

---

Box 36-4

Redbud Primary Care Center Violence Prevention/Security Assessment Checklist

Potential Weapons
Are sharp items (e.g., needles, scissors, scalpels) safely stored?

Is the staff kitchen area locked when not in use?

Hazardous Substances
Are hazardous substances that might be used to inflict harm secured?

Are drugs secured?

Are staff belongings stored in lockers, desks, or storage cabinets?

Clinic Entry
Are doors and windows to the outside in good condition?

Are doors and windows to the outside locked properly?

Is the alarm system functional? Do staff members remember to set the alarm as they leave for the day?

Is lighting to and from the clinic and in the parking areas adequate? Are broken bulbs or dim lighting reported?

Emergency Notification
Is the security alarm (help button) working properly?

Is the security telephone number prominently displayed near all telephones?

Does the staff know the emergency code for an escalating situation?

Prevention/Management Procedure
Do all staff members know the procedure for defusing a situation where a threat of violence exists?

Is the prevention and management policy written down and accessible to all staff?

Do staff members participate in training related to violence in the workplace?

eliminated and safety precautions, including emergency notification systems, that can be added; (2) provision of training on prevention and response to violent situations, updated annually, to all employees; (3) management support during episodes of potential or actual violence and afterward to deal with posttraumatic stress; (4) education and support of a response team; and (5) motivation of employees.

Organizational training may be done internally (by inservice educators) or by outside agencies who specialize in violence prevention in the workplace. OSHA's *Guidelines for Preventing Workplace Violence for Healthcare and Social Service Workers* (2000), available at their website (www.osha.gov), are often used as a framework for training. This document includes appendices containing a workplace violence checklist useful for site analysis and assessment, as well as forms for documentation. There is also an extensive reference list. Katz (2000) suggests that training include the following components: a prevention policy and prevention behaviors; risk factors; profiles of perpetrators; appropriate responses; diffusion of difficult situations; diversity training; and record keeping.

IMPLICATIONS FOR MSN EDUCATION AND ADVANCED PRACTICE

Knowledge of organizational culture can be invaluable in assessing the prospective employment site before accepting a position. Some APNs have opportunities to work in a prospective practice site as part of their clinical learning in graduate school. Others may be able to negotiate several days of unpaid observations in a practice setting before accepting employment. These kinds of opportunities can be used to assess the cultural context of the organization. The nature of patient care can not be used as the solitary reason for selecting one agency over another for employment; often it is the climate or culture of the organization that serves as a "make or break" experience. An appropriate learning assignment for APN students would be a cultural assessment of a selected clinical site. This written account would not only serve student learning, it would provide faculty with an additional objective view of the environment as a learning resource for the future. It would be very helpful, for example, to know in advance that there is low staff participation in decision-making or that a "them versus us" attitude is the norm; it would also be useful to learn of any myths or stories that show evidence of caring—not only for patients but for staff.

Fansano (2000) lists five key management skills for the twenty-first century: (1) think like an owner, (2) think creatively and independently, (3) be flexible, (4) be willing to take risks (not with patient care), and (5) create a vision

and develop a plan to achieve it. These are certainly reasonable expectations of an APN in a management position. With those expectations in mind, APN educators should ensure that students are prepared accordingly. Organizational loyalty is a characteristic that cannot be discounted; APNs should be helped to appreciate its importance to the corporate culture. Furthermore, they need to understand the ethic of either striving to change settings to which they feel no loyalty or leaving those settings for a more congruent workplace.

New managers can use knowledge of organizational culture to contrast their division's subculture with the corporate culture to look for consonance and to make necessary changes when an assessment indicates that problems exist. Even experienced managers need to know how to conduct cultural assessment on their organizations at times of reorganization, when the culture is no longer apparent. Assessment data provides an impetus for APNs to make proactive decisions.

Clearly, as practice sites of the future become more diverse, APNs will need to understand the dynamics of organizational culture so that policies, procedures, and practices that embrace diversity can be employed. Different cultures perceive different factors as "cool" in an employment setting. Sensitivity to these factors and a willingness to ask questions to determine what colleagues or employees of a different cultural group want from a job or in a job environment can be valuable to decision-making.

Boss (2000) introduces cyberspace as a new culture and notes its ability to make heterogeneous individuals into a homogeneous group, with news groups serving as the "new century water cooler." "Cyberspace is a community a lot like the world—huge and messy, with some delightful places and some streets you don't want to walk down." Boss describes the language and unique problems of cyberspace as a culture and addresses what it can mean to education and a sense of membership in a global village. All higher education, including preparation of APNs, needs to integrate student use of cyberspace into their curricula and make sure that students understand this culture and how to interact appropriately within it. For example, course syllabi might include lists of website addresses related to topics under discussion in the course. For the educators themselves, the website www.cob.ohio-state.edu provides information on teaching diversity. Net etiquette should be an expectation of those communicating through cyberspace; graduate students new to the e-mail medium may need a review of Internet etiquette—called "Netiquette" by Virginia Shea (1994).

APNs must be educated to recognize red flags of violence potential and understand measures for prevention of workplace violence. They should be aware of OSHA requirements and know how to diffuse escalating situations to protect themselves and others, including the aggressor. Educators might use case scenarios to introduce students to the issue of workplace violence and have students analyze the situation using guidelines for prevention and management from the literature or from OSHA. Clearly, students need to recognize that workplace violence is not limited to patients who arrive accompanied by police, in handcuffs, or under the influence of alcohol and drugs; violent episodes may occur in response to any crisis situation.

PRIORITIES FOR RESEARCH

Most of the research related to organizational culture in health care settings focuses on hospital environments. Nursing staff culture is only generally considered, with little attention paid to particular nurse populations, such as hospital-based CNSs, certified registered nurse anesthetists (CRNAs), CNMs, and nurse practitioners (NPs). Do those groups perceive the organizational culture differently? Are they affected differently by the culture? For example, what effect does the corporate culture have on recruitment and retention of these groups of nurses? Are they represented on relevant committees? To what extent do they participate in decision-making? Do the same behavioral norms apply to them? Is their clinical expertise valued?

As APNs enter more primary care practice roles, the organizational context of the primary care clinic should be studied. Existing organizational assessment tools might be used to that end, or empirical study might determine that these tools are lacking in appropriateness for a nonhospital site. Instruments from business or management disciplines might serve more credibly in assessing primary care sites. This assessment would include workplace violence prevention, education, and management.

It is evident that leadership plays a prominent role in determining the cultural context of an organization. In primary care settings, APNs are not always the acknowledged leaders; physicians often are. The leadership dimension of the corporate culture deserves study. An ethnographical approach might be used with APNs in those sites where they are considered a subculture.

The cultural context of the higher education enterprise in nursing would also provide for interesting and instructive research. One might use the existing cultural assessment instruments to examine a particular Master's program or use Fisher's (1996) suggestions for determining whether the program has a functional or dysfunctional corporate environment. Higher education is gearing for a severe nursing faculty shortage in the near future. There is an acknowledged "graying of the professorate," as well as limited numbers of graduate students entering programs to become nursing faculty. Knowing the culture of a particular university might provide direction to the administration about how to design systems to recruit and retain qualified faculty. Learning what is not compelling about the nurse faculty role might lead to ways to make this aspect of nursing a more attractive option.

Evaluation research before, during, and after a major reorganization continues to be a legitimate area of research. As both change and resistance to change are inevitable, studies of processes and systems that might effect change positively would be of value to advanced practice.

Attridge (1995) refers to relationships as the glue that holds an organization together. Although there has been limited study of relationships between APNs and collaborating physicians, there has been little to no research about relationships among APNs and between them and nursing and other staff. This is a particularly provocative area of research because many novice APNs believe that the nursing staff in a practice determines in great measure how an APN is perceived by patients and other providers and staff.

DISCUSSION QUESTIONS

These questions can be used to promote critical thinking and encourage discussion.

1. Use the Hagberg and Heifetz (1998) questions listed here to structure a description of your workplace (organization) that will be shared in a small group setting.

   - What 10 words describe your organization?
   - What is really important around your organization?
   - Who gets promoted?
   - What behaviors get rewarded?
   - Who fits in and who does not?

2. State your organization's mission. Ask senior management and a middle manager their views on the organization's mission and compare their answers (privately).
3. In a small group, discuss the following: How can an organization dramatically increase its visible commitment to diversity? How can an organization best train employees to appreciate differences in gender, race, age, and culture? How should an organization go about selecting, developing, and promoting females and minorities for executive-level positions? What differences in culture do you see in your baccalaureate and Master of Science in Nursing (MSN) programs?
4. Boss (2000) introduces cyberspace as a culture. Do you agree or disagree with this? Support your answer.
5. In a group setting, answer the following questions: What evidence of workplace violence have you seen in practice? How was it handled? Have you seen situations escalate that might have resulted in violence if appropriate management had not been initiated? What happened?

Suggestions for Further Learning

- Read the following journal article: Mor-Barak, M.E., & Cherin, D.A. (1998). A tool to expand organizational understanding of workforce development: exploring a measure of inclusion-exclusion. *Administration in Social Work, 22*(1), 47-64.
- Consult the following website for business information from other countries: www.websofculture.com.
- Read Stewart, D. (1993). *The power of people skills.* J.Wiley & Sons, and then consult the website at www.smartbiz.com to view a corporate culture instrument.
- Refer to the Organizational Climate Questionnaire, which measures individuals' perceptions of the organizational climate in which they work (on a 4-point Likert scale). It may be found in Litwin, G., & Stringer, R. (1968). *Motivation and organizational climate.* Cambridge, MA: Harvard University Press
- Refer to the Nursing Organization Climate Descriptive Questionnaire, which examines leadership and subordinate behaviors to measure the organizational climate of nursing units. It may be found in Duxbury, M., Hanley, G., & Armstrong, G.D. (1987). Measurement of the nurse organization climate of neonatal ICUs. *Nursing Research, 31*(2), 83-88.
- Refer to the instrument, useful at all levels of an organization, found in Stewart, T.A. (1994, February 7). Rate your readiness to change. *Fortune,* 106-110.
- Refer to the Nursing Unit Cultural Assessment Tool (NUCAT-3) to be found in Byers, S. (1997). *The executive nurse.* Cincinnati, OH: Delmar.
- View the 1995 film *Cultural Diversity in Healthcare,* in which Dr. Joyce Giger discusses six cultural dimensions in diversity. Available from Lippincott, Williams, and Wilkins, 351 West Camden, Baltimore, MD 21201.
- View the 1993 film *Cultural Diversity in the Hospital Setting: Fostering Understanding and Developing Cross-Cultural*

Management Skills, available from Hospital Educational Services, PO Box 396, LaJolla, CA 92038; phone (800) 858-4478. This is a 2-hour training program related to valuing and effectively managing a multicultural workforce, presented by Sandra Thiederman, President of Cross-Cultural Communications, 4585 48th Street, San Diego, CA 92115-3236.
- Check out these practical guides pertaining to diversity in the workplace, available from Richard Chang Associates Inc., 41 Corporate Park, Suite 230, Irvine, CA 92714; phone (800) 756-8096. These guides include both individual activities and group-based activities:
  - *Capitalizing on Workplace Diversity*
  - *Successful Staffing in a Diverse Workplace*
  - *Team Building for Diverse Work Groups*
  - *Communicating in a Diverse Workplace*
  - *Tools for Valuing Diversity*
- Use either the organizational culture assessment instrument in the chapter or one found in the literature to assess the culture in either your present organization or a clinical site. What are the strengths and limitations of the instrument you used? How would you modify the instrument to make it more appropriate for assessing a similar site?
- Consult the following websites for additional information about workplace violence:
  - Occupational Safety and Health Administration (OSHA) at www.osha.org. (The direct web address for the written guidelines is www.osha.slc.gov/SLTC/workplaceviolence/guideline.html.)
  - Nurse Advocate Organization at www.nurseadvocate.org/nursewpv.html.
  - Crisis Prevention Institute at www.crisisprevention.com.

REFERENCES/BIBLIOGRAPHY

Alspach, G. (1993). Nurses as victims of violence. *Critical Care Nurse, 13*(5), 13-17.

Andrews, M.M. (1999). Cultural diversity in the health care work force. In M.M. Andrews & J.S. Boyle (Eds.), *Transcultural concepts in nursing care* (3rd ed.) (pp. 471-506). Philadelphia: JB Lippincott.

Andrews, M.M., & Boyle, J.S. (1999). Transcultural concepts in nursing care (3rd ed.). Philadelphia: JB Lippincott.

Attridge, N.I. (1995). Human resources. *Boston Business Journal, 15*(28), 10.

Blair, T., & New, S. (1991). Assaultive behavior. *Journal of Psychosocial Nursing, 29*(11), 25-29.

Blumenreich,P., Lippman, S., & Bacani-Oropilla, T. (1991). Violent patients: are you prepared to deal with them? *Postgraduate Medicine, 90*(2), 201-206.

Boss, C.M. (2000). Cyberspace: the new culture. In M.L. Kelley & V.M. Fitzsimons (Eds.), *Understanding cultural diversity: culture, curriculum, and community in nursing* (pp. 87-98). Boston: Jones & Bartlett and National League for Nursing Press.

Bruhn, J.G. (1996). Creating an organizational climate for multiculturalism. *Health Care Supervisor, 4*(4), 11-18.

Bruhn, J.G., & Chesney, A.P. (1998). Diagnosing the health of organizations. In E.C. Hein (Ed.), *Contemporary leadership behavior.* Philadelphia: Lippincott-Raven.

Byers, M. (1997). The executive nurse in corporate structure. In S. Byers (Ed.), *The executive nurse* (pp. 2-13). Cincinnati, OH: Delmar.

Caudron, S. (1998). Be cool: cultivating a cool culture gives human resources a staffing boost. *Workforce, 77*(4), 50-61. Available online at www.workforceonline.com.

Chang, R.Y. (1996). *Capitalizing on workplace diversity.* Irvine, CA: Richard Chang Associates.

Coeling, H.V. (1997). Organizational subcultures. In S. Byers (Ed.), *The executive nurse* (pp. 84-206). Cincinnati, OH: Delmar.

Cooke, R., & Lafferty, J. (1989). *Organizational culture inventory*. Plymouth, MI: Human Synergistics.

Cox, T. (1993). *Cultural diversity in organizations*. San Francisco: Berrett-Koehler.

Curran, C., & Miller, M (1990). Impact of corporate culture on nurse retention. *Nursing Clinics of North America, 25*(3) 537-548.

DiBenedetto, D.V. (1992). Occupational hazards of the healthcare industry: protecting healthcare workers. *AAOHN Journal, 43*(3), 131-137.

Fansano, C.A. (2000). Reengineering and the corporate culture. In M.L. Kelley & V.M. Fitzsimons (Eds.), *Understanding cultural diversity: culture, curriculum, and community in nursing* (pp. 79-86). Boston: Jones & Bartlett and National League for Nursing Press.

Fisher, M.L. (1996). *Quick reference to redesigning the nursing organization*. Cincinnati, OH: Delmar.

Flanner, R.B. (1995). *Violence in the workplace*. New York: Crossroad Press.

Flarey, D.L. (1993). The social climate of work environments. *Journal of Nursing Administration, 23*(6), 9-15.

Fleegler, M.E. (1993). Assessing organizational culture: a planning strategy. *Nursing Management, 24*(2), 39-41.

Hagberg, R. & Heifetz, J. (1998). *Corporate culture/organizational culture: understanding and assessment*. Hagberg Consulting Group Home. Available online at www.hcgnet.com/html/articles/understanding-culture.html.

Harris, A.W., & Myers, S. (1996). *Tools for valuing diversity*. Irvine, CA: Richard Chang Associates.

Hughes, L. (1990). Assessing organizational culture: strategies for the external consultant. *Nursing Forum, 25*(1), 15-19.

Hunt, P.L. (1994, December). Leadership in diversity. *Health Progress*, 26-29.

Katz, E.L. (2000). *Workplace violence: a summary paper* (Unpublished paper). Atlanta, GA: WorkCultures, LLC.

Kinkle, S.L. (1993). Violence in the emergency department: how to stop it before it starts. *American Journal of Nursing, 93*(7), 22-24.

Koch, M.W. (1998). Diversity in the workforce. In. S. Price, M. Koch, & S. Bassett (Eds.), *Health care resource management* (pp. 283-288). St. Louis: Mosby.

Kuga, L.A. (1996). *Communicating in a diverse workplace*. Irvine, CA: Richard Chang Associates.

Marquis, B.L., & Huston, C.J. (2000). *Leadership roles and management functions in nursing* (3rd ed.). Philadelphia: Lippincott, Williams, & Wilkins.

Occupational Safety and Health Administration (2000). *Guidelines for preventing workplace violence for healthcare and social service workers* (OSHA 3148). Washington, DC: US Department of Labor. Available online at www.osha.gov.

Ouchi, W.B. (1981). *Theory Z*. Reading, MA: Addison-Wesley

Peters, T., & Waterman, R. (1982). *In search of excellence*. New York: Harper & Row.

Rakoczy, R. (2000a, August). Psychological training: increased security may help curb violent incidents in hospitals. *Pulse: For the Health Care Professional* (a publication of *The Atlanta Journal Constitution*), 7, 12.

Rakoczy, R. (2000b, August). When the health care setting becomes a battleground: stop potential violence before it escalates. *Pulse: For the Health Care Professional* (a publication of *The Atlanta Journal Constitution*), 8-9.

Rizzo, J.A., Gilman, M.P., & Mesermann, C.A. (1994). Facilitating care delivery redesign using measures of unit culture and work characteristics. *Journal of Nursing Administration, 24*(5), 32-37.

Rowland, H.S., & Rowland, B.L. (1997). *Nursing administration handbook* (4th ed.). Gaithersburg, MD: Aspen Publishers.

Salmond, S.W. (2000). Culture learning and unlearning: creating a culture supporting the development of transcultural nurse managers. In M.L. Kelley & V.M. Fitzsimons (Eds.), *Understanding cultural diversity: culture, curriculum, and community in nursing* (pp. 149-160). Boston: Jones & Bartlett and National League for Nursing Press.

Schein E.H. (1992). *Organizational culture and leadership*. San Francisco: Jossey Bass.

Shea, V. (1994, September-October). Core rules of etiquette. *Educom Review*, 58-61.

Sorrel-Jones, J. (1999). Organizational dynamics. In J. Lancaster (Ed.), *Nursing issues in leading and managing change*. St. Louis: Mosby.

Sovie, M.D. (1993). Hospital culture—why create one? *Nursing Economics, 11*(2), 69-75.

Speer, R.A. (1997). *Workplace violence: moving beyond the headlines*. Available online at www.wprkplacelaw.com/article1.htm.

Stewart, T.A. (1994, February 7). Rate your readiness for change. *Fortune*, 106-110.

Trice, H.M.T., & Beyer, J.M.B. (1993). *The culture of work organizations*. Englewood Cliffs, NJ: Prentice-Hall.

Vestal, K., Fralicx, R., & Spreier, S. (1997). Organizational culture: the critical link between strategy and results. *Hospital and Health Services Administration, 42*(3), 339-365.

Veninga, R.L. (1994, December). Valuing our differences. *Health Progress*, 30-34.

Wilkoff, M., & Ziegenfuss Jr., J.T. (1995, May). Culture audits: a tool for change. *Health Progress*, 34-38.

Chapter 37

Racial/Ethnic Group Issues and Health Care

Sue E. Meiner

Cultural influences are powerful determinants of health care behaviors. Racial and ethnic groups exhibit behaviors influenced by common beliefs, ideologies, knowledge, institutions, religion, and governance. Interventions that require health-related behavioral changes must be presented with cultural awareness and sensitivity. Encouraging activities that address health promotion and illness prevention in diverse groups or communities can be challenging for many health care providers (Huff & Kline, 1999).

Examining issues of diversity and of the unique culture of the health care provider is essential to the multicultural population of America (Huff & Kline, 1999). Many health care professionals' lack of knowledge about health beliefs and practices of culturally diverse groups has led to significant challenges in the provision of health care services (Brislin & Yoshida, 1994; Geissler, 1998). The intent of this chapter is to examine the racial and ethnic diversity issues that affect health care provided by advanced practice nurses (APNs).

DEFINITIONS

Race is a biological term referring to members of a group who share distinguishing physical traits such as skin color, hair, or genetic patterns (Torres, 1993). Zackerman (1990) defines race as "an inbreeding group of individuals with a specific geographic locus . . . Superficial physical similarity can coexist with drastic differences in cultural behavioral patterns." Genetic study indicates that there is more difference within each race than between the usually established races (Ramer, 1992).

Racism refers to the belief that individuals representative of one race are superior to those of another race. Kortak (1991) wonders if the public often confuses social behavior and diverse lifestyles with genetic or biological race, thereby contributing to racial discrimination. *Discrimination* is the "limiting of opportunities, choices, or life experiences because of prejudices about individuals, cultures, or groups" (Leininger, 1995).

According to Andrews and Boyle (1999), an *ethnic group* is a group of people within a larger social system whose members have common ancestral, racial, physical or national characteristics and who share cultural symbols such as language, lifestyle, religion, and other characteristics that are not fully understood or shared by outsiders. Ethnic characteristics shared by members of a particular group are distinctive. Leininger (1995) clarifies that *ethnicity* refers to "social identity and past origins of a social group due largely to a language, religion, and national origins," but she prefers the term *culture*, which she sees as more inclusive and specific because it refers to "holistic patterned lifeways" rather than "selected ethnic features or origin aspects." A *lifeway* "is more than a person's lifestyle. It is the totality of all the person is and does, which includes cultural values, beliefs, and practices" (Ramer, 1992).

CRITICAL ISSUES: RACIAL AND ETHNIC ISSUES IN HEALTH CARE

During the first century of U.S. history, the diverse ethnic and cultural groups were thought to be heading toward assimilation into a single American culture. However, during the last half of the twentieth century, this thought has diminished into obscurity. Today, many groups cling to and identify more closely with their ethnic heritage than with any newly created culture associated with combining racial or ethnic groups (May, 1992; Paniagua, 1994). This continued separation of cultures has created the need for a multicultural health care environment that addresses the needs of all Americans, whatever their race.

Despite recent improvements in the health status of all Americans, significant differences remain between racial and ethnic groups. Access to health care services can significantly influence health care use and outcomes (Kagawa-Singer & Chung, 1994). Health insurance plays a critical role in ensuring that Americans obtain timely medical care and have protection against expensive health care costs. A survey sponsored by the U.S. government examined the health status, access to health care, and health insurance conditions of three of the five major racial/ethnic groups. The study was financed through the Medical Expenditure Panel Survey (MEPS) from the Agency for Health Care Policy and Research (Kass, Weinrick, & Monheit, 1998). The survey consisted of multiple rounds of interviews with persons and households that were nationally representative of the civilian noninstitutionalized population. The racial category "white/other" (referred to in the Statistics discussion on this page as "Caucasian") used in the MEPS reports includes a number of individuals identified as Asians, American Indians, Aleuts, Eskimos, or other races. A statement regarding these groups was included in the report. The MEPS data present too few individuals to adequately represent health information of these groups. However the information is of interest, and the following material was obtained from that survey.

Health Status Reports

The self-reporting of health status has shown to be a reliable measure of an individual's health condition. In the MEPS survey, Hispanics and African Americans were more likely than Caucasians to report their health status as fair or poor. In the age group of 18 to 64, Hispanics reported a 17% rating of fair or poor health, while African Americans reported a 16% rating. Less than 10% of Caucasians reported such a status. The reporting of excellent health status was found to be nearly 35% in the Caucasian group, 29% in the African-American group, and only 27% in the Hispanic group (Kass et al, 1998).

Health Access Reports

Health outcomes are significantly influenced by the adequacy of access to health care services. The MEPS survey asked participants if they used a regular source of health care when they were sick or needed to talk to someone about a health concern. Quality and continuity of care are affected by the inconsistency of health services. If regular health services are used, barriers to receiving services because of financial or insurance restrictions remain. Another area is the lack of availability of providers at night or on weekends.

Caucasians used office-based health care services most often (76.3%), followed by African Americans (63.6%) and Hispanics (57.9%). Hospital-based health services were more frequently used by African Americans (16.2%), followed by Hispanics (12.5%). The Caucasian group used this source at a rate of 8.1%.

Barriers to health care included inability to afford care and lack of insurance benefits to cover basic or extended health care needs. Barriers to receiving health care were identified the most by Hispanics (15.1%). Caucasians noted barriers at a rate of 11.4%, with the African-American group noting barriers at 9.9% (Kass et al, 1998).

Health Insurance Reports

When all age groups within the selected racial or ethnic groups were surveyed regarding health insurance coverage, the three areas examined were private insurance, public insurance, and the uninsured. African Americans were the most likely to be publicly insured, while Caucasians were the most likely to have private coverage. African Americans and Hispanics were more likely than Caucasians to be uninsured (Kass et al, 1998). Job-related insurance was noted in 77.4% of the Caucasian group, 66% of the African-American group, and 54.9% of the Hispanic group. The following lists shows non–older adult uninsured Americans, represented by percentage of the total American population and then identified by uninsured racial or ethnic group percentage:

- Hispanics—11.6% of the U.S. population; 21.2% uninsured
- African Americans—13.1% of the population; 16.9% uninsured
- Caucasians—75.3% of the population; 61.9% uninsured (Kass et al, 1998)

Health promotion may require health-related behavior changes through ecological or environmental approaches intended to create change or support policies, regulations, and expanded access to resources that affect people where they live or work (Richard, Potvin, Kishchuk, Prlic, & Green, 1996).

Health Care Concepts and Perceptions

A major problem in caring for culturally diverse people in America involves matching of patients' perceptions of health problems to a health care provider's concept of health and treatment for illness. Knowing the cultural or racial background of a patient is as important in the selection of treatment options as the understanding of the disease process. Ignoring an individual's belief system and the role that health and illness plays within a racial or ethnic group can negatively affect the course of treatment (Kass et al, 1998).

Modern medicine, as taught and practiced in Western civilization, is the product of the North American health care provider. This mindset was created though decades of socialization with the belief that modern medicine is the answer to all of humankind's needs (Spector, 1996). However, this thinking does not answer questions related to missed appointments, failure to follow medication and treatment regimens, or failure to see a health care provider steeped in the scientific practice of medicine. A more sensitive approach to health issues must be practiced if the multiracial makeup of the American people is to be served appropriately. This can only be achieved through an awareness of culture-bound definitions of the state of health, the nature of health maintenance, and illness prevention (Kass et al, 1998).

The Health Belief Model

Although this model is presented in detail elsewhere in this text, an overview is provided here as a context for understanding racial and ethnic issues in health care. Spector (1996) says the socialization of health care providers into the health care profession creates a unique provider culture. When the provider culture clashes with traditional perceptions and beliefs regarding health issues, no-show clinic visits, failure to follow prescribed therapies, and failure to seek health care services may result. An example of a health belief is the idea that a common cold is treated by fasting, while the presence of a fever requires hot foods.

With few exceptions, health care providers rarely sanction alternative methods of protection and healing that are not based on a scientific foundation. When it does happen, approval of alternative providers usually includes formal educational preparation with certification of the practice by knowledge validation.

To perceive the relationship between personal well-being and health care behaviors, a susceptibility to illness needs to be present. If the perception of susceptibility is high and the seriousness of the illness is known, action may or may not be taken. Reasons for taking or not taking action can heavily depend upon the racial or cultural effects of a health-belief system. Six cultural phenomena have been identified by Giger and Davidhizar (1995): communication issues, personal space, social organization, time orientation, environmental control, and biological variations.

Communication issues

Language differences are only one of the communication obstacles. Nonverbal communication can also influence care both negatively and positively, depending upon the choices made by health care providers. Knowledge, education, dialect, and silence are elements of the communication process. When language differences are identified, a skilled interpreter is mandatory for effective communication.

Personal space

Territoriality is the term frequently used for the desire for personal space surrounding an individual. Culture influences the manner in which people perceive and react to the encroachment of others into their space. During health care encounters, the intimate zone is fre-quently encroached upon, and this is the most sensitive spatial dimension. Permission must be obtained through effective communication when cultural differences are known. Personal distance ranging from 18 inches to 4 feet is the norm for a health interview. The closer the proximity to the patient, the more appropriate is communication on the actions to be taken. The use of an ophthalmoscope is within the intimate zone, while the use of a handheld Rosenbaum eye chart can be in either intimate or less personal space. Social and public distances do not normally affect health care visits (Giger & Davidhizar, 1995).

Social organization

The family unit, community, and social organization produce an effect on entering the health care system. Often barriers arise from within and outside these diverse groups. For example, a particular family may wish for a daughter to try home remedies before seeing a physician, or a Navajo family may ask a shaman to complete a sand painting to cure their son instead of sending him to a traditional Western health care setting.

Time orientation

Reflection upon the passage of time and the effect of living within a specific time orientation varies among different cultural groups. The viewing of time as past-, present-, or future-oriented affects the setting of health care goals (Giger & Davidhizar, 1995). For example, past-oriented cultures make decisions based upon ancestral practices. Often a state of mistrust exists when past practices are ridiculed or brushed aside in communications.

Present orientation can be seen in patients who are consistently late for appointments or treatments; the time sequence needed to prepare for or travel to the appointment is given little attention. Taking medication after the symptoms have disappeared is another present orientation that causes problems with drug regimens that require completing a cycle after symptoms are gone. An example is a prescription for 10 days of antibiotic therapy in cases when the fever and other symptoms are gone after 2 days; chances are not good that a full course of antibiotics will be taken by a present-oriented patient.

Long-term goals are important to establish in health care practices with a future orientation. Prevention of future illnesses is affected directly on the belief that action now will have rewards in the future. Time orientation must not be seen as stereotypical for specific cultural groups; it is a way to work within the cultural phenomena that influence health care behaviors (Giger & Davidhizar, 1995). Health care providers need to identify the traditions and cultural differences of people in their care.

Environmental control

The environmental control issue relates to the use of folk medicine and healers within a culturally specific group of people. Health-related experiences can directly affect health-seeking behaviors (HSBs) when illness is present. Trust in folk medicine may overshadow Western practices or may supplement more traditional Western approaches. Alternative approaches to healing are so widely used today that they earn billions of dollars for the companies who deliver them.

Biological variations

Biological variations can be infinite. Color of skin; body structure; disease risks and manifestations associated with a higher mortality; nutritional differences and preferences; and genetic differences that may cause reactions to certain foods or drugs must be identified to provide effective health care.

Experience of Illness

As health is defined according to the experiences of individuals and groups with differing racial and cultural orientations, illness is determined by a sick person's definition and belief system. The sick role must be sanctioned by the family, community, or social organization of the sick person. According to Spector (1996), a four-stage illness experience is common; it includes the following stages: (1) onset (onset is slow or insidious, rapid or acute), (2) diagnosis (illness identified and sanctioned), (3) patient status (patient takes on the social aspects and physical limitations of illness), and (4) recovery (patient gives up patient status and resumes prepatient role).

Before the identification and sanctioning of the illness, knowledge of entry into the health care system is required. This HSB signifies a choice by the patient not to use a "lay" practitioner for health care needs at this time. While in the presence of the provider of care, barriers may become an issue that negates his or her choice of care. Acceptance of the plan of care with prescribed treatments can repel an ambivalent patient, and such unwillingness to comply with the treatment plan may be rooted in racial or ethnic health beliefs (Spector, 1996).

Experience of Suffering

The ways in which individuals respond to pain and suffering vary within and across cultures; pain is a complex, highly personal phenomenon. "Pain is a very private experience and is influenced by cultural heritage" (Ludwig-Beymer, 1999). In some cultures, expressing pain vocally is thought to bring dishonor to the suffering person and his or her family. For example, Asians and Native Americans would be humiliated to have their emotive expressions of pain witnessed by others. In contrast, Middle Eastern cultures find it acceptable to cry, moan, and show pain through expressive body language. The way in which individuals respond to pain is neither right nor wrong—it just is. McCaffery (1979) asserts as much in her

comprehensive and provocative definition of pain—pain is whatever the patient says it is and occurs whenever the patient says it does.

Pain is a subjective experience; therefore, its presence cannot be proved by those who are suffering, even though they may have objective signs of pain. This subjectivity, says one nurse practitioner (NP), "places the suffering person at the mercy of the nurse with the narcotic keys." There is some indication that nurses in this country expect patients experiencing pain to respond silently and use self-control. "Partly as a result of the nursing subculture, nurses often expect people to be objective about the very subjective experience of pain" (Ludwig-Beymer, 1999). It seems, at times, that nurses expect patients to report, describe, and endure pain, all using self-control.

To be culturally competent in situations involving suffering patients, APNs must confront their own personal beliefs about pain and the attitudes they possess as a result of their cultural backgrounds and personal experiences (Martinelli, 1987). They must respect patients' rights to express pain in whatever way they wish without being judgmental, even when the patients' reactions are different than the APNs' might be. APNs need to know ways to assess pain, including using words and a pain scale for adults and using other measures for children, such as "smiley faces." They need an expansive repertoire of pain management measures including, but not limited to, pharmacotherapeutics. Alternative or nontraditional measures like acupressure and imagery should be comfortable ones for APNs to accept, support, and possibly employ. Finally, APNs need an ability to evaluate the effectiveness of both traditional and nontraditional measures and to revise the management plan accordingly, giving patients permission to seek relief from suffering. In response to suffering, caring and culturally competent providers will not just do something and leave; they will sit with a patient and willingly listen as he or she talks about the suffering.

Barriers to Health Promotion and Illness Prevention

A number of cultural barriers exist that are not associated with an inability to afford care or a lack of insurance benefits to cover health care needs. Potential barriers that need to be identified at the earliest possible moment include educational level and literacy; primary language spoken and English fluency; traditional health beliefs and practices; communication patterns and customs; dietary preferences and practices; and orientation to preventive health services. This list is not an exhaustive example of multicultural barriers to health care; it represents areas of concern for health care providers and teams during planning of services for culturally diverse populations (Lester, 1998; Huff & Kline, 1999).

Racial and Ethnic Identification

While the African-American, Hispanic, Asian, and Native American populations are young and growing, the Caucasian majority is shrinking and aging (Spector, 1996). This trend is leading toward an ever-increasing multicultural American society. The U.S. Department of Health and Human Services (DHHS) defines the major racial and ethnic groups in America as African (Black) American, Asian/Pacific Islander, Native American/Alaska Native (e.g., Aleuts, Eskimos), Hispanic (can be from any other group), and European (Caucasian) American.

To a large extent race or ethnicity and health issues are directly tied to the ability to access health resources in America. Hispanics and African Americans are more likely than Caucasian Americans to lack private job-related health insurance coverage; be uninsured; lack a usual source of care; have a hospital-based usual source of care, and be in fair or poor health (Kass et al, 1998).

African-American issues

Cultural diversity is important in relation to the varied origins of African Americans. Diverse backgrounds comprising different languages, learned behaviors (including illness behaviors), and beliefs and values contribute to the diversity within the African-American population. The places of origin for this racial group include Africa, the Caribbean, and the Americas, and the languages spoken reflect these multifaceted origins. The commonalities of dark skin and similar features have placed all members of this racial group into an aggregate for health and social policies.

Attempts to identify or assess the access to health care services, the use of those services, and the measurement of the health status of African Americans have been difficult. The reasons for the underuse of health services among African Americans, even though they bear a heavier burden of disease, are complex and represent an intersection among economic, cultural, and historical factors. These factors included increased poverty, limited access to health insurance, and a health belief system that is not entirely steeped in the biomedical model (Jack, 1994; Lassiter, 1995; Bayne-Smith, 1996; Geissler, 1998).

Many African Americans retain a holistic philosophy of health and perceive the mind and body as inseparable. Folk healing is a common practice in many African-American communities. Two belief systems practiced in some African-American communities containing immigrants from West Africa are voodoo, which is associated with the practice of magic, and JuJu, a complex magical practice blended with medicinal procedures and superstitions. These practices often involve the use of charms and the burial of objects on the property of those wishing to ward off evil spirits. Unnatural illnesses are considered a punishment from God that requires the removal of the evil, which is not considered within the capabilities of Western medicine (Jack, 1994; Geissler, 1998).

Hispanic issues

Hispanics are defined by the U.S. DHHS (1994) as persons who consider themselves Mexican, Mexican American, Puerto Rican, or Cuban, or as persons who are born in or descended from those born in Central or South America, Spain, or selected locations in the Caribbean. This definition includes persons from more than 20 countries of the world. Hispanics comprise one of the youngest population groups in the United States. Hispanic women are more likely to live in poverty than are African-American or Caucasian women.

The definition of health in many Hispanic families is a holistic view of health and illness. Good health means that a person is behaving in accordance with his or her conscience, God's mandate, and the norms and customs of the church, family, and local community. The Hispanic family is generally a strong, loyal, and supportive group. Family members rally around a family member in crisis to provide full support and protection (Bayne-Smith, 1996; Geissler, 1998).

Cubans believe in the concepts of equilibrium and balance between individuals and the environment. They also believe in the germ theory of disease, although other causes can include stress, evil spells, and voodoo-type magic. This folk medical system is called *curanderismo*. It has evolved from spiritualistic, homeopathic, Aztec, Spanish, and Western elements of illness treatment (Lassiter, 1995; Hilfinger Messias, 1996; Geissler, 1998).

Native American/Alaska Native issues

The definition of health by Native Americans greatly differs from that of other racial groups in America. Native Americans define health as the balance or beauty of all things physical, spiritual, emotional, and social. When illness occurs, balance and harmony are absent in the life of the individual, and healing requires that this balance and harmony be restored. Traditional healing practices encompass a holistic and wellness-oriented approach that may involve one or more of the following:

- Prayer and chanting
- Dancing rituals
- Purification ceremonies
- Botanical medicines
- Physical manipulations to restore harmony

These healing practices may be carried out by a healer that incorporates a multitude of roles: doctor, psychiatrist/psychologist, religious consultant and diviner, and arbitrator (Lyon, 1996).

The health status of Native Americans and Alaska Natives is affected by long-standing socioeconomic conditions. According to the 1990 census, 35% of these two ethnic groups live below the federal poverty level; an unemployment rate of 21% was also reported. Poverty has created a pervasive attitude of helplessness among Native American populations. Economic issues addressed by a federal welfare system for this group have led to low self-esteem among tribal communities. Political issues are in disarray in most tribal communities, and the cause for this has been discussed as a conflict between federal representatives and a lack of tribal empowerment.

Cultural issues stem from the lack of traditional roles for men while women have maintained the caregiver role. This role confusion for men has been seen as one reason for their domestic violence against tribal women, and lifestyle issues include having a safe and nonviolent environment for the women and children. Changes in lifestyle toward the elimination of alcoholism and alcohol abuse have failed throughout the past century (Geissler, 1998).

Asian/Pacific Islander issues

Americans from Asia number more than 10 million according to Zhan (1999). Of these millions of people, 53 subgroups have retained much of their language, culture, and history among the elders. However, as each generation becomes Westernized, their health beliefs and health care practices begin to vary more.

Specific American health issues have rarely been identified for Asian cultures. Chen (1996) studied health beliefs among Chinese older adults living in America. Conformity with nature through harmonizing with the environment and listening to heaven were identified with health maintenance. Other cultural beliefs that emerged from Southeast Asia included kinship solidarity and the search for equilibrium.

Underlying traditional Chinese medicine is a concept that exists on the harmony between heaven and earth, Yin and Yang, and the five elements of wood, fire, earth, metal, and water. Following the path of Tao, a person can remain in balance with the laws of the universe. The major forces are Yin—the passive or negative female force (representing moon, earth, water, poverty, and sadness)—and Yang—the active male force (representing sun, heaven, fire, wealth, and goodness). If the balance of these forces is not observed, harmony will not be maintained and chaos will result. Manifestations of illness are directly associated with chaos from an imbalance of the forces (Lassiter, 1995; Chen, 1996; Spector, 1996; Geissler, 1998).

European (Caucasian) American issues

The Caucasian American population originates in many European countries. Major ethnic groups within the Caucasian American population migrated from Germany, Poland, Italy, the United Kingdom, Ireland, Austro-Hungary, and Russia, mainly over a period of 180 years. Therefore any discussion of the diversities within each of the major Caucasian groups can not be exhaustive or fully representative of each group. The following information is presented to identify the diversity of beliefs that are frequently but not universally represented within the selected ethnic groups.

German and Polish ancestry. These two ethnic groups have great similarities in health beliefs. The most common description of health is as a state of physical and emotional well-being. Health includes the ability to do one's duty, to maintain positive energy to do things, and to do, think, and act the way one would like. Health also means the ability to congregate and enjoy life. This description of health has only a few elements of being ill.

The germ theory of infection and certain stress-related theories are held by this group, as are other theories that include environmental changes, the evil eye, and punishment from God (Spector, 1996; Geissler, 1998). To prevent illness, they believe in proper nutrition, wearing clothing according to the seasons of the year, taking cod-liver oil daily, exercising daily, and working hard. Other means of illness prevention included wearing asafetida bags around the neck in the cold months; fresh air; and cleanliness.

Italian ancestry. Beliefs about health and illness traditionally identify the winds and currents as carriers of disease, along with contamination. Heredity is seen as an influencing factor in some diseases, while supernatural or human causes are factors in others. Explanations involving psychosomatic elements are also accepted as causes of illnesses; this belief is founded on the recognition that emotions are related to illness and that if emotions are bottled up and suppressed, harm will result.

Illness prevention includes practices like placing garlic cloves on a string around the neck of infants and children to prevent colds. Other preventive practices include staying out of wind drafts and the avoidance of washing one's hair before going out or during a menstrual period. The traditional belief in the evil eye, or *mal occhio*, remains common in some segregated Italian communities. If a person receives evil spirits by way of the evil eye, remedies must be applied according to the type of evil spirit thought to have invaded the person (Spector, 1996; Geissler, 1998; Huff & Kline, 1999).

English ancestry. Americans with English ancestry have the smallest adaptations to make to the American health care system. An illness is seen as the need for medical assessment and treatment. Community-based health care centers around a district nurse, with referrals to physicians as needed. Hospital stays are for special cases, with home care the predominant and expected form of care during illness or rehabilitation. Western medicine has its roots in the English system; therefore differences in health beliefs are more individualized than collective.

Irish ancestry. The Irish ethnic group demonstrates the tendency to use defense mechanisms such as denial, delaying, or completely ignoring signs and symptoms of illness. This refrain from expressing illness-related complaints has been identified with their view of life—an experience that has expectations of periodic suffering (Zola, 1966).

For some Irish Americans, illness behavior can be linked to sin and guilt ideology. It can be a self-fulfilling prophecy of something earned, and it must be accepted as fact with little treatment (Spector, 1996; Geissler, 1998). A common practice is for them to seek health care in emergencies only. This reactive rather than preventive view of health care contributes to the fatalistic beliefs about illness.

Russian ancestry. Russian Americans who practice Russian Orthodox beliefs assign responsibility for the length and depth of illnesses to the strength of their spirituality. Illness can be seen as punishment for a person not having enough faith. Other Russian Americans exhibit a highly developed self-care approach to illness and disease treatment. The emphasis is on aerobic exercise and nutritional observances of lowered intakes of salt, fat, and calories (Geissler, 1998). Alternative health modalities are practiced regularly. A strong belief in the properties of hot mineral waters, massage, spine and back manipulation, and corrective shoes prevails (Spector, 1996). (Figure 37-1 provides migration patterns to the United States over the past 500 years.)

Cultural Competence for Advanced Practice Nurses

Cultural competence can be defined as the ability of a system, organization, or individual to respond to the unique needs of peoples whose cultures are different from that of the dominant culture. A culturally competent system of health care recognizes and integrates the importance of culture on multiple levels, including policy-making, administration, and practice (Cross, 1997).

Malone (1998) notes that the goal of cultural competency remains a challenge to the profession of nursing in America. Nursing has been and continues to be a patient-centered caring profession. Providing care to an ever-changing multicultural and multilingual population while maintaining a patient-specific, personal delivery of health services may seem overwhelming to APNs (American Nurses Association, 1998), and in fact, achieving cultural competence is a lifelong learning process.

It is not necessary to know everything about one or more different racial or ethnic groups to provide health care services effectively. Being culturally competent is an ongoing process learned over time through a continued search for self-awareness concerning health beliefs. To achieve this, health care providers should embrace a self-awareness that includes cultural knowledge about illness and healing practices, intercultural communication skills, and behavioral flexibility (Lester, 1998).

While health care providers are seeking to become more culturally aware, the profession of health care has its own cultural content. A review of the beliefs, practices, habits, likes, dislikes, rituals, and customs of health care professionals shows they have an interesting similarity to a unique cultural group. When compared with various other ethnic and cultural groups, the health care provider culture exhibits similar characteristics. (Box 37-1 summarizes the cultural characteristics of typical health care providers.)

As health care providers are learning about multicultural health-related behaviors, they must be aware of their own unique cultural attributes. Providers must also understand the effect of the medical and nursing culture upon recipients before a crosscultural approach to health care can be realized (Stewart, 1998).

IMPLICATIONS FOR MSN EDUCATION AND ADVANCED PRACTICE

APNs need to be aware that cultural forces are powerful determinants of health-related behaviors in any group or subpopulation. Nurses also need to appreciate that those elements of a racial or ethnic group's beliefs and practices that can be modified to cause the desired health-related change may be associated with interventions.

Providers of health care to the American population must develop the ability to transcend language during patient encounters, while fostering an understanding of the racial or ethnic heritages existing in a multicultural society. Awareness of the cultural needs of others is a necessity for all health care providers to achieve the highest possible quality of health for all Americans. Providers must attempt to enter a patient's world to understand rationalization for and about the illness being presented. The ability to see each patient without being influenced by personal biases and judgments is a worthy goal for APNs seeking to understand, respect, and adapt to racial and ethnic differences.

APN students should have opportunities to learn about the genetic and biological variations in individuals of diverse racial and ethnic groups. They should understand the pathophysiology of disease entities; pharmacology and the diversity of individual response to drug therapy; variations in laboratory testing and clinical significance; and the aspects of disease risk. There should be ample opportunities to perform comprehensive physical assessments of culturally diverse patients to teach biological variations. Students should also have experiences with assessment and management of pain among culturally diverse patients to begin to fully appreciate the cultural aspects of suffering.

APN education should include content on the dietary management of disease, with opportunities to perform

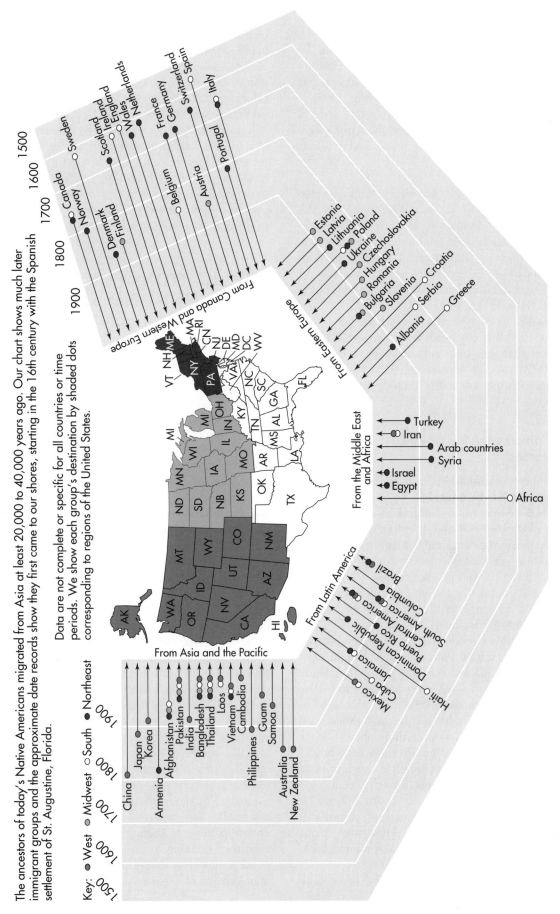

Figure 37-1 Migration patterns in the United States. (From Ebersole, P., & Hess, P. [1998]. *Toward healthy aging: human needs and nursing response.* St. Louis: Mosby.)

Box 37-1

Characteristics of the Culture of the Typical Health Care Provider

Beliefs
- Standardized definitions of health and illness
- Omnipotence of technology

Practices
- Maintenance of health and prevention of illness
- Annual physical examinations and screenings

Habits
- Charting
- Constant use of jargon
- Use of a systematic approach and problem-solving methodology

Preferences
- Promptness
- Neatness
- Organization
- Compliance

Dislikes
- Tardiness
- Disorganization
- Noncompliance

Customs
- Professional deference and adherence to the hierarchy found in autocratic and bureaucratic systems
- Handwashing
- Employment of certain procedures in birth and death

Rituals
- Physical examinations
- Surgical procedures
- Limitation of visitors and visiting hours

dietary assessments and suggest interventions that are culturally appropriate. An interesting approach for learning about culturally diverse diets is to invite international students and faculty to bring in a cultural dish that would be perceived as healthy in their culture and discuss how this diet would be modified in cases of illness.

Torres (1993) suggests that it might be helpful to have a basic understanding of these areas of cultural diversity: family structure; important events in the family life cycle; family roles; rules of interpersonal relations; decorum and discipline; standards of health and hygiene; education and teaching methods; perspectives of work and play; dress and personal appearance; and history and traditions for holidays and other celebrations. Linking with a patient from another culture, especially one who will agree to a home visit by the student, enables collection of these kinds

of details about a culture. If each student in a class were assigned to a different cultural representative, the collective learning experience (through group sharing) would provide an extremely comprehensive view of several cultures. In some programs, patients agree to be on a panel to answer questions about their culture; such panelists often wear representative clothing and bring arts and crafts for a higher education version of "show and tell."

Barriers to health care services must be removed for groups who are racially and ethnically diverse. As APNs design strategies for managing health care, they should consider the ways in which a clinic's location, hours, and current appointment system may affect certain racial or ethnic groups, then accommodate their needs to the extent possible. Taking health care into the community and creating settings where multiservice care is possible is advantageous. Furthermore, a culturally sensitive approach on the part of APNs and other providers and staff is invaluable in providing quality care for racial and ethnic populations. Every effort must be made to eliminate distrust in underserved communities in order to encourage HSBs for men and women of all ages and races.

PRIORITIES FOR RESEARCH

Understanding health promotion and illness prevention programs in a multicultural population requires research and planning. A properly fitting framework that can provide the blueprint for planning must be selected, one that addresses the target group and the provider of services. Involving a member of the target group is extremely important to the success of the program. One frequently used framework is PRECEDE-PROCEED (Green & Greuter, 1991; Lancaster, Onega, & Forness, 1992). The planner needs to identify the intended outcome, and this is done through an assessment process to collect culture-specific information about the target group. The five-step PRECEDE (**P**redisposing, **R**einforcing, and **E**nabling **C**onstructs in **E**ducational **D**iagnosis and **E**valuation) process requires some systematic diagnoses of social factors, epidemiological factors, behavioral factors, environmental factors, and educational factors.

The four-step PROCEED (**P**olicy, **R**egulatory, and **O**rganizational **C**onstructs in **E**ducational and **E**nvironmental **D**evelopment) component includes health education interventions, policy, organization, and regulation. Using this framework in the design of research projects directed at community assessment might be the vehicle to give future practitioners identification and intervention strategies for achieving change at all levels of a multicultural community.

Exploration through qualitative research of the experience of illness from the perspective of individuals in varied racial and ethnic groups can provide rich, meaningful data to enhance the APN's ability to plan appropriate inter-

Suggestions for Further Learning

- Complete a media search. Review racial or ethnic newspaper articles, novels, documentary films or videos, and ethnographies that can be used to further your understanding of racial and ethnic diversity.
- Visit markets, shops, and restaurants in diverse racial or ethnic neighborhoods. Examine the role that ethnic foods play in health and illness.
- Attend religious ceremonies, weddings, baptisms, and funerals at ethnic places of worship different than your own. Consider the role of rituals and religion in health and illness.
- Tour ethnic communities to learn about the cultural symbolism embodied in arts and crafts.
- Make classroom visits to an ethnic school to learn about competitiveness and cooperation in the playing of games.
- Interview diverse racial or ethnic families to learn about their beliefs concerning health and illness prevention.
- Review U.S. Department of Health and Human Services (1996). *PATCH: planned approach to community health—guide for the local coordinator.* Washington, DC: Centers

for Disease Control and Prevention. This is a framework for community assessment.
- Review specific racial/ethnic sections of Geissler, E.M. (1998). *Pocket guide to cultural assessment* (2nd ed.). St. Louis: Mosby. This pocket guide discusses approximately 200 countries in regard to their languages, sick care practices, endemic diseases, dominance patterns, life rituals, food practices, and more.
- Conduct a physical assessment and document the features of the objective data that are racial or ethnic variations.
- Consult the following: Ramer, L. (1992). *Culturally sensitive caregiving and childbearing families: module 1, series 4. Nursing for the 21st century.* White Plains, NY: March of Dimes Birth Defects Foundation. This module is available from the March of Dimes Birth Defects Foundation, 1275 Macaroneck Avenue, White Plains, NY 10605. The cost is $15.00 for the module and $35.00 for contact hours.
- To better understand the cultural aspects of bereavement, consult Parry, J.K., & Ryan, A.S. (1995). *A cross-cultural look at death, dying, and religion.* Chicago: Nelson-Hall.

---

ventions. Qualitative approaches may also be designed to determine how members of a particular racial or ethnic group perceive health and what factors are associated with their HSBs. To the extent possible, all research studies deigned by APNs should seek inclusion of subjects who are racially and ethnically diverse.

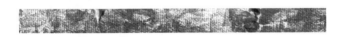

DISCUSSION QUESTIONS

These questions can be used to promote critical thinking and encourage discussion.

1. Remember a time in your nursing education or practice when the fact that a patient was from a different racial or ethnic background than you complicated care. Discuss that experience in a small group setting. Be specific about the problem that existed. How was the problem solved at the time? Now having more experience, would you solve the problem differently today? If so, in what way would you manage it differently and why?
2. Reflect on your own expectations of the sick role and specific experiences that show evidence of that role. How is your sick role like or unlike that of your life partner? Your children? What happens when sick role expectations in your family clash?

3. Reflect on your own pain experiences. How do you respond to pain? To what extent do you believe your response to pain matches the traditional response to pain by the racial or ethnic group to which you belong? How has being a nursing professional changed your view of pain and your reaction to pain?

REFERENCES/BIBLIOGRAPHY

American Nurses Association (1998). ANA addressing cultural diversity in the profession. *American Nurse, 30*(1), 25.

Andrews, M.M., & Boyle, J.S. (1999). *Transcultural concepts in nursing care* (3rd ed.). Philadelphia: JB Lippincott.

Bayne-Smith, M. (1996). *Race, gender, and health.* Thousand Oaks, CA: Sage Publications.

Brislin, R., & Yoshida, T. (Eds.). (1994). *Improving intercultural interactions: modules for cross-cultural training programs.* Thousand Oaks, CA: Sage.

Chen, Y.L. (1996). Conformity with nature: a theory of Chinese American elders' health promotion and illness prevention processes. *Advances in Nursing Science. 19*(2), 17-26.

Cross, I. (1997, February 7). Towards a culturally competent system of care. *Caring Headlines.*

Douglas, M.K. (1991). Cultural diversity in the response to pain. In K.A. Puntillo (Ed.), *Pain in the critically ill.* Gaithersburg, MD: Aspen Publishers.

Ebersole, P., & Hess, P. (1998). *Toward healthy aging: human needs and nursing response.* St. Louis: Mosby.

Geissler, E.M. (1998). *Pocket guide to cultural assessment* (2nd ed.). St. Louis: Mosby.

Giger, J.N., & Davidhizar, R.E. (1995). *Transcultural nursing: assessment and intervention* (2nd ed.). St. Louis: Mosby.

Green, L.W., & Greuter, N.W. (1991). *Health promotion planning: an educational and environmental approach* (2nd ed.). Mountain View, CA: Mayfield.

Hilfinger Messias, D.K. (1996). Brazilians. In J.G. Lipson, S.L. Dibble, & P.A. Minarik (Eds.), *Culture and nursing care: a pocket guide.* San Francisco: UCSF Nursing Press.

Huff, R.M., & Kline, M.V. (1999). *Promoting health in multicultural populations: a handbook for practitioners.* Thousand Oaks, CA: Sage.

Jack Jr., L., Harrison, I.E., & Airhihenbuwa, C.O. (1994). Ethnicity and the health belief systems. In A.C. Matiella (Ed.), *The multicultural challenge in health education.* Santa Cruz, CA: ETR Associates.

Kagawa-Singer, M., & Chung, R. (1994). A paradigm for culturally based care in ethnic minority populations. *Journal of Community Psychology, 22,* 192-208.

Kass, B., Weinrick, R., & Monheit, A. (1998). *Racial and ethnic differences in health—1996* (Publication No. 99-0001; chartbook No. 2). Rockville, MD: Agency for Health Care Policy and Research.

Kortak, P. (1991). *Anthropology: the exploration of human diversity.* New York: McGraw-Hill.

Lancaster, J., Onega, L., & Forness, D. (1992). Educational theories, models, and principles applied to community health in nursing. In M. Stanhope & J. Lancaster (Eds.), *Community health nursing: Process and practice for promoting health* (3rd ed.) (pp. 247-264). St. Louis: Mosby.

Lassiter, S.M. (1995). *Multicultural clients: a professional's handbook for health care providers and social workers.* Westport, CT: Greenwood.

Leininger, M. (1995). *Transcultural nursing: concepts, theories, research, and practices.* New York: McGraw-Hill.

Lester, N. (1998). Cultural competence: a nursing dialogue. *American Journal of Nursing, 98*(8), 26-33.

Ludwig-Beymer, P. (1999). Transcultural aspects of pain. In M.M. Andrews & J.S. Boyle (Eds.) *Transcultural concepts in nursing care* (3rd ed.). Philadelphia: JB Lippincott.

Lyon, W.S. (1996). *Encyclopedia of Native American healing.* Santa Barbara, CA: ABC-CLIO.

Malone, B.L. (1998). Diversity, divisiveness and divinity. *American Nurse, 30*(1), 5.

Martinetti, A.M. (1987). Pain and ethnicity. *AORN Journal, 46*(2), 273-281.

May, J. (1992). Working with diverse families: building culturally competent systems of health care delivery. *Journal of Rheumatology, 19*(33), 46-48.

McCaffery, M. (1979). *Nursing management of the patient with pain* (2nd ed). Philadelphia: JB Lippincott.

Paniagua, R.A. (1998). *Assessing and treating culturally diverse clients: a practical guide* (2nd ed.). Thousand Oaks, CA: Sage.

Parry, J.K., & Ryan, A.S. (1995). *A cross-cultural look at death, dying, and religion.* Chicago: Nelson-Hall.

Ramer, L. (1992). *Culturally sensitive caregiving and childbearing families: module 1, series 4. nursing for the 21st century.* White Plains, NY: March of Dimes Birth Defects Foundation.

Richard, L., Potvin, L., Kishchuk, N., Prlic, H., & Green, L.W. (1996). Assessment of the ecological approach in health promotion programs. *American Journal of Health Promotion, 10,* 318-328.

Spector, R.E. (1996). *Cultural diversity in health & illness* (4th ed.). Stamford, CT: Appleton & Lange.

Stewart, M. (1998). Nurses need to strengthen cultural competence for the next century to ensure quality patient care. *American Nurse, 30*(1), 26-27.

Torres, S. (1993, July). Cultural sensitivity: A must for today's primary care provider. *ADVANCE for Nurse Practitioners,* 16-18.

U.S. Department of Health and Human Services (1994). *Health-United States, 1994* (DHHS Pub. No. [PHS] 95-1232). Hyattsville, MD: Public Health Service.

U.S. Department of Health and Human Services (1996). *PATCH: planned approach to community health—guide for the local coordinator.* Washington, DC: Centers for Disease Control and Prevention.

Zackerman, M. (1990). Some dubious premises in research and theory on racial differences. *American Psychologist, 45*(12), 1297-1303.

Zagorsky, E.S. (1993). Caring for families who follow alternative health care practices. *Pediatric Nursing, 19*(10), 71-75.

Zhan, L. (1999). *Asian voices: Asian and Asian-American health educators speak out.* Sudbury, MA: Jones & Bartlett and National League for Nursing Press.

Zola, I. (1966). Culture and symptoms: an analysis of patient's presenting complaints. *American Sociological Review, 31,* 615-930.

Chapter 38

Women's Issues in Health Care

Sue E. Meiner & Cheryl Pope Kish

Women's health issues have traditionally centered on reproductive functions. However, today women are no longer seen as synonymous with their reproductive capacity, and the study of women's health has taken on a much broader meaning. The current interest in women's health is creating intense scientific, political, and commercial interest. Women's health issues are complex, and the social implications cannot be separated from the personal events in women's lives.

Not the least significant reason for the contemporary focus on women's health is that women now represent the gender majority in this country and are the predominant health care consumers. "From women's health courses in universities to mainstream magazine articles, from legislation in Congress to community self-help groups, and from managed care to grassroots activism, women's health has captured the attention of everyday individuals, legislators, and policymakers, health care providers, pharmaceutical manufacturers, and insurance companies" (Kasper, 1998).

For advanced practice nurses (APNs) to recognize the manner in which health risks and concerns affect diverse groups of women and to design responsive care, the nurses must understand how women relate to the world and how their health interfaces with their cultural, economic, and sociopolitical circumstances. This chapter examines multiple dimensions that affect the experience of health and illness in women and the responsive role of APNs.

DEFINITIONS

Gender refers to one's classification as either male or female in society, while *sex* refers to the biological factor of being either male or female. One's sex is determined at conception; gender, as a reference to the unique experience of being either a female or male person, develops over time and begins at birth, when parents begin to treat girl children and boy children differently.

Sexism is a belief that one gender is superior to the other; this accounts for gender discrimination. In many cultures, the male gender is considered superior; male children in such cultures are preferred and female children are less valued. In some cultures, the lives of female children are even sacrificed because of the slight esteem they hold in society.

CRITICAL ISSUES: HEALTH CARE FOR WOMEN

When statistics are reviewed, the role of women in society must be appropriately acknowledged. Approximately 52% of the total U.S. population is female, and 59% of those over age 65 are women. Women also make over 60% of all visits to physicians (Braus, 1997). Given these statistics, it is clear that all APNs will have women as patients; two specialty groups—the certified nurse midwife (CNM) and the women's health nurse practitioner (WHNP)—have female patients as their exclusive domain of practice.

Historically, the health care of women was fragmented, with one medical specialty responsible for care related to childbirth and the reproductive system and others responsible for meeting primary care needs. However, emerging models in contemporary practice are more holistic in nature and often include a multidisciplinary approach. The understanding of women as health care consumers is also increasing with shifts in research initiatives. Until the 1990s, with the exception of reproductive research, the majority of health care recommendations for women were based primarily on research conducted on men (Star, Lommel, & Shannon, 1995). In the 1970s, the Food and Drug Administration (FDA) forbade clinical trials in pregnant women; moreover, health care researchers often excluded women because they found the menstrual cycle and pregnancy to be prohibitive variables. The absence of statistics on women's responses to medical or surgical treatment over the past 30 years has created a significant gap in understanding diseases that contribute to illness and death among American women. It has also limited understanding of pharmacotherapeutics and their use and effect in women. The National Institutes of Health (NIH) began to take steps to improve the dearth of information available for the care and treatment of women's heath problems in 1990. This effort continues through the NIH's Women's Health Initiative (WHI), the largest clinical trial ever undertaken to answer questions regarding heart disease, breast cancer, and osteoporosis in women (Kasper, 1998).

The Society for the Advancement of Women's Health Research, created in 1990, was instrumental in the work of the NIH and in getting both the federal government and private industry to increase spending on women's health research. In 1993, the FDA reversed its former policy banning pregnant women from being included in clinical trials, and they subsequently developed a policy of inclusion for women in most clinical trials (Sarto, 1998).

Women are also being recognized for their power as consumers, not only by virtue of their numbers but also because they make three fourths of the health care decisions for American families and spend two of every three health care dollars annually, which amounts to an annual expenditure of nearly $500 billion (Smith Barney Research, 1998). Not surprisingly, with these provocative data health care providers and suppliers have begun to reshape the health care industry to capitalize on the fact that "women are the largest growing niche market in U.S health care history" (Phillips, Himwich, & Fitzgerald, 1999a).

Patterns of Health, Illness, and Death in Women

Women experience health and illness within the context of their social and cultural situation and their life circumstances. Cultural influences seem particularly significant to the way in which women view and prioritize preventive care. Racial and ethnic differences and the way in which people are assigned to an ethnic group confound gender diversity; few human beings can be neatly categorized into a specific box, and this makes interpreting epidemiological studies more complex (Sarto, 1998). There are some differences in the patterns of certain illness along racial, ethnic, and gender lines.

Domestic violence, which is covered extensively in Chapter 40, crosses all racial and ethnic populations, and heart disease and cancer are two primary causes of death in women of all ethnic groups; cancer is first for Asians, while heart disease ranks first as a cause of death in the other groups. As can be seen in Table 38-1, African-American, Hispanic, and Native American women are far more likely to die from diabetes than Caucasian women, but Caucasian women are more likely to die of chronic obstructive pulmonary disease (COPD). Although both African-American and Asian women have lower mean calcium intakes over their lifetimes, they have fewer osteoporotic fractures; there appears to be a genetic predisposition to osteoporosis in Caucasian women (Sarto, 1998). Unintentional injuries are a common killer of Native American women, and human immunodeficiency virus (HIV) is a common cause of death for African-American and Hispanic women. Asian and Native American women are more likely to die from suicide.

Age strongly influences causes of death in all women. For example, women from 25 to 64 years of age are more likely to die from cancer; for older women, the number-one cause of death is heart disease. The major causes of death among women ages 15 to 24 include unintentional injuries, homicide, and suicide. The majority of accidental

Table 38-1

Leading Causes of Death in Women by Ethnic Group

	CAUCASIAN	AFRICAN AMERICAN	HISPANIC	NATIVE AMERICAN/ ALASKA NATIVE	ASIAN/PACIFIC ISLANDER
1.	Heart disease	Heart disease	Heart disease	Heart disease	Cancer
2.	Cancer	Cancer	Cancer	Cancer	Heart disease
3.	Stroke	Stroke	Stroke	Unintentional injuries*	Stroke
4.	COPD	Diabetes mellitus	Diabetes mellitus	Diabetes mellitus	Unintentional injuries*
5.	Pneumonia/ influenza	Unintentional injuries*	Unintentional injuries*	Stroke	Pneumonia/influenza
6.	Unintentional injuries*	Pneumonia/influenza	Pneumonia/influenza	Chronic liver disease/ cirrhosis	Diabetes mellitus
7.	Diabetes mellitus	HIV infection	COPD	Pneumonia/influenza	COPD
8.	Atherosclerosis	Perinatal conditions†	Perinatal conditions†	COPD	Suicide
9.	Nephritis‡	COPD	HIV infection	Nephritis‡	Congenital anomalies
10.	Septicemia	Homicide¶	Congenital anomalies	Suicide	Homicide¶

*Includes motor vehicle accidents.
†Defined as "certain conditions originating in the perinatal period."
‡Includes nephrotic syndrome and nephrosis.
¶Includes legal intervention.
Data extracted from *Health, United States, 1995.*

deaths are caused by motor vehicle accidents, and women ages 25 to 34 die from motor vehicle accidents more often than any other cause. However, during these childbearing years, cancers of the breast, uterus, brain, and nervous system rank next in frequency, with leukemia and Hodgkin's disease causing the most cancer deaths. Again, homicide and suicide rank high on the list of causes of death in this age group (Fogel & Woods, 1995). Cardiovascular disease remains high in rank order, with most deaths caused by active rheumatic fever, chronic rheumatic heart disease, ischemic heart disease, acute myocardial infarction, and cerebrovascular disease (Fogel & Woods, 1995).

Although the major causes of death for women between age 35 and 44 are quite similar to the previous group, some cancers present more often than others. The main neoplasia involves the breast, lung, uterus, ovary, colon, and rectum. Additionally, leukemia and neoplasms of the lymphatic and hematopoietic systems account for significant deaths. Cardiovascular disease ranks second, with all other major disease states following accidents, suicide, and cerebrovascular disease (Fogel & Woods, 1995).

Cardiovascular disease is the number-one killer of women between the ages of 65 to 74 years. Neoplasms rank second. The next three causes, in order, are cerebrovascular disease, COPD, and pneumonia. This pattern continues for women 75 years of age and older (Fogel & Woods, 1995). Some diseases are more prevalent for women in general, including osteoporosis, arthritis, migraine headaches, fibromyalgia, lupus erythematosus, and thyroid disease. Urinary incontinence, a major factor for quality of life for older women, is disproportionately more common in women.

Some diseases present differently in women (e.g., heart disease). After menopause, a woman's risk of heart disease increases dramatically. "Heart disease takes a considerably greater toll on women than any other illness, including breast cancer, which, with its annual death toll of approximately 44,000 women, frightens them far more but kills them far less frequently" (Queenan & Beauregard, 1997). Following angina, which may not present in the same way as in men, the most frequent signs of heart disease for women are abdominal or epigastric pain, shortness of breath, nausea, vomiting, and fatigue (Cerrato, 1998). When sudden deaths in women were studied, three fourths of the women that died from myocardial infarction did not present with chest pain (Burke, Farb, Malcolm, Liang, Smialek, & Vermani, 1998).

Since coronary heart disease occurs in women some 10 to 15 years later than in men, informed asymptomatic women can alter their cardiovascular risks. However, symptomatic women often wait a while to see a health care provider, thus delaying diagnosis and treatment options that might reduce the severity of the disease (Halm & Penque, 1999). Women are less likely than men to be offered aggressive management of heart disease.

Osteoporosis is more common in women; bone loss is

more common among women who are fair skinned, of slender build, small in stature, and of northern European or Asian backgrounds. Treatment for osteoporosis has only been available for a few years, mainly because previous research had not been extensive enough to determine the cause and curative therapies. During the past decade, research found that treatment with estrogen replacement therapy in postmenopausal women was beneficial in the prevention of osteoporosis.

Women's Self-Care Activities

Unsafe lifestyle behaviors often lead to chronic or fatal health outcomes. The personal choices that may be amended when health teaching provides new information for receptive women need to be a goal of all APNs. Some of the behaviors that lend themselves to potential change are shown in Box 38-1.

Women contribute significantly to their own health through the practice of initiating self-care behaviors. These behaviors include taking vitamins, using contraceptives, taking prescription medications, and following dietary alterations when necessary for health maintenance (Fogel & Woods, 1995).

African-American Women

The reasons for the underuse of health services among African-American women, despite the fact that they bear a

---

Box 38-1

Lifestyle Behaviors that Contribute to Morbidity and Mortality in Women

- Cigarette smoking or a secondhand smoke environment
- Substance use or abuse (e.g., of alcohol, nicotine, caffeine, cocaine, or marijuana)
- Long-term use of prescription or nonprescription tranquilizers or pain medications
- Overuse of medication due to a failure to read or understand warnings or instructions for use
- Sedentary lifestyle and a lack of exercise or personal fitness
- Nutritional excesses and deficits (binging, purging, and anorexia more common among women)
- Unsafe automobile driving (e.g., inattention to the road or road conditions, not using seatbelts)
- Violence toward women (e.g., abuse or battering, rape, suicide, homicide, emotional traumas)
- Exposure to STDs, HIV, or hepatitis
- Lack of personal health care (e.g., no immunizations, no breast self-examinations, no Pap smears, unprotected sexual intercourse)
- Poor sleep habits or patterns

From Youngkin, E.Q., & Davis, M.S. (1998). *Women's health: a primary care clinical guide*. Upper Saddle River, NJ: Prentice-Hall.

heavier burden of disease, are complex. A combination of economic, cultural, and historical factors, including increased poverty, limited access to health insurance, and a health belief system that is not entirely steeped in the biomedical model, all contribute to such underuse (Bayne-Smith, 1996).

According to Duelberg (1992), African-American women are more likely to be obese and less likely to exercise than their Caucasian counterparts. They are more likely, however, to have cancer screening, possibly because several educational initiatives have targeted African-American women. More African-American women than Caucasian women die each year as a result of cancer (of the breast, lung, colon, rectum, ovary, uterus, and esophagus); cardiovascular and cerebrovascular disease; chemical dependency; cirrhosis of the liver; diabetes mellitus; homicide; and accidents (Bayne-Smith, 1996). More African-American women also die in childbirth each year than do Caucasian women. Following childbirth, African-American infants are three times more likely to die during the first year of life (Johnson, 1999). The National Cancer Institute (NCI) identified African American women in the age group of 65 to 74 years as having a higher rate of lung cancer than breast cancer. Lifestyle issues of increased smoking or living in conditions with secondary smoke are seen as contributing factors.

Bayne-Smith (1996) studied young African-American adolescent mothers to learn the cost of their diminished education and the possible lifetime loss of earnings. Keeping young mothers in school or providing for home education has become a priority in many major cities to combat teenage mothers becoming school dropouts and the cycle of poverty dropping out engenders. Infant mortality among teenage mothers and babies has been linked to a lack of prenatal care early in the pregnancy; nutritional deficiencies; poor environmental conditions; and a lack of social or family support.

African-American women are among the poorest of the poor. They are less likely than women of other races to finish high school or attend college. The majority of young African-American women are employed in low-paying, unskilled jobs. They have marginally benefited from public health programs for teenage pregnancies. African-American women experience proportionately higher numbers of health problems than all other minority populations (Johnson, 1999).

Hispanic Women

Hispanic women comprise one of the youngest population groups in the United States. Hispanic women are more likely to live in poverty than are African-American or Caucasian women. The definition of health in many Hispanic families is holistic. Good health for a woman means that she is following a role determined by the customs of her church, family, and local community. Illness is absent in the definition.

A dearth of research information is available on health patterns among Hispanic women. While major diagnostic groups have been noted by the National Center for Health Statistics (NCHS) (1995), sparse details have been published on the reasons for these patterns. The leading causes of death among Hispanic women are cardiovascular disease; cancer (in the following order of occurrence: lung, colorectal, breast, uterine); cerebrovascular disease; diabetes mellitus; accidents (non–motor vehicle); pneumonia and influenza; motor vehicle accidents; perinatal complications; COPD; and asthma (NCHS, 1995). While the incidence of breast cancer is lower in Hispanic women than in non-Hispanic Caucasian women, the death rate is higher. This fact is likely related to the stage at which breast cancer is diagnosed. Fewer Hispanic women have professional breast examinations, mammograms, and Pap smears than do non-Hispanic women.

Diabetes mellitus has reached an epidemic proportion among the Hispanic population. Hispanic women who experience gestational diabetes have a 30% to 40% chance of developing type 2 diabetes by midlife.

Lifestyle-related health problems include sexually transmitted diseases (STDs), domestic violence, and reproductive health problems associated with STDs (Bayne-Smith, 1996). Among Hispanic women, there are higher rates of chlamydia, gonorrhea, and trichomoniasis than in most other groups. Primary and secondary syphilis has increased in teenage Hispanic females at a similar rate to African-American teenage females.

Hispanic women continue to have difficulties in securing health care; financial, cultural, and institutional barriers are seen as reasons for this problem. Medical and nursing research with this population as a sample is so limited that specific disease information is difficult to obtain. Shortages of bilingual and bicultural health care providers also add to the continuing problem of health care access (Torres, 1996).

Native American/Alaska Native Women

Health in relation to the Native American culture greatly varies from Western medicine. Native American cultures for centuries understood health to "mean simply the balance or beauty of all things physical, spiritual, emotional, and social. Sickness was seen as something out of balance, the absence of harmony" (Kauffman, 1992). Women in the Native American culture are an integral force for balance and harmony. According to Niethammer (1977), women are seen in the roles of sacred lifegivers, teachers, caregivers, herbalists, "doctors," political voices, spiritual messengers, and warriors.

The health status of Native American and Alaska Native women is affected by long-standing poverty (below the federal poverty level) and poor socioeconomic conditions. These conditions have added to some of the chronic conditions that affect women. The leading causes of death among Native American and Alaska Native women include heart disease, accidents, cancer (cervical cancer being the most common in Alaska Native women), chronic liver disease/cirrhosis, cerebrovascular disease, and pneumonia and influenza (U.S. Indian Health Service, 1993). Although the leading causes of death in Native American women are heart disease and cancer, these diseases appear at a statistically lower rate than that for Caucasian women. Alcoholism and alcohol abuse continue to be major concerns, with patterns of alcoholism varying from tribe to tribe and region to region (Bayne-Smith, 1996).

Native American women have the highest incidence of both type 1 and type 2 diabetes of all races in America. Amputation of the lower extremities is common in Native American women. Likewise, gestational diabetes is quite common in young women and leads to the risk of developing type 2 disease within 2 decades (Bayne-Smith, 1996).

Among Alaska Native women, cancer is the leading cause of death. Native American women of the Northern Plains states and Alaska Native women have the highest rates of cancer (of all types) of all races in the United States. The poor survival rate of cervical cancer among Alaska Native women is attributed to late diagnoses.

The birthrate for women of these groups was higher than for all other races in America during the early 1990s; teenage pregnancy accounted for nearly 25% of the births. Chlamydia and gonorrhea account for the most STDs in these populations (Bayne-Smith, 1996).

Depression, with or without attempted or completed suicide, has been studied for 2 decades in these populations. Kauffman (1992) suggests that any diagnosis of mental health problems in Native American and Alaska Native women needs to consider their life circumstances in terms of economic, political, cultural, and lifestyle issues.

The balance of health for Native American and Alaska Native women is believed to be emotional, physical, spiritual, and social harmony, and this belief has been partially responsible for these women's neglect of preventive and screening health services. However, the poor economic conditions and the intense poverty they have created have also prevented sufficient health care services from being readily available to all Native American and Alaska Native women.

Asian/Pacific Islander Women

Common health problems with significant incidence and prevalence rates among Asian and Pacific Islander women include cardiovascular disease, cancer (of the breast, colon, rectum, lung, and cervix), hepatitis B infection, and tuberculosis (Zhan, 1999). Stroke and cerebrovascular disease are initially more common among Asian and Pacific Islander women than coronary artery disease (CAD); however, after one or two generations in America, the rate

of CAD increases, while the rate of cerebrovascular disease decreases (Zhan, 1999). The patterns in Asian women for the incidence and prevalence of breast, colorectal, and lung cancer are similar to other racial groups in America. However, cervical cancer is higher in the Asian and Pacific Islander women.

Tobacco and alcohol are not seen as significant health problems among Asian and Pacific Islander women when compared to their use by Caucasian women. Domestic violence in this population seems to increase as a health problem when the male authority as the patriarchal family head is damaged due to wives finding employment and expressing themselves in a nontraditional assertive manner (Choi, 1996).

Many Asian and Pacific Islander women identify fear related to misconceptions of federal policies on citizenship as a major factor in not seeking health care. The fear of being deported for seeking health care when public assistance is the only method of payment for services is identified as a main reason for reduced health care (Mayeno & Hirota, 1994). Health promotion programs must be culturally and linguistically appropriate, and health care providers must be knowledgeable of this population's cultural background (Zhan, 1999).

Women with Disabilities

Disabilities can be placed in basic categories such as sensory deficits, chronic musculoskeletal diseases, and cognitive or mental impairments; certainly they have the potential to affect every aspect of a woman's life through limiting her independence and functional status. Accessibility of health care may also be affected. For example, the physical design of a clinic space may include barriers and make visits more challenging; transfer to an examination table or positioning for an optimal gynecological examination may also be difficult. APNs need to assess patients' special needs before initiating care and accommodate the needs as much as possible (Bergman & Welner, 1994). APNs need to appreciate that wheelchairs, crutches, and other such items are part of a patient's personal belongings and personal space (Sawin, 1998).

Like other women, women with disabilities want to be valued as women. They need to be able to voice their needs and concerns and be treated nonjudgmentally. Often, they have greater knowledge about the medical aspects of their disabilities than the APN; this should not cause defensiveness on the part of the APN. Instead, this knowledge can be used to make the patient more of a partner in her care (Sawin, 1998).

Lesbian Women

For women who are lesbians, there is a "predominant sexual and affectional attraction for members of their own gender that remains over a significant period of time, whether or not they are sexually involved with women at a behavioral level" (Alexander, 1996). Like disabled women, patients who are lesbians share more commonalities with other women than differences. Surely such a patient needs and deserves the same level of health care. Too often, though, a lesbian patient will delay seeking care and enter the system only when necessary because of illness—not for preventative care. Often this is because of previous negative experiences with health care providers who have caused them embarrassment or been patronizing or outright hostile. Sometimes a lesbian patient has been made to feel uncomfortable by a provider who dwelled on the issue of her sexual orientation rather than treating her as a person with unique needs. A young lesbian patient who has not yet disclosed her sexual orientation may be worried that there will be visible signs of her sexual preference. Some lesbian patients will even hide their sexual orientation during clinic visits at the risk of not getting their health care needs met.

Although it is difficult to know with certainty the percentage of women who are homosexual, estimates suggest that between 2% and 10% of women in the United States are lesbians. According to Alexander (1996), 4% to 7% of all women have had a same gender partner at some point in time. Given this, APNs who believe that they will not encounter this aspect of human diversity in their practice sites are mistaken. Lesbian women are at risk for breast cancer secondary to nulliparity; moreover, because they are less likely to perform breast self-examination, tumors may not be found until the later stages. Lesbian women are also at risk for alcohol abuse, depression, obesity, vaginal candidiasis, and bacterial vaginosis. With exclusive female sexual partners, lesbian patients are less likely to have abnormal Pap smears; in fact, some providers suggest that Pap smears may be done every 3 years in such cases without undue risk.

A lesbian couple may decide they want to become parents through adoption or one partner becoming pregnant. In such cases it should be noted that some people in society tolerate or accept lesbianism but are troubled by those with a same-gender sexual preference bearing and rearing children. APNs who care for childbearing families need to examine their own feelings about this topic before being asked to provide sensitive care for such a diverse couple. Those working in pediatric settings might encounter children with same-gender parents.

APNs should never make assumptions about a patient's sexual orientation. APNs understand that heterosexual relationships can exist outside a conventional marriage and are careful to use the word "partner" (not "husband"); this same approach, used with all women, will show sensitivity for the partnered relationships of lesbian patients. There are many ways to frame assessment questions that do not make assumptions. Questions may include: Are you in a committed relationship? Are you in a relationship that involves intercourse? When was your last sexual contact

(not your last sexual intercourse)? Which safe-sex practice have you adopted? Has it been consistently used? Who do you consider your immediate family? Who would you want involved in your care if you became ill or needed to be hospitalized?"

If a lesbian patient does disclose her orientation to an APN, it is important to act nonjudgmentally and not surprised or shocked. Perhaps a question such as "Do others know?" or "Does that cause you special concern?" would be sensitive at the moment of disclosure.

APNs need to be able to talk to lesbian patients about gender-appropriate safe sex (e.g., not mixing sex with alcohol or drugs that would limit inhibitions and cause risky behavior; talking with a partner before engaging in sexual behavior; using barriers [condoms, dental dams, plastic wrap, latex gloves, or finger cots] with sexual devices and between all organs or orifices where there is a chance of exchanging body fluids with sexual devices). If an individual is bisexual, other aspects of safe sex need to be added.

Physical examination proceeds as usual for lesbian patients. A gentle vaginal examination is important. Allowing partners to be present during the examination and any discussion should be an option if it is the wish of the patient.

Designing Health Care for Women

Recommendations for optimizing the health care of women have been made by an expert panel from the American Academy of Nursing (1997). Box 38-2 provides an overview of these eleven recommendations.

In designing interventions to meet the health care needs of women, one must also consider what women want from the health care system. Phillips et al (1999a) identify the following substantive features that most women want in their health care:

1. To be taken seriously as they voice concerns about various aspects of their health, describe their symptoms, and seek information to answer pressing questions or provide additional details about their problem. Being taken seriously implies being "heard" and not rushed in the description of symptoms.
2. To be able to communicate with a clinician who can provide accurate and complete answers to questions and does not hold stereotypes about women as barriers to the provider-patient relationship.
3. To be treated with respect, with privacy and confidentiality ensured.
4. To have a caregiver they can trust within a provider-patient relationship that is empathic and caring.
5. To be treated holistically. Women prefer to be clothed and have their initial encounter with a clinician in an office, not an examination room. They also prefer to have time with the clinician in the office setting after the examination for a discussion of findings and the management plan.

Recommendations for Optimizing Women's Health Care

1. Provide health care to all women, regardless of their ability to pay.
2. Provide access to comprehensive health services, including health promotion and maintenance, restoration of health, and prevention of disease.
3. Provide access to a range of providers for primary care and specialty services, including APNs such as NPs, CNMs, and CNSs and medical specialists such as gynecologists and obstetricians.
4. Create access to services in a number of sites (e.g., schools, workplaces, homes, churches, public health settings such as community clinics, family planning clinics, birthing centers, nursing homes, intergenerational day care programs for young and old, and senior centers).
5. Provide funding for educational programs for APNs and retraining for nurses who have practiced in hospital settings to meet anticipated needs for primary care providers (PCPs).
6. Expand educational programs to prepare all health care providers to care for women in ways that enhance the acceptability of care and reduce gender bias in delivery of services.
7. Appoint women to boards that govern health care at all levels and to provider panels in MCOs.
8. Expand research and research training that will extend nursing's knowledge of women's health.
9. Enhance the public health infrastructure necessary to support population-based services.
10. Include in the evaluation of health care quality the availability of gender-specific health services.
11. Seek and apply for resources for international collaborative projects specific to women's health.

From Expert Panel on Women's Health (1997). Women's health and women's health care: recommendations of the 1996 AAN expert panel on women's health. *Nursing Outlook, 45*(1), 7-15.

6. To have a comfortable, "homey" environment. The decor in the waiting areas and examination rooms is important to female patients, as is a warm, comfortable, and quiet setting. Small comforts like padded stirrups and reading materials in the examination room are valued by women.
7. To have convenience. A clinic that is open at convenient hours, including evenings and weekends, is a real advantage to working women or those who must wait for a working partner to care for children so that she can visit her health care provider. Nearby parking with a well-lighted lot lends security and convenience. Clear previsit instructions and an understandable billing system are also important features.

Responses to surveys conducted by managed care organizations (MCOs) reveal that women in all age groups also want the following features in their health care (Nikkel 1998): follow-up on both positive and negative test results, reminders of routine follow-up needs (e.g., cards announcing that it is time for an annual gynecological examination), access to advice by telephone, and access to health education. Warner (1996) would add that women also want a choice between a male and female provider and the type of provider (physician or APN).

IMPLICATIONS FOR MSN EDUCATION AND ADVANCED PRACTICE

Women's health research and clinical practice need to be given the attention necessary to maintain movement toward equity in health care. Women, as informed consumers, need to be given information concerning health care issues that affect themselves and all members of their families. Scientists and providers from all health-related disciplines need to take part in gender-specific education and practice.

Understanding women's health needs requires an awareness of the life experiences and context of their lives. APNs are a national resource for providing primary health education and health care to all women. Comprehensive health care services must be made available to all women throughout their lifespans. Designing and marketing such comprehensive services presupposes that one understands what women prefer in their health care experiences and incorporates these preferences into making programs and services appealing to female patients. As women continue to represent a growing market niche, the ability to market gender-specific care will be an important advantage for health care organizations. Inclusive women's services include outpatient care with a focus on information, education, and health resources (e.g., support groups; ambulatory and diagnostic centers for breast, bone, continence, heart, menopause management, and infertility; maternity centers) and inpatient specialty care for gynecological care, breast problems, and urogynecology. Success in women's health care requires more than attractive rooms or clever advertising campaigns; success depends on services with substance and on care programs that emphasize "care" (Phillips, Himwich, & Fitzgerald, 1999b).

Numerous communities are initiating sexual assault nurse examiner (SANE) programs that ensure the presence of gender-specific providers in emergency settings for patients who experience rape. Many health care agencies are offering wellness care options, such as weight management, smoking cessation, and other counseling programs appealing to women as part of their gender-specific programs. As the numbers of women experiencing perimenopausal symptoms increase (to over 20 million by 2010), more programs related to aging and managing menopause will be needed. With more bone-density testing for osteoporosis and multichannel urodynamic testing for continence-related problems being done, support services can be added that relate to these specialty area of women's health. Preconception care is another attractive service option for women in the context of wellness management. APNs who have an awareness of the context of women's lives and understand the holistic needs of women will be ideally positioned to manage or provide care in innovative ambulatory programs and services such as these.

According to Nikkel (1998), care for women requires consideration of certain fundamental features, including "awareness of women's lives, reflective of the diversity of women, oriented to comprehensive care across the life-span, incorporated in a range of services, delivered by a range of health care providers, and accessible to all women." Because APNs tend to embrace a holistic as opposed to a biomedical view of women, they will appreciate that programs need to address health promotion, maintenance, and restoration of women's health across the lifespan and incorporate "treatment for diseases unique to women, more prevalent in women, or for which there are different risk factors for women" (Nikkel, 1998).

APNs should understand that health care for women begins with school-aged girls, who need to learn about good nutrition, healthy lifestyle behaviors that promote health, and the transitions of puberty. Body image and nutrition education may help to prevent the eating disorders so common in young women. APNs may address these care issues in their practice sites, or they may engage young girls in programs offered in school-based clinics or after hours in such places as churches, scouts, and clubs.

For the teen population, APNs must set a health care agenda that promotes good nutrition and healthy behavior, prevention of pregnancy and STDs, avoidance of risky behaviors that lead to injury and date rape, and avoidance of drug and alcohol abuse. Pregnancy-related care, including childbirth and parenting education, should be available (with an adolescent focus).

A common problem for adolescent girls is misinformation about sexuality. Because more than half of teenage girls are sexually active before they graduate from high school, a clear goal for APNs whose practices include teens and preteens is education about sexuality. Sexuality education for this group must focus on issues of safety and self-respect and present a clear message that they do not have to become sexually active until they are ready for the emotions such a relationship entails. Help in knowing how to offer a convincing "no" and roleplaying responses can be really helpful.

Childbirth still accounts for the highest incidence of hospital admissions in this country (Welsh & Ludwig-Beymer, 1998). Consequently, women of childbearing age need a full range of pregnancy-related services that are family centered, including preconception, prenatal, labor and delivery, and postpartum care. APNs in practice sites with pregnant women need a skill and knowledge base to promote healthy pregnancy, recognize complications, and either co-manage or refer women with complications. Assessment of fetal well-being is an important dimension of care, as is family planning services. One in six couples of childbearing age also needs access to infertility services. Educational programs that support childbearing and parenting are invaluable; these might include Lamaze, breast-feeding, and parenting classes for the couple (as well as classes for siblings and grandparents).

While women at midlife may still need childbearing services, meeting their health needs also requires a focus on self-care, early detection and treatment of chronic illness, management of perimenopause, and understanding of the pros and cons of hormone replacement. For many women, issues of employment and the challenges of being "sandwiched" between the competing needs of children and aging parents also need attention.

As women age, they experience the accumulative changes that come with growing older. They may need help in dealing with multiple changes in the areas of sexual function; ill health or death of spouse and friends; vision; hearing; and mobility; some will need help with a transition to new living arrangements with their children or in residential communities or nursing homes. Home health care services will likely be increasingly important for aging women. Many aging women need care related to incontinence and osteoporosis; some, because of dementia or Alzheimer's disease, have special needs related to memory loss. APNs working with aging women need to be comfortable with assessments of functional status as a basis for many decisions about health care.

Women of all ages need access to a full range of gynecological services (including assessment and treatment or referral for gynecological malignancy), as well as primary care that addresses appropriate age-specific screening tests for health maintenance. Issues of sexuality, violence, contraception, menstrual disorders, and STDs continue throughout all life stages. Access to mental health care should also be ensured. A knowledge base in pharmacology, including drug safety during pregnancy and lactation, is essential for APNs working with women, especially those APNs who are prescribing.

The extent to which Master of Science in Nursing (MSN) programs are accountable for educating APNs for roles involving women depends on the kinds of specialists being prepared. Obviously, a Master's program educating CNMs will have a very different educational focus with regard to women's care than will programs preparing pediatric nurse practitioners (PNPs) or neonatal nurse practitioners (NNPs). However, all APNs work with women in some capacity and will need to understand the context of women's lives. For example, PNPs and NNPs encounter women as mothers and grandmothers of their child patients. Family nurse practitioners (FNPs), even if their practice sites do not manage pregnant patients, provide primary and gynecological care for women; indeed, over half of their patients will likely be female. The extent to which the clinical nurse specialist (CNS) cares for women is very dependent on the practice site. One need only examine a comprehensive textbook for women's health to appreciate the range of topics applicable to women across the lifespan and the inherent content necessary in programs that prepare specialists to work in women's health.

For many graduate students, a course on women's health provides the first requirement for feeling comfortable with sexual assessment and counseling. This sensitive topic should not be overlooked in programs educating students for roles with female patients, because sexuality is a topic applicable to women across the lifespan. APNs need to be knowledgeable about sexuality and comfortable in discussions about it. Since many patients will have questions or concerns they are uncomfortable discussing, APNs should be familiar with strategies that encourage dialogue—for example, "giving voice" by saying something like, "Most of the women I work with have questions about how their pregnancy will affect their sexual relationship. What questions do you have?" or "Women often wonder how having genital herpes will affect their sex life. What concerns do you have about how this diagnosis will affect you?"

The educational program's philosophy, conceptual underpinnings, and program objectives will determine the extent to which topics pertinent to women's health are covered in a particular curriculum. With more than half of all patients being female, attention to the health problems and concerns of women will be addressed to some extent in most Master's programs. Classroom and clinical experiences should be designed to be congruent with the mission, philosophy, and objectives of the program.

In the last decade, there has been some discussion about the need for specialist practitioners in the area of men's health. There are currently some gaps in the health care services marketed to men and some compelling patterns of morbidity and mortality among men that necessitate reevaluation of men's health care. Bozett and Forrester (1989) noted a lack of skill on the part of many clinicians to get behind the male facade to deal with problems and concerns that men have difficulty voicing. Men have higher morbidity rates for unintentional injuries, coronary heart disease, emphysema, peptic ulcer, and hernia. Men also die more often than women from lung cancer, COPD, myocardial infarction, cirrhosis of the liver, homicide, and suicide (Forrester, 2000). Men seek care less than women; in fact, American women "see their health care providers approximately 150 million times more than American men" (Peters, 1999). Men often deny their physical symptoms and are less likely to disclose concerns to strangers out of fear of appearing emotionally vulnerable. "Fear, denial, threats to masculinity, and embarrassment are all impediments to men seeking health

care" (Peters, 1999). Contraception is not "held ransom" for men; unlike women, men do not have to undergo annual examination to access birth control pills. Hence, many men do not undergo routine health screening, even when they are at risk for particular illnesses. For example, Dan, age 42, has never had his cholesterol checked, even though his father died at age 51 from myocardial infarction. Also, Joe, whose father died from colon cancer, keeps putting off his screening test. "Although some men seek care for their hearts from cardiologists or treatment for their prostates from urologists, problems requiring a nonspecialist or more holistic approach often go unattended" (Forrester, 2000).

According to Dr. Kenneth Goldberg, urologist and author of *How Men Can Live as Long as Women* (1993), the Summit Group (cited in Peters, 1999), an analogy of automotive preventive maintenance, can be used successfully to help men understand the importance of preventive care. Men are socialized to messages like "no pain, no gain," "grin and bear it," and other such "macho" phrases that cause them to avoid health care. Education and aggressive marketing of health care options for men are needed, and some believe a men's health curriculum and men's health practitioners may be required to remedy what is perceived as a gap in men's health care and to optimize health care for this gender.

Whether APNs work with patients of either or both genders, they should continue to assess their own respective capacities to interact in culturally sensitive ways. In working with female patients, APNs need to consider a person's life stage, actual age, health status, socioeconomic position, race and ethnicity, sexual orientation, and baseline ability or disability. APNs need to stay informed and politically active to ensure that women receive equal representation in law and policy decisions.

PRIORITIES FOR RESEARCH

Any research with the potential to answer questions about health care problems that affect both genders should include both males and females in the sample. Without such research efforts, the imbalance in research that has existed over time will not be redressed. There should be gender-specific study of illnesses, diagnostic testing, and treatments, as well as answers to questions related to gender differences in response to teaching methods and materials used in health promotion and disease management.

Research should continue to focus on the experience of health and illness in women of all ages and racial, ethnic, and socioeconomic groups. Both urban and rural groups should be sampled. Qualitative studies need to expose the "voice" of women about experiences that are unique to women. For example, what is it like to lose both parents in a period of 1 year? What is the experience of losing a baby at age 35, only to try unsuccessfully to get pregnant again? Evaluation studies should address best practices in

Suggestions for Further Learning

- Search the literature for information about how to address the sexuality concerns of female patients at different ages in a sensitive manner. Give attention to women of diverse cultures. Investigate the PLISSIT model (**Per**mission, **L**imited **I**nformation, **S**pecific **S**uggestions, **I**ntensive **T**herapy).
- Consult Sawin, K.J. (1998). Health care concerns for women with physical disability and chronic illness. In E.Q. Youngkin & M.S. Davis (Eds.). *Women's health: a primary clinical guide* (pp. 905-941). Stamford, CT: Appleton & Lange. This is an exemplary chapter and includes numerous resources and references.
- Communication patterns between men and women are different, which helps, in part, to explain the way in which nurse-patient or workplace relationships between the genders are affected by communication. To learn more, read Tanner, D. (1990). *You just don't understand: women and men in conversation*. New York: William Morrow.
- Read Fisher, S. (1995). *Nursing wounds: nurse practitioners, doctors, women patients and the negotiation of meaning*. New Brunswick, NJ: Rutgers University Press.
- Interact with a woman from a culture different than your

own. Discuss her cultural experiences of puberty, childbirth, parenting, illness, and death.
- Investigate the following websites for additional information related to gender:
  - www.library.wisc.edu/libraries/womenstudies/native.htm
  - Women's Study Database at the University of Maryland at www.inform.umd.eduwww.wwwomen.com
  - Agency for Healthcare Research and Quality at ahcpr.gov
  - American College of Obstetrics and Gynecology at www.acog.org
  - Association of Women's Health, Obstetrics, and Neonatal Nursing at www.awhonn.org
  - American College of Nurse Midwifery at www.acnm.org
  - American Medical Women's Association at www.amwa-doc.org
  - Health Information for Minority Women at www.4women.gov/minority/index.htm (available through this site is *Closing the Gap: Minority Women's Health Initiative*, a monthly newsletter)

health promotion, disease prevention, and health maintenance for women. Furthermore, it is critical that findings from these studies be shared for the advantage of women everywhere. For example, is there a particular successful strategy for teens in Hawaii that might be transported to Alabama to lower the rate of STDs? Has a NP in Texas, working in a clinic with a population of Hispanic teens, found an intervention to help young women say "no" to sexual intercourse that would work with Hispanic youths in New York?

Adolescent pregnancy continues to be an area in need of research. The article "Practitioners Can Reduce Teen Pregnancies" (2000) cites a British study (Hippisley-Cox, Allen, Pringle, Ebdon, McPhearson, Churchill, & Bradley, 2000) that found that younger female physicians were associated with reductions in teen pregnancy for the particular practice that was studied. This study should be replicated with APNs.

Studies should address those women of all ethnic groups currently underserved by the health care system. What is their reason for not seeking care? How might this be remedied? How might the needs of special populations of women (e.g., the disabled) be met?

The human experiences of birth, illness, disability, and death are embedded within women's cultural contexts. Studies that would help APNs who represent the majority population understand childbearing, childrearing, and other aspects of womanhood for women of diverse cultures will add significantly to the way in which those women can be helped by the health care system.

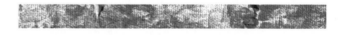

DISCUSSION QUESTIONS

These questions can be used to promote critical thinking and encourage discussion.

1. In every racial and ethnic group, according to sociologist Judith Lorber (1997), women "live longer but not better." Do you agree with this statement? If so, provide your rationale. If not, what is the basis of your disagreement?
2. Lorber asserts that the menstrual cycle has been "medicalized." Do you agree or disagree with this statement? Support your answer with examples.
3. Consider the desire by some people that a specialty in men's health be initiated. Do you believe such a specialty is justified? Support your answer. If you believe such a specialty is justified, what would a curriculum for a Master's degree in men's health include? How would you suggest marketing this kind of educational program? This kind of practice?
4. Starting from the front door, walk throughout the entire clinic setting or unit in which you work. Speculate on how this environment would serve the needs of a disabled patient. What changes would need to be made to make the setting more "friendly" for a female patient with a disability? Consider particularly those persons

who are hearing or visually impaired and those in wheelchairs.

5. Revisit the clinic setting as in #4, but assess the general atmosphere or milieu for the attitudes that would be encountered by lesbian patients. Speculate on how welcome these individuals would feel. How might changes be made to ensure a more warm and welcome atmosphere for patients with diverse sexual orientations?

REFERENCES/BIBLIOGRAPHY

Abbey, A., Andrews, F., & Halman, J.L. (1991). Gender's role in responses to infertility. *Psychology of Women Quarterly, 15,* 295-316.

Alexander, E. (1996). Sexual orientation. In C.A. Johnson, B.E. Johnson, J.L. Murray, & B.S. Apgar (Eds.), *Women's health care handbook* (pp. 53-56). Philadelphia: Hanley & Belfus.

Allen, K.M., & Phillips, J.M. (1997). *Women's health across the lifespan.* Philadelphia: JB Lippincott.

Allen, M. (1994). The dilemma for women of color in clinical trials. *Journal of the American Medical Women's Association, 47,* 105-107.

Auerbach, J.D., & Figert, A.E. (1995). Women's health research: public policy and sociology. *Journal of Health and Social Behavior* (extra issue), 115-131.

Avery, B.Y. (1992). The health status of Black women. In R.L. Braithwaite & S.E. Taylor (Eds.), *Health issues in the Black community* (pp. 35-51). San Francisco: Jossey-Bass.

Bair, B., & Cayleff, S.E. (1993). *Wings of gauze: women of color and the experience of health and illness.* Detroit: Wayne State University.

Bartman, B.A. (1996). Women's access to appropriate providers within managed care: implication for the quality of primary care. *Women's Health Issues, 6,* 45-50.

Bayne-Smith, M. (1996). *Race, gender, and health.* Thousand Oaks, CA: Sage.

Bergman, S., & Welner, S. (1994). *Guidelines for the care of women with disabilities for the primary care practitioner.* New York: McGraw-Hill.

Bergman-Evans, B. (1996). The prevalence of clinical preventive services utilization by older women. *Nurse Practitioner, 21,* 88-106.

Bozett, F.W., & Forrester, D.A. (1989). The men's health nurse practitioner: a proposal. *Image: Journal of Nursing Scholarship, 21*(3), 158-161.

Bransen, E. (1992). Has menstruation been medicalized? Or will it never happen . . . ?. *Sociology of Health and Illness, 14,* 98-110.

Braus, P. (1997). *Marketing health care to women.* Ithaca, NY: American Demographics Books.

Brink-Muinen, A. (Ed). (1998). Principles and practice of women's health care. *Women's Health Issues, 8*(2), 123-130.

Burke, A.P., Farb, A., Malcolm, G.T., Liang, Y., Smialek, J., & Vermani, R. (1998). Effect of risk factors on the mechanism of acute thrombosis and sudden coronary death in women. *Circulation, 97*(21), 2110.

Centers for Disease Control and Prevention. (1999). *Reported tuberculosis cases by race/ethnicity in the United States, 1997.* Atlanta, GA: Centers for Disease Control and Prevention.

Cerrato, P. (1998). Women & heart disease. *RN, 61*(11), 40-44.

Chen, Y.L. (1996). Conformity with nature: a theory of Chinese American elders' health promotion and illness prevention processes. *Advances in Nursing Science, 19*(2), 17-26.

Choi, P. (1996). Tuberculosis concerns for Asian Americans and Pacific Islanders. *Asian American and Pacific Islander Journal of Health, 4*(1-3), 127.

Corea, G. (1992). *The invisible epidemic: the story of women and AIDS.* New York: Harper Perennial.

Costello, C., Stone, A.J., & Women's Research and Education Institute (1994). *The American women, 1994-1995. Where we stand: women and health.* New York: Norton and Company.

Dan, A.J. (1994). *Reframing women's health: multidisciplinary research and practice.* Thousand Oaks, CA: Sage.

Davis, L.J., Okuboye, S., & Ferguson, S.L. (2000). Healthy people 2010: examining a decade of maternal and infant health. *AWHONN Lifelines, 4*(3), 26-33.

Dickerson, B.J. (1995). *African-American single mothers: understanding their lives and families.* Thousand Oaks, CA: Sage.

Dimond, M. (1995). Older women's health. In C.I. Fogel & N.F. Woods (Eds.), *Women's health care: a comprehensive handbook.* Thousand Oaks, CA: Sage.

Doyal, L. (1995). *What makes women sick: gender and the political economy of health.* New Brunswick, NJ: Rutgers University Press.

Duelberg, S.I. (1992). Preventive health behavior among Black and White women in urban and rural areas. *Social Science Medicine, 34*(2), 191-198.

Expert Panel on Women's Health. (1997). Women's health and women's health care: recommendations of the 1996 AAN Expert Panel on Women's Health. *Nursing Outlook, 45*(1): 7-15.

Fee, E., & Krieger (Eds.). (1994). *Women's health, politics, and power.* Amityville, NY: Baywood.

Fennema, K., Meyer, D.L., & Owen, N. (1990). Sex of physicians: patients' preferences and sterotypes. *Journal of Family Practice, 30,* 441-446.

Fisher, S. (1995). *Nursing wounds: nurse practitioners, doctors, women patients and the negotiation of meaning.* New Brunswick, NJ: Rutgers University Press.

Fogel, C.I., & Woods, N.F. (1995). *Women's health care: a comprehensive handbook.* Thousand Oaks, CA: Sage.

Forrester, D.A. (1986). Myths of masculinity: impact upon men's health. *Nursing Clinics of North America, 21*(1), 15-23.

Forrester, D.A. (2000). Revisiting the men's health curriculum. In M.L. Kelley & V.M. Fitsimons (Eds.), *Understanding cultural diversity: culture, curriculum, and community in nursing* (pp. 169-175). Boston: Jones & Bartlett & National League for Nursing Press.

Franks, P., & Clancy, C.M. (1993). Physician gender bias in clinical decision-making: screening for cancer in primary care. *Medical Care, 31,* 213-218.

Galindo, D.J., & Mintzer, M.J. (1998). Comprehensive geriatric assessment of the frail older woman. In L.A. Wallis (Ed.), *Textbook of women's health.* Philadelphia: Lippincott-Raven.

Gannon, L., & Ekstrom, B. (1993). Attitudes toward menopause: the influence of sociocultural paradigms. *Psychology of Women Quarterly, 17,* 275-288.

Geary, A.S. (1995). An analysis of the women's health movement and its impact on delivery of health care within the United States. *Nurse Practitioner, 20,* 24-35.

Goldstein, N. (1993). Lesbians and the medical profession: HIV/AIDS and the pursuit of visibility. *Women's Studies, 24,* 531-552.

Hall, J.A., & Roter, D.L. (1995). Patient gender and communication with physicians: results of a community-based study. *Women's Health: Research on Gender, Behavior, and Policy, 1,* 77-95.

Halm, M.A., & Penque, S. (1999). Heart disease in women. AJN, 99(4): 26-32.

Harding, S. (1991). *Whose science? Whose knowledge? Thinking from women's lives.* Ithaca, NY: Cornell University Press.

Hippisley-Cox, J., Allen, J., Pringle, M., Ebdon, D., McPhearson, M., Churchill, D., & Bradley, S. (2000). Association between teenage pregnancy rates and the age and sex of general practitioners cross sectional survey in Trent 1994-7. *British Medical Journal 320,* 842-845.

Hsia, J. (1993). Gender differences in diagnosis and management of coronary heart disease. *Journal of Women's Health, 2,* 349-352.

Hueppchen, N.A., & Pressman, E.K. (1999). Preconception care: planning for a healthy pregnancy. *Women's Health in Primary Care, 2*(4), 259-262, 265-278.

Hunt, W.G. (1996). Postreproductive gynecology: meeting the present and future needs of women. *American Journal of Obstetrics and Gynecology, 175*(2), 243-247.

Johnson, C.A., Johnson, B.E., Murray, J.L., & Apgar, B.S. (1996). *Women's health care handbook.* Philadelphia: Hanley & Belfus.

Johnson, R.W. (1999). *African American voices: African American health educators speak out.* Sudbury, MA: Jones and Bartlett & National League for Nursing Press.

Jones, W., Snider, D.E., & Warren, R.C. (1996). Deciphering the data: ethnicity and gender as critical variables. *Journal of the American Medical Women's Association, 51,* 137-138.

Kasper, A.S. (1998). Understanding women's health: an overview. In L.A. Wallis (Ed.), *Textbook of women's health.* Philadelphia: Lippincott-Raven.

Kauffman, J.A. (1992). *Indian women's health issues roundtable final report.* Washington, DC: U.S. Department of Health and Human Services, U.S. Indian Health Service.

Kemp, A.A., & Jenkins, P. (1992). Gender and technological hazards: women at risk in hospital settings. *Industrial Crisis Quarterly, 6,* 137-152.

Lahita, R.G. (1998). Fibromyalgia. In L.A. Wallis (Ed.), *Textbook of women's health.* Philadelphia: Lippincott-Raven.

LaRosa, J.H. (1998). Recent initiatives in women's health: a federal perspective. In L.A. Wallis (Ed.), *Textbook of women's health.* Philadelphia: Lippincott-Raven.

Lazarus, E. (1994). What do women want? Issues of choice, control, and class in pregnancy and childbirth. *Medical Anthropology Quarterly, 8,* 25-46.

Leafgren, F. (1990). Being a man can be hazardous to your health: Life-style issues. In D. Moore & F. Leafgren (Eds.), *Problem solving strategies and interventions for men in conflict* (pp. 265-275). Alexandria, VA: American Association for Counseling and Development.

Link, B.G., & Phelan, J. (1995). Social conditions as fundamental causes of disease. *Journal of Health and Social Behavior* (extra issue), 80-94.

Lorber, J. (1997). *Gender and the social construction of illness.* Thousand Oaks, CA: Sage.

Mansfield, P.K., & Voda, A.M. (1997). Women-centered information on menopause. *Health Care for Women International, 18,* 55-72.

Matthews, K.A., Shumaker, S.A., & Bower, D.J. (1997). Women's health initiative: why now? What is it? What's new? *American Psychologist, 52,* 101-116.

Mastroianni, A.C., Faden, R., & Federman, D. (Eds.). (1994). *Women and health research: ethical and legal issues of including women in clinical trials.* Washington, DC: National Academy Press.

Mayeno, L., & Hirota, S.M. (1994). Access to health care. In N.S. Zane, D.T. Takeuchi, & K.J. Young (Eds.), *Confronting critical health issues of Asian and Pacific Islander Americans* (pp. 347-375). Thousand Oaks, CA: Sage.

McAllister, M. (1998). Menopause: providing comprehensive care for women in transition. *Lippincott's Primary Care Practice, 2*(3), 256-270.

Mouton, C.P., & Espino, D.V. (1999). Health screening in older women. *American Family Physician, 59*(7), 1835-1842.

Muller, C. (1990). *Health care and gender.* New York: Russell Sage.

National Center for Health Statistics (1995, March 22). Advance report of final mortality statistics, 1992. *Monthly Vital Statistics Report, 43*(6; supplement). Hyattsville, MD: Centers for Disease Control and Prevention, National Center for Health Statistics.

Niethammer, C. (1977). *Daughters of the earth: the lives and legends of American Indian women.* New York: Macmillan.

Nikkel, M. (1998). Women's health care: roots to recommendations. *Lippincott's Primary Care Practice, 2*(3), 205-209.

Nosek, M.A. (1992). Primary care issues for women with severe disabilities. *Journal of Women's Health, 1,* 245-248.

Peters, S. (1999). Machismo and mortality. *ADVANCE for Nurse Practitioners, 7*(4), 51-52.

Phillips, C.R., Himwich, D.B., & Fitzgerald, C. (1999a, April-May). The business of women's health: what nurses need to know now and in the 21st century. *AWHONN Lifelines,* 23-29.

Phillips, C.R., Himwich, D.B., & Fitzgerald, C. (1999b, June-July). The business of women's health: building a successful women's health practice: part two. *AWHONN Lifelines,* 31-36.

Pinn, V.W. (1999). Women's health research on cardiovascular disease: an agenda for the 21st century. *Women's Health in Primary Care, 2*(12), 930-936.

Practitioners can reduce teen pregnancies. (2000, July). *Clinician Reviews, 10*(7), 51.

Queenan, R.A., & Beauregard, L. (1997). Diseases that are more prevalent in women. In F.P. Haseltine & B.G. Jacobson (Eds.), *Women's health research.* Washington, DC: Health Press International.

Rusek, S.B. (1998). Demographic changes that impact on women's health. In L.A. Wallis (Ed.), *Textbook of women's health.* Philadelphia: Lippincott-Raven.

Rusek, S.B., Olesen, V.L., & Clarke, A.E. (1997). *Women's health: complexities and differences.* Columbus, OH: Ohio State University Press.

Rusk, A., & Plum, F. (1998). Neurologic health and disorders. In L.A. Wallis (Ed.), *Textbook of women's health.* Philadelphia: Lippincott-Raven.

Sabo, D., & Gordon, D.F. (Eds.). (1995). *Men's health and illness: gender, power, and the body.* Thousand Oaks, CA: Sage.

Sarto, G.E. (1998). How race, ethnicity, and culture influence women's health. *Women's Health in Primary Care, 1*(10; supplement), 7-14.

Sawin, K.J. (1998) Health care concerns for women with physical disability and chronic illness. In E.Q. Youngkin & M.S. Davis (Eds.), *Women's health: a primary clinical guide* (pp. 905-941). Stamford, CT: Appleton & Lange.

Sherwin, S. (1992). *No longer patient: feminist ethics and health care*. Philadelphia: Temple University Press.

Siu, A.L., Reuben, D.B., & Moore, A.A. (1994). Comprehensive geriatric assessment. In W.R. Hazzard, E.L. Bierman, & J.P. Bloss (Eds.), *Principles of geriatric medicine and gerontology*. New York: McGraw-Hill.

Smith-Barney Research (1998). *The new women's movement: women's health care*. Available online at www.smithbarney.com/index-.html.

Solarz, A. (1999, October-November). Lesbian health care issues: exploring options for expanding research and delivering care. *AWHONN Lifelines,* 13-14.

Star, W.L., Lommel, L.L., & Shannon, M.T. (1995). *Women's primary health care: protocols for practice*. Washington, DC: American Nurses Publishing.

Tanner, D. (1990). *You just don't understand: women and men in conversation*. New York: William Morrow

Taylor, D.L., & Wood, N.F. (1996). Changing women's health, changing nursing practice. *Journal of Obstetrics, Gynecology, and Neonatal Nursing, 25*(9), 791-802.

Tong, M.F. (1996). The impact of hepatitis B infection in Asian Americans. *Asian American and Pacific Islander Journal of Health, 4*(1-3): 125-126.

Torres, S. (1996). *Hispanic voices: Hispanic educators speak out*. New York: National League for Nursing Press.

U.S. Department of Health and Human Services, National Center for Health Statistics (1994). *Health—United States, 1994* (DHHS Publication No. (PHS) 95-1232). Hyattsville, MD: Public Health Service.

U.S. Department of Health and Human Services, National Institutes of Health (1992). *Reports of the National Institutes of Health: opportunities for research on women's health* (NIH Publication No. 92-3457A). Washington, DC.

U.S. Indian Health Service (1993). *Trends in Indian health*. Washington, DC: U.S. Department of Health and Human Services.

Velkoff, V.A., & Lawson, V.A. (1998). *Gender and aging* (IB/98-3). Washington, DC: U.S. Department of Commerce, Economics and Statistics Administration, U.S. Bureau of the Census.

Wallis, L.A. (1998). *Textbook of women's health*. Philadelphia: Lippincott-Raven.

Warner, C.K. (1996). Planning for women's health care service. *Women's Health Issues, 6*(1), 60-63.

Warshaw, L.J., Lipton, R.B., & Silberstein, S.D. (1998). Migraine: a "woman's disease"? *Women Health, 28*(2), 79-99.

Welner, S. (1998). Caring for the woman with a disability. In L.A. Wallis (Ed.), *Textbook of women's health*. Philadelphia: Lippincott-Raven.

Welsh, C., & Ludwig-Beymer, P. (1998). Shortened lengths of stay: ensuring continuity of care for mothers and babies. *Lippincott's Primary Care Practice, 2*(3), 284-291.

Wenger, N.K. (1994). Coronary heart disease in women: gender differences in diagnostic evaluations. *Journal of the Medical Women's Association, 49,* 181-185.

Wenger, N.K. (1998). Coronary heart disease in women. In L.A. Wallis (Ed.), *Textbook of women's health*. Philadelphia: Lippincott-Raven.

Youngkin, E.Q., & Davis, M.S. (1998). *Women's health: a primary care clinical guide*. Upper Saddle River, NJ: Prentice-Hall.

Zhan, L. (1999). *Asian voices: Asian and Asian-American health educators speak out*. Sudbury, MA: Jones and Bartlett and National League for Nursing Press.

Chapter 39

Age Issues in Health Care

Sue E. Meiner

Cultural pluralism in the United States has become the accepted norm. This multicultural country demonstrates that different cultures can function side by side in some contexts and retain cultural uniqueness in other contexts. However, while younger members of ethnic groups often fit this scenario, older members, especially first-generation immigrants, have not readily accepted the side-by-side multicultural experience. Older adults are more likely to have been socialized in family and community groups where ethnic beliefs and values permeated everything in their daily lives (Holmes & Holmes, 1995). This is not to say that all ethnic older adults have remained within their community of ethnic origin and not ventured into other diverse environments. Change does occur following immigration to the United States. However, customs, rituals, language, and group cohesiveness remain intact within many cultural groups (Holmes & Holmes, 1995).

Older adults have become a new and flourishing minority group in the United States (Spector, 1996). Every week, more than 200 Americans celebrate turning 100 years of age, and it is estimated that the number of persons over age 85 will increase to nearly 24 million in the next 40 years; this group is now the fastest-growing segment of society. Persons ages 65 and over will number greater than 87 million in the next 40 years (American Association of Retired Persons, 1998). With numbers such as these, advanced practice nurses (APNs) will clearly see more aging individuals in their practices. This chapter examines the health issues of older adults and how they affect the culturally competent care provided by APNs in varied settings.

DEFINITIONS

Older adults, sometimes referred to as *elderly* or *aged adults*, are those individuals who have lived to an age of 60 years or older. A fast-growing subgroup has been identified as the **oldest old**—those individuals age 85 or older. The aging population in the United States is a particularly heterogeneous group, but many stereotypes exist to the contrary—stereotypes that present a negative view of aging that leads to **ageism,** or the belief that people of certain ages are inferior to others. The often distorted, negative view of aging that forms the belief framework of ageism promotes age discrimination.

Functional status, an important concept to the study of aging, refers to an individual's ability to perform those self-care measures that are considered **activities of daily living** (ADLs). Activities of daily living generally include self-care behaviors associated with health and hygiene needs. **Instrumental activities of daily living** (IADLs) include physical performance behaviors needed to remain independent. (Box 39-1 provides a listing of the elements of ADLs and IADLs.) An important role for APNs working with aging adults is the ability to assess functional status.

CRITICAL ISSUES: AGING AMERICANS AND HEALTH CARE

Today's older adult Americans are viewed as the survivors of epidemics, communicable diseases, and infections; this view includes surviving the influenza epidemic in 1918 and 1919 and the early-century lack of immunizations for communicable diseases. Immunizations were not common until the mid-1930s, although immunization against smallpox became routine after 1914 (Top, 1979). Another factor that emphasizes survivorship is the lack of antibiotics during the teenage and young adult years for this cohort. Even health education during the 1920s and 1930s described health quite differently than it is today defined by the World Health Organization (WHO). Corish (1923) described the elements of health as follows:

- General expression of vigor by facial expression
- Not having any painful or unpleasant sensations
- Maintaining a body temperature of 98.4° Fahrenheit (F).
- Having a regular (in force and time) pulse of 72 beats per minute
- Having good appetite and digestion of food with a daily bowel movement
- Having skin and kidneys that are working in a normal manner
- Having a balanced nervous system with clear eyes.

> ## Box 39-1
>
> Functional Status of Older Adults as Measured by Activities
>
> **ACTIVITIES OF DAILY LIVING**
> Bathing activities
> Dressing activities (including attire and laundry)
> Transferring activities (from bed to chair to standing)
> Toileting ability and associated hygiene
> Bowel continence and control
> Self-feeding
>
> **INSTRUMENTAL ACTIVITIES OF DAILY LIVING**
> Telephone use
> Preparation and administration of medications
> Ability to go outside, with or without help
> Driving within legal and physical limitations
> Housework and home maintenance
> Food preparation (including planning, shopping, and preparing meals)
> Ability to pay bills and manage finances

For many older adults, this definition was a part of their understanding of health. However, in striking contrast, today the WHO (1947) defines health as "a state of complete physical, mental, and social well-being and not merely the absence of disease or infirmity." Spector (1996) expands the WHO definition to include "the ability of a system to respond adaptively to a wide variety of environmental challenges." This addition is particularly relevant in defining health in the aging adult population.

Demographics with Implications for Health Care of the Aging

The cohort of "baby boomers" will begin to turn 65 in the year 2010, and this increase in older adults will challenge the service sector and entitlement programs. By 2030, there should be stabilization of the proportion of older adults in the United States population (Siegel, 1996). Health care planners appreciate that more primary health care programs are becoming necessary for older women than older men, reflecting the existing gender difference. The projected gender imbalance in the over-65 group will level out some as mortality rates converge, but women are expected to continue to outnumber men, especially in the over-85 group (Burke & Laramie, 2000).

The racial mix in the U.S. population over age 65 is projected to change significantly. In 2050, the Hispanic proportion of the over-65 group will have increased to more than 17% (from its 4.5% in 1995). The African-American proportion will have increased from 8% in 1995 to almost 11% in 2050. Asian/Pacific Islanders will increase significantly as well. The proportion of Caucasians in the over-65 group is projected to decrease from about 90% in 1995 to 82% in 2050 (U.S. Bureau of Census, 1993). Racial factors have implications for primary health care policy because of the prevalence of certain diseases within racial groups. For example, hypertension, diabetes mellitus, and arthritis are more common in African Americans, while hypertension and diabetes are more common in Hispanics.

The majority of older individuals rate their health status as good to excellent, though African Americans are more likely than Caucasians to assess their health as fair or poor (Burke & Laramie, 2000). Many older adults do have at least one chronic health problem; the most common chronic diseases in noninstitutionalized older adults are arthritis, hypertension, heart disease, hearing impairments, cataracts, orthopedic impairments, sinusitis, and diabetes (U.S. Department of Health and Human Services [DHHS], 1993).

The probability of having a disability increases with aging. Those over age 65 account for 43% of people with severe disabilities. *Severe disability* is defined by the U.S. Bureau of the Census (1993) as a person requiring a wheelchair or some other special aid for 6 months or longer, being unable to perform one or more functional activities or needing assistance with ADLs or IADLs, being prevented from working at a job or at housework, or having a condition such as autism, cerebral palsy, Alzheimer's disease, senility or dementia, or mental retardation. Strokes, hip fractures, coronary heart disease, congestive heart failure, pneumonia, diabetes mellitus, and dehydration account for a significant share of disability in older adults (Burke & Laramie, 2000).

Older adults account for approximately 73% of the annual deaths in this country. Heart disease, cancer, and stroke are the leading causes. Other significant causes include pneumonia, influenza, and chronic obstructive pulmonary disease (COPD). Deaths related to acquired immune deficiency syndrome (AIDS) in older adults more than doubled between 1987 and 1993. Data from the National Center for Health Statistics (1996) indicate that deaths related to human immunodeficiency virus (HIV) are higher in older adults than in the 20-year-old age group.

Physician office visits and drug costs increase as one ages. Home health services and durable medical equipment expenses are also more likely to be necessary. According to Burke and Laramie (2000), physician contact for those over age 65 breaks down as follows: physician's office, 53%; hospital outpatient department, 10%; telephone, 9%; and home health, 19%. These data suggest the way in which the services of APNs in primary care will be required to meet the needs of the aging population.

Where individuals live as they age is determined in part by their health status and economic resources. Availability of family support is also a factor, and preference for living arrangements may be culturally determined to some extent. The ability to stay in one's own home is dependent on access to primary health care support services; consequently, assisted living arrangements, including onsite nursing services, have greatly increased to reflect the population trends. Community-based services have also increased to support the growing number of older adults. APNs need information about residential and community-based services as sites for potential employment and in order to advocate for older adults.

Age is an important factor affecting health beliefs and illness behaviors. Older people are less likely than younger people to discuss technology and a scientific view on health matters. Beliefs and values about health and illness are commonly formed early in life and are often resolute (Barker, 1997). These old beliefs can clash when a health care provider plans a highly technological intervention within a short period. This gap in health and illness beliefs can foster a generation gap that may not be clearly understood by the health care provider. When ethnic differences are added to cohort differences, the outcome may be rejection of the plan of care. The potential for problems between the health care provider and an older patient needs to be a consideration. Sometimes a disparity exists between provider values and the realities of older people's lives, which can create incongruities (Barker, 1997).

Health care is generally founded upon individual values and practices. When older patients from diverse cultural backgrounds enter the health care arena, the likelihood of misinterpretation can be predictable. The following factors have the potential to become problematic: referral to a specialist by a general practitioner (e.g., family physician or practitioner); requirement of services at multiple locations and by providers with unfamiliar credentials (e.g., physician assistant [PA], nurse practitioner [NP]); lack of an immediate answer to health problems; and placement of the responsibility for follow-up and for obtaining third-party payment for care on the older adult.

Comparison of Life Expectancy and Mortality in Ethnic Groups

Older adults make up a smaller proportion of ethnic minority populations (African Americans, Hispanics, Asian/Pacific Islanders, and Native American/Alaska Natives) than they do in the Caucasian population. However, small population groups pose special problems for epidemiologists. Multiple confounding variables exist, including

socioeconomic status, education, immigration patterns, and policy initiatives. The U.S. Bureau of the Census (1990) reported the following percentages of older adults within the major racial and ethnic groups:

- African (Black) Americans—8.4 %
- Asian/Pacific Islanders—6.2 %
- Native American/Alaska Natives—5.8 %
- Hispanics—5.2 %
- European (Caucasian) Americans—13.9 %

As mentioned, Caucasians have the largest percentage of older adults in their ethnic group. Hispanics have the smallest percentage of older adults in their group (National Institute on Aging, 1997).

Functional Status of Older Americans

One of the most important gauges of a person's ability to remain independent is the maintenance of physical and mental functioning. When functional impairment of an older adult is assessed, underlying and contributory causes are important to establishing a plan of treatment. Differences have been found in the expectations of activity and function among ethnic groups, and when the same sets of activities are examined for performance, these differences are also apparent.

Western medicine assesses a reduction or absence of activities (e.g., ADLs, IADLs) as being an indicator of frailty in older adults. However, in some cultures the performance of some ADLs and most IADLs is assigned to younger family members as a legacy of respect toward the elders. This is especially true with Native American populations (Reuben, Wieland, & Rubenstein, 1993).

When assessing these measures, an APN needs to separate a lack of performance from an inability to perform the specific task. If living arrangements provide for most of the IADLs, this must be taken into account before documenting the lack of performance as an inability. If family members expect to assist with ADLs as a sign of respect or for other ethnic or cultural reasons, this attitude needs to be identified and documented. When an assessment identifies the inability to perform any or all of either ADLs or IADLs, the self-care deficit needs to be addressed in the plan of care and with the patient and family or caregivers.

Diseases and Disorders Common in Older Ethnic Americans

Chronic health conditions are nearly four times as prevalent in older adults as in any other age group. Several chronic illnesses coexist in nearly half of persons over age 65, and these conditions require medications or treatments that must be examined frequently. In order of prevalence, the U.S. Department of Commerce (1993) identified the top four major chronic illnesses in older adults as asthma, hypertension, hearing impairment, and heart conditions. The leading causes of death in persons over age 65 are heart disease, cancer, and stroke (Eliopoulos, 1999). Accidents are a major concern, as are the sensorineural deficits that can predispose older adults to falls and other accidents. Falls are the most common cause of fatal injury for all older persons (Eliopoulos, 1999). Moreover, injuries related to falls significantly affect older adults' functional status.

Several chronic conditions that are managed differently across racial and ethnic groups are hypertension, Alzheimer's disease, diabetes mellitus, and tuberculosis. A brief discussion of these chronic conditions is presented here.

Hypertension and heart disease

Isolated systolic hypertension is more commonly associated with older adults and is identified as a rise in systolic blood pressure disproportional to diastolic pressure. The cause is thought to be the rigidity or stiffness of the arteries that develops over time.

Variances in drug metabolism contribute to different responses in various racial groups to the treatment of hypertension. The leading cause of death in older African Americans is heart disease, especially hypertension. African Americans with hypertension respond poorly to drugs in the beta-blocker category, while Chinese Americans have been found to be twice as sensitive to beta blockers as Caucasians. Lower renin levels and plasma volume are found in older adults with hypertension, and this factor is important to note when selecting an antihypertensive therapy for older patients (Spector, 1996; Ebersole & Hess, 1998; Lueckenotte, 2000).

Older adults with mild to moderate hypertension may be asymptomatic. Consequently, they may not seek treatment or may not comply with medication because their cultural beliefs associate medication with symptoms. Headache, vertigo, palpitations and fatigue are common symptoms with progressive hypertension. Severe hypertension is frequently manifested by throbbing occipital headache, confusion, epistaxis, and coma (Lueckenotte, 2000). Untreated hypertension can lead to the following complications: ventricular hypertrophy; congestive heart failure; myocardial infarction; angina; transient ischemic attack or cerebral vascular accident; sudden death; azotemia, proteinuria, and/or microalbuminuria (kidney failure); peripheral vascular disease; aneurysm; retinal hemorrhage or exudates; and papilledema (Lueckenotte, 2000).

Alzheimer's disease

The caregiving experience differs for family members of different racial and ethnic groups when faced with an elder with Alzheimer's disease. Cox and Monk (1996) studied 76 African-American and 86 Hispanic caregivers of Alzheimer's relatives. The two items examined were personal stress and role strain. Both groups of caregivers, in attempting to meet the demands of caregiving, became vulnerable to extreme stress and feelings of being overwhelmed.

Differences in the ages of caregivers demonstrated that younger caregivers often experience conflict due to the demands of the caregiver role and its interference with their own goals and plans (Cox & Monk, 1996). Hispanic caregivers were significantly younger than the African-American caregivers.

Both groups coped with the older adult's memory loss and disruptive behavior. The Hispanic group experienced more exhaustion from performing daily physical caregiving. Religion and prayer served as the mechanism for dealing with the physical and emotional stress in both groups (Cox & Monk, 1996).

When African-American caregivers of Alzheimer's patients were compared with Caucasian caregivers, Haley, Roth, Coleton, Ford, West, Collins, and Isobe (1996) identified that no evidence of psychological distress was noted in the African-American families, while the Caucasian caregivers experienced significant rates of depression and a lower life satisfaction. The researchers concluded that race had a significant effect on appraisal and coping responses, which in turn influenced well-being. Caucasian and African-American caregivers reported similar social network satisfaction, and no racial differences were found in the practice of religion and prayer by the caregivers.

Diabetes mellitus

Persons over the age of 65 account for 38% of those with both type 1 and type 2 diabetes mellitus. Many older adults do not have common signs or symptoms. In many of them, type 2 disease is associated with memory problems and an increase in depression. Other signs and symptoms experienced by older patients include numbness and/or tingling in fingers, toes, or elsewhere; blurred vision, with or without a headache; desensitization to temperatures of either extreme, especially in the lower extremities; and infections of the urinary tract, vagina, or areas of skin subject to breakdown (Lueckenotte, 2000).

Within Hispanic groups, Mexican Americans have a significantly higher rate of diabetes mellitus. It is listed as the sixth leading cause of death for Native Americans living on reservations and the ninth leading cause of death for African-American men (U.S. DHHS, 1993). Obesity and insulin resistance are prevalent in the older members of each of these groups.

Tuberculosis

An increase in the incidence of tuberculosis has created concern for both independent older adults and those in long-term care (LTC) facilities. When adults over age 65 were studied, the Centers for Disease Control and Prevention (1999) found Asian/Pacific Islander men had the highest incidence of tuberculosis (225 cases per

100,000 men), while the lowest incidence was among Caucasian women (6 per 100,000).

Tuberculosis can remain inactive for decades and become reactivated when an aging person's immune system becomes less effective. Often an older adult may complain of weight loss, anorexia, and fever. When classic signs and symptoms are present, they include purulent sputum positive for acid-fast bacilli (AFB); fatigue and weakness; night sweats with a low-grade fever; and hemoptysis, crackles, wheezes, and lung consolidation (Lueckenotte, 2000).

Drug therapy must be carefully selected for older patients. Isoniazid rapidly inactivates in African Americans, Asians, and Native Americans, though combining it with pyridoxine (vitamin B$_6$) can partially slow the inactivation (Giger & Davidhizar, 1999). The use of skin tests for detection of sensitivity to tuberculosis bacilli has been proven unreliable in older persons; reduced immune system activity causes frequent false-negatives. If skin testing is required, the standard 5-TU Mantoux technique test can be given in a two-test approach to older patients who have not been tested for greater than 5 years. The second test serves as a booster and should be administered within a 2-week period after the first. If a positive finding occurs with the second skin test and a follow-up chest radiograph confirms a destructive process, a sputum culture for AFB should be done for a definitive diagnosis (Lueckenotte, 2000).

Racial and Ethnic Views on Aging and the Aged

There are differences in how growing old is viewed by members of different racial and ethnic populations. Knowing how different groups view aging can be helpful to APNs.

African Americans

Among older African Americans born in the United States, the view of getting old can be generalized by the following statements, noted by Holmes & Holmes (1995). Old age is a reward to a long life, so there are fewer anxieties concerning being old, and a high morale is expressed most of the time. The family structure includes the older adult, and support is present in mutual assistance from neighbors and family. The older adult maintains a useful and acceptable place in family functions, and most behavior is tolerated by family members in spite of exhibited peculiarities. Religious behaviors are continued, while economic and political action is left to the younger generation. Although socioeconomic and class differences exist within this racial group, repeated measures of similarities have been presented over the last 30 years (Holmes & Holmes, 1995).

The role of the grandmother is important to African-American families, as the matrifocal family relies heavily on the grandmother as an authority figure. The number of intergenerational families is much larger in the African-American communities of America (Holmes & Holmes, 1995).

The most prevalent health problems or diseases of older African Americans are cardiovascular/heart disease, stroke, cancer, diabetes mellitus, and cirrhosis of the liver (Ebersole & Hess, 1998).

Asian/Pacific Islanders

The Chinese and the Japanese have the longest history of immigration of the multiple cultures included under the classification of Asian/Pacific Islanders. The diversity of cultural practices among the Asian groups has created problems for scientists who have grouped diverse Asian people into a like category. Asian older adults are not homogeneous. According to the U.S. Bureau of the Census (1993), older adults represent about 8% of the total Chinese-American population.

In the past, more men than women immigrated to the United States. However, a shift occurred in the last 30 years, and there are now more older Chinese women than men. Holmes and Holmes (1995) found that older Chinese people have spent most of their lives in a culture (America) they do not understand. Many never learned the English language, which leads to self-imposed isolation in Chinese communities.

Mainly due to the lack of communication skills, Chinese Americans often refrain from seeking legal advice, health care, or financial assistance from the government. According to Holmes and Holmes (1995), Chinese older adults exhibit the following coping behaviors: (1) acceptance of reality and endurance of the circumstances, (2) frugal living, (3) independent living within young families who will be present when needed, and (4) coping by faith in God.

Among Japanese Americans, the traditional birthday that ushers in the beginning of old age is the sixtieth. However, babies in this culture are born on their first birthday, so their actual age at this time is 59 years by the Western determination. A community holiday is held on September 15 of each year to celebrate Respect-the-Aged Day. This respect is rooted in a belief in Confucian ideals that include filial piety and respect for hierarchy. The family pattern in Japan calls for the eldest son to care for his aging parents. Aging women are expected to dominate the daughter-in-law with the blessing of the son. Until the age of 60, fathers hold status as head of their households.

Following immigration, cohort-specific behaviors have been identified among Japanese Americans. Using the terms *first*, *second*, *third*, and *fourth generation* to discuss cohorts, labels have been applied to these immigrant families, and the following terms have been given to these Japanese Americans (Giger & Davidhizar, 1999). The Issei (first generation) arrived before 1924, experienced relocation to camps during World War II, and were unable to own property, become citizens, or intermarry. These people worked hard after release from the camps, but rarely escaped the emotionally crippling experience. The Nisei (second generation) were born and educated in America. They sought opportunities for education in the professions or in highly skilled occupations. Most are now bicultural and bilingual. The Sansei (third generation) are being raised in bicultural, but not always bilingual, homes. The Yonsei (fourth generation) were only infants and small children during the 1990s.

When providing care to an Asian older adult, an APN should understand certain characteristics that are commonly shared among the diverse Asian ethnic groups. Ebersole and Hess (1998) identify these characteristics as a cyclic view of time, organization of space with careful planning, the importance of ancestry and traditional practices, a written language with subtle imagery, a belief that collective goals are greater than individual ones, and a view of health as a vital balance.

Hawaiian and Samoan natives are classified as Pacific Islanders for most census data. However, the Older Americans Act of 1961 placed these two ethnic groups under the Native American/Alaska Natives category, and the debate over classification of people from these two locations is ongoing. When a Samoan seeks health care from a non-Samoan health care provider, an elder or the most educated family member is involved as the family spokesperson (Ishida, Toomata-Mayer, & Mayer, 1996).

Ebersole and Hess (1998) list the following as the most common health conditions or diseases among specific older Asian/Pacific Islander groups:

- Hawaiian Natives—hypertension, coronary heart disease, cancer, and diabetes mellitus.
- Chinese—hypertension, cancer, and diabetes mellitus
- Japanese—hypertension, coronary heart disease, cancer, and diabetes mellitus
- Filipinos—hypertension and diabetes mellitus

Native American/Alaska Natives
The heritage of Native American/Alaska Natives is impossible to describe as a unit. O'Leary and Levinson (1991) identify 307 officially recognized tribes, bands, nations, and other group designations within this classification. Languages are different, and beliefs and customs are not similar across the classification. This diversity within the cultural group can pose problems when attempting to identify commonalities to all. An example is the differing focus on food-gathering by older members of these groups; Sokolovsky (1997) identifies the following:

- Caribou hunting in the subarctic regions
- Salmon fishing in the Northwest Coastal area
- Acorn and pine nut collecting in the Great Basin region of California
- Bison hunting on the Plains
- Intense agriculture in the Southwest and Southeast Woodlands (Sokolovsky, 1997).

Although food-gathering activities are influenced by region, customs, and tradition, other characteristics do have some similarities. Cultural characteristics taught by the elders to the children are considered consistent across all Native American groups; these include respect for individual freedom and autonomy; seeking of group consensus rather than majority rule; respect for the land and all living things; demonstrations of hospitality and respect for all; avoidance of bringing shame to self, family, clan, or tribe; and belief in a supreme being (Holmes & Holmes, 1995).

Of all the factors relating to the state of Native Americans as an ethnic group, the most debilitating and oppressive is their poverty. As a people, they have for many generations experienced the worst poverty known to any ethnic group in the United States (Holmes & Holmes, 1995). The most common health conditions or diseases of older Native American/Alaska Natives are heart disease, cancer, accidents, chronic liver disease and cirrhosis, diabetes mellitus, and pneumonia/influenza (Ebersole & Hess, 1998).

Hispanics
This ethnic group has strong cultural ties to their older adults. They exhibit a strong sense of obligation and support of older family members and demonstrate a sense of shame if family responsibilities are not properly handled (Holmes & Holmes, 1995). Often misunderstandings occur between a health care provider and a Hispanic family when medical protocols clash with family values and traditions. Medical treatment may be given to an older patient, but the family is an integral part of the treatment; establishing communication with the family and the older patient is essential for treatment plans to be implemented. Holmes and Holmes (1995) identify these factors as being associated with the Hispanic extended family:

- Familism (centrality of the family, with social status derived from family status)
- Age hierarchy
- Male leadership
- Mutual aid and support

The most common health conditions and diseases among older Hispanics are hypertension, diabetes mellitus, and cancer (Ebersole & Hess, 1998).

European (Caucasian) Americans
To generalize Caucasian Americans by their heritage consistency, the elements of the family and of the care of their older adults need to be similar. To assess heritage consistency, one must determine ethnic group differences in health beliefs and practices. Spector (1996) describes factors for heritage consistency as continuous exposure to the group's ethnic culture, language, foods, and customs; continuous exposure to the group's religion and religious practices, including social activities and educational pro-

grams; celebration of ethnic cultural events, such as holidays and festivals in the country of origin; maintenance of close contact with all generations of an ethnic group; and continuous expressions of pride that are identified with people from the country of origin.

An example of the concept of heritage consistency as it pertains to the role of older adults is that of Italian Americans. This ethnic group represents the practice of strong family ties, and the family is the most important asset in their value system. Respect is reciprocal from generation to generation; the youngest son is expected to care for aging parents, and dutiful daughters are expected to provide day-to-day care. Guilt is the tool used to maintain parental control (Holmes & Holmes, 1995).

Another example of heritage consistency is that of Irish Americans. This group exhibits several different relational orientations to family that include older adults as important, if not equal, members; the orientations are lateral, lineal, and individualistic. These relational orientations pertain to the goals and welfare of all members of the family, young and old alike. The lateral orientation includes the care of siblings and older adults before extending responsibility to others. The lineal orientation supports the entire family group and places primary importance on kinship support despite age differences. The most contrasting is the individualistic orientation, in which individual goals are of primary importance, but each member is held responsible for personal behavior that supports the extended family.

Health Issues and Senior Centers across the Nation

The Older Americans Act provided the foundation for the development of today's senior centers, where men and women over the age of 60 can come to share many activities and a meal 5 to 7 days a week. A senior center is managed by an employee of an area agency on aging (AAA), but it is directed by a site board composed of senior members attending the center. Each center selects its own programmed activities. (Box 39-2 indicates programs included in senior centers.) Some centers have ongoing health screening programs provided by neighborhood health centers; others rely upon local students in programs for health professionals. During annual influenza immunization periods, most senior centers welcome health department nurses or nursing students and their teachers to provide the injections and educational support.

Older adults often find that the variety of activities provides abundant opportunities to help others and do volunteer work. Age homogeneity among center participants stimulates pride in aging, and parties, especially birthday parties, are among the favorite festivities of many centers. The oldest members become the celebrities when visitors are present (Tsuji, 1997).

Box 39-2

Programs Common in Senior Citizen Centers

- Health screening activities
- Immunizations (seasonal or episodic need)
- Workshops for arts and crafts
- Seminars on gardening or house plants
- Literature groups (for reading or writing)
- Dance and exercise groups
- Education (computer classes)
- Local travel events

IMPLICATIONS FOR MSN EDUCATION AND ADVANCED PRACTICE

Older Americans that experienced their youth in remote areas of other countries or in rural America generally encountered few health services. Health practices were predominately folk remedies or nontraditional (non-Western) health practices. APNs need to be aware of their own cultural roots while maintaining the proper prospective in nurse-patient relationships. Supporting the needs of an older adult within the belief system of a specific racial or ethnic group is a significant goal for clinicians. Accepting alternative healing methods along with traditional ethnic practices, while still including Western medicine, may seem an enormous goal. Maintaining awareness that explanations of the nature and source of a disease can lead to crosscultural misinterpretations is also important; these misunderstandings can result from the absence of a germ theory or from a belief in evil spirits or God's anger. Seeking to understand how an older adult views health, sickness, and death is important in planning interventions that will be accepted and followed by the patient and family. Knowing how aging adults view growing older can also enhance planning. For example, the oldest old may be more interested in quality of life than in adherence to a special diet, exercise, or screening tests (Resnick, 1998). Others between the ages of 60 and 85 may have similar preferences. For example, Walt, at age 69, has early kidney failure. However, he believes he has lived a rich, full life and is less interested in "buying a few more years" than in enjoying his remaining time. So Walt eats foods not on his special diet, fully knowing the implications.

APNs whose roles include working with older individuals must remain politically active and advocate at every opportunity for policy directed to remedying the problems associated with aging. Primary health care with a holistic approach must be designed to meet the needs of growing numbers of older patients. Primary care for older adults must consider the life transitions with which they are faced; their social and physical conditions; prevention, early diagnosis, and treatment of illness and injury; and health promotion. Health screening and provision of services in community settings (e.g., senior centers, health fairs) can be an invaluable adjunct to health care for older adults.

Although Americans ages 65 and older account for 12% of the total population, this group uses 20% of physician services, 40% of hospital days, and more than 90% of nursing home days, all of which accounts for 36% of the nation's total expenditures on health care (Pawlson, Infield, & Lastinger, 1997). These statistics clearly demonstrate the need for APNs to be educated to provide care for geriatric patients and perhaps find a creative practice niche with that group. The ability to refer appropriately to community resources and to work in interdisciplinary teams with other providers to improve health for older adults is an invaluable asset for APNs.

APN students need multiple and varied experiences caring for older patients in both health promotion and health care settings. Students also need experience with prescribing drugs appropriate for older adults; the basic concepts of prescription differ significantly from those for people in other age groups because of the effects of aging and alterations in absorption, metabolism, and excretion of drugs.

PRIORITIES FOR RESEARCH

Because of the sheer numbers of aging individuals as potential patients for APNs, it would be difficult to argue against the conducting of well-designed, cost-efficient research related to aging individuals and their needs. To effect a holistic approach, APNs need a practice informed by a clear understanding of who makes up this current cohort of older adults, including information on how they perceive aging, the many transitions they face, and what brings them satisfaction in life. Cultural variations continue to be of such importance that researchers are encouraged to design studies with multiethnic samples, samples of both genders, and samples of urban versus rural populations.

Research needs to continue to focus on the mobility of older adults to provide evidence-based practice interventions on ways to reduce frailty and prevent the falls that account for so much morbidity and mortality. Other aspects of health promotion and the way health interfaces with particular lifestyles should continue to be studied, with emphasis on quantity and quality of life. Studies also need to address chronic diseases in older adults and the new trend of AIDS in this population.

In the last 2 decades, several studies have focused on caregiver burden and stress when caring for aging parents; most have concluded that the caregiver experiences were negative, skewing perceptions of the coping behaviors of caregivers. Louderbach (2000) describes the positive aspects of caregiving: feelings of pride and self-worth, closer relationships with those cared for, and pleasure in a job well done. One's caregiving experience may be determined in part by culture and educational level. Qualitative studies of caregiving should continue to provide understanding of that role for both the caregiver and the one cared for. Although most caregivers are women, the experience of both genders and of different ethnic groups should be studied. Access to this information will help APNs work more effectively with their aging patients and provide more anticipatory guidance, training, and support to family caregivers.

At the other end of the spectrum is an aging individual responsible for rearing a grandchild and what that experience holds. According to the Gerontological Society of America (1997), 1 in 10 grandparents rears a child for a minimum of 6 months—often for longer. Clearly such arrangements have the potential to affect life satisfaction and interface with the other challenges facing aging individuals. Research should address not only what this experience of parenting a grandchild is like for the older adult and the child but also explore possible roles for APNs in meeting the unique needs of this group.

Empirical and evaluation studies should be designed to look to the best practices in adult day care, respite care, and other senior community care sites where health promotion and health care are being provided. For some older individuals, care provided by an APN may be a new experience. Study of patient satisfaction with and preference for APN providers would be both interesting and instructive. Addressing what aging individuals seek in health care and health care providers would serve to inform the design, implementation, and evaluation of creative services for this population of patients.

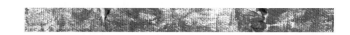

DISCUSSION QUESTIONS

These questions can be used to promote critical thinking and encourage discussion.

1. Describe the manner in which an initial interview could be handled in a primary care setting with an older Vietnamese man who does not speak English.
2. Due to an older Hispanic woman's diagnosis of chronic dyspepsia, you must prepare and teach a dietary plan to reduce acidic foods. What are your initial actions? What types of follow-up will be planned? How will you evaluate the success of this intervention?
3. Plan continuing care with home rehabilitation for an older adult patient living alone and existing on social security and supplemental security income. Select a

patient that is from a racial or ethnic group unfamiliar to you. Consider the following:

- Cost of services
- Interpretation of services
- Cultural or religious beliefs

4. Reflect on your own view of aging. How has it changed over time?
5. Reflect on the following scenario: At your present age and with your current life circumstances, it becomes necessary that you assume caregiving responsibility for an aging parent. How would you feel about this

---

Suggestions for Further Learning

- Conduct a community assessment of all the resources available to the aging population. If yours is a large community, it may be helpful to undertake this as a group activity. Make a chart with salient information for your future practice. For each agency, include name, address, telephone number, contact's name, service provided, eligibility, and cost (if applicable).
- Using the data obtained in the previous activity, determine where there are gaps in service and discuss in a small group how those gaps might be remedied. Explore the ways in which this gap in services might serve as a "market niche" for a creative APN.
- Interview a grandparent who has assumed a parenting role for a grandchild about what the experience has been like. Ask about the greatest joys, greatest challenges, and greatest surprises of the endeavor. What does the person perceive as the most pressing need now? What was the most pressing need initially? After the interview, reflect on how an APN might have made a difference for this family.
- Interview a family member who has assumed a caregiving role for an aged individual. Ask about the greatest joys, greatest challenges, and greatest surprises of the endeavor. What does the person perceive as the most pressing need now? What was the most pressing need initially? After the interview, reflect on how an APN might have made a difference for this family.
- Consult Burke, M.M., & Laramie, J.A. (2000). *Primary care of the older adult: a multidisciplinary approach.* St. Louis: Mosby. This book provides a comprehensive view of aging adults to inform advanced and other professional nursing practice.
- Employ the following resources to inform your practice with aging adults:
  - American Society on Aging, 833 Market Street, San Francisco, CA 94103
  - Multicultural Studies Catalog, 10200 Jefferson Boulevard, PO Box 802, Culver City, CA 90232-0802
  - National Council on Aging (also the National Center on Rural Aging), 409 3rd Street, SW, Washington, DC 20024
  - National Association of Area Agencies on Aging, 1112 16th Street, NW, Washington, DC 20024
  - U.S. Department of Health and Human Services/Public Health Service/Health Services Administration/Indian Health Service, 5600 Fishers Lane, Rockville, MD 20857
  - U.S. Department of Health and Human Services/Public Health Service/Office of Minority Affairs, Room 118-F/HHH Building, 200 Independence Avenue, SW, Washington, DC 20201
- Employ the following Internet sites to inform your practice regarding aging adults:
  - Administration on Aging (www.aoa.dhhs.gov)
  - Ageline Database (www.research.aarp.org)
  - AGENET Falls Prevention (www.agenet.com/fall_prevention.html)
  - Alzheimer's Association (www.alz.org)
  - Alzheimer's Caregiving Page (www.alzwell.com)
  - American Academy of Ophthalmology (www.eyenet.org)
  - American Association of Retired Persons (www.aarp.org)
  - American Diabetes Association (www.diabetes.org)
  - American Heart Association (www.americanheart.org)
  - American Lung Association (www.lungusa.org)
  - American Foundation for Suicide Prevention (www.afsp.org)
  - Arthritis Foundation (www.arthritis.org)
  - Arthritis Net (www.arthritisnet.com)
  - Better Hearing Institute (www.betterhearing.org)
  - Brain Attack Coalition (www.stroke-sit.org)
  - Caregiving Online Newsletter (www.caregivers.com)
  - Elderweb Online Eldercare Sourcebook (www.elderweb.com)
  - Ethics in Aging (www.grants.cohpa.ucf.ed/age-ethics)
  - Family Caregiver Alliance (www.caregiver.org)
  - Health Care Financing Administration (www.hcfa.gov)
  - Healthwise Handbook—Neck and Back Pain (www.betterhealth.com)
  - National Center on Elder Abuse (www.gwjapan.com/ncea/)
  - National Coalition for Adult Immunization (www.nfid.org.ncai)
  - National Institute on Aging (www.nih.gov/nia)
  - National Parkinson's Foundation, Inc. (www.parkinson.org)
  - Rx List Internet Drug Index (www.rxlist.com)
  - Self-Help for Hard of Hearing People (www.shhh.org)
  - Senior InfoSite (www.senior-infosite.com)
  - Skin Cancer Zone (www.melanoma.com)
  - www.diabetes.org/internetresources.asp
  - www.seniorlaw.com/elderabuse.htm
- Use the functional status assessment instrument in this chapter to assess an aging patient's functional level.

obligation? What modifications would be necessary in your life? Where would you turn for help? What do you imagine would be the greatest challenges of such an endeavor? The greatest satisfactions?

REFERENCES/BIBLIOGRAPHY

American Association of Retired Persons (1998). *A profile of older Americans 1998*. Washington, DC: American Association of Retired Persons.

Andrews, M., & Boyle, J. (1999). *Transcultural concepts in nursing care* (3rd ed.). Philadelphia: JB Lippincott.

Angel J.L., & Hogan, D.P. (1991). *The demography of minority aging populations: minority elders—longevity, economics, and health*. Washington, DC: Gerontological Society of America.

Barker, J.C. (1997). Between humans and ghosts. In J. Sokolovsky (Ed.), *The cultural context of aging* (2nd ed.). Westport, CT: Bergin and Garvey.

Burke, M.M., & Laramie, J.A. (2000). *Primary care of the older adult: a multidisciplinary approach*. St. Louis: Mosby.

Carman, M. (1997). The psychology of normal aging. *Psychiatric Clinics of North America, 20*(1), 15-24.

Centers for Disease Control and Prevention (1999). *Reported tuberculosis cases by race/ethnicity in the United States, 1997*. Atlanta, GA: Centers for Disease Control and Prevention.

Corish, J.L. (Ed.) (1923). *Health knowledge*. New York: Domestic Health Society.

Cox, C., & Monk, A. (1996). Strain among caregivers: comparing the experiences of African American and Hispanic caregivers of Alzheimer's relatives. *International Journal of Aging and Human Development, 43*(2), 93-105.

Ebersole, P., & Hess, P. (1998). *Toward healthy aging: human needs and nursing response* (5th ed.). St. Louis: Mosby.

Eliopoulos, C. (1999). *Manual of gerontologic nursing* (2nd ed.). St. Louis: Mosby.

Fisher, J. (1993). A framework for describing developmental changes among older adults. *Adult Education Quarterly, 43*, 76-89.

Gelfand, D., & Yee, B.W. (1991). Trends and forces: influence of immigration, migration, and acculturation on the fabric of aging in America. *Generations: Journal of the American Society on Aging, 15*(4), 7-10.

Giger, J.N., & Davidhizar, R.E. (1999). *Transcultural nursing* (3rd ed.). St. Louis: Mosby.

Haley, W.E., Roth, D.L., Coleton, M.I., Ford, G.R., West, C.A., Collins, R.P., & Isobe, T.L. (1996). Appraisal, coping, and social support as mediators of well-being in Black and White family caregivers of patients with Alzheimer's disease. *Journal of Consulting and Clinical Psychology, 64*(1), 121-129.

Holmes, E.R., & Holmes, L.D. (1995). *Other cultures, elder years* (2nd ed.). Thousand Oaks, CA: Sage.

Ishida, D.N., Toomata-Mayer, T.F., & Mayer, J.F. (1996). Samoans. In J.G. Lipson, S.L. Dibble, & P.A. Minarik (Eds.), *Culture and nursing care: a pocket guide*. San Francisco: UCSF Nursing Press.

Lueckenotte, A.G. (2000). *Gerontologic nursing* (2nd ed.). St. Louis: Mosby.

Louderback, P.L. (2000). Elder care: a positive approach to caregiving. *American Academy of Nurse Practitioners, 12*(3), 97-99.

Lynch, S.A. (1998). Who supports whom? How age and gender affect the perceived quality of support from family and friends. *The Gerontologist, 38*(2), 231-238.

McGoldrick, A. (1994). The impact of retirement on the individual. *Reviews in Clinical Gerontology, 4*(2), 151-160.

Miller, C.A. (1999). *Nursing care of older adults: theory and practice*. Philadelphia: JB Lippincott.

National Center for Health Statistics (1996). *Health United States, 1996, with socioeconomic status and health chartbook*. Hyattsville, MD: Public Health Service.

National Institute on Aging (1997). *Aging in the United States: past, present, and future* (chart). Washington, D.C., US Department of Commerce, Economics and Statistics Administration, Bureau of the Census.

O'Leary, T.J., & Levinson, D. (Eds.). (1991). *Encyclopedia of world cultures: volume 1. North America*. Boston: GK Hall.

Pawlson, G., Infield, D., & Lastinger, D. (1997). The health care system. In R.J. Ham, & P.D. Sloane (Eds.), *Primary care geriatrics* (3rd ed.). St. Louis: Mosby.

Peterson, M. (1994). Physical aspects of aging: is there such a thing as "normal"? *Geriatrics, 49*, 45-49.

Resnick, B. (1998). Health promotion practices of the old-old. *Journal of the American Academy of Nurse Practitioners, 10*(4), 147-153.

Reuben, S., Wieland, D., & Rubenstein, L. (1993). Functional status assessment of older adults: concepts and practical implications. *Annals of Gerontology, 7*, 367-378.

Sieleg, J. (1996). *Aging into the 21st century* (National Aging Information Center HHS-100-95-0017 with the Administration on Aging). Washington, DC: US Department of Health and Human Services.

Sokolovsky, J. (1997). *The cultural context of aging: worldwide perspectives* (2nd ed.). Westport, CT: Bergin & Garvey.

Spector, R.E. (1996). *Cultural diversity in health & illness* (4th ed.). Stamford, CT: Appleton & Lange.

Top, F.H. (1979). *Communicable and infectious diseases* (5th ed.). St. Louis: Mosby.

Tsuji, Y. (1997). An organization for the elderly, by the elderly: a senior center in the United States. In J. Sokolovsky (Ed.), *The cultural context of aging: worldwide perspectives* (2nd ed.) (pp. 350-361). Westport, CT: Bergin & Garvey.

U.S. Bureau of the Census. (1990). *Population estimates by age, sex, race, and Hispanic origin*. Washington, DC: US Government Printing Office.

U.S. Bureau of the Census. (1993). *Population profile of the United States: 1993* (Publication number 23-185). Washington, DC: Government Printing Office.

U.S. Department of Health and Human Services. (1990). *Minority aging* (DHHS Pub. No. HRS [P.DV90-4]). Washington, DC: US Department of Health and Human Services.

U.S. Department of Health and Human Services (1993). *Health United States 1992* (DHHS Publication No. [PHS] 93-1232). Washington, DC: US Government Printing Office.

World Health Organization (1947). Constitution of the World Health Organization. *Chronicles of WHO, 1*, 1-2.

Chapter 40

Domestic Abuse and Violence

Sandra L. Cromwell

Domestic violence, or the abuse of children, adults, and older adults, is one of America's most severe social and public health problems. For decades, domestic violence was predominately a private tragedy, hidden from the view of others. Today, however, it is recognized as a severe social problem that severely damages all of the people involved (Anderson & Cramer-Benjamin, 1999). Domestic violence is estimated to result in over 100,000 days of hospitalization, 40,000 office visits, and 30,000 emergency room visits annually (National Victims Center, 1995). Domestic violence robs many individuals—children and adults of all ethnic groups—of the right to live with dignity and respect, free of fear. In today's society, nurses have a critical role in the identification and treatment of cases of domestic violence; however, Tilden and Limandri (1994) discovered that many practicing nurses did not have any coursework on violence issues in their basic nursing programs.

Advanced practice nurses (APNs) have an especially critical role because they are often the first health care providers (and frequently the only health care providers) to see abused patients. They are in a position to initially diagnose abuse and initiate interventions to address domestic violence. However, there is some evidence that APNs may have difficulty identifying cues to domestic violence and formulating appropriate interventions for their patients. Gagan (1996) studied the accuracy of diagnostic and intervention performance of 118 adult nurse practitioners (ANPs) and family nurse practitioners (FNPs). She had the APNs formulate diagnoses and plan interventions based on 10 patient vignettes. Five of the vignettes contained evidence of domestic violence; the other five served as a control. Gagan found that the APNs correctly identified 57% of the total violence diagnoses in the vignettes; they identified less than 20% of the acceptable violence interventions.

Therefore the purpose of this chapter is to address: (1) violence and abuse in society, (2) useful theories explaining violent and abusive behavior, (3) the diagnosis of potential and actual abuse, (4) the nurse's role in intervention, reporting, and referral, and (5) services provided in society to prevent violence and treat individuals involved in violent or abusive events.

DEFINITIONS

Violence is the unjust exercise of power by one person or group against another person or group. *Domestic violence* is a learned pattern of behaviors used by one person in a relationship to control another person or persons. Child abuse and neglect, spouse/partner abuse, and older adult abuse and neglect are examples of domestic violence in society. *Child abuse and neglect* is defined as demonstrated harm or child endangerment that is nonaccidental, avoidable, and committed by the child's caretaker (National Center on Child Abuse and Neglect, 1996). *Spouse/partner abuse* refers to deliberate and repeated physical or sexual assault inflicted within an intimate adult relationship for the purposes of coercive control (Campbell, 1989; Campbell & Humphreys, 1993). *Older adult abuse and neglect* is behavior by a caregiver that results in unmet or increased needs for physical or emotional support on the part of the older adult. Such behavior may be intentional abuse, or it may be unintentional abuse in the form of neglect by the caregiver (O'Malley, 1986).

Abuse comes in many forms, including physical abuse, emotional and psychological abuse, sexual abuse, neglect, abandonment, and exploitation. Box 40-1 presents a generally accepted definition for each of these terms.

CRITICAL ISSUES: DOMESTIC VIOLENCE AND ABUSE

Domestic violence is a worldwide problem. International studies have found that wife beating occurs in 84% of the world's societies; physical punishment of children occurs in 74% (Levinson, 1989). In families that believe wife beating and physical punishment of children are appropriate and necessary ways for shaping behavior, the suggestion that such behavior is abusive is rejected. Each culture includes a set of beliefs about what a family "should be" and the responsibilities of each of its members to the family as a whole (Anetzberger, Korbin, & Tomita, 1996). Cultural beliefs and role practices can influence the occurrence of domestic violence. Cultural beliefs identify the role each individual is to play in the family and the way in which

Terms Related to Domestic Violence and Abuse

Physical abuse—Use of physical force that may result in bodily injury and/or physical pain; this may involve overt acts of violence, such as forcible restraint, force-feeding, and the use of medications to control the actions of another.

Psychological abuse—Infliction of anguish, emotional pain and distress on another, including verbal assaults, threats and intimidation, and humiliation of the other person.

Sexual abuse—Nonconsensual sexual contact with another adult, or sexual contact with an individual unable to give consent (e.g., children, noncompetent adults); this includes forced nudity and sexually explicit photography.

Neglect—Failure to provide the basic necessities of life (e.g., food, water, clothing, shelter, medical care), emotional support and affection (e.g., nurturance, praise), and/or physical and psychological safety and security.

Abandonment—Desertion of a person for whom one is legally and ethically responsible to provide physical and psychological care.

Exploitation—Illegal use of the funds or property of another; this includes stealing money or property, cashing checks of another without permission, forging a signature or deceptively misleading another into signing a document (e.g., will, sales agreement), and disposing of the property of another without permission; it also includes misuse of a conservatorship, guardianship, or power of attorney

other members "should" react when a member does not fulfill role expectations. Although these role expectations are learned in childhood and known by all family members, verbal discussions are rare except when an individual does not meet expectations. This can make identification of families in need of assistance with domestic violence difficult (Count, Brown, & Campbell, 1999).

The absence of others who share the family's culture can also influence the occurrence of domestic violence. Families can be geographically separated from their extended families and socially isolated from the community in which they live due to racial or language barriers. Although this is especially true for recent immigrants to this country, there are many long-term residents who choose to maintain their primary language and/or ethnic practices within the home. The absence of a social network that shares and is supportive of such a family's culture and values can lead to increased stress and a feeling of social isolation. This lack of a culturally appropriate support network for all family members can encourage the family to hold tightly to their beliefs and practices out of fear of losing their cultural heritage. When the family's cultural values are known to be inconsistent with the beliefs of the dominant culture in which the family lives, this isolation

can also encourage secrecy and guardedness when discussing family matters with "outsiders." This can make identification of violence and helpful intervention with minority families difficult to achieve.

The stress and frustrations of poverty can also put great pressure on all family members, and this pressure can lead to domestic violence. In the United States, a disproportionately large number of those identified as poor are members of ethnic minority groups (U.S. Department of Health and Human Services [DHHS], 1991). Disentangling the influences of poverty and culture is a difficult task. However, it is important to remember although the incidence of domestic violence is higher in minority groups in this country, only a portion of the causes for this higher level can be attributed to cultural factors. Poverty, irrespective of culture, is also a powerful contributor to the occurrence of domestic violence and societal violence of all forms.

Child Abuse and Neglect

Child abuse is a severe social problem that appears to be increasing in the United States. The National Center on Child Abuse and Neglect (NCANDS) (1996), a section of the U.S. DHHS, reported that over 1 million children experienced abuse or neglect in 1996, an 18% increase since 1990. These cases included physical abuse (24%), sexual abuse (12%), neglect (52%), emotional abuse (6%), medical neglect (3%), and other forms of abuse (14%). (NCANDS, 1996). The abuser was almost always a parent, guardian, other family member, or caretaker.

The actual number of abused children is probably considerably higher because many cases are not reported. It is estimated that over 2000 children die from abuse or neglect annually, which amounts to 5 children every day. Most are under the age of 5 (U.S. Advisory Board on Child Abuse and Neglect, 1995). The number of children reported to child protective services or other agencies has been rising steadily at a rate of about 3% per year, suggesting that the problem is getting worse and/or reporting is getting better.

Forms of child abuse

Physical abuse is the most visible form of child mistreatment and involves physical injury from such events as hitting, punching, kicking, biting, or burning a child. All children do have accidents and get bumps and bruises during play. However, physical abuse is suspected when the explanations for injuries do not fit the physical findings or when a repeated pattern of injuries in differing stages of healing is identified.

Interestingly, corporal punishment (e.g., spanking, slapping, hitting a child) is not generally considered child abuse in America. For many observers, a child must be really physically injured for such punishment to be included in the definition of physical child abuse. However, research has shown that corporal punishment is generally ineffective for changing a child's behavior, and it may teach the child that violent behavior is acceptable. Other forms of discipline, such as timeouts, removal of privileges, and parental disapproval are far more effective in fostering acceptable behavior in children, yet corporal punishment continues.

Child neglect, or the failure to provide age-appropriate care, is the most common form of child mistreatment and involves failure to provide food, clothing, shelter, and assistance with proper hygiene and personal care. It may also include failure to send the child to school regularly. Poverty often contributes to child neglect; however, a distinction is drawn between parents who are unable to provide adequate care due to lack of financial resources and parents who are unwilling to provide this care. One form of neglect, medical neglect, involves failure to obtain medical care to prevent illness (e.g., immunizations, even when offered free in the community) and failure to obtain medical care for illnesses and injuries. Neglected children may display poor physical hygiene, low weight gain, signs of malnutrition, and low self-esteem. Neglected children are more frequently seriously ill and miss school more often than other children.

Emotional or psychological abuse of children involves behaviors that impair a child's emotional development. This kind of abuse may involve everything from ignoring or rejecting the child to threatening or terrorizing the child verbally. Failure to provide warmth and nurturance is emotional abuse, as is shaming or humiliating a child. Children who experience this form of abuse suffer at least as much as children who are physically abused. This form of abuse can lead to poor self-esteem, alcohol and drug use, and suicide. Severe emotional neglect in infants can lead to death.

Sexual abuse of children involves both parents and others (e.g., relatives, adult friends). Usually the perpetrator of sexual abuse is known by the child; rarely is it a stranger. This kind of child abuse may involve nontouching behaviors (e.g., exposing genitals to the child, exposing the child to pornography or to the sexual acts of others, masturbation in front of the child), touching behaviors (e.g., fondling, directing the child to touch adult genitalia, penetration of the child by penis or other forms of sodomy), and exploitative behaviors (e.g., use of the child in pornography or prostitution). Sexual abuse may be disclosed by the child or may be suspected by the attending parent. Genital injuries are surprisingly rare; 80% of examinations are negative, even with admitted sexual assault by the perpetrator. The child may experience dysuria, enuresis, encopresis, pelvic pain, or undue irritation of the area. Behavioral changes are also commonly associated with sexual abuse in children; these include: depression, regressive behaviors, sleep and appetite problems, aggression with acting out, conduct problems at home and school, poor academic performance and truancy,

drug use, and sexualized behavior or a knowledge level of sexual matters beyond the child's developmental level.

Children who have experienced sexual abuse should be assessed and treated in a child advocacy center where there are specially trained providers who can collect evidence to help substantiate abuse in addition to providing appropriate treatment and follow-up. If there is a history of child sexual abuse occurring less than 72 hours before a clinic visit, the child is immediately referred; if the most recent incident occurred more than 72 hours earlier, nonemergent referral is appropriate (Kish, 2000).

Research has identified numerous factors as contributing to parental child abuse, including young and immature parents with few parenting skills and unrealistic expectations about the level of acceptable behavior a child is capable of displaying (Chalk & King, 1998). Sometimes parents attempting to discipline their child using physical punishment are unaware of the force with which they are striking the child and the damage that can occur; also, they often punish in anger, making the spanking more forceful. Parents' own childhood experiences of abuse may contribute to poor parenting behaviors, and alcohol and drug use (Widom, 1992; Nair, Black, Schuler, Keane, Snow, Rigney, & Magder, 1997) and the stress of frequent family crises also are known to contribute to child abuse.

The long-lasting effects of damage to children, even from psychological abuse alone (e.g., verbal aggression and threats by a parent) have been shown to significantly lower the self-esteem of children and to negatively affect their school grades (Solomon, 1999); lifelong difficulties with self-esteem often occur. Children who have experienced abuse are also more likely, as adults, to be arrested and to commit violent crimes than nonabused children (Widom, 1992). (Note that long-term treatment of a child who has been sexually abused is beyond the scope of this chapter.)

Spouse/Partner Abuse

Although both men and women can be abusers, 97% of all abusers are men; therefore this chapter is limited to a discussion of abuse of women. Every 15 seconds in America a woman is abused by her spouse or partner. It has been estimated that between 4 and 8.7 million women of all races and classes are battered by an intimate partner (Roberts & Burman, 1998), and that 50% of women will be victims of domestic violence at some point in their lives (Mahoney, 1991). The rule of thumb, an old English law that stated it was all right for a man to beat his wife as long as he used a stick no bigger than his thumb, is still in evidence in today's society. Clearly attitudes about the devastating effects of domestic violence change slowly.

Forms of spouse/partner abuse

Physical abuse involves not only assault and beatings but also includes being confined to the home, with the woman becoming a virtual prisoner of her abuser. This social isolation is often combined with psychological abuse in the form of verbal derogation and threats and financial exploitation in the form of restriction of access to family assets (Erchak & Rosenfeld, 1994). Feelings of powerlessness and hopelessness in such abused women are common. Rape, sexual abuse, and sexual humiliation are also common in domestic violence relationships and further erode a woman's self-esteem as she begins to believe the derogatory statements made by the abuser.

The effects of abuse on women are extensively described in the next section on theories of violence and abuse. However, it is important to note at this point that mothers who are abused are twice as likely to abuse their children. Sometimes this is a woman's response to her own abuse, but other times it is an attempt to control children's behavior, thereby preventing her own abuse by the man. For the children, the effects of witnessing domestic violence between parents can be devastating and result in severe behavioral problems. Withdrawal and anxiety are common, and some children exhibit aggressive behavior toward others and engage in delinquency in response to their experiences (Anderson & Cramer-Benjamin, 1999). The effect of observing parental abuse on a child is very similar to and equally as damaging as the effect of personally experiencing child abuse (Echlin & Marshall, 1995).

Factors contributing to the continuation of spouse/partner abuse

Why does an abused woman not just leave the relationship? The answer is complex. The most dangerous time for a woman is when she attempts to leave a violent relationship. Homicide rates, with the abuser killing the woman who is trying to leave or has left, escalate during this time (Russell, 1990). Many abused women are stalked by their abusers as they seek to escape from the violence (Federal Bureau of Investigation, 1998). Even changing one's name is not always adequate protection. One critical factor influencing a woman's decision to leave an abusive relationship is whether she can financially survive without the abuser. Poverty levels are five times higher for female heads of households than for married families in America, with nearly one half of such female-led households living in poverty. Abused women may not be able to find jobs for several reasons. They may have no marketable skills and need training before employment or, for those who have been employed, their abuser may have ruined their work record through harassment at work or forced frequent absences, which makes future employment more difficult to obtain.

Older Adult Abuse, Neglect, and Exploitation

Currently over 44 million Americans are over the age of 60 years. Public policies addressing retirement, long-term care (LTC) services, and quality of life are being developed to address the unique needs of the aging population. However, the abuse and neglect of older Americans living in their homes has been largely unidentified and unnoticed by society. Congress, through the Family Violence Prevention and Services Act of 1992, directed that a national study of the incidence of older adult abuse and neglect be conducted. The results of this study show the magnitude of this problem in society. The study estimated that approximately 450,000 older adults living in the community were abused or neglected in 1996. The cases included neglect (49%), emotional abuse (35%), physical abuse (26%), exploitation (financial abuse) (30%), and abandonment (3%). Older women were more frequently abused than men, and the oldest-old (those 85 years and over) were more frequently abused than their younger counterparts. In 90% of cases, the perpetrator was a family member; in two thirds of the cases, the perpetrator was a spouse or adult child of the older adult. The 1996 study also found that 84% of abused older adults were Caucasian, 8.3% were African American, 5.1% were Hispanic, 2.1% were Asian/Pacific Islander and 0.4% were Native American/Alaska Native, indicating that older adult abuse is a problem for all cultures (Administration on Aging, 1998). Sadly, only about 20% of the cases identified in this study had been reported to Adult Protective Services agencies for investigation.

Older adult abuse has some similarities to the other forms of domestic violence already discussed. Older adult abuse is often spouse/partner abuse in older people. Older adult abuse has also been compared to child abuse, and there are some similarities. Often, much like a child, an older adult is frail and in need of physical care and assistance with everyday activities of living, like eating, cooking, and cleaning. However, there are some significant differences. Older adults are indeed adults, and their abusers, whether spouses or adult children, have long-standing relationships with them. Phillips (1988) has argued that this long-standing relationship and any problems that have occurred during it can lead to older adult abuse. For example, a wife who has been abused by her spouse may retaliate when he becomes physically unable to resist, or an abused child may abuse or neglect aged parents.

Neglect, the most common form of older adult abuse, involves a failure to meet the physical and psychological needs of the person. Neglect can be an intentional act, but it also can occur because the caregiver is ignorant of or incapable of providing the necessary care and assistance. The care provider may be as old and infirm as the person who is being neglected. In addition, even the most well-meaning adult children may not have the necessary knowledge or financial resources to assist aging parents appropriately.

Financial or material exploitation of older adults is committed more frequently by younger family members. Taking funds from social security checks, selling property (both personal and real) without consent and keeping the proceeds, and taking savings from bank accounts all occur. Older adults are often frail and unable to manage their own finances without assistance, making them extremely vulnerable to exploitation and unable to protect themselves from it. According to former Vice President Al Gore, telemarketing fraud also qualifies as older adult exploitation. Each year 14,000 illegal telemarketing groups take $40 billion from Americans. Half of these people are 50 years of age or older. This form of exploitation often robs older adults of their life savings through intentionally misleading them into voluntarily giving their money to another.

Self-neglect is a form of abuse discussed in the literature only in relationship to older adults. It involves failure to provide such things as food, shelter, clothing, hygiene, and medical care for oneself. Estimates of as many as 100,000 older adults experiencing self-neglect have been reported (Administration on Aging, 1998). Self-neglect usually involves the oldest-old and older adults who are confused, depressed, or extremely frail; such people are often incapable of providing all of their own self-care and may have no one to ask for assistance, or they may be unwilling to ask for assistance from a formal service agency or family and friends.

Contributing factors and effects of older adult abuse

Older adults with physical or mental frailties are more vulnerable to abuse and neglect. Approximately 14% of older adults have difficulties with one or more activity of daily living (ADL) (e.g. bathing, dressing, eating, toileting) and need assistance from another person; three out of four older adults who suffer abuse have these difficulties with self-care activities. Some older adults are difficult to provide physical care for, as all nurses know, and the ongoing daily burden of providing assistance to someone can be very stressful for family caregivers. The "sandwich generation," women providing care for both their children and their aged parents, has a great deal of responsibility and often shows the strain through irritability, illness, and fatigue. This strain may precipitate abuse or neglect.

About 10% of older adults suffer from some form of dementia, and six out of ten older adult abuse victims suffer from some form of confusion or dementia. Such mental impairment may frustrate a caregiver, leading to violence, or it may contribute to the caregiver seeing the older adult as "less than a person" and feeling justified in controlling and abusing him or her. However, the caregiver may also be totally lacking in knowledge of how to assist such an person and may restrain or confine him or her out of fears for the person's safety. Finally, aggression by the older adult against the caregiver may precipitate retaliation through controlling behaviors designed to protect the caregiver from harm during caregiving encounters.

Depression is common in abused older adults, although whether this is a precipitating factor for abuse or the outcome of being abused is unclear. However, providing care to depressed older adults takes additional time and patience on the part of caregivers, increasing the stress they experience.

The relative invisibility of older adults in society can also contribute to their abuse. As older adults become more frail, they withdraw from social contact with others in the community. The spouse or adult child providing care and assistance may be the only other person an older adult sees, and this lack of social support and community assistance places a greater burden on the caregiver to meet all of the older adult's needs. Older adults rarely report abuse or neglect, thereby remaining invisible to the community of helping agencies. They are often afraid to report abuse for fear of retaliation and increased abuse or of withdrawal (by the abusers) of needed assistance with critical ADLs. They may also wish to remain in their own homes and fear institutionalization if the contact an "official" agency for assistance. Finally, for many, it is humiliating to admit that their own children are abusing them.

Abuse of Marginal Groups in Society

Homosexual relationships, gay or lesbian, also involve domestic violence at approximately the same rate as heterosexual relationships in society. Abused lesbian women are often reluctant to seek assistance for fear that others will learn of their sexual orientation, resulting in loss of friends, rejection by family, discrimination at work, and the danger of losing custody of children. These are very real concerns, and many communities have established gay and lesbian hotlines to enable individuals to get assistance while maintaining relative anonymity in the dominant culture (Brand & Kidd, 1988).

The physically disabled in society are also at increased risk for abuse and neglect. Abuse by family and professional caregivers may involve control and isolation through removal of wheelchair ramps, wheelchairs, or telephones. It may also involve physical abuse and neglect of basic physical and psychological needs. Exploitation in the form of taking money from disability checks has been reported in this group. Because of their physical limitations, this group is often poorly connected to others in the community, making abuse difficult to detect. Fear of withdrawal of physical assistance discourages the physically disabled from reporting abuse and neglect, especially if caregivers are family members.

Statistics document that individuals in society who are developmentally disabled or mentally ill, whether in institutions, group homes, or private homes, are more frequently abused than others in society. Adults and children in institutions are also known to be at increased risk for violence and abuse from their professional caregivers.

These individuals are largely invisible to most of society and are generally unable to draw public attention to their plight.

Theories Addressing Abuse

Why do individuals abuse other people? Theories of domestic violence, family violence, spousal abuse, child abuse, and older adult abuse can be divided into three groups: theories that focus on motivational factors leading the abuser to engage in violent and abusive behaviors, theories focusing on the interpersonal relationship dynamics within violent and abusive relationships, and societal theories that propose a subculture of violence within a society. Each group is described here, and salient factors useful to APN interventions are identified.

Theories addressing motivational factors

The earliest psychological theory to account for violent behavior is the Frustration-Aggression Theory (Dolland, Doob, Miller, Mowrer, & Sears, 1939; Berkowitz, 1978). It proposes that aggression is the result of frustration in attaining a goal. When an individual is unable to attain a goal, anger results; the anger builds and the desire to perform an aggressive act increases. If aggression against the source of frustration is blocked (e.g., by fear of punishment or disapproval), the aggression may be redirected toward another object or person.

A common example of this theory in operation is what often occurs when an individual puts money in a vending machine and receives no product. The goal was to obtain the desired item, and the person did his part by inserting money. The machine, however, did not do its part by supplying the desired item. Not infrequently, it is therefore kicked, hit, or shaken in an attempt to obtain the desired item. If a friend passes by at this instant, they may be greeted with a hostile or derogatory remark. Obviously, no one really believes that a machine is intentionally frustrating attainment of a goal, and certainly the friend did not cause the frustration felt. However, humans do often respond in irrational ways to the frustration of having a desired goal blocked.

This theory is the basis for most family violence theories and has been extensively used to explain why parents hit children, partners abuse partners, and adult children abuse their aging parents. This theory has also been used to explain the means through which the frustrations of poverty, lack of education, unemployment, poor housing, and discrimination can be transferred to abuse of a family member. It suggests that interventions to teach abusers effective nonviolent ways of dealing with interpersonal frustrations may be effective, along with assistance with the social and economic hardships causing the frustration.

The Theory of Power and Control (Pence & Paymar, 1993) views abuse as a means for the abuser, usually a man, to gain power and control over the abused, usually a woman, through fear; it is used extensively to explain the dynamics of spouse/partner violence and abuse. It describes how verbal attacks, intimidation, coercion, and threats are used for control. A man may threaten to leave the woman, take the children, report her to authorities, destroy her property, hurt her pet, or harm other family members. Insults and humiliating remarks are made. Additionally many male abusers attempt to isolate women by controlling who they see and talk to, what they read, and where they go. Economic abuse is another common form of power and control. Not allowing a woman to have money or access to money, or taking her pay and giving her an allowance, are common. Taking the role of "master of the house" and making all decisions, treating the woman like a servant, is also a part of power and control, as is minimizing a woman's injuries and denying responsibility for them. If the woman raises concerns abut the violence, the concerns are dismissed, minimized, and blamed on her by the abuser (Dutton & Golant, 1995).

Role relationship expectations (e.g., who is the "master of the house") and expectations for the allocation of power within relationships are culturally based. These role expectations are normatively supported by other individuals in the family (e.g., parents, grandparents), by friends and social acquaintances, and by the overall societal norms and influences within the culture. This theory suggests interventions to decrease violence would require a change in normative social values and need to increase the individual abuser's awareness of other, less violent ways to have successful family relationships.

Theories addressing the interpersonal dynamics of violence and abuse

Walker (1984) developed the three-phase Cycle of Violence Theory from her program of research with battered women. It is useful in understanding the process of domestic abuse, the reasons it is difficult to leave an abusive relationship, and the guilt so often felt by the abused individual. The theory states that during the first phase, the initial tension-building phase, the man seems irritable and lashes out at the woman verbally. He may be emotionally abusing, tell her that she is stupid, incompetent, and unconcerned about him. In response, the women, becoming anxious, apologizes for her faults, attempting to calm and please him. The woman is not angry at the man's behavior; she feels helpless and unworthy, assuming personal responsibility for his anger. The man fears rejection or abandonment, and that fear heightens his anger toward the woman.

The next phase, the violence phase, involves physical abuse by the man. The woman's children may also be a target of abuse at this time. Many women are severely injured or killed during the violent beating that follows. However the man usually underestimates her injuries and is reluctant to summon medical help. Typically, the man blames her for the abuse. For example, he might say, "If you had my dinner on the table on time, I wouldn't have had to hit you."

The third phase, seduction, involves the man apologizing and saying he will never repeat this pattern of behavior again. He may shower her with loving praise and bring her gifts to "apologize." His gentleness and support convince the woman that she has a strong loving relationship and the violence will not reoccur, especially if she is careful not to provoke him. Seeking outside assistance at this point is unthinkable for the woman. Then the cycle is repeated, often getting worse over time. Interventions based on this theory attempt to teach more effective ways of coping with the tensions of life within the relationship.

This theory helps to explain findings from studies of both abused children and abused adults, explaining why a parent abuses a child and why a man engages in partner abuse. However, abused women are known to remain in or return to abusive relationships time after time, and this theory offers only limited help in understanding why women do so.

A recent theoretical model, the Heart of Intimate Abuse (Mill, 1998), offers insights into why men and women remain or return to abusive relationships. This theory identifies five reasons why it is difficult for an abused woman to leave an abusive relationship: love for the batterer; love for the children; religion, culture, and race; fear; and financial dependency. The abused woman loves the batterer when he is not abusive, and she is committed to the relationship. She may also feel empathy for him, based on his previous history of abuse or her own. She may have learned through her past history that love and violence are intertwined. She also loves her children and believes that they love and need their father and that he loves them.

There are also pressures to remain based on religion, culture, and race. Divorce is an unacceptable alternative in many religions, and religious leaders often encourage an abused woman to stay in the relationship. For some, maintaining the two-parent nuclear family is imperative at any cost. Culture defines the nature of the family unit and the roles each member is expected to play. Culture also defines what is viewed as abusive and how abuse is to be handled. For example, culturally, it is known that many African-American women are reluctant to involve outsiders (e.g., police, agencies) for fear of the response to them and to their batterer (White, 1994). The Mexican-American culture is patriarchal, which usually defines family roles as the man making the decisions and the woman acting as peacemaker and mediator within the family unit (Rivera, 1994). Asian Americans also often define the family as a patriarchy, with emphasis on harmony and saving face or preventing family shame by hiding abusive events (Lee & Au, 1998). Native American people tend to avoid discussing family violence openly for fear of reinforcing negative societal stereotypes about "savages," and Native American women may fear tribal intervention

and possible child removal if they acknowledge abuse (Bohn, 1993).

Fear is a strong motivator for remaining in an abusive relationship. The woman may fear retaliation, and the risk of violence does increase when a women attempts to leave an abusive home. She may fear that she is inadequate to make it on her own and support and care for her children. She may also fear that the male partner can not survive without her or will commit suicide if she leaves.

Finally, financial dependency is a very real problem in today's society. Men can earn far more than women, and if a woman has little education or few job skills, she may quite realistically question her ability to obtain adequate housing, child care, and food for herself and her children if she leaves. With several children needing day care, women who earn limited wages can not afford to work. Losing her children due to her inability to adequately provide for them is an issue that plagues a woman contemplating leaving an abusive relationship. Lack of friends, family, and personal self-esteem only compound her fears that life will be no better, and may be worse, if she leaves.

Mill's theory (1998) also provides additional insights into the experience of the abuser. The abuser has learned that violence and love are intertwined. He loves the woman but fears rejection by her. He attempts to control her as well as manipulate her using his own violent past history. How could he behave differently, given his past acts of violence? He loves his children but uses them to control her. His belief in a patriarchal family structure justifies his violence to control the family.

This theory suggests many potential interventions, including: (1) counseling to assist in redefinition of the family structure as a democratic group where family problems are solved through the nonviolent use of conflict-resolution techniques; (2) open discussion of cultural and religious values and modification of these values or finding of alternative nonviolent means to express important values; and (3) providing information about a "safe" place to go initially when leaving an abusive relationship and arranging for initial financial assistance coupled with job training and employment assistance.

Theories addressing violent cultures and subcultures

Anthropologists have known for some time that some cultures are basically peaceful and nonviolent toward all their members while others display abuse of women and children, frequent interpersonal confrontations, and warlike behaviors. Sociologists were the first to propose that a subculture of violence exists within our society (Wolfgang & Ferracuti, 1967). Members of this violent subculture were said to share many of the values of the dominant society, but they differ from it in their views on appropriateness of aggression and violence as the means to deal with conflicts or disputes. The acquisition of these subculture values is usually attributed to early childhood learning of appropriate responses in given situations, as well as parental role modeling.

The theory of a violent subculture was tested in American high school boys (Felson, Liska, South, & McNulty, 1994). Researchers found that the level of interpersonal violence displayed was related to the shared contextual values within the boys' subculture. Another test of this theory involved the reanalysis of data on wife abuse collected from186 different cultures (Erchak & Rosenfeld, 1994). This analysis found that those cultures with normative patterns of violence to address conflicts had significantly higher rates of wife abuse than cultures that resolved their conflicts nonviolently.

Is America a violent culture, or is there a violent subculture in America? Our legal structure certainly does not overtly condone violence in any form; however it does sanction the use of power, force, and violence by police to a greater extent than some other cultures. For example, Great Britain does not allow uniformed police officers to carry weapons during usual daily activities. The existence of gang violence seems to support the subculture contention, and it seems that the American culture as a whole reflects at least an interest in, if not tacit approval of, violence. One has only to review the headlines in daily newspapers or listen to local or national television news to recognize the number of violent events Americans are exposed to on a daily basis. There is an ongoing debate in America about the number of violent and sexually explicit movies and television shows and their effect on the culture; even some contemporary music and video games present a violent message. However, it is clear these examples of violence would not continue unless a significant number of Americans were involved with them, suggesting that Americans enjoy violence at least vicariously. Another current controversy relates to Internet violence and abuse and its potential effects on both adult citizens and children. At the very least, American culture seems conflicted in its desire to both protect freedom of speech and protect vulnerable members of society from harmful influences.

Research to date has been generally inconclusive regarding the effects of exposure to violent content on long-term violent outcomes in adults and children. However, there is substantial evidence that it is harmful for children to watch violent television at early ages. Viewing of violent television by children has been directly related to aggressive behavior in preschool children (Singer & Singer, 1980) and to future aggression during adolescence (Eron, 1980).

If, in fact, Americans live in a moderately violent culture, then it is important to know whether negative sanctions from this culture—clear messages that certain modes of behavior are not acceptable—can decrease the occurrence of violence. Count et al (1992) found that sanctions from the community against domestic violence were powerful in keeping occasional wife abusers from increasing the frequency of their abuse. This study suggests that initiating sanctions against violence within a culture or subculture could also be effective in controlling or diminishing violence.

The culture of violence theory suggests that interventions to diminish abuse and violence need to be targeted at the community level. For example, national and local dissemination of information on violence and abuse, town-hall meetings, and meetings with local religious, parent, or school groups to discuss alternatives may yield some solutions. Offering widely available classes on parenting and management of conflict within the family are also supported by this theory, as are campaigns to decrease the media portrayal of violence as attractive.

Assessing Domestic Violence

APNs are in a unique position to identify cases of domestic violence. They are often the initial contact for victims, and they need to be aware of cues to violence and abuse. Many patients may be initially unwilling to admit to domestic violence; however, a history of any of the factors in Box 40-2 should alert APNs to further explore this possibility.

Reports of traumatic injuries or sexual abuse in the past are clear indications of a high risk for future abuse. However, many patients will not directly provide this evidence. Vague stories explaining their previous injuries should alert an APN to potential abuse, especially when the explanation for the injury fails to match the evidence (Moss & Taylor, 1991). For example, Mrs. Jiminez explained to the nurse that the burn on the top of her daughter Carmen's hand was caused by reaching over a pressure cooker, but a burn from that source would likely be on the underside of the arm and would not have defined pointed marks in the shape of the tip of an iron.

Evidence from a physical assessment may also provide important data. An APN should observe for evidence of current bruising or lacerations and for untreated wounds or injuries in various stages of healing. As described earlier, abused individuals are often not able to receive immediate

---

Box 40-2

Cues to Abuse and Violence

- Traumatic injuries or sexual abuse
- Multiple old and unexplained injuries
- Delay in seeking medical attention following injury
- Problems or injuries during pregnancy
- Evasiveness or reluctance to speak in front of a partner or parent
- Suicide attempts
- Drug overdoses
- Vague complaints
- Physical symptoms related to stress
- Overly protective or controlling parent or spouse

medical assistance for their injuries. APNs should look for evidence of old fractures and other musculoskeletal injuries, abdominal injuries, and missing teeth. As mentioned, APNs should also be alert for inconsistencies between the explanations of these injuries and the physical findings (Moss & Taylor, 1991; Campbell & Humphreys, 1993; Fishwick, 1995).

A history of suicide attempts may be indicative of the helplessness and despair experienced by abuse victims. A relationship between domestic abuse and abuse of alcohol and street drugs by the abuser has been well documented (McFarlane, Parker, & Soeken, 1996; Nair et al, 1997). Alcohol and drugs impair judgment and control, disrupt normal sleep, and diminish higher cortical functioning. It is not clear from the research whether the drugs and alcohol cause the abuse, or whether situational and personality factors lead to alcohol and drug abuse and to domestic violence (Bushman & Cooper, 1990).

Abuse victims often present with vague complaints and physical symptoms related to stress. Headaches, stomach aches, back and shoulder pain, problems with sleep, and fatigue are only a few of these vague symptoms (Moss & Taylor, 1991; Campbell & Humphreys, 1993; Fishwick, 1995). The appearance of such symptoms without any apparent cause should alert an APN to potential abuse.

Based on the evidence that power and control are primary ingredients in abusive relationships, APNs should observe the relationships between family members whenever possible. They should watch for signs of overt control by the potential abuser and of discomfort or reticence to speak by the potential abuse victim. Because of the role of social and economic hardships in domestic violence, it is also important to collect data about these factors. (A list of critical factors is presented in Box 40-3.)

When evidence of abuse is present, a complete assessment following the recommendations of the Family Violence Prevention Fund is indicated. These assessment guidelines, sponsored by the American Nurses Association (ANA) and 10 other health care organizations, are summarized in Table 40-1. Additionally, APNs should be sure to ask about actions taken by patients in the past to deal with previous violence and abuse and the consequences of these actions. It may be helpful for APNs to make copies of this table as a reminder during assessment interviews.

This assessment interview should be conducted in a safe area and without other family members present to ensure the patient's safety and enable free discussion. Many clinicians are reticent to ask questions about abuse for fear of alienating a patient; these are, after all, not casual questions. Furthermore, even though clinicians realize that violence crosses all racial, ethnic, and socioeconomic lines, it is sometimes difficult to believe it is happening to women the clinicians see in their practices day after day. This reticence contributes to the large number of unreported cases of violence and abuse seen each year. It is generally easier for patients to tell a health professional about abuse if the professional brings up the subject.

Box 40-3

Assessment of Social and Economic Factors Related to Abuse

- Employment status and recent unemployment
- Income adequacy to meet requirements of dependents
- Housing conditions and adequacy
- Education and skill training levels
- Social support network and available forms of assistance
- Use of any community resources for assistance

Table 40-1

Assessment of Victims of Abuse or Violence

TARGET AREAS FOR ASSESSMENT	SPECIFIC ACTIONS
Take a domestic violence history.	• Record past history of domestic violence events. • Record past history of sexual assault.
Send important supportive messages to the patient.	• You are not alone. • You are not to blame. • There is help available. • You do not deserve to be treated this way.
Assess the patient's immediate safety.	• Are you afraid to go home? • Have there been threats of homicide or suicide? • Are there weapons present? • Can you stay with family or friends? • Do you need access to a shelter? • Do you want police intervention?
Make referrals and ensure follow-up visits.	• Involve social workers (if available). • Provide lists of shelters, resources, and hotline numbers. • Schedule a follow-up appointment.
Document all findings clearly.	• Use the patient's own words regarding the injury or abuse. • Document the time, place and order of events leading to the injury. • Legally document all injuries using a body map. • Take photographs of the injuries.

Practice sites should have an expectation that all women be screened for domestic violence as part of their routine care. APNs can normalize this screening and possibly make patients and themselves feel more comfortable about the necessary questions by saying something like, "In our practice, we are very concerned about what is happening to so many women who are being hurt by someone, so we ask all women questions about it." Then an APN may proceed with the screening. Figure 40-1 shows an example of a commonly used screening instrument. Feldhaus, Koziol-McLain, Amsbury, Norton, Lowenstein, and Abbott (1997) designed three screening questions that they used in emergency settings to detect significant abuse: (1) "Have you been hit, kicked, punched or otherwise hurt by someone within the past year? If so, by whom?" (2) "Do you feel safe in your current relationship?" and (3) "Does a partner from a previous relationship make you feel unsafe now?"

Victims of abuse are more likely to disclose it in private settings. They may be more likely to talk about their abuse when there are posters or brochures in the clinic setting that refer to violence, suggesting the safety of telling staff about abusive relationships. Some clinics have placed these in bathrooms where they can be seen in private; having telephone numbers available, especially on "tear-offs," can be helpful, but it is important that the help numbers not be advertised as such, lest an abuser, who might find the telephone numbers, retaliate against the victim for seeking help.

At times, an APN will notice a patient's vagueness about symptoms or that the patient has numerous symptoms that cannot be connected in any way to form a diagnostic possibility. Sometimes this indicates domestic violence and a woman having conflict about disclosure. In such cases, the APN is advised to ask, "How are things going at home?" or some similar open-ended question to give the woman an option of disclosing abuse.

Interventions for Abuse and Violence

Interventions to assist abuse victims are aimed at the prevention of future violence and abuse. There is little or

---

1. **Within the last year**, have you been hit, slapped, kicked, or otherwise physically hurt by someone?   YES   NO

   If YES, by whom? _____

   Total number of times _____

2. **Since you have been pregnant**, have you been hit, slapped, kicked, or otherwise physically hurt by someone?   YES   NO

   If YES, by whom?_____

   Total number of times_____

   MARK THE AREA OF INJURY ON THE BODY MAP. SCORE EACH INCIDENT
   ACCORDING TO THE FOLLOWING SCALE: SCORE

   1 = Threats of abuse including use of a weapon
   2 = Slapping, pushing; no injuries and/or lasting pain
   3 = Punching, kicking, bruises, cuts and/or continuing pain
   4 = Beating up, severe contusions, burns, broken bones
   5 = Head injury, internal injury, permanent injury
   6 = Use of weapon; wound from weapon

   If any of the descriptions for the higher number apply, use the higher number.

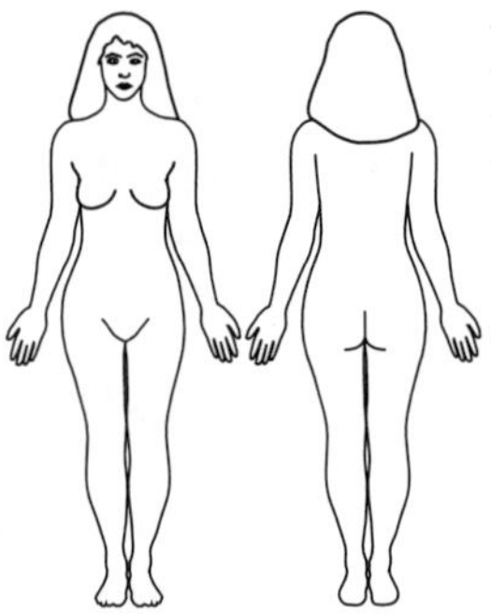

   Within the last year, has anyone forced you to have sexual activities?

3. If YES, by whom?_____   YES   NO

   Total number of times _____

Figure 40-1 Abuse Assessment Screen. (Developed by the Nursing Research Consortium on Violence and Abuse.)

no research on the effectiveness of specific intervention strategies on domestic violence. However, theories of violence do give guidance for interventions; most of the suggestions for actions for addressing abuse are based on these theories and the empirical evidence of risk factors for abuse discussed in the previous sections.

Interventions are often categorized into primary, secondary, and tertiary levels of prevention. Consistent with the definition of prevention proposed by Shemansky and Clausen (1980), primary prevention of abuse involves actions taken before abuse that decrease the probability of future violent events in at-risk families or individuals. Primary prevention of abuse includes both the community interventions previously discussed and interventions with individuals and families to alleviate poverty, lack of education, unemployment, substance abuse, and poor housing conditions. Assistance with social and economic hardships may also decrease the frustration that leads to violence. Services for referrals to assist with these problems are discussed in an upcoming section.

Primary prevention also includes identification of families with ineffective communication patterns for resolving conflicts and managing frustration, as well as those with rigid patriarchal family roles. Frustration-aggression and power theories suggest the use of interventions to teach abusers alternative nonviolent ways to deal with interpersonal frustrations. Assertiveness training for women may also be of value. Parenting classes may help prepare young persons for the responsibilities of parenting (Campbell & Humphreys, 1993), as may individual discussions with an APN about effective childrearing practices and anticipated problems. Interpersonal theories of violence suggest family counseling to explore family communication patterns and family role relationships, as well as teaching of nonviolent anger management strategies and coping skills.

Secondary prevention involves actions taken when some dysfunction is known or suspected in an effort to halt or reverse the dysfunction; this includes early diagnosis and intervention in cases of abuse to assist in preventing future abuse and violence. This level of intervention may dictate temporary removal of a child or separation of spouses or partners from a joint environment. Individual and family counseling are strongly indicated to assist in the development of more effective communication and coping skills. However, this can occur only when all individuals are in a "safe place," both physically and psychologically. The first step in this counseling is often to get all parties to admit to the violence and abuse (Taylor & Campbell, 1993; McFarlane & Parker, 1994). This is essential before more effective means of coping can be developed. Secondary prevention also includes referrals to local agencies for assistance with social and economic problems.

Clinicians must guard against the pitfall of being a "rescuer" of someone experiencing domestic violence. The victim must be given options by the health care team, including access to safe places, legal recourse, education,

and hotline numbers (e.g., 800-779-SAFE). It must be a woman's own decision to leave the setting, and many women will leave several times before staying away. APNs can assist patients to develop an exit plan that includes what the family will need once the decision is made to leave (Box 40-4).

Patient safety continues to be the priority. APNs must explore with patients how to remain safe in the home and at work, irrespective of their decision about leaving the abuser or staying in the home. APNs must understand that an abused woman is often at greatest risk when she is preparing to leave or has recently left the home. (Box 40-5 provides examples of parts of a safety plan used by one clinic.) Campbell (1986) determined that certain behaviors in the abuser are associated with increased risk for homicide: violence increasing in frequency or severity, especially with use of a weapon; presence of a gun in the home; forced sex acts; drug or alcohol abuse; abuse during pregnancy; control of daily activities; consistent jealousy; and violence toward children and outside the home.

Tertiary prevention occurs when a disability is fixed, unchangeable, and irreversible. For abuse and violence, tertiary prevention involves rehabilitation with the goal of restoring each individual to an optimal level of functioning. For children, this may mean permanent relocation of a child to a safe environment and counseling for the child to overcome the psychological damage from previous abuse.

Box 40-4

Packing List—What You Need to Take When You Leave

If it is safe to do so, you should take the following items when leaving an abusive home:

- Identification (e.g., social security card, passport, immigration papers)
- Aid to Families with Dependent Children (AFDC) and food stamp statements
- Birth certificates
- Marriage license
- Proof of spouse's income
- Bank records, credit cards, checks, cash, and automatic teller machine (ATM) card
- Clothing for 5 days
- Insurance papers
- Medications
- Address/phone book
- Children's school records and immunization forms
- Medicaid or Medicare card
- Copies of keys
- A few small, familiar toys for children
- A few small sentimental items or personal treasures (e.g., photographs, letters)
- Driver's license

Box **40-5**

Safety in Explosive Situations (Part of a Domestic Violence Safety Plan at Redbud Clinic)

- If an argument can not be avoided, try to get the angry person into a room where you have an exit to safety and where there are no weapons nearby.
- Practice how you and your children will exit the house in an emergency, just as you would practice for a fire. Know which doors and windows are the best exits. Know where you will go from your home to be safe.
- Have extra keys and a packed bag ready and in an undisclosed place you can get to quickly.
- Alert someone who lives nearby about the violence so that they will know to call the police if a disturbance is heard coming from your home.
- Make up a code word that you can use with your children and others that says "I need help—call the police."
- Do not put yourself in the way of more harm.
- Review your safety plan frequently so that when you decide it is time to leave you will be ready. Remember that leaving is the most dangerous time for a woman. Be cautious!

Box **40-6**

Assistance for Abused and Neglected Children

- Legal removal of a child from the home and placement in foster care or group homes
- Food and clothing
- Medical care and treatment
- Parental counseling
- Parental job training and employment assistance
- Reestablishment of a community support base for the family

new number. An APN will be able to provide some of this documentation.

Community Services for Domestic Violence

The initial goal of intervention is to ensure the immediate safety and protection of the victim of violence and abuse. It is essential that APNs be aware of specific services and contacts within their immediate community. Appropriate use of referrals may significantly enhance future outcomes for individuals involved in domestic violence. However, the services to assist with domestic violence and abuse are still quite fragmented and uncoordinated in many communities. Some programs only seek to treat the victim (e.g., child, adult partner, older adult), others target the family as a unit, and still others target the abuser. It is critical for APNs to be knowledgeable of the services available locally. The following is a review of services for children, adults, and older adults available in many communities.

Assistance for child abuse

Although anyone can report a suspected case of child abuse or neglect, most states legally require that teachers, nurses, and other health care and social service workers report all suspected cases. Each state law specifies one or more organizations to receive reports of suspected child abuse and investigate each case (e.g., the child welfare agency). It is important for health care professionals to identify the appropriate reporting mechanism in their state. However, concerned individuals can call the local police department, child protective services, the county health department, the department of social services, the district attorney's office, family and children's services, or the local welfare office and be referred to the appropriate agency. (Forms of child assistance that should be available in any community are summarized in Box 40-6.)

There has been a good deal of criticism of state reporting systems in recent years, including criticisms of underinvestigation, overinvestigation, and underreporting

Maintaining a relationship on some level with the parents is desirable but not always possible. The physical and psychological safety of the child in the future is of paramount concern at this stage.

For abused women, psychological, social, and economic assistance is usually needed at this point. Support for the woman's decision to leave the relationship is critical because, in many cases, she needs to totally redesign her entire life. Although many agencies are available to assist with aspects of this process, she needs consistent support and counseling. An APN can provide problem-solving interventions aimed at assisting her to make decisions about housing and employment and developing a new social network for herself and her children. The APN can also assist by teaching effective strategies for child discipline and control. Most abused women with children have had no opportunity to develop these skills.

In many cases, a woman also needs protection from her abuser. Assistance with the process of changing her name or social security number is warranted. In a move designed to assist victims of domestic violence evade their abusers, the Social Security Administration has recently made it easier for women to obtain a new social security number. In the past, a woman had to show that her abuser had misused her social security number, which is guaranteed to be private, in order to locate her. The new change only requires that the women provide evidence (e.g., police reports, medical treatment evidence) of abuse to obtain a

Box 40-7

Assistance for Abused Women and their Children

- A safe temporary shelter, with food and clothing for herself and her children
- Counseling
- Police protection and assistance
- Medical assistance
- Financial assistance for her or her children (e.g., welfare, aid to adults with dependent children)
- Legal assistance with restraining orders or prosecution
- Job training and employment counseling

Box 40-8

Assistance for Abusers

- Counseling for both individuals and couples
- Assistance with job training and education
- Employment counseling
- Legal means to maintain relationships with children (under supervision)

due to overly complex or redundant systems (Van Voorhis & Gilbert, 1998). National studies have shown that although the numbers of abused or neglected children are rising in the United States, the proportion of reported cases investigated has declined from 44% in 1986 to 28% in 1993. The Secretary for Health and Human Services, Donna Shalala, commented on this trend by stating, "It is a shame and startling to see that so many more children are in danger and that proportionately fewer incidents are investigated" (Vobejda, 1996).

Assistance for abused women

Individuals who observe domestic violence should contact the local police and adult protective services agencies. Most states legally require nurses and other health care and social service workers to report all suspected cases. It is therefore important for APNs to determine state and local legal requirements for reporting suspected abuse.

The list in Box 40-7 includes services offered to abused women in most communities. An APN must identify specific agencies offering each of these services and refer patients appropriately. Some agencies accept only certain patients. Referral processes are sometimes quite easy, but they are also sometimes rather complex, requiring the collection of material and documents before acceptance of the woman into the service. APNs can assist patients by understanding the requirements for services and assisting with this process.

Assistance for abusers

Many in society believe that abusers should simply be prosecuted and then "locked up" to protect society, and many abusers are incarcerated every year. However, there is some evidence that counseling of abusers can be helpful. Research on intervention programs with abusers has shown a small but significant reduction in the reoccurrence of domestic violence (Babcock & Steiner, 1999). Prison systems are beginning to offer classes to inmates convicted of violent crimes in an attempt to decrease the likelihood

of their reoffending when released. (Box 40-8 lists services that may be of use to abusers.)

Assistance for older adults

Reporting suspected older adult abuse or neglect is also mandated for nurses and other health care and social service workers. Every state legislature has passed some form of legislation to protect older adults from abuse and neglect. Three fourths of states have made provisions for local adult protective services agencies through the state's Social Services Department. In the other states, the State Units on Aging are assigned this task. These groups are responsible for receiving reports of older adult abuse and neglect and investigating them. Abuse hotlines are available in some states 24 hours a day, and services available in most communities to address older adult abuse, neglect, and exploitation are summarized in Box 40-9.

In many cases, this assistance is sufficient to allow an older adult to remain in the home. Furthermore, the family caregiver, spouse, or adult child may, with this assistance, be able to continue to provide adequate care. However, in some cases, relocation of the abused older adult is necessary. Sheltered care or nursing home placement may be needed to protect the person from future abuse or neglect.

IMPLICATIONS FOR MSN EDUCATION AND ADVANCED PRACTICE

All APNs need to appreciate the pervasiveness of violence in this country, which necessitates that all women be screened for domestic violence and all children and older adults for whom there is evidence of abuse be carefully evaluated and treated. APNs should know how to assess for domestic violence and how to manage patients experiencing abuse, including what local and national resources are available for them. Working with domestic violence can be frustrating because APNs, concerned about the safety of their patients, often believe that a patient cannot be safe in an abusive home. It is difficult to see a woman's assessment of her safety vacillate over time and have her remain in a potentially unsafe environment. An APN new to handling

> ### *Box* 40-9
>
> ### Assistance for Abused and Neglected Older Adults
>
> - Case investigation and referral to local police
> - Admission to a hospital
> - Food and clothing
> - Provision of heat and electricity
> - Provision of needed medications
> - Arrangement for home health care
> - Arrangement for homemaker services
> - Referral of the case to an attorney
> - Older adult care education for caregivers

patients in violent situations needs support regarding this frustration and the common desire to be a "fixer" at any cost. The APN may need to be reminded of why women often stay in abusive homes.

Having opportunities to work with patients in abusive situations and to hear their stories firsthand can be of inestimable value for informing practice and learning to be an advocate. There might be possibilities for clinical hours in a shelter or child advocacy center as part of Master's education. Case studies can be valuable adjuncts to education, and Campbell (1992) suggests that novels or movies like *The Color Purple* and *The Prince of Tides* can be used to learn at a distance about violence. Nonfiction descriptions of abuse can also be helpful. (See the Suggestions for Further Learning box at the end of this chapter.)

APNs, because of their knowledge of domestic violence and actual experiences with victims, can have an invaluable place in political advocacy and community initiatives for prevention and education. For example, APN students in one community hold classes for teenagers on dating relationships that include the topic of violence. In another example, groups of APNs formed a primary prevention network that conducted parenting classes so that new parents would have more realistic expectations of children and their developmental abilities. APN students and those in practice can have an informed voice in changing societal attitudes about abuse and violence and in campaigns that increase public awareness of the incidence, prevalence, and damaging outcomes of abuse and violence in any form.

PRIORITIES FOR RESEARCH

Additional research on domestic violence is critically needed, especially studies of the effects of specific interventions to reduce the abuse involved in all forms of domestic violence. Although some recommendations for culturally sensitive interventions exist in the literature (Torres, 1991; Bohn, 1993; Fishwick, 1993; Rodriguez, 1993), no tests of these interventions have been published

to date. Practicing APNs or graduate students with faculty supervision are in an excellent position to initiate some of these studies.

Studies of domestic violence can be difficult. The National Institute of Mental Health (1993) cautions that researchers studying domestic violence must take care that subjects are clearly informed about the consequences of agreeing or refusing to participate in a research study. The Institute cautions that subjects sometimes believe that they must participate in the study if they are receiving free treatment, or that if they refuse to participate negative consequences will occur that affect their court decision or probation status. Additionally, subjects may refuse to participate in research involving interventions because they fear that their circumstances as victims of violence will become known to others in the community (e.g. employers, friends, the police, child protective services) who could use the knowledge in a way that would harm the family. Some subjects, especially abused adults, may be placed at increased risk for future abuse from their partner because they have chosen to "tell" a researcher about their situation through participation in a violence intervention study. Finally, research studies often offer a variety of services to members of families identified as having problems of domestic violence; services include counseling, health screening and care, and additional social services support. The ethics of withdrawal of these services at the completion of the study must be considered, because the family may suddenly lose the support that made it possible for them to function more effectively. Ethically, intervention studies should include a realistic plan involving ways for the community to assume responsibility for the services provided by a research program after its completion (Thomas, 1995).

Both quantitative and qualitative methods have a place in research design related to domestic violence. When possible, studies should include representatives of diverse racial and ethnic groups so that insights may be gained about prevention and management of victimization in diverse cultural groups.

DISCUSSION QUESTIONS

These questions can be used to promote critical thinking and encourage discussion.

1. Why do you think it is so difficult for some providers, including APNs, to ask about domestic violence?
2. Think about your present clinical setting. What message, if any, is conveyed about how domestic violence is viewed by those practicing in your setting? What measures could be implemented that would increase the probability that battered individuals would be more

Suggestions for Further Learning

- Go to the Nurse Advocate website at www.nursadvocate.org and review the purposes of this nursing organization.
- Identify the appropriate organization for reporting of cases of child abuse, spouse/partner abuse, and older adult abuse in your community. Write down their phone numbers for future reference. Collect written materials from each that you can place in clinic waiting rooms or give to patients as needed.
- Review the lists of community services for the abused in this text. Identify the organizations in your community that provide each of these services. Divide the list of organizations among a group of fellow students and each of you contact your given organizations and identify all services offered and appropriate methods for patient referral. Meet as a group and share your findings. Identify gaps in services within your community. Discuss these gaps and develop a plan suitable for your community to fill one of these gaps.
- Consider reading one of the following nonfiction books about personal experiences with violence: Kehol, L. (1995). *In this dark house: a memoir*. New York: Schocken Books; and Rhodes, R. (1990). *A hole in the world: an American boyhood*. New York: Simon & Schuster.
- Visit the following Internet sites related to domestic violence for additional information, and conduct a search for other sites:
  - Commission on Domestic Violence at www.abanet.org/domviol/home.html
  - National Center on Elder Abuse at www.gwjapan.com/ncea/
  - National Coalition against Domestic Violence at www.ncadv.org
  - Domestic Violence Institute at www.dviworld.org/
  - Web resources on elder abuse at www.seniorlaw.com/elderabuse.htm
- For those working with abused children, consider the following *Portable Guides to Investigating Child Abuse*, available from the U.S. Department of Justice, Office of Juvenile Justice and Delinquency Prevention, Washington, DC 20531:
  - *Battered Child Syndrome: Investigating Physical Abuse and Homicide*
  - *Burn injuries in Child Abuse*
  - *Child Neglect and Munchausen Syndrome by Proxy*
  - *Criminal Investigation of Child Sexual Abuse*
  - *Diagnostic Imaging of Child Abuse*
  - *Interviewing Child Witnesses and Victims of Sexual Abuse*
  - *Law Enforcement Response to Child Abuse*
  - *Photodocumentation in the Investigation of Child Abuse*
  - *Recognizing When a Child's Injury or Illness Is Caused by Abuse*
  - *Sexually Transmitted Diseases and Child Abuse*
  - *Understanding and Investigating Child Sexual Exploitation*
- View the 3 CD-ROMs on domestic violence called *Understanding Partner Abuse,* available from Echo Bridge Productions, 1632 Pennsylvania Avenue, Miami Beach, Florida 33139; phone (800) 738-0786
- Investigate these information resources on domestic violence:
  - American Academy of Pediatrics, Section on Child Abuse & Neglect, 141 Northwest Point Boulevard, Elk Grove Village, IL 60009-0927
  - Battered Women's Justice Project; phone (800) 903-0111; fax (612) 824-8965
  - EMERGE: A Counseling and Education Service to Stop Male Violence, 2380 Massachusetts Avenue, Suite 101, Cambridge, MA 02140; phone (617) 422-1852; fax (612) 547-0904
  - National Committee to Prevent Child Abuse, 332 S. Michigan Avenue, Chicago, IL 60604; phone (312) 663-3520; fax (312) 939-8962
  - National Council on Child Abuse & Family Violence, 1155 Connecticut Avenue NW, Suite 400, Washington, DC 20036; phone (202) 429-6695; fax (800) 222-2000
  - National Organization of Victim Assistance, 1757 Park Road NW, Washington, DC 20010; phone (202) 232-6682 or (800) TRY-NOVA (879-6682)
  - National Resource Center on Domestic Violence, Pennsylvania Coalition against Domestic Violence, 6400 Flank Drive, Suite 1300, Harrisburg, PA 17112; phone (800) 537-2238; fax (717) 545-9456
  - Resource Center on Child Protection and Custody; phone (800) 527-3223; fax (702) 784-6160

comfortable disclosing their circumstances in your setting?

3. What experiences have you had with victims of domestic violence? Did those persons leave their violent homes or remain there? If they remained in abusive situations, how did that make you feel? Why might they have stayed?

4. In a group with other APNs, discuss the existing services for victims of domestic violence in your community. Where do gaps exist? What might be done to fill those gaps?

REFERENCES/BIBLIOGRAPHY

Administration on Aging (1998). *The national elder abuse incidence study: final report*. Available online at www.aoa.dhhs.gov/abuse/report/default.htm.

Anderson, S., & Cramer-Benjamin, D. (1999). The impact of couple violence on parenting and children: An overview and clinical implications. *American Journal of Family Therapy,* 27(1), 19.

Anetzberger, G., Korbin, J., & Tomita, S. (1996). Defining elder mistreatment in four ethnic groups across two generations. *Journal of Cross Cultural Gerontology, 11,* 187-212.

Babcock, J., & Steiner, R. (1999). The relationship between treatment, incarceration, and recidivism of battering: a program evaluation of Seattle's coordinated community response. *Journal of Family Psychology, 13,* 46-59.

Berkowitz, L. (1978). What happened to the frustration-aggression hypothesis? *American Behavioral Scientist, 21,* 691-708.

Brand, P., & Kidd, A. (1988). Frequency of physical aggression in heterosexual and female homosexual dyads. *Psychological Reports, 59,* 1307-1313.

Bohn, D. (1993). Nursing care of Native American battered women. In J. Campbell (Ed.), *AWHONN's clinical issues in perinatal and women's health nursing* (pp. 424-36). Philadelphia: JB Lippincott.

Brandt, E.N., Hadley, S., & Holtz, H. (1996, September 15). Family violence: a covert health crisis. *Patient Care,* 138-166.

Buel, S.M., Candib, L.M., Dauphine, J., & Sugg, N.K. (1993, November 15). Domestic violence: it can happen to anyone. *Patient Care,* 63-95.

Bushman, B., & Cooper, H. (1990). The effects of alcohol on human aggression: an integrative review. *Psychological Bulletin, 107,* 341-354.

Campbell, J.C. (1986). Nursing assessment for risk of homicide in battered women. *Advances in Nursing Science, 8,* 36-51.

Campbell, J.C. (1989). A test of two explanatory models of women's responses to battering. *Nursing Research, 38,* 18-24.

Campbell, J.C. (1992). Ways of teaching, learning, and knowing about violence against women. *Nursing & Health Care, 13*(9), 464-470.

Campbell, J.C. (Ed.). (1995). *Assessing dangerousness: violence by sexual offenders, batterers, and child abusers.* Thousand Oaks, CA.: Sage.

Campbell, J.C., & Campbell, D. (1996). Cultural competence in the care of abused women. *Journal of Nurse Midwifery, 41*(6), 457-469.

Campbell, J.C., & Humphreys, J. (1993). *Nursing care of survivors of family violence.* St. Louis: Mosby.

Campbell, J.C., Pliska, M.J., Taylor, W., & Sheridan, D. (1994). Battered women's experiences in the emergency department. *Journal of Emergency Nursing, 20,* 280-288.

Chalk, R., & King, P. (Eds.). (1998). *Violence in families: Assessing prevention and treatment programs.* Washington, DC: National Academy Press.

Chaney, S. (2000). Child abuse: clinical findings and management. *Journal of the American Academy of Nurse Practitioners, 12*(11): 467-471.

Coeling, H., & Harmon, G. (1997). Learning to ask about domestic violence. *Women's Health Issues, 7,* 263-268.

Count, D., Brown, J., & Campbell, J. (1992). *Sanctions and sanctuary: cultural analysis of the beating of wives.* Boulder, CO: Westview.

Count, D., Brown, J., & Campbell, J. (1999). *To have to hit: cultural perspectives on wife beating.* Champaign, IL: University of Illinois Press.

Dill, B., Dill, J.E., Sibcy, G.A., & Brende, J.O. (1997). The registered nurse's role in the office treatment of patients with histories of abuse: a proposed treatment model. *Gastro-enterology Nursing, 20*(5), 162-166.

Dolard, J., Doob, L., Miller, N., Mowrer, O., & Sears, R. (1939). *Frustration and aggression.* New Haven, CT: Yale University Press.

Domestic violence: ending the cycle of abuse. (1998). *Clinician Reviews, 8*(1), 55-69.

Dutton, D., & Golant, S. (1995). *The batterer: a psychological profile.* New York: Basic Books.

Echlin, C., & Marshall, L. (1995). Child protection services for children of battered women. In E. Peled, P. Jaffe, & J. Edleson (Eds.), *Ending the cycle of violence: community responses of battered women* (pp. 170-185). Thousand Oaks, CA: Sage.

Erchak, G., & Rosenfeld, R. (1994). Social isolation, violence norms, gender relations: a reexamination and extension of Levinson's model of wife beating. *Cross-Cultural Research, 28,* 111-33.

Eron, L. (1980). Prescription for reduction of aggression. *American Psychologist, 35,* 244-52.

Family Violence Prevention Fund (1999). *Domestic violence guidelines.* Available online at www.igc.org/fund.

Federal Bureau of Investigation (1998). *Uniform crime reports for the United States.* Washington, DC: US Department of Justice.

Feldhaus, K.M., Koziol-McLain, J., Amsbury, H.L., Norton, I.M., Lowenstein, S.R., & Abbott, J.T. (1997). Accuracy of 3 brief screening questions for detecting partner violence in the emergency department. *Journal of the American Medical Association, 277,* 1357-1361.

Felson, R., Liska, A., South, S., & McNulty, T. (1994). The subculture of violence and delinquency: individuals vs. school context effects. *Social Forces, 73,* 155-73.

Fishwick, N. (1993). Nursing care of rural battered women. In J. Campbell (Ed.), *AWHONN's clinical issues in perinatal and women's health nursing* (pp. 441-448). Philadelphia: JB Lippincott.

Fishwick, N. (1995). Getting to the heart of the matter: nursing assessment and interventions with battered women in psychiatric mental health settings. *Journal of the American Psychiatric Nursing Association, 1,* 48-54.

Fishwick, N.J. (1998). Assessment of women for partner abuse. *Journal of Obstetric, Gynecologic, & Neonatal Nursing, 27*(6), 661-670.

Furniss, K., Torchen, C., & Blakewell-Sachs, S. (1999, July-August). Learning to ask (editorial). *Journal of Obstetric, Gynecologic, & Neonatal Nursing,* 252.

Gagan, M. (1996). *Correlates of nurse practitioner diagnosis and intervention performance for domestic violence* (unpublished doctoral dissertation). Iowa City, IA: University of Iowa.

Hamberger, L.K., Saunders, D.G., & Hovey, M. (1992). Prevalence of domestic violence in community practice and rate of physician inquiry. *Family Medicine, 24*(2), 283-287.

Hendricks-Matthews, M.K. (1993). Survivors of abuse—health care issues. *Primary Care, 20*(2), 391-406.

Holz, E., & Boyce, M. (1997). Responding to family violence. *Journal of the Medical Association of Georgia, 86,* 221-222.

Holz, K. (1994). A practical approach to clients who are survivors of sexual abuse. *Journal of Nurse Midwifery, 39*(1), 13-18.

Humphreys, J. (1995). The work of worrying: battered women and their children. *Scholarly Inquiry for Nursing Practice, 9*(2), 127-145.

Jensen, L.A. (2000). The cycle of domestic violence and the barriers to treatment. *The Nurse Practitioner, 25*(5), 26, 29.

Jezierski, M. (1994). Abuse of women by male partners: Basic knowledge for emergency nurses. *Journal of Emergency Nursing, 20*(5), 361-372.

Kish, C.P. (2000). Determining sexual abuse in children and adolescents. In D.L. Robinson & C.L. McKenzie (Eds.), *Procedures for primary care providers* (pp. 381-390). Philadelphia: JB Lippincott.

Landenburger, K.M. (1998). The dynamics of leaving and recovering from an abusive relationship. *Journal of Obstetric, Gynecologic, & Neonatal Nursing, 27*(6), 700-705.

Lazzaro, M.V., & McFarlane, J. (1991). Establishing a screening program for abused women. *Journal of Nursing Administration, 21*(10), 24-29.

Lee, A. (1993). Does a history of sexual abuse in childhood play a role in women's health problems: a review of the literature. *Journal of Women's Health, 2*(2), 165-172.

Lee, M., & Au, P. (1998). Chinese battered women in North America: their experiences and treatment. In A. Roberts (Ed.), *Battered women and their families* (pp. 448-482). New York: Springer.

Levinson, D. (1989). Family Violence: a cross cultural perspective. Newbury Park, CA: Sage.

Limandri, B.J., & Tilden, V.P. (1996). Nurses' reasoning in the assessment of family violence. *Image: Journal of Nursing Scholarship, 28*(3), 247-252.

Mahoney, M. (1991). Legal images of battered women: redefining the issue of separation. *Michigan Law Review, 90,* 1-93.

McFarlane, J., Christoffel, K., Bateman, L., Miller, V., & Bullock, L. (1991). Assessing for abuse: self report versus nurse interview. *Public Health Nursing, 8,* 245-250.

McFarlane, J., Parker, B. (1994). Preventing abuse during pregnancy: an assessment and intervention protocol. *Maternal Child Nursing, 19,* 321-24.

McFarlane, J., Parker, B., & Soeken, K. (1996). Physical abuse, smoking, and substance abuse during pregnancy: prevalence, interrelationships and effects on birth weight. *Journal of Obstetric, Gynecologic, & Neonatal Nursing, 25,* 313-320.

Mills, L. (1998). *The heart of intimate abuse: new interventions in child welfare, criminal justice, and health settings.* New York: Springer.

Moore, M.L., Zaccaro, D., & Parsons,L.H. (1998). Attitudes and practices of registered nurses toward women who have experienced abuse/domestic violence. *Journal of Obstetric, Gynecologic, & Neonatal Nursing, 27,* 175-182.

Moss, V., & Taylor, W. (1991). Domestic violence: identification, assessment, intervention. *American Operating Room Nurses, 53,* 1158-62.

Nair, P., Black, M., Schuler, M., Keane, V., Snow, L., Rigney, B., & Magder, L. (1997). Risk factors for disruption in primary caregiving among infants of substance abusing women. *Child Abuse and Neglect, 21,* 1139-1051.

National Center on Child Abuse and Neglect (1996). *The Third National Incidence Study on Child Abuse and Neglect.* Washington, DC: US Department of Health and Human Services.

National Institute of Mental Health (1993). *Ethical considerations in violence-related research* (unpublished document). Bethesda, MD: National Institute of Mental Health.

National Victims Center (1995). *Crime and victimization in America: statistical overview.* Arlington, VA: National Victims Center.

Nudelman, J., Durvorow, N., Grambs, M., & Lettellier, P. (1997). *Best practices: innovative domestic violence programs in health care settings.* San Francisco: Family Violence Prevention Fund.

O'Malley, T. (1986). Abuse and neglect of the elderly: the wrong issue? *Pride Institute Journal of Long Term Home Health Care, 5,* 25-28.

Pence, E., & Paymar, M. (1993). *Educating groups of men who batter.* New York: Springer.

Phillips, D.S.H. (1998). Culture and systems of oppression in abused women's lives. *Journal of Obstetric, Gynecologic, & Neonatal Nursing, 27*(6), 678-683.

Phillips, L.R. (1988). The fit of elder abuse with the family violence paradigm and implications of a paradigm shift for clinical practice. *Public Health Nursing, 5,* 222-239.

Poirier, L. (1997). The importance of screening for domestic violence in all women. *The Nurse Practitioner, 22*(5), 105-122.

Quillian, J.P., & Dempster, J.S. (1995). Domestic violence. *Journal of the American Academy of Nurse Practitioners, 7*(7), 351-356.

Ragozine, J.E. (1998, Spring). Abuse during pregnancy: the role of the nurse practitioner. *Contemporary Nurse Practitioner,* 3-10.

Rivera, J. (1994). Domestic violence against Latinas by Latino males: an analysis of race, national origin, and gender differentials. *Boston College Third World Law Journal, 14,* 231-257.

Roberts, A., & Burman, S. (1998). Crisis intervention and cognitive problem-solving therapy with battered women: a national survey and practice model. In A. Roberts (Ed.), Helping battered women: new perspectives and remedies (pp. 13-70). New York: Oxford University Press.

Roberts, S.J., Reardon, K.M., & Rosenfeld, S. (1999). Childhood sexual abuse: surveying its impact on primary care. *AWHONN Lifelines, 3*(1), 39-45.

Rodriguez, R. (1993). Violence in transition: nursing care of battered migrant workers. *AWHONN's Clinical Issues, 4,* 437-40.

Russell, D. (1990). *Rape in marriage.* Bloomington, IN: Indiana University Press.

Ryan, J., & King, C. (1997). Child witnesses of domestic violence: principles of advocacy. *Clinical Excellence for Nurse Practitioners, 1*(1), 47-57.

Sampselle, C.M. (1991). The role of nursing in preventing violence against women. *Journal of Obstetric, Gynecologic, & Neonatal Nursing, 20*(6), 481-487.

Sampselle, C.M. (Ed.). (1992). *Violence against women.* New York: Hemisphere.

Sampselle, C.M., Peterson, B.A., Murtland, T.L., & Oakley, D.J. (1992). Prevalence of abuse among pregnant women choosing certified nurse midwife or physician providers. *Journal of Nurse Midwifery, 37*(4), 269-273.

Sassetti, M.R. (1993). Domestic violence. *Primary Care, 20*(2), 289-305.

Shemansky, S., & Clausen, C. (1980). Levels of prevention: examination of the concept. *Nursing Outlook, 28,* 104-108.

Sheriden, D.J. (1993). The role of the battered woman specialist. *Journal of Psychosocial Nursing, 31*(11), 31-37.

Singer, J., & Singer, D. (1980). Television viewing, family style and aggressive behavior in preschool children. In M.R. Green (Ed.), *Violence and the family* (pp. 23-36). Boulder, CO: Westview.

Solomon, C.R. (1999). Effects of parental verbal aggression on children's self-esteem and school marks. *Child Abuse and Neglect, 23,* 339-351.

Stewart, J. (2000). Becoming advocates for battered women. *Clinician Reviews, 10*(6), 25-28.

Taylor, W., & Campbell, J. (1993). Treatment protocols for battered women. *Response, 14,* 52-57.

Tilden, V., & Limansdri, B. (1994). Factors that influence clinicians' assessment and management of family violence. *American Journal of Public Health, 84,* 628-633.

Thomas, J. (1995). *Child protective services responses to child mistreatment. Service provider perspectives on family violence interventions* (proceedings of a workshop by the Committee on the Assessment of Family Violence Interventions). Washington, DC: National Academy Press.

Torres, S. (1991). A comparison of wife abuse between two cultures: perceptions, attitudes, nature and extent. *Issues in Mental Health Nursing, 12,* 113-31.

U.S. Advisory Board on Child Abuse and Neglect (1995). *A nation's shame: fatal child abuse and neglect in the United States.* Washington, DC: US Government Printing Office.

U.S. Department of Health and Human Services (1991). *Health status of minorities and low-income groups.* Rockville, MD: US Government Printing Office.

Valente, S.M. (2000). Evaluating and managing intimate partner violence. *The Nurse Practitioner, 25*(5), 18-19, 23-33.

Van Voorhis, R., & Gilbert, N. (1998). The structure and performance of child abuse reporting systems. *Children and Youth Services Review, 20,* 207-221.

Vobejda, B. (1996, Sept 19). Child abuse increasing. *The Washington Post,* A08.

Walker, B., Jones, J.S., & Krohmer, J. (1991). To report or not to report emergency services' response to elder abuse. *Prehospital Disaster Medicine, 6,* 380.

Walker, L. (1984). *The battered wife syndrome.* New York: Harper & Row.

Warshaw, C. (1996). *Improving the health care response to domestic violence: a resource manual for health care providers* (2nd ed). San Francisco: Family Violence Prevention Fund.

White, E. (1994). The psychology of abuse. In E.C. White (Ed.), *Chain, chain, change: For black women in abusive relationships* (pp. 19-32). Seattle, WA: Seal Press.

Widom, C. (1992). Child abuse and alcohol use and abuse. In P. Martin (Ed.), *Alcohol and interpersonal violence: fostering multidisciplinary perspectives* (pp. 291-314). Rockville, MD: National Institute on Alcohol Abuse and Alcoholism.

Wolfgang, M., & Ferracuti, F. (1967). *The subculture of violence.* London: Travistock Press.

Section VIII

Health Promotion and Disease Prevention

Cheryl McKenzie

Health promotion is the wide array of personal, clinical, and community-based interventions that influence the goal of achieving health. The development of social policies and their application can also influence health. Health promotion includes encouraging healthy lifestyles, creating supportive environments for health, strengthening community action, reorienting health services, and building health-related public policy. Today, people are demanding a health care system that extends lives, provides information needed to extend productive years, and helps make those years of high quality. As the health care delivery system changes, there needs to be more widespread access to health promotion activities and services. Nursing has focused on health by supporting prevention of illness and identifying other factors that may influence the person's definition of health. Concepts such as holism, quality of life, self-care, and healthy lifestyle have been important concepts related to nursing education for many years, and these concepts should transcend individual patients and include families and communities. This section presents information related to health promotion and disease prevention by advanced practice nurses (APNs).

Chapter 41 provides information related to the theoretical background needed for health promotion. The historical roots of health promotion are presented, along with the most influential theoretical models. Prominent nursing models by Pender and Orem are highlighted. This chapter provides the basis for the remaining chapters in the section.

The health of individuals, families, and groups is the focus of Chapter 42. This chapter extends the notion of health promotion from individual patients to an aggregate or community application. Tools such as the ecomap, the genogram, and community assessment are presented as ways that APNs can develop a complete picture of the health promotion needs of individuals, families, and communities.

An important part of health promotion is a healthy lifestyle. Chapter 43 examines the specifics of a healthy lifestyle in detail. Suggestions are provided on how to implement healthy lifestyle recommendations within an APN's practice. Multiple resources are identified, and a sample case is included.

Another important piece of health promotion is stress reduction and relaxation; Chapter 44 details the physiological basis of both of these. The relationships between stress and disease are examined, and the influence of spirituality on health is discussed.

Risk reduction plays an important part in how much needs to be done for a particular patient. The scope of risk reduction (also known as *health protection*) is limited to those interventions that may prevent specific diseases or injuries, limit or prevent illness or disability, and increase years of productive life. Risk reduction is based on current scientific knowledge of specific disease and injury. It employs primary, secondary, and tertiary prevention and is believed to affect morbidity, mortality, and disability among all populations. Chapter 45 stresses the concepts of risk reduction in primary care, and an example is provided of how an APN used the concepts to develop specific interventions for patients.

A newer concept is that of disease management. Chapter 46 is devoted to exploring this concept in depth. Disease management utilizes evidence-based medicine in the form of clinical guidelines to monitor the care a patient is receiving. Evidence exists that effective disease management programs are achieving better outcomes than standard care. Patient outcome data are being used by insurance companies as a way to identify providers that give high-quality care, and APNs need to use this data to promote the quality and effectiveness of their own care.

Chapter 47 presents a summary of the alternative and complementary therapies that have become so prominent. Specifics of each type of therapy are described, and ways in which APNs can incorporate these techniques into their practices are shared.

Chapter 41

Health Promotion and Disease Prevention across the Lifespan

Irene S. Morgan

Thousands of Americans suffer from chronic conditions such as heart disease, cancer, cerebrovascular disease, chronic obstructive pulmonary disease, diabetes mellitus, and liver and renal disease. America is burdened with the high costs of caring for complications from these conditions. Sophisticated medical technology for the diagnosis and treatment of disease conditions has surpassed society's ability to pay for such services (US Department of Health and Human Services [DHHS], 1991; Woolf, Jonas, & Lawrence, 1996). Mobilizing the creative efforts of the nation in the interest of disease prevention and health promotion has become an economic imperative. Advanced practice nurses (APNs) are ideally suited to take active leadership in advancing the nation's health.

A major role within advanced practice is that of health educator and health promotion advocate. Quality health promotion programs are not created by chance; they are the product of much effort and should be based on sound theoretical models. Theoretical models are the means by which health care practitioners can give structure and organization to disease prevention and health promotion programs. Applying theory in health promotion practice can play a critical role in the success of a particular program. Theory can be helpful during the various stages of planning, implementing, and evaluating an intervention.

DEFINITIONS

Based on the explanation provided by the Ottawa Charter (discussed in this chapter), *health promotion* is the process of enabling individuals and communities to increase control over and improve their health. The key word, as Green & Raeburn (1990) emphasize, is *enabling*. Enabling signifies a recent philosophical stance in health promotion to transfer control of important resources in health, namely knowledge, skills, authority, and money, to people and their communities. Health promotion is not only concerned with enabling the development of life skills and individual competence to influence factors determining health, it

is also concerned with environmental intervention to reinforce factors supporting healthy lifestyles and change factors that prevent or prohibit good health. Health promotion has been summarized in the following way:

> Health promotion works *with* people, not *on* them; it starts and ends with the local community; it is directed to the underlying as well as immediate causes of health; it balances concern with the individual and the environment; it emphasizes the positive dimensions of health; and it concerns and should involve all sectors of society and the environment. (Nutbeam, 1996)

In contrast to the concept of disease prevention, health promotion is considered a more general term. Generally excluded from the concept of health promotion are all clinical activities (e.g., medical diagnosis, treatment, patient care) (Noack, 1987). Health promotion does not take its primary stimulus from medicine; in fact, early health promotion literature was prompted by a rejection of some of the traditional medical definitions of health. The departure from the security of medicine left an ideological gap and created confusion over who owns health promotion and what discipline has the right to define the parameters of health promotion (Green & Raeburn, 1990). After decades of emphasis on disease care, nursing began to redefine the concepts of health and health promotion into a broader context. Brubaker's (1983) linguistic analysis of health promotion advanced the construct that health promotion is: "care directed toward high-level wellness through processes that encourage alteration of personal habits or the environment in which people live. It occurs after health stability is present and assumes disease prevention and health maintenance as prerequisites or by-products." Laffrey (1985) defined health promotion as any action taken for the purpose of achieving a higher level of health and well-being. In 1996, Pender suggested that health promotion was directed toward increasing the level of well-being and self-actualization of a given individual or group. Health promotion focuses on efforts to approach a positively balanced state of high-level health and well-being. Although the concept of health promotion from a nursing perspective has evolved over the past several decades, the definitions remain broad.

Health promotion is a relatively new term and not clearly defined. The meaning of *health promotion* overlaps considerably with the meaning of *prevention*. The main difference between the concepts of disease prevention and health promotion seems to be one of focus. Prevention is a disease-related concept; health promotion is a health-related one. The term *disease prevention* is normally used to represent strategies designed either to reduce risk factors for specific diseases or enhance personal factors that reduce susceptibility to disease. Disease prevention is essentially an activity grounded within a traditional medical perspective that concentrates on individuals or particularly defined groups at risk. Disease prevention aims to conserve health; it does not represent a positive vision of health that moves ahead. Rather, disease prevention is concerned with maintaining the status quo. Customarily, three levels of prevention are distinguished (Noack, 1987; Nutbeam, 1996):

Primary prevention can be defined as those activities that seek to prevent the initial occurrence of a disease or disorder. Primary prevention is the promotion of health by personal and community-wide efforts of improving nutritional status, physical fitness, emotional well-being, immunization against infectious diseases, and provision of a safe environment.

Secondary prevention seeks to arrest or retard existing disease through early detection and appropriate treatment. Secondary prevention involves those measures available to individuals and populations for early detection, as well as prompt and effective interventions to correct deviations from good health. Annual physical examinations incorporating diagnostic procedures for detecting cervical, breast, prostrate, or rectal cancer would be an example of secondary prevention.

Tertiary prevention is aimed at reducing complications. Tertiary measures consist of those interventions that reduce impairments and disabilities, minimize suffering caused by existing deviations from good health, and promote a patient's adjustment to an altered, chronic condition. The art and science involved in rehabilitation care is an example of tertiary prevention.

CRITICAL ISSUES: DEVELOPMENT OF HEALTH PROMOTION AND DISEASE PREVENTION THEORIES

Theories and models should serve as the foundation for planning successful health promotion programs. They can be used to examine the reasons why a specific population may or may not be taking good care of their health. Theories and models can help pinpoint what APNs need to know before developing and planning disease prevention and health promotion programs. They can also provide valuable insight into how APNs might design program strategies to reach a target population so that nursing interventions will make a positive difference. Finally, theories and models are important in determining what should be measured, monitored, and compared to evaluate the outcomes of an intervention. Theories and models explain behavior and suggest ways to achieve behavior change. Before introducing some of the major theories and models related to health promotion and disease prevention, a look back at the historical roots of the health promotion and disease prevention movement is worthwhile in gaining an appreciation for the pioneering efforts that have preceded present-day thinking.

Historical Roots of Health Promotion and Disease Prevention

Many threads have been woven into the pattern of health promotion and disease prevention as it now appears. An especially significant influence was the long-standing partnership of public health programs and health education agencies to gain the cooperation of the public. Health promotion and disease prevention emerged from public health approaches and health education programs of the 1950s and 1960s that were initiated to gain public acceptance and cooperation for immunization and tuberculosis screening programs (Green & Raeburn, 1988; Macdonald & Bunton, 1992). Concern over the widespread failure of people to participate in low- or no-cost programs in prevention and early detection of disease motivated a group of U.S. Public Health Service social psychologists to develop a model of health behavior (Rosenstock, 1990). The well-known health belief model (HBM) became a significant development in predicting individual preventive health behavior.

Additional impetuses in the health promotion movement included: (1) the improvements in technology and mass communication in the 1950s and 1960s, which enlightened the public and encouraged grassroots initiatives; (2) the self-care, women's rights, and self-help movements of the 1960s, which demanded that individuals be provided with increased knowledge and authority to decrease their dependency on others; (3) the soaring costs of delivering health care and the cost-containment concerns of the 1970s that led to caps on expenditures for high-tech medical care; (4) the growing recognition of lifestyle as a contributor to chronic disease risks; (5) the support of social, behavioral, and educational sciences applied to health; and (6) the growing dissatisfaction and impatience of the lay public with conventional biomedical approaches to health, approaches that often ignored the mind/body/spirit connection (Green & Raeburn, 1988). The term *health promotion* was first used in 1974 when Canadian Health Minister Marc Lalonde issued *A New Perspective on the Health of Canadians* (Stone, 1986;

Macdonald & Bunton, 1992; McIntyre, 1992; Terris, 1992). As a response to the concerns of many who had become critical of the constricted view of health associated with the biomedical model, Lalonde's report advanced the perspective that people's health was affected by a broad range of factors, including human biology, lifestyle, the organization of health care, and the social and physical environments in which people live. As a result of his report, the Canadian government shifted its emphasis in public health policy from the treatment of disease to illness prevention and, subsequently, health promotion (Macdonald & Bunton, 1992). The Lalonde perspective has been widely credited in furthering understanding of how lifestyle factors affect health (Minkler, 1989), and it was the instrumental evidence that prompted the World Health Organization (WHO) to issue a series of initiatives, beginning with the Alma Ata Declaration in 1978. This declaration outlined the WHO commitment to the principles of health for all by the year 2000 (Macdonald & Bunton, 1992).

By 1979, Julius Richmond, the U.S. Surgeon General, adopted the lifestyle theory of illness etiology and submitted the first *Surgeon General's Report on Health Promotion and Disease Prevention* (US DHHS, 1991; Terris, 1992). This report established broad national goals that served as the blueprint for health improvement of Americans. Health promotion was conceptualized separately from disease prevention, and the two were assigned equal status. Health promotion was characterized by positive lifestyle changes; prevention was characterized as protection from environmental threats (US DHHS, 1991). In 1980, the Surgeon General issued a second report, *Promoting Health/Preventing Disease: Objectives for the Nation,* which established specific, quantifiable objectives necessary for the attainment of the national goals. Objectives were organized around each of the 15 priority areas identified in the first Surgeon General's report (US DHHS, 1991) and included such target areas as smoking cessation, reduction of alcohol misuse, positive dietary changes, exercise, periodical high blood pressure screening, cancer screening, and adequate immunizations (McIntyre, 1992). In 1984, the European Office of the WHO published another influential health promotion report entitled *Health Promotion: A Discussion Document on the Concepts and Principles* (1986). A central position in this document was health for all by promoting equity through the same opportunities for everyone to enjoy good health.

A significant advancement in health promotion occurred in 1986 when, in response to growing expectations for a new global public health movement, WHO, Health and Welfare Canada, and the Canadian Public Health Association convened the first International Conference on Health Promotion in Ottawa, Ontario, Canada; 212 participants from 38 countries met, exchanged experiences, and shared knowledge of health promotion. The Ottawa conference concluded with the production of a charter for "action to achieve health for all by the year 2000 and beyond" (Dines & Cribb, 1993). What has since become a broad definition of health promotion was first articulated in the Ottawa Charter:

> Health promotion is the process of enabling people to increase control over, and to improve, their health. To reach a state of complete physical, mental and social well-being, an individual or group must be able to identify and realize aspirations, to satisfy needs, and to change or cope with the environment. Health is, therefore, seen as a resource for everyday life, not the objective of living. Health is a positive concept emphasizing social and personal resources, as well as physical capacities. Therefore, health promotion is not just the responsibility of the health sector, but goes beyond healthy lifestyles to well-being. (WHO, 1987)

The following five major health promotion actions were outlined in the Ottawa Charter and targeted as the framework for delivery of health promotion programs: building healthy public policy, creating supportive environments, strengthening community action, developing personal skills, and reorienting health services (WHO, 1987).

Closely following the WHO report (1986), Jake Epp, Minister of National Health and Welfare in Canada, released *Achieving Health For All* (Epp, 1986). Proposing an approach to health promotion based on the concepts articulated in the Ottawa Charter, Epp (1986) advocated identifying health as a resource that gave people the ability to manage and change their surroundings. Strategies suggested for implementation included fostering public participation, strengthening community health services, and coordinating healthy public policy (Epp, 1986).

A recent national health strategy published by the U.S. DHHS is *Healthy People 2000*, a platform for action to help Americans fulfill their health potential. The report consists of three broad goals: (1) increasing the span of healthy life, (2) reducing health disparities, and (3) achieving access to preventive services (US DHHS, 1991). To support accomplishments toward these goals, *Healthy People 2000* established 300 measurable objectives in 22 priority areas for health promotion, health protection, and clinical preventive services to be accomplished by the year 2000. Health promotion strategies were described as:

> Those related to individual lifestyle/personal choices made in a social context that can have a powerful influence over one's health prospects. These priorities include physical activity and fitness, nutrition, tobacco, alcohol and other drugs, family planning, mental health and mental disorders, and violent and abusive behavior. Education and community-based programs can address lifestyle in a crosscutting fashion. (US DHHS, 1991)

The newest national agenda is called *Healthy People 2010*. This framework builds upon previous national efforts to outline health promotion and disease prevention objectives. The new 2010 guidelines are the United States' contribution to the WHO's plan. Development of the objectives for *Healthy People 2010* began through the efforts of an alliance of 350 national membership organizations and 250 state health, mental health, substance abuse, and environmental agencies known as the Healthy People Consortium. The consortium met regularly to discuss what improvements were needed from the year 2000 framework to make the next *Healthy People* guidelines relevant for the first decade of the twenty-first century. The focus of the *Healthy People 2010* guidelines is to continue working toward the elimination of health disparities among various racial and ethnic groups and to increase the quality and years of healthy life. Input for guiding the next set of objectives was received from people from every state, the District of Colombia, and Guam. The public made contributions to *Healthy People 2010* objectives through a series of regional and national meetings and an interactive website. Public comments can be found at www.health.gov/hpcomments., and two additional related Internet sites are for the Office of Disease Prevention and Health Promotion (odphp.osophs.dhhs.gov/) and *Healthy People 2010* (odphp.osophs.dhhs.gov/pubs/hp2010/).

Multidisciplinary Contributions

Many disciplines have contributed to theories related to health promotion. Social psychologists have contributed theoretical literature, emanating from value-expectancy theory, that attempts to explain behavior and the mechanisms of change (Becker, 1974; Bandura, 1977; Abramson, Seligman, & Teasdale, 1978; Ajzen & Fishbein, 1980). Sociology has provided theoretical insights into the nature and practice of health promotion by (1) evaluating the social variables that affect health promotion, such as class, gender, age, and culture; (2) defining the norms and values that underpin health promotion, and (3) critically evaluating the medical model (Thorogood, 1992). The discipline of education has contributed educational theory and methodology that health educators and promoters have incorporated into practice (Weare, 1992). The science of epidemiology, focusing on the distribution and determinants of disease in human populations, has contributed scientific information on disease etiology and associated risk factors (Tannahill, 1992). Economic theorists have expanded understanding of cost effectiveness and allocation of health promotion services (Hicks & Boles, 1994).

The earliest historical influences on health promotion and disease prevention in nursing can be traced to Florence Nightingale, who believed in creating environments that were conducive to the restoration and preservation of health. Nightingale described the nurse as a "guide and teacher of health to the individual in the home" (Moore & Williamson, 1984). Early images of public health nurses conducting child immunization clinics, case-finding, and providing health education for the prevention of communicable diseases are also part of

nursing's heritage in health promotion (Novak, 1988). Lillian Wald, famous for establishing the Visiting Nurse Service and Henry Street Settlement in the late 1800s, was remarkable for her early leadership in providing public health care to immigrant families and for her political involvement in working with the legislature to establish health and social policies (Backer, 1993).

Pivotal Health Promotion and Disease Prevention Theoretical Models

Cognitive-behavioral models

Contemporary models of health behavior at the individual and interpersonal levels usually fall within the broad category of cognitive-behavioral theories. Two key concepts cut across these theories:

1. Behavior is considered to be mediated through cognition (i.e., what we know and think affects how we act).
2. Knowledge is necessary but not sufficient to produce behavior change. Perceptions, motivation, skills, and factors in the social environment also play important roles.

This section discusses two of most prominent theories of behavior change; social cognitive theory and the theory of reasoned action. These theories are valuable not only for describing and predicting health-related behavior changes, but also for the effectiveness of interventions based upon them.

Social cognitive theory. The social learning theories of Rotter (1954) and Bandura (1977) have been renamed by Bandura (1986) as the social cognitive theory (SCT). A fundamental premise of this theory is that people learn not only through their own experiences, but also by observing the actions of others and the results of those actions. SCT combines concepts and processes from behaviorism and cognitive theories. Tenets of behavioral psychology propose that behavior is based on reinforcement. Reasoning is not needed to explain behavior. SCT is complex, and learning is explained through key concepts or constructs. Rosenstock, Strecher, and Becker (1988) and McKenzie and Smeltzer (1997) have provided additional explanations of some of the main concepts.

SCT states that reinforcement combined with an individual's expectations of the consequences of behavior determine the specific behavior. The environment shapes, maintains, and constrains behavior. However, people are not passive in the process. People can create and change their environments. The concept of *reciprocal determinism* states that there is a dynamic interaction among the person, the behavior, and the environment; change is bidirectional. The person can shape the environment, and the environment can shape the person. APNs can apply the concept of reciprocal determinism by involving the participants in changing environments that are not conducive to healthy living.

Expectancies and incentives or reinforcements are also important components of the theory. *Expectancies* are one's beliefs about the likely results of an action. The ability of human beings to think and thus to expect certain things describes the meaning of this construct. APNs can use the concept of expectancies in planning illness prevention and health promotion care by incorporating information about the likely results of a particular health-related action in advance. SCT proposes that expectancies may be divided into three types:

1. Expectancies about environmental cues and how events are connected
2. Expectancies about how one's own behavior is likely to influence outcomes
3. Expectancies about one's own competence to perform the necessary behaviors needed to influence outcomes

Incentives or *reinforcements* have been defined as the value of a particular object or outcome. Reinforcement can be accomplished directly, vicariously, or through self-management. Direct reinforcement can occur when a facilitator, such as a weight loss group, directly provides verbal feedback to participants. Vicarious reinforcement, also known as *social modeling*, refers to having participants observe someone else being reinforced to meet behavioral goals. A smoker who desires to give up the habit of smoking and observes an individual being heartily praised and respected for quitting cigarettes is an example of vicarious reinforcement. APNs can take advantage of the opportunities provided through observational learning by pointing out others' positive experiences and physical changes and identifying role models to emulate. When self-management reinforcement is used, participants keep a record of their own behavior. When that behavior was performed in an appropriate manner, participants reward themselves. Using an exercise diary with a predetermined

self-reward for meeting weekly exercise goals is an example of self-management reinforcement.

Behavioral capability is a construct conveying the notion that if individuals are to perform specific behaviors, they must first know what the behaviors are and be taught how to perform the behaviors. Skill mastery is very important. APNs can apply this concept by providing information and training about a particular action, such as how to ease into an exercise program that will fit within a person's daily routine. Writing a prescription for exercise and thoroughly explaining how to use the prescription is a method to increase behavioral capability.

One construct of SCT that has received special attention in health promotion models is the idea of *self-efficacy*. Beliefs that a person has about his or her ability to successfully engage in a desired behavior, also referred to as one's *perception of self-competence*, are central to SCT. Self-efficacy, not actual capability, is thought to be important in predicting behavior change and maintenance. *Outcome expectations* go hand-in-hand with self-efficacy. If a person does not expect that a health action will yield a beneficial result, he or she has little reason to attempt it. A person is most likely to perform some behavior when self-efficacy is high and outcome expectations are positive, and persons with positive outcome expectations are more likely to maintain positive behavior change (Skinner & Kreuter, 1997). It is important for APNs to assess self-efficacy for each specific behavior in question. They should be sure to point out a person's strengths, use persuasion and encouragement, and approach behavior changes in small steps so the person or group is able to achieve an initial goal and thus enhance self-efficacy (Figure 41-1).

Theory of reasoned action. Another theory that is relevant in understanding health behavior change is the theory of reasoned action (TRA) (Fishbein & Ajzen, 1975; Ajzen & Fishbein, 1980). While SCT is concerned with behavior, the TRA provides a model for understanding

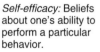

Self-efficacy: Beliefs about one's ability to perform a particular behavior.

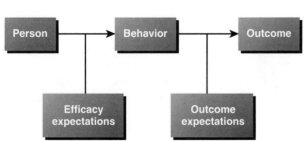

Outcome expectations: Beliefs about a particular behavior leading to some specific outcome.

Figure 41-1 Diagrammatic representation of the concept of self-efficacy and outcome expectations. (From Bandura, A. [1977]. *Social learning theory.* Upper Saddle River, NJ: Prentice-Hall.)

attitudes toward behaviors. The TRA introduces some important concepts that are similar to, but not specified, in other models. Ajzen and Fishbein postulate that there is a relationship among attitude, belief, behavioral intention, and behavior. According to this theory, behaviors are mainly determined by intentions. Individuals' intentions to perform a behavior are a function of their attitude toward performing the behavior plus subjective norms. The notion of subjective norms distinguishes this theory from other theories that try to explain human behavior. *Subjective norms* are the normative beliefs about what relevant others think the person should do. This concept suggests that a person's intent to perform desirable behaviors is dependent partly on what the person believes relevant others will think about him or her engaging or not engaging in a particular behavior and partly on the fact that the person cares about what these relevant others think (McKenzie & Smeltzer, 1997; Skinner & Kreuter, 1997). This theory suggests people are likely to engage in a behavior that they intend to do. Intent to engage in a particular behavior is determined by one's attitude about engaging in the behavior and what the person believes others might think about them doing the particular behavior. The potential value of this theory for APNs may lie in the importance of subjective norms, and application of this theory for APNs should include recognizing the value of the opinion of important others and the relative weight of those opinions on a person's behavioral intentions. Relevant others may include a person's parents, siblings, spouse, close friends, and coworkers, as well as health care professionals. For example, people who think that their significant others believe they should stop smoking will feel some social pressure to do so. This pressure is likely to have more effect if the person highly values and feels motivated to comply with the desires of others. Another example might be at the workplace, where employees who wish to please a boss or impress fellow coworkers might feel a greater intention toward, and thus be more likely to engage in, an onsite health promotion program (Figure 41-2).

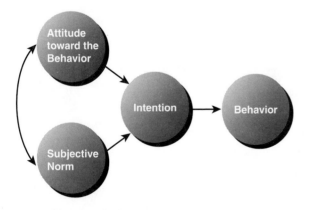

Figure 41-2 Diagrammatic representation of the theory of reasoned action. (From Ajzen, I. [1988]. *Attitudes, personality and behavior.* Chicago: Dorsey Press.)

Health behavior models

Several models have been developed to explain health behaviors. Some of these models are based upon aspects of the theories mentioned earlier in this chapter. This section presents the two best-known of the health behavior models, the HBM and the transtheoretical or stages of change model. The HBM addresses a person's perceptions of the threat of a health problem and the accompanying appraisal of a recommended behavior for preventing or managing the problem. The stages of change model describes an individual's readiness to change or attempt to change toward healthy behaviors. Both of these models should provide APNs with frameworks for providing health promotion, illness prevention, and maintenance-of-function care throughout the lifespan.

Health belief model. The HBM was one of the first models to adapt theory from the behavioral sciences to health problems. It remains one of the most widely recognized frameworks of health behavior explaining self-care activities, but it has a focus on behavior related to the prevention of disease (Becker, 1974; Rosenstock, 1974). During the 1950s, a group of social psychologists at the United States Public Health Service were influenced to develop the HBM after a widespread failure of people partaking in low-cost or free-of-charge programs (e.g., chest x-rays for tuberculosis screening, immunizations) to prevent or detect disease. The social psychologists who outlined the model believed that people feared diseases and that health actions were probably motivated by the amount of fear a person has, the amount of fear reduction possible by taking a particular health action, and the obstacles in the way of taking a action. They were strongly influenced by Lewin's decision-making model (Lewin, Dembo, Festinger, & Sears, 1944) and the view that a person's daily activities are guided by processes of attraction to positive valences and avoidance of negative valences. Illnesses are thought to be areas of negative valence that can be expected to exert a force to move a person away, while health-enhancing behaviors are strategies for avoiding the negatively balanced regions of a person's life space.

The HBM purports to explain why people do or do not engage in a preventive health action in response to a specific disease threat. Specifically, the HBM contends that whether an individual undertakes a recommended health action is dependent upon the following factors: an individual's perceptions of the level of personal susceptibility to the particular illness or condition (the perceived threat); the degree of severity of consequences that might result from contracting the condition (the perceived severity); the health action's potential benefits in preventing susceptibility (the perceived benefits); and the physical, psychological, financial, and other barriers related to the advocated behavior (the perceived barriers or costs). The model also suggests that a stimuli or cue to action must occur to trigger the appropriate behavior. Demographical, social-psychological, and structural variables are included in the theory as potential modifying factors that influence both individual perceptions and the perceived benefits of preventive actions.

The awareness of one's susceptibility to a disease believed to be serious is thought to provide a force leading to action. Rosenstock (1974) suggests behavior depends upon how beneficial an individual believes the various alternatives will be. If the level of readiness to act is strong and the negative aspects of taking an action are perceived as weak, the preventive action is likely to be taken. The amount of cue needed for action is related to the level of readiness. A somewhat high level of readiness requires a slight cue to action, whereas low psychological readiness requires a more intense stimulus (Rosenstock, 1974) (Figure 41-3).

The HBM has been the focus of considerable research and theoretical attention. Janz and Becker (1984) summarized a total of 46 studies related to parts of the HBM. Perceived barriers and perceived susceptibility have received some empirical support, but cues to action, perhaps due to a less-explicit definition, are rarely supported in the HBM research. Much of the research completed on the HBM has been through a shotgun method of selecting variables for study rather than a unified conceptual approach (Davidhizar, 1983). More studies are needed to uncover the generalizability of the HBM for people from different age groups and different cultural backgrounds. The HBM may have greater applicability to individuals who are future oriented and can defer immediate gratification in the interest of long-term goals (Davidhizar, 1983). The HBM will probably not be pertinent to the homeless or other lower socioeconomic groups that often live in the present in order to survive. Perceived susceptibility and perceived severity have a strong cognitive component that depends at least partly on knowledge. Application of the HBM to people who have completed little formal education is questionable. However, despite the limitations identified, the HBM is useful in suggesting that health promotion activities may depend upon each person's belief system.

The HBM has a good fit when the problem behavior or condition calls for health motivation because that is the central focus of the model. The HBM has applications for APNs in planning care that especially caters to increasing motivation. Before a person can accept a diagnosis of a silent health problem, such as hypertension, and follow through a prescribed treatment plan, the person must believe they can have the condition, even without symptoms (perceived susceptibility). APNs can be at the forefront in defining populations at risk. Whenever possible, APNs can personalize risk based on a patient's profile or behavior and heighten perceived susceptibility if it is too low. To reinforce perceived severity, APNs can

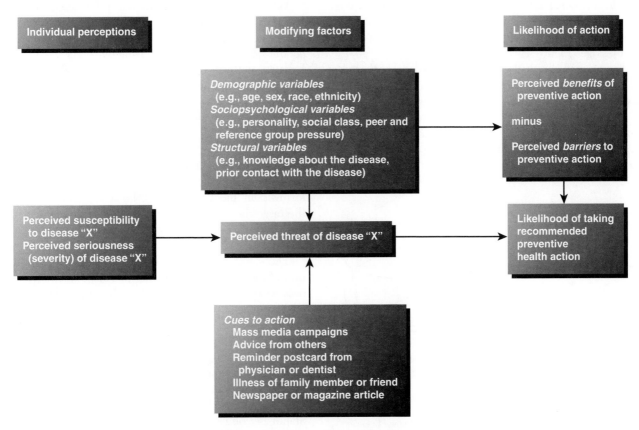

Figure 41-3 Diagram of the health belief model.

educate a patient about any consequences of the risk and the condition. To enhance perceived benefits, APNs can help patients define what actions can be taken and specify the expected positive effects. They can also help patients identify and reduce barriers through reassurance, incentives, and assistance; contribute cues to action by taking advantage of opportunities to promote awareness; provide step-by-step information; and deliver reminders. A most promising application for this model is to serve as a guide for APNs to develop messages that are likely to persuade individuals to make healthy decisions. An example would be offering free mammogram or prostate screenings to patients. APNs need to discuss the importance of preventative screenings with patients when applicable.

The transtheoretical or stages of change model. The transtheoretical model or, as it has been more commonly named, the stages of change model (Prochaska & DiClemente, 1982, 1992; Prochaska, DiClemente, & Norcross, 1992) evolved from work with smoking cessation and the treatment of drug and alcohol addiction. As its title implies, the model is transtheoretical; variables and concepts specified in other models can be applied across the stages of change. A basic premise of this theory is that behavioral change is a process and not an event. Individuals may be at varying levels of motivation or readiness to change, and persons at different points in the process of changing a health behavior can benefit from interventions specifically matched to their current stage of change. This is a spiral rather than a linear model. The model allows for people to enter and exit at any point, and relapse can occur at any stage (Figure 41-4).

The transtheoretical model conceptualizes that in changing an existing behavior or adopting a new one, people move through a series of stages. Five unique stages of change are identified in this model: precontemplation, contemplation, preparation, action, and maintenance. The *precontemplation stage* is defined as the phase at which there is no intention to change behavior in the foreseeable

future. Many people in this stage are not aware of having a problem, though significant others in a person's life are often well aware that there is a problem. "Resistance to recognizing or modifying a problem is the hallmark of pre-contemplation" (Prochaska et al, 1992).

A person is in the second stage, the *contemplation stage*, when the individual is aware that a problem exists and is seriously thinking about doing something about it in the next 6 months but has not yet made a commitment to take action. People can remain stuck in this stage for a long time. Smokers, for example, may consider quitting after weighing the pros and cons of their behavior, but they are not yet quite ready to do anything. During this stage people may struggle with the amount of energy, effort, and loss it would take to overcome the problem. Serious consideration of problem resolution is the central element of contemplation (Prochaska et al, 1992).

The third stage is called the *preparation stage* and combines intention and behavioral criteria. People in this stage are making a plan to change in the next month and have not been successful in taking action within the past year. Individuals in this stage who are prepared to take action report some small behavioral changes toward action, such as cutting back on the number of cigarettes they smoke in a day, purchasing exercise clothing, or buying a book on low-fat cooking. This stage was originally referred to as the *decision-making stage* or the *preparation for the action phase*.

When people are overtly making changes in their behavior, environment, or experiences in order to overcome their problems, they are considered to be in the *action stage*. This stage of change reflects a consistent behavior pattern. Individuals seeking to modify addictive behaviors are thought to be in the action stage if they have successfully performed a desired behavior for a period of from 1 day to 6 months. Modifications of the behavior made in this stage tend to be more obvious, such as a person meeting their criterion of cutting back by 50% on the amount of cigarettes smoked per day. In the action phase people are working hard to change and are actively involved in meeting a target behavior. Modification of the target behavior to an acceptable criterion and significant overt efforts to change are the hallmarks of action (Prochaska et al, 1992).

The *maintenance stage* is considered to be a continuation of the action stage. During this stage people work to prevent relapse and continue the gains attained during the previous stage. Maintenance is not a static stage; it is a continuation of change. For addictive behaviors this stage is thought to extend from 6 months to an indefinite period. A goal of health promotion and disease prevention is to encourage lifetime maintenance of health-enhancing behaviors. People during this stage may need a boost to help them maintain the changes they have already made. Stabilizing behavior change and avoiding relapse are the hallmarks of maintenance (Prochaska et al, 1992).

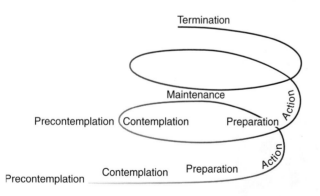

Figure 41-4 A spiral model of the transtheoretical or stages of change model. (From Prochaska, J., DiClemente, C., & Norcross, J. [1992]. In search of how people change: applications to addictive behaviors. *American Psychologist, 47,* 1104.)

The transtheoretical model can be useful to APNs in several ways. First, it serves as a reminder that not everyone is ready for change at the same time. APNs using this framework to understand that people may proceed through behavior change at different paces can design a health promotion program that may better meet a person's present state of change. During the precontemplation stage, when the person is unaware of a problem or has not thought about change, an APN could increase awareness of the need for change and personalize information on the risks and benefits of the present behavior. Recognizing that someone may be in the contemplation stage (i.e., thinking about change in the near future), an APN could assist a person by motivating the individual and encouraging him or her to make specific plans. When assessing someone who is making a plan to change, as in the preparation stage, an APN can assist a person in developing concrete action plans and setting gradual, obtainable goals. An APN working with someone who is in the action stage can assist that person by providing feedback, social support, reinforcement, and problem-solving as issues come up. Finally, when working with a person in the maintenance stage, an APN can teach coping skills, develop a system of reminders to keep the behavior up, and assist the person to avoid relapse. If relapse does occur, an APN can be available to support the person back into one of the change stages, such as the precontemplation or contemplation stage, until the person eventually succeeds in maintaining change.

Prominent nursing models

Health promotion model. When the HBM was introduced and tested as a major theoretical development in explaining preventive health behavior, the health promotion movement was just beginning. Finding that the HBM explained preventive but not health promotion behavior was the impetus that led Pender (1982, 1987, 1996) to develop and refine a health promotion model (HPM) for nursing. Expectancy value (Feather, 1982), social cognitive theory (Bandura, 1986), and the HBM (Becker, 1974; Rosenstock, 1974) were some of the theoretical influences contributing to the construction of the HPM. Pender advanced the HPM in an effort to synthesize the features from many theories that had the most relevance for nursing.

Pender's model (1996) proposes relationships among behavior-specific cognition and affect, behavioral outcome, and individual characteristics and experiences. Individual characteristics and experiences include personal biological, psychological, and sociocultural factors. Pender submits that although personal factors are thought to influence the likelihood of engaging in health promoting behavior, some personal characteristics, such as age, gender, and ethnicity, can not be changed and thus are seldom incorporated into nursing interventions.

The core of the HPM model accentuates the impor-

tance of behavior-specific cognition and affect as the primary motivators of behavior. Pender (1996) emphasizes that these variables could be especially significant for nurses to consider, as they are subject to modification through nursing interventions. The six elements of behavior-specific cognition and affect considered to be of major motivational significance in encouraging one to engage in health-promoting behaviors have been identified as: perceived benefits of action, perceived barriers to action, perceived self-efficacy, activity-related affect, interpersonal influences, and situational influences. Actions that increase personal health status are hypothesized to be related to positive perceptions of the anticipated expected outcome, minimal barriers to action, feeling efficacious and skilled, positive feelings about the health behavior, presence of family and peer social support, positive role models, and availability of environments that are compatible, safe, and interesting (Pender, 1996).

Behavioral outcomes are proposed to be influenced by a person's sense of commitment to a plan of action with identified specific strategies, as well as the capacity of the person to repress competing demands and preferences. Health-promoting behavior is the action outcome in the model. Pender (1996) highlights that health-promoting behavior is ultimately directed toward attaining positive health outcomes that should result in a positive health experience throughout a person's lifetime (Figure 41-5).

The HPM is quite complex, with many subcomponents. Some aspects of the model could use further clarification; all concepts should be defined, and the gaps explaining the direction of the relationships between the concepts should be closed. Although several dissertations and research reports have been published that use the HPM or have tested components of the model, some of the hypothesized relationships in this framework have yet to be tested or reported. The HPM is broad in scope and has the potential to guide nursing in providing a comprehensive approach to health promotion. Social, contextual, and developmental factors that may contribute to the deliberate engagement of health promotion behaviors are not well explained by the HPM.

Self-care theory. Self-care, as a theoretical framework for understanding and studying health promotion, is useful as a guide in understanding factors that may contribute to people engaging in activities to maintain and improve their health. The words *self-care*, *self-help*, and *health promotion* have been used interchangeably. Orem (1995) has been instrumental in proposing a nursing theory of self-care. Orem submits that a relationship exists between deliberate self-care actions and the development and functioning of individuals and groups. Self-care is viewed as a learned, deliberate behavior based on cultural aspects of groups. Self-care agency reflects the ability of an individual to provide for his or her self-care needs. Orem has defined self-care as activities that individuals initiate

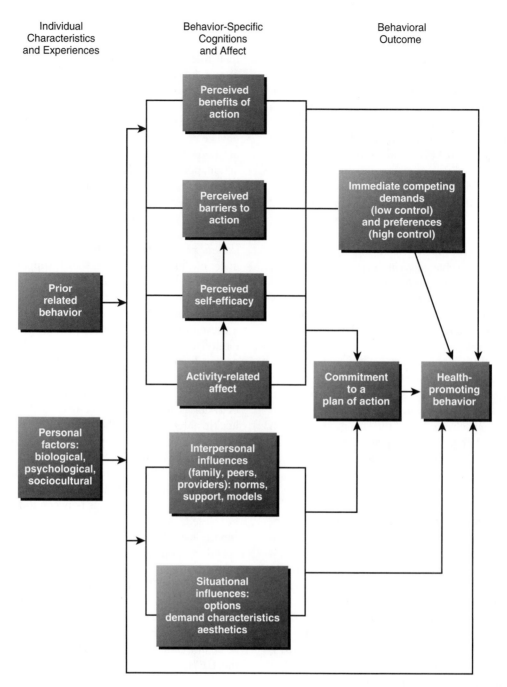

Figure 41-5 The health promotion model. (From Pender, N. [1996]. *Health promotion in nursing practice* [3rd ed.]. Upper Saddle River, NJ: Prentice-Hall.)

and perform on their own behalf in maintaining life, health, and well-being. Orem connected self-care needs, self-care agency, and self-care deficits to three types of nursing systems: those that are wholly compensatory, those that are partially compensatory, and supportive-educative systems. The purpose of nursing, from Orem's perspective, is to identify self-care needs and design interventions to assist the individual or family members to meet those self-care requirements. Individuals are seen as active participants of professional health care, not merely as passive recipients.

Orem (1995) offered that people have three types of self-care needs: universal, developmental, and health deviation self-care. Universal self-care needs are those that are common to everyone and are associated with life processes and maintenance of health. Universal self-care requisites consist of maintenance of a sufficient intake of air, water, and food; maintenance of elimination; a balance between rest and activity and solitude and social interaction; avoidance of hazards to human life; and promotion of human functioning and development within social groups.

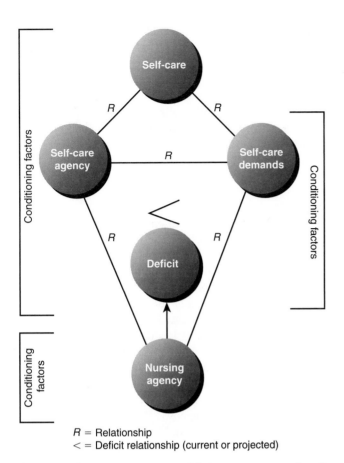

R = Relationship
< = Deficit relationship (current or projected)

Figure 41-6 Orem's Self-Care Model. (From Orem, D. [1995]. *Nursing: concepts of practice*. St. Louis: Mosby.)

Developmental self-care requisites are those care needs associated with human developmental processes that occur during various stages of the life cycle. Developmental self-care requisites include the bringing about and maintenance of living conditions that support life processes and promote the processes of development (Orem, 1995). Also included under this type of self-care is the provision of care either to prevent the occurrence or harmful effects of conditions that can affect human development or to relieve or overcome the effects of such conditions as educational deprivation and oppressive living circumstances (Figure 41-6).

Health deviation self-care needs come forth from human structural and functional deviations and their effects, as well as from associated medical diagnostic and treatment procedures. Health deviation self-care requisites include seeking and securing appropriate medical assistance, attending to the effects of pathologic conditions, carrying out medically prescribed therapeutics, regulating harmful effects of medical care measures, modifying the self-concept, and learning to live with the effects of pathological conditions. Orem's framework has guided descriptive research documenting the universal and illness-related self-care practices of young adult women in several studies (Woods, 1985; Maunz & Woods,

1988; Lawrence & Schank, 1995) and has been combined with the transtheoretical model to form a theory of exercise (Ulbrich, 1999). (Orem's framework was discussed in greater detail in Chapter 30.)

Health promotion planning models

Models that support program-planning processes include the newly developed Health Promotion Matrix (Gorin & Arnold, 1998) and the well-established and popular PRECEDE-PROCEDE model by Green and Kreuter (1991). These two theories can be useful in directing interventions and providing effective programs. Health promotion planning models increase the odds of success by examining health and behavior at multiple levels. Generally speaking, health promotion interventions involve two basic changes: changes within people themselves and changes within the environment. The most powerful health promotion planning approaches combine both options. Both of the models presented here focus on meeting patients' self-determined needs within the context of their environments.

Health Promotion Matrix. The most recent HPM to be developed by nurses is one that focuses on health promotion planning. It is called the Health Promotion Matrix (Gorin & Arnold, 1998). The authors describe this model as a clinical tool to be used by health professional and patient as partners in health promotion care. The role of the health care professional is as one who transfers knowledge and skill so the patient can make an informed and deliberate decision about taking actions that may enhance health. Health image is a central concept. Gorin and Arnold (1998) propose that the image of an authentic ideal, including that of health, exerts a strong force on the patient's life. The health care professional can encourage the patient to move toward reaching the patient's ideal image of health. APNs can use the matrix to personalize care for patients by identifying patients' unique health images, strengths, and capabilities, then enabling patients to engage in specific behaviors according to their individual needs.

The Health Promotion Matrix consists of three major components that lead to health: patient systems, dimensions, and healthy behaviors. There are four patient systems, five dimensions for maximizing health-promoting interventions, and nine positive health behaviors. Patient systems may vary to include individuals, families, groups, or communities. Strategies unique for each of the possible patient systems are offered. Entry into the matrix begins with a health care professional assisting a patient through the five dimensions. The first dimension is image creation. During image creation the patient begins to construct an ideal image of health. Intervention by the APN during this phase could be in the form of helping the patient to clarify his or her image of health, the many aspects of his or her health, and the value of health for the patient. After image creation comes the second dimension, image appraisal.

Using the matrix as a guide, image appraisal occurs as the APN examines the patient's current health status, compares it to the patient's stated ideal image, and recognizes the gap. While in this dimension the patient and APN determine whether the patient's personal image of health is realistic and achievable. Intervention strategies necessary to achieve the patient's personal image of health are then considered. The third dimension, minimizing health-depleting patterns, begins as the patient is assisted in analyzing present patterns that are health depleting and in beginning to change them. Together the patient and APN can prioritize the interventions. At the same time as health-depleting behaviors are being modified, the patient can be supported to continue through the matrix and optimize health-supporting patterns. The APN should identify the patient's strengths and encourage the continuation of health-supporting patterns. An important role for the APN during this period is to praise any movement toward narrowing the gap between the ideal healthy self and the present actual self. The final dimension is internalizing the ideal image. At this point, the gap has become narrower as health behavior changes have become part of the patient's routine. Health is viewed as a process rather than a goal. "The process of moving from image creation and image appraisal, through minimizing depleting patterns and optimizing health supportive patterns toward internalizing an idealized image of health is repetitive, involving re-evaluations and re-formulation of intervention foci" (Gorin & Arnold, 1998).

The last major component of the matrix is the nine positive health behaviors. The nine behaviors were derived from major national policy literature and from a review of health promotion literature. The nine behaviors are: smoking cessation, eating well, physical activity, sexual awareness, injury prevention, substance safety, oral health, self-development, and productivity. The APN and the patient devise interventions (moving from creating an ideal image through to the internalizing process) within each of the nine positive health behaviors. All of the behaviors are interconnected, with each behavior influencing every other behavior. The Health Promotion Matrix "operationalizes health as the confluence of the nine healthy behaviors" (Gorin & Arnold, 1998) (Figure 41-7).

PRECEDE-PROCEED. A discussion of theoretical models for health promotion, disease prevention, and maintenance of function throughout the lifespan would be incomplete without including the PRECEDE-PROCEED framework (Green & Kreuter, 1991), which is a popular and comprehensive model developed specifically for health promotion planners. An overriding principle of this model is that most enduring health behaviors are voluntary in nature. This principle is reflected in the model as it seeks to empower individuals with understanding, motivation, skills, and active engagement to improve the quality of their lives. PRECEDE-PROCEED has nine phases; the first five phases are diagnostic (social, epidemiological, behavioral and environmental, educational and organizational, and administrative and policy); the remaining four phases are devoted to implementation and evaluation. The five diagnostic phases serve to identify objectives and set priorities based on their importance, immediacy, and changeability. The result of all of these diagnoses is a plan with specific objectives and strategies; strategies are based

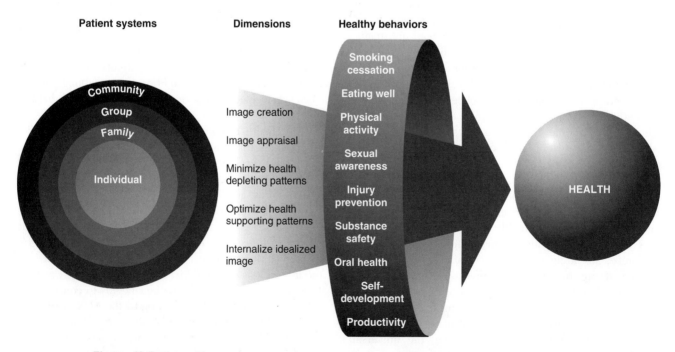

Figure 41-7 The Health Promotion Matrix. (From Gorin, S., & Arnold, J. [1998]. *The Health Promotion Matrix health promotion handbook*. St. Louis: Mosby).

on information learned in the diagnostic phases about key causes and factors contributing to the identified problem.

PRECEDE-PROCEED begins by identifying the desired outcome (based on patient needs), determining what will cause the desired outcome, and finally designing an intervention aimed at reaching it. Phase 1 in the model is called *social diagnosis*. The purpose of this phase is to subjectively define quality of life by encouraging the target population to engage in a self-study of their own needs. In phase 2 the health promotion planner develops an epidemiological diagnosis by ranking the health goals or problems that may contribute to the needs identified during the first phase. Phase 3 involves determining and prioritizing the behavioral and environmental factors that are thought to be associated with the health goals or problems identified in phase 2. Behavioral factors are related to individual practices such as adherence, consumption patterns, coping skills, self-care, preventive behaviors, and utilization. Environmental factors are those factors outside of an individual that can be modified to support health and quality of life.

The PRECEDE-PROCEED model is most likely to be informative to the APN during phase 4, the educational and organizational diagnosis. This phase focuses on examining factors that shape behavioral actions and environmental factors. Behavioral actions such as improving one's diet, participating in an exercise program, and obtaining regular Pap smears are shaped by predisposing, reinforcing, and enabling factors. Environmental factors, such as the availability of prevention services or workplace hazardous material safety measures, are influenced primarily by enabling factors.

Predisposing factors are those that can facilitate or hinder a person's motivation to change and may include knowledge, attitudes, values, cultural beliefs and readiness to change. The APN can alter predisposing factors through direct communication. Enabling factors are those that can support or hinder a person's efforts to make the desired behavior change and could include skills, access to health care facilities, supportive policies, assistance, services, or barriers. APNs could help change enabling factors by working with communities and organizations to reduce barriers and improve resources. Reinforcing factors are those factors that come into play after a behavior has begun and can encourage or discourage continuation of the desired behavior. Social support, praise, reassurance, symptom relief, and negative feedback following a behavior are examples of reinforcing factors. APNs can affect reinforcing factors by communicating with family, friends, peers, employers, teachers, and others who are in a position to offer social reward.

Phase 5 of the model addresses administrative and policy diagnosis. During this phase, health promotion planners determine if capabilities and resources are available to develop and implement the program. Phase 5 ends the PRECEDE portion of the model. The final four phases, phases 6 through 9, make up the PROCEED half

of the framework. During phase 6, if appropriate resources are available, the health promotion planner selects the methods and strategies for the intervention; program implementation now begins. Phases 7, 8, and 9 focus on evaluation, effects, and outcomes and are based on objectives determined earlier in the model. All three of the final phases may not be necessary. The evaluation requirements of the program determine which ones would be most helpful (Figure 41-8).

PRECEDE-PROCEED's systematic approach to diagnosing health-related problems facilitates critical thinking by APNs regarding intervention points and strategies. The framework allows for broad analysis on multiple levels, such as individual cognitive, situational, sociopolitical, and environmental. A primary application of using this complex model is as an aid in identifying factors, both behavioral and environmental, that influence health-related behaviors in the population of interest.

IMPLICATIONS FOR MSN EDUCATION AND ADVANCED PRACTICE

Studying and discussing theories in an academic setting with colleagues and mentors is a stimulating activity that enhances understanding and promotes enthusiasm. However, applying theories to the "real world" setting can be challenging and sometimes even discouraging. Although suggestions have been offered on steps APNs can take in applying each of the theories presented in this chapter, planning interventions for people never seems to be quite so straightforward as the models might suggest. People are complex and live in a variety of contexts. Theories may have to be twisted and tweaked a bit so that they will work for a particular situation.

Health educators in particular have paid attention to this phenomenon. An investigation published in the health education literature by Burdine and McLeroy (1992) explored why health care professionals were not using the theories they learned during their professional preparation. The research revealed three main concerns: (1) theory taught in school fails to adequately guide clinical practice in specific settings or unusual situations, (2) most of the theories are individualistic and lack guidance for community-oriented interventions, and (3) once out of an academic setting, it is difficult to transfer theories to the practice environment. Burdine and McLeroy (1992) suggest that some of these concerns are probably due to the origins of the early health behavior theories. Health promotion and disease prevention was created primarily from the behavioral and social sciences, where the popular notion of changing individual behavior as the means to improve health has long been accepted. Many of the foundational theories from which other theories have been built did not concern themselves with the larger contextual

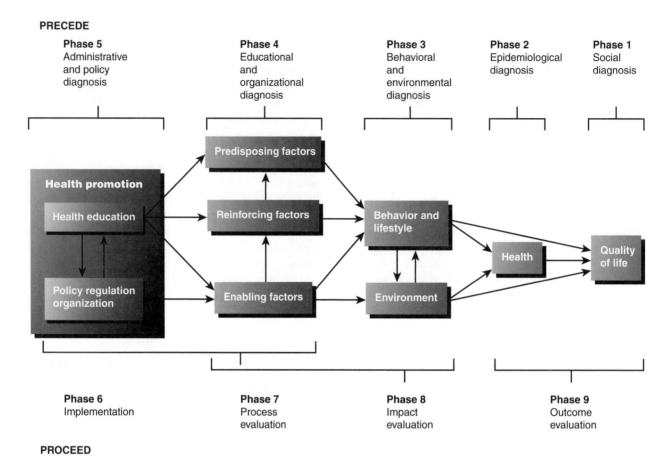

Figure 41-8 PRECEDE-PROCEED model for health promotion planning and evaluation. (From Green, L.W., Marshall, W., & Kreuter, M.W. [1999]. *Health promotion planning: an educational and environmental approach* [3rd ed.]. Mountain View, CA: Mayfield Publishing Company.)

issues affecting health, such as poverty; pollution; lack of health insurance; and the commercialization of fast food, tobacco, and alcohol. Another possible contributor to why theories are not being applied in clinical settings may have to do with the way theories are taught. Instead of teaching theories in isolation from life situations, Burdine and McLeroy (1992) urge academicians to teach theory by starting with a specific health problem and asking students to critically think through how each of the theories can help to improve understanding of the problem.

McKenzie and Smeltzer (1997) have examined theory application research and provided a summary of ideas that should help health care practitioners apply theory to their clinical practices:

1. APNs need to take the time to learn theories by truly understanding each theory as a whole rather than memorizing the parts. By becoming comfortable with theories and their interrelationships, an APN will be better prepared to take the next step, which is to examine the applicability of the theories for specific problems that arise in the clinical setting.

2. The scientific literature should be reviewed to see what theoretical approaches have been successfully tried in the past for a particular health issue.

3. Another approach to discovering which theory is suited for a particular problem is to look at the goals of an APN-initiated activity and then match a theory that will assist the APN in meeting his or her goals; several theories may be applicable.

4. Seldom does a single theory address all of the complex issues of a problem. Parts of theories can be synthesized and customized to fit a particular situation; however, if parts of a theory are removed, the original theory is not the same and its effectiveness cannot be ensured.

5. APNs must know their own philosophies of care and beliefs surrounding a particular issue. APNs will be more comfortable using a theoretical framework that matches their own views and values.

PRIORITIES FOR RESEARCH

Health promotion in the United States from 1979 to the present day has been narrowly defined, focusing on health

Leading Health Indicators of *Healthy People 2010*

Physical activity	Tobacco use
Overweight and obesity	Substance abuse
Responsible sexual be-haviors	Mental health
	Environmental quality
Injury and violence	Access to quality health
Immunizations	care

behavior, chronic disease risk factors, and lifestyle issues. The United States' view depicts health promotion as those actions people can undertake for themselves; this reflects the strong individualism so deeply ingrained in American culture. Individual behavior is considered the most important influence on health, and the disease prevention factor is considered the most responsive to change. Changing individual lifestyles is assumed to be necessary to reduce health care expenditures and other morbidity- and mortality-related economic losses (Morgan & Marsh, 1998).

The lifestyle approach to health promotion is housed within a Western ideology that values the individual and recognizes the importance of personal responsibility for individuals' successes and failures. This approach frequently results in a "blaming the victim" mentality and can exonerate health care providers of accountability (Crawford, 1977). The lifestyle approach represents health as converted into a marketplace commodity and does not adequately account for the social, economic, political, and environmental factors that affect a person's way of living. Becker (1993) questions whether the individual lifestyle approach to health promotion actually decreases the level of health in our society because of the focus on individual health rather than societal well-being. Research that examines the extent of the "blame the victim" mentality is vital. Self-efficacy and accountability are important concepts that need further research. Many of today's diseases can be positively affected by lifestyle changes, but these are the changes that are most difficult to make. Intervention studies that focus on outcomes and the effectiveness of APN teaching and their focus on health promotion will be important to conduct in the future.

The *Healthy People 2010* objectives have identified leading health indicators (Box 41-1) that reflect the major public health concerns in the United States. Data will soon be available to indicate progress on these leading health indicators and the success that organizations have had in reaching *Healthy People 2010* goals. Strategies and action plans that address one or more of the indicators will likely be very strong competitors for research grant monies. It will be interesting to see if the proposed strategies and

interventions can help equalize the health disparities currently seen in underserved populations.

Muhlenkamp, Brown, and Sands (1985) found several predictors of health-promoting behavior in a study they conducted in a nursing clinic. Those patients who had more education, were younger, were female, or who perceived their own health status were more likely to engage in health-promoting behaviors. The authors also found a negative relationship between an external locus of health control and healthy behavior. These factors were similar to those found by Weitzel (1989) and Duffy (1988). Frauman and Nettles-Carlson (1991) examined predictors of health-promoting behaviors in a clinical population of patients who had chosen to see a nurse practitioner (NP) who focused on health maintenance. Most of the patients (80%) had an internal locus of control and ranked their health as their highest value. Patients with higher scores on the Health Promoting Life Style Profile had higher educational levels and income. The authors' interpretation of this data indicates that a patient's concept of what being healthy means influences behavior. The message to APNs from this research is that patients with higher educational levels and incomes are more likely to need factual information about health risks and guidance on how to achieve lifestyle changes. Patients with less education and income need more assistance in getting motivated to make necessary lifestyle changes.

Research conducted by Lemley, O'Grady, Rauckhorst, & Russell (1994) evaluated the effectiveness of NPs in clinical preventive services based on *Healthy People 2000*. The survey data, which regarded the percentage of patients who routinely receive specified assessment and intervention services, was completed by 892 NPs. In the majority of cases, NPs provided care that exceeded the *Healthy People 2000* objective targets. Future research needs to expand studies such as that by Lemley et al. In part, as increased quality outcome data is collected, these answers will become part of the routine evaluation of APNs' effectiveness of services.

DISCUSSION QUESTIONS

These questions can be used to promote critical thinking and encourage discussion.

1. Why are theoretical frameworks important to use when planning illness prevention and health promotion care?
2. What concepts seem to be common across the models? How does that help or hinder their application?
3. Of the eight models presented, which one is most appealing to you? Name the different phases of the model and defend why you chose this model.

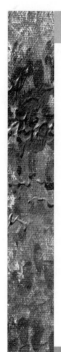

Suggestions for Further Learning

- Get the following article: Lemley, K., O'Grady, E., Rauckhorst, L., Russell, D., & Small, N. (1994). Baseline preventive data provided by nurse practitioners. *Nurse Practitioner, 19*(5), 57-63. What are areas of the *Healthy People 2000* objectives in which APNs excel? What areas need improvement? What are some strategies that would improve health promotion in those areas?
- Get the article: Bergman-Evans, B., & Walker, S. (1996). The prevalence of clinical preventive services utilization by older women. *Nurse Practitioner, 21*(4), 88, 90, 99-100. How well do older women do in attaining preventive services? What implications does this research have for APNs who serve older adult patients?
- Get the article: Burn, C. (1994). Toward Healthy People 2000: the role of the nurse practitioner and health promotion. *Journal of American Academy of Nurse Practitioners, 6*(1), 29-35. What recommendations does Burn have for APNs in terms of health promotion? Are they

realistic for use in practice? Will the strategies work for APN students?
- Go to the *Healthy People 2010* website (www.health.gov/healthypeople) for an update on its progress.
- Get the *Healthy People 2010 Toolkit* at www.bookstore.phs.org to obtain examples of state and national examples of setting objectives.
- Visit the following internet resources:
  - www.umich.edu/~nursing/faculty/pender_nola.html (contains links to information about health promotion models)
  - www.who.int/ (contains information on health promotion and disease prevention from a global perspective)
  - www.monash.edu.au/health/IJHP/index.htm (an online journal from Australia's Monash University Faculty of Medicine Health Promotion Unit)
  - web.health.gov/healthypeople/prevagenda/whatishp.htm

4. Take your favorite model or one of the others and, using a hypothetical health problem with a target population of your choice, discuss how that model would guide your care.
5. After reviewing the models presented in this chapter, were there any major concepts missing? How would your own model look based on your perspective of the elements necessary in a health promotion and illness prevention theoretical framework? Draw a diagram of your model so you can explain it.
6. Where should the majority of health promotion and disease prevention money, time, and effort be aimed: individual level, family level, community level, or national level? What goals and responsibilities should APNs have in promoting health and preventing disease?
7. How can the work of APNs promote the national agenda for the twenty-first century? Should APNs develop their own guidelines for health promotion care, based on the underlying beliefs from which nursing was originally founded? If so, what principles would be most important to you in drafting such a document?
8. As an APN, will you be prepared to be a leader in guiding the future of health promotion and illness prevention care? What strengths do you have in terms of health promotion? What are areas in which you think you need more experience?

REFERENCES/BIBLIOGRAPHY

Abramson, L., Seligman, M., & Teasdale, J. (1978). Learned helplessness in humans: critique and reformulation. *Journal of Abnormal Psychology, 87*, 49-74.

Ajzen, I. (1988). *Attitudes, personality and behavior.* Chicago: Dorsey Press.

Ajzen, I., & Fishbein, M. (1980). *Understanding attitudes and predicting behavior.* Englewood Cliffs, NJ: Prentice Hall.

Backer, B. (1993). Lillian Wald: connecting caring with activism. *Nursing & Health Care, 14*(3), 122-129.

Bandura, A. (1977). *Social learning theory.* Upper Saddle River, NJ: Prentice-Hall.

Bandura, A. (1986). *Social foundations of thought and action.* Englewood Cliffs, NJ: Prentice Hall.

Becker, M. (1974). The health belief model and personal health behavior. *Health Education Monographs, 2*, 324-508.

Becker, M. (1993). A medical sociologist looks at health promotion. *Journal of Health and Social Behavior, 34*(3), 1-6.

Brubaker, B. (1983). Health promotion: a linguistic analysis. *Advances in Nursing Science, 5*, 1-14.

Burdine, J., & McLeory, K. (1992). Practitioners' use of theory: examples from a workgroup. *Health Education Quarterly, 19*(3), 331-340.

Crawford, R. (1977). You are dangerous to your health: the ideology and politics of victim blaming. *International Journal of Health Services, 7*(4), 663-680.

Davidhizar, R. (1983). Critique of the health belief model. *Journal of Advanced Nursing, 8*, 467-472.

Dines, A., & Cribb, A. (1993). Ottawa Charter for health promotion. In A. Dines & A. Cribb (Eds.), *Health promotion: concepts and practice.* London: Blackwell Scientific.

Duffy, M. (1988). Determinants of health promotion in midlife women. *Nursing Research, 37*, 358-362.

Epp, J. (1986). *Achieving health for all: a framework for health promotion.* Ottawa, Canada: Department of National Health and Welfare.

Feather, N. (1982). *Expectations and actions: expectancy-value models in psychology.* Hillsdale, NJ: Lawrence Erlbaum.

Fishbein, M., & Ajzen, I. (1975). *Belief, attitude, intention, and behavior: an introduction to theory and research*. Reading, MA: Addison-Wesley.

Frauman, A., & Nettles-Carlson, B. (1991). Predictors of a health promoting lifestyle among well adults clients in a nursing practice. *Journal of the American Academy of Nurse Practitioners, 3*(4), 174-179.

Gorin, S., & Arnold, J. (1998). The Health Promotion Matrix. In S. Gorin & J. Arnold (Eds.), *Health promotion handbook* (pp. 91-113). St. Louis: Mosby.

Green, L., Marshall, W., & Kreuter, M. (1991). *Health promotion planning: an educational and environmental approach* (2nd ed.). Mountain View, CA: Mayfield.

Green, L., & Raeburn, J. (1988). Health promotion. What is it? What will it become? *Health Promotion, 3*(2), 151-159.

Green, L., & Raeburn, J. (1990). Contemporary developments in health promotion: definitions and challenges. In N. Bracht (Ed.), *Health promotion at the community level* (pp. 29-43). Newbury Park, CA: Sage.

Hicks, L., & Boles, K. (1994). Why health economics? In C. Harrington & C. Estes (Eds.), *Health policy and nursing: crisis and reform in the U.S. health care delivery system*. Boston: Jones & Bartlett.

Janz, N., & Becker, M. (1984). The health belief model: a decade later. *Health Education Quarterly, 11*(1), 1-47.

Laffrey, S. (1985). Health promotion: relevance for nursing. *Topics in Clinical Nursing, 7*, 29-38.

Lawrence, D., & Schank, M. (1995). Health care diaries of young women. *Journal of Community Health Nursing, 12*(3), 171-182.

Lemley, K., O'Grady, E., Rauckhorst, L., Russell, D., & Small, N. (1994). Baseline preventive data provided by nurse practitioners. *Nurse Practitioner, 19*(5), 57-63.

Lewin, K., Dembo, T., Festinger, L., & Sears, P. (1944). Level of aspiration. In J. Hunt (Ed.), *Personality and the behavior disorders* (pp. 333-378). New York: Ronald Press.

Macdonald, G., & Bunton, R. (1992). Health promotion: discipline or disciplines? In R. Bunton & G. Macdonald (Eds.), *Health promotion: disciplines and diversity* (pp. 1-19). London: Routledge.

Maunz, E., & Woods, N. (1988). Self-care practices among young adult women: influence of symptoms, employment, and sex-role orientation. *Health Care for Women International, 9*, 29-41.

McKenzie, J., & Smeltzer, J. (1997). *Theories and models commonly used for health promotion interventions: planning, implementing, and evaluating health promotion programs*. Needham Heights, MA: Allyn & Bacon..

McIntyre, L. (1992). The evolution of health promotion. *Probe, 26*(1), 15-22.

Minkler, M. (1989). Health education, health promotion and the open society: an historical perspective. *Health Education Quarterly, 16*(1), 17-30.

Moore, P., & Williamson, G. (1984). Health promotion: evolution of a concept. *Nursing Clinics of North America, 19*(2), 195-206.

Morgan, I., & Marsh, G. (1998). Historic and future health promotion contexts for nursing. *Image: Journal of Nursing Scholarship, 30*(4), 379-383.

Muhlenkamp, A., Brown, N., & Sands, D. (1985). Determinants of health promotion activities in nursing clinic patients. *Nursing Research, 34*, 327-332.

Noack, H. (1987). Concepts of health and health promotion. In T. Abelin, Z. Brzezinski, & V. Carstairs (Eds.), *Measurement in health promotion and protection* (European series no. 22) (pp. 5-28). Copenhagen: World Health Organization Regional Publications.

Novak, J. (1988). The social mandate and historical basis for nursing's role in health promotion. *Journal of Professional Nursing, 4*(2). 80-87.

Nutbeam, D. (1996). Health promotion glossary. In *Health promotion: an anthology* (Scientific publication no. 557) (pp. 343-358). Washington: Pan American Health Organization.

Orem, D. (1995). *Nursing: concepts of practice* (5th ed.). St Louis: Mosby.

Pender, N. (1982). *Health promotion in nursing practice*. Norwalk, CT: Appleton & Lange.

Pender, N. (1987). *Health promotion in nursing practice* (2nd ed.). New York: Appleton-Century-Crofts.

Pender, N. (1996). *Health promotion in nursing practice* (3rd ed.). Upper Saddle River, NJ: Prentice-Hall.

Prochaska, J., & DiClemente, C. (1982). Transtheoretical therapy: toward a more integrative model of change. *Psychotherapy: Theory, Research, and Practice, 20*, 161-173.

Prochaska, J., & DiClemente, C. (1992). Stages of change in the modification of problem behaviors. In M. Hersen, R. Eisler, & P. Miller (Eds.), *Progress in behavior modification* (pp. 184-214). Sycamore, IL: Sycamore Press.

Prochaska, J., DiClemente, C., & Norcross, J. (1992). In search of how people change: applications to addictive behaviors. *American Psychologist, 47*, 1102-1114.

Rosenstock, I. (1974). Historical origins of the health belief model. In M. Becker (Ed.), *The health belief model and personal health behavior*. Thorofare, NJ: Charles B. Slack.

Rosenstock, I. (1990). The health belief model: explaining behavior through expectancies. In K. Glanz, F. Lewis, & B. Rimer (Eds.), *Health behavior and health education: theory, research and practice* (pp. 39-59). San Francisco: Josey-Bass.

Rosenstock, I., Strecher, V., & Becker, M. (1988). Social learning theory and the health belief model. *Health Education Quarterly, 15*(2), 175-183.

Rotter, J. (1954). *Social learning theory and clinical psychology*. New York: Prentice Hall.

Skinner, C., & Kreuter, M. (1997). Using theories in planning interactive computer programs. In R. Street, W. Gold, & T. Manning (Eds.), *Health promotion and interactive technology: theoretical applications and future directions* (pp. 39-65). Mahwah, NJ: Lawrence Erlbaum.

Stone, D. (1986). The resistible rise of preventive medicine. *Journal of Health Politics, Policy and Law, 11*(4), 671-695.

Tannahill, A. (1992). Epidemiology and health promotion. In R. Bunton & G. Macdonald (Eds.), *Health promotion: disciplines and diversity* (pp. 86-107). London: Routledge.

Terris, M. (1992). Concepts of health promotion: dualities in public health theory. *Journal of Public Health Policy, 13*(3), 267-276.

Thorogood, N. (1992). What is the relevance of sociology for health promotion? In R. Bunton & G. Macdonald (Eds.), *Health promotion: disciplines and diversity* (pp. 42-65). London: Routledge.

Ulbrich, S. (1999). Nursing practice theory of exercise as self-care. *Image: Journal of Nursing Scholarship, 31*(1), 65-70.

U.S. Department of Health and Human Services (1991). *Healthy people 2000: national health promotion and disease prevention objectives* (DHHS publication no. [PHS] 91-50213). Washington, DC.

Weare, K. (1992). The contribution of education to health promotion. In R. Bunton & G. Macdonald (Eds.), *Health promotion: disciplines and diversity*. London: Routledge.

Weitzel, M. (1989). A test of the health promotion model with blue collar workers. *Nursing Research, 38,* 99-104.

Woods, N. (1985). Self-care practices among young adult married women. *Research in Nursing & Health, 8,* 227-233.

Woolf, S., Jonas, S., & Lawrence, R. (1996). *Health promotion and disease prevention in clinical practice*. Baltimore: Williams & Wilkins.

World Health Organization (1986). A discussion document on the concepts and principles of health promotion. *Health Promotion, 1*(1), 73-76.

World Health Organization (1987). Ottawa Charter for health promotion. *Health Promotion, 1*(4), iii-v.

Chapter 42

Health Promotion of Individuals, Families, Groups, and Communities

Leslie Cooper, Cheryl McKenzie, & Denise Robinson

As people enter the twenty-first century, the pursuit of optimal health is a growing trend. By some estimates, at least 70% of major health problems are attributed to health-damaging lifestyles (Pender, 1996). Society and the environment have nearly as significant an effect on the health of an individual as do personal choices and family influence. Culture (both ethnic and popular) and environment contribute to an individual's and family's health practices. Consumers are bombarded with a variety of messages regarding their health choices and how they can improve their lifestyles. Media stars appear on afternoon talk shows to discuss the latest discovery that will help viewers retain their youth. Athletes write syndicated columns advising readers about diet and exercise. Advertisements tout vitamins, herbal remedies, diet aids, and food supplements designed to relieve stress, improve memory, induce weight loss, or promote a good night's sleep. Organizations such as the American Cancer Society and the American Heart Association compete with cigarette and alcohol manufacturers for the attention of the American public, using the same slick advertising campaigns as their "competitors."

Advanced practice nurses (APNs) must understand the concepts of health promotion and be knowledgeable of the health trends and messages bombarding health consumers. In addition to traditional health care, APNs in clinical practice must be able to discuss alternative and complementary therapies and assist their patients in making the best health choices. Most importantly, all APNs must take a leadership role in creating an atmosphere that promotes positive health behaviors for individuals, families, and communities.

DEFINITIONS

To *promote* is to help or encourage to exist or flourish. Pender (1996) defines *health promotion* as being "motivated by the desire to increase well-being and actualize human health potential." Health promotion is not disease or problem specific; it is an approach seeking to expand the positive potential for health. Effective health promotion requires a shift in emphasis from illness to wellness. Individuals must move away from the idea of seeking health care to fix their health problems and accept responsibility for their own health. This kind of change requires that health care providers shift from a paternal approach to a partnership approach, which requires that health care providers be prepared to look beyond traditional treatment modalities and health care delivery systems as they assist patients in achieving optimal health. It also requires that health care workers move beyond traditional provider-patient relationships and form partnerships with groups and agencies within the community to provide effective, comprehensive health promotion. Health promotion includes five aspects: building health-promoting public policy, creating supportive environments, strengthening community action, developing personal skills, and reorienting health services (Stanhope & Lancaster, 1996). These five aspects of health promotion demonstrate how close the links are between community health nursing, health promotion, and primary health care. Each incorporates community-based practice, involvement in community health care decisions and goal-setting, a focus on disease prevention and health promotion, and the use of an interdisciplinary and multisectoral approach in planning and implementing solutions to health problems. Changes in one area affect the others.

Stanhope and Lancaster (1996) define a ***group*** as "a collection of interacting individuals who have a common purpose or purposes. Each member influences and is in turn influenced by every other member to some extent." Health behavior is influenced by the groups to which people belong and in which they value membership. A ***partnership*** is the informed, flexible, and negotiated distribution and redistribution of power among all participants in the process of change for improved community health (Stanhope & Lancaster, 1996). Some people use the term **aggregate** instead of *group* when referring to a particular population. Examples of aggregates might include patients who smoke, diabetics, or pregnant adolescents. The people in the aggregate share a common variable that is identifiable.

Community is defined as "people and the relationships that emerge among them as they develop and use in common some agencies and institutions and a physical environment" (Stanhope & Lancaster, 1996). The Coalition for Healthier Cities and Communities (www.healthycommunities.org) defines *community* as "all persons and organizations within a reasonable circumscribed geographic area in which there is a sense of interdependence and belonging." The World Health Organization (WHO) defines a healthy city or community as one that is safe, with affordable housing and accessible transportation systems, work for all who want to work, a healthy and safe environment with a sustainable ecosystem, and access to health care services that focus on prevention and staying healthy.

CRITICAL ISSUES: HEALTH PROMOTION AND ADVANCED PRACTICE NURSES

National health policy continues to focus on health promotion, health protection, and preventive health services. The documents *Healthy People 2000* and *Healthy People 2010* continue to provide national health objectives that drive health policy in the United States. The Centers for Disease Control and Prevention (CDC) worked (and continue to work) with state and local governments to use the national health objectives as their framework for health promotion and prevention activities. (This information is discussed in greater detail in Chapters 41 and 45.)

A health promotion model was proposed by Palank (1991) and Simmons (1990) that complements some of the other health-promoting models that are currently available. This model (Box 42-1) uses three categories of determinants for health-promoting behavior: cognitive perceptual

---

Box 42-1

Three Categories of Determinants of Health-Promoting Behavior

COGNITIVE-PERCEPTUAL FACTORS

Definition of health
Importance of health
Perceived health status
Perceived control of health
Perceived self-efficacy
Perceived benefits of health-promoting behaviors
Perceived barriers to health-promoting behaviors

MODIFYING FACTORS

Demographic factors
- Age
- Gender
- Race
- Ethnicity
- Education
- Income
Biological characteristics
- Body weight
- Body fat
- Height
Interpersonal influences
- Expectations of significant others
- Family patterns of health care
- Interactions with health professionals
Situational (environmental) factor
- Access to care
Behavioral factors
- Cognitive and psychomotor skills necessary to carry out healthy behaviors

VARIABLES AFFECTING THE LIKELIHOOD OF INITIATING ACTIONS

Depend on internal and external cues:
- Desire to feel well
- Individualized health teaching
- Mass media health promotion campaigns

Data from Palank, C.L. (1991). *Nursing Clinics of North America, 26*(4), 815-832; and Simmons, S.J. (1990). *Journal of Advanced Nursing, 15*(10), 1162-1166. Reprinted with permission from Stanhope, M. & Lancaster, J. (Eds.). (1996). *Community health nursing: promoting health of aggregates, families, and individuals* (4th ed.). St. Louis: Mosby.

factors, modifying factors, and variables affecting the likelihood of initiating action. These categories are similar to the health belief model (HBM); however, this newer model expands each of the areas. APNs can use this model to help determine if patients are likely to make health-promoting changes in lifestyle. Many patients engage in health-promoting behaviors for different reasons. Laffrey (1990) conducted research to determine subjects' five most important health behaviors and why they usually performed those behaviors. Responses indicated that there were generally three reasons why they engaged in health behaviors. For one individual, exercise was necessary because he had heart disease and the exercise was an illness-preventing behavior. For another person, exercise made him feel better and more energetic, so the exercise could be considered a health-promoting behavior. One woman described her exercise as a way to keep her weight under control; in this instance, the exercise was a health maintenance behavior. APNs can take this information and discuss what role exercise or other health behavior might play in his or her patients' lives. Hitting upon the "right" reason may be enough to make the behavior more important to a patient. For example, in Jean's case, she knows that exercising is a vital part of her care to address her hypertension. It really serves two purposes: to help keep her weight stable and to keep her heart and body as fit as possible, even in the presence of heart disease. While she might be tempted to stop exercising, she knows that it helps her in numerous ways and therefore is less likely to stop.

Health Promotion for Individuals

Health promotion is an aim of APNs; however, many times it is not differentiated from disease prevention or health maintenance. Brubaker (1983) believes that health promotion and disease prevention are two sides of the same coin. Health promotion of individuals many times incorporates principles of health promotion, risk appraisal, and risk reduction. Information supplied by patients about their health behaviors, family health history, personal health history, and personal demographics is compared to data from epidemiological studies and vital statistics. These comparisons are used to make predictions about an individual's morbidity and mortality, as well as the strategies that can be used to reduce risks. (Chapter 45 presents more information related to risk reduction and preventative services for individuals.)

In addition to calling for individual actions and policy changes, previous research and reports have emphasized the link between physical and mental health, the link between health and the environment, and the need for strong family and community support systems. Although few research studies have been done on the importance of screening for mental health disorders in the ambulatory

care setting, screening is an essential component of health promotion. In the past, small studies reviewed the effectiveness of mental health screenings with unclear results. The problems may have been related to the screening tools used in the studies, which may have been too narrowly focused. Another hypothesis is that health care providers may have not screened for mental health disorders due to lack of time or interest. The U.S. Preventive Services Task Force did not find sufficient documentation to support screening for depression, suicide, drug abuse, or dementia (1996), but it still recommends health care providers be aware of signs and symptoms in patients.

There are compelling arguments related to screening for all mental health disorders in the ambulatory care setting. Patients with depression tend to have increased rates of heart disease and reduced bone mineral density (Dinan, 1999). Also, health care costs may be increased if mental health disorders go unrecognized. One study looked at health care costs in patients without a previous diagnosis of a mental health disorder in the ambulatory setting. During the research study, the patients screened positive for either depression or anxiety. The study found that although the costs of health care in those patients who screened positive for depression and anxiety were higher, it was not related to increased mental health services, but to an increased use of medical services (Simon, Ormel, & VonKorff, 1995). Patients with mental health disorders do not usually make a health care visit for a specific condition, such as anxiety or depression. They may be evaluated for a physical problem that has an etiology related to mental health. Also, mental health problems can increase the severity of some physical problems.

APNs should also have a role in the community in relation to sexual health. Of particular importance is the adolescent population. Approximately 1.1 million adolescent girls become pregnant in the United States annually. These adolescents are at high risk for multiple problems as a result of being a teen mother. There is also an increased incidence of sexually transmitted diseases (STDs) in the teen population (CDC, 1998). APNs need to identify those patients who are considered to be at high risk to provide teaching, counseling, and treatment. Sexual health is also important in the adult population. Screenings can be offered in the community for women and men. Research has shown that women are now living 6 years longer than men, which is related to the attention they give to their overall health. Women in the United States are seen 150 million more times by their health care providers than men each year according to the Men's Health Network. Many of the deaths from diseases related to sexual health might be prevented if men and women participated in health promotion activities. Services such as prostate and mammogram screenings can be offered in the community. Also, education about self-testicular and self-breast exami-

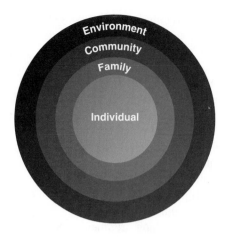

Figure 42-1 Subsystems that exist within the environment.

nations would assist in decreasing the amount of misinformation regarding sexual health.

Health Promotion for Families

Health promotion should focus on the family as well as the individual. Certainly, individuals play a critical role in the determination of their own health. However, individuals do not exist in a vacuum, free of contact with others and their influence. Individuals exist as subsystems within the family. The family exists as a subsystem within the community, which is a subsystem within the environment (Figure 42-1). The first step to begin looking at the health promotion needs of a family is to conduct a family assessment. Family assessment can be utilized in the ambulatory care setting. There are many tools available that provide information regarding the family structure and function. Two of the most common and usable tools are the genogram and the ecomap (Hitchcock, 1999). The genogram (Figure 42-2) allows APNs to visually depict the family structure. It includes information about family history related to genetic diseases and family illnesses; examples of illnesses that might be depicted include diabetes, coronary disease, cystic fibrosis, mental illness, and tuberculosis. The genogram needs to include data from three generations in chronological order. As the genogram is being mapped out, family risk factors can be assessed; this helps identify potential health problems and demonstrate to the family the need for intervention (Hitchcock, 1999).

The ecomap (Figure 42-3) visually depicts the family and their relationship to the external environment. It provides information related to the strengths, conflicts, and resources available to the family (Hitchcock, 1999). The ecomap is a valuable tool when assessing a family's involvement in the community. The genogram and ecomap can both be completed in collaboration with the family during an initial family interview. Examples of information that may be assessed utilizing the ecomap are the

relationships the family has with their church, school, health care facilities, extended family, and work.

After completing a family assessment using the genogram and ecomap, APNs can use the nursing process to identify the health risks for the family and identify the appropriate nursing diagnoses. The major health risks for families arise in several areas: biological, social, economic, lifestyle, and life events leading to crisis (Table 42-1). In most cases, it will take more than a single threat to affect family health, and a combination of factors from two or three categories is more common. For example, John has a family history of myocardial infarction (MI). His father had a MI at age 42, but John compounds the issue of genetic risk by smoking a pack of cigarettes a day. Numerous family assessment tools are available to help identify health risks and family stressors, and Robinson (1997) uses family theory as a way to identify a family under stress and identify possible strategies the family can use to address the stressors.

Nursing diagnoses related to the family are not well developed. Diagnoses more often deal with the individual patient within a family. For an APN focusing on a family as the patient, some nursing diagnoses may need to be modified to the clinical situation. Box 42-2 identifies possible nursing diagnoses that could be used in the ambulatory setting when providing care for a family.

Kang, Barnard, and Oshio (1994) described the practice of APNs who provide care for families at risk in rural Washington. They conducted a retrospective review of the records of patients seen and found that the most frequently occurring nursing diagnoses assigned to parents were altered parenting, altered family processes, fear, noncompliance, and knowledge deficit. For children, the most frequently used nursing diagnoses were impaired physical mobility, impaired verbal communication, altered nutrition (less than body requirements), sensory-perceptual alteration, and altered thought processes. Box 42-3 provides an example for utilizing the nursing process when providing care for a family in the ambulatory care setting.

Burr, Klein, and Burr (1994) examined changes experienced during family life in nine separate areas. They found that families did use various strategies to address life stresses and also found significant differences between men and women. Women used more strategies, while men were more likely to use harmful strategies. These findings are helpful for APNs to keep in mind when a family is undergoing crisis. Discussion of helpful and nonhelpful strategies that a family might use when under stress might be instrumental in what choice of strategies the family makes. For example, John, when he is stressed (as he was when laid off from work), tends to self-medicate with alcohol to reduce his anxieties about not working and contributing to the family. For the APN to discuss this tendency with him during his last visit was important so that he became aware of his use of nonhelpful strategies. Lisa, the APN, used an interactive, collaborative style to

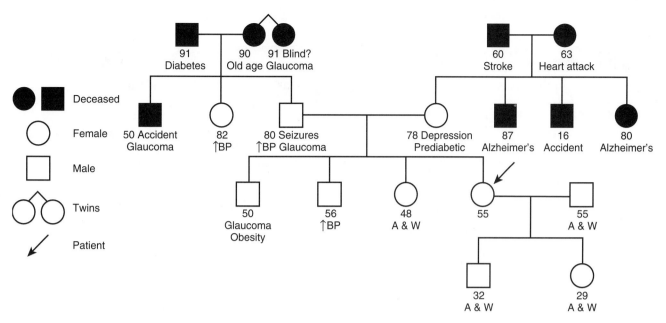

Figure 42-2 Sample genogram. *A & W*, Alive and well; *BP*, blood pressure. (From Seidel, H. [1999]. *Mosby's guide to physical examination*. St. Louis: Mosby.)

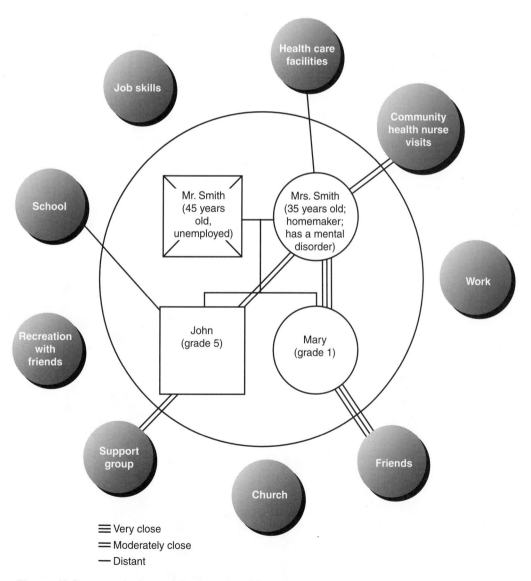

Figure 42-3 Ecomap for the Smith family. (Adapted from Swanson, J.M., & Nies, M.A. [1997]. *Community health nursing* [2nd ed.]. Philadelphia: WB Saunders.)

Table 42-1

Types of Family Risks

TYPE OF RISK	EXAMPLES OF RISK
Biological	This involves illnesses that have a familial component or a genetic basis, including cardiovascular disease, obesity, diabetes, hypertension, some types of cancer, and gallbladder disease.
Social	This includes things such as living in a high-crime neighborhood; living in a community with inadequate recreational or health resources; environmental issues, such as noise or contamination by chemicals; high stress; and discrimination.
Economic	Poverty places people at higher risk for health problems. Economic risk is determined by the relationship between family financial resources and the demands on those resources.
Lifestyle	This includes things such as amount of sleep, diet, smoking, risky sexual behaviors, amount of exercise, substance abuse, and violence.
Life event	Movement from one stage of development to another within the family involves life events, and these are potential risks for families. Life events include things such as marriage, divorce, birth of a child, death of a family member, graduation, starting school, moving, or loss of a job.

Box 42-2

Potential Nursing Diagnoses for Use with Family Issues

Altered family processes
Altered parenting
Anticipatory grieving
Family coping
Ineffective health-seeking behaviors
Ineffective family coping
Compromised family coping

Box 42-3

Case Scenario Utilizing the Nursing Process for a Family

Parents bring their 6-month-old infant in for a well-child care visit. They also have a 3-year-old child who is developmentally delayed. History reveals the home is not "childproof" and the parents do not always use a car seat.

Nursing Diagnoses
Potential for altered health maintenance related to safety hazards in the home

Interventions
- Assess the age and developmental level of all family members.
- Stress the importance of health promotion.
- Provide education and anticipatory guidance related to hazards (e.g., car seats, seatbelts, motor vehicle safety, fire hazards, choking hazards).

Evaluation
- Is the family keeping appointments for well-care visits for both children?
- At the next well-care visit, have they instituted safety precautions in the home and car?
- Do they have access to resources available in the community?

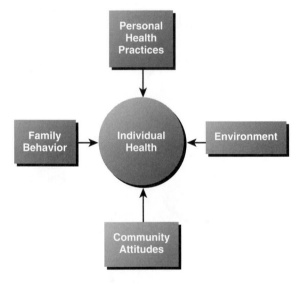

Figure 42-4 Factors affecting the health of an individual.

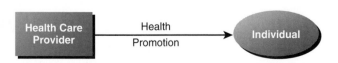

Figure 42-5 Individual approach to health promotion.

discuss various strategies John might use. Lisa had John contract with her on the maximum number of beers he would drink a day, and John was willing to do this because he had not been aware he was using alcohol as a stress reducer.

Empowerment of families may be a good option when working with families on health risks. Empowerment gives the family access and control over needed resources and provides them decision-making and problem-solving abilities to deal with the issues that are affecting them. Families may need help to learn how to identify sources of help and even on when they might need help. They need to know the critical questions to ask to obtain the information that gives them mastery over their affairs.

Health Promotion for the Community

Effective health promotion must extend beyond the boundaries of the individual and family. Traditionally, nurses have provided care to individuals and families, and even in community settings, the nursing role has been limited to traditional care in clinics. Flynn (1997) points out that whether people have livable wages, safe streets, affordable housing, good schools, and a clean and green environment affects the community's health. It is important for APNs to realize that a community is more than the sum of the individuals, families, and aggregates within it; for any change to occur, the larger community must be considered (Stanhope & Lancaster, 1996). The notion of community as patient has been difficult to integrate into practice, and multiple levels of intervention are needed to make meaningful changes in the community.

Pender (1996) states that health is both an individual and a societal issue. Personal practices are only one factor affecting the health of an individual. Comprehensive health promotion also recognizes and assesses the influences of family behaviors, community attitudes, and the environment on health. To be successful, individual behavioral changes must have the support of the family, the community, and the environment (Figure 42-4).

Effective, comprehensive health promotion can be challenging for APNs practicing within the framework of managed care. One-on-one assessment of health behaviors, provision of health information, and reinforcement of positive health practices is costly and time consuming. This approach rarely addresses subsystems beyond the level of the individual, and traditionally, this is how most nursing care is delivered (Figure 42-5).

APNs must be involved in a partnership approach to health promotion. A partnership approach includes members of the various subsystems working with health workers to create an atmosphere that promotes and supports good health practices and healthy lifestyles (Figure 42-6). This approach is critical for APNs working as population-focused case managers with high-risk groups. Flynn (1997) notes that APNs bring community leadership,

community assessment, research, and policy advocacy expertise to the process of building healthy communities. Changes aimed at improving the health of a community involve partnerships among its residents and health workers from a variety of disciplines. Partnership is important because health is not given; it is generated through new and increasingly effective forms of collaboration (Stanhope & Lancaster, 1996).

Traditional roles have limited nursing's involvement in changing the health status of the community. The nursing process (assessment, planning, implementation, and evaluation) has been used to provide care for individuals and, in some cases, families. However, in the community health arena, nurses are usually informed of desired changes and become involved only during the implementation phase (Stanhope & Lancaster, 1996). The power for inducing significant change through assessment and planning has traditionally belonged to health workers such as physician health officers and health planners, but nurses today must understand the concept of providing care in a population-focused practice (PFP) in order to be fully included in the process.

Rather than providing nursing care to individual patients in a clinical setting, priorities in a PFP are to develop and maintain organized mechanisms for the provision of care to defined populations. In a PFP, the emphasis should be on the relationships between the health status of the population, the factors that influence health status, and the responses and effectiveness of the care system in dealing with the population's health (Figure 42-7). Nurses engaged in a PFP collaborate with patients to identify needs and develop solutions. They participate actively in system-level decisions and influence other decision-makers to implement solutions (Stanhope & Lancaster, 1988). APNs must be leaders in identifying health problems of the entire community and advocating partnership approaches in which all involved are assessing, planning, implementing, and evaluating community changes. Clearly, nurses whose practice is population focused are involved in health pro-

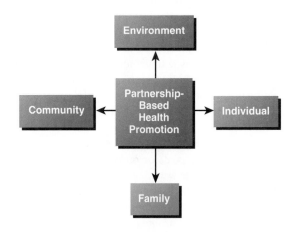

Figure 42-6 Partnership approach to health promotion.

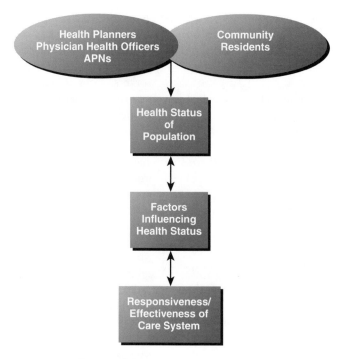

Figure 42-7 Population-focused practice.

motion. This is an advanced practice role, and many graduate programs have incorporated a community focus.

APNs can utilize the nursing process when focusing on health promotion in the ambulatory care setting. The nursing process works when applied to the community as well as when applied to an individual (see Figure 42-4). The first step occurs with the assessment of an individual, family, or community. Assessment includes obtaining a thorough history and other pertinent data about health risks. Assessment of a community will indicate how community subsystems are functioning to meet the health needs of the community. For example, an outbreak of hepatitis A may mean a breakdown in sanitation measures by health personnel. Any changes found on the assessment may mean that readjustments need to be made in health services. At the Redbud Family Health Center, for example, APNs noted an increase in the number of Hispanics who were coming to the center. The clinic administration and APNs got in touch with the local government to determine if there was actually an increase in the demographics of Hispanics in the community. An increase in this population was identified, and it was noted that many of the Hispanics were not able to speak English, thus limiting their ability to seek care at Redbud.

The next step in community assessment is the planning phase, when realistic goals or outcomes are determined. Planning may include teaching, counseling, and health screening. Nursing interventions related to health promotion are based on the type of prevention applicable. With health promotion in the ambulatory care setting, interventions may happen over a longer period. At Redbud, a goal was made to increase by 50% the number of Hispanics who

used the center as their primary care center. Once a goal is determined, intervention strategies to address the goal and problem should be identified and put into motion. The intervention strategy at Redbud was to initiate a Spanish-speaking health team, consisting of a nurse practitioner (NP), a licensed practical nurse, and a receptionist. A pamphlet in Spanish was developed and distributed to the part of the community where most of the Hispanic people lived. Information about the new service was also shared with social services and the organization that normally supplied interpreters.

The plan and intervention should be evaluated on a regular basis to determine if the goals have been achieved or if modification is needed. When dealing with health promotion in the community setting, evaluation should involve reviewing data to see if rates of illness are declining as a result of health promotion screening or activities. At Redbud, it is still too early to tell how the Spanish-speaking team is affecting the health of the patients. It is clear that the number of Spanish-speaking patients has tripled since the service was begun, but further data must be collected to see how the intervention affects the health of the community.

Since many APNs continue to provide care for individuals within a community, it might be helpful to see the differences in the levels of intervention for an individual, family, and community. For example, with disease prevention, an individual intervention might be teaching a mother the specifics of a well-balanced diet for a 2-year-old toddler. A family intervention might consist of counseling the whole family on nutritious food choices to avoid anemia; using play food, each family member could describe what a well-balanced diet would look like for 24 hours. A community focus would address aggregates; in this situation, this would involve assessment of children at a school for signs of malnutrition, examination of baseline health data, and work with others to reduce the children's risk of malnutrition.

In terms of health promotion, a comparison of individual, family, and community might look like this. For the individual, health promotion might mean working with a mother to incorporate healthy activities into a child's day. At the family level, it might mean identification of health activities (e.g., biking, hiking) and incorporation of them into the family's lifestyle. At the aggregate level, it might be teaching a class of first and second graders about dental hygiene and the importance of brushing twice daily and receiving regular dental checkups; pamphlets could be sent home to the family describing the same information. A community as patient approach might include dental screening activities or the establishment of community exercise activities to encourage the integration of healthy behaviors into everyday activities.

IMPLICATIONS FOR MSN EDUCATION AND ADVANCED PRACTICE

Nursing education must include a community focus at both the graduate and baccalaureate levels, and education for APNs needs to incorporate content related to community health at the graduate level. This means subjects such as epidemiology principles, models applicable to community health, and research specific to community health issues must be presented.

Interest in health promotion is a growing trend, not a passing fad. Community partnerships in health promotion empower communities by helping community members gain power over their own lives. These partnerships have the potential to bring about policy changes that affect many people. Nursing's role in helping patients achieve optimal health status is shifting from institutional care to self-care. However, Pender (1996) warns that any strategy for health promotion that focuses only on individual behavioral change is doomed to failure without simultaneous efforts to alter the environment and collective behavior. Involvement in community partnerships insures nurses a voice in health decision-making.

First and foremost, an APN needs to do a community assessment of the area in which he or she will be practicing. This means knowing the risks affecting patients that will be seen. It also means knowing the resources that are available to patients within that community. Knowing how to get a cab voucher for a patient who can not take the bus and does not have personal transportation may mean the difference between follow-up and no follow-up.

Abraham and Fallon (1997) worked with a large

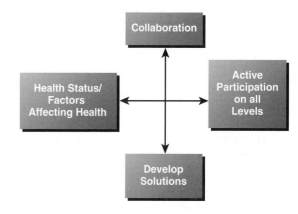

Figure 42-8 Starting point for healthy community initiatives.

metropolitan hospital in Boston to deliver care to a small urban community. The APNs attended health care delivery meetings, met community leaders, visited various community sites, and became familiar with the community and its residents. In effect, the APNs conducted a community assessment. Their assessment became the cornerstone for the development of proposed intervention strategies and a model, based on Orem's Self-Care Model, of enhancing the delivery of care. The authors believe that the use of a community assessment enabled them to become health care leaders in the community.

APNs engaged in primary practice must work with their colleagues to identify community partnerships that will expand their health promotion efforts beyond individual patients. A successful community initiative relies on participation from many different individuals. However, in most instances, healthy community initiatives start because a single person or organization within the community takes the initiative. (Figure 42-8 shows the starting point for most healthy community initiatives.)

APNs must identify and use strategies that help patients achieve optimal levels of health. The development of nursing centers may be one way to serve people within a community that are without health resources. Barger and Rosenfield (1993) looked at the more than 80 nursing centers around the country. They found most of the centers were associated with a parent organization, such as a school of nursing, and provided care for a high proportion of disadvantaged patients.

APNs in administrative roles must provide leadership to other health professionals and be prepared to practice in a population-focused manner. Nurse-researchers can provide leadership and examples through community-based health promotion demonstration projects and population-based intervention projects aligned with the current, national health objectives. Of special interest will be projects focusing on low-income families, immigrant populations, and blue-collar workers; these populations are often overlooked in health promotion efforts. They are also the very populations often served by APNs in primary practice.

APNs must be knowledgeable regarding national health policy because policy drives funding for health services as well as research. APNs need to be familiar with the current national health objectives and ensure that strategies to achieve those objectives are reflected in their interactions with patients, families, and the community. This includes being aware of all aspects of physical and psychological health.

PRIORITIES FOR RESEARCH

Significant research topics can be generated for health promotion of the individual, family, and community. Many times, APNs can identify research topics just through observations made as part of everyday practice. Research questions might focus on cost effectiveness, accessible health care, community involvement, disease prevention and health promotion, and a multiorganizational approach. For example, how cost effective are health promotion activities? What is the best way to integrate health promotion into primary practice? How well do APNs do at health promotion activities? What is the best way to determine outcomes related to heath promotion? How effective are health promotion interventions among low-income, older adult, immigrant, and blue-collar worker populations who are at more risk? What are the best health promotion interventions related to children, adolescents, and young, middle, and older adults?

Rickelman and Gallman (1994) looked at the use of quality-of-life assessments for older adults who are independent. They found that a strong level of attachment to a significant other was significantly and positively correlated with quality of life and self-rated health. Ahljevych

and Bernhard (1994) looked at health-promoting behaviors among African-American women, but the authors concluded that the tool they used might have a middle-class bias and may not truly indicate a low interest by the women in health promotion for healthy lifestyles. Results from studies like this do provide much useful information to APNs in practice. For example, if it was noted on a number of studies that a particular ethnic group did not usually engage in health-promoting behaviors, it would make a difference in what strategies APNs might use when discussing plans of care with patients.

Miovech (1996) conducted a study looking at the nursing time and activities of APNs who provided care to women with unplanned cesarean deliveries. She used the Community Health Intensity Rating Scale to classify nursing encounters. While the data was not normally distributed, Miovech believes that the scale is applicable for APNs because it addresses anticipatory guidance and the holistic view of patients.

Ockene, Adams, and Hurley (1999) describe a study looking at the effect of brief counseling given by physicians or NPs to high-risk drinkers. Randomized into this study were 530 patients. The intervention group got a health booklet with advice on general health issues, and a 5- to 10-minute counseling session at the time of their routine visit. The usual care group received the same health booklet and were encouraged to ask any questions of their health care provider. Outcomes were determined by self-report of weekly alcohol intake and binge drinking episodes. After adjusting for age, baseline alcohol consumption, and sex, patients who received the counseling session had a lower alcohol consumption (mean reduction

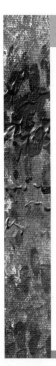

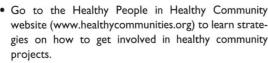

Suggestions for Further Learning

- Go to the Healthy People in Healthy Community website (www.healthycommunities.org) to learn strategies on how to get involved in healthy community projects.
- A national resource to help with the development of healthy communities is The Coalition for Healthier Cities and Communities, c/o Hospital Trust and Educational Trust, 1 North Franklin, Chicago, IL, 60606; website www.healthycommunities.org. Visit the coalition website for information about various states' healthy community projects
- Reece (1998) describes the process of community analysis and needs assessment for comprehensive health promotion. While helpful to APNs in general, this article specifically addresses APNs in primary practice in the community. Is this approach something that would provide you with helpful data?
- Polivka and Ryan-Wenger (1999) use a population-focused approach in their survey of health promo-

tion behaviors among school-age children. Their findings suggest that there are different health promotion needs among different subgroups of children. Are these needs similar to what you have found in practice?
- Effectiveness, both in terms of cost and behavioral change, is critical in determining the success of health promotion efforts. Lugo (1997) discusses the cost savings enjoyed by a company with a nurse-managed corporate employee wellness center. How does this information translate to primary care?
- Pohl and Caplan (1998) look at a smoking cessation program for low-income women. They present group intervention as an effective method for providers in primary care. How can you use this information in your care of individuals, families, and your community?
- Fenton, Rounds, and Anderson (1991) propose the merging of NPs and community health nurses. Do you support this idea? Why or why not?

of 5.8 versus 3.4 drinks a week; p = 0.001). There were no differences in the binge drinking episodes per month between the groups. While this study needs to be replicated, brief counseling may be an intervention strategy that APNs want to consider using in their practice for patients at higher risk for alcohol consumption.

Many more researchable issues related to health promotion of individuals, families, and communities exist. APNs need to contribute to the advancement of nursing science by identifying researchable problems and conducting research within their nursing practice.

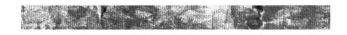

DISCUSSION QUESTIONS

These questions can be used to promote critical thinking and encourage discussion.

1. Describe the types of partnerships that exist within a community. What effect do these partnerships have on the health status of the community?
2. What effect does current health funding have on health promotion efforts?
3. Identify nurses or nursing roles that have or should have a population focus. Why should they have this focus?
4. How does culture (popular or ethnic) influence a family or individual's health practices?

REFERENCES/BIBLIOGRAPHY

Abraham, T., & Fallon, P. (1997). Clinical exemplar: caring for the community: development of the advanced practice nurse role. *Clinical Nurse Specialist, 11*(5), 224-230.

Ahljevych, K., & Bernhard, L. (1994). Health promoting behaviors of African American women. *Nursing Research, 43*(2), 86-89.

Barger, S. (1997). Building healthier communities in a managed care environment: opportunities for advanced practice nurses. *Advanced Practice Nursing Quarterly, 2*(4), 9-14.

Barger, S., & Rosenfield, P. (1993). Models in community health care: findings from a national study of community nursing centers. *Nursing and Health Care, 14*(8), 426-431.

Barker, J., Bayne, T., & Higgs, Z. (1994). Community analysis: a collaborative community practice project. *Public Health Nursing, 11*, 113-118.

Bilsborrow, R., DeGraff, D., & Anker, R. (1993). *Rapid assessment surveys of poverty* (Monograph). Geneva, Switzerland: International Labor Office.

Brubaker, B. (1983). Health promotion: a linguistic analysis. *Advances in Nursing Science, 5*(3), 1-14.

Bunkers, S., Michaels, C., & Ethridge, P. (1997). Advanced practice nursing in community: nursing's opportunity. *Advanced Practice Nursing Quarterly, 2*(4), 79-84.

Burr, W., Klein, S., & Burr, R. (1994). *Reexamining family stress: new theory and research*. Thousand Oaks, CA: Sage.

Centers for Disease Control and Prevention (1991). *A guide to the selection and utilization of selected health assessment and planning models to improve community health and to contribute to the achievement of the year 2000 objectives*. Washington, DC: Department of Health and Human Services.

Centers for Disease Control and Prevention. (1998). Trends in sexual risk behavior among high school students in the United States: 1991-1997. *Morbidity Mortality Weekly Report, 47*(36), 749-752.

Dinan, T. G. (1999). The physical consequences of depressive illness. *British Medical Journal, 318*, 826.

Eisenberg, D. M., Davis, R.B., & Ettner, S.L. (1998). Trends in alternative medicine use in the United States, 1990-1997: results of a follow-up national survey. *Journal of the American Medical Association, 280*(18), 1569-1575.

Fenton, M., Rounds, L., & Anderson, E. (1991). Combining the role of the nurse practitioner and the community health nurse: an educational model for implementing community-based primary health care. *Journal of the American Academy of Nurse Practitioners, 3*(3), 99-105.

Flick, L, Reese, C., Rogers, G., & Sonn, J. (1994). Building community for health: lessons from a seven-year-old neighborhood/university partnership. *Health Education Quarterly, 21*(3), 369-380.

Flynn, B. (1997). Partnerships in health cities and communities: a social commitment for advanced practice nurses. *Advanced Practice Nursing Quarterly, 2*(4), 1-6.

Glisson, J., Crawford, R., & Street, S. (1999). Review, critique, and guidelines for the use of herbs and homeopathy. *The Nurse Practitioner, 24* (4), 44-66.

Hacker, K., & Wessel, G. (1998). School based health centers and school nurses: cementing the collaboration. *Journal of School Health, 68*(10), 409-414.

Hitchcock, J.E., Schubert, P.E., & Thomas, S.A. (1999). *Community health nursing*. Albany, NY: Delmar.

Holt, F. (2000). Challenges of community based practice. *Clinical Nurse Specialist, 14*(1), 39

Jenkins, M., & Sullivan-Marx, E. (1994). Nurse practitioners and community health nurses: clinical partnerships and future visions. *Nursing Clinics of North America, 29*(3), 459-470.

Kang, R., Barnard, K., & Oshio, S. (1994). Description of the clinical practice of advanced practice nurses in family centered intervention in two rural settings. *Public Health Nursing, 11*(6), 376-384.

Kullig, J., & Wilde, I. (1996). Collaboration between communities and universities: completion of a community needs assessment. *Public Health Nursing, 13*, 112-119.

Laffrey, S. (1990). An exploration of adult health behaviors. *Western Journal of Nursing Research, 12*(4), 434-447.

Lugo, N. (1997). Nurse-managed corporate employee wellness centers. *The Nurse Practitioner, 22*(4), 104-113.

Mayer, T., & Cates, R. (1999). Service excellence in health care. *Journal of the American Medical Association, 282*(13), 1-9.

Meininger, J. (1997). Primary prevention of cardiovascular disease risk factors: review and implications for population based practice. *Advanced Practice Nursing Quarterly, 2*(4), 70-79.

Meng, A. (2000). A school based asthma clinic: a partnership model for managing childhood asthma. *Nurse Practitioner Forum, 11*(1), 38-47.

Miovech, S. (1996). *Determining nursing intensity of advanced practice nurse (APN) care using the community health intensity rating scale* (Unpublished doctoral disseration). Philadelphia: University of Pennyslvania.

Moody, N., Smith, P., & Glenn, L. (1999). Client characteristics and practice patterns of nurse practitioners and physicians. *Nurse Practitioner, 24*(3), 94-96, 99-100, 102-103.

Morrisey-Ross, M., & Greiner, P. (2000, January-February). Hitting the mark in community health outreach: what counts? *Journal of Healthcare Quality,* 1-12.

Nokes, K. (2000). Exploring the clinical nurse specialist role in an AIDS community based organization. *Clinical Nurse Specialist, 14*(1), 8-11.

Nurse practitioners to lead border health teams. (1994). *Texas Nursing, 68*(8), 6-7.

Ockene, J., Adams, A., & Hurley, T. (1999). Brief physician and nurse practitioner delivered counseling for high risk drivers. Does it work? *Archives in Internal Medicine, 159,* 2198-2205.

Palank, C. (1991). Determinants of health promotive behavior: a review of the current research. *Nursing Clinics of North America, 26*(4), 815-832.

Pender, N.J. (1996). *Health promotion in nursing practice* (3rd ed.). Stamford, CT: Appleton and Lange.

Pohl, J., & Caplan, D. (1998). Smoking cessation: using group intervention methods to treat low-income women. *The Nurse Practitioner, 23*(12), 13-37.

Polivka, B., & Ryan-Wenger, N. (1999). Health promotion and injury prevention behaviors of elementary school children. *Pediatric Nursing, 25*(2), 127-134.

Reece, S. (1998). Community analysis for health planning: strategies for primary care practitioners. *The Nurse Practitioner, 23*(10), 46-59.

Rickelman, B., & Gallman, L. (1994). Attachment and quality of life in older, community-residing men. *Nursing Research, 43*(2), 68-72.

Rivo, M. (1998). It's time to start practicing population-based health care. *Family Practice Management.* Available online at www.aafp.org/fpm/980600fm/popbased.html.

Robinson, D. (1997). Family theory: application to primary care. *Journal of the American Academy of Nurse Practitioners, 9*(1), 17-23.

St. Martin, E. (1996). Community health centers and quality of care: a goal to provide effective health care to the community. *Journal of Community Health, 13*(2), 83-92.

Simon, G., Ormel, J., & VonKorff, M. (1995). Health care costs associated with depressive and anxiety disorders in primary care. *American Journal of Psychiatry, 152,* 352-357.

Simmons, S. (1990). The health promoting self care system model: directions for nursing research and practice. *Journal of Advanced Nursing, 15*(10), 1162-1166.

Stafford, R., Saglam, D., Causino, N., Starfield, B., Culpepper, L., Marder, W., & Blumenthal, D. (1999). Trends in adult visits to primary care physicians in the United States. *Archives in Family Medicine, 8*(1), 26-32.

Stanhope, M., & Lancaster, J. (Eds.). (1988). *Community health nursing: process and practice for promoting health* (2nd ed.). St. Louis: Mosby.

Stanhope, M., & Lancaster, J. (Eds.). (1996). *Community health nursing: promoting health of aggregates, families, and individuals* (4th ed.). St. Louis: Mosby.

Taylor, D. (1998). Crystal ball gazing: back to the future. *Advanced Practice Quarterly, 3*(4), 44-51.

Tessaro, I. (1997). The natural helping role of nurses in promoting health behaviors in community. *Advanced Practice Nursing Quarterly, 2*(4), 73-78.

US Department of Health and Human Services (1990). *Healthy people 2000: national health promotion and disease prevention objectives* (DHHS Publication # [PHS] 91-50212.). Washington, DC: US Public Health Service.

US Department of Health and Human Services (2000). *Healthy people 2010: national health promotion and disease prevention objectives.* Washington, DC: US Public Health Service.

US Preventive Services Task Force (1996). *Guide to clinical preventive services* (2nd ed.). Baltimore, MD: Williams & Wilkins.

US Public Health Service (1979). *Healthy people: the Surgeon General's report on health promotion and disease prevention* (Publication # [PHS] 79-55071). Washington, DC: US Department of Health, Education, and Welfare.

US Public Health Service (1980). *Promoting health/preventing disease: objectives for the nation.* Washington, DC: US Department of Health, Education, and Welfare.

Vezeau, T., Peterson, J., Nakao, C., & Ersek, M. (1998). Education of advanced practice nurses: serving vulnerable populations. *Nursing and Health Care Perspectives, 19*(3), 124-131.

White, S. (1997). Schooled in primary care. *Hospitals and Health Networks, 71*(17), 80.

Yano, E., Fink, A., Hirsch, S., Robbins, A., & Rubenstein, L. (1995). Helping practices reach primary care goals. *Archives of Internal Medicine, 155,* 1146-1156.

Zapka, J., Pbert., L., Stoddard, A., Ockene, J., Goins, K., & Bonollo, D. (2000). Smoking cessation counseling with pregnant and postpartum women: a survey of community health center providers. *American Journal of Public Health, 90*(1), 78-84.

Chapter 43

The Healthy Lifestyle

Karen D. Agricola & Denise Robinson

Health care professionals have always known the benefits of illness prevention. However, over the past 30 to 40 years, the value of preventive practices has truly been displayed. Childhood immunizations have made epidemics of deadly infectious diseases like poliomyelitis, rubella, diphtheria, and pertussis obsolete in industrialized countries. Furthermore, preventive services for early detection of disease have resulted in decreased morbidity and mortality from cerebrovascular accidents secondary to untreated hypertension, cervical cancer, phenylketonuria, and congenital hypothyroidism (US Preventive Services Task Force [US PSTF], 1996). Today, providing immunizations and preventive services continues to be an important part of primary care, and ongoing research has shown the effect of personal lifestyle behaviors on health. Heart disease, cancer, cerebrovascular disease, chronic obstructive pulmonary disease (COPD), unintentional and intentional injuries, and human immunodeficiency virus (HIV) infection are some of the leading causes of death in the United States, and they are all associated with unhealthy personal lifestyle behaviors (US PSTF, 1996). Tobacco, alcohol, and illicit drug use; diet and exercise practices; and motor vehicle and sexual conduct were linked to almost 50% of the (potentially preventable) deaths in the United States in 1990 (McGinnis & Foege, 1993).

Unfortunately, delivery rates for preventive services in the United States are low, often falling below 50% (US Public Health Service, 1994). Bergman-Evans and Walker (1996) examined the prevalence of clinical preventive services (CPS) used by older women. Data for 5574 women was obtained from the 1991 *Health Promotion and Disease Prevention Supplement of the National Health Interview Survey.* Of these women, 78% reported having had a physical examination in the past 2 years. However, fewer than 1% reported receiving all of the recommended screening services, and only 5.3% of the women were current with recommended immunizations. While these data are not specific to advanced practice nurses (APNs), APNs are primary care providers (PCPs) and must claim some responsibility for the lack of adequate preventive services.

APNs in the patient care setting are in the perfect position to assist patients and their families in learning about and adopting healthy lifestyle behaviors. Individuals and groups have a tremendous capacity for change. Pender (1996) explains:

> The power and skill to change health behaviors or modify health-related lifestyles are within the domain of the patients. The expertise to provide educative-developmental care facilitative of behavior change and to foster environmental conditions supportive of health behaviors are within the domain of the professional nurse. The nurse can promote a positive climate for change, serve as a catalyst for change, assist the patient with various steps of the change process, and develop the patient's capacity to maintain change.

CRITICAL ISSUES: IMPLEMENTING CLINICAL PREVENTIVE SERVICES

Over 20 years ago, an extensive review of literature pertaining to the effectiveness of preventive services began when the Canadian government commissioned the Canadian Task Force on Periodic Health Examination. The group consisted of experts on health care and policy who systematically reviewed published studies of preventive services and rated the services' effectiveness for different populations at varying risks for disease. Recommendations of the panel were published in 1982 and updated in 1994, when recommendations were published in the *Canadian Guide to Clinical Preventive Health Care.*

The effort continued in the Unites States. In 1984, the U.S. Public Health Service commissioned the U.S. PSTF. Their findings and recommendations were published in the 1989 *Guide to Clinical Preventive Services.* This guide was updated in 1996 (US PSTF, 1996) to include CPS not previously examined and to make current recommendations based on new findings in the scientific literature. Over 6000 articles were reviewed in order to make recommendations for 70 topics and hundreds of preventive services. Each recommendation was rated to indicate the strength of the panel's recommendation for or against the service (Box 43-1).

The quality of the evidence was given a grade by systematically applying three criteria: the burden of suffering of the U.S. population from the target condition (e.g., heart disease), the characteristics of the intervention, and the effectiveness of the intervention as shown in published clinical research. Other factors that could influence the recommendations by the task force were cost and policy issues. (The ratings for the quality of evidence are listed in Box 43-2.) This guide is a wonderful resource to help to provide thorough and effective care to patients. It has a companion text called *Put Prevention into Practice: Clinician's Handbook of Preventive Services*, which gives practical tips on how to apply the data in the guide to practice (US Department of Health and Human Services [DHHS], Public Health Service, Office of Public Health and Science, & Office of Disease Prevention and Health Promotion, 1998). The text contains federal information produced by the U.S. DHHS that does not endorse any particular organization or its activities, products, or services. The American Nurses Association (ANA) and the National Alliance were two of the many organizations who reviewed and contributed to the materials in the handbook. Principal findings were published in the second edition of *Guide to Clinical Preventive Services* (US PSTF, 1996).

Interventions that address a patient's personal health practices are crucially important. Effective interventions that address personal health habits like tobacco use, physical inactivity, poor nutrition, alcohol and illicit drug use, and poor attention to safety measures lower the incidence and severity of the leading causes of death and illness in the United States more than screening for disease can. Clinicians and patients should discuss and decide upon the type of preventive services indicated so that services may be tailored to a patient's needs and value system. The risk to benefit ratio (known and unknown) for each intervention should be discussed. Clinicians should be selective in ordering tests and providing preventive services, and tests should be done in a manner to reduce the chances of false positives. Outcomes for an intervention must be clear or the intervention should not be recommended. Clinicians should take every opportunity to deliver preventive services, especially for those with limited access to care. Some people at the highest risk for preventable diseases like tuberculosis (TB), HIV, and cervical cancer often do not receive preventive services because they only seek care in times of illness. People who are ill do not absorb information as well as they do when healthy, but if a sick visit is the only opportunity to address health promotion, a clinician must take advantage of it. Sometimes a sick visit is the perfect time to address health promotion issues (e.g., a patient who smokes presents to the office with bronchitis, a patient who is overweight and sedentary presents to the office with knee pain).

For some health problems, interventions in the community may be more effective than preventive services in the office. Examples of problems better addressed in a community setting include youth and family violence, initiation of tobacco use, unintended pregnancy in adolescents, and certain unintentional injuries. A more effective role for the clinician may be to refer individuals to existing community programs, become a consultant for an existing community program, support existing community pro-

---

Box 43-1

Strength of Recommendations for Preventative Services

- Good evidence to support a recommendation that a condition be specifically considered in a periodic health examination
- Fair evidence to support a recommendation that a condition be specifically considered in a periodic health examination
- Insufficient evidence to recommend for or against inclusion of the condition in a periodic health examination (recommendations may be made on other grounds)
- Fair evidence to support a recommendation that a condition be excluded from consideration in a periodic health examination
- Good evidence to support a recommendation that a condition be excluded from consideration in a periodic health examination

Data from U.S. Preventive Services Task Force. (1996). *Guide to clinical preventive services* (2nd ed.). Baltimore: Williams & Wilkins.

Box 43-2

Quality of Evidence for Preventative Services*

- Evidence from at least one properly randomized controlled trial.
- Evidence from well-designed controlled trials without randomization.
- Evidence from well-designed cohort or case-control analytical studies, preferably from more than one center or research group.
- Evidence from multiple time series, with or without the intervention. Dramatic results in uncontrolled experiments (e.g., the results of the introduction of penicillin treatment in the 1940s) could also be regarded as this type of evidence.
- Opinions of respected authorities, based on their clinical experience; descriptive studies and case reports; or reports of expert committees.

Data from U.S. Preventive Services Task Force (1996). *Guide to clinical preventive services* (2nd ed.). Baltimore: Williams & Wilkins.
*Beginning with the highest quality.

grams, and support or introduce legislation regarding community health issues.

Nursing and Clinical Preventive Services

Illness prevention through health promotion is potentially more beneficial than treatment of disease and must be effectively addressed at each patient encounter in the office. APNs need to focus on health promotion in their practices and incorporate recommended topics into every visit. This means that even if a child or adult comes into the office for a sick visit, the APN should address other issues that are relevant for that patient because the patient may not return for a well visit. Children are more likely to come for well visits than adolescents or adults, so it is even more crucial to emphasize health promotion activities or interventions at all visits for adolescents and adults.

There are a number of barriers that may interfere with the incorporation of preventive services into practice (Box 43-3). Some barriers that have been identified

---

Box 43-3

Barriers to Clinical Prevention

Patient Barriers
- Ignorance of benefits
- Doubts about a PCP's ability to detect a hidden disease
- Cost of procedures
- Discomfort
- Conscious or unconscious desire not to change unhealthy habits
- Social and cultural norms
- Fear

Health System Barriers
- Inadequate reimbursement
- Lack of health insurance
- Population mobility
- Patients with multiple providers
- Categoric, sporadic screening programs (e.g., health fairs)

Provider Barriers
- Lack of knowledge
- Uncertainty about conflicting recommendations
- Uncertainty about the value of tests or interventions
- Disorganized medical records
- Delayed and indirect gratification from screening
- Lack of time
- Attitudes and personal characteristics
- Belief that a patient is not interested in changing, or a lack of compliance on part of patient

Adapted from Lang, R., & Shainoff, J. (1993). Integrating clinical preventive service into office practice. In R. Matzen & R. Lang (Eds.), *Clinical preventive medicine* (p. 128). St. Louis: Mosby.

---

include lack of time, lack of reimbursement, insufficient staff support, insufficient organizational support to keep track of needed services, inadequate training and skills, and an emphasis on illness in the health care system. In addition, there are numerous recommendations by different organizations, so it is difficult to know what preventive services should be done and when and how often to do them. The development of evidence-based guidelines helps in removing some of the disparities between organizations' recommendations. Using these guidelines decreases the uncertainty of what should be done and hopefully increases commitment to the delivery of CPS.

Griffith (1994a, 1994b) feels the lack of involvement of nursing and nursing organizations in the development of the preventive guidelines has been problematic. She feels that nursing is not seen as a national authority on CPS because of this lack of involvement and the lack of development of published guidelines by nursing organizations. APNs must use the guidelines of other organizations that do not have a nursing perspective. The ANA feels it would be advantageous to develop its own preventive guidelines or make a recommendation of support or nonsupport of other guidelines, based on a nursing perspective. Having CPS guidelines developed does not mean they are implemented in practice. The Put Prevention into Practice (PPIP) program was developed to improve the delivery of CPS by providing PCPs with a kit of materials to assist them in implementing CPS with their patients. An example of how the PPIP might assist APNs in delivering CPS follows.

Sara is a 42-year-old woman who is waiting for an appointment with Rachel, a nurse practitioner (NP) at Redbud Community Health Center. As she sits in the waiting room she notices a poster on the wall that says "We Put Prevention Into Practice—please ask us for details." This poster informs Sara that the office is focused on prevention. While Sara waits, she is also given a copy of *The Personal Health Guide*, a document that identifies CPS needed and provides a place to mark which services have been completed. (This is similar to the immunization and growth books given to parents of newborns to record immunizations and other data, such as height and weight.) From the office perspective, the receptionist pulls up a copy of the PPIP flow sheet to identify what CPS have been completed and those that might need to be done. She marks the chart with a removable sticker identifying services that need to be discussed. In the examination room, a poster with a timeline of CPS is mounted on the wall, again emphasizing its importance. Once Sara is in the examination room, Rachel addresses the acute problem but also takes a few minutes to discuss Sara's preventive needs. The flow sheet reveals that Sara has not had a cholesterol screen done in over 5 years, so Rachel recommends that the test be done during this visit. Sara also needs a gynecological examination, so Rachel recommends that Sara schedule that for her next visit in the

Data from U.S. Department of Health and Human Services, Public Health Service, Office of Public Health and Science, & Office of Disease Prevention and Health Promotion (1998). *Put prevention into practice: clinician's handbook of preventive services* (2nd ed.). Washington DC: US Government Printing Office. Available online at www.ahcpr.gov/ppipindes.html.

Box 43-4

Guidelines on Effective Clinical Counseling

- Organize teaching strategies to match patient perceptions.
- Inform a patient of the reason and expected outcomes of an intervention. Be complete and include a possible timeline.
- Suggest small changes instead of large ones.
- Be specific.
- Remember that it may be easier to add a healthy behavior than eliminate an unhealthy one.
- Link new behaviors to old behaviors.
- Use the power of the profession.
- Get explicit commitment from the patient.
- Use a combination of education strategies.
- Involve the office staff.
- Refer as needed.
- Establish regular follow-ups.

upcoming weeks. After Sara leaves, Rachel marks the PPIP flow sheet. A postcard is also completed to remind Sara of the need for an appointment for a gynecological examination.

Incorporating a Healthy Lifestyle into Primary Care Practice

Knowledge alone will not motivate a patient to change. However, if a patient is considering a change in health behavior, it is more appropriate to provide accurate information about the benefits of change than to provide specific details on how to change behavior. (Some general guidelines for effective clinical counseling are included in Box 43-4.) Preventative strategies must be customized to each patient. Patients need specific details and support to make lifestyle changes. APNs should organize teaching strategies to match a patient's perceptions, because if information is presented in a familiar way, it is more likely to be understood. A thorough assessment of "factors in promoting health" and other variables in the history is necessary to establish appropriate intervention techniques. The patient's beliefs and concerns about behavior change should also be assessed. A patient with debilitating arthritis of the knees may not be able to walk for 30 minutes four times a week without some specialized instruction. It is also imperative to know a patient's literacy level; a person's reading level may be five grades below the grade

completed. In general, public education materials should be written at a fifth grade to seventh grade reading level. To enhance communication with a patient with low literacy, everything extraneous should be eliminated, and the APN should only instruct on the correct way to do the intervention, breaking content into small parts and speaking in short sentences and words with few syllables. Then the APN should have the patient demonstrate or repeat what they learned (Redman, 1997).

APNs should completely inform patients of the reasons for and expected outcomes of intervention, as well as when to expect the outcomes. For example, it is important for someone embarking on a smoking cessation program to know that it will take at least 2 weeks for the craving for nicotine to subside. Lifestyle changes are not easy, and small changes should be suggested over large ones. Success with small changes improves a patient's self-efficacy so that he or she will be more confident with future attempts to change behavior. APNs should be specific when making healthy lifestyle suggestions; for example, recommending, "Lose 10 pounds at a rate of 1 or 2 pounds per week" is more helpful to a patient than, "Lose weight." Sometimes it is easier to add a healthy behavior than to eliminate an unhealthy one (e.g., effectively encouraging someone who smokes to exercise may help him or her to stop smoking). More success is realized when APNs can help patients link new behaviors to old behaviors. If a patient normally takes time away from work for lunch, an APN might suggest that the patient take a walk after lunch.

When providing information to a patient, an APN should use a combination of education strategies. Individual counseling can be integrated with group classes, audiovisual aides, written materials, and community resources. Written materials are more effective when they are personalized and at the patient's reading level. However, handouts do not replace personal attention given to a patient by the clinician. Patients respect health professionals' advice, so the power of the profession may be used when making suggestions. Patients are also more likely to follow advice if the clinician follows it too, so APNs should be good role models.

APNs should involve the other members of the office staff in healthy lifestyle promotion activities. A team approach makes patient education more effective. Office staff can direct patients to office displays of preapproved educational materials. APNs should also remember to refer when a situation would be better handled by other entities. There are four major sources of referral: community agencies (e.g., hospitals and insurance companies offering health promotion programs), national voluntary health organizations (e.g., the American Heart Association), instructional references (e.g., books and videotapes), and other patients.

A patient must be willing to make changes if lifestyle modification is to be successful. Therefore, an APN must get an explicit commitment from the patient. It should be noted that the goal of patient education is not regimen compliance, but patient empowerment for change. A patient may need to change multiple lifestyle behaviors. If possible, a patient should be allowed to choose the one he or she would like to address initially. APNs should also establish regular follow-up and encouragement (e.g., a soon-to-be ex-smoker can be called on the "quit date" to congratulate him or her). Regular follow-up is important to evaluate progress, reinforce successes, and identify and respond to problems. Patients with low self-efficacy need more positive reinforcement from their health care providers, and health provider follow-up contact is more effective than patient-initiated calls. Taking the time to make a phone call reinforces the importance of change taking place. *Guide to Clinical Preventive Services* (US PSTF, 1996) and *Put Prevention into Practice: Clinician's Handbook of Preventive Services* (US DHHS et al, 1998) are excellent tools to assist APNs in providing patients with current information and practical approaches for behavior change.

Exercise

Children

According to a 1996 report by the Surgeon General on physical activity and health, only about 50% of children and young adults ages 12 to 21 exercise regularly, and the amount of exercise decreases as age and grade level increase. The benefits of exercise include building and maintaining healthy bones, muscles, and joints; controlling weight; reducing body fat; and preventing or delaying the development of hypertension and diabetes. Furthermore, the exercise habits of childhood usually carry over into adulthood (US DHHS et al, 1998). APNs can use their role to promote exercise in children. (Box 43-5 outlines basic guidelines for exercise counseling.) APNs should use every office visit to assess a child's and parent's activity level in relationship to other events of the day like commuting, watching television, and playing on the computer. Promotion of physical activity should begin in the early school years and continue throughout life. Active children are more likely to become active adults.

Activities should be selected based on the age of a child. Preschool children need a safe place to be active and not structured activity, whereas school age children may enjoy participating in structured activities like ballet, karate, or gym class. Whatever activity is chosen, the main goal should be enjoyment rather than competition. An unpleasant experience in competitive sports can cause a general distaste for physical activity.

Many times, children get exercise through organized sports, and most APNs have the opportunity to conduct preparticipation sports examinations. The purpose of the preparticipation sports examination is to identify individuals at risk for worsening preexisting medical conditions, to identify general health, and to identify those at risk for

> ### Box 43-5
>
> ## Guidelines on Exercise Counseling for Children
>
> - Assess the child's and parents' activity level in relation to other events of the day during every office visit.
> - Choose age-appropriate physical activities.
> - Encourage activities for enjoyment rather than competition.
> - Encourage a variety of activities that can be practiced year round.
> - Encourage activities that can easily fit into a child's daily routine.
> - Stress the importance of safety equipment (e.g., helmets, wrist guards).
> - Counsel that the use of cigarettes, alcohol, and other drugs interferes with performance and can increase the chances of injury.
> - Encourage children with disabilities to participate fully after appropriate medical evaluation and consideration of the appropriateness of the activity.
> - Advise children that injuries can be reduced by following proper training advice, avoiding sudden changes or increases in activity, and treating injuries appropriately before starting or resuming play.
> - Advise adolescents of the dangers of anabolic steroids and other performance-enhancing drugs.
> - Create an office environment that includes posters, pamphlets and displays that promote physical activity.
>
> Data from U.S. Department of Health and Human Services, Public Health Service, Office of Public Health and Science, & Office of Disease Prevention and Health Promotion (1998). *Put prevention into practice: clinician's handbook of preventive services* (2nd ed.). Washington DC: US Government Printing Office. Available online at www.ahcpr.gov/ppipindes.html.

future medical problems. Ideally the examination should take place at least 6 weeks before the sports event to allow for follow-up if needed. Only about 1.7% of all athletes are disqualified from participating in sports, regardless of age, and the most common reasons for restriction with follow-up include musculoskeletal problems, asthma, vision difficulty, heart murmur, and elevated blood pressure (Rifat, Ruffin, & Gorenflo, 1995). Adolescents are more at risk for developing injuries because of an imbalance of strength and flexibility. In addition, significant changes are taking place in children's biochemical properties, which leads to increased stiffness in bone and decreased resistance to impact.

When a child comes for a sports physical examination, it is important for an APN to utilize the opportunity to obtain more information than that needed for the examination. In many instances, this will be the only opportunity for the APN to see the child for a well-child examination because access and cost may be issues. (Information related to medical conditions and sports participation for children can be accessed at the American Academy of Pediatrics website at www.aap.org.)

Adults

Morbidity and mortality for cardiovascular disease (CVD) has decreased over the last 25 years because of improvement in its recognition and treatment; however, CVD continues to be the leading cause of death in adults in the United States. According to the 1996 report on physical activity and health given by the Surgeon General, 60% of adults do not exercise regularly, and 25% do not exercise at all. The amount of physical inactivity is greater in women than men, in African Americans and Hispanics than Caucasians, in older adults than younger adults, and in the less affluent than the affluent. It is not clear why these discrepancies exist, although several viable reasons could be postulated. One reason why fewer women than men exercise may be the lack of organized sports for women (especially those now ages 35 or older) to participate in as children and teens. Many women over age 35 also did not have mothers who were physically active to serve as role models. Having one's family involved in sports activities increases the likelihood that all family members will be physically active. In addition, for those with limited economic resources, fewer choices exist for sports activities due to equipment needs. Biking, for example, requires a bike, which is expensive. This limits the lower socioeconomic group to activities that do not require costly equipment.

Sedentary lifestyle is a major risk factor for CVD, type 2 diabetes mellitus (DM), colon cancer, obesity, osteoporosis, and falls. The benefits of regular exercise include a lower risk for the development of the aforementioned problems; decreased stress; and improvement in musculoskeletal functioning and weight loss and control. Regular exercise is the only way to maintain weight loss. Considering the effect of regular exercise on health, counseling about activity is an essential component of high-quality primary care. Unfortunately, only 30% of clinicians surveyed routinely advise patients who are sedentary to exercise (USDHHS et al, 1998).

To devise an exercise plan, APNs should use every office visit to assess the activity level of adults. APNs should ask about structured exercise as well as the type of activity involved with an adult's occupation and hobbies. They should ask about the number of hours of television watched in a 24-hour period, because time for exercise may be available in the time spent watching television. APNs should assess an adult's time spent commuting and going through fast food lanes. The goal of these questions is to discover what the patient's lifestyle is like so an APN can offer better advice. The APN should also determine if a patient's current activity level is sufficient. *Sufficient activity level* is defined as exercise of moderate intensity for 30 minutes a day at least 4 days a week. *Moderate intensity* is defined as an activity resulting in 50% to 69% of maximal

heart rate. Maximal heart rate is calculated by subtracting one's age from 220.

APNs should help patients select appropriate exercise activities. An activity must be medically safe, enjoyable, convenient, realistic, and structured. The National Institutes of Health (NIH) recommend a medical evaluation for people with CVD, as well as men over the age of 40 or women over the age of 50 with multiple risk factors for CVD (e.g., hypertension, hyperlipidemia, type 2 DM, current smokers, obesity) before beginning an exercise program. The American College of Cardiology and the American Heart Association (AHA) recommend that people with two or more risk factors for CVD have a cardiac stress test.

To ensure safety, patients should be advised to increase the intensity of exercise gradually, alternate days of exercise, and do stretching exercises before activity to decrease the risk of injuries. Enjoying an exercise makes it more likely to become a habit. A patient's effort should go into the exercise, not traveling to or preparing for the exercise, and goals for exercise must be achievable to enhance a patient's self-efficacy. An APN and patient should plan what the exercise will be, what time of day it will be practiced, the duration spent doing it, and how many days a week it will be practiced. If a patient is unable or unwilling to exercise regularly, he or she should be encouraged to increase daily activity by parking farther away from store entrances, using the steps instead of elevators, or walking places instead of driving.

Many barriers to exercise for children also apply to adults. Many leisure activities today revolve around watching television, playing on the computer, and staying near air conditioning when it is hot. Children also tend to be busier now than in years past, so participation in spontaneous activity is less likely. For many children and adults, one of the best ways to get them to exercise is to involve the parents and family in the same activity. Having the whole family go for a bike ride or play a game of pickup basketball conveys the message that exercise is fun and an important family activity. Organizations such as the Boys Club often have programs available for children who can afford it.

It is important for APNs to be aware of exercise and sports options in the communities in which they practice. Having handouts describing how to get started with an exercise program or family activity may also be a good way to provide information to patients. Many people believe they do not have time to engage in exercise, so it may come as a relief to them that 10 to 15 minutes of exercise several times a day can provide the same benefits as a sustained exercise period. Office and nursing staff should be involved in providing information and support to patients. APNs should also consider starting a patient education committee in the office and using multiple resources (e.g., posters, pamphlets, videos, displays) to promote a healthy atmosphere. Exercise should include aerobic training, resistance training, and flexibility training.

As an example of all of this, Steve and Marsha, APNs at Redbud Community Health Center, recognized that many of their patients, both children and adults, did not get enough exercise. They decided to have an exercise fair at their local health center. They chose a night, involved sponsors from their area health education center, and demonstrated various exercise techniques that did not require extensive equipment. While the turnout was not as good as they had hoped, they did have 10 patients who attended. Several of the women in particular were interested in attending exercise classes if offered on site. Since Marsha did aerobic weight training herself, she was interested in leading the classes. She also knew that by serving as a role model she might influence her patients.

Nutrition

Children

Proper nutrition in childhood is essential for adequate growth and development. The most common deficiencies in childhood are related to iron and calcium. Poor dietary habits in childhood translate into poor dietary habits as adults, leading to increased risk for CVD, hypertension, type 2 DM, certain types of cancer, and other diseases (USDHHS et al, 1998) (Box 43-6).

Nutritional guidelines are different for children of different ages. For infants, breast milk is the best source of nutrition. APNs should educate parents about the benefits and techniques of successful breastfeeding. Barriers to breastfeeding include maternal time restraints, temperament of an infant, decreased milk supply, maternal discomfort, poor maternal nutrition, drug and alcohol use, and inadequate suckling ability of an infant. An APN should discuss breastfeeding with a mother and identify problems from the mother's point of view. A problem-oriented examination should also be conducted. It is important for the APN to provide the mother with education, and encouragement. A support person (e.g., husband, mother, friend) is helpful in getting the breast-feeding started, and local support groups such as the La Leche League and the Nursing Mothers Counsel may also provide a helpful resource.

When a child is around the age of 4 to 6 months, solid food may be introduced. The child should be developmentally ready; he or she should be able to sit up, have adequate head and neck control, and take baby food from a spoon. Infant rice cereal mixed with breast milk or formula is a good first choice. Foods should be introduced one at a time every 5 days to assess for intolerances. Foods should be introduced in the following order: rice, cereal, vegetables, fruit, and meat.

APNs should encourage iron-rich foods that promote adequate growth and development and protect against lead poisoning. They should consider screening for anemia at the age of 6 to 12 months in high-risk infants (e.g., infants living in poverty, African Americans, Native American/Alaska Natives, immigrants from developing

---

Box 43-6

Guidelines on Nutrition Counseling for Children

Under 2 Years Old

- Advise parents that breast milk is the best source of nutrition for infants.
- Introduce solid food at 4 to 6 months when the child is developmentally ready.
- Encourage iron-rich foods.
- Advise parents not to give infants cow's milk; it will not meet their nutritional needs.
- Advise parents not to give honey to infants for fear of botulism.
- Counsel parents not to limit fat in the first 2 years of life.
- Counsel parents that vitamin supplements are not usually needed for healthy children who eat a balanced diet.
- Advise parents that children who live in areas with an inadequate amount of fluoride in the water may need supplementation to prevent dental caries.

Over 2 Years Old

- Counsel parents that children and adults need to eat a wide variety of foods.
- Advise parents that the amount of total fat in the diets of children and adults should be limited to 30% of the total daily caloric intake; saturated fat should be limited to 10%.
- Counsel parents to avoid foods with excessive amounts of added sugar and salt.
- Counsel families to include foods rich in calcium (e.g., milk, yogurt) and iron (e.g., lean meats, legumes, fortified cereals, whole grain products) in their diets.
- Counsel families on the importance of maintaining a healthy weight.
- Advise parents that weight reduction through dieting is not appropriate for children and adolescents because they are still growing.
- Advise parents that healthy children who eat well-balanced diets do not need diet supplements. Children living in areas with inadequate fluoridation of the water supply may need fluoride supplements to prevent dental caries.
- Advise adolescent women to consume an adequate amount of folic acid to prevent neural tube defects in pregnancy.

Data from U.S. Department of Health and Human Services, Public Health Service, Office of Public Health and Science, & Office of Disease Prevention and Health Promotion (1998). *Put prevention into practice: clinician's handbook of preventive services* (2nd ed.). Washington DC: US Government Printing Office. Available online at www.ahcpr.gov/ppipindes.html.

---

countries, premature and low–birth weight infants, infants whose primary source of nutrition is unfortified cow's milk) (US PSTF, 1996). It is important for APNs to advise parents that cow's milk will not meet a child's nutritional needs. Similarly, children less than 2 years old should not be given reduced-fat milk. In fact, parents should be counseled not to limit fat in a child's first 2 years of life. APNs should also make sure to ask the parents how they make formula. It is not unheard of for parents to inadvertently overdilute or underdilute formula. For example, Rachel, the NP at Redbud Community Health Center, had the unpleasant experience of doing a well-baby check for a 7-month old baby girl who laid listlessly on the examination table. Her height and weight were completely below the growth chart percentages. When Rachel questioned the mother about the type of formula she was feeding her daughter, the mother indicated that she was feeding low-fat milk, even though she had Women, Infants, and Children (WIC) vouchers for formula. Rachel sent the baby to the emergency room for further evaluation and hydration and called Children's Protective Services. Even more disconcerting was the fact that 2 years later, the same mother began feeding her 10-month-old child whole milk instead of formula. Rachel learned in this instance that one can not assume a mother is feeding a baby the recommended foods unless one asks very specific questions.

Vitamin supplements are not usually needed for healthy children who eat a balanced diet. However, infants who are exclusively breastfed may need a vitamin D supplement if they are not exposed to sunlight on a regular basis. Children who live in areas with inadequate amounts of fluoride in the water may need supplementation to prevent dental caries.

Both children and adults need to eat a wide variety of foods. Children are less finicky if foods are offered to them consistently during the toddler years. Types of foods and suggested amounts of each are presented in the Food Pyramid, which most school age children learn about. After age 2, the amount of total fat in a healthy diet should be limited to 30% of the total daily caloric intake; saturated fat should be limited to 10%. Fried and fatty foods should be avoided.

APNs should counsel families on the importance of maintaining healthy weight. Utilizing pediatric growth charts helps with this task, though immigrant children from developing countries may be of shorter stature and lesser weight. Because children and adolescents are still growing, weight reduction through dieting is not appropriate. If a child is overweight, the weight should be maintained while the child grows by having the child be more physically active and nutrition conscious. APNs should obtain a dietary history for patients and pay particular attention to women and children playing sports that have weight requirements (e.g., wrestling, gymnastics) for evidence of anorexia or bulimia.

Many children in the United States are significantly overweight, physically inactive, and consuming diets excessive in total fat, saturated fat, and carbohydrates. More than one fourth of children in America are obese. Keller and Stevens (1996) note that childhood is a critical time for the initiation of obesity associated morbidities, especially re-

garding the risk of CVD in both childhood and adulthood. Prevalence of obesity estimates range from 25% to 30% in prepubertal children and 18% to 25% in adolescents. More Hispanic children (56%) and African-American children (41%) are obese than Caucasian children (28%). Determination of obesity in children is difficult due to variations in physical size and growth, even among children of the same chronological age. Keller and Stevens (1996) recommend using a combination of skin folds, circumferences, body mass index (BMI), and waist to hip ratio.

An APN should complete an assessment to identify what factors have influenced the development of obesity in a particular child. An exercise and activity assessment (described previously) would be helpful. Physical activity among American children has decreased, creating an imbalance between food intake and energy expenditures. Also, there certainly appears to be a parental and genetic tendency toward obesity, with approximately a 35% genetic transmission across generations (Keller & Stevens, 1996). Families also influence nutrition and obesity in ways besides genetics. The family sets a child's lifestyle and establishes the normal behaviors expected regarding nutrition. Parents serve as role models of behaviors, good or bad, and the ability to make appropriate choices is learned in the home.

There are many APN interventions to address childhood obesity, though there is no currently accepted standard method for treatment of obesity in children. APNs should determine the emotional effect of obesity on a given child, and assessment using a number of anthropometric measurements will determine which children are actually obese. Many children and adolescents may think they are fat but actually are not. Recent research has focused on family involvement, behavioral and problem-solving techniques, and the mother's attendance at weight loss classes; exercise is a crucial component of any weight loss plan. School-based intervention plans are having some success in that children are learning positive eating habits through social support and behavioral counseling. An emphasis on healthy eating habits, exercise, and open communication may go a long way in assisting overweight children. Parents can be enlisted to help keep low-calorie snacks and foods available; since children do not have direct control over the eating style of their families, interventions must be family based.

Adults

CVD, type 2 DM, stroke, and certain types of cancers are four of the leading causes of death related to dietary intake in the United States; these diseases account for two thirds of the 2 million annual deaths. Health conditions related to diet cost up to $250 billion annually. Over one third of the adult population is overweight. Overconsumption of calories is linked to obesity, hypertension, type 2 DM, and CVD; increased intake of alcohol is linked to stroke, hypertension, heart disease, and certain cancers; and increased intake of sodium is linked to hypertension. Under-consumption of folic acid in women of childbearing age is related to neural tube defects in the children they bear; foods with folic acid include breakfast cereals, and policies to fortify the general food supply are being developed. Underconsumption of calcium is related to osteoporosis. Therefore a healthy diet is an important component of prevention and treatment of diseases, and offering specific advice about a proper diet to patients is an important role for APNs (US DHHS et al, 1998) (Box 43-7).

APNs should weigh patients on a regular basis and suggest an appropriate weight for each. A BMI equal to or greater than 27.8 for men and 27.3 for women has been

---

Box 43-7

Guidelines on Nutrition Counseling for Adults

- Weigh patients on a regular basis and suggest an appropriate weight for each patient.
- Assess patients' dietary habits.
- Counsel patients to eat a wide variety of foods, including fruits, vegetables, and grain products.
- Encourage patients to limit the amount of total fat to 30% of their daily caloric intake, limit saturated fat to 10%, and limit cholesterol to 300 mg per day.
- Encourage patients to limit intake of foods with excessive amounts of added sugar and salt.
- Counsel patients who drink alcohol to do so in moderation.
- Teach patients the food pyramid, which is a useful tool regarding healthy nutrition.
- Counsel women to consume adequate amounts of calcium to produce and maintain high-quality bone, with the goal of preventing osteoporosis. Advise men to consume adequate calcium as well.
- Counsel women of childbearing age to consume 0.4 mg to 1 mg of folic acid per day to prevent neural tube defect if they should become pregnant.
- Counsel patients who are overweight to increase physical activity and reduce their intake of calories and fat.
- Counsel patients with hyperlipidemia on a cholesterol-lowering diet recommended by the National Cholesterol Education Program (NIH, 1993).
- Provide ongoing follow-up and support.
- Include family members to provide additional support for patients.
- If necessary, contact the American Dietetic Association at (800) 366-1655 for advice on the management of patients with severe dietary deficiencies.

Data from U.S. Department of Health and Human Services, Public Health Service, Office of Public Health and Science, & Office of Disease Prevention and Health Promotion (1998). *Put prevention into practice: clinician's handbook of preventive services* (2nd ed.). Washington DC: US Government Printing Office. Available online at www.ahcpr.gov/ppipindes.html.

---

equated with obesity (NIH, 1996). A waist to hip ratio greater than 1 in men and 0.9 in women is associated with a substantial increase in the risk for hypertension, stroke, and diabetes. Patients' heights should be measured once a year to screen for osteoporosis. During a visit, an APN should assess a patient's dietary habits, and when reviewing medications, the APN should be sure to inquire about dietary supplements. Using a questionnaire can help to identify patients at high risk (Figure 43-1). Patients should be encouraged to eat a wide variety of foods each day, including fruits, vegetables, and grain products, while limiting the amount of total fat to 30% of daily caloric intake, saturated fat to 10%, and cholesterol to 300 milligrams (mg) per day. The APN should review self-help materials and sample labels with the patient to ensure that the patient understands these calculations. Listing specific types of food to avoid while on the current diet for patients with low literacy is more effective than teaching calculations.

APNs should counsel patients who drink alcohol to do so in moderation. Women should limit intake to one serving a day, and men should limit servings to two per day. A serving equals 12 ounces (oz) of regular beer, 5 oz of wine, or 1.5 oz of 80-proof distilled spirits.

Women (in particular) need to make sure they consume adequate amounts of calcium to produce and maintain high-quality bone and prevent osteoporosis. Women ages 11 to 24 should consume 1200 to 1500 mg a day, while those ages 25 to 50 years should consume 1000mg a day. Women who are pregnant or nursing should consume 1200 to 1500 mg a day, postmenopausal women should consume 1500 mg a day, and women over the age of 65 should consume 1500 mg a day. Dairy products are the best sources of calcium, with 300 to 400mg in every 8 oz of milk or yogurt. Other sources of calcium include canned fish with soft bones, vegetables like broccoli and spinach, and fortified cereals and grains. Orange juice with added calcium can be purchased. For those who are unable to consume enough calcium, a supplement should be recommended. Men should also be advised on adequate calcium consumption. Males from ages 11 to 24 years should consume 1200 to 1500 mg of calcium a day, men ages 25 to 65 years should consume 1000 mg, and men over 65 should consume 1500 mg.

APNs should counsel women of childbearing age to also consume 0.4 mg to 1 mg of folic acid per day to prevent neural tube defects if they should become pregnant. Folic acid supplements can be purchased over the counter. Good dietary sources of folic acid include dry beans, leafy green vegetables, citrus fruits, and fortified foods like breakfast cereals.

APNs should counsel patients who are overweight to increase physical activity and reduce calorie and fat intake. A goal of 1 pound of weight loss per week is reasonable. Patients should be reminded that the only method proven to keep weight off is exercise. Lifelong healthy eating habits should be encouraged, while fad diets should be

Determining Your Nutritional Health: Checklist for Older Adults*	
	Yes
I have an illness or condition that made me change the kind and/or amount of food I eat.	2
I eat fewer than two meals per day.	3
I eat few fruits and vegetables or milk products.	2
I have three or more drinks of beer, liquor, or wine almost every day.	2
I have tooth or mouth problems that make it hard for me to eat.	2
I don't always have enough money to buy the food I need.	4
I eat alone most of the time.	1
I take three or more different prescribed or over-the-counter drugs a day.	1
Without wanting to, I have lost or gained 10 pounds in the last 6 months.	2
I am not always physically able to shop, cook, or feed myself.	2
	TOTAL

* Instructions: Read the statements above. Circle the number in the "yes" column for those that apply. For each "yes" answer, score the circled number. Total your nutrition score. If it is:

0-2	Good! Recheck your nutritional score in 6 months.
3-5	You are at moderate risk. See what can be done to improve your eating habits and lifestyle. Your office on aging, senior nutrition program, senior citizens center, or health department can help. Recheck your nutritional score in 3 months.
≥6	You are at high nutritional risk. Talk with your clinician, dietitian, or other qualified health or social service professional about this checklist. Ask for help to improve your nutritional health.

Figure 43-1 Nutrition questionnaire. (Reprinted with permission from The Nutrition Screening Initiative, a project of the American Academy of Family Physicians, The American Dietetic Association, and the National Council on the Aging, and funded in part by a grant from Ross Products Division, Abbott Laboratories.)

discouraged. Very low calorie diets (less than 800 calories a day) should be considered only for the severely or morbidly obese. Family members can provide additional support for the patient; ideally, the rest of the family should be eating similarly to the patient or following the diet will become very difficult and the patient will be less likely to continue. Barriers for adult patients are very similar to those experienced by children, except an adult has the ability to control his or her behaviors. Behavioral modification programs have some success in helping individuals with weight loss. Also, although weight loss medications are available, they must be combined with exercise and healthy eating to be effective. The medications are not covered on insurance plans, so patients must pay for them out of pocket.

The family role in healthy eating can not be overemphasized. Verbal and nonverbal reinforcement of weight loss is crucial to success. APNs should recognize that most efforts at weight loss are not successful. The most successful are those that are self-directed, and these have the best long-term results. Most of the people that have been successful—72% of them—in maintaining significant weight loss have done so on their own, while 20% enrolled in commercial programs, 3% used diet pills, and 5% enrolled in a medically managed program (Foreyt & Goodrick, 1993).

Smoking Cessation

Children

Cigarette smoking remains the leading cause of preventable morbidity and mortality in the United States. Tobacco use is linked to CVD, hypertension, lung and esophageal cancer, and chronic lung disease. Smokeless tobacco is associated with cancers of the gum, mouth, larynx, pharynx, and esophagus. If parents smoke, children are twice as likely to smoke. The decision to smoke is often made in the teenage years; 22% of high school age children smoke, and 10% to 25% of children try cigarettes by the sixth grade. Of high school age children, 11% use smokeless tobacco, some starting at the age of 4 or 5 years. Teens become addicted to nicotine quickly and consequently develop into adults with tobacco-related health problems, which cost $50 billion in health care costs in 1993.

Passive cigarette smoke is a potential health threat to over 30% of children younger than age 10 in the United States. Environmental cigarette smoke increases the likelihood of allergies, asthma, lower respiratory infection, otitis media, and decreased pulmonary function. Each year, 300,000 children suffer the consequences of passive cigarette smoke (US DHHS et al, 1998).

With all of the potential health risks associated with smoking during the adolescent years, smoking cessation is a priority for promoting a healthy lifestyle (Box 43-8).

Box 43-8

Guidelines on Smoking Cessation Counseling for Children

- Establish a smoke-free office or clinic environment.
- Obtain a smoking history for the child and significant others in the home, day care, or school settings.
- Counsel parents who smoke in the home that smoking in another room of the home, blowing smoke away from the child, and opening a window in a room are not effective ways to reduce the child's exposure to smoke.
- Educate school age children about the perils of tobacco use.
- Obtain information from the child or adolescent in a nonthreatening manner.

Data from U.S. Department of Health and Human Services, Public Health Service, Office of Public Health and Science, & Office of Disease Prevention and Health Promotion (1998). *Put prevention into practice: clinician's handbook of preventive services* (2nd ed.). Washington DC: US Government Printing Office. Available online at www.ahcpr.gov/ppipindes.html.

APNs should obtain a smoking history for children and significant others in their home, day care, or school settings. Those who smoke around children should be advised to quit. Communicating the consequences for children exposed to environmental tobacco smoke to their parents can be helpful, and APNs should offer support (e.g., counseling, referral) to parents who desire to quit.

APNs should educate school age children about the perils of tobacco use, emphasizing the cosmetic (e.g., bad breath, smelly clothes, stained teeth, oral sores) and athletic (e.g., reduced endurance, shortness of breath) consequences of cigarette smoking. When obtaining information from a child or adolescent, an APN should do so in a nonthreatening manner. Parents should be asked to leave the room, and it may help to ask a patient about friends' and parents' tobacco habits before asking the patient about his or her own habits.

Adults

Cigarette smoking is the leading cause of preventable morbidity and mortality in the United States, with tobacco-related deaths numbering 400,000 per year. Nonsmokers exposed to tobacco smoke have an increased risk for CVD and lung cancer. Children exposed to cigarette smoke have higher rates of lower respiratory infections, allergies, asthma, and otitis media. Unlike counseling for exercise, nutrition, and safety, there actually is evidence that counseling patients to stop smoking helps them quit (Figure 43-2). Simple interventions like asking about a patient's smoking status and advising him or her to quit can result in long-term quit rates of 5% to 10%. If all practitioners

did this, the national smoking cessation rate could double (Box 43-9). Recent studies show that less than 50% of patients receive assistance from their health care providers to stop smoking (US DHHS et al, 1998). Barriers to smoking cessation include such factors as smoking cues and triggers, peer pressure, emotional dependence, oral gratification, relaxation and stress, and physiological addiction to nicotine.

APNs should identify patients who smoke and indicate that information in the medical chart. Information about smoking cessation efforts and strategies can be organized in the chart (or possibly on a flow sheet) so it can be easily accessed. Patients who smoke may be required to complete a smoking assessment form to identify their common characteristics (Figure 43-3). APNs should advise all smokers to stop smoking, and advice should be clear, strong, and personalized. An APN should clearly state, "I think it is important for you to quit smoking now, and I will help you. Cutting down when you are sick is not enough." The advice must be strong: "As your health care provider, I need you to know that quitting smoking is the single most important thing you can do to protect your current and future health." Finally, the advice should be personalized; smoking may be tied to the patient's current health or illness, to effects on others in the household, to the economic effect, and to the person's readiness to quit.

APNs should be a resource to help patients who want to quit smoking, encouraging patients to set a quit date within 2 weeks. Patients who are ready to quit should inform friends, family and coworkers so that their support may be recruited. Cigarettes must be removed from the environment. APNs should review the circumstances around previous attempts of quitting and specifically try to identify what helped and what caused patients to start smoking again, coming up with a plan to address these challenges this time. If a relapse in the past was preceded by anger at a coworker, the patient should be helped to more effectively deal with anger (e.g., through simple relaxation exercise). APNs may discuss the use of medicinal aids like nicotine replacement therapy or Zyban/Wellbutrin. Studies have shown that these medications are more effective in reducing cravings for nicotine when used together than when used separately. APNs should provide advice on successful cessation, and total abstinence from cigarettes is crucial. Drinking alcohol is greatly associated with restarting cigarette smoking, and it is also more difficult to quit with other smokers in the household. Referring patients to a formal smoking cessation program may be helpful.

When a patient is ready to begin a smoking cessation program, educational materials can be provided to prepare him or her for smoking cessation success. Data show that even in old age, survival improves if patients quit smoking. The message needs to be clear—whenever a patient quits smoking, it is worthwhile, but the sooner, the better. Even though smokers do suffer damage to their health, when it

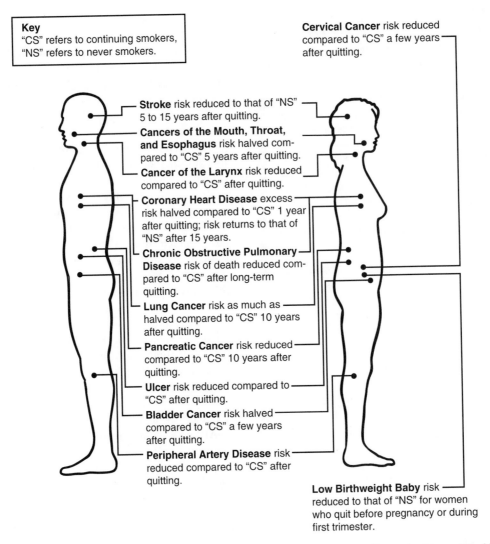

Figure 43-2 Benefits of smoking cessation. (From Centers for Disease Control, Office on Smoking and Health. [1990]. *The health benefits of smoking cessation: a report of the Surgeon General* [USDHHS publication CDC 90-8419]. Rockville, MD.)

comes to future potential health problems, someone who quits is better off (Ask the Professor, 1999). Also, most smokers try to stop smoking more than once; this fact may be used to support a patient (not to blame or accuse him or her) and show that a past experience in quitting could help the next time.

Safety

Children

Accidents, the leading cause of death for children in the United States, are often preventable. One half of accidents are related to motor vehicles; other causes of injury include drowning, burns, choking, firearms, falls, poisoning, and sports. Accidental injuries result in 20,000 deaths; 60,000 hospitalizations; 16 million emergency department visits; and $165 billion in costs each year. Characteristics of children at higher risk include male gender, low income, pre-

vious severe injury, and children in families with young mothers. Barriers to preventing accidents in children include cost (e.g., for outlet covers, car seats), ignorance of causes of accidents, poor planning, being in a hurry, and a sense of invulnerability. Alcohol and drug use are often implicated in injuries in adolescents (US DHHS et al, 1998).

It is critical for APNs to conduct a safety assessment as part of well-child care. A documentation form addressing the following areas brings up the subject and starts a discussion related to safety (e.g., use of seat belts and bicycle helmets, how to call 911 and Poison Control); it can also address the previously identified barriers. APNs can help parents keep children safe by offering advice and resources. Parents should be encouraged to learn cardiopulmonary resuscitation (CPR) and to educate their children about why, when, and how to dial 911. APNs should discuss the role of a child's self-esteem in dealing with peer pressure. If a child's good behavior has been consistently

Box 43-9

Guidelines on Smoking Cessation Counseling for Adults

- Consider designating one person to coordinate the smoking cessation program in the office. That person would then obtain and maintain patient education materials and be a support person for other providers in the office.
- Identify patients who smoke and indicate such information in the medical chart.
- Advise all smokers to stop smoking.
- Ask every smoker if he or she is ready to quit.
- Help patients who desire to quit.
- Discuss the use of medicinal aids like nicotine replacement therapy or Zyban/Wellbutrin.
- Give patients pertinent advice on successful cessation.
- Consider referring patients to a formal smoking cessation program. Call the National Cancer Institute Information Service (800-4-CANCER) for high-quality programs in the area.
- Give patients educational materials to prepare them for smoking cessation success.

Data from U.S. Department of Health and Human Services, Public Health Service, Office of Public Health and Science, & Office of Disease Prevention and Health Promotion (1998). *Put prevention into practice: clinician's handbook of preventive services* (2nd ed.). Washington DC: US Government Printing Office. Available online at www.ahcpr.gov/ppipindes.html.

reinforced, the child will be more likely to possess skills to choose appropriate behavior in a situation involving peer pressure. Parents should be encouraged to be good role models for safe behavior; children are more likely to imitate behavior that they see consistently reinforced. Finally, APNs must be aware of and prepared to give information about available community resources to families with limited access to resources for child safety (US DHHS et al, 1998).

About 50% of all accidents involving children are related to motor vehicles. Car seats are required by law in all 50 states. In some states, citations can be written against a driver solely on the basis of a child passenger who is not properly restrained. It is important that car seats are carefully and properly installed. Instructions for the use of a safety seat must be read and followed. The seat must then be properly attached to the car, preferably in the center of the vehicle's rear seat. It is important for APNs to review when a child should ride in a safety seat. For infants, safety seats must be placed backwards until the child weighs 20 pounds or is 1 year old, and safety seats must be used until a child weighs 40 pounds and is 40 inches tall. When a child no longer needs a safety seat, booster seats should be used until the child is tall enough that the lap belt fits securely at hip level and the shoulder harness crosses at shoulder

level, or until the child's ears come up above the vehicle seat back. APNs should also stress to parents to make sure others who are transporting their children also use car seats and seat belts.

Rachel, the NP at Redbud, likes to make a game of seat belt use. She encourages parents to emphasize that the car will not start until all its occupants have on seat belts. If parents model this behavior, it is more likely that children wear the belts. Parents should be advised that children should ride in the appropriate seat, not in the storage area of a pickup, sports utility vehicle, or station wagon.

Infants and children should never ride in a seat equipped with an airbag. Parents should ask their auto manufacturer about specific height restrictions regarding air bag use for older, taller children. Children and adolescents should also be counseled not to ride with anyone who is under the influence of drugs or alcohol.

Children may also be injured by choking on small objects or foods (e.g., hot dogs, carrots, hard candies) and subsequently suffocating. Parents should be advised to keep objects small enough to fit through the barrel of a toilet paper roll away from children. Small objects such as carrots and hot dogs should not be cut into small circles because this increases the likelihood of choking. APNs should recommend that such circles be cut in half again to make sure they do not pose a choking risk. Emphasis should be placed on the necessity to chew foods adequately before swallowing. APNs should also encourage parents to discuss these tips with other child care providers. In case a child does aspirate an object, parents and other child care providers should learn the Heimlich maneuver.

While most parents know that children are in danger of drowning when around large bodies of water, children can also drown in shallow depths of water like buckets and toilets. Children should have no access to such objects. Buckets and wading pools should be put out of reach after being used. Parents should also be warned to never leave a child unattended in the bathtub. Similarly, children should never be allowed to swim alone; parents should be sure that swimming pools are surrounded by a fence at least 4 feet tall with a self-closing gate.

Children can encounter numerous safety hazards within the home. APNs should advise parents to use plastic guards to cover electrical outlets that are not being used. Ground fault interrupter circuits should be installed in kitchens and bathrooms and anywhere else that water may come in contact with bare skin.

Safety gates (not the accordion type) should be used to prevent children from climbing up and falling down steps. Furniture should be kept away from windows so children can not climb onto the windowsill, and window guards should be installed on windows above the first floor. It should also be noted that baby walkers are linked to more injuries per year than any other baby product; parents who choose to use these must be advised to closely supervise children so they do not fall down steps.

Smoking Assessment Form

Name: _____ Date: _____
1. Do you smoke cigarettes?   _____ Yes _____ No
2. Does the person closest to you smoke cigarettes? _____ Yes _____ No
3. How many cigarettes do you smoke a day?   _____ cigarettes
4. How soon after you wake up do you smoke your first cigarette?
   _____ Within 30 minutes _____ More than 30 minutes
5. How interested are you in stopping smoking?
   _____ Not at all _____ A little _____ Some _____ A lot _____ Very
6. If you decided to quit smoking completely during the next 2 weeks, how confident
   are you that you would succeed?
   _____ Not at all _____ A little _____ Some _____ A lot _____ Very

---

Figure 43-3 Smoking assessment form. (From Glynn, T.J., & Manley, M.W. [1995]. *How to help your patients stop smoking: a National Cancer Institute manual for physicians* [NIH Publication NIH 95-3064]. Bethesda, MD: National Institutes of Health.)

Parents should be advised to keep the water temperature setting of the water heater at 120° Fahrenheit (F) (49° Celsius [C]). Anti-scald devices can be placed on kitchen and bathroom faucets.

In all households, each level of the home and each bedroom should have a functioning smoke detector. If battery-operated, the batteries should be changed every 6 months (with the time change), and the detectors should be checked every month. A family fire escape plan should be created and practiced. Each floor of a home should also have a carbon monoxide detector.

It is important for APNs to ask parents about guns during each well-child visit. APNs should counsel parents on the dangers of keeping firearms; over 90% of firearm incidents involving children occur in the home (US PSTF, 1996). This is a staggering statistic that may encourage parents to rethink the way they keep their guns. If parents choose to have firearms in the home, they should keep the unloaded gun out of reach in a locked location separate from the ammunition. Gun locks have been suggested as a way to prevent unintentional deaths, and many police stations are offering free gun locks to gun owners. Parents should tell children that they are not allowed to touch or look at a gun without a parent's supervision. Parents should also be advised to interview their child's friends' parents about gun access before their child visits friends' homes.

When childproofing a home, parents should keep medicines in child-resistant containers and locked up out of reach, keep the number of the Poison Control Center within easy access of the phone, and keep a current 1 oz bottle of syrup of ipecac at home. (Parents should not administer ipecac unless advised to do so by the Poison Control Center or health care provider.) APNs should distribute the Poison Control Center telephone number to parents as needed.

When a child leaves the home, there are also safety precautions to be considered. Parents should demonstrate to children how to cross the street safely, and children less than age 9 to 12 years old need supervision when crossing. Parents should insist that safety helmets be worn by children who bicycle, roller skate, in-line skate and skateboard. The helmet should be approved by the American National Standards Institute (ANSI) or the Snell Memorial Foundation of the American Society for Testing Materials (ASTM). Wrist guards, elbow pads, and knee pads should also be worn by children using roller skates, in-line skates and skateboards. Personal flotation devices that fit properly should be worn by children participating in boating activities.

The primary role of APNs related to safety is initiating discussion. This means that an assessment of safety issues needs to be conducted on a routine basis; a well-child visit is a logical choice. During the assessment of safety, an APN has the opportunity to address any barriers or preconceived notions that parents may identify related to safety. Handouts or safety checklists are useful to give to parents to help them remember potential accident-causing factors.

Adolescents

Violence and firearms are major health threats to school age and adolescent children. While safety related to firearms and violence occurs in children as well as teens, murder is the second-leading cause of death in persons ages 15 to 24 years old. It is the leading cause of death for African-American men and women and for Hispanic men ages 15 to 24 years old. One out of every four households has a gun, and two thirds of homicides in children and adolescents involve handguns. Adolescent males have a much higher risk of dying or being victimized than adolescent females. Female adolescents are more likely to be victims of date violence, sexual assault, and rape. Other risk factors for violence include living in an urban household, low socioeconomic status, poor school performance, juvenile detention or imprisonment, alcohol or other drug use, access to firearms, mental illness, homelessness, lack of social support, and a history of violence in the home (US DHHS et al, 1998).

APNs should assess a patient's and family's risk for violence with the goal of preventing it. First, an adolescent should be asked about the violence in his or her surroundings and then asked about any personal experiences with violence. Parents, as mentioned with children, should be advised of the dangers of keeping a gun in the home. If they choose to keep a gun in the home anyway, they should be advised to keep the firearm and its ammunition in separate areas and out of the reach, to always handle the firearm as if it were loaded, and to have a gunsmith check antique guns for safety and fix these guns so they can not be fired. APNs should encourage parents to find out about the availability of firearms at places where their children spend time (e.g., friend's houses, school, recreational facilities) and keep their children away from places where they may have access. APNs should find out the circumstances of any injury that may have been the result of violence; it is especially important to find out if the conflict leading to the injury is settled or not and if a patient feels safe. Maintaining confidentiality is important, but not if a patient's safety is at risk. Sometimes parents, police, and other authorities need to be consulted.

APNs should explore with patients how they manage their feelings of anger. Multiple office resources about violence (e.g., videos, pamphlets, posters) may encourage patients and parents to participate in community activities aimed at preventing violence.

Again, the role of APNs is to initiate discussion related to safety. It is hard to discuss safety with adolescents because they have a high sense of invulnerability (i.e., "it always happens to someone else"). Using threats and intimidation also does not work because of this invulnerability. Instead, an interactive discussion about safety and using "what if" questions to stimulate conversation may prove effective. Having this discussion with parents out of the room is probably helpful so an adolescent does not feel obliged to protect them. Sometimes, use of a confidential adolescent survey is a good way to initiate or identify topics of concern to a teen. Rachel the NP uses one of these at Redbud. She is very careful to describe to the patient what the form is used for and how the information will be kept confidential (unless someone is in danger). Rachel reviews the completed sheet with the teen patient and then rips the form up in front of them to maintain her credibility.

Adults and older adults

Two safety issues that affect adults include unintentional injuries and domestic violence. Accidental injuries are the fifth-leading cause of death for all age groups in the United States and the leading cause of death in persons ages 1 to 44 years old (Box 43-10). Motor vehicle accidents are the cause of 50% of accidental injuries; 20% of nonfatal and 40% of fatal motor vehicle accidents are linked with alcohol. It is estimated that 68% of people in the United States wear their seat belts, but in cases of fatal car accidents, seat belt use is only 50%. Other causes for deaths from unintentional injury include falls, poisoning, drowning, and house fires (US DHHS et al, 1998).

Falls are the second-leading cause of injury death in adults ages 65 to 84 years and the leading cause of injury death in adults over age 85. People ages 65 to 84 have twice as many falls resulting in death than the general population; people over age 85 have 15 times the number of falls resulting in death. Hip fracture is the most common consequence of falling, and many older adults who sustain hip fractures never completely recover. The annual cost for

---

> ### *Box* **43-10**
>
> ## Guidelines on Injury Prevention Counseling for Adults
>
> - Include safety counseling as part of routine primary care.
> - Advise all patients to wear safety belts when driving or riding as a passenger in a motor vehicle.
> - Advise patients not to drink alcohol when driving a motor vehicle, boating, swimming, or using motorized tools or firearms. Encourage delegating a designated driver.
> - Advise patients to wear safety helmets while driving or riding as a passenger on a motorcycle.
> - Encourage the use of a mouth guard if patients are participating in contact sports.
> - Counsel all patients to have operational smoke detectors in their homes, change the batteries every 6 months (at the transitions to and from Daylight Savings Time in the spring and fall), and check the function every month. Each floor of the home should also have a carbon monoxide detector.
> - Advise patients of the dangers of keeping guns in the home. Many more children, family members, and friends are killed than are intruders in homes where there are guns. Counsel patients on the importance of keeping guns and ammunition locked up separately if guns are kept in the home.
> - Counsel patients to be aware of safety hazards at the workplace and utilize recommended prevention techniques.

Data from U.S. Department of Health and Human Services, Public Health Service, Office of Public Health and Science, & Office of Disease Prevention and Health Promotion (1998). *Put prevention into practice: clinician's handbook of preventive services* (2nd ed.). Washington DC: US Government Printing Office. Available online at www.ahcpr.gov/ppipindes.html.

---

hip fractures in the United States is estimated as $10 to $20 billion (US DHHS et al, 1998).

APNs should counsel older adults and their caretakers to inspect the home for efficient lighting and hazards that could predispose one to tripping (e.g., electrical wires, loose rugs, toys); to install handrails and traction strips in stairways and bathtubs; to keep the hot water temperature below 120° F, or 49° C. Using a checklist for home safety during a home visit can also be an effective intervention (Figure 43-4). APNs should check the visual acuity and mobility of their adult patients on a regular basis. An APN should not prescribe medications that could predispose a patient to fall (e.g., long-acting benzodiazepines, tricyclic antidepressants, major tranquilizers, other sedatives), and he or she should review a patient's medications (including vitamins and nutritional supplements) each visit. Many falls for older adults are due to polypharmacy. Older adults should exercise unless it is medically contraindicated. Regular exercise maintains muscle and bone strength, mobility, and flexibility and therefore reduces the risk of

---

Home Safety Checklist for Older Adults

Place a check mark next to each question if the answer is yes. Discuss unmarked items with patient.

Housekeeping

_____ Do you clean up spills as soon as they occur?

_____ Do you keep floors and stairways clean and free of clutter?

_____ Do you put away books, magazines, sewing supplies, and other objects as soon as you are through with them and never leave them on floors or stairways?

_____ Do you store frequently used items on shelves that are within easy reach?

Floors

_____ Do you keep everyone from walking on freshly washed floors before they are dry?

_____ If you wax floors, do you apply two thin coats and buff each thoroughly or use self-polishing wax?

_____ Do all area rugs have nonslip backings?

_____ Have you eliminated small rugs at the tops and bottoms of stairways?

_____ Are all carpet edges tacked down?

_____ Are rugs and carpets free of curled edges, worn spots, and rips?

_____ Have you chosen rugs and carpets with short, dense pile?

_____ Are rugs and carpets installed over good quality, medium-thick pads?

Lighting

_____ Do you have light switches near every doorway?

_____ Do you have enough good lighting to eliminate shadowy areas?

_____ Do you have a lamp or light switch within easy reach of every bed?

_____ Do you have night lights in your bathrooms and in hallways leading from bedrooms to bathrooms?

_____ Are all stairways well lighted with light switches at both top and bottom?

Bathrooms

_____ Do you use a rubber mat or nonslip decals in tubs and showers?

_____ Do you have a grab bar securely anchored over each tub and shower?

_____ Do you have a nonslip rug on all bathroom floors?

_____ Do you keep soap in easy-to-reach receptacles?

Traffic Lanes

_____ Can you walk across every room in your home, and from one room to another, without detouring around furniture?

_____ Is the traffic lane from your bedroom to the bathroom free of obstacles?

_____ Are telephone and appliance cords kept away from areas where people walk?

Stairways

_____ Do securely fastened handrails extend the full length of the stairs on each side of the stairways?

_____ Do the handrails stand out from the walls so you can get a good grip?

_____ Are handrails distinctly shaped so you are alerted when you reach the end of a stairway?

_____ Are all stairways in good conditions with no broken, sagging, or sloping steps?

_____ Are all stairway carpeting and metal edges securely fastened and in good condition?

_____ Have you replaced any single-level steps with gradually rising ramps, or made sure such steps are well lighted?

Ladders and Step Stools

_____ Do you always use a step stool or ladder that is tall enough for the job?

_____ Do you always set up your ladder or step stool on a firm, level base that is free of clutter?

_____ Before you climb a ladder or step stool, do you always make sure it is fully open and that the stepladder spreaders are locked?

_____ When you use a ladder or step stool, do you face the steps and keep your body between the side rails?

_____ Do you avoid standing on the top step of a step stool or climbing beyond the second step from the top on a stepladder?

Outdoor Areas

_____ Are walks and driveways in your yard and other areas free of breaks?

_____ Are lawns and garden free of holes?

_____ Do you put away garden tools and hoses when they are not in use?

_____ Are outdoor areas kept free of rocks, loose boards, and other tripping hazards?

_____ Do you keep outdoor walkways, steps, and porches free of wet leaves and snow?

_____ Do you sprinkle icy outdoor areas with de-icers as soon as possible after a snowfall or freeze?

_____ Do you have mats at doorways for people to wipe their feet on?

_____ Do you know the safest way of walking when you can't avoid walking on a slippery surface?

Figure 43-4 Safety home checklist. (From National Safety Council [1982]. *Falling—the unexpected trip: a safety program for older adults. Program leader's guide.* Chicago: National Safety Council.)

Home Safety Checklist for Older Adults—Cont'd

Place a check mark next to each question if the answer is yes. Discuss unmarked items with patient.

Footwear

_____ Do your shoes have soles and heels that provide good traction?

_____ Do you avoid walking in stocking feet and wear house slippers that fit well and don't fall off?

_____ Do you wear low-heeled oxfords, loafers, or good quality sneakers when you work in your house or yard?

_____ Do you replace boots or galoshes when their soles or heels are worn too smooth to keep you from slipping on wet or icy surfaces?

Personal Precautions

_____ Are you always alert for unexpected hazards, such as out-of-place furniture?

_____ If young children visit or live in your home, are you alert for children playing on the floor and toys left in your path?

_____ If you have pets, are you alert for sudden movements across your path and pets getting underfoot?

_____ When you carry packages, do you divide them into smaller loads and make sure they do not obstruct your vision?

_____ When you reach or bend, do you hold onto a firm support and avoid throwing your head back or turning it too far?

_____ Do you always move deliberately and avoid rushing to answer the phone or doorbell?

_____ Do you take time to get your balance when you change position from lying down to sitting and from sitting to standing?

_____ Do you keep yourself in good condition with moderate exercise, good diet, adequate rest, and regular medical checkups?

_____ If you wear glasses, is your prescription up to date?

_____ Do you know how to reduce injury in a fall?

_____ If you live alone, do you have daily contact with a friend or neighbor?

Figure 43-4, cont'd

falls. Older women may be assessed for the appropriateness of estrogen replacement therapy, with the goal of preventing hip fracture secondary to osteoporosis. APNs should also assess their need for weight-bearing exercise and calcium and other nutritional supplementation.

Domestic violence can be a deadly health hazard for many women. Partner abuse also affects a small percentage of men. Sources say that from 1 to 4 million women a year suffer from partner abuse, and they are often treated for their injuries in general medical practices, prenatal clinics, urgent care centers, and emergency departments. The risk for domestic violence increases during pregnancy and after separation or divorce. The consequences of domestic violence can range from injury to death. Of women murdered each year, 30% are victims of someone they knew intimately. Studies show that clinicians need to improve their skills in assessment and counseling related to domestic violence (US DHHS et al, 1998).

Evidence for violence can sometimes be assessed on physical examination. The areas of the body most typically injured include the head, neck, chest, abdomen, breasts, and upper extremities. Burns and bruises in the shape of handprints, belts, cords, or other weapons may be seen. An APN should suspect partner violence in a patient with recurrent somatic complaints like headaches; insomnia; choking sensations; hyperventilation; gastrointestinal symptoms; and pain in the chest, back, and pelvis. Each patient should be asked, in a caring and nonjudgmental manner, for any history of physical abuse (Box 43-11). If a woman says she is being abused, the APN should acknowledge the problem and explain that it is unacceptable and could happen again. The APN should also let the patient know that abuse is a common problem and that help is available. APNs should have a plan prepared for women who disclose being the victims of abuse and inform patients of community, social, and legal resources; advise

them they have legal rights; and provide a plan for dealing with the abusive partner. APNs may call the National Council on Child Abuse and Family Violence at (800) 222-2000 for phone numbers for local resources. Most importantly, APNs should make sure that they routinely screen for domestic violence and then document their findings. These screenings should be as commonplace as those for potential pregnancy (see Chapter 40).

PRIORITIES FOR RESEARCH

Little research has been devoted to determining what interventions are effective in addressing individual lifestyle behaviors (with the exception of reducing smoking and alcohol problems). Effective counseling for other health behaviors has only been studied in highly specialized settings (e.g., sexually transmitted disease [STD] clinics) and in cases where multiple visits with a specialist have occurred (e.g. with some cholesterol-lowering interventions). Whether a brief intervention for health promotion during a routine office visit is as effective as an office visit exclusively for health promotion is unknown. Many patients do not have well or preventive visits, so it is vital for an APN to conduct a well or preventive visit when a patient is in the office. Research looking at the efficacy of the method of prevention delivery would be important, and outcomes related to specifically scheduled well visits versus prevention done at every visit could be compared.

Nurses are well known for counseling patients. Diabetes education began in the 1930s; it is one of the most formally structured and well-developed types of counseling programs and is often practiced by nurses. APNs need to describe and substantiate effective counseling strategies in the office setting for wellness and prevention in clinical research. Unfortunately, there is evidence that APNs do

Recommended Questions for Clinicians to Ask Potential Victims of Abuse

- Have you been hit, kicked, punched, or otherwise hurt by someone in the past year? If so, by whom?
- Are you currently in a relationship in which you have been physically hurt or threatened by your partner? Have you ever been in such a relationship?
- Are you in a relationship in which you are treated badly? In what way?
- Has your partner ever destroyed things that you cared about?
- Has your partner ever threatened or abused your children?
- Has your partner ever forced you to have sex when you didn't want to? Have you been forced to engage in sex that makes you uncomfortable?
- We all fight at home. What happens when you and your partner fight or disagree?
- Do you ever feel afraid of your partner?
- Has your partner ever prevented you from leaving the house, seeking friends, getting a job, or continuing your education?
- How does your partner act when drinking or on drugs? Is your partner ever verbally or physically abusive?
- Do you have guns in your home? Has your partner ever threatened to use them when angry?
- Have the police been called to your home because of a dispute with your partner?

Adapted from American Medical Association (1992). *Diagnostic and treatment guidelines on domestic violence*. Chicago: American Medical Association.

not provide CPS as often as recommended. For example, the Office of Disease Prevention and Health Promotion, U.S. Public Health Service (1992) found that evaluation of alcohol consumption was provided to 81% to 100% of patients by only 45% of NPs. The range of assessment for all PCPs was 29% to 63%. NPs were the lowest of all primary providers in the area of referral to Alcoholics Anonymous (19% of NPs providing referral to 19% to 33% of patients needing intervention). In other areas of CPS, NPs were found to be in the low to middle range of all providers for such areas as assessment of physical activity, tobacco use, pneumococcal vaccination and cholesterol screening. These results are just not acceptable given advanced practice's claim of emphasis on preventive services and counseling. As these results are almost 10 years old and a new edition of the preventive services guidelines has been published, one hopes that the percentage of CPS offered by APNs has improved; however, little scientific evidence has been published to counteract the older data.

Knowledge of a lifestyle change needed by a patient is not enough. It is a beginning step but does not necessarily lead to compliance. Research evaluating the best ways to encourage lifestyle changes is needed. In addition, research is necessary to determine what steps APNs can take to encourage patients to assume more self-responsibility in making the needed changes so that the changes become long term. Use of lifestyle questionnaires may prove helpful in gathering data about patients (Hutchins, 1988).

APNs should use *The Guide to Preventive Services* (US PSTF, 1996) as a resource document for research on CPS. However, the authors of the book were frequently not able to find adequate evidence to evaluate effectiveness because studies were not done or findings were unreliable. APNs should use this source as a basis on which to begin their own research related to CPS. APNs can identify where there is insufficient evidence and design studies to target those areas. In addition, APNs need to collaborate with other researchers to improve the overall quality of preventive research. Griffith and Diguiseppi (1994) believe that APN involvement in the development, dissemination, implementation, and evaluation of nursing guidelines for CPS is essential.

IMPLICATIONS FOR MSN EDUCATION AND ADVANCED PRACTICE

It is important that APNs learn about CPS in their educational programs. Nursing faculty should model incorporation of these services into their practices, and preceptors should also model ways in which preventive services can be offered on a consistent basis. APN students then see the importance of the services and will use them on a regular basis. Keller (1993) suggests a model for a course in preventive medicine, and while the recommendations are for medical students, much if not all the content is applicable for APNs. The important thing to note is the integration of preventive medicine with pathophysiology and clinical care; these courses serve as the framework on which all other courses can be based. (Table 43-1 identifies content that is important when considering preventive care.) Ways in which APNs can incorporate CPS into their practices are numerous. The recommendation of a clinician using a prescription pad can be a powerful motivator in such areas as exercise (Ades, Waldmann, & McCann, 1992). If APNs do not address patients' lack of activity, patients may interpret this as a sign that inactivity or sedentary behavior is acceptable; the same line of reasoning can be used with other preventive services such as those for obesity or smoking. APNs should address CPS during as many office visits as possible. They can ask patients what their goals are regarding a preventive service and help patients identify short-term goals that are realistic and attainable. Tips to assist patients in adopting lifestyle

Table 43-1

Model for Course in Preventive Medicine

CONCEPT FOCUS	CONTENT
What does this case or disease represent in the community?	• Concepts of causality • Agents of disease • Persons at risk (e.g., profile of a high-risk person) • Interaction of agent, host, and environment • Course of the disease • Strategies of prevention (primary, secondary, and tertiary) • Illustration of the natural history of selected diseases of current concern
Who is normal?	How do we determine the normal range of test results? • Selected screening tests: sensitivity, specificity, predictive value, and effect of prevalence on predictive value • Ruling in and ruling out • Serial and parallel testing • Current thinking regarding routine screening tests
How well do you know the odds?	How do we make decisions from data? • Role of probability in medical decision-making • Descriptive statistics • Testing hypotheses • Type I and type II errors • Understanding of statistical statements in the literature • Examples of the use of statistics in nursing and medicine
How long do I have? Thoughts on prognosis?	• Distinction between risk factors and prognostic factors • Survival analysis • Cohort studies to assess prognosis • Biases that may affect cohort studies • Combinations of factors affecting prognosis
What shall we do for the patient?	• Thoughts on the choice of treatments • Clinical trials: selection of study population, allocation of patients to treatment and control groups, randomization, and double blind studies • Types of biases and methods of reducing bias • Ethical considerations • Examples of past and present clinical trials
Is there is a lot of it going around?	• Description of the occurrence of a disease • Incidence, prevalence, secular trends, crude rates, cause-specific rates, and proportional and standard mortality rates • Relative and attributable mortality ratios • Methods of rate adjustment • Investigation of an outbreak of disease, including examples of such investigations
Are you a case or control?	• Retrospective and prospective studies: advantages and disadvantages • Odds ratio and relative risk • Concurrent and historical cohort studies • Illustrative examples of case-control and cohort studies
Who is the patient?	• Realization of numerous subsets of the general population: genetic, cultural, occupational, and other demographic subsets (e.g., age, sex) • Notion that demographics affect the probability of occurrence of certain diseases and also affect health knowledge, attitudes, and behaviors.

Reproduced with permission from *Pediatrics, 97*, 757-780. (1994).

changes might include group exercise or group support for weight loss; spouse/partner support for the lifestyle change; and encouragement for patients to reward themselves for achieving certain goals. APNs and patients should share decision-making related to CPS. For example, if a 52-year-old man comes in to the office, based on his age a rectal and prostate exam should be done; the APN should discuss the merits and disadvantages of prostate antigen screening (PSA) and let the patient decide if this is a test he wants to have done. Patients should be given the information and then encouraged to make an informed decision. Self-care principles form the basis of staying healthy from the patient's perspective, and letting patients know that they play a major role in staying healthy is important. (Figure 43-5 shows an algorithm for a stepped care approach to counseling patients in self-care.)

Research indicates that there are a variety of ways to increase CPS. These methods include computerized reminders for patients, flow sheets, monthly summary feedback, chart reminders, chart audits and feedback, and nurse-administered screening protocols (Griffith & Diguiseppi, 1994; Yano, Fink, Hirsch, Robbins, & Rubenstein, 1995; Shea, Dumouchel, & Bahamonde,

1996). APNs may also want to start using PPIP kits to improve preventive services. These kits include such items as waiting room posters, chart alerts, reminder stickers, and prevention prescription pads.

It will also be critical for APNs to increase access to CPS for those who are most often in need of the services—the underserved. Those patients who normally seek care in the emergency room are missing preventive services because they are not usually available or offered in the emergency department. Since NPs are a key source of care for the underserved, incorporating CPS into NP care will increase delivery of these services. APNs also needs to be selective in ordering tests and providing services. For example, a TB test is not warranted for the general popula-

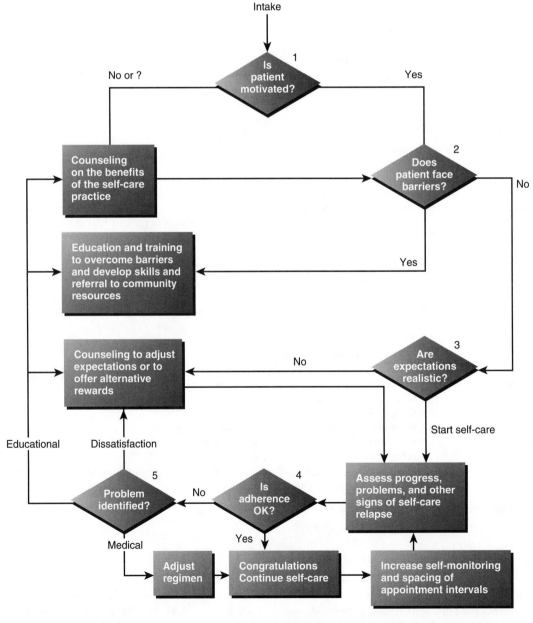

Figure 43-5 Stepped care approach to counseling patients. (From Green, L.W. [1987]. How physicians can improve patient's participation and maintenance in self-care. *Western Journal of Medicine, 147*, 346-349.)

tion. However, a TB test may be prudent for all underserved, low-income patients as part of the CPS protocol because these are patients that are at increased risk.

Many articles have been written about the periodic health examination (Frame, 1995; Luckmann & Melville, 1995). Frame (1995) wrote an editorial about how the annual physical examination refuses to die, even though extensive evidence is available supporting the notion of selective longitudinal health maintenance. Recommendations to this effect were made by both the American College of Physicians and the American Medical Association in the early 1980s, yet many people persist in believing that an annual examination is warranted. APNs should use each visit to get the most "bang for the buck," which means only doing testing that is warranted based on a patient's history and risk profile.

Because not all preventive services are covered by private or public health insurance, it is important for APNs to be aware of low-cost, high-quality service delivery settings that offer tests at a reasonable cost and refer patients to them. Financial concerns may limit what tests patients choose to receive, but it should not limit what APNs discuss with patients or what is ordered; patients will make the decisions based on their finances. APNs should discuss the pros and cons of each test, letting patients know how the test fits into the preventive plan and where the patients fall in terms of level of risk relative to the test.

Most studies indicate that PCPs overestimate the amount of CPS provided. Given this, it is vital for APNs to conduct reviews of the preventive services provided to get objective feedback of actual compliance. (As computerized medical records become more prevalent, this will become a less labor-intensive job.) APNs that precept students may want students to conduct miniature quality assurance reviews of how well preventive services are delivered. This may serve both clinicians and students well; it provides

data to a clinician and also provides a meaningful research project for the student, a project that will probably be implemented into his or her practice upon graduation.

Since counseling is a major part of CPS, review of principles to facilitate culturally appropriate counseling is necessary. The environment of the office can be tailored to promote preventive care, and using a variety of resources is helpful, as is having pamphlets and other materials easily accessible for patients to browse through. It is important for APNs and patients to have a therapeutic relationship before counseling. This makes the counseling less like a sermon and more like a discussion, and the more a patient is involved in decision-making, the more likely it is that change will occur. Even brief (quality) interventions can be effective.

DISCUSSION QUESTIONS

These questions can be used to promote critical thinking and encourage discussion.

1. Describe how you would share decision-making about CPS with a patient.
2. How do you determine which patients are at high risk and therefore need more screening?
3. A 22-year-old woman comes in to your office for the first time with a 2-week history of productive cough with green sputum. She has smoked one pack of cigarettes a day for 10 years. Her past medical history is negative, and her only medication is oral contraceptives. She is single and lives with her boyfriend. Other than fever of 100° Fahrenheit (F) and reddened nasal mucosa, her physical examination, including her lungs, is normal.

Suggestions for Further Learning

- Get one of the following articles on exercise: Anderson, R., Franklin, B., & Trotto, N. (1999). Exercise for optimum health. *Patient Care for the Nurse Practitioner, 11*, 13-28; Fletcher, G. (1997). How to implement physical activity in primary and secondary prevention: a statement for healthcare professionals from the Task Force on Risk Reduction, American Heart Association. *Circulation, 96*, 355-357; or Pinto, B., Goldstein, M., & Marcus, B. (1998). Activity counseling by primary care physicians. *Preventive Medicine, 27*, 506-513. What recommendations do these articles make related to exercise and primary care? Are there exercise modifications for specific patient populations?
- Get the article: Lemley, K., O'Grady, E., & Rauckhorst, L. (1994). Baseline data on the delivery of clinical preven-

tive services provided by nurse practitioners. *Nurse Practitioner, 19*(5), 57-63. What implications does this article have related to CPS? What barriers and facilitators are identified for CPS?
- Find one or more of the following resources for patients and APNs, all published by the American Academy of Pediatrics, PO Box 927, Elk Grove Village, IL 60009-0927; phone (800)433-9016; website www.aap.org:
  - *Nutrition in Children: The Gift of Love*
  - *Feeding Kids Right Isn't Always Easy*
  - *Tips for Preventing Food Hassles*
  - *Growing Up Healthy: Fat, Cholesterol and More*
  - *Right from the Start: ABC's of Good Nutrition for Young Children*
  - *What's to Eat? Healthy Foods for Hungry Children*

Continued

- Browse the following:
  - *Nutrition and Sports Performance: A Guide for High School Athletes*. American College of Sports Medicine, PO Box 1440, Indianapolis, IN 46202-1440; phone (317) 634-7817
  - *Nutrition and Your Health; Dietary Guidelines for Americans; The Food Guide Pyramid* (all booklets). Cooperative Extension System or contact the Superintendent of Documents, US Government Printing Office, Washington, DC 20402; phone (202) 783-3238
  - *The Food Guide Pyramid: Beyond the Basic 4*. Food Marketing Institute, 800 Connecticut Avenue, NW, Washington, DC 20006
  - *A Food Guide for the First Five Years*. Education Department of the National Live Stock and Meat Board, 444 North Michigan Avenue, Chicago, IL 60611
  - *Nutrition in Adults: An Eating Plan for Healthy Americans*. American Heart Association; phone (800) 611-6083
  - *The American Cancer Society Cookbook*. American Cancer Society; phone (888) 227-5552; website: www.cancer.org
- Find a copy of *Eating Smart: Even When You're Pressed for Time* from the National Cattlemen's Beef Association, 444 North Michigan Avenue, Suite 1800, Chicago, IL 60611. This book was reviewed favorably by the American College of Sports Medicine, Shape Up America!, and the American Academy of Family Physicians Foundation and consists of details on how to use the food pyramid.
- Review the following:
  - *A Good Start: Nutrition During Pregnancy*. Education Department of the National Live Stock and Meat Board, 444 North Michigan Avenue, Chicago, IL 60611
  - *CHATS: A Guide to Sensible Eating* (scripted slide show); *Osteoporosis in Women: Keeping Your Bones Healthy and Strong*. American Academy of Family Physicians, 8880 Ward Parkway, Kansas City, MO 64114-2797; phone (800) 944-0000; website: www. aafp.org
  - *Diet, Nutrition and Cancer Prevention: The Good News*. Office of Cancer Communications, National Cancer Institute, Building 31, Room 10A24, Bethesda, MD 20892; phone (800) 4-CANCER; website: www.nci. nih.gov
  - *Choosing a Safe and Successful Weight-Loss Program; Physical Activity and Weight Control; Very Low Calorie Diets*. The National Institute of Diabetes and Digestive and Kidney Disease, 1 WIN Way, Bethesda, MD 20892-3665; phone (800) 946-8098; website: www. niddk.nih.gov/NutritionDocs.html
- Look for information at the National Health Information Center (NHIC). NHIC is a health information referral service that links consumers and health care professionals who have questions about health to organizations who can best answer them. It was established in 1979 by the Office of Disease Prevention and Health Promotion within the U.S. Public Health Service, U.S. DHHS. The NHIC provides a variety of health information resource materials, a toll-free telephone service, and a database of health-related organizations.

- Review one of the following sources on exercise:
  - *Exercise in Children; Better Health and Fitness Through Physical Activity; Sports and Your Child*. American Academy of Pediatrics, PO Box 927, Elk Grove Village, IL 60009-0927; phone (800) 433-9016; website: www.aap.org
  - *Get Fit: A Handbook for Youth Ages 6-17; Kids in Action: Fitness for Children Ages 2-17; Presidential Sports Awards: 4-Month Qualifications for Anyone Ages 6 and Up; The Physician's RX: Exercise*. The President's Council on Physical Fitness and Sports, 701 Pennsylvania Avenue, SW, Suite 250, Washington, DC 20004; phone (202) 272-3421
  - *Anabolic Steroids and Athletes; Nutrition and Sports Performance: A Guide for High School Athletes; Weight Loss and Wrestlers; Youth Fitness*. Available through the American College of Sports Medicine; website: www.acsm.org/sportsmed
  - *Exercise in Adults; Exercise and Your Heart* (37-page booklet), *Walking for a Healthy Heart* (11-page booklet). American Heart Association; phone (800) 611-6083
  - *Fitting Fitness In: Even When You're Pressed for Time*. National Cattlemen's Beef Association, 444 North Michigan Avenue, Suite 1800, Chicago, IL, 60611.
  - Shape Up America! 6707 Democracy Blvd., Suite 306, Bethesda, MD 20817; fax (301) 493-9504; website: www.shapeup.org
  - *Weight Control: Losing Weight and Keeping It Off*. American Academy of Family Physicians, 8880 Ward Parkway, Kansas City, MO 64114-2797; phone (800) 944-0000; website: www.aafp.org
  - *Women and Exercise* (educational bulletin 173); *Exercise and Fitness: A Guide for Women*. American College of Obstetricians and Gynecologists, 409 12th Street, SW, Washington, DC 20024; phone (800) 762-2264; website: www.acog.com
  - *Weight Control: Eating Right and Keeping Fit*. American College of Obstetricians and Gynecologists; phone (800) 762-2264; website: www.acog.com
  - *Check Your Healthy Heart IQ; Check Your Physical Activity and Heart Disease IQ; Exercise and Your Heart; Aprenda a Reconocer un Corazon Sano*. National Heart, Lung and Blood Institute Smoking Education Program, PO Box 30105, Bethesda, MD 20824-0105; phone (301) 251-1222 (available in English and Spanish); website: www.nhlbi.nih.gov/nhlbi/nhlbi.html
  - *Provider Resources: Physician-Based Assessment and Counseling for Exercise*. Project PACE, San Diego State University, San Diego, CA 92182-0567; phone (619) 594-5949
- Check out the following resources on smoking cessation:
  - *Smoking Cessation in Children; Clearing the Air: How to Quit Smoking and Quit for Keeps; Chew or Snuff Is Real Bad Stuff; Smoking: Facts and Tips for Quitting; Why Do You Smoke?* National Cancer Institute, U.S. Superintendent of Documents, Consumer Information Center-3C, PO Box 100, Pueblo, CO 81002

- *Stop Smoking Kit; Smoking Cessation in Adults; Smoking: Steps to Help You Break the Habit.* American Academy of Family Physicians, 8880 Ward Parkway, Kansas City, MO 64114-2797; phone (800) 944-0000; website: www.aafp.org

- *Through with Chew.* American Academy of Otolaryngology, 1 Prince Street, Alexandria, VA 22314; phone (703) 836-4444

- *Smoking: Guidelines for Teens; Tobacco Abuse—A Message to Parents and Teens; Straight Talk about Smokeless Tobacco; Smoking: Straight Talk for Teens; Environmental Tobacco Smoke: A Danger for Children.* American Academy of Pediatrics, PO Box 927, Elk Grove Village, IL 60009-0927; phone (800) 433-9016; website: www.aap.org

- *Smoking and Reproductive Health; Smoking in Women.* American College of Obstetricians and Gynecologists, 409 12th Street, SW, Washington, DC 20024; phone (800) 762-2264; website: www.acog.com

- *Smokeless Tobacco: Think before You Chew; Smoking Can Really Do A Number on Your Health.* American Dental Association, Department of Salable Materials, 211 E Chicago Avenue, Chicago, IL 60611; phone (800) 947-4746

- *You Can Quit Smoking: Smoking Cessation Consumer Guide* (clinical practice guideline number 18; publication number 96-0695); *Helping Smokers Quit: A Guide for Primary Care Clinicians* (clinical practice guideline number 18; publication number 96-0693). Agency for Health Care Policy and Research, Publications Clearinghouse, PO Box 8547, Silver Spring, MD 20907; phone (800) 358-9295; website: www.ahcpr.gov

- *Bright Futures: Guidelines for Health Supervision of Infants, Children and Adolescents; Bright Futures Pocket Guide; Bright Futures Anticipatory Guidance Cards.* National Center for Education in Maternal and Child Health, 2000 15th Street North, Suite 701, Arlington, VA 22201-2617; phone (703) 524-7802; website: www.brightfutures.org

- Center for Disease Control and Prevention Information and Prevention Source Page; website: www.cdc.gov/tobacco

- *Clinical Interventions to Prevent Tobacco Use by Children and Adolescents.* National Cancer Institute; phone (800) 4-CANCER; website: wwwicic.nci.nih.gov.

- *Doctors Helping Smokers* (smoking cessation program and video). Doctors Helping Smokers at Blue Plus, PO Box 64179, R3-11, St. Paul, MN 55164; phone (800) 382-2000, ext 1975

- *How to Help Your Patients Stop Smoking: A National Cancer Institute Manual for Physicians; How to Help Your Patients Stop Using Tobacco: A National Cancer Institute Manual for the Oral Health Team.* Office of Cancer Communications, National Cancer Institute, Building 31, Room 10A16, Bethesda, MD 208292; phone (800) 4-CANCER; website: wwwicic.nci.hih.gov.

- *Nurses: Help Your Patients Stop Smoking.* National Heart, Lung, and Blood Institute Smoking Education Program, PO Box 30105, Bethesda, MD 20824-0105; phone (301) 251-1222 (available in English and Spanish); website: gopher://fido.nhlbi.hih.gov:70/11/nhlbi/health/lung/other/prof/nrsmk

- *On the Teen Scene: Young People Talk with the FDA Commissioner about Smoking.* FDA Office of Consumer Affairs, HFE 88, Room 1675, 5600 Fishers Lane, Rockville, MD 20857; phone (800) 532-4400. Contact the American Lung Association at (800) 586-4872 to receive an order form

- *How to Quit Cigarettes: The Fifty Most Often Asked Questions about Smoking and Health and the Answers.* American Cancer Society; phone (800) 227-2345; website: www.cancer.org

- *Check Your Smoking I.Q.: An Important Quiz for Older Smokers.* National Heart, Lung, and Blood Institute Smoking Education Program, PO Box 30105, Bethesda, MD 20824-0105; phone (301) 251-1222 (available in English and Spanish); website: www.nhlbi.hih.gov/nhlbi/nhlbi.html

- Check out one of the following sources on safety:

- Safety in Children Auto Safety Hot Line. National Highway Traffic Safety Administration; phone (800) 424-9393

- *Child Safety: How to Keep Your Home Safe for Your Baby.* American Academy of Family Physicians, 8880 Ward Parkway, Kansas City, MO 64114-2797; phone (800) 944-0000; website: www.aafp.org

- *Reduce the Risk of Sudden Infant Death Syndrome (SIDS)* (available in English and Spanish). Back to Sleep, PO Box 29111, Washington, DC 20040; phone (800) 505-2742

- *Safe Kids Gear Up Guide; How to Protect Your Child from Injury.* National SAFE KIDS campaign, 1301 Pennsylvania Avenue, NW, Suite 1000, Washington, DC 20004; phone (202) 662-0600

- U.S. Consumer Product Safety Commission, Publication Requests. Washington, DC 20207. Available in English and Spanish; phone (800) 638-2772

- *Raising Children to Resist Violence: What You Can Do; Child Sexual Abuse: What It Is and How to Avert It; Fun in the Sun: Keep Your Baby Safe; 1995 Family Shopping Guide to Car Seats: Guidelines for Parents; A Guide to Safety Counseling in Office Practice; Physician's Resource Guide for Bicycle Safety Education; Injury Prevention for Children and Youth.* American Academy of Pediatrics, 141 Northwest Point Boulevard, PO Box 927, Elk Grove Village, IL 60009-0927; phone: (800) 433-9016; website: www.aap.org

- *STOP: Steps to Prevent Firearm Injury.* Center To Prevent Handgun Violence, 1225 I Street, NW, Suite 1100, Washington, DC 20005; phone (202) 289-7319.

- *Provider Resources Identification and Prevention of Youth Violence: A Protocol for Health Care Providers; Assessment and Treatment of Hospitalized Adolescent Victims of Interpersonal Violence.* Adolescent Wellness Program, Department of Health & Hospitals, 1010 Massachusetts Avenue, 2nd Floor, Boston, MA 02118; phone (617) 534-5196

- Centers for Disease Control and Prevention, National Center for Injury Prevention and Control; website: www.cdc.gov/ncipc

- The Injury Prevention Program, American Academy of Pediatrics, PO Box 927, Elk Grove Village, IL 60009-0927; phone (800) 433-9016; website: www.aap.org

Continued

Suggestions for Further Learning—cont'd

- *Safety in Adults.* National Highway Traffic Safety Administration, Office of Occupant Protection, NTS-13, 400 7th Street, SW, Washington, DC 20590; phone (202) 366-2727
- *Injury Control News.* Association for the Advancement of Injury Control, 888 17th Street, NW, Suite 1000, Washington, DC 20006; phone (202) 296-6161
- *Age Page—Accident Prevention and the Elderly; Age Page—Preventing Falls and Fractures.* National Institute on Aging, Building 31, Room 5C27, 31 Center Drive, MSC 2922, Bethesda, MD 20892-2922; phone (310) 496-1752; website: www.nih.gov/nia/health/pubpub/pubpub.htm
- *The Abused Woman; Domestic Violence* (Technical bulletin # 209). American College of Obstetricians and Gynecologists, 409 12th Street, SW, Washington, DC 20024-2188; phone (202) 638-5577; website: www.agog.com
- *Your Home Safety Checklist; Preventing Falls: A Safety Program for Older Adults; Facts About Backs; Playing it Safe: A Pocket Guide to Fitness.* National Safety Council, 444 N Michigan Avenue, Chicago, IL, 60601; phone (800) 621-7619, ext 1300
- *Diagnostic and Treatment Guidelines on Domestic Violence; What Can You Do About Family Violence?* (#NC110992). American Medical Association, 515 N State Street, Chicago, IL 60610; phone (800) 621-8335; website: www.ama-assn.org
- *Understanding Violence against Women.* National Academy Press, 2101 Constitution Avenue, NW, Washington DC 20418; phone (800) 624-6242

Would it be appropriate to address health promotion issues at this visit? What health promotion issues would you address? What would be the most effective way to address these issues? What kind of follow-up would you arrange?

REFERENCES/BIBLIOGRAPHY

Ades, P., Waldmann, M., & Polk, K.D. (1992). Referral patterns and exercise response in the rehabilitation of female coronary patients aged greater than or equal to 62 years. *American Journal of Cardiology, 69,* 1422-1425.

Andersen, R., Blair, S., & Cheskin, L. (1997). Encouraging patients to become more physically active: the physician's role. *Annals of Internal Medicine, 127,* 395-400.

Andersen, R., Franklin, B., & Trotto, N. (1999). Exercise for optimum health. *Patient Care for the Nurse Practitioner, 11,* 13-28.

Ask the Professor (1999). Smoking cessation interventions: making them work in your practice. *Consultant, 39*(12), 3384-3392.

Bandura, A. (1992). Exercise of personal agency through the self-efficacy mechanism. In R. Schwarzer (Ed.), *Self efficacy: thought control of action* (pp. 4-32). Washington DC: Hemisphere Publishing.

Bergman-Evans, B., & Walker, S. (1996). The prevalence of clinical preventive services utilization by older women. *Nurse Practitioner, 21*(4), 88, 90, 99-100.

Byrd, J. (1994, November). The VA preventive medicine program. *Federal Practitioner,* 11-17.

Canadian Task Force on Periodic Health Examination (1994). *Canadian guide to clinical preventative services.* Ottawa: Canadian Communication Group.

Cogswell, B., & Eggert, M. (1993). People want doctors to give more preventive care: a qualitative study of health care consumers. *Archives of Family Medicine, 2,* 611-619.

Curtis, P., & Goldstein, A. (1998). Helping your patients stay healthy. In P. Sloane, L. Slatt., P. Curtis, & M. Ebell (Eds.), *Essentials of family medicine* (3rd ed.). Baltimore: Williams & Wilkins.

Foreyt, T., & Goodrick, G. (1993). Weight management without dieting. *Nutrition Today, 28*(2), 4-9.

Frame, P. (1995). The complete annual physical examination refuses to die. *The Journal of Family Practice, 40*(6), 543-545.

Frame, P., Berg, A., & Woolf, S. (1997). US Preventive Services Task Force: highlights of the 1996 report. *American Family Physician, 55*(2), 567-577.

Griffith, H. (1994a). Nursing's role in the delivery of clinical preventive services. *Journal of Professional Nursing, 10,* 69.

Griffith, H. (1994b). Resources to put more prevention into your practice. *Journal of American Academy of Nurse Practitioners, 6*(4), 253-256.

Griffith, H., & Diguiseppi, C. (1994). Guidelines for clinical preventive services. *Nurse Practitioner, 19,* 25-35.

Hutchins, E.B. (1988). *Healthier people: health risk appraisal programs* (5 volumes). Carter Center, Emory University, PO Box 109050, Chicago, IL 60610.

Janis, I.L., & Mann, L. (1977). *Decision-making: a psychological analysis of conflict, choice and commitment.* London: Cassell & Collier Macmillan.

Keller, M. (1993). Teaching preventive medicine. In R. Matzen and R. Lang (Eds.), *Clinical preventive medicine.* St. Louis: Mosby.

Keller, C., & Stevens, K. (1996). Assessment, etiology and intervention in obesity in children. *Nurse Practitioner, 21*(9), 31-42.

Kotthoff-Burrell, E. (1992). Health promotion and disease prevention for the older adult: an overview of the current recommendations and a practical application. *Nurse Practitioner Forum, 4,* 195-209.

Lang, R., & Shainoff, J. (1993). Integrating clinical preventive service into office practice. In R. Matzen & R. Lang (Eds.), *Clinical preventive medicine* (pp. 127-137). St. Louis: Mosby.

Lemley, K., O'Grady, E., Rauckhorst, L., Russell, D., & Small, N. (1994). Baseline data on the delivery of clinical preventive services provided by nurse practitioners. *Nurse Practitioner, 19,* 57-63.

Luckmann, R., & Melville, S. (1995). Periodic health evaluation of adults: a survey of family physicians. The *Journal of Family Practice, 40*(6), 547-554.

Matzen, R., & Lang, R. (1993). *Clinical preventive medicine.* St. Louis: Mosby.

McGinnis, J.M., & Foege, W.H. (1993). Actual causes of deaths in the United States. *Journal of the American Medical Association, 270,* 2207-2212.

National Institutes of Health (1993). *Second report of the National Cholesterol Education Program Expert Panel on Detection, Evaluation & Treatment of High Blood Cholesterol in Adults (Adult Treatment Panel II)* [NIH Publication 93-3095]. Bethesda, MD: National Institutes of Health.

Office of Disease Prevention and Health Promotion, U.S. Public Health Service (1992). *Survey of preventive care practices of primary care providers* (Unpublished).

Pender, N. (1996). *Health promotion in nursing practice* (3rd ed.). Stamford, CT: Appleton & Lange.

Redman, B. (1997). *The practice of patient education.* St. Louis: Mosby.

Rifat, S., Ruffin, M., & Gorenflo, P. (1995). Disqualifying criteria in a preparticipation sports evaluation. *Journal of Family Practice, 41,* 42-50.

Shea, S., DuMouchel, W., & Bahomonde, L. (1996). A meta analysis of 16 randomized controlled trials to evaluatecomputer based clinical reminder systems for preventive care in the ambulatory setting. *Journal of the American Medical Informatics Association, 3*(6), 399, 409.

Sox, H. (1994). Preventive health services in adults. *New England Journal of Medicine, 330*(22), 1589-1595.

Sox, H., & Woolf, S. (1993). Evidence based practice guidelines from the US Preventive Services Task Force. *Journal of the American Medical Association, 269,* 2678.

U.S. Department of Health and Human Services, Public Health Service, Office of Public Health and Science, & Office of Disease Prevention and Health Promotion (1998). *Put prevention into practice: clinician's handbook of preventive services* (2nd ed.). Washington DC: US Government Printing Office. Available online at www.ahcpr.gov/ppipindes.html.

U.S. Preventive Services Task Force (1996). *Guide to clinical preventive services* (2nd ed.). Baltimore: Williams & Wilkins.

U.S. Public Health Service (1994). Put prevention into practice. *Journal of the American Academy of Nurse Practitioners, 6*(6), 257-265.

Woolf, S., Jonas, S., & Lawrence, R. (1996). *Health promotion and disease prevention in clinical practice.* Baltimore, MD: Williams and Wilkins.

Yano, E., Fink, A., Hirsch, S., Robbins, A., & Rubenstein, L. (1995). Helping practices reach primary care goals. *Archives of Internal Medicine, 155,* 1146-1156.

Chapter 44

Relaxation and Stress Management

Jean E. DeMartinis

There have been many recent advances in the diagnosis and treatment of illness, all coming within a tighter, more cost-conscious health care environment. However, there are inherent difficulties in trying to maintain innovative quality care at the lowest cost, and the advances made have been overshadowed by increased provider frustration and patient dissatisfaction. Patients are concerned about issues ranging from questions of quality management to the dehumanization of treatment. This predicament is more troublesome and costly due to an increased number of patients making additional return visits to providers because they are still not feeling well, regardless of having received conventional medical treatment. However, the American Institute of Stress estimates that 60% to 90% of all primary care visits involve stress-related complaints, which may explain this increase (Benson & Friedman, 1996).

CRITICAL ISSUES: RECOGNIZING THE BENEFITS OF RELAXATION AND STRESS MANAGEMENT

Research evidence accumulated over the last 20 years has profoundly implicated stress as associative in both the development and continuation of disease; it produces many deleterious effects, including anxiety, burnout, depression, suicide, and other physiological problems. However, traditional medicine has little to offer in terms of treatment for many complaints related to chronic stress and pain (Benson & McKee, 1993). Providers have been trying to treat stress-related complaints with traditional pharmaceutical and surgical methods; providers also persistently fail to consider the potential influence of psychophysiological stress on patients' health status. For the last 150 years, the medical profession has fostered the bias that diagnosis and treatment of patients' health problems should come solely from the body of knowledge attributable to the results of rigorous scientific clinical trials (the "hard sciences" approach to treatment). This philosophy leaves no room for consideration of the placebo response or encouragement of belief as a valid therapeutic intervention. Many providers are resistant to fostering spiritual beliefs in combination with more traditional treatment modalities. Finally, many providers have also failed to consistently and adequately recognize that individual personality characteristics affect behavior and thus affect health, illness, and recovery.

Mind-Body Behavioral Medicine

Recently, the medical community began a huge paradigm shift toward recognition of the benefits of inquiry into and use of treatment models derived from the "soft sciences." Qualitative studies are becoming more popular, and their results are viewed as more valid and reliable. Patient outcomes have become the center of scientific study, and quality of life and life satisfaction are key determinants of positive outcomes. More practitioners are including both hard science and soft science interventions in their treatment protocols. Therefore stress management interventions should no longer be considered an alternative treatment modality to conventional medical practice, but rather a complementary therapy (Benson & McKee, 1993; Weil, 1995; Benson & Friedman, 1996; LaForge, 1997; Benson & Stark, 1998). Stress management can best be implemented through the integration of mind-body behavioral medicine and self-care practices targeted to tap the powerful influence of the mind on the body.

Multidisciplinary, multifactorial management plans have recently been accepted as essential foundations for treatment protocols designed to assist patients with positive lifestyle changes, and advanced practice nurses (APNs) are the most broadly educated and trained practitioners in the health care field (Wells-Federman, 1996). They embraced the paradigm shift toward holistic health promotion even before the national mandates of *Healthy People 2010* (US Department of Health and Human Services [DHHS], 1999). Therefore they are key personnel on multidisciplinary teams and are in a pivotal position to take the leadership roles.

Currently, a growing coalition within the medical community is looking at traditional medical practice dogma and suggesting that it be rethought and expanded to involve patients more in their own health care so they can mobilize their physical and mental resources for health and healing. This shift in paradigmatic thinking is known as *mind-body medicine* (Benson, 1979; Wells-Federman, Stuart, Deckro, Mandle, Baim, & Medich, 1995; Epperby, 1997; Benson & Stark, 1998). The central premise of mind-body medicine is that the power of the mind can be used to help heal the body, and strategies designed to influence perspectives or appraisals that assist patients in altering the perception of or response to a threat are the basis of mind-body practices. Benson and McKee (1993) encourage practitioners, including physicians and APNs, to include mind-body medicine interventions in traditional medicine as complementary, synergistic, integrative therapeutic approaches that can maintain or restore health. According to Wells-Federman et al (1995), APNs are well suited to understanding the mind-body connection because they typically view patients holistically and in terms of their relationships to the environment. For example, an APN seeing a patient for a neck strain may incorporate massage therapy as a complementary therapy to traditional nonsteroidal anti-inflammatory drugs (NSAIDs).

Physiological Basis for Stress and the Stress Response

Understanding of the physiological basis for the stress response has its roots in the work of the forerunners in this field: Claude Bernard, Walter Cannon, and later Hans Selye (Selye, 1956; Lazarus, 1966; Everly, 1989; Blonna, 1996; Hubbard & Workman, 1998; McCance & Huether, 1998). Bernard, a French physiologist working in the late nineteenth century, described the body's internal environment and how living organisms were constantly seeking balance. Nearly 50 years later, in the early 1900s, Bernard's work was expanded upon and refined by Cannon, a Harvard physiologist, who renamed this balance-seeking process *homeostasis* and used the term *stress* for the psychological and physical strains on homeostasis.

Selye, a Canadian endocrinologist, confirmed Cannon's findings in the 1940s and 1950s and went further by describing a phenomenon that he noticed in conjunction with the processes activated to maintain homeostasis (1956). He discovered laboratory animals not only adjusted to the demands of stress created by the need to adapt to external stimuli, but that their responses were the same, regardless of the source of the demand. Selye then developed his model, the General Adaptation Syndrome (GAS) (Selye, 1956), to describe this nonspecific response to a demand. The model has three distinguishable sequential phases that last a variable length of time (from seconds to days or more): (1) alarm ("fight-or-flight"), (2) resistance (the crux of the stress response), and (3) recovery or exhaustion (successful adaptation or coping, or maladaptation and illness or death). Although

Selye's work has been regarded as a framework for study of the stress response, it describes a purely physiological phenomenon. Moreover, other researchers working in the 1950s and 1960s clearly showed evidence that there is a psychosocial context in which individuals respond to stressors (Lazarus, 1966). Today, it is widely accepted that individuals' physical responses to stressors are intrinsically interwoven with their interaction or transaction with the environment.

Shelby and McCance (1998) describe a modern, more comprehensive theoretical basis from which to investigate stress. *Psychoneuroimmunology* is the study of the interaction of consciousness with the action of the brain and central nervous system (CNS) and the body's defenses against endogenous and exogenous stressors. Psychoneuroimmunology assumes that all immune-related disease is multifactorial, the result of interrelationships among psychosocial, emotional, genetic, neurological, endocrine, immune systems, and behavioral factors. Stressors (e.g., noise, infection, inflammation, pain, decreased oxygen supply, heat, cold, trauma, prolonged exertion, responses to life events, obesity, old age, drugs, disease, surgery, medical treatment) can elicit the stress response. These noxious stimuli are appraised by an individual as a threat capable of causing harm, and a subsequent psychophysiological response is initiated in the body.

Ultimately, stress response systems function to reestablish the state of dynamic equilibrium or homeostasis in the body, a process that can be termed *adaptational responses* (Everly, 1989; Engler & Engler, 1995; Blonna, 1996; Hubbard & Workman, 1998; Shelby & McCance, 1998). These responses are characterized by central adaptation that leads to arousal, alertness, vigilance, enhanced cognition, focused attention, aggression, and inhibition pathways that subserve vegetative functions. Peripherally, stress adaptation is geared toward mobilizing energy to the CNS and muscles. Increased heart rate, blood pressure, respiratory rate, blood glucose, and protein and fat catabolism aid in delivery of substrates and oxygen to the tissues and vital organs and increase production of energy to fight the stressors. Stress response mechanisms must be effective and efficient at restraining their own activity through negative feedback via the cortisol and cognitive/perceptive feedback inhibition pathways.

For example, as Figure 44-1 depicts, once a stressor is psychophysiologically recognized as a threat to the system, the hypothalamus begins secreting corticotropin-releasing factor (CRF), and a whole cascade of neuroendocrine hypothalamic-pituitary-adrenal (HPA) axis events begin. The activation of the noradrenergic neurons in the locus ceruleus leads to a release of norepinephrine during activation of the sympathetic nervous system (SNS), which also directly stimulates the adrenal medulla to release epinephrine. These catecholamines (norepinephrine and epinephrine) work individually and synergistically directly and through the liver and pancreas to produce cardiovas-

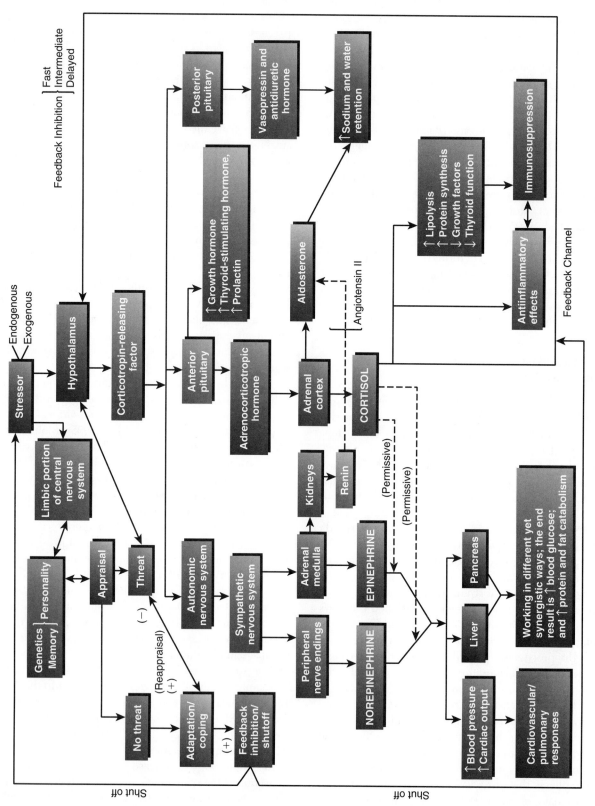

Figure 44-1 Cascade of psychoneuroimmunological events that are generated when the stress response is initiated.

cular, pulmonary, and primary metabolic effects. Stimulation of the renin-angiotensin II-aldosterone mechanism further increases blood pressure.

The posterior pituitary, stimulated by CRF, secretes vasopressin/antidiuretic hormone (ADH), which is responsible for water retention. Concomitantly, the adrenal cortex releases aldosterone, and the effects of sodium ion (NA^+)–withholding further enhance sodium and water retention. Cortisol is secreted secondary to the activation of the adrenal cortex by adrenocorticotropic hormone (ACTH) from the anterior pituitary. Cortisol mobilizes the substances (carbohydrates, fats, and proteins) needed for cellular metabolism through lipolysis; protein synthesis and catabolism; and gluconeogenesis (increasing blood glucose), while producing a direct effect in reducing the immune and inflammatory responses. In addition, cortisol enhances or potentiates the effects of other neuroendocrine and endocrine hormones. Whether cortisol-induced effects are adaptive or destructive depend on the intensity, type, and duration of the stress response and the ability of the feedback inhibition pathway to function properly.

Glucocorticoid feedback inhibition occurs at multiple locations in both the brain and the pituitary and is a direct response to the rate of rise and plasma levels of glucocorticoids, primarily cortisol. As chronic stress, inactivity, and deconditioning persist, the feedback loop that shuts off the stress response is blocked, thereby fostering continuation of the response and perpetuation of the physical decline. As the physical decline continues, waste products build and certain hormones, particularly cortisol and serotonin, circulate in excess. Secondary psychophysiological consequences result, including insomnia, depression, sadness, hyperglycemia, weight gain, and muscle wasting. Ultimately, this is a downward-spiraling phenomenon, and its repeated aggravation of existing physical and emotional instability will finally end in complete physical and mental decompensation and collapse.

Environmental events may either cause or set the stage for mobilization of the stress response. The cognitive-affective domain is the critical causal phase in most stress reactions. Since stress is a matter of perception, individuals' interpretations of events are what create most stressors and stress responses. For example, some people are bothered by driving in the city (with all of its traffic), while others do it on a daily basis and consider it normal. The nervous system serves as the foundation of the stress response. The perception of a threat from a noxious stimulus generates the initiation of a cascade of biochemical events by the CNS that is integrated through the hypothalamus activating the HPA axis and stimulating the manufacture and secretion of many neuroendocrine biochemical mediators. The hypothalamus attempts to regulate homeostasis and responds to the continuous feedback between the body and the mind as it modifies the integration of the response to the stressors. The limbic portion of the CNS, on the other hand, organizes and

responds to thoughts, feelings, and emotions and is guided by personality characteristics and ingrained behavior and memory. The adaptive, or coping, abilities of the individuals are superimposed upon and affect this process throughout, moderating the response or ameliorating the effect over time. Should stress arousal be excessive or prolonged, target organ dysfunction and/or pathology will result.

For example, a patient may present to the clinic with an exacerbation of a condition that had previously been under control for some time. Conditions such as irritable bowel, angina, headaches, hypertension, asthma, and diabetes may fall into this category. When a patient presents to the clinic with complaints of shortness of breath secondary to an "asthma attack," the APN should recognize that the stress response has been activated and that both emotional and physiological triggers were aggravated. A good history will reveal that the patient had some unexpected, overwhelming, surprising or taxing event occur in his or her life that preceded the "attack." The history may reveal that the patient just began graduate education, started a new job, is having relationship difficulties, has an upcoming competitive sports event, or has had a recent loss. Also, it may be that an acute physical illness such as the flu, pneumonia, trauma from a car accident, or a fall preceded the office visit. Any of these emotional or physical factors can trigger the stress response and exacerbate an existing condition. When an APN sees that a patient is stressed, a complete work-up should be accomplished, goals for stress management should be designed (with the patient's input), and a supervised plan of accomplishing the goals should be set, with appropriate follow-up visits to check progress.

APNs should be aware of the physiology behind the neuroendocrine responses during stress because they must know when and where to intervene and with what medication or other intervention. For instance, should the APN change asthma medication or increase the dosage to aid in a stressful time for a patient? Or should the APN increase a patient's blood pressure medication because of a persistent increase in secretion of epinephrine and norepinephrine during a stressful time? Or should that APN wait and see if other interventions will help stop the current increase in stress and let the patient's blood pressure return to its previous stable state without changing the regimen?

Stress and Disease

A strong relationship has been found between excess stress and an exacerbation of disease in patients with trauma-induced severe acute pancreatitis (Levy & DeMartinis, 1996), premenstrual symptoms (Woods, Lentz, Mitchell, & Kogan, 1994), essential hypertension (Engler & Engler, 1995), fibromyalgia and chronic fatigue syndrome (Crofford & Demitrack, 1996), back pain, headache, irritable bowel syndrome, reflux disorder, and many other conditions (Benson & McKee, 1993; Hubbard &

Workman, 1998; McCance & Huether, 1998). In fact, there have been so many accounts over the past 20 years that "stress-related disorders" has become its own category of diseases, catalogued by body system and with the names of stress-related conditions included for each system.

Becker, Pepine, Bonsall, Cohen, Goldberg, Coghlan, Stone, Forman, Knatterud, Sheps, and Kaufmann (1996) recently investigated stress and its effects on the mind and body. They documented the cardiovascular response of mental stress among 29 middle-aged healthy individuals who had no coronary risk factors or disease and a negative stress test. The authors found that a significant sympathetic response occurred, resulting in increases in plasma levels of norepinephrine and epinephrine, heart rate, blood pressure, and heart muscle work. Another important finding was that although left ventricular volume increased, the blood volume pumped (the ejection fraction) decreased secondary to the increased blood pressure (the afterload). Because the amount of blood that leaves the heart with each beat (carrying essential nutrients and oxygen to organs and tissues) is so important, the results of this study, showing a decrease in blood pumped when the body is under stress, is directly relative to patients with chronic stress and cardiovascular disease. Likewise, all individuals with prolonged psychophysiological problems will suffer from the effects of a decreased ejection fraction over time.

Researchers continue to find evidence that psychoneuroimmunological factors are associated with the development of chronic disease and that people influence their own health outcomes by their emotional and psychological responses to the disease, even though causality has been harder to prove. Although many potentially new psychoneuroimmunological response mechanisms have yet to be discovered, there is an increasing body of evidence showing that the healthy mind is capable of mobilizing the immune system, while the troubled mind can dampen the function of the immune system and contribute to disease.

Altered Consciousness and the Relaxation Response

Western medicine has typically concentrated on the more impersonal, objective scientific theoretical approach to practice, with exclusive emphasis on logic and analysis. Therefore it is often difficult for health care practitioners to understand and embrace practice grounded in critical study of a more intuitive, gestalt mode of thought (Benson, 1976; Everly, 1989; Wells-Federman et al, 1995; MacLean, Walton, Wenneberg, Levitsky, Mandarino, Wazial, Hillis, & Schneider, 1997; Roth & Creaser, 1997; Benson & Stark, 1998; Hubbard & Workman, 1998). However, for years health care practitioners have used operant conditioning, via B.F. Skinner, and biofeedback, via Neil Miller, to demonstrate behavioral control of involuntary bodily

responses through rewarding a desirable performance and conducting visceral learning, respectively. Also, for over 2500 years of recorded history, mind control of physiological function has been documented in the East. Some of the oldest and most well-known archetypes of mind control are seen by those trained in the ancient art of meditation, the Hindu and Buddhist traditions of ancient India, the Taoist practices in China, and the Zen forms in Japan. Transcendental meditation (TM) is the Westernized version of these ancient arts and was brought to this country by Maharisha Mahesh Yogi.

TM, which gained popularity in the 1960s, began the Western movement toward such practices, and numerous methods of meditation, practiced alone or in combination with other forms of mind-body work (e.g., yoga, hypnosis, biofeedback, autogenic training, progressive relaxation, mindfulness meditation, guided imagery, acupuncture, acupressure) have become popular since. The common link in all of these practices is the emergence of an altered state of consciousness effected through use of a focal device. Consciousness is a part of a continuum that ranges from coma through sleep, drowsy, awake, alert, and on to hyper-alert. There is a place, or "space," one can get to using TM that is between awake and asleep and is called "reverie"; it is where the conscious mind is quiescent and the subconscious mind is extensively open to suggestion. This altered state of consciousness induces a profound psychological and physiological relaxation that usually does not occur spontaneously, but rather must be consciously and purposely evoked. It is described subjectively as a feeling of peace of mind, a sense of well-being or restfulness, and total relaxation. This reaction is also called the *relaxation response*, an involuntary response of the SNS. While the "fight or flight" response is associated with an overactivation of the SNS, the relaxation response leads to a quieting of the same system. It is an innate protective mechanism against stressors and can lessen the harmful effects of stress through changes in the autonomic, endocrine, immune, and neuropeptide systems.

Like Selye, who is known for his work in physiological stress research, Benson is considered a leader in the field of mind-body medicine, and he has been investigating the relaxation response and the power of belief for over 30 years. Wallace, Benson, and Wilson (1971) first described the relaxation response from their investigation of recorded changes in the physiological responses of 36 participants who practiced TM for 20 to 30 minutes while being monitored. Specific physiological changes related to a hypometabolic state occurred that were consonant with a decrease in central and peripheral adrenergic excitation and hormonal feedback. Table 44-1 compares the objective, measurable physiological and psychological changes that occur during the stress response with those that are the result of the initiation of the relaxation response in relation to heart rate, blood pressure, blood lactate, rate of

Table 44-1

Objective Evidence Identifying the Differences in Psychophysiological Responses

VARIABLES	STRESS RESPONSE	RELAXATION RESPONSE
Heart rate	↑	↓
Blood pressure	↑	↓
Respiratory rate	↑	↓
Basal Metabolic rate	↑	↓
O_2 consumption	↑	↓
CO_2 production	↑	↓
Blood lactate levels	↑	↓
Muscle tension	↑	↓
Brain waves	↑ excitation ↓ alpha waves	↓ excitation ↑ alpha waves
Psychological factors	↑ anxiety, anger, hostility	↓ calmness, ↓ anxiety

The stress response increases hormonal release and the effects of adrenergic excitation, while the relaxation response moderates hormonal release and decreases adrenergic excitation.

breathing, oxygen consumption, carbon dioxide production, brain wave activity, muscle tone, metabolism, and level of arousal.

Recorded accounts of individuals who regularly benefited from relaxation resulting from achieving an altered state of consciousness have appeared in documents across Eastern and Western cultures for centuries. There appear to be certain common elements necessary to evoke the relaxation response. Benson (1976) described the components he had observed to be essential in eliciting this response, and these components are outlined in Box 44-1.

According to Benson, if these basic components come into being over time, science occurs in the form of measurable, predictable, and reproducible physiological change. Many avenues are possible to initiate the relaxation response, providing that the basic two steps are present (see Box 44-1).

Because the relaxation response can be objectified, physiological changes can be documented in clinical trials. The number of follow-up office or hospital visits, the number and strength of medications consumed, and the number of referrals to specialists can be documented as objective results and compared to a control group. Self-report data, although not a totally objective information base, is quite helpful in assessing persons' perceptions of the efficacy of treatment. For example, reports of decreased anxiety, depression, anger, hostility, irritability, and pain, as well as reports of an increased sense of well-being, calm, or hardiness, can be recorded. Data analysis of an individual's changes in perception over time or of perceptions within and among groups of individuals can provide meaningful results, even though this data is partially "soft science." Additionally, entirely qualitative analyses of in-depth patient interviews are productive,

Box 44-1

Elements to Set the Stage for Relaxation

General Elements
- Locate a quiet environment.
- Focus on a mental device or obtain an object to dwell on.
- Adopt a passive attitude.
- Assume a comfortable position.

Elements of Transcendental Meditation
- Repetition of a word, sound, phrase, or prayer
- Passive disregard for other thoughts and gradual return to the repetition

beneficial, and more widely accepted in the "new world view." Rich results can be obtained through understanding what patients think and feel about themselves, their lives, and their lifestyles. Mandle, Jacobs, Arcari, and Domar (1996) reviewed 37 investigations that used a combination of qualitative and quantitative methods to investigate the efficacy of relaxation response interventions and found that the relaxation response is effective in reducing hypertension, insomnia, anxiety, pain, and medication use across multiple populations, diagnostic-related groups (DRGs), and settings.

Using the suggestions just given, APNs are challenged to document patient progress during stress management interventions. Conducting practice-based research is feasible, easily done, and rewarding because outcome data to support APNs' work with patients is essential. In addition, APNs are challenged to conduct interviews of patients to find out what they really think and feel.

Stress, Relaxation, and Health

Optimal wellness is a correlate to a positive balance between stress and relaxation in individuals' physical, cognitive, emotional, spiritual, cultural, social, occupational, and environmental spheres. People experience health/illness in different ways. Each person brings to it a singular set of values, beliefs, expectations, and fears. The degree to which people function ideally in each sphere and across spheres, the amount of stress in their lives, their perception of the stressors as threats, and the magnitude of belief they have in their ability to adapt to or cope with the stressors, strongly influence this delicate balance. APNs must understand these concepts so that they can use this information to form trusting and effective therapeutic relationships. For example, Julie is an APN practicing in both a private office and an inner-city housing project. Most of her patients in the housing project are young, single mothers receiving welfare, and with many of the families, a woman's mother and grandmother all live in the same housing project. This culture of poverty has a major effect on the patients. Julie knows that the perspectives of these patients are different then the perspectives of the patients she sees in her private office.

Person-Environment Transaction

People—individuals, family, friends, and colleagues, groups, and communities—form social networks as they engage in communication and activities over time. This social sphere for each individual can either be a source of nurturing human interaction or a source of negativity and stress. A total absence of a social foundation in one's life produces isolation and despair. Series of investigations advocate that individuals with a supportive social network and successful social relationships are better able to adapt and cope with problems, manage stress, and prevent disease (Houston-Miller & Taylor, 1995; US DHHS, 1995). The opposite is also true; evidence suggests that a lack of social support is a contributing factor in the development of disease or lack of ease (Case, Most, Case, McDermott, & Eberly, 1992; King & Martin, 1993). Julie, the APN, finds that many of her patients in the housing project lack social support. Sometimes, mothers who are sick have no one to help watch their children. One of her patients, Tammie, had an asthma exacerbation and was admitted to the hospital. Less than 8 hours after her admission, Tammie left the hospital (against medical advice) because she had no one she could depend on to watch her daughter.

Personality and interaction

Inherited characteristics and life experiences form the foundation of peoples' personalities, which are a unique compilation of thoughts, attitudes, values, beliefs, perceptions, and behaviors that define who they are as individuals (Everly, 1989; US DHHS, 1995; Blonna, 1996). Although there is a genetic predisposition to a personality pattern, individuals' personalities are constantly evolving and redefining over time and make up the sum of everything they have experienced in life. There are five common theories of personality development:

- Behaviorists believe that personalities develop through interaction with the environment.
- Freud proposes that personality development is intricately enmeshed in a struggle between the conscious and unconscious mind.
- Erickson describes personality development as a cognitive progression, in stages, throughout life as a person ages.
- Kohlberg purports that personality evolves and refines itself as moral development, moral thinking, and moral reasoning are acquired.
- Maslow theorizes that personality development is hierarchical and eventually transcendent in response to basic human needs.

Presumably, personality develops in all of these ways simultaneously and within several spheres of a person's life. Take yourself, for example. You are a compilation of your life experiences, parents' genes, career choices, relationships, and other factors. Can you trace how you developed the personality you have today? Have you ever taken a personality inventory?

The growing body of theoretical and empirical evidence suggests that personality patterns may be uniquely important factors when considering diagnosis and treatment of many stress-related disorders (US DHHS, 1995). Patients who have a tendency to persistently interpret their transaction with the environment as stressful are more likely to exhibit a personality-based predisposition toward stress (Lazarus & Folkman, 1984). Researchers have proven that certain personality types and personality behavior patterns are associated with increased stress and illness levels. The type A behavior pattern has received more attention than any other behavioral or psychological variable as a risk factor for the development of disease because of the propensity of these individuals to be more aggressive, hostile, competitive, and urgent. Conversely, the type B behavior pattern has been documented as calm, more easily able to cope, and less urgent and overtly aggressive; such a person is therefore less likely to develop disease. However, recent research has produced inconsistent findings relative to type A versus type B behavior patterns and subsequent disease, particularly coronary heart disease and myocardial infarction. It appears that many type A individuals never develop problems, and many type B individuals do develop stress-related conditions. Currently, after distilling all of the factors inherent in the type A personality pattern, evidence suggests it is the higher levels of anger and hostility that are associated with adverse outcomes; type B individuals who "bottle-up" these emotions may suffer from adverse outcomes as well. The prognostic value of psychosocial characteristics (e.g., life stress, social isolation, type A and B behavior, depression) on adverse outcomes is highly correlational and must be considered when assessing levels of stress and designing any stress management protocol. In other words, APNs need to take time to talk with patients about their emotions and whether they have an avenue to vent these emotions.

Spirituality

Spirituality is a basic human phenomenon that helps individuals create meaning beyond the self and into a worldlier connectedness (Fuller, 1989; Kaye & Robinson, 1994; Sumner, 1998). Spirituality is a way of being that comes about through awareness of a transcendent dimension characterized by certain identifiable values in regard to self, nature, life, and whatever one considers to be "ultimate." Belief in a relationship with some higher power, creative force, divine being, or infinite source of energy is the transcendent dimension for many people. Others may find that spirituality includes some of the following behaviors: finding purpose and meaning in life; sharing the joys of living; talking to friends about spiritual matters; prayer; reading; being part of a community; working to save the environment; helping to feed the needy; or committing to the cause of world peace.

Religion is a part of spirituality, but spirituality is much broader and may not include belief in an organized religion at all. Spirituality is so much a part of persons' belief systems that it plays a major role in their everyday lives. This role becomes heightened when adversity, lack of ease, or disease strikes. To ignore spirituality's potential positive influence on healing is paramount to negligence in caregiving. Fostering patients' spiritual beliefs is what is important, not trying to force one's own beliefs onto the patient. Providers must, in many cases, set aside their diverse belief systems, particularly regarding spiritual matters, and encourage patients' spirituality if that is something important to them. For example, an APN may discuss this with his or her patient by saying, "There is some research that suggests evaluating your religion or faith is helpful to the healing process. Is your religion or faith helpful to you in handling problems in your life or with your health?" If the answer is yes, a further question is, "Is there anything that I can do to facilitate this?" An APN should let patients know that he or she cares about them and is there for them.

Patients' belief systems and the provider-patient relationship

Throughout Benson's work, opponents criticized that mind-body practices only elicited the placebo effect, so Benson and his colleagues began to study the placebo response (Wells-Federman et al, 1995; Benson &

Friedman, 1996). This is a powerful force, effective in about 50% to 90% of cases. Nearly 80% of symptoms reported during a primary care visit are self-limiting, will go away without any treatment, or will have a nonspecific response to treatment. It is a matter of belief—belief can kill you or keep you alive. This concept is important because it leads providers to the assumption that mind-body medicine practices or complementary or alternative medicine practices may be as or more effective in treatment regimens as traditional practices using drugs, procedures, and surgeries.

Benson and Friedman (1996) describe three components to the placebo effect: belief on the part of the individual, belief on the part of the healer, and shared beliefs that arise from the relationship between the individual and the healer. These factors are important toward understanding the role of the placebo effect in healing. Before the mid-1800s, the placebo effect *was* medicine. Providers had next to nothing else, so they utilized "faith." Then the work of Pasteur, Koch, and others, including Fleming, revolutionized medicine. Their new drugs and procedures worked in most cases, regardless of belief. The placebo effect, or having faith, paled in comparison to these awesome cures that modern medicine brought about. So, after the Flexner report in 1911, allopathic medicine was created, and it has molded the field of medicine toward the hard sciences and toward drugs, procedures, and surgeries ever since. Today, the problem with encouraging use of the placebo effect is the medical dogma that surrounds its use, which criticizes that it is not hard science.

However, APNs have seen the placebo effect work firsthand in watching people walk across hot coals and not burn their feet, watching someone lying on a bed of nails without a puncture wound, and taking care of a dying patient that has suffered from what he believes is the result of a spell. Also, numerous double-blind clinical trials have been documented that produced hard-science results, results scientists are confounded by and cannot refute, that show evidence of the power of belief. Studies of patient satisfaction with mind-body medicine treatment practices show that patients display increased satisfaction with care, increased senses of well-being, and greater compliance with treatment when they believe in their provider. There have been reports of decreased preoperative anxiety and better postoperative courses of recovery for patients when providers strongly support the surgery, are trusted, and have supportive relationships with patients.

The cases are too numerous to discuss separately, but the message is clear—if a patient's belief system is fostered, with unbiased support of that belief system by the provider and with a supportive provider-patient relationship, healing happens. APNs working closely with patients, building therapeutic relationships while subtly fostering self-efficacy, and teaching self-help relaxation techniques encourage patients to become active partners in their health care, improving their coping ability even when cure is unlikely (Moser & Dracup, 1995).

Stress Management

Choosing the most effective interventions

In addition to the general health promotion, personality development, adaptation and coping, and environmental transaction theories previously discussed, there a few noteworthy theories, discussed in this section, that are heavily grounded in persons' belief systems and behavioral change. Of the many models of behavioral change, social cognitive theory, developed by Bandura (1977), is one of the most influential exemplars of human behavior change. The model describes three factors that are associative and influence one another: behavior, cognition and other personal factors, and the environment. The relative influence of these three factors varies from one activity to another and from one person to another, but each factor must be considered in developing a behavior change program. The theory also focuses on how people learn and emphasizes the importance of self-efficacy as a mediator of behavioral change. Self-efficacy reflects an individual's self-confidence in judgment about how successful he or she will be in performing certain tasks or managing change. It is shaped by four principal sources of information: successful performances, vicarious experiences of others' performances, verbal persuasion and other types of social influences, and a person's perception of his or her own physiological state. Also, the perceived effects of a behavior change affect the likelihood that it will be maintained.

For a long time, Becker (1974), in his health belief model (HBM), has emphasized the importance of belief in behavioral change. Becker proposes that individuals are likely to change when they believe the recommended changes will improve their condition or reduce their risk of problems, and when they believe they have the ability and resources to accomplish the desired change. The HBM focuses on patient compliance and preventive health care practices.

More recently and more specifically, Prochaska and DiClemente (1983) expanded upon the work of Bandura (1977) and Becker (1974) among others and defined a model for change based on observations of smokers. Their original transtheoretical or stages of change model describes three stages that an individual progresses through on the way to successful behavioral change: precontemplation (considering change, but not strongly committed), contemplation (willing to change and can be influenced to do so), and action (highly committed to change, with change having begun). This model is dynamic and cyclical across and between stages and does not follow a set time plan. It may take an individual a long time to pass from precontemplation to contemplation and beyond, and there

may be many setbacks in the process because many individuals must make several attempts at behavioral change before goals are realized. Various extraneous factors can affect the progression toward change and set a person back one or more stages. Also, this process is begun anew with each new idea for or area needing change. This model has become a popular framework for assisting patients with behavioral change as researchers test its reliability and validity across populations.

Esther Hellman (1997) conducted one of the first studies in cardiac rehabilitation, testing the validity of the stages of change model as applied to exercise adherence. She used the most current form of the model, which now contains five stages: precontemplation, contemplation, preparation (starting to participate, but inconsistent), action, and maintenance (more than 6 months of continuing change). She tested the model with older patients following their discharge from a cardiac rehabilitation inpatient program and found that it is a valid measure as applied to assessing exercise adherence behavior.

Role of relaxation in stress management

When individuals do not feel "whole," they do not function efficiently and have fewer resources from which to draw emotional, physical, and spiritual strength. These stressful concerns lead them to believe that they can not cope effectively. However, through stress management, individuals can return to their maximum efficiency and will have more resources at their disposal to assist them to manage stress effectively (Blonna, 1996; Chiaramonte, 1997; Hubbard & Workman, 1998). When people are physically healthy, in touch with and in control of their emotions, socially active with a strong support network, and spiritually "full" with a strong faith or belief system, they perceive a sense of order that they subsequently display as a positive attitude toward the future.

Breath and relaxation. The goal of all relaxation interventions is to provide the means for individuals to consciously achieve psychophysiological adjustment of the autonomic nervous system by bringing involuntary responses under voluntary control. All relaxation methods begin with getting in touch with the pace and depth of the breath (Beary & Benson, 1974; Benson, 1976; Benson & Friedman, 1996; Benson & Stark, 1998). Breathing is rhythmic and cyclical and involves downward movement of the diaphragm with each breath. Benson teaches the concept of the "perfect breath," which includes four phases: (1) a refreshing, slow deep inhalation (4 to 6 seconds), (2) a pause (holding the breath for another 3 to 4 seconds), (3) a cleansing, slow exhalation (4 to 6 seconds), and (4) another short pause. The entire breath should take a minimum of 14 to 20 seconds and a maximum of 32 seconds (if 2 seconds are added to each pause) to complete. The perfect breath can be the center of concentration for extended periods.

The two most common types of regular breathing are thoracic and abdominal breaths. Thoracic breathing, or chest breathing, is autonomic and involves, primarily, the thoracic cage rising while the lungs force the diaphragm downward with each breath; it includes some movement of the abdomen outward. Abdominal breathing is also autonomic and involves, primarily, the abdomen expanding outward, drawing the diaphragm downward with less movement of the thoracic cage. Either breathing pattern can stimulate a satisfactory diaphragmatic breath. The secret to the perfect breath is the conscious slowing and deepening of the breath, with adequate pauses to ensure good oxygen transfer.

The tone of the SNS and parasympathetic nervous system (ParaNS) is greatly affected by the process of breathing. As the diaphragm becomes involved in breathing and its movement stimulates the solar plexus and the right vagus nerve, the ParaNS is stimulated. The major function of the ParaNS is one of inhibition; therefore, when stimulated, the antithesis of the SNS is actualized, and relaxation is facilitated. A diaphragmatic breath can be taught in which both types of breathing are consciously used simultaneously, with concentration on flattening the diaphragm as much as possible during the breath and including longer pauses. No more than 15 minutes of this type of deep breathing should be done during any kind of relaxation practice. Hyperventilation should be avoided and can cause palpitations, dizziness, shortness of breath, syncope, chest pain, tetany, weakness, tachycardia, and epigastric pain. Therefore, after beginning with deep diaphragmatic breathing, patients should be taught to simply concentrate on the perfect breath and the mantra—a word, phrase, prayer, object, or progression of body muscle relaxation.

Consciously concentrating on breathing slowly and deeply produces a calming effect on the body and mind that Benson has termed *conscious calming*. This sets the stage for the release of tension and unconsciously harbored psychophysiological stress. Conscious calming involves the belief that breathing is essential and nourishing and can be consciously stimulated, as with the perfect breath. After this, using Benson's (1976) essential components for and steps in evoking the relaxation response, total mental and physical relaxation can occur. The focal device of the perfect breath and the repetition of the mantra work synergistically to enhance relaxation and open the subconscious mind to suggestion. Together, they stimulate the intuitive mind (or subconscious) to dominate consciousness or stimulate the dominant, analytical ego-centered mode of thought-processing of the left hemisphere to shift and stimulate the right hemisphere to engage and become dominant, producing an extraordinary awareness potential of the mind (Everly, 1989). In other words, the altered state of consciousness that promotes the best restorative power for the body has been reached.

Relaxation techniques. Relaxation can be initiated in a passive manner as with concentration on the perfect breath, either alone or as it is involved with meditation, visualization, guided imagery, autogenic training, or hypnosis. Active relaxation is also accomplished with initial concentration on the perfect breath, but then some form of physical participation, including systematic muscle relaxation, yoga, and various forms of moving meditation, is added. Massage, therapeutic touch, and acupuncture and acupressure also fall into the category of active relaxation; even though the physical body is not moving, the spiritual body forces called chakras (Bruyere, 1987) are being stimulated into realignment. Combining these forms of relaxation may provide for the ultimate in psychophysiological relaxation. Getting the mind and body working together to reduce effects of a stress response is key. Biofeedback has long been considered effective in stress reduction and is a common, if costly, method for patients to get in touch with their stressors and learn to turn them off. Being cost prohibitive, it may not be many patients' first choice of relaxation method unless it is paid for by insurance.

Research has also shown that the use of various relaxation methods as a basis for stress management intervention is internationally accepted and successful in a wide range of populations: older African Americans with hypertension (Alexander, Schneider, Staggers, Sheppard, Clayborne, Rainforth, Salerno, Kondwani, Smith, Walton, & Egan, 1996; Barnes, Scheider, Alexander, & Staggers, 1997), men with human immunodeficiency virus (HIV) disease (McCain, Zeller, Cella, Urbanski, & Novak, 1996), patients with coronary heart disease from the United Kingdom (Trzcieniecka-Green & Steptoe, 1994), Dutch patients with coronary heart disease after angioplasty (Appels, Bar, Lasker, Flamm, & Kop, 1997), American patients with coronary artery disease (Ornish, Brown, Scherwitz, Billings, Armstrong, Ports, McLanahan, Kirkeide, Brand, & Gould, 1990; Rutledge, Hyson, Garduno, Cort, Paumer, & Kappagoda, 1999), patients after acute myocardial infarction (Nelson, Baer, Cleveland, Revel, & Montero, 1994), patients with headaches (Blanchard, Appelbaum, Nicholson, Radnitz, Morrill, Michultka, Kirsch, Hillhouse, & Dentinger, 1990), patients with chronic orofacial pain in the dentist's office (Logan, Risner, & Muller, 1996), patients with schizophrenia (Stein, 1989), children experiencing pain or distress (Kleiber, 1999), Latino women in an inner-city clinic (Roth & Creaser, 1997), and many more.

The research just given and many more documented studies have led us to understand that there is no single best relaxation technique, nor has any one technique been hallmarked as curative for any one stress-related disorder. The answer to this seeming paradox resides in the concept of individual differences. How does a provider know which stress management or relaxation technology to employ as the most effective intervention for a patient? If the relaxation response can be elicited in a variety of ways, with none showing generic superiority, then the provider should select the relaxation method or methods that best meet the interacting requirements of the patient, the provider, and the situation. Unfortunately, there are no established protocols to guide providers in this regard. Taking into consideration a patient's personality characteristics—beliefs, values, attitudes, and patterns of behavior—may be the singlemost important determinant to choosing the best treatment measure (Everly, 1989). For example, structured, somewhat compulsive, tightly wound individuals may benefit more from structured therapy and a set routine, with more directive step-by-step instructions. More laid back, flexible, less-structured individuals may benefit most from being given choices and general instructions, then being let go to modify and use the choices in any way they want, making up their own routine or purposeful lack of routine. Therefore it may be best to instruct patients regarding the variety of interventions to choose from, then make the decision a shared decision. However, APNs may want to teach patients the "fun and easy" self-help approaches discussed in this chapter, even if they eventually choose a supervised and/or more costly approach to stress management.

Crying and laughing

Laughter is important in taking oneself lightly while taking work seriously (Blonna, 1996). Laughter creates a physiological state that is incompatible with stress. It decreases muscle tension post-laugh, resulting in a sense of well-being similar to that of deep relaxation. Crying also has powerful stress-reducing powers. Crying, like laughing, involves several major muscle groups and is followed by a more relaxed state. This is admittedly hard to prove scientifically, except that tears have been shown to contain enkephalins, which are a form of natural opiate and have pain-relieving effects. The point is that one should not suppress a good cry; it is nature's way of managing the stress of sadness, grief, and disappointment. Both APNs and patients should support expressions of joy (through laughter) and sadness or grief (through tears).

Exercise

Becoming fit or using physical activity to relieve stress is an essential part of any stress management program. Exercise, in itself, causes an initiation of the stress response, but it is its short-term psychological benefit and long-term fitness benefit that support it as restorative, healing, and health promoting. Exercise for stress management should include aerobic activity contained in rhythmic movements of large muscle groups that do not overly stress the muscles or joints. The choice of exercise should conform to an individual's lifestyle and routine and be noncompetitive.

Physical fitness varies with each individual, and it is not necessary to become an athlete to benefit from the stress-reducing effects of exercise. Daily life satisfaction increases if people feel healthy and can be more active and involved. High levels of physical well-being are directly related to people's positive attitudes about themselves and the world around them; physical well-being means people have more energy stores to do more and enjoy the days. People have fewer aches and pains, sleep better, and become less fatigued; subsequently the stress response is shut off and people become less stressed, both physiologically and psychologically. Indirectly, exercise and postexercise benefits relax the body in the forms of active relaxation and effective breathing.

The central objective of an appropriate exercise prescription is for a patient to achieve a change in personal health behavior to include habitual physical activity (American College of Sports Medicine [ACSM], 1995). Exercise is intended to improve physical and cardiopulmonary fitness and promote health by reducing risk factors for chronic disease. The optimal exercise prescription is determined by a trained provider from an objective evaluation of a patient's response to exercise (Box 44-2).

The exercise regimen should be designed with careful consideration of an individual's heath status, risk factor profile, behavioral characteristics, personal goals, and exercise preferences. Another important consideration is the medications that a patient may be taking, either prescribed or over the counter and including herbal therapy, because medications can significantly alter the way the body responds to exercise. Medications can significantly affect heart rate and blood pressure during exercise, which affect exercise outcomes and can actually produce negative outcomes. Even using the American Heart Association guidelines for encouraging patient exercise without knowledgeably individualizing the prescription is inappropriate and can be dangerous. Referral to properly trained practitioners, physical therapists, or exercise physiologists for determination of the best prescription for a patient is essential.

Aerobic exercise may be performed at 55% to 90% of the maximal heart rate (maximal heart rate is often estimated as 220 minus a person's age) or 40% to 85% of the maximal oxygen uptake reserve (VO_2R) or heart rate maximal reserve (HRR). The threshold for most people is likely to lie between 55% and 65% of maximal heart rate

---

Box 44-2

Essential Components of an Individualized Exercise Prescription

- *Mode*—Choice of exercise method (e.g., jogging, walking, dance, swimming, biking, calisthenics, strength training)
- *Intensity*—Level of difficulty
- *Duration*—Length of time per exercise session
- *Frequency*—How often in a day or week, reflecting the progression of physical activity or advancement at an individual's own pace

or 40% and 50% of VO_2R or HRR. The lower intensity values apply primarily to patients who are physically unfit or not conditioned. Calculating aerobic exercise via VO_2R increases accuracy in the prescribed target heart rate and relative exercise intensity, as well as in the calculation of net caloric expenditure. Patients can measure the intensity of the exercise routine by performing the "talk test"—a person should be able to converse while engaged in moderate-intensity exercise. Patients should be advised to use large muscle groups during activity, and the activity should be rhythmical, continuous, and aerobic. Examples include jogging, rowing, stair climbing, swimming, skating, and cross-country skiing (Trotto, 1999).

Traditional approaches to developing the best exercise routine had previously been based on the premise that individuals should strive to increase exercise participation in order to improve physical fitness and muscle development (ACSM, 1995). Furthermore, augmenting physical fitness, whenever possible, is always a desirable goal of exercise prescription. However, the exact nature and level of the augmentation needs differ for each individual (US DHHS, 1995). For example, the quantity of exercise necessary to achieve positive results in the reduction of risk for disease has been shown to be considerably less than that needed to develop and maintain higher levels of physical and muscle fitness. This new knowledge bears important implications for health care providers when improvement in health status for a patient with chronic disease is the primary outcome goal. To illustrate this point, for the sedentary person compromised by or at risk for premature chronic disease, adoption of only a moderately active lifestyle may produce important health benefits and represent a realistic and attainable goal. APNs may find that even patients with chronic obstructive pulmonary disease or heart failure respond well to exercise producing 30% to 40% of HRR and exhibit enough physical gains to improve their activities of daily living and life satisfaction.

PRIORITIES FOR RESEARCH

Until the late 1980s, Benson (1984) primarily recommended the relaxation response to combat the harmful or uncomfortable effects of stress on the mind and body. However, his investigations began to reveal that the relaxation response could be used as a catalyst to assist individuals to change habits to improve their health. Evoking the relaxation response may be the most important first step in any self-help, personal-control program (Benson, 1984; Benson, 1987; Benson & Friedman, 1996). Over the years, people develop patterns or pathways of thought that control the way they think, act, and feel. These patterns can become so fixed that, according to Benson, they become almost impossible to transform. However, through multifactorial multidisciplinary approaches to eliciting the relaxation response while practicing meditation, prayer, and other stress management techniques, one can

coordinate electrical activity between the left and right sides of the brain, thus producing a level of combined arousal that stimulates the mind. This sets the stage for teaching habit-altering brain changes toward remembered wellness. Initially, this can be time consuming; time is needed to teach and work with patients until the chosen technique is learned, but once it is learned, follow-up takes much less time.

Results of recent multifactorial risk-reduction trials of patients with established coronary heart disease show significant positive effects on reducing the rate of progression of atherosclerosis; in many cases, the results show stabilization of the plaque and even lumen-blockage reversal (Ornish et al, 1990; Houston-Miller & Taylor, 1995). While the evidence clearly shows that lifestyle modification is often beneficial, most people find it difficult to discard lifelong habits and adopt and maintain unfamiliar practices. It is suggested by Houston-Miller and Taylor (1995) and Ornish et al (1990) that a multidisciplinary approach to this multifactorial intervention protocol be used. A combination of methods or the use of multiple methods is more powerful than exercise alone or exercise and health teaching regarding lifestyle change alone.

Houston-Miller and Taylor (1995) suggest that a provider trained specifically in how to manage multiple disciplines efforts, such as an APN case manger, can become a major player in the primary care arena where multifactorial cardiovascular disease preventive services are offered. A case manager can coordinate a team's efforts to ensure effective treatment, education, and counseling while fostering the support of family and friends. Continued feedback and reinforcement from the team and family and friends increases the likelihood of individuals successfully changing their lifestyles.

Insurance companies are beginning to understand the financial advantages in reimbursing many types of mind-body therapies previously denied. American Western Life Insurance and Kaiser Permanente both accept some mind-body choices, and Oxford Health Care is reimbursing a full range of services provided by qualified practitioners, including massage, acupuncture, and yoga (Benson & McKee, 1993). However, only a small percentage of alternative therapies are entirely reimbursed by third-party payers. Health insurance is most likely to cover herbal therapists, providers of biofeedback, physical therapists, occupational therapists, chiropractors, and providers of vitamin therapy regimens. Many health maintenance organizations (HMOs) cover at least chiropractic care and physical therapy, where a patient can receive massage, myofascial manipulation, and acupuncture or acupressure in addition to traditional skeletal and muscle manipulation with heat or cold therapy; most third-party payers are less inclined to pay for acupuncture and massage therapy not performed by a physical therapist or chiropractor. This is a start, however, and tangible possibilities are just over the horizon. The Health Care Financing Administration (HCFA) is currently exploring the prospect of reimbursement for Medicare patients who enter the Ornish Heart Disease Reversal Program. The HCFA is currently supporting research by Ornish programs across the country to investigate the reproducibility of the programs' investigational findings regarding the positive effects of multifaceted risk reduction and stress management on the reversal of heart disease.

Areas that warrant increased research include the mind-body interaction/transaction and its influence on health and illness. The National Center for Complementary and Alternative Medicine (NCCAM) (nccam.nih.gov/nccam/research/grants/rfb/grant-1.html) has recognized the importance of researching this connection, and they have awarded $350,000 to an investigator to research the effects of meditation on coronary heart disease. Other studies in process are evaluating areas such as acupuncture and hypertension, biofeedback for pain, and intercessory prayer. Once the results of current investigations indicate efficacy, studies related to how these interventions can be integrated into practice will become popular.

Research is ongoing to look at the ability of relaxation to affect diabetes and pain. The relationships among patients' inherent personalities; their thoughts, feelings and beliefs; and their subsequent psychophysiological responses are very closely tied to both wellness and the ability to invoke a relaxation response. The role, use, and fostering of personal spiritual beliefs in health promotion and healing needs further research; preliminary research is being conducted now on the effect of prayer on recovery, but much more research needs to be conducted to provide adequate data for skeptical providers.

One area that has seen quite a bit of research is the use of aerobic exercise, dietary control, relaxation, and cognitive-behavioral interventions to reduce and manage stress. The efficacy of a multifactorial approach to risk factor management through relaxation and stress management is currently under intense investigation through large, longitudinal, federally funded projects. However, much more needs to be done in this key area. Again, the ways in which APNs can incorporate the research findings into their practices need to be explored in further detail, particularly in light of the current limited reimbursement modalities.

IMPLICATIONS FOR MSN EDUCATION AND ADVANCED PRACTICE

APNs are prime targets for the negative effects of stress as they carve out their practice and incorporate it into people's daily lives (Wells-Federman, 1996; Kivisto & Couture, 1997). Stress, like the wind, cannot be seen directly, but its effects are often fully visible. Nurses are encouraged to practice relaxation response techniques and engage in other stress-reducing and health-promoting

behaviors to decrease physical tension and anxiety and increase effective adaptation and coping. Practicing conscious calming to experience a more focused mind and a relaxed body will help nurses to become centered. Also, many authorities believe that providers should practice various methods of relaxation before suggesting them to patients. If APNs expect patients to "buy into" teaching, it is helpful for them to believe it themselves. APNs are better role models and more knowledgeable teachers of those experiences they have lived.

There are implications therein for APNs in both independent and collaborative roles in acute and primary care positions for consulting with staff, accessing a personal caseload, designing the best therapeutic options, and conducting research. The American Nurses Association's *Code of Ethics* (Sumner, 1998) specifies that a nurse caring for individuals must promote an environment in which the individuals' values, customs, and beliefs are respected. APNs can provide enhanced psychological and spiritual support to patients by establishing trust and unconditional acceptance.

Once a therapeutic relationship is secure, an APN can be a patient's most informed advocate, responsive teacher, and guide. Patients want to know which methods or techniques can help them the most, what is reliable and safe, and how they can live well despite disease and work toward optimum wellness. APNs need to explore various ways to incorporate relaxation strategies into their practices, promoting the use of these techniques by patients. APNs also need to be advocates for their patients and lobby for alternative treatment methods (e.g., stress relaxation) to be covered by insurance. Patients who are medically underserved need additional support and information to be willing to pay out of pocket for such therapies. APNs should not pass up this golden opportunity to become leaders in the health care arena by becoming the best providers of assessment and management for patients' stress.

APNs combine theory, research, and practice to assist them in understanding patients holistically or in terms of wholeness of mind, body, and spirit within the context of the interrelationship of these spheres to the environment. Understanding how these theoretical constructs synergistically blend should form the foundation for advanced practice education curricula.

Medical curricula have undergone some changes over the past decade, and further improvements could equip physicians to address more fully the goals of *Healthy People 2000* and *Healthy People 2010* (US DHHS, 1999). However, although provider awareness of effective screening tests has increased over the past decade, attitudes and skills related to preventive services continue to vary based on specialty training and practice setting. According to *Healthy People 2010*, insufficient training continues to contribute to inadequate delivery of recommended services, particularly of lifestyle counseling by clinicians. Perceived efficacy of counseling is strongly correlated with the delivery of health promotion messages about stress, relaxation, diet, exercise, and smoking. For example, providers who do not regularly offer lifestyle counseling commonly cite their belief that they cannot effectively counsel patients to change behavior.

It is imperative that nurse educators take notice and seize the opportunity to respond quickly to the mandates set forth by *Healthy People 2010*, tailoring their curricula to emphasize the education and training of APNs in health promotion and disease prevention. By concentration of content on comprehensive strategies to effect stress reduction and risk management, graduates can emerge as leaders in delivering quality primary and secondary preventive services at the best cost.

Creighton University, School of Nursing in Omaha, Nebraska recently initiated an exemplary dual track Master's program specifically designed to address the education and training deficiencies just described. The school created an innovative dual-degree curriculum model by expanding their existing Cardiac Health and Rehabilitation/Clinical Nurse Specialist major to include a broader focus in health promotion, cardiac health, and wellness and adding this concentration to the Adult Nurse Practitioner (ANP) curriculum. They are educating APNs to have the appropriate comprehensive advanced education in assessing risk and counseling for stress management, risk factor management, and exercise to help fill a huge gap in primary care, where there is a real need for these services. It is suggested that more Master's programs consider a paradigm shift from a disease-based curriculum to a health promotion–based curriculum.

As APNs enter the new millennium, it is apparent that the health care environment in which APNs and other providers practice is more technologically advanced than ever before, complicated by mega-organizations who govern decision-making using the "quality at the best cost" principle. One of the most important challenges facing APNs today is to create a healing "space" for each patient within the context of this fast-paced, ever-changing health care environment. It has been proven that caregiving strategies geared toward potentiating the mind-body connection can produce significant positive lifestyle changes and other health outcomes for patients, despite the increased environmental stress in their lives. APNs have the responsibility to understand this interaction/transaction and to choose a cadre of interventions that best suit patients' belief systems, elicit relaxation, and ultimately foster self-managed stress reduction.

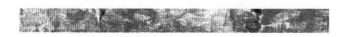

DISCUSSION QUESTIONS

These questions can be used to promote critical thinking and encourage discussion.

1. Discuss the effects of the stress response in short-term and long-term daily life situations. Imagine how you would react if you were almost in a car accident on your way to work, and describe the stress response you would experience. Describe the stress effects you might experience if you face a malpractice care in the future, perhaps 1 to 1½ years from now. Periodic meetings will have to be held with your lawyer and the claimant's lawyer. How would this experience differ from that of the car accident? Describe how the usual psychophysiological responses to stress can negatively affect the body over time. Identify common triggers of your stress response.

2. Discuss the components of the relaxation response and various ways to elicit the response. Using a variety of methods discussed in this chapter, demonstrate the induction and progression of the relaxation response in a laboratory setting, measuring temperature pulse rate and rhythm, blood pressure, and breathing rate and rhythm. Use electroencephalogram (EEG) and/or electromyogram (EMG) measurements if possible to illuminate this response further. Practice various methods of relaxation before suggesting any to patients. How would you incorporate relaxation exercises into your patients' regimens? What would be the best way to teach these exercises?

3. Explain how APNs could/would/should foster the power of belief in themselves and their patients to assist with stress management and illness prevention; this may include the following steps:

- Explore your own beliefs and values.
- Explore examples of various patients' beliefs and values, considering culture, religion, and enculturation.
- Prepare a list of questions that can be used when inquiring about patients' beliefs and whether spirituality is important to them.
- Discuss ways to foster a "shared" belief system, especially when divergent belief systems exist between an APN and patient.
- Discuss the potential positive health outcomes of this practice.
- Design a lifestyle change or stress reduction contract and work through it (with instructor guidance) over the course of a semester or two.
- Explore ways and means to realistically incorporate this stress-reducing behavior into daily practice in an efficient and cost-effective manner. Design potential care plans, treatment protocols, teaching tools, and follow-up plans.
- Discuss when, how, and to whom to refer patients for relaxation and stress management.
- Identify how or if your preceptor uses stress management strategies in his or her practice. If he or she does not, why is this not a part of the practice? How would you envision the practice if these components were included?

Suggestions for Further Learning

- Go to the National Center for Alternative Medicine at nccam.nih.gov. Look at the funded research. Which of the projects relate to stress and its effects?
- Get the article: Kelly, G. Nutritional and botanical interventions to assist with the adaptation to stress *Alternative Medical Review, 4(4):249-265.* What recommendations can you glean from this article, and how would you integrate these ideas into your practice?
- For more information on relaxation and stress management, check out the following resources. What information can you glean from these sources that would be helpful for your patients? Would you recommend these book to your patients?
  - Benson, H., Stewart, E., & Medical Institute Staff (1993). *The wellness book: the comprehensive guide to maintaining health and treating stress-related illness.* New York: Fireside
  - Brennan, B. (1987). *Hands of light: a guide to healing through the human energy field.* New York: Bantam
  - Caudill, M. (1995). *Managing pain before it manages you.* New York: Guilford
  - Chopra, D. (1999). *Ageless body, timeless mind.* New York: Three Rivers
  - Davis, M., Eshelman, E., & Mckay, M. (1988). *The relaxation & stress reduction workbook.* Oakland, CA: New Harbinger
  - Hanh, T.N. (1991). *The miracle of mindfulness: a manual of meditation.* Boston: Beacon
  - Kabat-Zinn, J. (1990). *Full catastrophe living: using the wisdom of your body and mind to face stress, pain, and illness.* New York: Delacorte
  - Kabat-Zinn, J. (1994). *Wherever you go, there you are: mindfulness meditation in everyday life.* New York: Hyperion
  - Stein, D. (1995). *Essential reiki: A complete guide to an ancient healing art.* Freedom, CA: The Crossing Press
  - Weil, A. (1997). *Eight weeks to optimum health.* New York: Alfred A. Knopf
- Check out the following Internet resources:
  - www.HealthGate.com
  - www.meditationcenter.com
  - www.AskDr.Weil.com
  - www.LifeMatters.com
  - www.MindBody&SoulNetwork.com
  - www.WellspringMedia.com
  - www.NIHOfficeofAlternativeMedicine.com
  - www.chopra.com
  - www.health.net/cmbm,aquariusproductions.com
- For additional information, contact the following organizations:
  - Biofeedback Society of America, 4301 Owens Street, Wheat Ridge, CO 80033
  - International Society for the Study of Subtle Energies & Energy Medicine, 356 Coldco Circle, Golden, CO 80403; phone (303) 278-2228
  - Mind/Body Medical Institute, 110 Francis Street, Suite 1A, Boston, MA 02215; phone (617) 632-9530 (stress reduction/relaxation tapes available)
  - Nurse Healers-Professional Associates, Inc., PO Box 444, Allison Park, PA 15101-0444; phone (412) 355-8476
  - National Resource Center, Center for Mindfulness in Medicine, Health Care, and Society, Stress Reduction Clinic, University of Massachusettes Medical Center, 55 Lake Avenue North, Worcester, MA 01655-0267; phone (508) 856-2656
  - The Barbara Brennan School of Healing, PO Box 2005, East Hampton, NY 11937; phone (516) 329-0951
- You many also want to examine the following journals:
  - *Advances: The Journal of Mind-Body Health,* John E. Fetzer Institute, Kalamazoo, MI; phone (616) 375-2000
  - *Brain, Behavior, and Immunity,* Academic Press Inc., San Diego, CA; phone (619) 230-1840
  - *Spirituality & Health,* Spirituality & Health Publishing, Inc., New York, NY
  - *Mind-Body Medicine,* Decker Periodicals, Hamilton, Ontario, Canada; phone (800) 568-7281
- Relaxation tapes are available through Emmett Miller, MD, and Steven Halpern, PhD, PO Box W, Stanford, CA 94309; phone (800) 52-TAPES. They provide excellent tapes and have many to choose from, including *Letting Go of Stress* (with four different techniques for deep relaxation)

REFERENCES/BIBLIOGRAPHY

Alexander, C., Schneider, R., Staggers, F., Sheppard, W., Clayborne, B., Rainforth, M., Salerno, J., Kondwani, K., Smith, S., Walton, K., & Egan, B. (1996). Trial of stress reduction for hypertension in older African Americans: part II. Sex and risk subgroup analysis. *Hypertension, 28*(2), 228-237.

American College of Sports Medicine (1995). *ACSM's guidelines for exercise testing and prescription* (5th ed.). Baltimore: Williams & Wilkins.

Appels, A., Bar, F., Lasker, J., Flamm, U., & Kop, W. (1997). The effect of a psychological intervention program on the risk of a new coronary event after angioplasty: a feasibility study. *Journal of Psychosomatic Research, 43*(2), 209-217.

Bandura, A. (1977). *Social learning theory.* Englewood Cliffs, NJ: Prentice Hall.

Barnes, V., Schneider, R., Alexander, C., & Staggers, F. (1997). Stress, stress reduction, and hypertension in African Americans: an updated review. *Journal of the National Medical Association, 89*(7), 464-476.

Beary, J., & Benson, H. (1974). A simple psychophysiologic technique which elicits the hypometabolic changes of the relaxation response. *Psychosomatic Medicine, 36,* 115-120.

Becker, L.C., Pepine, C.J., Bonsall, R., Cohen, J.D., Goldberg, A.D., Coghlan, C., Stone, P.H., Forman, S., Knatterud, G., Sheps, D.S., & Kaufmann, P.G. (1996). Left ventricular, peripheral vascular, and neurohumoral responses to mental stress in normal middle-aged men and women. *Circulation, 94*(11), 2768-2777.

Becker, M. (1974). *The health belief model and personal health behavior.* Thorofare, NJ: Charles B. Slack.

Benson, H. (1976). *The relaxation response.* New York: Avon.

Benson, H. (1979). *The mind/body effect: How behavioral medicine can show you the way to better health.* New York: Simon & Schuster.

Benson, H. (1984). *Beyond the relaxation response: How to harness the healing power of your personal beliefs.* New York: Times Books.

Benson, H. (1987). *Your maximum mind.* New York: Times Books.

Benson, H. (1997). *Spirituality and healing in medicine IV.* Boston: Harvard Medical School Department of Continuing Education.

Benson, H., & Friedman, R. (1996). Harnessing the power if the placebo effect and renaming it "remembered wellness." *Annual Review of Medicine, 47,* 193-199.

Benson, H., & McKee, M. (1993). Relaxation and other alternative therapies. *Patient Care, 27*(20), 75-86.

Benson, H., & Stark, M. (1998). *Timeless healing: the power and biology of belief.* London: Pocket Books.

Blanchard, E., Appelbaum, K., Nicholson, N., Radnitz, C., Morrill, B., Michultka, D., Kirsch, C., Hillhouse, J., & Dentinger, M. (1990, May). A controlled evaluation of the addition of cognitive therapy to a home-based biofeedback and relaxation treatment of vascular headache. *Headache,* 371-376.

Blonna, R. (1996). *Coping with stress in a changing world.* St. Louis: Mosby.

Bruyere, R. (1987). *Wheels of light.* Glendale, CA: Healing Light Center.

Case, R., Moss, A., Case, N., McDermott, M., & Eberly, S. (1992). Living alone after myocardial infarction: impact on prognosis. *Journal of the American Medical Association, 267,* 515-519.

Chiaramonte, D. (1997). Mind-body therapies for primary care physicians. *Primary Care, 24,* 787-808.

Collins, J., & Rice, V. (1997). Effects of relaxation intervention in phase II cardiac rehabilitation: replication and extension. *Heart & Lung, 26*(1), 31-44.

Crofford, L., & Demitrack, M. (1996). Evidence that abnormalities of central neurohormonal systems are key to understanding fibromyalgia and chronic fatigue syndrome. *Rheumatic Disease Clinics of North America, 22*(2), 267-284.

Engler, M.B., & Engler, M.M. (1995). Assessment of the cardiovascular effects of stress. *Journal of Cardiovascular Nursing, 10*(1), 51-63.

Epperly, B.G. (1997). *Spirituality and health, health and spirituality: a new journey of spirit, mind, and body.* Mystic, CT: Twenty-Third Publications.

Everly, G. (1989). *A clinical guide to the treatment of the human stress response.* New York: Plenum.

Fuller, R. (1989). *Alternative medicine and American religious life.* New York: Oxford University Press.

Hellman, E. (1997). Use of the stages of change in exercise adherence model among older adults with a cardiac diagnosis. *Journal of Cardiopulmonary Rehabilitation, 17,* 145-155.

Houston-Miller, N., & Taylor, C. (1995). *Lifestyle management for patients with coronary heart disease* (Monograph number 2). Champaign, IL: Human Kinetics.

Hubbard, J., & Workman, E. (Eds.). (1998). *Handbook of stress medicine: an organ system approach.* Boca Raton: CRC Press.

Kaye, J., & Robinson, K. (1994). Spirituality among caregivers. *IMAGE: Journal of Nursing Scholarship, 26*(3), 218-221.

King, A., & Martin, J. (1993). Exercise adherence and maintenance. In J.L. Durstine (Ed.), *Resource manual of guidelines for exercise testing and prescription* (pp. 443-454). Philadelphia: Lea & Febiger.

Kivisto, J., & Couture, R. (1997). Stress management for nurses: controlling the whirlwind. *Nursing Forum, 32*(1), 25-33.

Kleiber, C., & Harper, D. (1999). Effects of distraction on children's pain and distress during medical procedures: a meta-analysis. *Nursing Research, 48*(1), 44-49.

LaForge, R. (1997). Mind-body fitness: encouraging prospects for primary and secondary prevention. *Journal of Cardiovascular Nursing, 11*(3), 53-65.

Lazarus, R. (1966). *Psychological stress and the coping process.* New York: McGraw Hill.

Lazarus, R., & Folkman, S. (1984). *Stress, appraisal, and coping.* New York: Springer.

Levy, J., & DeMartinis, J. (1996). Trauma-induced severe acute pancreatitis: conceptual review of pathophysiological events. *Gastroenterology Nursing, 19*(1), 18-24.

Logan, H., Risner, A., & Muller, P. (1996). Anticipatory stress reduction among chronic pain patients. *SCD Special Care in Dentistry, 16*(1), 8-14.

MacLean, C., Walton, K., Wenneberg, S., Levitsky, D., Mandarino, J., Wazial, R., Hillis, S., & Schneider, R. (1997). Transcendental meditation program on adaptive mechanisms: changes in hormone levels and responses to stress after 4-months of practice. *Psychoneuroendocrinology, 22*(4), 277-295.

Mandle, C., Jacobs, S., Arcari, P., & Domar, A. (1996). The efficacy of relaxation response interventions with adult patients: a review of the literature. *Journal of Cardiovascular Nursing, 10*(3), 4-26.

McCain, N., Zeller, J., Cella, D., Urbanski, P., & Novak, R. (1996). The influence of stress management training in HIV disease. *Nursing Research, 45*(4), 246-253.

McCance, K., & Huether, S. (1998). *Pathophysiology: the biologic basis for disease in adults and children.* St. Louis: Mosby.

Moser, D., & Dracup, K. (1995). Psychosocial recovery from a cardiac event: the influence of perceived control. *Heart & Lung, 24*(4), 273-280.

Nelson, D., Baer, P., Cleveland, S., Revel, K., & Montero, A. (1994). Six-month follow-up stress management training versus cardiac education during hospitalization for acute myocardial infarction. *Journal of Cardiopulmonary Rehabilitation, 14,* 384-390.

Ornish, D., Brown, S., Scherwitz, T., Billings, J., Armstrong, W., Ports, T., McLanahan, S., Kirkeide, R., Brand, R., & Gould, K. (1990). Can lifestyle changes reverse coronary heart disease? *Lancet, 336,* 129-133.

Prochaska, J., & DiClemente, C. (1983). Stages and processes of self-change of smoking: toward an integrative model of change. *Journal of Consulting and Clinical Psychology, 51,* 390-395.

Roth, B., & Creaser, T. (1997). Mindfulness meditation-based stress reduction: experience with a bilingual inner-city program. *The Nurse Practitioner, 22*(3), 150-176.

Rutledge, J., Hyson, D., Garduno, D., Cort, D., Paumer, L., & Kappagoda, C.T. (1999). Lifestyle modification program in management of patients with coronary artery disease: the clinical experience in a tertiary care hospital. *Journal of Cardiopulmonary Rehabilitation, 19,* 226-234.

Schrader, K. (1996). Stress and immunity after traumatic injury: the mind-body link. *AACN Clinical Issues, 7*(3), 351-358.

Selye, H. (1956). *The stress of life.* New York:McGraw-Hill.

Shelby, J., & McCance, K. (1998). Stress and disease. In K. McCance & S. Huether (Eds.), *Pathophysiology: the biologic basis for disease in adults and children* (pp. 286-298). St. Louis: Mosby.

Stein, F. (1989). Teaching stress management techniques to a schizophrenic patient. *The American Journal of Occupational Therapy, 43*(3), 162-169.

Sumner, C. (1998). Recognizing and responding to spiritual distress. *American Journal of Nursing, 98*(1), 26-31.

Trotto, N. (1999). Exercise for optimum health. *Patient Care, 33*(18), 97-104.

Trzcieniecka-Green, A., & Steptoe, A. (1994). Stress management in cardiac patients: a preliminary study of the predictors of improvement in quality of life. *Journal of Psychosomatic Research, 38*(4), 267-280.

U.S. Department of Health and Human Services (1995). Cardiac rehabilitation (Clinical practice guideline number 17, AHCPR Publication No. 96-0672). Rockville: MD: US Department of Health and Human Services.

U.S. Department of Health and Human Services (1999). *Healthy People 2010: national health promotion and disease prevention objectives.* Washington, DC: US Public Health Services.

Wallace, R., Benson, H., & Wilson, A. (1971). A wakeful hypometabolic physiologic state. *American Journal of Physiology, 221,* 795-799.

Weil, A. (1995). *Spontaneous healing: how to discover your body's natural ability to maintain and heal itself.* New York: Ballintine Publishing Group.

Wells-Federman, C. (1996). Awakening the nurse healer within. *Holistic Nurse Practitioner, 10*(2), 13-29.

Wells-Federman, C., Stuart, E., Deckro, J., Mandle, C., Baim, M., & Medich, C. (1995). The mind-body connection: the psychophysiology of many traditional nursing interventions. *Clinical Nurse Specialist, 9*(1), 59-66.

Woods, N., Lentz, M., Mitchell, E., & Kogan, H. (1994). Arousal and stress response across the menstrual cycle in women with three perimenstrual symptom patterns. *Research in Nursing & Health, 17,* 99-110.

Zamarra, J., Schneider, R., Besseghini, I., Robinson, D., & Salerno, J. (1996). Usefulness of the transcendental meditation program in the treatment of patients with coronary artery disease. *The American Journal of Cardiology, 77,* 867-870.

Chapter 45

Risk Reduction: Preventive Services

Mollie R. Poynton & Denise Robinson

Health promotion has long been an objective of nursing care, encompassing prevention of disease and illness but also addressing a patient's health and wellness as a whole, considering mind, body, and spirit. Health promotion seeks to assist individuals, families, and communities in obtaining a general state of health, and it employs basic public health measures such as hygiene and sanitation. It also involves education of individuals, families, and communities on safety, healthy lifestyles and behaviors, and child rearing. These measures are intended to assist patients in achieving optimal health and wellness from a holistic viewpoint (Edelman & Milio, 1994).

Risk reduction differs from health promotion in its objective. Risk reduction is consistent with health promotion's process and goals, but its objective is significantly more narrow. The scope of risk reduction (also known as *health protection*) is limited to those interventions that may prevent *specific* disease or injury; limit or prevent illness or disability; and thus increase years of productive life (Pender, 1996). Risk reduction is based on current scientific knowledge of specific disease and injury and employs primary, secondary, and tertiary prevention, as it is believed to affect morbidity, mortality, and disability among populations. Interventions for risk reduction are based on an understanding of epidemiological knowledge. Although health care providers have yet to fully understand the relationship between certain diseases or injuries and demographic characteristics (e.g., age, race, occupation, lifestyle), the prevalence of or exposure to these diseases and injuries among different demographic groups is often clear. This knowledge allows for patient-specific intervention for risk reduction (U.S. Preventive Services Task Force [PSTF], 1996).

For example, intravenous drug users have been identified as a population with significant exposure to hepatitis B, and an important (and proven) risk reduction intervention for this group is vaccination against hepatitis B. Provision of the vaccine as a preventive measure to all intravenous drug users encountered by the health care delivery system reduces the likelihood of individual intravenous drug users contracting hepatitis B. This intervention may prevent persons from experiencing devastating illness, lost years of productive life, and even death. It may also prevent those exposed to the drug users' blood and body fluids in the future from exposure to hepatitis B and subsequent infection (US PSTF, 1996).

Theoretically, avoidance of unnecessary illness related to risk reduction decreases total health care costs. In other words, money directed at preventive services today may result in greater savings in the future through avoidance of expensive medication, therapies, and hospitalizations. Evidence of this potential benefit is demonstrated in several economic analyses (Wagner, 1997; People who quit smoking are much less likely to be hospitalized than those who don't, 1998). Risk reduction and preventive services may yield other economic benefits as well. Employees able to avoid illness or disability may fuel the economy with greater productivity, more years of productivity, and fewer sick days due to illness or injury. This benefit is, as of yet, unproven.

DEFINITIONS

Health promotion is "a process undertaken to increase the levels of wellness in individuals, families, and communities" (DeLaune & Ladner, 1998). *Illness* is considered "the inability of an individual's adaptive responses to maintain physical and emotional balance that subsequently results in an impairment in functional abilities" (DeLaune & Ladner, 1998). *Levels of prevention* refers to the ability to intervene at various stages of an illness. It is possible to interrupt illness processes so as to influence health in a positive direction. *Primary prevention* refers to interventions to prevent disease or injury. This may involve interventions such as increasing a patient's resistance or decreasing the resistance of the disease agent. These actions are done to prevent the onset of a targeted condition, and an example would be routine immunizations for children. *Secondary prevention* refers to interventions for early detection and treatment of illness states in order to optimize clinical outcomes. These are for patients who have already developed risk factors or preclinical disease but in whom the condition is not apparent. Examples of secondary prevention are Pap smears and screening activities. *Tertiary prevention* refers to interventions to prevent or limit illness and disability due to a disease or injury. These are preventive measures that are part of the treatment and management of a clinical illness that is already present. An example would be a person following a low-fat diet after having a myocardial infarction.

Healthy People 2010 is the report of the national health objectives published by the U.S. Public Health Service in 2000. *Healthy People 2010* addresses issues of primary, secondary, and tertiary prevention. It also addresses risk reduction. **Risk reduction** involves interventions to decrease an individual's risk of illness or death due to disease or injury. The objectives of *Healthy People 2010* and risk reduction are a major focus of primary care. **Primary care** is the provision of health care services including assessment, diagnosis, treatment, coordination of care, preventive services, and education at the point of entry into the health care system (DeLaune & Ladner, 1998). **Planned change** is change that is "intentional and thought out, occurs over time, and includes mutual goal setting, an equal power distribution, and deliberation" (Lancaster, 1999).

CRITICAL ISSUES: UNDERSTANDING THE NEED FOR RISK REDUCTION AND PREVENTIVE SERVICES

The American health care delivery systems of the early twentieth century clearly focused on the treatment of symptomatic illness and disease (DeLaune & Ladner, 1998). Risk reduction was limited and consisted mainly of periodic physical examinations with general laboratory testing, in addition to immunization for the prevention of communicable diseases (US PSTF, 1996; DeLaune & Ladner, 1998). Many early health promotion and disease prevention initiatives were led by nursing leaders such as Lillian Wald and Margaret Sanger.

The shift in America's health care focus to include health promotion and risk reduction is traced by many to the release of the initial *Healthy People* report in 1979—*Healthy People: The Surgeon General's Report on Health Promotion and Disease Prevention,* along with the accompanying *Health Promotion–Disease Prevention: Objectives for the Nation.* The intent was to create a "public health revolution" wherein disease prevention was emphasized (Office of Disease Prevention and Health Promotion, 1998). Health agencies began to adopt the reports' objectives, which targeted specific illnesses for improved prevention and control by the year 1990 (Edelman & Milio, 1994; Pender, 1996; Office of Disease Prevention and Health Promotion, 1998). Another document that helped point out the need for risk reduction and preventive services was the report of the U.S. PSTF, first published in 1989. The U.S. PSTF reviewed research for evidence of the effectiveness of various interventions that could help prevent over 60 illnesses and conditions. The *Guide to Preventive Services* (1996) offers the task force members' recommendations, based on a standardized review of current evidence, for the clinical preventive services a prudent clinician should provide. As the *Guide* points out, the benefits of incorporating prevention into medical care have become increasingly apparent over the past 30 years. Although screening and immunizations play an important part in prevention, it is becoming apparent (as reflected in the *Healthy People 2000* and *2010* goals) that the most promising role of prevention and risk reduction lies in changing personal health behaviors before clinical disease develops.

Progress reviews of the *Healthy People 2000* objectives shaped the *Healthy People 2010* objectives, which are widely used and included in the textbooks of many health care disciplines (Maiese & Fox, 1998). The 2000 objectives have also been incorporated into the Health Plan Employer Data and Information Set (HEDIS) measures of health care quality (Office of Disease Prevention and Health Promotion, 2000). Almost all states currently operate their own *Healthy People* plans, and the progress of some taxpayer-funded health programs (e.g., the Indian Health Service) is currently measured according to the *Healthy People 2000* objectives (Office of Disease Prevention and Health Promotion, 1998). The purpose of the 2000 objectives was to battle against premature death and disability. Abundant evidence is available that shows that the majority of deaths among Americans below the age of 65 are preventable. The 2000 and 2010 goals set benchmarks against which progress can be measured. The whole notion of having *Healthy People* goals makes a risk reduction focus much more important; it also makes it the goal of the nation, assisting in consistency from one part of the country to another and helping with education of both patients and primary care providers (PCPs).

Healthy People 2010 was released with two goals in mind. The first is to increase the quality of life and the years of healthy life. This goal aims to increase life expectancy for individuals of all ages; however, the goal is not only an increase in the number of years that one lives; it also expects those years to be of high quality, permitting a person to do the activities that he or she wants to do without limitations of illness or disability. An example of increasing the quality and length of healthy life would relate to a person who stops smoking after 25 years; making this lifestyle change would help prevent the development or worsening of chronic obstructive pulmonary disease (COPD), which would have a major effect on quality of life and length of life. The second goal is to eliminate health disparities. *Health disparities* refers to the poor health experienced by some segments of the population who are more at risk for various diseases. Examples would include the increased incidence of tuberculosis (TB) for low-income, underserved populations and the increased incidence of certain diseases for some ethnic groups (e.g., hypertension for African Americans).

Healthy People 2010 Focus Areas

Access to quality health services	Injury and violence prevention
Arthritis, osteoporosis, and chronic back conditions	Maternal, infant, and child health
Cancer	Mental health and mental disorders
Chronic kidney disease	Nutrition and overweight
Diabetes	Occupational safety and health
Disability and secondary conditions	Oral health
Educational and community-based programs	Physical activity and fitness
Environmental health	Public health infrastructure
Family planning	Respiratory diseases
Food safety	Sexually transmitted diseases
Health communication	Substance abuse
Heart disease and stroke	Tobacco use
HIV	Vision and hearing
Immunization and infectious diseases	

From Office of Disease Prevention and Health Promotion (2000). *Healthy people 2010: what is it?* Available online at web.health.gov/healthypeople/PrevAgenda/whatishp.htm.

The *Healthy People 2010* document will most likely shape preventive health services and measurement of preventive health services over the next 10 years. Its focus areas (identified in Box 45-1) target both primary and secondary prevention through attention to areas such as injury and violence prevention, tobacco use, and nutrition (Office of Disease Prevention and Health Promotion, 2000). If the goals set by *Healthy People 2010* are obtained, more people will have a longer, higher quality life, and the incidence of illness affecting certain segments of the population will be lessened. Probably the most important part of the *Healthy People* objectives is the lifestyle and behavior changes, which generally are the most difficult changes to make.

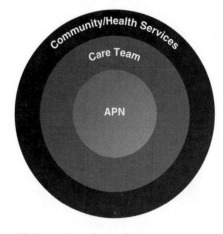

Figure 45-1 Interdependence of primary care team members.

Advanced Practice Nursing and Risk Reduction

Advanced practice has situated many advanced practice nurses (APNs) in primary health care settings. In these settings, APNs may independently initiate and deliver some preventive services (e.g., health behavior counseling). However, other services require collaboration with health care teams for delivery of services. For example, a mammogram is discussed with a patient and ordered by a nurse practitioner (NP). Another team member then assists the patient in making financial and operational arrangements for the mammogram. Still another team member provides education about mammography as well as preprocedure instructions. A radiology technician guides the patient through the actual mammogram, and a radiologist views and interprets the results. Finally, the NP counsels the patient regarding the results and implications of the mammogram.

An APN in a position of leadership and authority collaborates closely with other members of the health care team for effective delivery of preventive services but generally serves as the coordinator (Figure 45-1). APNs are particularly well suited to serve in this position; they have the skills, knowledge, and resources to prevent disease and promote health in addition to curing disease. This is important considering that the process by which a patient receives preventive care and addresses risk factors has never been more complex. Gone are the days of the routine annual physical examination, which was a simple process but relatively ineffectual. In its place is a stepped-care approach based entirely on the risk factors that a person has. Counseling now plays a large role in preventive care, based on the identification of those risk factors. APNs are good at emphasizing wellness, patient education, and counseling, making them logical choices to coordinate preventive services. Yano, Fink, Hirsch, Robbins, and Rubenstein (1995) found that nurse implementation of prevention protocols increased the performance of the protocols. Evidence from a five-site community health center revealed that at the site where NPs saw the majority of patients (physician provided care was available there only 4 out of 28 of the total clinic hours per week), the quality assurance (QA) data showed more preventive care, teaching, and counseling objectives being met than at the other offices. While this data is not an experimental intervention study, it does provide support for the notion of APNs as team leaders in providing preventive care.

Risk Reduction and Preventive Services Delivery in the Primary Care Setting

Sifri and Wender (1996) note that physicians routinely overestimate the amount of preventive care they provide to patients. A 1998 study showed primary care patients were current with only a mean 63% of recommended preventive services according to the U.S. PSTF's guidelines (Flocke, Stange, & Zyzanski, 1998). However, many third-party payers are now measuring the performance of PCPs on preventive care and risk reduction measures, sometimes as a basis for setting capitation. For example, HEDIS, a commonly used monitoring tool, evaluates provider networks' childhood immunization rates, cholesterol screenings, mammography screenings, and cervical cancer screenings (Sifri & Wender, 1996). According to Buppert (2000), health plan accreditation by the National Committee for Quality Assurance (NCQA) is now mandated by Medicare, some Medicaid programs, and some employers. NCQA accreditation considers performance on HEDIS measures, and Buppert anticipates performance on HEDIS measures will also soon determine inclusion on health plan provider panels, an important practice issue for many APNs. APNs must make sure to audit their own records to get objective data related to risk reduction and prevention; APNs can not rely on how they "think" they are doing. For example, Linda, an APN at Redbud Community Health Center, was putting a lot of emphasis on childhood immunizations. The registered nurse (RN) that worked with Linda reviewed all charts before seeing patients and sent out cards for those patients who needed immunizations. Linda felt they were doing all they could to get children under the age of 3 immunized. However, a NP student she was precepting was working on a research project and did a quick record review of 50 charts of kids between 20 and 36 months. Linda was very disappointed when she realized that this spot check showed an immunization rate of 79%. This really brought home the need for routine QA reviews and objective data. The team then began working on another strategy to get the rate up to at least 90%.

The health of primary care patients and third-party payer expectations of quality care both demand improvement in the delivery of risk reduction and preventive services. However, current research fails to clearly describe factors influencing delivery of these services. A 1998 study found that the quality of primary care delivery (characterized by good interpersonal communication with patients, patients' preferences for their usual providers, accumulated knowledge of patients, and coordination of care) is associated with the delivery of preventive services (Flocke, Stange, & Zyzanski, 1998). Good communication between PCPs and patients is strongly associated with the delivery of health habit counseling, an important component of preventive services. NPs, prepared through both basic and graduate nursing programs to communicate, educate, and establish therapeutic nurse-patient relationships, seemingly hold great potential for improving the delivery of preventive services via health habit counseling (DeLaune & Ladner, 1998).

Periodic health examinations have also been found to be strongly associated with the delivery of preventive services—a significant finding in light of the recent deemphasis of the periodic physical examination (Sox, Dietrich, Tosteson, Winchell, & Labaree, 1997). Indeed, the U.S. PSTF recommendations are intended for inclusion in a periodic health examination; however, a frequency for such visits is not recommended or discussed (US PSTF, 1996). Alternatively, the U.S. PSTF has created aids such as checklists, postcards, educational materials, and chart flow sheets to assist providers in incorporation of systematic preventive services delivery into both episodic and periodic health visits.

Limited research exploring factors associated with risk reduction in the primary care setting suggests the following factors may be important in the effective delivery of risk reduction and preventive services:

- Periodic health examination
- Established relationship between the provider and patient
- Efficient coordination of care
- Knowledge of the patient's health history

APNs should strive to establish strong relationships with their patients. A periodic health examination should be conducted based on thorough knowledge of a patient's health history. As various tests and other services are needed, an APN should coordinate the care so that the patient is seen efficiently and cost effectively. At Redbud Family Health Center, Linda works to establish a caring relationship with all her patients. One patient is Kim, a 38-year-old woman. She is fair haired and slight with freckles. Her mother has had several basal skin cancers removed from her face, so Linda conducts a thorough skin assessment on a yearly basis. Linda also knows that Kim's father died very suddenly of a myocardial infarction at the age of 51. Kim does not smoke, and she is diligent about exercising. Linda has checked Kim's cholesterol, which has a high-density lipoprotein (HDL) of 85, low-density lipoprotein (LDL) of 95, and total cholesterol of 156. Therefore both the cardiovascular risk factor and the skin cancer risk have been addressed. The only other risk factor Linda has identified for Kim is her diet. Kim does not like fruits or vegetables, and she also does not drink milk. Linda counseled Kim to take a multivitamin and calcium supplement. Kim's mother has osteoporosis, but that risk factor is addressed by Kim's weight-bearing exercises and the calcium supplement. Kim is married and in a monogamous relationship, so she is not considered at high risk for sexually transmitted diseases (STDs), but Linda does mail Kim a card every year to remind her about her yearly gynecological examination. Kim is a health care worker and has had the hepatitis B series and yearly TB tests. Her latest tetanus-diphtheria toxoid (Td) was given in 1997. This example of Linda and Kim shows how an APN tailors preventive care, based the risk factors identified. Such care is cost efficient because no extraneous tests (e.g., chest x-ray, Venereal Disease Research Laboratory [VDRL]) are ordered; in the example, Kim's health history and risk factors did not support such testing.

Implementation of a Preventive Services Program

Screening, health behavior counseling, and immunization are the three cornerstones of a focused preventive services program (US PSTF, 1996). Delivery of these services must be systematic and patient-specific to ensure effective delivery to all patients encountered by PCPs. This implies an approach that allows for individual variations such as age, culture, socioeconomic status, and environmental factors. Interventions are also based on the leading causes of morbidity and mortality for a given population. For example, when counseling a 56-year-old female patient during the last few minutes of an office visit, information related to cardiovascular disease would be more important to discuss than human immunodeficiency virus (HIV) or other STDs, because the woman is more likely to die from cardiovascular disease.

The addition of preventive services to periodic and episodic health care visits requires appropriate time and resources. Efficient and cost-effective delivery of preventive services also demands a redistribution of the time allotted for each patient-provider encounter. Time spent in conversation with patients and time spent performing physical assessment techniques may be reduced to allow for preventive service delivery, and research shows that this reduction may minimize the increased time allotted for a health care encounter due to delivery of preventive services (Flocke, Stange, & Goodwin, 1998). For example, when Sherry, a 48-year-old hypertensive patient of Linda's, comes in for a visit, the physical examination part of the visit is relatively short. The visit is primarily spent on discussing ways that Sherry can reduce her blood pressure via diet and exercise. She has lost 5 pounds in the last 3 months but has hit a plateau recently. Linda emphasizes the need for exercise and talks about various exercise options. She gives Sherry an exercise diary, and they then discuss specific ways that Sherry can start exercising.

Cost-effectiveness must be considered in implementation of a risk reduction program. With the growth of capitation and other cost pressures (driven by third-party payers), PCPs are challenged to deliver comprehensive risk reduction services to all patients with little or no additional reimbursement. To minimize the cost of additional preventive service delivery while ensuring delivery to all patients, a formal organizational approach may be utilized within individual practice settings. Organized delivery increases the efficiency and quality of the preventive services delivered and ensures that services are routinely delivered to all patients (Leininger, Finn, Dickey, Dietrich, Foxhall, Garr, Stewart, & Wender, 1996). Many risk reduction strategies focus on lifestyle changes; lifestyle changes are the least expensive areas to address but also the most difficult because of the necessary long-term behavioral changes. It makes sense to emphasize services that have been proven to be effective and tailor the content of the periodic health examination to the individual needs of a patient. This is even more important when time constraints limit how much can be done in one visit. Therefore the two most important factors to consider when deciding on clinical interventions are the potential effectiveness of the interventions and the leading causes of morbidity and mortality. For example, Linda from Redbud uses information related to morbidity and mortality when she counsels John. He is 44 years old and smokes 1½ packs of cigarettes a day; he has not been in the office for about 10 years. The most significant risk factor for John is that of coronary artery disease (CAD). His father had his first heart attack at age 42 and died at age 51. Since CAD risk can be reduced, it is critical for John to stop smoking as soon as possible. John is a bodybuilder and very active, so exercise does not appear to be a risk factor. He has not had his cholesterol checked in over 20 years, so that must be checked during the visit today. Linda also finds that when she assesses for alcohol intake, John may have a drinking problem. He drinks at least six cans of beer (12 ounces each) a day. He usually wears his seat belt when driving, and has smoke detectors in his home. He is married with two children. Given his past medical and family history, Linda concentrates on the two biggest risk factors for John: beer drinking and smoking. She conducts a quick screening physical and spends the majority of the time discussing John's health goals and what he is willing to do to reduce his risk for heart disease. John has tried to quit smoking before, cold turkey and with the nicotine patch; he would like to try Zyban. Linda describes to John how the product works and writes him a prescription. John sets a quit date of 2 weeks, and he will return to the office in about 3 to 4 weeks to reassess how the smoking cessation is going.

Implementation of a Risk Reduction and Clinical Preventive Services Program

A clinical preventive services program is a program practiced in the clinical setting that is concerned with the maintenance and promotion of health and the reduction of risk factors that result in injury and disease (Matzen, 1993). Murphy (1995) notes that most health promotion and disease prevention strategies are aimed at encouraging the reduction of risk factors for adverse health outcomes. To identify risk factors, APNs utilize a variety of health risk assessment methods. Risk factors are considered those characteristics or exposures that have been associated with a higher risk of a given disease. It is important to remember that risk factors are not the cause of a disease. Even for risk factors that are presumed to be negative, such as smoking, the presence of a risk factor does not guarantee a poor outcome. A single risk factor rarely is sufficient to cause disease; in most cases, it is the complex interaction between multiple risk factors, genetics, and immunological susceptibility that contributes to a "web of causation." How do health care providers prevent disease? They identify those risk factors that can be changed on an individual level, which are generally risky choices made in daily life. Health-promoting activities are aimed at curtailing risky choices. Strategies then usually address these choices by presenting healthier choices, such as healthy eating, smoking cessation, stress reduction, and avoidance of drug abuse. Risk reduction is an integral component of the preventive services program because it is the assessment of risk factors for disease and injury that determines what preventive interventions are applied. One way to look at the relationship of risk reduction and clinical preventive services is to consider risk reduction as the cornerstone or framework for the preventive services. (Figure 45-2 shows the relationship of the two.) Two terms are important to know describing risk. One is *relative risk*. This is the ratio of the frequencies of exposed and unexposed individuals who develop the disease and who do not develop the disease. If the risk is the same in the exposed and unexposed group, the relative risk is 1. If the risk of disease is greater in the exposed than in the unexposed group, the relative risk is greater than 1 and this exposure may be considered a risk factor. If the relative risk is less than 1, exposure reduces the risk of the disease (a protective function). Attributable risk is the difference between the incidence in the exposed and unexposed groups. This identifies the absolute percentage of individuals who develop the disease following exposure, after subtracting out the disease in those not exposed.

Beck (1993) uses the hypothetical example of cigarette smoking and facial wrinkles. Data are given where smokers and nonsmokers are followed in a prospective study to determine whether facial wrinkling appears. Wrinkling appears in 80% of smokers and 20% of nonsmokers.

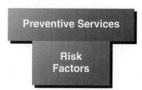

Figure 45-2 Relationship of preventive services program and risk reduction factors.

Therefore the relative risk is 80% divided by 20%, or 4. Thus smokers have four times the risk of developing facial wrinkles that nonsmokers do. The attributable risk is 80% minus 20%, which equals 60%. The attributable risk percentage is 60% of 80%, or 75%. Thus if all smoking ceased, the percentage of persons with facial wrinkling would be reduced 75%. These measures of risk apply to the population as a whole and not to the individual. Individuals are not the same, so even if they have the same level of exposure to a risk factor, they may not develop the problem. This means an individual's risk and a population's risk are not the same. When an APN finds an association between a risk factor and disease, he or she needs to decide what this association means for patients. The patients also need to decide what it means for them. Their decisions will influence what preventive services will be used in their plans of care.

Implementation of a risk reduction program within health care organizations requires planned organizational change. Change is a demanding process that requires thoughtful planning and execution. (This was discussed in detail in Chapter 8.) APNs educated in leading and managing change may play an important role in successful implementation of a risk reduction program. Table 45-1

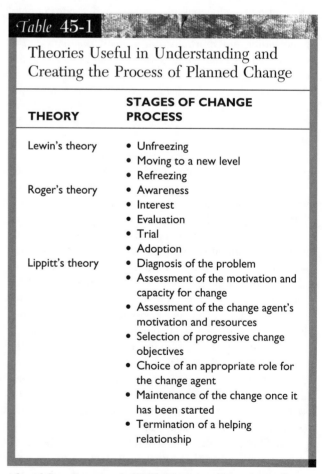

Table 45-1

Theories Useful in Understanding and Creating the Process of Planned Change

THEORY	STAGES OF CHANGE PROCESS
Lewin's theory	• Unfreezing • Moving to a new level • Refreezing
Roger's theory	• Awareness • Interest • Evaluation • Trial • Adoption
Lippitt's theory	• Diagnosis of the problem • Assessment of the motivation and capacity for change • Assessment of the change agent's motivation and resources • Selection of progressive change objectives • Choice of an appropriate role for the change agent • Maintenance of the change once it has been started • Termination of a helping relationship

Adapted from Lancaster, J. (1999). Managing change. In J. Lancaster (Ed.), *Nursing issues in leading and managing change.* St. Louis: Mosby.

outlines several theories useful in understanding the process of planned change.

Leininger et al (1996) also outline eight steps towards the organization of preventive services within individual primary care settings that are useful for APNs (Table 45-2).

Guidelines for Risk Reduction and Preventive Services

In 1984, 5 years after the initial *Healthy People* report, the U.S. PSTF was commissioned to reevaluate health protection and promotion practices according to current scientific

---

Table 45-2

Organization of Preventive Services in Primary Care

STEPS TO ORGANIZE SERVICES	EXAMPLE
Development of a written practice policy for preventive services and establishment of outcome criteria for successful delivery of preventive services	Metropolis Family Practice formed a committee composed of one NP, one physician, one RN, and one office manager to develop a preventive service delivery system for its patients. They reviewed HEDIS measures and the recommendations of the U.S. PSTF and chose to deliver preventive services according to the U.S. PSTF recommendations. They chose NCQA/HEDIS benchmark data as their comparison criteria for successful delivery of services. Satisfactory delivery of services was characterized as services meeting or exceeding the 75th percentile according to last year's NCQA/HEDIS measures. Goal delivery of services was characterized as services meeting or exceeding the 90th percentile according to last year's NCQA/HEDIS measures. They formalized a written policy prioritizing preventive services and adopting the U.S. PSTF's recommendations as their practice guidelines.
Baseline data collection and utilization of chart review to assess baseline provision of preventive services	QA audits were conducted for three selected areas: influenza vaccinations in older patients, counseling for smoking cessation, and Pap smears for women ages 21 to 64.
Development of a written plan for all steps of preventive services delivery (to be developed by both clinicians and information managers)	The committee reviewed U.S. PSTF, PPIP, and NCQA materials, then planned implementation of a preventive service delivery system. The plan included implementation of a flow sheet for all preventive services, chart flags for smoking, and review of preventive services at each visit. (Reminder postcards for Pap smears and well-child examinations were already in place.) The plan then identified the team member responsible for developing each component of the system.
Identification of an individual as coordinator of the system for preventive services delivery	The office manager was identified as the system coordinator and given release time for that purpose. The NP was designated as the system coordinator's primary resource for clinical issues.
Development or adaptation of tools necessary for implementation of the delivery system (e.g., flow sheets, chart flags, educational materials)	The committee developed a flow sheet addressing preventive issues for adults, based on the U.S. PSTF recommendations. Additionally, a chart flag system was selected for smoking, alerting providers to their patients' smoking status. (A bright green sticker was selected for this purpose.) Educational materials were currently in use, and these were judged appropriate by the committee. The system coordinator made arrangements for printing and purchase of materials.
Setting of a date for initial implementation	The committee chose October 1 as their implementation date. One week before implementation, all clinic staff and providers were oriented to their role in the new delivery system. Upon implementation, the office staff asked each patient about their smoking status and flagged charts accordingly. They also clipped a blank preventive services flow sheet to each chart. The RN documented immunizations and screening tests for each patient during triage. The PCPs (NP and physician) reviewed and updated the flow sheets upon each patient's visit and planned for any needed services.

Continued

Table 45-2	

Organization of Preventive Services in Primary Care—cont'd

STEPS TO ORGANIZE SERVICES	EXAMPLE
Performance of periodic evaluation of the delivery system and modification as necessary	The committee met 3 weeks after implementation to review their progress. While documentation of immunizations had been relatively smooth, the RN expressed concern that documentation of screening tests was slowing triage. Since the results of screening tests must be reviewed by a PCP, the committee decided to delegate documentation of screening tests on the flow sheet to the NP and physician. The NP and physician had found that limited visit time made provision of adequate health habit counseling difficult. To limit the amount of time necessary to discuss recommended counseling topics, the committee decided to prepackage educational materials according to age group and provide them to patients as they waited for appointments. The NP or physician could then reinforce the material and answer questions or make recommendations as necessary. The flow sheet was adapted to allow for documentation of each patient's receipt of a packet. The NP was assigned the task of securing and adapting appropriate materials for the packets, and the educational packets were implemented 2 weeks later.
Performance of periodic outcome measurement as an evaluation tool and modification of the plan as necessary	At 6 months, a chart audit was conducted, examining the three previously selected target measures: immunization of older adults for influenza, counseling for smoking cessation, and Pap smears for women ages 21 to 65. The audit revealed significant improvement in Pap smears and influenza vaccination, slightly exceeding the NCQA's 75th percentile. There was also a small improvement in smoking cessation, which had initially exceeded the NCQA's 75th percentile.

evidence (US PSTF, 1996). Its subsequent recommendations initiated a transition from generic risk reduction measures to targeted intervention according to evidence-based guidelines. In developing a program for primary care risk reduction and preventive services, one of the most important steps is deciding which services will be provided, to whom, and how often. Fortunately, several well-respected guidelines are available for adaptation to clinical settings (Box 45-2). APNs should use these resources to help direct the preventive care given to patients. These resources should be readily available in the clinical area, either in written format or via the Internet.

The recommendations outlined in the *Guide to Clinical Preventive Services* (US PSTF, 1996) and *Put Prevention into Practice: Clinician's Handbook of Preventive Services* (U.S. Department of Health and Human Services [DHHS], Public Health Service, Office of Public Health and Science, & Office of Disease Prevention and Health Promotion, 1998) are perhaps the most widely referenced guidelines in publication today. Based on a comprehensive review and analysis of current scientific knowledge, the guides offer evidence-based guidelines for screening tests, immunizations, and counseling throughout the lifespan. The guides emphasize "tailored" provision of preventive health care services to individual patients based on age,

Box 45-2	

Currently Available Preventive Service Guidelines

- U.S. PSTF's *Guide to Clinical Preventive Services* (1996)
- U.S. Public Health Service's *Put Prevention into Practice: Clinician's Handbook of Preventive Services* (US DHHS et al, 1998)
- The American Medical Association's *AMA Guidelines for Adolescent Preventive Services: Recommendations and Rationale* (1994). Available at www.ama-assn.org
- National Center for Education in Maternal and Child Health's *Bright Futures: Guidelines for Health Supervision of Infants, Children, and Adolescents* (Green & Palfrey, 2000)

Data from Pender, N.J. (1996). *Health promotion in nursing practice* (3rd ed.). Stamford, CT: Appleton & Lange.

sex, lifestyle, and other risk factors demanding appropriate intervention (US PSTF, 1996).

Age-specific charts (also including pregnant women) for recommended primary and secondary preventive interventions from the *Guide to Clinical Preventive Services*

(US PSTF, 1996) are provided in Tables 45-3 to 45-7. (Definitions of the high-risk codes used in these tables are provided in Box 45-3.) Using the chart for ages 65 and older (see Table 45-8), Linda (from Redbud) sees Dorothy, a 67 year-old woman, for a follow-up visit. Dorothy is in good health, though her past medical history reveals hypertension, hypothyroidism, and osteoporosis. Dorothy used to smoke four packs of cigarettes a day but stopped 12 years ago when her husband was diagnosed with lung cancer. Specific interventions recommended that apply to Dorothy based on her age include screening for skin cancer due to her fair skin and hair. Dorothy has had several basal cell cancers removed from her face, so whole body screening for cancer is also a priority. Dorothy has had a dual-energy x-ray absorptiometry (DEXA) scan, which revealed osteoporosis (her mother also had it), and she takes Fosamax and daily calcium for it. Dorothy is not sexually active. There do not appear to be any risk factors for problem drinking. Dorothy walks 2 to 3 miles 5 days a week. She has also done some weight training recently. She takes hormone replacement therapy because she had a hysterectomy about 20 years ago. She gets yearly mammograms and pelvic examinations. Most of the visit with Linda is spent talking about preventive testing that she needs. Dorothy has never had a sigmoidoscopy or colonoscopy, so Linda discusses what the tests are for and makes a referral for Dorothy to get the tests. Linda also reviews safety issues with Dorothy, such as seat belts, smoke detectors, and fall prevention. The emphasis is placed on counseling rather than physical examination and testing because there is good evidence that clinicians can change behavior through simple counseling interventions in the primary care setting for important areas such as smoking and problem drinking (Kottke, Battista, & DeFriese, 1988; Lichtenstein & Glasgolo, 1992; Bien, Miller, & Tonigan, 1993). (Suggestions to improve the efficacy of patient counseling are included in Table 45-8.)

The program titled *Put Prevention into Practice* (PPIP) (US DHHS et al, 1998) to implement the guidelines developed by the U.S. PSTF in primary care settings has been published by the U.S. Public Health Service. PPIP contains suggested tools and materials to implement simple tracking and documentation systems. An example of one such tool is given in Figure 45-3, and this may be easily adapted to suit individual practices. Figure 45-4 shows an adaptation of the PPIP flow sheet currently used by one primary care organization. Addition of simple office tools such as those offered by the PPIP program may significantly improve preventive service delivery.

Bright Futures, a program of the National Council for Maternal and Child Health Education, provides guides to preventive service delivery and health supervision for children. Bright Futures includes sample provider forms that incorporate important preventive services—tailored to the child's age and development—into each periodic well examination. All the Bright Futures materials have been developed with the goal "to respond to the current and emerging preventive and health promotion needs of infants, children, and adolescents" (Green & Palfrey, 2000). The materials were developed by a multidisciplinary panel of experts and are based on a combination of scientific evidence and expert opinion. Box 45-4 provides an example of Bright Futures health supervision guidelines for a 4-month well-child visit with "Bobby." Figure 45-5 provides a sample provider form. Box 45-5 identifies developmental assessment questions to use during a well-child examination (with "Jerome" as an example), and Box 45-6 provides a guide for APNs concerning parent-child interactions and identifies the physical examination components that should be included in the well-child examination for a 4-month old. Available as a free download from the Bright Futures website, the provider forms are easily adapted to different periodicity schedules. Guidelines and corresponding provider forms are available for all periodic well examinations, from infancy through adolescence (0 to 21 years). Linda from Redbud uses the Bright Futures forms to help make her well-child visits more efficient. She has found the forms stimulate questions on the part of parents and help her ask important questions and screen for such things as child abuse and discuss anticipatory guidance issues. In addition, because the physical examination form is a flow sheet, she can rapidly document her findings. Each form is individualized, based on the age of the child, and the receptionist at Redbud prints these forms before each child's scheduled appointment.

Issues for the Future of Risk Reduction and Preventive Services

The role of the periodic health examination in risk reduction needs to be clearly determined. Evidence exists that the complete physical examination (CPE) is not money well spent for APNs or patients. Frame (1995) discusses how the annual physical examination refuses to die despite data that shows the CPE is not the best way to deliver preventive care. These ideas were broached by Frame and Carlson in 1975, when they said that longitudinal health maintenance for adults is appropriate. This health maintenance should include only those interventions for which a patient was determined to be at risk for, the idea being that many of the health maintenance objectives could be accomplished during acute visits. A thorough update of the history (or new history if needed) and a review of systems (ROS) would be included, with the history and ROS dictating what parts of the physical examination or testing were necessary. In addition, the health maintenance visit should concentrate mainly on counseling interventions. Given these 1975 recommendations, it is surprising to find that in the 1995 study done by Luckmann and Melville, most family physicians (80%) felt that the CPE was their primary mechanism for delivering preventive services. Reasons for why physicians

Text continued on p. 652

Table 45-3

Interventions Considered and Recommended for the Periodic Health Examination: Birth to 10 Years

Leading Causes of Death

Conditions originating in perinatal period
Congenital anomalies
Sudden infant death syndrome (SIDS)
Unintentional injuries (non–motor vehicle)
Motor vehicle injuries

Interventions for the General Population

SCREENING

Height and weight
Blood pressure
Vision screen (age 3-4 yr)
Hemoglobinopathy screen (birth)[1]
Phenylalanine level (birth)[2]
Thyroxine (T_4) and/or thyroid-stimulating hormone (TSH) levels (birth)[3]

COUNSELING

Injury Prevention

Child safety car seats (age <5 yr)
Lap-shoulder belts (age ≥5 yr)
Bicycle helmet; avoid bicycling near traffic
Smoke detector, flame retardant sleepwear
Hot water heater temperature <120-130° F
Window/stair guards, pool fence
Safe storage of drugs, toxic substances, firearms & matches
Syrup of ipecac, poison control phone number
CPR training for parents/caretakers

Diet and Exercise

Breastfeeding, iron-enriched formula and foods (infants & toddlers)
Limit fat & cholesterol; maintain caloric balance; emphasize grains, fruits, vegetables (age ≥2 yr)
Regular physical activity

Substance Use

Effects of passive smoking*
Anti-tobacco message*

Dental Health

Regular visits to dental care provider*
Floss; brush with fluoride toothpaste daily*
Advise about baby bottle tooth decay*

IMMUNIZATIONS

Diphtheria-tetanus-pertussis (DTP)[4]
Oral poliovirus (OPV)[5]
Measles-mumps-rubella (MMR)[6]
H. influenzae type B (Hib) conjugate[7]
Hepatitis B[8]
Varicella[9]

CHEMOPROPHYLAXIS

Ocular prophylaxis (birth)

Interventions for High-Risk Populations

POPULATION	POTENTIAL INTERVENTIONS
Preterm or low birth weight	Hemoglobin/hematocrit (HR1)
Infants of mothers at risk for HIV	HIV testing (HR2)
Low income; immigrants	Hemoglobin/hematocrit (HR1); purified protein derivative (PPD) (HR3)
TB contacts	PPD (HR3)
Native American/Alaska Native	Hemoglobin/hematocrit (HR1); PPD (HR3); hepatits A vaccine (HR4); pneumococcal vaccine (HR5)
Travelers to developing countries	Hepatitis A vaccine (HR4)
Residents of long-term care (LTC) facilities	PPD (HR3); hepatitis A vaccine (HR4); influenza vaccine (HR6)
Certain chronic medical conditions	PPD (HR3); pneumococcal vaccine (HR5); influenza vaccine (HR6)
Increased individual or community lead exposure	Blood lead level (HR7)
Inadequate water fluoridation	Daily fluoride supplement (HR8)
Family history of skin cancer; nevi; fair skin, eyes, hair	Avoid excess/midday sun, use protective clothing* (HR9)

For a description of the high risk (HR) codes used in this table, see Box 45-3.
From U.S. Preventive Services Task Force (1996). *Guide to clinical preventive services* (2nd ed.). Baltimore: William & Wilkins.
[1]Whether screening should be universal or targeted to high-risk groups will depend on the proportion of high-risk individuals in the screening area, and other considerations. [2]If done during first 24 hr of life, repeat by age 2 wk. [3]Optimally between day 2 and 6, but in all cases before newborn nursery discharge. [4]2, 4, 6, and 12-18 mo; once between ages 4-6 yr (DTaP may be used at 15 mo and older). [5]2, 4, 6-18 mo; once between ages 4-6 yr. [6]12-15 mo and 4-6 yr. [7]2, 4, 6 and 12-15 mo; no dose needed at 6 mo if PRP-OMP vaccine is used for first 2 doses. [8]Birth, 1 mo; or, 0-2 mo, 1-2 mo later, and 6-18 mo. If not done in infancy: current visit, and 1 and 6 mo later. [9]12-18 mo; or any child without history of chickenpox or previous immunization. Include information on risk in adulthood, duration of immunity, and potential need for booster doses.
*The ability of clinician counseling to influence this behavior is unproven.

Table 45-4

Interventions Considered and Recommended for the Periodic Health Examination: 11-24 Years

Leading Causes of Death	
Motor vehicle and other unintentional injuries	Suicide
Homicide	Malignant neoplasms
	Heart diseases

Interventions for the General Population

SCREENING

Height and weight
Blood pressure[1]
Papanicolaou (Pap) test[2] (females)
Chlamydia screen[3] (females <20 yr)
Rubella serology or vaccination history[4] (females >12 yr)
Assess for problem drinking

COUNSELING

Injury Prevention

Lap/shoulder belts
Bicycle/motorcycle/ATV helmets*
Smoke detector*
Safe storage/removal of firearms*

Substance Use

Avoid tobacco use
Avoid underage drinking and illicit drug use*
Avoid alcohol/drug use while driving, swimming, and boating*

Sexual Behavior

STD prevention; abstinence; avoid high-risk behavior*;
    condoms/female barrier with spermicide*
Unintended pregnancy; contraception

Diet and Exercise

Limit fat & cholesterol; maintain caloric balance; emphasize
    grains, fruits, and vegetables
Adequate calcium intake (females)
Regular physical activity*

Dental Health

Regular visits to dental care provider*
Floss; brush with fluoride toothpaste daily*

IMMUNIZATIONS

Tetanus-diphtheria (Td) boosters (11-16 yr)
Hepatitis B[5]
MMR (11-12 yr)[6]
Varicella (11-12 yr)[7]
Rubella[4] (females >12 yr)

CHEMOPROPHYLAXIS

Multivitamin with folic acid (females planning or capable
    of pregnancy)

Interventions for High-Risk Populations

POPULATION	POTENTIAL INTERVENTIONS
High-risk sexual behavior	Rapid plasma reagin (RPR)/venereal disease research laboratory (VDRL) (HR1); screen for gonorrhea (female) (HR2), HIV (HR3), chlamydia [female] (HR4); hepatitis A vaccine (HR5)
Injection or street drug use	RPR/VDRL (HR1); HIV screen (HR3); hepatitis A vaccine (HR5); PPD (HR6); advice to reduce infection risk (HR7)
TB contacts; immigrants; low income	PPD (HR6)
Native American/Alaska Native	Hepatitis A vaccine (HR5); PPD (HR6); pneumococcal vaccine (HR8)
Travelers in developing countries	Hepatitis A vaccine (HR5)
Certain chronic medical conditions	PPD (HR6); pneumococcal vaccine (HR8); influenza vaccine (HR9)
Settings where adolescents and young adults congregate	Second MMR (HR10)
Susceptible to varicella, measles, and mumps	Varicella vaccine (HR11); MMR (HR12)
Blood transfusion between 1975-1985	HIV screen (HR3)
Institutionalized persons; health care/lab workers	Hepatitis A vaccine (HR5); PPD (HR6); influenza vaccine (HR9)
Family history of skin cancer; nevi; fair skin, eyes, hair	Avoid excess/midday sun, use protective clothing* (HR13)
Prior pregnancy with neural tube defect	Folic acid 4.0 mg (HR14)
Inadequate water fluoridation	Daily fluoride supplement (HR15)

For a description of the high risk (HR) codes used in this table, see Box 45-3.
From U.S. Preventive Services Task Force (1996). *Guide to clinical preventive services* (2nd ed.). Baltimore: William & Wilkins.
[1]Periodic BP for persons aged ≥21 yr. [2]If sexually active at present or in the past; q≤3 yr. If sexual history is unreliable, begin Pap tests at age 18 yr. [3]If sexually active. [4]Serologic testing, documented vaccination history, and routine vaccination against rubella (preferably with MMR) are equally acceptable alternatives. [5]If not previously immunized: current visit, 1 and 6 mo later. [6]If no previous second dose of MMR. [7]If susceptible to chickenpox.
*The ability of clinician counseling to influence this behavior is unproven.

Table 45-5

Interventions Considered and Recommended for the Periodic Health Examination: 25-64 Years

Leading Causes of Death
Malignant neoplasms
Heart diseases

Motor vehicle and other unintentional injuries
HIV infection
Suicide and homicide

Interventions for the General Population

SCREENING
Blood pressure
Height and weight
Total blood cholesterol (men age 35-64, women age 45-64)
Pap test (women)[1]
Fecal occult blood test[2] and/or sigmoidoscopy (≥50 yr)
Mammogram ± clinical breast exam[3] (women 50-69 yr)
Assess for problem drinking
Rubella serology or vaccination history[4] (women of child-bearing age)

COUNSELING

Substance Use
Tobacco cessation
Avoid alcohol/drug use while driving, swimming, and boating*

Diet and Exercise
Limit fat & cholesterol; maintain caloric balance; emphasize grains, fruits, and vegetables
Adequate calcium intake (women)
Regular physical activity*

Injury Prevention
Lap/shoulder belts
Motorcycle/bicycle/ATV helmets*
Smoke detector*
Safe storage/removal of firearms*

Sexual Behavior
STD prevention; abstinence; avoid high-risk behavior*; condoms/female barrier with spermicide
Unintended pregnancy; contraception

Dental Health
Regular visits to dental care provider*
Floss; brush with fluoride toothpaste daily*

IMMUNIZATIONS
Td boosters
Rubella[4] (women of childbearing age)

CHEMOPROPHYLAXIS
Multivitamin with folic acid (females planning or capable of pregnancy)
Discuss hormone prophylaxis (peri- and postmenopausal women)

Interventions for High-Risk Populations

POPULATION	POTENTIAL INTERVENTIONS
High-risk sexual behavior	RPR/VDRL (HR1); screen for gonorrhea (female) (HR2), HIV (HR3), chlamydia [female] (HR4); hepatitis A vaccine (HR6)
Injection or street drug use	RPR/VDRL (HR1); HIV screen (HR3); hepatitis B vaccine (HR5); hepatitis A vaccine (HR6); PPD (HR7); advice to reduce infection risk (HR8)
Low income; TB contacts; immigrants; alcoholics	PPD (HR7)
Native American/Alaska Native	Hepatitis A vaccine (HR6); PPD (HR7); pneumococcal vaccine (HR9)
Travelers in developing countries	Hepatitis B vaccine (HR5); hepatitis A vaccine (HR6)
Certain chronic medical conditions	PPD (HR7); pneumococcal vaccine (HR9); influenza vaccine (HR10)
Blood product recipients	HIV screen (HR3); hepatitis B vaccine (HR5)
Susceptible to measles, mumps, or varicella	MMR (HR11); varicella vaccine (HR12)
Institutionalized persons	Hepatitis A vaccine (HR6); PPD (HR7); pneumococcal vaccine (HR9); influenza vaccine (HR10)
Health care/lab workers	Hepatitis B vaccine (HR5); hepatitis A vaccine (HR6); PPD (HR7); influenza vaccine (HR10)
Family history of skin cancer; fair skin, eyes, hair	Avoid excess/midday sun, use protective clothing* (HR13)
Previous pregnancy with neural tube defect	Folic acid 4.0 mg (HR14)

For a description of the high risk (HR) codes used in this table, see Box 45-3.
From U.S. Preventive Services Task Force (1996). *Guide to clinical preventive services* (2nd ed.). Baltimore: William & Wilkins.
[1]Women who are or have been sexually active and who have a cervix; q≤3 yr. [2]Annually. [3]Mammogram q1-2 yr, or mammogram q1-2 yr with annual clinical breast examination. [4]Serologic testing, documented vaccination history, and routine vaccination (preferably with MMR) are equally acceptable.
*The ability of clinician counseling to influence this behavior is unproven.

Table 45-6

Interventions Considered and Recommended for the Periodic Health Examination: 65 and Older

Leading Causes of Death
Heart diseases
Malignant neoplasms (lung, colorectal, breast)

Cerebrovascular disease
Chronic obstructive pulmonary disease
Pneumonia and influenza

Interventions for the General Population

SCREENING
Blood pressure
Height and weight
Fecal occult blood test[1] and/or sigmoidoscopy
Mammogram ± clinical breast exam[2] (women ≤69 yr)
Pap test (women)[3]
Vision screening
Assess for hearing impairment
Assess for problem drinking

COUNSELING

Substance Use
Tobacco cessation
Avoid alcohol/drug use while driving, swimming, and
    boating*

Diet and Exercise
Limit fat & cholesterol; maintain caloric balance; emphasize
    grains, fruits, vegetables
Adequate calcium intake (women)
Regular physical activity*

Injury Prevention
Lap/shoulder belts
Motorcycle and bicycle helmets*

Fall prevention*
Safe storage/removal of firearms*
Smoke detector*
Set hot water heater to <120-130° F*
CPR training for household members

Dental Health
Regular visits to dental care provider*
Floss; brush with fluoride toothpaste daily*

Sexual Behavior
STD prevention; avoid high-risk sexual behavior*; use
    condoms*

IMMUNIZATIONS
Pneumonococcal vaccine
Influenza[1]
Td boosters

CHEMOPROPHYLAXIS
Discuss hormone prophylaxis (peri- & postmenopausal
    women)

Interventions for High-Risk Populations

POPULATION	POTENTIAL INTERVENTIONS
Institutionalized persons	PPD (HR1); hepatitis A vaccine (HR2); amantadine/ rimantadine (HR4)
Chronic medical conditions; TB contacts; low income; immigrants; alcoholics	PPD (HR1)
Persons ≥75 yr; or ≥70 yr with risk factors for falls	Fall prevention intervention (HR5)
Cardiovascular disease risk factors	Consider cholesterol screening (HR6)
Family history of skin cancer; nevi; fair skin, eyes, hair	Avoid excess/midday sun, use protective clothing* (HR7)
Native American/Alaska Native	PPD (HR1); hepatitis A vaccine (HR2)
Travelers in developing countries	Hepatitis A vaccine (HR2); hepatitis B vaccine (HR8)
Blood product recipients	HIV screen (HR3); hepatitis B vaccine (HR8)
High-risk sexual behavior	Hepatitis A vaccine (HR2); HIV screen (HR3); hepatitis B vaccine (HR8); RPR/VDRL (HR9)
Injection or street drug use	PPD (HR1); hepatitis A vaccine (HR2); HIV screen (HR3); hepatitis B vaccine (HR8); RPR/VDRL (HR9); advice to reduce infection risk (HR10)
Health care/lab workers	PPD (HR1); hepatitis A vaccine (HR2); amantadine/ rimantadine (HR4); hepatitis B vaccine (HR8)
Persons susceptible to varicella	Varicella vaccine (HR11)

For a description of the high risk (HR) codes used in this table, see Box 45-3.
From U.S. Preventive Services Task Force (1996). *Guide to clinical preventive services* (2nd ed.). Baltimore: William & Wilkins.
[1]Annually. [2]Mammogram q1-2 yr, or mammogram q1-2 yr with annual clinical breast exam. [3]All women who are or have been sexually active and who have a cervix. Consider discontinuation of testing after age 65 yr if previous regular screening with consistently normal results.
*The ability of clinician counseling to influence this behavior is unproven.

Table 45-7

Interventions Considered and Recommended for the Periodic Health Examination: Pregnant Women†

Interventions for the General Population

SCREENING

First Visit
Blood pressure
Hemoglobin/hematocrit
Hepatitis B surface antigen (HBsAg)
RPR/VDRL
Chlamydia screen (<25 yr)
Rubella serology or vaccination history
Rh typing, antibody screen
Offer chorionic villi sampling (CVS) (<13 wk)[1] or
    amniocentesis (15-18 wk)[1] (age ≥35 yr)
Offer hemoglobinopathy screening
Assess for problem or risk drinking
Offer HIV screening[2]

Follow-Up Visits
Blood pressure
Urine culture (12-16 wk)

Offer amniocentesis (15-18 wk)[1] (age ≥35 yr)
Offer multiple marker testing[1] (15-18 wk)
Offer serum α-fetoprotein[1] (16-18 wk)

COUNSELING
Tobacco cessation; effects of passive smoking
Alcohol/other drug use
Nutrition, including adequate calcium intake
Encourage breastfeeding
Lap/shoulder belts
Infant safety car seats
STD prevention: avoid high-risk sexual behavior*; use
    condoms*

CHEMOPROPHYLAXIS
Multivitamin with folic acid[3]

Interventions for High-Risk Populations

POPULATION	POTENTIAL INTERVENTIONS
High-risk sexual behavior	Screen for chlamydia (1st visit) (HR1), gonorrhea (1st visit) (HR2), HIV (1st visit) (HR3); HBsAg (3rd trimester) (HR4); RPR/VDRL (3rd trimester) (HR5)
Blood transfusion 1978-1985	HIV screen (1st visit) (HR3)
Injection drug use	HIV screen (HR3); HBsAg (3rd trimester) (HR4); advice to reduce infection risk (HR6)
Unsensitized Rh-negative women	Rh antibody testing (24-28 wk) (HR7)
Risk factors for Down syndrome	Offer CVS[1] (1st trimester), amniocentesis[1] (15-18 wk) (HR8)
Prior pregnancy with neural tube defect	Offer amniocentesis[1] (15-18 wk), folic acid 4.0 mg[3] (HR9)

For a description of the high risk (HR) codes used in this table, see Box 45-3.
From U.S. Preventive Services Task Force (1996). *Guide to clinical preventive services* (2nd ed.). Baltimore: William & Wilkins.
[1]Women with access to counseling and follow-up services, reliable standardized laboratories, skilled high-resolution ultrasound, and, for those receiving serum marker testing, amniocentesis capabilities. [2]Universal screening is recommended for areas (states, counties, or cities) with an increased prevalence of HIV infection among pregnant women. In low-prevalence areas, the choice between universal and targeted screening may depend on other considerations. [3]Beginning at least 1 mo before conception and continuing through the first trimester.
*The ability of clinician counseling to influence this behavior is unproven.
†See Tables 45-4 and 45-5 for other preventive services recommended for women of this age group.

are reluctant to stop doing the CPE include inadequate knowledge of the benefits and risks of screening tests; patients' expectations for receiving CPEs; feelings that the CPEs help physician-patient relationships; old habits being hard to change; fear of malpractice suits if CPEs are not done; and the ability to code a preventive visit higher so that more income is generated. Since

Luckmann and Melville's study (1995) was completed before the second edition of the *Guide to Clinical Preventive Services* (US PSTF, 1996) was published, one hopes that the number of PCPs who believe a CPE is the only way to deliver preventive care has decreased. No data is currently available on how APNs approach the issue of CPEs.

Box 45-3

High Risk Code Definitions

HR1—HIV positive, close contacts of persons with known or suspected TB, health care workers, persons with medical risk factors associated with TB, immigrants from countries with high TB prevalence, medically underserved low-income populations (including homeless), alcoholics, injection drug users, and residents of long-term care facilities

HR2—Persons living in, traveling to, or working in areas where the disease is endemic and where periodic outbreaks occur (e.g., countries with high or intermediate endemicity; certain Alaska Native, Pacific Islander, Native American, and religious communities); men who have sex with men; injection or street drug users. Consider for institutionalized persons and workers in these institutions, and day-care, hospital, and laboratory workers. Clinicians should also consider local epidemiology.

HR3—Men who had sex with men after 1975; past or present injection drug use; persons who exchange sex for money or drugs, and their sex partners; injection drug-using, bisexual, or HIV-positive sex partner currently or in the past; blood transfusion during 1978-1985; persons seeking treatment for STDs. Clinicians should also consider local epidemiology.

HR4—Consider for persons who have not received influenza vaccine or are vaccinated late; when the vaccine may be ineffective due to major antigenic changes in the virus; for unvaccinated persons who provide home care for high-risk persons; to supplement protection provided by vaccine in persons who are expected to have a poor antibody response; and for high-risk persons in whom the vaccine is contraindicated.

HR5—Persons ages 75 years and older; or ages 70-74 with one or more additional risk factors including: use of certain psychoactive and cardiac medications (e.g., benzodiazepines, antihypertensives); use of four or more prescription medications; impaired cognition, strength, balance, or gait. Intensive individualized home-based multifactorial fall prevention intervention is recommended in settings where adequate resources are available to deliver such services.

HR6—Although evidence is insufficient to recommend routine screening in elderly persons, clinicians should consider cholesterol screening on a case-by-case basis for persons ages 65-75 with additional risk factors (e.g., smoking, diabetes, or hypertension).

HR7—Persons with a family or personal history of skin cancer, a large number of moles, atypical moles, poor tanning ability, or light skin, hair, and eye color.

HR8—Blood product recipients (including hemodialysis patients), persons with frequent occupational exposure to blood or blood products, men who have sex with men, injection drug users and their sex partners, persons with multiple recent sex partners, persons with other STDs (including HIV), travelers to countries with endemic hepatitis B.

HR9—Persons who exchange sex for money or drugs and their sex partners; persons with other STDs (including HIV); and sexual contacts of persons with active syphilis. Clinicians should also consider local epidemiology.

HR10—Persons who continue to inject drugs.

HR11—Healthy adults without a history of chickenpox or previous immunization. Consider serological testing for presumed susceptible adults.

PRIORITIES FOR RESEARCH

The efficacy and cost-effectiveness of nursing (specifically, of APNs) in risk reduction and preventive service delivery is an area that needs further exploration. Lemley, O'Grady, Rauckhorst, and Russell (1994) conducted a study to see how well NPs do in providing preventive services. The survey was based on 17 of the *Healthy People 2000* objectives. Data was obtained from 892 NPs who completed a survey. The data indicated that NPs already exceed the targets in some areas and are close in some other areas. However, in other areas, the provision of preventive services was below the targets. While this research provides some data related to preventive services, a number of researchers have found that PCPs overestimate the amount of preventive services that are done. It will be important for APNs to conduct chart reviews to determine how well they are doing at risk identification. For example, Mullins (2000) conducted a study looking at how well NPs do at screening for osteoporosis in at-risk women. She reviewed 52 charts of postmenopausal women ages 35 to 86 and found that

77% of the women received counseling regarding hormone replacement therapy, while far fewer women got counseling related to exercise, calcium, and vitamin D. Only 29% of the population received bone mineral density testing. While these results are somewhat disappointing, they serve as a starting point to focus on risk reduction for menopausal women.

Larger, more prospective studies are also needed for areas of preventive care such as smoking cessation, exercise and weight loss, and counseling. It is not until APNs are willing to examine their current patterns of care related to risk reduction and prevention that they will know where care needs to be strengthened. A focus on the outcomes of care, both for chronic illness treatments and for risk reduction and preventive care measures, will force APNs to look at practice patterns.

Another necessary area of research relates to the identification of barriers to providing preventive care. Many factors have been identified, such as inadequate reimbursement, fragmentation of health services, insufficient time with patients, and lack of knowledge related to

Table 45-8

Strategies to Improve the Efficacy of Patient Counseling

STRATEGY	EXAMPLES
Frame the teaching to match the patient's perceptions	Identifying the beliefs of a patient related to the topic (e.g., "What gets in the way of you . . . ?")
Fully inform patients of the purposes and expected effects of interventions and when to expect these effects	Letting a patient know when to expect any changes based on the intervention, which increases compliance with the change
Suggest small changes rather than large ones	Using self-efficacy theory, because a goal that is accomplished, even if small, is positive and tends to encourage continuation of the activity
Be specific	Giving very specific instructions (e.g., begin walking around the block five times a week for 1 week, then walk around the block two times each day)
Remember that it is sometimes easier to add new behaviors than to eliminate established behaviors	If losing weight is difficult, having the patient exercise is a way to accomplish the same goal
Link new behaviors to old behaviors	Suggesting a patient ride an exercise bike while watching the news
Use the power of the profession	Remembering that clinicians are seen as health experts and not being afraid to say "I want you to stop smoking," because direct messages are effective if they are short and specific
Get explicit commitments from patients	Asking a patient how he or she will integrate the new activity into his or her life, then having the patient sign a contract or indicate what his or her commitment level is
Use a combination of strategies	Using whatever seems to work (e.g., individual counseling, group counseling, written handouts, other community resources)
Involve office staff	Having the front office staff member hand out reading material before the appointment, which the nursing staff can discuss or reinforce through teaching
Refer	Remembering that it is not always possible to provide all education for a patient and that it is sometimes best to refer to someone else who can do the teaching; knowing areas of strength and getting assistance for weaker areas
Monitor progress through follow-up visits	Calling or scheduling a visit may help keep the patient on track; it also gives them an opportunity to ask questions as they begin the lifestyle changes. Proactive calls help reinforce the behavior change

From U.S. Preventive Services Task Force (1996). *Guide to clinical preventive services.* Baltimore: Williams & Wilkins.

specific preventive services needed. However, much of the available research was conducted in the 1980s, perhaps before most PCPs were familiar with the U.S. PSTF guidelines. Now with the wide availability of guidelines via the Internet, PCPs should be aware of screening and risk factor counseling measures. Research to determine how well APNs do with screening and identification of barriers to providing care would provide guidance for both advanced practice and APN education.

Clinical and economic outcomes of risk reduction and preventive service delivery in primary care settings are important to determine. In many cases, effectiveness may be due to counseling, and the effects of counseling on specific behaviors have not been examined in appropriately designed studies. Small changes in behavior would be difficult to prove in prospective studies, yet they could have an important effect when applied to populations at risk. Since the cost is low to do counseling in the office, the U.S.

PSTF recommends counseling even though evidence is not available to support it. Many APNs have anecdotal evidence that counseling makes a difference, as evidenced by one APN who was counseling a patient regarding obesity. The patient indicated that in all the years she had gone to that practice, no one had ever told her that she was obese. For this patient, it made all the difference, and when the patient was 50 pounds lighter, the APN knew that her counseling did indeed make a difference. Researching the effects of brief, directed counseling regarding health behaviors on patient outcomes is a research area that APNs need to address.

Research related to the clinical outcomes of preventive service delivery in specific groups (based on ethnic group, sex, age, socioeconomic status, and other factors) is another important area of research for APNs. There is disparity among American ethnic groups in terms of morbidity, mortality, and participation in preventive services.

Text continued on p. 658

Name
D.O.B.
No.

Adult Preventive Care
Flow Sheet

PUT PREVENTION
INTO PRACTICE

ALLERGIES:

Health Counseling

(Circle if appropriate)
1. Alcohol and Drugs
2. Aspirin
3. Dental and Oral Health
4. Hormone Replacement Therapy
5. Domestic Violence
6. Family Planning
7. Folate
8. Injuries (e.g., seat belts, falls)
9. Nutrition
10. Occupational Health
11. Osteoporosis
12. Physical Activity
13. Polypharmacy
14. Self-Exams (skin, breast, testicular)
15. STDs/HIV Infection
16. Tobacco
17.____________________
18.____________________

Date							
Type(s)							
Date							
Type(s)							
Date							
Type(s)							
Date							
Type(s)							
Date							
Type(s)							
Date							
Type(s)							

Screening and Tests

Suggested Examinations and Tests:*

BLOOD PRESSURE
BREAST EXAM
CHOLESTEROL
COGNITIVE AND FUNCTIONAL IMPAIRMENT
DEPRESSION
DIGITAL RECTAL EXAM
FECAL OCCULT BLOOD
GLAUCOMA
HEARING
HEIGHT/WEIGHT
MAMMOGRAPHY
ORAL CAVITY EXAM
PAP SMEAR/PELVIC EXAM
PLASMA GLUCOSE
PROSTATE EXAM/PSA
SIGMOIDOSCOPY
SKIN EXAM
TESTICULAR EXAM
THYROID FUNCTION/EXAM
TUBERCULIN SKIN TESTING
URINALYSIS
VISION

*Specific preventive protocols should be tailored to the patient's risk factors and based on discussion between the patient and provider

Examinations and Tests	Schedule									
		Date								
		Result								
		Date								
		Result								
		Date								
		Result								
		Date								
		Result								
		Date								
		Result								
		Date								
		Result								

Immunizations

Immunizations/Frequency

Immunization					
Influenza ≥ 65 YRS. OR IMMUNOCOMPROMISED YEARLY	Date Manuf. & Lot No.				
Pneumococcal ≥ 55 YRS. OR IMMUNOCOMPROMISED ONE DOSE	Date Manuf. & Lot No.				
Varicella NON-IMMUNE ADULTS TWO DOSES DELIVERED 4-8 WEEKS APART IF IMMUNIZED AFTER AGE 13 YEARS	Date Manuf. & Lot No.				
Hepatitis B ADULTS AT INCREASED RISK 3 OR 4 DOSE SERIES	Date Manuf. & Lot No.				
Tetanus and Diphtheria ALL ADULTS EVERY 10 YEARS	Date Manuf. & Lot No.				
Rubella WOMEN OF CHILDBEARING AGE AND HEALTH CARE WORKERS WITHOUT EVIDENCE OF IMMUNITY OR PRIOR IMMUNIZATION ONE DOSE	Date Manuf. & Lot No.				

Other Immunizations

	Date Manuf. & Lot No.	
	Date Manuf. & Lot No.	
	Date Manuf. & Lot No.	
	Date Manuf. & Lot No.	
	Date Manuf. & Lot No.	
	Date Manuf. & Lot No.	

Figure 45-3 Adult preventative care flow sheet (From U.S. Preventive Services Task Force [1996]. *Guide to clinical preventive services*. Baltimore: Williams and Wilkins.)

REDBUD FAMILY HEALTH CENTER
PREVENTIVE CARE FOR LOW-RISK ASYMPTOMATIC ADULTS

Name   DOB

Recommendation	Date	Date	Date	Date	Date	Date	Date	Date	Date	Date
BP. Ht. Wt. q yr										
Cholesterol q 5y 20-75										
Fecal occult blood q 1y >50										
Sigmoidoscopy q 5y >50										
Fasting glucose q 3 yr >45 if asymptomatic										
Dental visit 1-2 ×/yr (floss/brush)										
Hear/eye q 2yr unless DM then q 1y >65										
Breast exam q 1-3 y 19-39 then q 1yr										
Mammogram q 2y >40, q 1 yr >50										
Pap smear q 1-3 yr (q 1 yr for high risk)										
Rectal exam/prostate q 1y >50										
Assess alcohol/tobacco/drugs q 1yr										
Assess depression (high risk patient)										
Assess family violence										
Counseling										
Safety/injury prevention/falls										
Exercise										
Nutrition										
HRT/osteoporosis/folate										
Tobacco/drug abuse cessation										
Unintended pregnancy/STD										
Advance directives										
Skin										
Immunizations										
Td										
Influenza										
Pneumovax										
Hepatitis B										
Lyme/Varicella										
TB										

A

Figure 45-4 A, Redbud Family Health Center adult preventative flow sheet. (Developed from data from U.S. Preventive Services Task Force [1996]. *Guide to clinical preventive services*. Baltimore: Williams and Wilkins.)

REDBUD FAMILY HEALTH CENTER
Chronic Illness Follow-Up

Name   DOB
Diabetes Care

Action	Date	Date	Date	Date	Date	Date	Date	Date	Date	Date
Glucose control (q visit)										
Hgb A1C (q 3-4 mos)										
U/A, microalbuminuria (q 1yr)										
Fasting lipids (q 1yr unless 1)										
BUN/creatinine/lytes (q 1 yr)										
ECG (q 1 yr)										
Dilated eye exam (q 1 yr)										
Foot exam (at least q 1 yr)										
Smoking cessation										
Education (include referrals)										

Hypertension/CV Disease

Action	Date	Date	Date	Date	Date	Date	Date	Date	Date	Date
BP control (q visit)										
U/A, microalbuminuria (q 1yr)										
Fasting lipids (q 1yr or q 6 mos if 1)										
BUN/creatinine/lytes/LFTs (q 1 yr)										
ECG/echo at diagnosis										
Eye exam (q 1yr)										
Smoking cessation										
Education										
DM/CHF ACE inhibitor										
Post MI beta blocker/ASA										
Positive family history CAD folate										

Asthma

Action	Date	Date	Date	Date	Date	Date	Date	Date	Date	Date
PEFR/PFT (q 1 yr)										
Instructions for self-care (q 1 yr)										
Review use of MDI (q 6 mos)										
Smoking cessation										
Antiinflammatory/beta agonist										

B

Figure 45-4, cont'd B, Redbud Family Health Center chronic illness follow-up form. (Developed from data from U.S. Preventive Services Task Force [1996]. *Guide to clinical preventive services.* Baltimore: Williams and Wilkins.)

Health Supervision: 4 Months

The following questions are intended to be used selectively to invite discussion, gather information, address the needs and concerns of the family, and build partnerships. Use of the questions will vary from visit to visit and from family to family. Questions can be modified to match the health professional's communication style.

Questions for Parents

- How are you?
- How are you feeling?
- How is your family getting along?
- What do you enjoy most about Bobby?
- What questions or concerns do you have about Bobby?
- What new things is he doing?
- Have there been any major stresses or changes in your family since the last visit?
- Who helps you out with Bobby?
- How do you know what Bobby wants or needs? Is it easy or difficult to tell?
- What have you found to be the best way to comfort Bobby?
- Do you have any questions about feeding Bobby? What are you feeding him at this time?

- Does Bobby sleep through the night?
- Do you put Bobby to sleep on his back?
- Is Bobby fastened securely in a rear-facing infant safety seat in the back seat every time he rides in the car?
- Do you think Bobby hears all right? Sees all right?
- Are you reading to Bobby or singing to him?
- Have you returned to work or school, or do you plan to do so? What are your child care arrangements?
- Have you and your partner been getting out without the baby? Who takes care of the baby when you go out?
- Do you know what to do in case of an emergency?
- Do you know first aid and infant cardiopulmonary resuscitation (CPR)?
- Do you know how to reduce Bobby's risk of exposure to lead hazards if you live in an older home or one that has been renovated recently?
- Does anyone in your home have a gun? If so, is the gun unloaded and locked up? Where is the ammunition stored?
- Have you considered not owning a gun because of the danger to children and other family members?

This may result from limited access to risk reduction and preventive services. Research related to how specific interventions work with specific groups will help improve the ability to provide preventive care. For example, knowing that hypertension is more commonly found in African Americans, an APN begins research that examines the genetic markers for hypertension in that population. Another APN, whose office is located in a low-income housing project, knows that low-income adolescent girls are more at risk for early pregnancy. She institutes a program known as "Girls' Night Out" for girls ages 11 and older. The girls come to the office, have pizza, and discuss issues related to early pregnancy. Research comparing preprogram pregnancy rates with those after the program will provide feedback as to the effectiveness of this program, and while it is obvious that there are many more factors involved in teenage pregnancy, this can be just one part of the interventions that this APN uses.

IMPLICATIONS FOR MSN EDUCATION AND ADVANCED PRACTICE

APN programs designed around the information needed in actual practice are important. Pickwell (1993) identified the 20 most common family physician and family nurse practitioner (FNP) diagnoses, and this research is helpful when designing or retooling an APN curriculum. Clinical experience in risk reduction and preventive services comes with an adequate number of clinical practica hours, and exposure to a wide variety of common diseases (not the unusual ones) helps students gain self-confidence in their abilities. Many times, a student's clinical experience is concentrated only on patient care and not administrative issues, such as serving on organization committees; however, this too is a learning experience and should be an integral part of APN education. APN education is dynamic and must be redesigned on a regular basis to remain current with the changing needs of patients and the health care system. It is also critical that faculty who teach in APN programs be experienced and participate in the care of patients.

It is important for APNs to systematically incorporate preventive services into primary care delivery, both episodic and periodic. Many adults do not seek well visits, so an APN must deliver preventive services and risk reduction interventions whenever a patient is seen. This necessitates being vigilant to the process and using mechanisms to remind and keep track of any preventive interventions done. It also means telling a patient when health maintenance visits are recommended and why the CPE may not be the best time for getting those services. Frame (1995) states that, "No one can predict the future but there are a number of things that you can do that will decrease your risk of premature death or disability." A health maintenance handout describing the vital self care-interventions a

4-Month Visit	ID#:			Date:	
Name:		DOB:		Sex:	
Parent Name:		Phone:			
Wt. (__%)	Length (__%)	HC	T	P	R	BP

Questions for Parent
- How is your family getting along?
- Who helps you out with _____?
- Is it easy or difficult to tell what _____ wants or needs?
- Does _____ sleep through the night?
- Have you returned to work or school, or do you plan to do so? What are your child care arrangements?
- Have you and your partner been getting out without the baby?

Developmental Observation
- How does _____ move around?
- Tell me about _____'s typical play.

Circle all that apply:
Babbles and coos; smiles, laughs, and squeals; on stomach, holds head erect and raises body on hands; rolls over from stomach to back; opens hands, holds own hands; grasps rattle; controls head well; reaches for and bats objects; recognizes parent's voice and touch.

Family's Questions
- What questions or concerns would you like to discuss today?

Anticipatory Guidance
Healthy habits
- [ ] Car seat
- [ ] Sleep on back
- [ ] Water temperature < 120°
- [ ] Keep hand on baby
- [ ] Smoke-free environment
- [ ] Hot liquids/cigarettes
- [ ] Sun exposure
- *[ ] Childproof home
- *[ ] Syrup of Ipecac
- [ ] No baby walkers
- [ ] Know signs of illness
- [ ] Breastfeed or iron-fortified formula
- *[ ] Introduce solid food
- [ ] Avoid honey

Parent/infant interaction
- [ ] Hold, cuddle, rock
- [ ] Talk, sing, read, play music
- [ ] Games and toys
- [ ] Bedtime routine
- [ ] Comfort objects

Family relationships
- *[ ] Partner and sibling involvement
- [ ] Attention to siblings
- [ ] Time for self and with partner
- [ ] Contact with friends/family

Interval History

Medications:

Allergies:

Recent injury/illness:

Special health care needs:

Visits to other health care providers/facilities:

Changes/stressors in family or home:

Physical Examination

	Normal		Normal
General	[ ]	Heart	[ ]
Skin	[ ]	Abdomen	[ ]
Head	[ ]	Back	[ ]
Eyes (red reflex, strabismus)	[ ]	Genitalia	[ ]
		Hernia	[ ]
Ears	[ ]	Extremities	[ ]
Nose/throat	[ ]	Feet	[ ]
Mouth	[ ]	Neurologic	[ ]
Neck	[ ]	Reflexes	[ ]
Lungs	[ ]	Signs of abuse	[ ]

If abnormal, explain:

Community interaction
- [ ] Referrals
- [ ] Play and parent support groups
- *[ ] Community involvement

Immunizations
Immunizations up to date? _____
Side effects discussed? [ ]
Hepatitis B # _____   [ ]
Diphtheria, tetanus, pertussis # _____   [ ]
H. influenzae type B # _____   [ ]
Polio # _____   [ ]

Summary
- Summarize visit
- Arrange continuing care _____
  _____
  _____

Referral   Phone Numbers
Health insurance _____ [ ]
SSI _____ [ ]
WIC _____ [ ]
Food Stamps _____ [ ]
Social Services _____ [ ]
Housing _____ [ ]
Other:

Notes:

Signature:_____

Bright Futures is sponsored by **MCHB, HRSA,** and, in part, supported by unrestricted educational grants from **Pfizer Pediatric Health**. Bright Futures material is produced by **NCEMCH** and is not copyrighted.

Figure 45-5 Bright Futures 4-month visit form.

Box **45-5**

Developmental Surveillance and Milestones

Questions and Possible Responses

Do you have any specific concerns about Jerome's development or behavior?

How does Jerome communicate what he wants?

- Demonstrates range of feelings (e.g., pleasure, displeasure, sadness)
- Vocalizes (e.g., babbles, "aaaa," "eeee," "oooo")

What do you think Jerome understands?

- Recognizes parent's voice

How can Jerome move his body?

- Controls head well
- In prone position, holds head upright and raises body on hands
- Sits with support
- Rolls over from front to back
- Opens hands and holds own hands

How does Jerome act around family members?

- Babbles and coos
- Smiles, laughs, and squeals
- Recognizes parent's voice and touch
- Has spontaneous social smile

Tell me about Jerome's typical play.

- Mouths objects
- Blows bubbles
- Imitates a cough or razzing noises
- Reaches for and bats at objects
- Grasps rattle

Milestones

- Babbles and coos
- Smiles, laughs, and squeals
- In prone position, holds head upright and raises body on hands
- Rolls over from front to back
- Opens hands, holds own hands, and grasps rattle
- Controls head well
- Begins to bat at objects
- Looks at and may become excited by mobile
- Recognizes parent's voice and touch
- Has spontaneous social smile
- May sleep for at least 6 hours
- Able to comfort himself (e.g., fall asleep without breast or bottle)

Box **45-6**

Parent-Child Interactions and Examination Components

Observation of Parent-Infant Interaction

Are the parent and infant interested in and responsive to each other (e.g., gazing, talking, smiling)? Does the parent hold and cuddle the infant? How does the parent attend to the baby when he or she is being examined? How does the parent comfort the baby when he or she cries?

Physical Examination

Measure and plot on a standard chart (e.g., the revised CDC/NCHS growth charts) the infant's head circumference, length, weight, and weight for length. Share the information with the family.

As part of the complete physical examination, the following should be particularly noted:

- Developmental hip dysplasia
- Cardiac murmurs
- Neurological problems
- Evidence of possible neglect or abuse

Additional Screening Procedures

Vision

- Examine eyes; assess for red reflex and strabismus

Hearing

- Conduct or arrange for inital hearing screening if not previously done with follow-up screening, evaluation, and referral as needed.

Immunizations

Hepatitis B virus (Hep B) vaccine

- Administer once at age 1 to 4 months per dosage schedule

Diphtheria, tetanus, pertussis (DTaP) vaccine
***Haemophilus influenzae* type b (Hib) vaccine**
Inactivated polio virus (IPV) vaccine

- Discuss possible side effects of the immunizations, what to do about them, and when to call the health professional.

---

patient can do to contribute to this process is important. Having a specific written health maintenance plan that patients can see and understand also goes a long way toward getting them to "buy in" to the process. This also means sharing decision-making with patients by fully

informing them about the potential consequences of interventions (e.g., screening and possible invasive follow-up). Determining what a patient's goal is for his or her health and what he or she is willing to put into the equation is helpful. It does not do much good to spend 30 minutes

Suggestions for Further Learning

- Obtain the article: Lemley, K., O'Grady, E., Rauckhorst, L, & Russell, D. (1994). Baseline data on the delivery of clinical preventive services provided by nurse practitioners. *Nurse Practitioner, 19*(5): 57-63. On which areas, based on this study, do APNs need to concentrate? In what areas are the preventive services they provide below the recommendations of *Healthy People 2000*? Why do you think these areas are below the levels of most of the other areas? How would you address these areas in your practice?

- Go to the Bright Future website (www.brightfutures. org) and obtain the resource *Health Supervision Guidelines that Incorporate Primary and Secondary Preventive Services Essential in Childhood, from Infancy through Late Adolescence* (from the National Center for Education in Maternal and Child Health, Georgetown University). These guidelines and other materials are available free as downloads; printed copies may be ordered from the website or from the National Maternal and Child Health Clearinghouse, 2070 Chain Bridge Road, Suite 450, Vienna, VA 22182-2536; phone (703) 356-1964; fax (703) 821-2098. How would you anticipate putting these to use in your clinical area? Describe the process you would go through to use these. Discuss barriers that you might need to overcome to adapt them.

- Go to the website for the *Guide to Clinical Preventive Services* at odphp.osophs.dhhs.gov/pubs/guidecps/. Published in 1996, this is the most widely recognized and referenced guide to risk reduction and preventive services. The text may be viewed or printed (free of charge) at the website just given, or a printed copy may be ordered from the Superintendent of Documents, U.S. Government Printing Office, at (202) 512-1800 (stock # 017001005258, with a single copy price of $35 [shipping included]). Does your current preceptor use this book in practice? Why or why not?

- Consult the following: U.S. Department of Health and Human Services, Public Health Service, Office of Public Health and Science, & Office of Disease Prevention and Health Promotion (1998). *Put prevention into practice: clinician's handbook of preventive services* (2nd ed.). Washington DC: US Government Printing Office. Available online at www.ahcpr.gov/clinic/ppipix.htm. As discussed in this chapter, this is a handbook and program

for implementation of the U.S. PSTF guidelines for primary care office settings. This resource is available to view or print (free of charge) at the website just given, or printed materials may be ordered from AHCPR Publications Clearinghouse, PO Box 8547, Silver Spring, MD 20907; phone (800) 358-9295. The handbook in available at a single copy price of $20. A free information packet, including sample tools, is also available.

- Visit the *Healthy People* website at web.health.gov/ healthypeople/. Sponsored by the Office of Disease Prevention and Health Promotion, U.S. DHHS, this site includes comprehensive information regarding the 2000 and 2010 initiatives, including progress reviews and current news.

- Visit the Office of Disease Prevention and Health Promotion website at odphp.osophs.dhhs.gov/. An office of the U.S. DHHS, their website provides a variety of information, publications, and links to other relevant websites.

- Obtain the book *Clinical Evidence*, published by the British Medical Journal Publishing Group. This book presents the current evidence available for a variety of conditions; it is published every 6 months so that it may remain current. It is available online at www. clinicalevidence.org.

- Obtain a copy of Lancaster, J. (Ed.). (1999). *Nursing issues in leading and managing change*. St. Louis: Mosby. This book holds a wealth of information regarding the change process as it pertains to the current health care delivery system. It is helpful for an agency planning to implement a preventive services program.

- Other helpful Internet resources include:
  - Agency for Health Research and Quality (www. ahrw.gov)
  - American Academy of Pediatrics (www.aap.org)
  - American College of Preventive Medicine (www. acpm.org)
  - Centers for Disease Control and Prevention Guidelines (www.cdc.gov/prevguid.htm)
  - Guidelines for Adolescent Preventive Services (www. ama-assn.org/adolhlth/adolhlth.htm)
  - National Coalition for Adult Immunization (www. medscape.com/affiliates/ncai)

talking about how to stop smoking if a patient is not willing to stop. By being given information and a choice, a patient may decide that walking is something he or she is willing to do, even if quitting smoking is not. For people who seek sporadic care or who have limited access, APNs must deliver preventive care at every visit, no matter what the visit is for. Establishment of effective interpersonal communication between nurses and patients serves as a foundation for health behavior counseling, and communication is an area where APNs usually excel. Talking with

patients in a language they can understand is critical, and using written material to enhance the conversation helps focus patients on the important points (and it is available for patient review once they leave the office). An established relationship with patients helps them feel that APNs care for them as individuals. Caring is also demonstrated by listening, touching, and using effective communication.

Leadership by APNs in the collaborative delivery of risk reduction and preventive services will be important. Opportunities to serve on medical record committees or

QA committees provides data to improve practice. APNs seem willing to get involved and contribute to the development of practice protocols, so if no process is in place for risk reduction or preventive services, APNs need to take a leadership role in instituting these programs. It will also be vital for APNs to keep up with the explosion of evidence available regarding health maintenance. APNs can expect expansion of the knowledge base surrounding the delivery of risk reduction and preventive services every 4 to 5 years. As more emphasis gets placed on patient outcomes, there will be more emphasis on preventive services.

The important point about risk reduction and preventive services is that they need to be considered at every visit; if all issues can be addressed, a separate visit need not be made, thus saving the patient and the APN time and money. Selective longitudinal health maintenance based on research evidence should be routinely offered to all patients in an APN's practice.

DISCUSSION QUESTIONS

These questions can be used to promote critical thinking and encourage discussion.

1. Using the U.S. PSTF recommendations, identify the appropriate preventive services for one or more of the following patients:

   - 5-year-old African-American male from a low-income family and living in an urban area
   - 19-year-old Caucasian female, 12 weeks pregnant with a history of high-risk sexual activity (e.g., multiple partners, no barrier use)
   - 48-year-old Asian male who is a practicing NP
   - 32-year-old Caucasian male, a sexually active homosexual
   - 30-year-old Hispanic male, a migrant farm worker
   - 80-year-old African-American female, a resident of a long-term care facility

2. Discuss potential aids and barriers to risk reduction and preventive services according to the following:

   - Age
   - Sex
   - Lifestyle
   - Socioeconomic status
   - Religious beliefs
   - Cultural identification

3. Analyze the risk reduction and preventive services in your current practice setting. Are services delivered systematically to all patients? What aids are used to

track the provision of preventive services? Are outcome measures tracked for preventive services? Outline a plan for implementation or improvement of preventive service delivery in your practice setting.

REFERENCES/BIBLIOGRAPHY

Beck, G. (1993). The clinical application of epidemiology and the interpretation of diagnostic tests. In R. Matzen & R. Lang (Eds.), *Clinical preventive medicine* (pp. 97-108). St. Louis: Mosby.

Bien, T., Miller, W., & Tonigan, J. (1993). Brief interventions for alcohol problems: a review. *Addiction, 88,* 315-336.

Branch, W., & Crouch, M. (1998). Periodic health exams: what really matters. *Patient Care.* Available online at www.patientcare.com.

Buppert, C. (2000). Measuring outcomes in primary care practice. *The Nurse Practitioner, 25*(1), 88-98.

Delaune, S.C., & Ladner, P.K. (1998). *Fundamentals of nursing standards and practice.* Albany, NY: Delmar Publishers.

Edelman, C.L., & Milio, N. (1994). Health defined: objectives for promotion and prevention. In C.L. Edelman & C.L. Mandle (Eds.), *Health promotion throughout the lifespan* (3rd ed.). St. Louis: Mosby.

Flocke, S.A., Stange, K.C., & Goodwin, M.A. (1998). Patient and visit characteristics associated with opportunistic preventive services delivery. *The Journal of Family Practice, 47*(3), 202-208.

Flocke, S.A., Stange, K.C., & Zyzanski, S.J. (1998). The association of attributes of primary care with the delivery of clinical preventive services. *Medical Care, 36*(8), AS21-AS30.

Frame, P. (1995). The complete annual physical examination refuses to die. *The Journal of Family Practice, 40*(6), 543-545.

Green, M., & Palfrey, J.S. (Eds.). (2000). *Bright futures: guidelines for health supervision of infants, children, and adolescents* (2nd ed.). Arlington, VA: National Center for Education in Maternal and Child Health.

Kottke, T., Battista, R., & DeFriese, G. (1988). Attributes of successful smoking cessation interventions in clinical practice: a meta analysis of 42 controlled trials. *Journal of the American Medical Association, 259,* 2882-2889.

Lancaster, J. (1999) Managing change. In J. Lancaster (Ed.), *Nursing issues in leading and managing change.* St. Louis: Mosby.

Leininger, L.S., Finn, L., Dickey, L., Dietrich, A.J., Foxhall, L., Garr, D., Stewart, B., & Wender, R. (1996). An office system for organizing preventive services. *Archives of Family Medicine, 5,* 108-115.

Lemley, K., O'Grady, E., Rauckhorst, L., & Russell, D. (1994). Baseline data on the delivery of clinical preventive services provided by nurse practitioners. *Nurse Practitioner, 19*(5), 57-63.

Lichtenstein, E., & Glasgolo, R. (1992). Smoking cessation: what have we learned over the past decade? *Journal of Consulting Clinical Psychology, 60,* 518-527.

Luckmann, R., & Melville, S. (1995). Periodic health evaluation of adults: a survey of family physicians. *Journal of Family Practice, 40,* 547-554.

Maiese, D.R., & Fox, C.E. (1998). Laying the foundation for healthy people 2010—the first year of consultation. *Public Health Reports, 113,* 92-95.

Matzen, R., & Lang R. (1993). *Clinical preventive medicine.* St. Louis: Mosby.

Mullins, D. (2000). *Osteoporosis prevention patterns: are nurse practitioners following the current national osteoporosis foundation guidelines?* (Unpublished Master's thesis). Highland Heights, KY: Northern Kentucky University.

Murphy, P. (1995). Assessing risk vs. assessing blame. *Nurse Practitioner, 20,* 15-16, 21.

Office of Disease Prevention and Health Promotion (1998). *Healthy People 2010 fact sheet.* Available online at web.health.gov/healthypeople/2010fctsht.htm.

Office of Disease Prevention and Health Promotion (2000). *Healthy people 2010: what is it?* Available online at web.health.gov/healthypeople/PrevAgenda/whatishp.htm.

Pender, N.J. (1996). *Health promotion in nursing practice* (3rd ed.). Stamford, CT: Appleton & Lange.

People who quit smoking are much less likely to be hospitalized than those who don't. (1998, March 5). (Media advisory). Rockville, MD: Agency for Health Care Policy and Research. Available online at www.ahcpr.gov/news/press/smokepr.htm.

Pickwell, S. (1993). The structure, content and quality of family nurse practice. *The Journal of the American Academy of Nurse Practitioners, 5*(1), 6-9.

Sifri, R., & Wender, R.C. (1996). Preventive care steps towards implementation. *Primary Care 23*(1), 127-140.

Sox, C.H., Dietrich, A.J., Tosteson, T.D., Winchell, C.W., & Labaree, C.E. (1997). Periodic health examinations and the provision of cancer prevention services. *Archives of Family Medicine, 6,* 223-230.

U.S. Department of Health and Human Services, Public Health Service, Office of Public Health and Science, & Office of Disease Prevention and Health Promotion (1998). *Put prevention into practice: clinician's handbook of preventive services* (2nd ed.). Washington DC: US Government Printing Office. Available online at www.ahcpr.gov/clinic/ppipix.htm.

U.S. Preventive Services Task Force (1996). *Guide to clinical preventive services* (2nd ed.). Baltimore: Williams & Wilkins.

Wagner, J.L. (1997). Cost-effectiveness of screening for common cancers. *Cancer Metastasis Review, 16*(3-4), 281-194.

Yano, E., Fink, A., Hirsch, S., Robbins, A., & Rubenstein, L. (1995). Helping practices reach primary care goals. *Archives Internal Medicine, 155,* 1146-1156.

Chapter 46

Disease Management: Maximizing the Quality of Life

Mollie R. Poynton

Disease management (DM) has recently emerged as a significant movement in health care. Although the literature offers multiple definitions of DM, every DM program has certain characteristics in common. While DM programs span the continuum of care from hospitals and rehab facilities to primary care facilities and pharmacies, primary care is central. DM programs are focused on prevention, working to prevent both the disease and its complications through patient involvement and empowerment and ongoing and periodic evaluation of outcome measures. Such programs are based on a disease's natural history and require knowledge-based care.

The availability of clinical practice guidelines and outcome measures combined with computer-facilitated information management has effectively spurred DM to the forefront of managed care. Under ever-increasing pressure to reduce costs and improve patient outcomes, providers turn to comprehensive DM systems to minimize costs and improve patient quality-of-life. They believe DM reduces costs by decreasing hospitalization and emergency visits and preventing or controlling costly complications such as diabetic nephropathy (Gerber & Stewart, 1998). They also believe DM programs improve outcomes for patients by preventing disease or disease complications (e.g., nephropathy and retinopathy in diabetic patients), minimizing or avoiding patient hospitalization, and improving the quality of care (Hunter & Fairfield, 1997).

Proponents laud DM's potential for improving clinical economic outcomes. However, the effectiveness of DM in reducing costs and improving outcomes has not been clearly demonstrated (Hunter & Fairfield, 1997). Evidence of improved outcomes lies only in case studies and anecdotes rather than randomized controlled trials. If the input cost of DM is not rewarded with significant health care savings, some managed care professionals predict it will quickly vanish.

Although true DM entails systemwide implementation, many providers are integrating elements of DM programs into their everyday practice. Outcomes measurement, goal-setting, and clinical practice guidelines are all components of DM that may contribute to improvement of clinical and economic outcomes within individual practice settings (Kibbe & Johnson, 1998). Providers challenged with the care of chronically ill patients find clinical practice guidelines a useful tool in improving quality of life and preventing complications (Richman, Scott, & Kornberg, 1998).

DEFINITIONS

Although no single definition exists, for the purpose of a primary care discussion it is sufficient to define *disease management* as a knowledge-based, comprehensive approach to management of health care based on specific disease states. DM focuses on specific diseases, typically high-cost chronic diseases like diabetes, asthma, and human immunodeficiency virus (HIV)/acquired immune deficiency syndrome (AIDS) (Hunter & Fairfield, 1997). Patients suffering from a particular disease or patients at significant risk of contracting that particular disease are the targets of the DM program. The goal of a DM program is optimization of outcomes, both clinical and economic (Ellrodt, Cook, Lee, Cho, Hunt, & Weingarten, 1997). Financial resources are directed towards interventions that produce improved clinical outcomes for a population at the lowest possible cost. The interventions are chosen based on clinical practice guidelines and outcomes research.

In general, *disease prevention* or *health management* can be defined as "the optimization of clinical, financial, and quality-of-life outcomes accomplished by management of the entire range of health risks for a population" (Peterson & Kane, 1997). Clinical practice guidelines frequently are the mainstay for developing a DM program. *Clinical practice guidelines* are guidelines, algorithms, or pathways for the care of patients with similar disease states or health characteristics. They are generally developed through professional consensus and scientific trials. *Care process mapping* is the plan for implementation of a DM program across all areas of care.

Outcomes are the results of medical care. Outcomes fall into three categories: medical, service and cost. (Table 46-1 shows the components of each category.) Inherent in looking at outcomes is a patient's quality of life. **Quality of life** is a person's overall sense of well-being (Doyle, 1997). Another factor that influences the incidence of disease is a person's health risks. A **health risk** is a factor that increases the likelihood that a person will experience disease, injury, or illness.

CRITICAL ISSUES: DEVELOPMENT OF DISEASE MANAGEMENT PROGRAMS

Zitter (1997) traces the origin of DM to initiatives by the Mayo Clinic in the late 1980s and early 1990s. Eicher, Wong, and Smith (1997) relate DM's more recent development to the market transition presently occurring in health care—specifically, growth in capitation and domi-

nance of managed care organizations (MCOs). Eicher et al view DM as a stage in health care's evolution towards "population-based health management," in which an integrated health care system provides management of a population's overall health and wellness, as opposed to specific disease states.

Today, most MCOs have adopted DM programs in some form. Many have established departments devoted entirely to development and implementation of DM programs (Cassidy, 1997). A variety of commercial DM programs are available, and the services offered range from consultation to companies that upload all data and perform all calculations. While some primary care providers (PCPs) are initiating DM programs independently, the majority have been initiated by MCOs as a way to decrease cost expenditures and avoid disease complications. Programs initiated by individual primary care practices are seldom implemented on a systemwide basis. Thus the importance of MCOs related to DM lies in their power and initiative to implement protocols and information systems across the continuum of care.

The DM concept's emergence has been both a catalyst and a beneficiary of a boon in clinical practice guidelines and outcomes research. Many clinical practice guidelines in existence were developed during the last 10 years. In fact, the unprecedented demand for these guidelines in the past few years prompted the U.S. Agency for Health Care Policy and Research (AHCPR) (now the Agency for Health Care Research and Quality [AHRQ]), in cooperation with the American Association of Health Plans and the American Medical Association (AMA), to develop an internet clearinghouse to facilitate the dissemination of clinical practice guidelines—The National Guideline Clearinghouse (www.ahrq.gov). Also, in June 1998, then Vice President Al Gore launched the planning committee that created the Forum for Health Quality Measurement and Reporting in the private sector. This forum serves to endorse core sets of measures for standardized reporting of health quality. APNs need to keep apprised of the developments and recommendations of this committee relative to patient care outcomes.

Likewise, outcomes research is quickly becoming the priority of many health care researchers, including nurse researchers. Using guidelines based on outcomes research, DM programs tailor limited resources to the interventions and programs that most significantly affect patient outcomes (Doyle, 1997). Third-party payers will likely base reimbursement practices on outcome data in their on-going attempt to minimize the cost-benefit ratio of health care services. In fact, the Health Plan Employer Data and Information Set (HEDIS), used by the National Committee on Quality Assurance (NCQA) (a consumer-driven, nonprofit organization that accredits health plans) to evaluate the quality of both public and private health plans, incorporated some clinical outcome measures into its 2000 data set (Buppert, 2000). These outcome

Table **46-1**

Types of Outcomes and Components

TYPE OF OUTCOME	COMPONENTS
Medical outcomes	• Rate of complications • Attainment of therapeutic goals • Improvement of functional status measures • *Worst case*—death
Service outcomes	• Patient satisfaction • Patient waiting times • Cycle times (i.e., time from entrance into the office until discharge) • Prompt follow-up of abnormal data • Prompt attention to telephone calls • *Worst case*—loss of the patient from practice
Cost outcomes	• Reduction of the cost of treating an episode of illness • Amount of money spent on hospitalizations • Amount of money spent on emergency department visits • *Worst case*—bankruptcy of practice

Data from Buppert, C. (2000). *The primary care provider's guide to compensation and quality.* Gaithersburg, MD: Aspen Publishers.

Table 46-2

HEDIS 2000 Measures of Effectiveness of Care

Measures	Applicable to		
EFFECTIVENESS OF CARE MEASURES	**MEDICAID**	**COMMERCIAL**	**MEDICARE**
Childhood immunization status	X	X	
Adolescent immunization status	X	X	
Breast cancer screening	X	X	X
Cervical cancer screening	X	X	
Chlamydia screening in women (first year)	X	X	
Prenatal care (first trimester)	X	X	
Checkups after delivery	X	X	
Controlling high blood pressure (first year)	X	X	X
Beta-blocker treatment after a heart attack	X	X	X
Cholesterol management after acute cardiovascular events	X	X	X
Comprehensive diabetes care	X	X	X
Use of appropriate medications for people with asthma (first year)	X	X	
Follow-up after hospitalization for mental illness	X	X	X
Antidepressant medication management	X	X	X
Advising smokers to quit	X	X	X
Flu shots for older adults			X
Medicare health outcomes survey			X

Data from National Committee for Quality Assurance (2000). *HEDIS 2000 list of measures.* Available online at www.ncqa.org/pages/policy/hedis/h00meas.htm.

measures include control of blood pressure to less than 140/90 millimeters of mercury (mm Hg) in hypertensive patients, timely performance of Pap smear screening for cervical cancer, immunization of children, and counseling for smoking cessation (Buppert, 2000). (Table 46-2 lists the 2000 HEDIS measures related to effectiveness of care.)

Targeted Diseases and Populations

Generally, the most appropriate patients for DM programs are patients with chronic illness—patients requiring health care over an extended period. The choice of target population is commonly based on the most frequent diagnoses in a practice or organization and the diagnoses responsible for the most significant cost in a practice or organization (Hunter & Fairfield, 1997; Kibbe & Johnson, 1998). The knowledge base for the diagnosis and disease must be extensive to support knowledge-based clinical practice guidelines (Hunter & Fairfield, 1997). Box 46-1 provides examples of common targets for DM programs. Additionally, DM programs may target only patients suffering from a particular illness or condition who exhibit the greatest severity (Kibbe, 1998).

Development of a Disease Management Process

An APN interested in measuring patient outcomes should begin by reviewing the resources available. The process logically begins by reviewing background theory and

Box 46-1

Diseases and Conditions That Are Candidates for Disease Management Programs

Arthritis
Asthma
Chronic obstructive pulmonary disease
Congestive heart failure
Depression
Diabetes
Gastroesophageal reflux disease
HIV/AIDS
Hypertension
Hypercholesterolemia
Low back pain
Migraine headache

research related to outcomes measurement. Figure 46-1 shows the steps in the process to develop a DM program. Next, an APN should choose a problem area. The problem area should be one of particular interest to the APN or his or her practice, an outcome identified by HEDIS, or a disease that is difficult to manage (e.g., diabetes, depression). The use of published clinical practice guidelines is a good place to start in identifying the target outcomes.

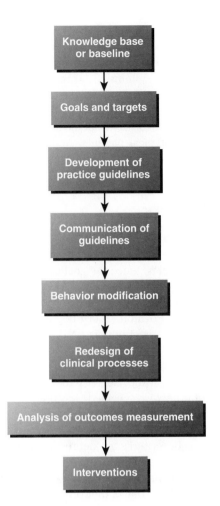

Figure 46-1 The disease management process. (From Hunter, D.J., & Fairfield,G. [1997]. Disease management. *British Medical Journal*, *315*, 50-53).

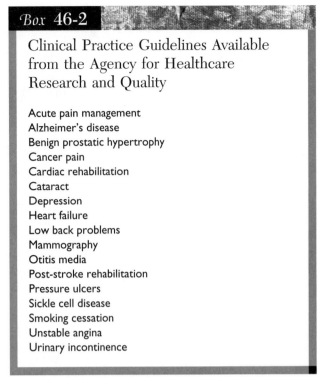

Data from Agency for Health Care Policy and Research (1999). *AHCPR clinical information*. Available online at www.ahcpr.gov/clinic/index.html.

Clinical practice guidelines

Defined as systematically developed statements intended to assist practitioners and others in determining appropriate health care for specific clinical situations, *clinical practice guidelines* are the central component of DM programs (Ellrodt et al, 1997). Generally, such guidelines seek to determine the best practices and reduce variations in care and treatment among providers. The desired outcomes of guideline implementation are those of DM, cost savings, and improved clinical outcomes.

Providers seeking clinical practice guidelines may adapt existing clinical practice guidelines or create their own based on a review of current literature. Existing clinical practice guidelines are available from a variety of resources (Ellrodt et al, 1997). They are most easily accessed on the Internet.

Particularly useful in locating guidelines is The National Guideline Clearinghouse, administered by the AHRQ (formerly the AHCPR). Accessed via the Internet, this database provides a current, searchable guide to clinical practice guidelines available from a variety of sources. The user may access synopses of guidelines with key recom-

mendations highlighted. The database enables the user to compare various guidelines in terms of source, basis, and other criteria. The user is also provided with information necessary to obtain full-text copies of guidelines or with hypertext links to full-text guidelines available on the web (AHCPR, 1999).

The AHRQ itself is also a reliable source for clinical practice guidelines. To date, this agency has sponsored the development of 17 clinical practice guidelines for chronic illness or problematic conditions (Box 46-2). Developed by multidisciplinary committees with patient representation, these guidelines are comprehensive, evidence-based, and readily available (at www.ahcpr.gov or www.guideline.gov).

Groups independently developing clinical practice guidelines should conduct a thorough search and review of current literature, using such databases as Medlars Online (MEDLINE) and the Cumulative Index of Nursing and Allied Health Literature (CINAHL). Guidelines should be based on strong evidence in the form of randomized controlled trials when possible. If guidelines applicable to the target population already exist, they may serve as a valuable guide and resource (Ellrodt et al, 1997).

Those adapting or developing guidelines should evaluate those guidelines for the following characteristics:

- Currency of information and research
- Evidence-based recommendations
- Recommendations graded according to the strength of evidence (randomized controlled trials versus retrospective and pilot studies)

- Applicability to intended setting and population
- Relevance for the specified patient population

An example of how a clinical practice guideline can be used to direct a DM program will be presented here, and each part of a DM program will be related to the DM of a specific guideline—that for depression. Box 46-3 identifies the selection of a clinical practice guideline.

Informatics and disease management

Crucially important in any DM program is clinical informatics, particularly clinical information systems. Identification of target patients; information management; and evaluation of outcomes require powerful manipulation of data (Armstrong, 1996). Technological tools such as computers, software, telecommunications media, and systemwide Intranets are essential for a successful DM endeavor. As patient advocates, APNs should critically analyze clinical information systems with attention to confidentiality and management of patient variations. They should also critically evaluate nursing taxonomies, so that the process of nursing care is adequately identified and described.

Clinical information systems designed for DM programs manage and manipulate extensive information about patients (Armstrong, 1996). The use of this information and access to this information are key areas of concern. Kibbe (1998) noted a recent incident wherein a marketing firm was contracted to supply DM program patients with educational materials on their prescriptions. The firm then used the patient information to market other drugs via mailed advertisements. Such blatant abuse of patient information threatens compliance and undermines trust.

Another issue that can be significantly influenced by clinical information systems is the treatment of variance. DM attempts to minimize variance in treatment and outcomes. However, clinical information systems, particularly protocols and algorithms, should allow for appropriate management of atypical patients. Additionally, DM programs should consider cultural and socioeconomic factors and issues of compliance (Armstrong, 1996). Advocacy in the development stages of a DM program can address these factors.

Determining a baseline

After a target population is identified, creation of the DM program itself begins. Since the goal of any DM program is to reduce costs and improve clinical outcomes, DM programs must begin by identifying current clinical and economic outcomes. Poynton (2000) researched the current practice of nurse practitioners (NPs) in a community health center in relation to the AHCPR/AHRQ guidelines for depression (1993). A list of all patients diagnosed with International Diagnostic Code (ICD-9) 311 (depressive disorder, not otherwise specified) was used to identify the patients. Fifty-one medical charts of four NPs were reviewed and compared to the guidelines. Comparison of the diagnostic criteria for depression with the chart documentation revealed that all patients were documented to have five of nine symptoms needed to diagnose depressive disorder. None of the patients had all diagnostic criteria addressed. Sixteen of the charts used a depression self-rating scale, and these charts indicated moderate or severe depression. Prescription of medications in 86% of the charts was consistent with the AHCPR guidelines. (Since the guidelines were published in 1993, a number of the drugs that were prescribed were not available when the guideline was written.) Lack of adherence to the guidelines was revealed in the area of follow-up, and review of the data indicated that patients did not keep their follow-up appointments once medication was started. In addition, there was not a good system in place to assist the NPs in tracking of the patients, either for counseling referrals or for needed follow-up. This pilot study provides data on which a DM program could be initiated.

Once baseline data is established, outcome measures and corresponding goal outcomes for a DM program can be developed (Doyle, 1997). Examples of possible outcome measures used in a depression study include:

- Annual hospitalization rate
- Average length of stay among patients admitted for tertiary care
- Annual number of emergency department visits
- Rate of absenteeism
- Quality of life (e.g., degree of interference with activity due to depression, signs of patient satisfaction)

Box 46-3

Example of Clinical Practice Guideline Selection: Disease Management Program for Depression

1. Depression guideline panel: U.S. Department of Health and Human Services, Public Health Service (1993, April). *Depression in primary care: volume 1. Detection and diagnosis* (Clinical practice guideline number 5, AHCPR Publication No. 93-0550). Rockville, MD: Agency for Health Care Policy and Research.
2. Depression guideline panel: U.S. Department of Health and Human Services, Public Health Service (1993, April). *Depression in primary care: volume 2. Treatment of major depression* (Clinical practice guideline number 5, AHCPR Publication No. 93-0550). Rockville, MD: Agency for Health Care Policy and Research.
3. Educational materials and topics: National Institutes of Health. *NIH Publication No. NIH-99-3561*. U.S. Department of Health and Human Services. (Contains information about depression for patients.)

- Percentage of patients who are treated with recommended antidepressants (e.g., selective serotonin reuptake inhibitors [SSRIs])
- Percentage of patients with depression that return for follow-up

Doyle (1997) provides a categorization for clinical outcomes according to knowledge of a disease's natural history (Table 46-3). Doyle also recognizes the importance of establishing process measures such as satisfaction, utilization, and compliance in addition to the outcome measures described previously.

Measurement of these outcomes can take many forms, including laboratory test results, chart reviews, abstraction of computerized patient information, surveys, and interviews. Ongoing as well as periodic measurement of these outcomes is necessary for appropriate evaluation. Such evaluation corresponds well to continuous quality improvement (CQI) techniques (Hunter & Fairfield, 1997). HEDIS measures are also an important consideration in measurement of outcomes. (Table 46-4 provides specific outcome measures identified by the NCQA for commercial managed care plans in 1999.) NCQA accreditation of health plans is based on HEDIS measures; thus acceptance to health plan provider panels may soon depend upon the performance of individual health care organizations according to HEDIS measures (Buppert, 2000a).

Setting goals
Goals within individual DM programs reflect the overall goal of improving economic and clinical outcomes and are stated in terms of the selected outcome measures. Since DM programs target the overall health of individuals with a common illness or characteristic, goals are set for the targeted population as a whole. This type of goal-setting represents a change for APNs accustomed to goal-setting for individuals or families.

Examples of DM program goals include:

- Decrease the number of annual inpatient days by 15% over 2 years
- Decrease the number of emergency department visits by 20% over 18 months
- Decrease the average low-density lipoprotein (LDL) level among participants by 15 milligrams/deciliter (mg/dl) over 6 months
- Increase the average score on a quality-of-life assessment tool by 10 points over 18 months

Goals for the sample DM program for depression are presented in Box 46-4.

Implementation and evaluation
Once clinical practice guidelines are selected and minimal outcome measures are established, the DM program may be implemented (Table 46-5). The magnitude and complexity of implementation depends on the magnitude and complexity of the DM program. Organizational or system-wide implementation of a DM program is a distinct organizational change that requires consideration of organizational dynamics and change theory for success. Anecdotal evidence indicates that significant involvement of an organization's respected clinicians and opinion leaders during

---

Table 46-3

Causes and Consequences of Disease States

DISEASE SEQUENCE	DEFINITION	ILLUSTRATIVE OUTCOME MEASURES (FOR CORONARY ARTERY DISEASE)
Health risk	Factors that increase the likelihood that a person will experience the onset or exacerbation of a health condition	Cigarette smoking
Physiological status	Description of a person's physical and chemical functioning	Degree of arterial blockage, as measured by angiogram
Symptoms	Subjective indications of disease as perceived by a patient	Chest pain
Signs	Objective indications of disease as perceived by an examiner	Sweating
Functional status	A person's ability to perform normal activities and roles	Ability to climb a flight of stairs
Quality of life	A person's overall sense of well-being	Self-reported satisfaction with physical, social, and financial aspects of life

From Doyle, J.B. (1997). Health outcomes: measuring and maximizing value in disease management. In T. Warren & D. Nash (Eds.), *Disease management: a systems approach to improving patient outcomes.* San Francisco: Jossey-Bass (a subsidiary of John Wiley and Sons, Inc.).

Table 46-4

Outcomes for Commercial Managed Care Plans

PERFORMANCE MEASURES	EXPECTED OUTCOMES	1999 NATIONAL OUTCOMES
Mammograms every 2 years for eligible women ages 52 to 69	81%	71%
Pap smears for eligible women ages 21 to 64	81%	71%
Yearly eye examinations for adult diabetics	57%	39%
Outpatient follow-up within 30 days of hospitalization for mental illness	87%	67%
Prenatal care within the first 13 weeks of pregnancy	95%	83%
Postnatal checkup within 6 weeks of delivery	87%	66%

Data from National Committee for Quality Assurance (2000). *HEDIS 2000 list of measures.* Available online at www.ncqa.org/pages/policy/hedis/h00meas.htm.

Box 46-4

Example of Goals for a Disease Management Program for Depression

- Increase the number of patients with major depressive disorder who are treated with antidepressants by 20 percentage points within 1 year.
- Increase the number of patients with major depressive disorder who are treated with antidepressants for at least 3 months by 20 percentage points within 1 year.
- Increase the number of patients who experience improvement in the severity of symptoms within 6 weeks of initial diagnosis by 30 percentage points.

Table 46-5

Disease Management Program for Depression: Summary of Clinical Guidelines

Screening	• Annual screening for symptoms of depression • Use of brief, 8-item survey to identify key symptoms of depression • Survey completed by each patient while waiting to be seen
Diagnosis	• Clinical interview for differential diagnosis of depressed mood • Documentation of symptoms according to DSM-IV criteria • Use of depressed mood flow sheet for documentation (Figure 46-2)
Referral criteria	• Suicidal intent and/or plan • Symptoms or history of mania • Severe personality disorder • Substance abuse or positive CAGE screening • Thought disorder, psychosis, or severe melancholic features • Age less than 18 years
Treatment	• All patients to receive counseling referrals and antidepressant medication • Antidepressant treatment continued for at least 4 months after first response to medication • Antidepressant treatment continued indefinitely for patients with three or more episodes of major depression • Patient education topics and written material for all patients (e.g., National Institutes of Health, 1999). • Follow-up visits and treatment modification per 1993 AHCPR guidelines for management of depression in primary care settings • Documentation of follow-up visits using depression follow-up form (Figure 46-3)

Redbud Family Practice	Depressed Mood Form

Date: _____ DOB: _____ MR#: _____
Name:
BP:_____ HR:_____ RR:_____ T:_____

Allergies:
Medications:
PMH:

SUBJECTIVE

HPI:

Symptom Inventory (Check all that apply):
___ Depressed mood
___ Duration:_____
___ Loss of interest or pleasure in almost all activities
___ Weight loss:_____
___ Weight gain:_____
___ Loss of appetite:_____
___ Increased appetite:_____
___ Sleep disturbance:_____
___ Diminished ability to concentrate
___ Indecisiveness
___ Recurrent thoughts of death or suicide
___ Significant distress or psychosocial impairment

Other Symptoms:

Severity of Symptoms: (check one):
___ Mild   ___ Moderate   ___ Severe

OR Zung score:_____ (Attach to patient record)

Differential Diagnosis: (Check all that apply):
___ Recent loss or traumatic event:_____
___ Psychotic symptoms:_____
___ Melancholic symptoms:_____
___ Anxiety/pain symptoms:_____
___ Manic symptoms:_____

CAGE Screening: (Check all "yes" responses):
___ CUT (Have you ever felt you ought to cut down on your drinking?)
___ ANNOYED (Have people ever annoyed you by criticizing your drinking?)
___ GUILTY (Have you ever felt bad or guilty about your drinking?)
___ EYE OPENER (Have you ever had a drink first thing in the morning to steady your nerves or get rid of a hangover?)

Substance/Street Drug Use:

Previous Mental Health History:
(Check all that apply):
___ History of manic episodes
___ Psychotic disorder
___ Schizoaffective disorder
___ Hospitalizations:_____
___ Suicide attempts:_____
___ Previous episodes of depression:_____

Family Mental Health History:

OBJECTIVE

General:

Grooming:

Affect:

Speech:

Mental Status (Include results of MMSE if administered):

Skin:

HEENT:

Neck/Thyroid:

Chest:

Heart:

Lungs:

Abdomen:

Extremities:

Neurological:

ASSESSMENT

1)

2)

3)

PLAN
___ TSH
___ H&H
___ Other diagnostic testing:_____
___ Counseling referral:_____
___ Antidepressant:_____
___ Exercise regimen:_____
___ Follow-up in 2 weeks
___ Educational materials given
___ Patient teaching per checklist

Other:

Signature: _____

Figure 46-2 Depression flow sheet. *MMSE,* Mini mental status examination.

the planning stages may contribute to successful implementation of a DM program (Richman et al, 1998).

Evaluation or analysis of process and outcome measures should take place on both an ongoing and a periodic basis. Evaluation is crucial; it provides the feedback necessary for adaptation and improvement of the original program (Ellrodt et al, 1997). DM programs necessarily respond to this ongoing feedback.

Evaluation of patient outcomes in DM programs requires seven steps (Table 46-6). In addition to periodic evaluation of outcomes, DM programs must respond to changes in the body of knowledge supporting the clinical practice guidelines, as well as changes in the health care system with which DM is intertwined. Goals should be reevaluated, outcome measures and guidelines critiqued, and processes changed (Ellrodt et al 1997). A truly dynamic process, responsive to change, should be fostered.

Redbud Family Practice	**Depression Follow-up Form**
Date: DOB: MR#: Name: BP:_____ HR:_____ RR:_____ T:_____	Allergies: Medications: PMH:

SUBJECTIVE

___ **Changes in symptoms:**

___ **Suicidal thoughts/thoughts of death:**

___ **Toleration of antidepressant:**

___ **Other:**

Severity of Symptoms: (check one):
___ Gone ___ Mild ___ Moderate ___ Severe

OR Zung score:_____ (Attach to patient record)

Social Changes/Events:

OBJECTIVE

General:

Grooming:

Affect:

Speech:

Mental Status (Include results of MMSE if administered):

Other:

ASSESSMENT

PLAN
___ Counseling:
___ Antidepressant:
___ Follow-up in 2 weeks
___ Follow-up in 3-4 weeks
___ Referral:
___ Other:

Signature: _____

Figure 46-3 Depression follow-up flow sheet.

Major Issues in the Development of Future Disease Management Programs

A critical issue related to DM will be the role of third-party payers in clinical decision-making. More third-party payers will soon expect the use of patient outcome data. It may even serve to identify which providers and practices are "invited" to participate in managed care companies. Those organizations that can say, "Our diabetic patients have an average glycosylated hemoglobin [HgbA1C] of 6.8, with fewer hospitalizations and complications" will be the practices that are put on provider panels. Employers will likely embrace the concept of DM because it has the potential to coordinate health care resources to optimize outcomes and, at the same time, keep costs under control. It makes more sense to treat a condition as well as possible from the beginning (e.g., modifying risky behaviors, reducing the occurrence of illness) than to pay for preventable and costly complications later. Proactive organizations and providers should recognize their role in managing conditions more cheaply and effectively.

Thus far, the role of pharmaceutical companies in DM programs has not been made clear. APNs can rest assured that if DM is found to be beneficial for these companies, initiatives started by pharmaceutical companies will appear. Ideas may range from the development of DM flow sheets for particular diseases (using their products) to computer software programs to assist in calculation of outcomes measures. Pharmacists may also play a more defined role in medication management and follow-up in the future.

Patient confidentiality within clinical information systems is an issue that needs to be addressed. The use of electronic medical records (EMRs) facilitates the DM process greatly, but ways to protect a patient's EMR is a much-debated issue. As more practices adopt EMRs, there will be more information available about this potential problem.

PRIORITIES FOR RESEARCH

It is important to conduct outcomes research in all areas and specialties. However, it makes sense to target the high-cost diagnoses initially and expect to see other diseases and preventive care included in the future. Outcomes measurement techniques will soon become commonplace. As DM programs become more sophisticated, the effect of DM programs on clinical and economic outcomes will be calculated. Utilization of clinical practice guidelines will be an integral part of conducting outcomes research, and the effect of such guidelines on the success of clinical outcomes will be an important factor to determine.

Depending on who the stakeholder is (e.g., payer, provider, policy-maker, researcher, regulatory organization, consumer, government) in the research, outcomes can be measured in a variety of ways. Outcomes measurement tools fall into three major categories: general health and

Table 46-6

Steps in a Disease Management Program for Depression

PROGRAM STEPS	APPLICATION
Identify clinical issue of interest.	• Poor follow-through for second appointments and little to no follow-up with counseling for depression • Pharmacological treatment of patients diagnosed with major depressive disorder and treated for a minimum of 4 months after diagnosis, with a noted decrease in symptoms within 6 weeks of initial diagnosis
Identify the source of data.	• Computerized database of prescriptions and refills • Chart reviews
Choose a sampling method.	50 patients diagnosed with ICD-9 code 311 (depression, not otherwise specified) in the last year, at least 4 months before data collection
Collect and analyze baseline data.	70% of patients with ICD-9 code 311 received prescriptions for antidepressants. However, only 25% received at least 4 months of medications. Of these patients, 30% showed an improvement of symptoms within 6 weeks of starting medication, but less than 10% had information or consultation related to counseling.
Compare baseline data to benchmark data, then set goal.	NCQA HEDIS data indicate the national average for treatment of depressed health plan members with antidepressants in 1998 was 54.4% (Buppert, 2000b). There is no benchmark data available for evaluation length of antidepressant treatment, improvement in symptoms, or follow-up.

Goals
- 90% of depressed patients treated with antidepressants
- 50% of depressed patients treated with antidepressants for at least 4 months
- 70% of depressed patients showing improvement in severity of symptoms within 6 weeks of initial diagnosis; if no improvement is seen, adjustment of medications warranted

Collect data periodically throughout implementation of the disease management program.

Data collected at 3, 6, and 12 months after implementation of the DM program for depression:

	BASELINE	3 MOS	6 MOS	12 MOS
Antidepressants	70%	80%	85%	95%
Treatment for 4 months	25%	27%	30%	40%
Improvement	30%	40%	62%	65%

	BASELINE	1 YEAR	GOAL
Use information to evaluate and amend the DM program.		
Antidepressants	70%	95%	Increase by 20% Actual increase 25% (goal met)
Treatment for 4 Months	25%	40%	Increase by 20% Actual increase 15% (goal not met*)
Improvement	30%	65%	Increase by 30% Actual increase 35% (goal met)

*A high treatment dropout rate was noted as an important contributing factor to early discontinuation of antidepressant treatment. The DM program was amended to include phone-call reminders for scheduled follow-up visits, revised patient education materials highlighting the importance of follow-up care in depression treatment, and a printed patient record of scheduled follow-up visits.

generic measures, disease-specific measures, and functional status measures.

General health and generic measures have historically been used to assess the health of a large population. Today, these tools look at the positive aspects of physical, social, and emotional well-being. An example of a general health outcome measure is the *Medical Outcomes Study Short Form 36* (Ware & Sherbourne, 1992). Disease-specific measurements are generally of the most interest to patients and providers. Examples of these types of measurement tools include the Adult Asthma Quality of Life Questionnaire, the Quality of Life after Myocardial Infarction Questionnaire, and the Kidney Disease and Quality of Life Short Form. Functional status measures focus on various aspects of a patient's performance of specific activities; an example would be the Functional Independence Measure. Outcomes that include patient satisfaction, clinical outcomes, functional health status, and cost provide a complete picture in assessing outcomes (Maloney & Chaiken, 1999). It will be important for APNs to use well-defined outcomes measurement tools in their research endeavors, and familiarity with the attributes of a well-defined instrument is important (Weaver, 1997).

As APNs collect data related to outcomes, it is important for the data to be collected and measured correctly. Developing clear standards for data collection does much to add reliability and validity to studies that are completed. Outcomes assessment can help answer the question, "What makes a difference?" (Maloney & Chaiken, 1999). Once information is collected and analyzed, it is important to go beyond the data and monitor the outcomes indicators. A glimpse in time is less compelling in its strength to support inferences than data collected through repeated measurements. Finally, once the "dust clears" after the measurements are completed, it is important to use the information to achieve optimal outcomes.

IMPLICATIONS FOR MSN EDUCATION AND ADVANCED PRACTICE

New APN graduates must have knowledge and experience with outcomes research. Programs might want to emphasize the importance of research, which evaluates the effectiveness of care. Many providers believe that they provide complete, quality care, but when the outcomes are actually measured, the results are disappointing. Students should get in the habit of evaluating their own level of care against national standards (e.g., HEDIS, AHQR guidelines). The process of doing this emphasizes how easy it is to miss important components of care, which could be overlooked without data collection, and develops the beginning of an excellent practice habit. It could even parlay into future employment possibilities when the APN graduate states "When I cared for diabetic patients, the average Hgb A1C of my patients was . . . ," or "When I cared for patients with depression, 96% completed a minimum of 4 months of drug therapy." These are strong indicators of quality and can impress most potential employers.

APNs will want to participate in the provision of knowledge-based care to maximize value. The time will come when an APN's individual performance data will be available to patients, and health-plan performance is already being measured and widely reported. NCQA data will be available not only to the specific health plan, but breakouts of individual PCP data are anticipated in the near future. The reporting of this data is a compelling reason for APNs to be active participants and leaders in the development of DM programs within their practices. In addition, APNs can serve as advocates for patients in the creation or adaptation of clinical practice guidelines and DM programs, as well as in the process of adopting EMRs.

The ideal system of care for DM includes several themes. First, patients need to be an integral part of the program. The focus needs to be on empowerment and not correction (e.g., providers telling patients what they need to change). A patient focus means that patients are given the information and responsibility to get involved in their own care. Patients should set self-management goals that *they* find meaningful and that they are able to accomplish. Asking a patient, "What is your goal for the visit today?" may be a place to begin a patient focus. The patient's answer may be surprising!

Second, the use of evidence-based care is important. This means using the latest data and clinical guidelines to guide care. Finally, population-based care should be provided. The goal of such care is to satisfy the health needs of all patients by knowing who patients are and what conditions they have; this means monitoring their care proactively (e.g., keeping patients from "falling through the cracks"). If a patient is not back in the office when expected, a phone call or letter may serve as a reminder to get him or her back into the system. Proactive care may also mean using a patient flow sheet to track needed services (White, 1999) (see Figure 45-4, *B*).

Many people are betting on DM as the process of the future, and if DM does all that is hypothesized, it will indeed become an established process for the care of patients. In this case, it will be important for APNs to lead the way as it becomes the standard of care. APNs have nothing to fear from DM; if anything, it will let APNs shine brighter, and the world will soon learn about the positive capabilities of APNs.

DISCUSSION QUESTIONS

These questions can be used to promote critical thinking and encourage discussion.

Suggestions for Further Learning

- Access The National Guideline Clearinghouse at www. ahrq.gov. Developed by the AHRQ, this site is a searchable database of available clinical practice guidelines. It provides summaries and comparisons of guidelines, as well as a forum for related discussion. What guidelines seem appropriate for use in developing a DM program?
- Obtain either of these articles: Kibbe, D.C. (1998, October). Disease management: who's caring for your patients? *Family Practice Management.* Available online at www.aafp.org/fpm/981000fm/disease.html; or Kibbe, D.C., & Johnson, K. (1998, November-December). Do-it-yourself disease management. *Family Practice Management.* Available online at www.aafp.org/fpm/

981100fm/disease.html. Do these articles make the case for DM? What are some barriers to implementing such a system? Why do you think some PCPs would not be very positive about implementing such a program?
- Go to the site for the AHRQ at www.ahrq.gov. This is a source for full-text copy and information about the AHRQ's own series of clinical practice guidelines.
- Obtain Warren, T., & Nash, D. (Eds.). (1997). *Disease management: a systems approach to improving patient outcomes.* Chicago: American Hospital Publishing. This book is a comprehensive source of information on the entire DM process. Would this book serve as a step-by-step guide in implementing DM in an APN practice? Why or why not?

---

1. Which patient populations in your practice area are most suitable for DM programs? Which would be least suitable? Why?

2. What changes in clinical informatics have occurred at your health care workplace in the last 5 years? What forces drove these changes? What new information is available? How can you use that information to better understand your practice?

3. Split students into seven pairs or groups and assign each group one of the following stakeholders: providers, patients, third-party payers, employers of patients, APNs, registered nurses (RNs), and pharmaceutical companies. Instruct each group to identify the benefits and disadvantages of DM for their particular stakeholder. What were the findings? What were the barriers identified?

4. What is the role of APNs or PCPs in systemwide DM of chronic illness?

5. How do you think that APNs would fare if outcomes research was done on their charts and patients? How do you think APNs would do when compared to other PCPs? Discuss what leads you to make these conclusions.

REFERENCES/BIBLIOGRAPHY

Agency for Health Care Policy and Research (1999). *AHCPR clinical information.* Available online at www.ahcpr.gov/clinic/index.html.

Armstrong, E.P. (1996). Monitoring and evaluating disease management: information requirements. *Clinical Therapeutics, 18*(6), 1727-1733.

Buppert, C. (2000a). Measuring outcomes in primary care practice. *The Nurse Practitioner 25*(1), 88-98.

Buppert, C. (2000b). *The primary care provider's guide to compensation and quality.* Gaithersburg, MD: Aspen Publishers.

Cassidy, J. (1997, November-December). Strategies for chronic disease management. *Health Progress,* 13-14.

Doyle, J.B. (1997). Health outcomes: measuring and maximizing value in disease management. In T. Warren & D. Nash (Eds.), *Disease management: a systems approach to improving patient outcomes.* San Francisco: Jossey-Bass.

Eichert, J.H., Wong, H., & Smith, D.R. (1997). The disease management development process. In T. Warren & D. Nash (Eds.), *Disease management: a systems approach to improving patient outcomes.* Chicago: American Hospital Publishing.

Ellrodt, G., Cook, D.J., Lee J., Cho M., Hunt D., & Weingarten, S. (1997). Evidence-based disease management. *Journal of the American Medical Association, 278*(20), 1687-1692.

Gerber, J.C., & Stewart, D.L. (1998). Prevention and control of hypertension and diabetes in an underserved population through community outreach and disease management: a plan of action. *Journal of the Association for Academic Minority Physicians, 9*(3), 48-52.

Horn, S. (1997). Clinical practice improvement: a methodology to improve quality and decrease cost in health care. *Oncology Issues, 12*(1), 16-20.

Hunter, D.J., & Fairfield, G. (1997). Disease management. *British Medical Journal, 315,* 50-53.

Joint Commission on Accreditation of Healthcare Organizations. (1997). *National library of healthcare indicators: health plan and network edition.* Chicago: Joint Commission on Accreditation of Healthcare Organizations.

Kibbe, D.C. (1998, October). Disease management: who's caring for your patients? *Family Practice Management.* Available online at www.aafp.org/fpm/981000fm/disease.html.

Kibbe, D.C., & Johnson, K. (1998, November-December). Do-it-yourself disease management. *Family Practice Management.* Available online at www.aafp.org/fpm/981100fm/disease.html.

Kozma, C., Kaa, K., & Reeder, C. (1997). A model for comprehensive disease management. *The Journal of Outcomes Management, 4*(1), 4-8.

Maloney, K., & Chaiken, B. (1999, November-December). An overview of outcomes research and measurement. *Journal of Healthcare Quality.* Available online at www.nahq.org.

Mowinski, B., & Staggers, N. (1997). The hazards in outcomes management. *The Journal of Outcomes Management, 4*(1), 18-22.

Nash, D. (1997). Disease management: a bumpy road ahead. *The Journal of Outcomes Management, 4*(1), 2.

National Committee for Quality Assurance (2000). *HEDIS 2000 list of measures*. Available online at www.ncqa.org/pages/policy/hedis/h00meas.htm.

National Institutes of Health (1999). *Patient education materials—depression* (Pub. No. 99-3561). Washington, DC: US Department of Health and Human Services.

Peterson, K.W., & Kane, D.P. (1997). Beyond disease management: population-based health management. In T. Warren & D. Nash (Eds.), *Disease management: a systems approach to improving patient outcomes*. Chicago: American Hospital Publishing.

Poynton, M. (2000). *Diagnosis and acute phase management of major depressive disorder by primary care nurse practitioners* (Unpublished Master's thesis). Highland Heights, KY: Northern Kentucky University

Prager, L. (1999, January 11). First disease specific report cared pushes improved care. *American Medical News*. Available online at www.ama-assn.org.

Richman, M.J., Scott, P., & Kornberg, A. (1998). Partnership for excellence in asthma care: evidence-based disease management. *Pediatric Annals, 27*(9), 563-568.

Roglier, J., Futterman, R., McDonough, K., Malya, G., Karwath, K., & Bowman, D. (1997). Disease management interventions to improve outcomes in congestive heart failure. *American Journal of Managed Care, 3*(12), 1831-1839.

Rosser, W. (1999). Application of evidence from randomized controlled trials to general practice. *Lancet, 353*, 661-664.

Ware, J., & Sherbourne, C. (1992). *The MDS 36-item short form health status survey (SF-36). Medical Care, 30*, 253-265.

Weaver, S. (1997). Issues in the measurement of satisfaction with treatment. *The American Journal of Managed Care, 3*, 579-589.

White, B. (1999). Improving chronic disease care in the real world: a step by step approach. *Family Practice Management*. Available online at www.aafp.org/fpm/991000fm/38.html.

Zitter, M. (1997). Disease management: maximizing quality of life—a new paradigm in health care delivery: disease management. In T. Warren & D. Nash (Eds.), *Disease management: a systems approach to improving patient outcomes*. Chicago: American Hospital Publishing.

Chapter 47

Complementary and Alternative Medicine

Elizabeth A. Lorenzi & Denise Robinson

According to the traditional American viewpoint, therapies such as medication, surgery, and psychotherapy are conventional, and the absence of disease is what is viewed as "healthy." Everything outside this mainstream is considered alternative medicine. However, today this view is changing, both in the United States and Europe. In France and Germany, the most common prescription drug is gingko biloba (Deloughery, 1998), and homeopathic treatments are commonly used in Western Europe. While most Americans feel that Western medicine is the dominant system of health care, in fact, only about 10% to 30% of all health care is provided by conventional providers. The alternative model stresses that health and disease are a continuum, with health being a positive state of physical, emotional, and mental well-being. Holistic medicine is an approach to health that deals with a patient as a whole and not merely with physical symptoms; it takes into account the psychological status of a person, as well as social and environmental factors and the individual's spirit. Table 47-1 compares the assumptions of conventional, or allopathic, medicine as opposed to those of other alternative systems.

Scientific evidence is mounting to support the notion that the brain and body are inextricably linked. Psychoneuroimmunology is the study of the interrelations between the nervous and hormone systems and the immune system. The means of communication within the body is via neurotransmitters or neuropeptides within the nervous system. Signals are sent from one body system to another via the transmitters to receptor sites on the surface of cells within the receiving system. Emotions such as stress can affect the immune system. (This was discussed in detail in Chapter 44.)

DEFINITIONS

Alternative therapies are therapy choices existing outside of conventional health delivery systems. Alternative therapies by definition (and definition *only*) are used *in-stead* of conventional medicine. ***Complementary therapies***, on the other hand, are used with conventional medicine (also known as *allopathic medicine*). A new word emerging on the scene is *integrative therapies*, because it involves the integration of different nontraditional therapies with allopathic care. Today, however, ***complementary/alternative medicine*** (CAM) is the most commonly used term.

A central theme in CAM is balance—balance of body, mind, and spirit. Disease, often referred to as "dis-ease," represents an imbalance in one or more of these areas. Essential to achieving balance is involvement on the part of a given individual, which means performing the necessary therapy on one's self, working with a therapist, or just consenting to having a therapist do the work.

CRITICAL ISSUES: THE PRACTICE OF COMPLEMENTARY/ ALTERNATIVE MEDICINE

Most of the CAM therapies have been around for years, some from the time before Christ. Most therapies practiced today evolved in other cultures, particularly those of China and India. Acupuncture and herbs have been used for thousands of years in China, and the principles of Ayurvedic medicine derive from the religious texts of Hinduism, which are thought to be approximately 5000 years old. Native American shamans believed physical illness was caused by a spiritual or mental imbalance, while healers from Eastern cultures focused on the concept of the life force within each person (Andrews, Angone, Cray, Lewis, & Johnson, 1999). It was not until the germ theory of disease evolved in the late nineteenth century that the relationship of disease with the mind-body-spirit balance became separated and fragmented. The holistic view of health and illness reemerged in Western medicine in the 1940s with Dunbar's work on psychosomatic medicine

Table 47-1

Comparison of Various Types of Medicine

CONCEPT	ALLOPATHIC MEDICINE (BIOMEDICINE)	CHINESE MEDICINE	AYURVEDIC MEDICINE	HOMEOPATHIC MEDICINE	OSTEOPATHIC MEDICINE
Origin	Until the mid-1800s, care was a combination of homeopathic, naturopathic, and botanical remedies; emergence of germ therapy heralded the era of biomedicine and a belief that all diseases could be eliminated once the microbe or chemical imbalance was discovered	Practiced for over 3000 years and used by 25% of the world's population; focus on prevention; metaphysical world based on the views of Taoism, Confucianism, and Buddhism; basic concept is ying/yang (interaction of opposing forces); qi is the vital energy necessary to maintain life	Means "science of life"; combines philosophical, religious, and scientific principles; derived from Vedas, a philosophy that encompasses whole human life	Based on "like cures like"; homeopathic preparations are doses of dilute substances that contain small portions of what causes a person's symptoms; preparations are used to heal the body or help the body heal itself; the more dilute a preparation, the more potent it is believed to be; another principle is that illness is specific to an individual	Believes in a correlation between body structure and bodily function; incorporates all the tools of allopathic medicine as well as a variety of manual, diagnostic, and manipulative techniques; closely aligned with conventional medicine
Definition of health	Absence of symptoms; a person is either healthy or not healthy	Positive state of physical, emotional, and mental vitality; health and disease are a continuum; optimal mind and body health depends on lifestyle, thoughts, and emotions	Cornerstones are the metabolic body type (doshas), of which there are three types: vatta (thin), pitta (muscular), and kapha (fat); each dosha associated with special body organs and two of the five elements (i.e., fire, earth, air, water, space); good health requires balance between the three doshas within each individual and between the body, mind, and spirit and the environment	Balance in the body's vital force	Structural integrity

View of the body	Works mechanistically as a biochemical, physiological entity; mind a secondary factor in illness	Not only a biomedical, physiological entity; also surrounded by and suffused with energy fields; mind and body connected, with mind a primary or equal factor in illness	Interconnectedness of body, mind, and spirit with individual and environment; balance and harmony of elements; personality determined by dominant dosha	Interconnectedness of body, mind, and spirit	Integrated unit consisting of body, mind, and spirit; body structure can not be separated from function; body is capable of healing itself
View of Disease	Disease or disability an entity in and of itself; pain and disease are negative	Evidence of body's defenses; illness signifies an excess or deficiency of qi or an imbalance of ying/yang; pain and disease may be signs of internal conflict	Disease is caused by imbalance of doshas, which can be influenced by unhealthy lifestyle, internal and external stressors, seasonal influences, genetic predisposition, and toxic substances	Disturbance in the vital force, manifested by a whole pattern of physical, mental, and emotional responses that are unique to each person; imbalance in the body's vital force could be restored with small stimulus balance	Any restriction in the spine or other bony structures can impair function of entire organs and body systems
Source of knowledge	Derives from laboratory tests and quantitative data	Derives initially and primarily from clinical practice and qualitative data; uses looking, asking, listening, smelling, and touching	Determined by the predominant dosha, detailed history, and physical examination; uses observation, questioning, palpation, and auscultation, with special attention to pulse, tongue, eyes, nails, and urine	Elicits symptoms from patient, even those that do not seem related to illness; emotional and mental symptoms especially relevant because they are a good indicator of how a patient feels	Musculoskeletal system is focus of diagnosis; using palpation and inspection, provider examination of the musculoskeletal system
Diagnostics	Symptom led; rational analysis of data using reductionistic interpretation. Diagnosis is based on the symptoms that fit a disease category and diagnostic reasoning (e.g., a person has irritable bowel disease; APN orders Bentyl)	Reliance on subjective data and holistic assessment; some of the following diagnostic frameworks may be used: eight principles, pathogenic factors (six evils), six stages, four levels of disease, and five phases theory; focus on detecting patterns of imbalance in a particular patient; two people with same symptoms may be treated differently due to different imbalances	Reliance on subjective data and holistic assessment; observing the tongue can provide insight into dosha imbalances	Reliance on subjective data	Reliance on both subjective and objective data

Continued

Data from Ullman, D. (1993). The mainstreaming of alternative medicine. *Healthcare Forum Journal*; Andrews, M., Angone, K., Cray, J., Lewis, J., & Johnson, P. (Eds.). (1998). *Nurse's handbook of alternative & complementary therapies.* Springhouse, PA: Springhouse; and Delougbery, G. (1998). *Issues and trends in nursing* (3rd ed.). St. Louis: Mosby.

Table **47-1**

Comparison of Various Types of Medicine—cont'd

CONCEPT	ALLOPATHIC MEDICINE (BIOMEDICINE)	CHINESE MEDICINE	AYURVEDIC MEDICINE	HOMEOPATHIC MEDICINE	OSTEOPATHIC MEDICINE
Treatment	Seeks to excise diseased tissue and infecting organisms and inhibit, manage, or control symptoms	Attempts to restore balance of elements; herbs, acupuncture, diet, massage, and qigong are therapies used	Treatment recommended to restore equilibrium and is usually some combination of diet, lifestyle changes, purification therapy (e.g., massage, enemas, steam treatments) and mental exercises	Homeopathic remedies from raw herbs and other natural substances derived from animal and mineral sources; substances crushed and dissolved in water or alcohol and then diluted many times	Holistic approach; uses manipulation techniques along with conventional therapies
Role of practitioner	The authority; the provider is emotionally neutral	A therapeutic partner with patient; provider's caring is a component of healing and he or she serves as a guide and role model that recommends measures to modify behavior; offers herbs, massage, or needles	Same as for Chinese medicine	Healing should proceed in reverse chronological order, from the most recent symptoms to the oldest; provider is responsible for healing	Provider's task is to assist the body in the process of healing
Role of patient	Dependent on health provider for help	Responsible for own well-being	Responsible for achieving prevention of disease through proper diet, exercise, sleep, and other lifestyle interventions	Not specifically identified	Self-care techniques designed to keep body functioning properly and use body more efficiently

Data from Ullman, D. (1993). The mainstreaming of alternative medicine. *Healthcare Forum Journal*; Andrews, M., Angone, K., Cray, J., Lewis, J., & Johnson, P. (Eds.). (1998). *Nurse's handbook of alternative & complementary therapies*. Springhouse, PA: Springhouse; and Deloughery, G. (1998). *Issues and trends in nursing* (3rd ed.). St. Louis: Mosby.

(Andrews et al, 1999), and the popularity of CAM has grown steadily since the 1970s. In 1980, the American Holistic Nurses Association was founded. Its focus is on "healing the healers" to help contribute to the failing health care system. In 1992, the National Institutes of Health (NIH) established the Office of Alternative Medicine (OAM) to study the efficacy and cost of alternative practices, and in 1998, the OAM became a freestanding center called the National Center for Complementary and Alternative Medicine (NCCAM).

Payment for Complementary/Alternative Medicine

Due to the results of studies from the OAM, as well as public pressure, insurance companies are slowly starting to pay for some CAM therapies (e.g., chiropractic, imagery, acupuncture, energy healing, massage) (Eisenberg, Davis, Ettnec, Appel, Wilkey, VanRompey, & Kessler, 1998). Weber (1997) found that some health plans are using accessibility to CAM therapies (with a copay or prenegotiated fee) as a way to entice patients and thus increase enrollment in the health plan. In addition, patients are demanding that CAM therapies be added as options in health care plans. Coverage varies from company to company and from state to state. However, the increased support from the NIH has certainly encouraged insurance companies to at least reevaluate reimbursement for CAM. Unfortunately, for the medically underserved, CAM is not a really viable option. For most insurance companies and institutions, the motivation in providing CAM is to generate revenue, and most services are provided via fee-for-service or as a health plan rider. Those without insurance or with catastrophic coverage only must pay out of pocket for these services. CAM, then, becomes medicine for the privileged few (Ananth, 1999).

A few organizations are beginning to make these services available to anyone, regardless of ability to pay. One such program is at Lincoln Hospital in New York. This hospital introduced acupuncture in 1974 as an alternative to methadone for treating heroin addiction. It has since become the largest medically supervised drug-free outpatient center for drug and alcohol addiction in the country (Ananth, 1999), and the success rate for this program is approximately 60%. Because CAM therapies are low tech and low cost, they rely on minimal intervention and more self-care. Thus, as a new model of health care delivery is developed, it will be imperative to include alternative therapies.

Use of Complementary/Alternative Medicine

A recent study in the *Journal of the American Medical Association* (Astin, 1998) confirmed that 4 in 10 persons in the United States use complementary therapies. These persons were not dissatisfied with conventional medicine; they were found to be well educated, possess a holistic philosophy of health, and be in poorer health than many other people, with at least one or more of the following: back problems, chronic pain, urinary tract problems, and anxiety disorders. Other studies, as reported by Starr (1997), have shown that persons with conditions that do not respond well to conventional treatment also frequently seek out CAM.

The use of CAM appeals to adolescents because it offers autonomy and a "natural" alternative to traditional medicine. The use of CAM (herbs in particular) is substantial among well-insured, healthy adolescent populations (Ernst, 1999). Among adolescent athletes, 29% of boys and 12% of girls report taking herbal supplements (Bates, 1999). Among patients with chronic illness, the number of adolescents who take herbal supplements is even higher (between 40% and 80%) (Sawyer, Ganoni, & Toogood, 1994). Among homeless teens, 70% report using CAM, with 74% of those using herbs (Breuner, Barry, & Kemper, 1998). Some of the reasons why teenage girls use supplements include premenstrual syndrome, urinary tract infections, obesity, and unwanted pregnancy (Gardiner, Conboy, & Kemper, 2000).

Borkan, Nehrer, Anson, and Smoker (1994) and Boucher and Lenz (1998) additionally reported that greater than 50% of all physicians, especially primary care physicians, made referrals to CAM providers in the preceding year. Referrals were made based primarily on patient demand and interest in CAMs, but also because of a failure of conventional treatment, a belief that a patient had an emotional illness, or a belief that there would be positive results from CAM therapies. In 1997, an estimated 4.8 million visits were made to homeopathic practitioners in the United States, with sales of homeopathic remedies estimated at $250 million in 1996 (D'epiro, 1999).

Safety of Complementary/Alternative Medicine

The biggest concern with CAM therapies is the lack of standardization and quality control. While drugs must comply with strict Food and Drug Administration (FDA) standards, herbs do not. There is no assurance that a product is all natural; pesticides and heavy metals may be present. Any assurance of quality is currently based on the word of the manufacturer. Also, the inherent variability of plants themselves (related to soil content, rain, maturity, and time of harvest) makes the very notion of standardization and precision out of the question (The analytical study of herbs: as yet a fledgling science, 2000). Another area that lacks sufficient information is the biochemical analysis of medicinal plant components and their actions and interactions. For example, even though St. John's wort has been thoroughly analyzed, no one knows exactly which of its active principles is responsible for the herb's action. Until more information becomes available, it is critical for APNs and patients to make efforts to educate themselves about any products they recommend or use. The Dietary Supplement Health and Education Act (DSHEA) of 1994 calls for the use of packaging that must include the name, the quality of each ingredient, if the product is of plant origin, and the part of the plant used. If any part of the components meet daily serving requirements, those percentages must also be identified. Even those products that are not ingested can pose toxic effects. In aromatherapy, essential oils are used in conjunction with massage. The most commonly used oils are seldom dangerous; however, some aromatherapists are introducing novel plant oils, extracts, and phytols into their massage routine. These chemicals have no odor and are potentially toxic, especially for people with previous sensitization (Lis-Balchin, 1999).

Types of Complementary/Alternative Medicine

There are many types of CAM therapies available to consumers. The theories and philosophies behind each of them are similar in many ways, and many of the therapies are used together. For purposes of discussion, the following categories will be used to present the most common CAMs: energy therapies, physical/manual therapies, combination energy/physical therapies, mind-body interventions, and miscellaneous therapies.

Energy therapies

Energy therapies, as well as many of the other CAM therapies, have the purpose of balancing the body's energy, which is called *chi, ki, qi* (all pronounced "chee") and *prana*, to either restore equilibrium or prevent illness. This is based on the belief that energy exists within and outside of the physical forms in which people live; people are surrounded by universal life energy. A basic concept in energy therapy is the existence of an energy system in the body called the *chakra system*. Chakras are the major energy centers of the body. There are seven major chakras, which are whirling, cone-shaped vortexes of energy located along the spinal column. There are also many minor chakras located throughout the body. The vibrational frequency of each chakra emits an electromagnetic field (EMF), and the EMF of each chakra blends with the others to create the human energy field, better known as the *aura*. A disruption in the flow of one's energy results in "dis-ease." People's energy connects and constantly interacts with the environment and the universal life energy to restore balance and promote self-healing for the body, mind, and spirit. Energy therapies are often accomplished through the ancient art of laying-on of hands (although no physical contact may actually take place). *Therapeutic touch* involves the manipulation of a patient's energy field to bring it into balance. The steps for therapeutic touch are centering, intention (for the highest good of the individual), assessment, unruffling, and transfer of energy. The technique was developed for nurses by nurses. *Healing touch* uses light touch to affect the human energy system on all levels (mind, body, and spirit); it encompasses a wide variety of energy techniques, including therapeutic touch. *Reiki* involves the laying-on of hands in a series of positions, with the flow of energy occurring in each position. (The strengths and weaknesses of these types of energy therapies are discussed in Table 47-2.)

Physical/manual therapies

Physical manual therapies involve some form of structural manipulation of the muscles, soft tissue, connective tissue, and spine. However, the effects of structural manipulation can go beyond the musculoskeletal system. Other effects often occur in the skin, blood, lymph system, and central nervous system, especially the autonomic nervous system. Effects are also often seen in the emotions. *Chiropractic therapy* deals with manipulation of the spine to promote

Table 47-2

Energy Therapies

THERAPY	STRENGTHS	WEAKNESSES
Therapeutic touch	• Relieves pain and anxiety • Promotes relaxation • Helps to alleviate stress-related disorders and headaches • No equipment needed	None are known, and complications are rare.
Healing touch	• Relieves pain and anxiety • Promotes relaxation • Helps to alleviate stress-related disorders and headaches • No equipment needed	None are known, and complications are rare.
Reiki	• Reduces a variety of physical problems • Improves psychospiritual well-being	None are known, and complications are rare.

overall structural integrity. *Massage therapy* involves manipulation of the muscles, soft tissues, and connective tissues, along with stimulation of the skin, nerves, blood, and lymph to restore the balance of qi. *Rolfing* involves the manipulation of the fascia to restore proper alignment of bones and muscles, which leads to improved overall functioning of the body. *Postural repatterning techniques* involve the reeducation of bodily movement to help individuals unlearn unhealthy habits of movement and posture. Postural repatterning techniques should not be used for patients who are uncomfortable with physical contact. (Table 47-3 discusses the strengths and weaknesses of each type of physical/manual therapy.)

Combination energy/physical therapies

Other therapies are a combination of the theories behind energy therapies and physical manual therapies. The underlying concept of Chinese theory is the concept of *qi*. Qi refers to the vital life force or energy that flows through the body along channels known as meridians. Qi is necessary to maintain life, and a balance is required to maintain health. A blockage of qi can cause disease. Qi is obtained from three sources: original qi (from the moment of conception), nutritional qi (from the foods people eat), and air qi (from the air people breathe).

Qigong consists of breathing exercises that originated in China and use the breath to unblock one's chi to promote health. These breathing exercises are combined with gentle exercise and meditation. Quiescent qigong is a meditative state; dynamic qigong is movement from one posture to another.

Craniosacral therapy is a gentle form of manipulative therapy used to affect the rhythm of the cerebrospinal fluid and the structures that enclose it. It is believed that bringing balance to the craniosacral system enhances overall well-being and disease resistance. However, there is little scientific evidence available.

Polarity is a type of energy balancing that uses physical and nonphysical touch techniques to balance another's energy. Techniques are used to unblock physical and emotional energy blocks and promote relaxation and healing.

Reflexology is the belief that areas of the feet, hands, and ears reflect major organs, glands, muscles, and bones of the body. Thumb or finger pressure is applied to the reflex points along the zones of the feet, hands, or ears to affect a corresponding body part and thus restore balance to the system. Again, there is little scientific evidence to support the effects of this therapy.

Acupuncture involves the use of fine needles along the meridian system's 12 pairs of pathways to balance one's chi. The meridian system of the body is closely associated with the autonomic nervous system and the organs affected by it. Chi flows towards these pathways and nourishes the organs of the body. There is scientific evidence to support the effectiveness of this therapy. *Acupressure* is closely associated with acupuncture, but it involves the use of finger pressure instead of needles along the meridian system to affect the body's energy system. (Table 47-4 evaluates the strengths and weaknesses of various combination energy/physical therapies.)

Mind-body therapies

Mind-body therapies take into consideration the holistic effects of mind-body-spirit balance. The purpose behind such therapies is to keep the systems open and in balance on all levels. Emotional and spiritual balance is seen to positively affect all of the physical systems, and vice versa. This concept is central to Ayurvedic and traditional Chinese medicine and is part of their guiding philosophies.

Many mind-body therapies are popular in the United States. *Tai chi chuan*, one of the many types of mind-body therapies, is a form of exercise that originates from the Chinese martial arts. It involves slow, purposeful, rhythmic

---

Table 47-3

Physical/Manual Therapies

THERAPY	STRENGTHS	WEAKNESSES
Chiropractic	• Relieves musculoskeletal pain and disability	This can cause nerve damage due to improper technique.
Massage	• Relieves stress and aids relaxation • Promotes circulation • Complementary therapy used with other therapies	A massage table is needed, but few complications are seen.
Rolfing	• Reduces pain and muscle spasms • Increases range of motion, flexibility, and energy • Reduces tension	The technique is painful at times, but there are no complications if it is done by a trained person.
Postural repatterning (Alexander, Feldenkrais, Traiger)	• Loosens tense muscles and stiff joints • Not a treatment in and of itself, it is best if used with other therapies	A padded table needed, but complications are rare.

Table 47-4

Combination Energy/Physical Therapies

THERAPY	STRENGTHS	WEAKNESSES
Qigong	• Suitable for all ages and physical conditions • Can be done while sitting or lying in bed • Promotes the relaxation response • No equipment needed	None are known, and there are no complications.
Craniosacral	• Used to treat chronic headaches and back pain • May promote relaxation and decrease stress and muscle tension	There is concern if this is done with infants or toddlers because their skull bones have not fused.
Reflexology	• Relieves stress and muscle tension • Produces relaxation	Healing crises consist of rash, fever, or worsening of symptoms related to the chief complaint, as well as signs of toxins being released. There is also no proof that the therapy is working
Acupuncture	• Relieves pain • Used to treat certain addictions	This requires extensive training and equipment, including fine, solid filiform needles. Complications are rare, but they can occur (e.g., pneumothorax).
Acupressure	• Relieves pain	None are known, and complications are rare.

Table 47-5

Mind-Body Therapies

THERAPY	STRENGTHS	WEAKNESSES
Tai chi chuan	• Complementary therapy • Increases balance, posture, and coordination • Promotes health and wellness	A patient can experience strains and sprains; falls and fractures are also possible.
Yoga	• Promotes relaxation • Enhances feeling of well-being • Complementary therapy	Muscle injury may occur if yoga is not properly performed.
Biofeedback	• Used for stress related disorders	Equipment is needed, and local skin irritation may be caused by electrodes.
Hypnosis	• Manages a number of medical and psychological problems • Helps to manage pain in childbirth • Decreases anxiety • Helps manage some addictions such as smoking	This may elicit disturbing emotions or memories
Meditation	• Reduces stress • Complementary therapy	This may elicit negative emotions or memories of bad experiences.
Imagery	• Helps to mobilize the immune system • Relieves pain and stress	There are only rare complications, though a patient may relive an unpleasant event.
Music	• Complementary therapy • Relieves anxiety	Few are known, and complications are rare.

movements used to restore balance and is often accompanied by QiGong exercises. *Yoga*, which means to join or yoke the body (e.g., mind-body-spirit balance) is a series of exercises including physical postures, breathing, and mental and spiritual reflection, that are used to promote balance. *Biofeedback* is a process that teaches one to have voluntary control of various bodily responses controlled by the autonomic nervous system through the use of electronic monitors.

Other mind-body therapies focus on mental centering. *Hypnosis* involves the use of suggestion to promote positive changes (physiological or psychological) in an individual. The suggestions are given when the person is in an altered state of consciousness, and some patients may become lightheaded after treatment. *Meditation* involves focusing one's attention on a single image, idea, or sound to promote physical-emotional-mental-spiritual balance of the system. Meditation is really a matter of being with one's self in quiet and paying attention. *Imagery* is the use of mental stimuli involving one or more of the five senses to promote relaxation and healing, relieve symptoms (such as pain), and induce sleep. *Music* may also be used as a mind-body therapy. Music promotes relaxation, decreases stress, and enhances healing. The type of music can be individualized to each person. *Flower essences* are made from flowers, and the essences are ingested in a liquid form (which is extremely dilute, with only minute quantities of flowers). Flowers are believed to contain earth energy and be able to balance and heal on all levels, especially the emotional level. It is believed that there are emotional precursors to physical disease, and flower essences are used to affect a person on this level. (Table 47-5 presents the strengths and weakness of mind-body therapies.)

Miscellaneous therapies

There are other therapies that fall into several of the above categories. They all involve restoring balance to the body, mind, and spirit and can be used alone or in conjunction with other therapies. The Chinese therapy *tui na* is a combination of massage, manipulation, and acupressure. *Biomagnetics* involves the use of magnetic fields to prevent and treat disease. Theories suggest that magnets increase blood supply, decrease inflammation, stimulate the release of certain neurotransmitters, and realign the body's own electromagnetic field to promote balance and healing. *Nutrition and diet therapies* may also be used; foods have been found to have therapeutic values as well as nutritional value. Certain foods can be used to prevent disease, heal the body, and provide a sense of well-being. Also included in this category is the use of vitamins and megavitamins for nutritional health.

Aromatherapy involves the use of essential oils and their vibrational energy to enhance healing on a physical and/or emotional level. Essential oils possess many properties and can be used as antibacterial agents, relaxants, and antiinflammatory agents, as well as to stimulate circulation and decrease spasms.

There are many types of herbs used for medicinal purposes. They are available in many forms, including infusions, decoctions, compresses, poultices, salves, capsules, and tinctures (Box 47-1). Problems associated with herbs, discussed briefly earlier in this chapter, are because the majority of them have not been tested through clinical studies. Most of the information circulated about herbs comes via word of mouth. *Crystal therapy* suggests that earth energy from crystals be used in conjunction with the energy of the human energy field to promote balance and healing. Different crystals are believed to have varying frequencies and uses, but there is no evidence available to support this therapy. (Table 47-6 describes the strengths and weaknesses of these miscellaneous therapies.)

Box 47-1

Types of Herb Preparations

Tincture—An herb placed in alcohol or liquid glycerin; has a strong taste.

Capsule/tablet—A ground or powdered form of an herb; less potent than a tincture.

Lozenge—A sweetened preparation that is dissolved in the mouth.

Tea—Made from most herbs; prepared by infusion (putting an herb in hot water to steep for 3 to 5 minutes) or decoction (putting an herb in boiling water for 15 to 20 minutes).

Poultice—A moist paste made from crushed herbs and applied directly to an area.

Compress—Made by soaking a cloth in a tea or tincture, wringing it out, and then applying it to the affected area.

Major Issues for the Use of Complementary/ Alternative Medicine

Many critical issues need to be addressed with the use of CAM. One issue is how to effectively integrate allopathic care with CAM. It will behoove APNs to be aware of the various types of CAM, and each APN needs to determine his or her comfort level with the various types of CAM before using them with patients. The use of CAM may not even be the choice of a particular APN, but patients may demand the use of CAM in their care. APNs certainly have to be aware that a significant number of patients use CAM therapies without discussing them with their providers, so APNs will need to get in the habit of asking patients if they use CAM. For those people with CAM insurance coverage, there will be little to no coordination of care between the CAM provider and the patient's primary care provider (PCP). The vast majority of CAM programs offer direct access, and it is unlikely that a CAM provider will notify a PCP of a patient's participation. Again, APNs can avoid missing patient participation in CAM therapies if they get in the habit of routinely asking patients. APNs also need to provide clear information to their patients about CAM therapies, especially herbs and other supplements. Since the number of adolescent patients who try herbs is so high, it will be vital for APNs to target teaching to teenage patients.

Legal Ramifications of Referral to Complementary/Alternative Medicine Practitioners

Another area that requires clarification is how to effectively and safely refer to CAM providers. APNs can not assume that health care plans have researched the credentials of a provider. Networks who must manage CAM services are more likely to have a thorough credentialing process. To be safe, an APN should check the credentials of a CAM

Table **47-6**

Miscellaneous Therapies

THERAPY	STRENGTHS	WEAKNESSES
Biomagnetics	• Relieves strains and sprains • According to anecdotal reports, possibly helps with back pain and other chronic disorders with pain components	Magnets should only be used under supervision due to possible overstimulation of the brain. Patients with pacemakers and defibrillators should not use them, and they are not recommended during pregnancy or for children under the age of 5.
Nutrition	• Ranges from avoiding processed food or certain chemicals to increasing the amount or types of healthy food	There is concern over toxicity related to megadoses of vitamins; inadequate intake of food (fasting); or electrolyte or other imbalances, depending on the type of diet.
Aromatherapy	• Promotes relaxation	Essential oils and other equipment may be needed. Irritation of skin may occur in people who are sensitive, and it should be avoided during pregnancy and by children under the age of 5. Some oils, such as wintergreen and savory, are not safe to use at home. Oils should be kept away from the eyes and other mucus membranes.
Herbs	• Inexpensive • Can create minor health problems such as colds, flu, and insomnia	Herbs are largely unregulated, with no quality control. There is also a need to assess for potential interactions between herbs and medications.
Crystal therapy	• Promotes relaxation	None are known.

provider before referring patients. There is also little relevant case law regarding CAM; there are some cases involving physicians who practice CAM themselves, but there are no cases involving physicians who referred to a CAM practitioner. It is likely that the CAM industry will continue to expand and that insurance coverage for such services will also grow. However, it is most likely that insurance coverage will only extend to those services where there is demonstrated clinical effectiveness and patient satisfaction (Grandinetti, 1999b). As CAM usage increases, more litigation is likely, and referring APNs could get involved in the cases. The first such cases will clarify how the courts view CAM practitioners and APNs who refer to CAM providers as part of their practices. Until such cases occur, it is difficult to discuss a risk reduction strategy.

In most cases, the courts will likely treat referrals to CAM practitioners as it has treated other referrals; APNs are generally not liable for harm inflicted by other practitioners, although there are some exceptions. Referral to a chiropractor instead of a needed surgeon, or to an incompetent practitioner or unlicensed practitioner, could cause an APN to be held liable for injuries the other practitioner causes the patient. APNs should make it clear to patients that they are not supervising care with regard to CAM therapies. Any referral should initiate a new and independent patient-provider relationship, and the CAM

practitioner to which an APN refers should carry his or her own malpractice coverage. Uninsured CAM practitioners may settle cases quickly or declare bankruptcy, leaving APNs to pay most of the awards.

If an APN does decide to use CAM therapies in practice, he or she should make sure to obtain all necessary tests and records from other providers and make a medical diagnosis before using CAM therapies. There is some reassurance in knowing that CAM practitioners are not sued as often as physicians (Grandinetti, 1999a). If an APN decides to refer to a CAM practitioner, he or she should keep up with the scientific literature. As knowledge of CAM expands, courts may determine APNs act negligently if they refer a patient to a therapy that they know (or should know) brings no benefits (Grandinetti, 1999a). If an APN decides not to use or refer to CAM practitioners, he or she is not totally in the clear; the APN must still assess diligently for the use of CAM therapies, particularly herbs, high-dose vitamins, and other supplements. Patients must be asked about alternative medicine usage, and APNs may want to include this information on new patient intake forms and then update it at every visit. Lastly, it is important for an APN to document conversations with patients regarding CAM, identifying when a patient says he or she does not use CAM supplements and making sure to document warnings to a patient regarding the use of alternative therapies.

PRIORITIES FOR RESEARCH

Topics for research for CAM are unlimited. A place to start might be why patients choose CAM. Fathman (2000) conducted a pilot study looking at whether hepatitis C patients use CAM therapies, because the conventional therapy is less-than-satisfactory in most instances. She developed a website with links to several hepatitis C resources for patients. Many subjects (284) completed the questionnaire, including 19 from outside the United States. Of the subjects, 76% (175) used some form of alternative therapy to treat their hepatitis C. All 8 of the subjects ages 21 to 30 reported using alternative therapy, while those in the 31 to 40 and over 60 age groups reported the lowest frequency of use, at 61% (27) and 60% (3), respectively. Of the largest sample age group, ages 41 to 50, 77% (101) reported using alternative therapy, while 90% (36) of the 51 to 60 age group reported use. The percentage of males and females using alternative therapy did not differ significantly. Also, few of the people who responded had insurance coverage for CAM. Only 9% of those who had private insurance had coverage for CAM therapies. Choices for CAM included Chinese therapies (27%), homeopathy (11%), relaxation (28%), and herbs (97%). Milk thistle was the most commonly used herb (by 149 subjects) among the choices.

The majority (54%) of patients who used CAM therapies chose the Internet as a source of knowledge about alternative therapy. The "Other" category was the next most prevalent choice at 43%. For this survey, subjects could type in an answer for this question, and responses generally included sources such as books and magazines. The four categories of health professionals listed were the least frequently selected options. Only 19% (33) of subjects using identified an alternative medicine practitioner as a source of knowledge, while 8% (14) chose their primary physician; 7% (12) chose a liver specialist, and only 2% (3) chose their nurse practitioner (NP).

The final research question addressed factors that influenced the decision to use alternative therapy as a means of treatment for hepatitis C. The choices listed were as follows: limited treatment options, quality of health, others who have used alternative therapy, concern with side effects of interferon or ribavirin, encouragement by friends or relatives, and encouragement by primary physician, NP, or other health professional. Subjects could select as many of the choices as applied to them. If none of the options applied, subjects could type their influence in a free text box labeled "Other." Of the respondents, 66% (116) chose limited options as a factor that influenced their decision. The next most common influences were quality of health (102) and side effects of interferon or ribavirin (101). The number of subjects who chose encouragement by friends or relatives and others using alternative therapy were 51 and 69, respectively. Encouragement by a health care provider was the least common choice (23). The last group of 39 subjects typed in other influences. Of those, 16

subjects indicated dissatisfaction with conventional medical treatment and 10 indicated that their personal philosophy influenced their decision to use alternative therapy. Other influences included personal research, a sense that "it can't hurt," and experience with alternative therapy before the diagnosis of hepatitis C.

This study has particular relevance for APNs. While not a large study, it indicates that patients are becoming knowledgeable consumers about their health, particularly when a chronic disease is involved. Patients will seek out alternative methods of treatment, whether or not APNs participate in or know about the decision. It is important for APNs to be aware of common CAM therapies for various diseases and make sure that they question the patients about their use. It may also be helpful for APNs to bring up the subject of CAM therapies with patients—especially those therapies with a strong research base—and recommend their use. Continued research along this line is important. While research by Astin (1998) identified that 4 in 10 people have used CAM, it does not specify with what illnesses. Future research should focus on the most commonly used CAM therapies and in what circumstances they are used.

Another area of research is patient satisfaction with the integration of CAM and allopathic care, or the safety and effectiveness of CAM therapies used alone or in conjunction with traditional allopathic care for common health problems. A study by Fawcett, Sidney, Riley-Lawless, and Hanson (1996) examined the relationship between alternative therapies, functional status, and symptom severity in people with multiple sclerosis (MS). All 16 subjects used both traditional and alternative therapies. Self-reported MS symptoms were less severe following the use of alternative therapies; however, the more therapies that were used, the lower their functional status. Other studies are currently in place to evaluate MS, and a phase I study looking at bee venom safety for MS patients is currently being conducted. Numerous studies will be conducted in the future to evaluate the credibility and effectiveness of various CAM therapies, so APNs should keep informed about the research and refer patients who might be eligible to participate.

Research that helps to determine what factors are associated with the choice of an alternative therapy is ongoing. Also, the effectiveness of the use of CAM therapies for illness prevention in high-risk individuals is an area where not much research has been conducted. Prevention in general is a difficult area to research; it may be even more difficult in patients who use nonstandardized therapies. As more becomes known about CAM, the potential for illness prevention and health promotion will be more fully explored.

The last area in which more research needs to be conducted is related to the issue of ethnicity and CAM. Initial work done by Lee, Lin, Wrensch, Adler, and Eisenberg (2000) reveals that alternative therapies and the factors influencing the choice of therapy varied by

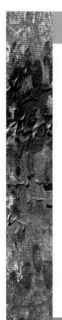

Suggestions for Further Learning

- Go to the website for the National State Boards of Nursing at www.ncsbn.org and find the link to your state. Look at the rules and regulations related to advanced practice. Does your state support the practice of CAM?
- Go to the website for the Office of Dietary Supplements at dietary-supplements.info.nih.gov to learn more about the optimal use of dietary supplements. Available via the website are 400,000 abstracts and publications on dietary supplements to assist both APNs and patients in educating themselves about the best way to use such supplements.
- The Food and Drug Administration/Center for Food Safety and Applied Nutrition provides reports and warnings against specific dietary supplements at the website vm.cfsan.fda.gov/~dms/supplmnt.html.
- Visit some of these other CAM websites:
  - www.healingtouch.net

- herbsthatheal.com
- qi.org/
- www.acupuncture.com
- nccam.nih.gov
- cpmcnet.columbia.edu/dept/rosenthal/factsheets.html
- www.therapeutictouch.com
- www.reiki.com
- www.reikilinks.com
- www.naturalhealthmag.com
- www.herbs.org
- ayurvedic.com
- www.floweressence.com
- www.drwhitaker.com
- www.holisticonline.com
- www.aromaweb.com
- www.ncbi.nlm.nih.gov/entrez/query.fcgi

ethnicity in women with breast cancer. African Americans used spiritual healing most often (36%), Chinese used herbal remedies most often (22%), Hispanic women used dietary methods (30%) and spiritual healing (26%) most often, and Caucasian women used dietary methods (35%) and physical methods such as massage and acupuncture most often (21%). APNs should be aware of future findings related to culture and CAM. As more data confirms the initial findings, this information can be helpful to APNs discussing CAM therapies with their patients.

IMPLICATIONS FOR MSN EDUCATION AND ADVANCED PRACTICE

With the public's increasing use of CAM therapies each year (Eisenberg et al, 1998), PCPs need to be more knowledgeable about the different types of CAM. This includes the implications for each type of therapy, the risks and benefits, and the possible side effects. For this reason, medical schools around the country (64% of them) have started to include course work on CAM in their curricula (Wetzel, Eisenberg, & Kaptchuk, 1998). Furthermore, with more and more advanced practice nurses (APNs) entering the primary health care provider arena, it is necessary for them to also be knowledgeable about CAM for the purpose of referrals and for integrative approaches to patient care. APN programs should include CAM content, either via required courses or electives. Pharmacology courses should address herbs and dietary supplements and their interactions with medications.

If PCPs demonstrate increased knowledge about CAM

therapies and make referrals, the general population may feel more comfortable discussing their use of such therapies with their PCPs. Currently, only about 39% of patients disclose this information (Eisenberg et al, 1998). Routine discussion of CAM therapies could increase trust between providers and consumers and ward off any untoward effects among different types of therapies.

DISCUSSION QUESTIONS

These questions can be used to promote critical thinking and encourage discussion.

1. What is the difference between the theoretical approach of CAM therapies when compared to conventional allopathic medicine? How might an APN incorporate various CAM therapies into his or her practice?
2. What are significant take-home messages related to access of CAMs, choice of CAMs, and ethnicity? Discuss how an APN might make CAM more approachable for patients.
3. Discuss the way CAM therapies might be utilized, either alone or in conjunction with other CAMs or allopathic medicine. What is the best way to present this information to your patients?
4. Discuss how PCPs should be prepared in CAM therapies. As a PCP, how would you feel most comfortable when using or referring for CAM?
5. What are the liabilities related to using or referring patients for CAM? How can you avoid the potential for negligence related to CAM?

REFERENCES/BIBLIOGRAPHY

Alternative therapy: what's a nurse to do?. (1999). *Arkansas Nursing News*, 16(1), 27-29.

The analytical study of herbs: as yet a fledgling science. (2000). *Patient Care for the Nurse Practitioner, 1*, 12-16.

Ananth, S. (1999). Alternative therapies for the medically underserved. *Health Forum Journal*. Available online at www.healthforum.com.

Andrews, M., Angone, K., Cray, J., Lewis, J., & Johnson, P. (Eds.). (1998). *Nurse's handbook of alternative & complementary therapies*. Springhouse, PA: Springhouse.

Astin, J. (1998). Why patients use alternative medicine: results of a national study. *Journal of the American Medical Association, 279*, 1548.

Bates, B. (1999, May). Teens using performance enhancing supplements. *Pediatric News*, 7.

Berman, B., Singh, K., Lao, L., Singh, B., Ferentz, K., & Hartnoll, S. (1995). Physicians' attitudes toward complementary or alternative medicine: a regional survey. *Journal of American Board of Family Practice*, 8(5), 361-366.

Borkan, J., Nehrer, J.O., Anson, O., & Smoker, B. (1994). Referrals for alternative therapies. *Journal of Family Practice, 39*, 545-50.

Boucher, T.A., & Lenz, S.K. (1998). An organizational survey of physicians' attitudes about and practice of complementary and alternative medicine. *Alternative Therapies*, 4(6), 59-65.

Brennan, B. (1987). *Hands of light: a guide to healing through the human energy field*. New York: Bantam.

Breuner, C., Barry, P., & Kemper, K. (1998). Alternative medicine use by homeless youth. *Archives of Pediatric Adolescent Medicine, 152*, 1071.

Cohen, M. (1998). *Complementary and alternative medicine: legal boundaries and regulatory perspectives*. Boston: The Johns Hopkins University Press.

Deloughery, G. (1998). *Issues and trends in nursing* (3rd ed.). St. Louis: Mosby.

D'epiro, N. (1999). Homeopathy: can we cure like? *Patient Care for the Nurse Practitioner, 12*, 7.

Eisenberg, D. (1993). Unconventional medicine in the U.S.—prevalence, costs, and patterns of use. *New England Journal of Medicine* 328(4): 246.

Eisenberg, D., Davis, R., Ettnec, S., Appel, S., Wilkey, S., VanRompey, M., & Kessler, R. (1998). Trends in alternative medicine use in the united states, 1990-1997: results of a follow-up national survey. *Journal of the American Medical Association*, 280(18), 1569-1575.

Ernst, E. (1998). Harmless herbs? A review of the current literature. *American Journal of Medicine, 104*, 170-178.

Ernst. E. (1999). Prevalence of complementary/alternative medicine for children: a systematic review. *European Journal of Pediatrics, 158*, 7.

Fathman, A. (2000). *Alternative therapy and hepatitis C: a quantitative study* (Unpublished Master's thesis). Highland Heights, KY: Northern Kentucky University.

Fawcett. J., Sidney, J., Riley-Lawless, K., & Hanson, M. (1996). An exploratory study of the relationship between alternative therapies, functional status, and symptom severity among people with multiple sclerosis. *Journal of Holistic Nursing, 14*(2), 115-129.

Fontanarosa, P., & Lundberg, G. (1998). Alternative medicine issue. *Journal of the American Medical Association, 280*, 18.

Gerber, R. (1988). *Vibrational medicine*. Santa Fe: Bear & Co.

Gardiner, P., Conboy, L, & Kemper, K. (2000). Herbs and adolescent girls: avoiding the hazards of self treatment. *Contemporary Pediatrics*. Available online at www.pdr.net/physician/static.htm?path=content/journals/k/data/2000/0301/kgardiner.html.

Grandinetti, D. (1999a). Will alternative medicine referrals get you sued? *Medical Economics*. Available online at www.pdr.net/memag/static.htm?path=docs/052499/article4.html.

Grandinetti, D. (1999b). Your newest competitors: alternative medicine networks. *Medical Economics*. Available online at www.pdr.net/memag/static.htm?path=docs/052499/article5.html.

Hover-Kramer, D., Mentgen, J., & Scandrett-Hibdon, S. (1996). *Healing touch: a resource for health-care professionals*. Albany, NY: Delmar.

Jonas, W., & Jacobs, J. (1996). *Healing with homeopathy: the doctor's guide*. New York: Warner Books.

Jonas, W., & Levin, J (1999). *Essentials of complementary and alternative medicine*. Hagerstown, MD: Lippincott, Williams, and Willkins.

Kass-Annese, B. (2000). Alternative therapies for menopause. *Clinic in Obstetrics and Gynecology*, 43(1), 162-183.

Keegan, L. (1998). Alternative and complementary therapies. *Nursing 98*, 28(4), 50-53.

Kelly, G. (1999). Nutritional and botanical interventions to assist with the adaptation to stress. *Alternative Medicine Review*, 4(4), 249-265. Available online at www.thorne.com/altmedrev/stress-ab4-4.html.

Kupecz, D. (1998). Drug news: St. John's wort—an alternative therapy in treating depression. *Nurse Practitioner*, 23(7), 110-112.

Lee, A., & Kemper, K. (2000). Homeopathy and naturopathy: practice characteristics and pediatric care. *Archives of Pediatric Adolescent Medicine*, 154(1), 75-80.

Lee, M., Lin, S., Wrensch, M., Adler, S., & Eisenberg, D. (2000). Alternative therapies used by women with breast cancer in four ethnic populations. *Journal of National Cancer Institute*, 92(1), 42-47.

Lis-Balchin, M. (1999). Possible health and safety problems in the use of novel plant essential oils and extracts in aromatherapy. *Journal of Research and Social Health, 119*(4), 240-243.

Mansour, A., Beuche, M., Laing, G., Leis, A., & Nurse, J. (1999). A study to test the effectiveness of placebo Reiki standardization procedures developed for a planned Reiki efficacy study. *Journal of Alternative and Complementary Medicine*, 5(2), 153-164.

McGregor, K., & Peay, E. (1996). The choice of alternative therapy for health care: testing some propositions. *Social Science and Medicine*, 43(9), 1317-1327.

Mitzel-Wilkinson, A. (2000). Massage therapy as a nursing practice. *Holistic Nursing Practice*, 14(2), 48-56.

O'Hara, M., Kiefer, D., & Farrell, K. (1998). A review of 12 commonly used medicinal herbs. *Archives in Family Medicine*, 7, 523-536.

Olsen, C. (1999). Alternative therapy: to teach or not to teach. *Perspective on Physician Assistant Education*, 10(1), 25-27.

Pelletier, K., Marie, A., Krasner, M., & Haskell, W. (1997). Current trends in the integration and reimbursement of complementary and alternative medicine by managed care, insurance carriers and hospital providers. *American Journal of Health Promotion*, 12, 112-123.

Sawyer, M., Ganoni, A., & Toogood, I. (1994). The use of alternative therapies by children with cancer. *Medical Journal of Australia, 160*(6), 320.

Skinn, B. (1994). The relationship of belief in control and purpose in life to adult lung cancer patients' inclination to use unproven cancer therapies. *Canadian Oncology Nursing Journal, 4*(2), 66-71.

Spicer, J. (1997). Embracing the alternative. *Family Practice Management.* Available online at www.aafp.org/fpm/970600fm/embrace/html.

Starn. J. (1998). The path to becoming an energy healer. *Nurse Practitioner Forum, 9*(4), 209-216.

Starr, C. (Ed.). (1997). Manual therapy: hands on healing. *Patient Care, 12,* 69-70.

Ullrich, S., & Hodge, P. (1999). The Ullrich Hodge alternative therapy assessment model: teaching students to evaluate pa-tients for use, motivation and risks. *Nurse Educator, 24*(6), 19-23.

Vickers, K.A., & Zollman, C. (1999). Herbal medicine. *British Medical Journal, 319,* 1050-1053.

Weber, D. (1997). The empowered consumer. *The Health Forum Journal.* Available online at www.healthforum.com.

Werbach, M. (2000). Nutritional strategies for treating chronic fatigue syndrome. *Alternative Medicine Review, 5*(2), 93-108. Available online at www.thorne.com/altmedrev/fatigue-ab5-2.html.

Wetzel, M.S., Eisenberg, D.M., & Kaptchuk, T.J. (1998). Courses involving complementary and alternative medicine at U.S. medical schools. *Journal of the American Medical Association, 280,* 784-87.

Index